Advanced Cardiac Imaging

Related titles

Biomaterials and Devices for the Circulatory System
(ISBN 978-1-84569-464-7)

Minimized Cardiopulmonary Bypass Techniques
(ISBN 978-1-84569-800-3)

Shape Memory Alloys for Biomedical Applications
(ISBN 978-1-84569-344-2)

Woodhead Publishing Series in Biomaterials: Number 99

Advanced Cardiac Imaging

Edited by

Koen Nieman, Oliver Gaemperli, Patrizio Lancellotti and Sven Plein

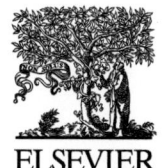

AMSTERDAM • BOSTON • CAMBRIDGE • HEIDELBERG
LONDON • NEW YORK • OXFORD • PARIS • SAN DIEGO
SAN FRANCISCO • SINGAPORE • SYDNEY • TOKYO
Woodhead Publishing is an imprint of Elsevier

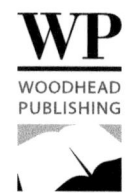

Woodhead Publishing is an imprint of Elsevier
80 High Street, Sawston, Cambridge, CB22 3HJ, UK
225 Wyman Street, Waltham, MA 02451, USA
Langford Lane, Kidlington, OX5 1GB, UK

© 2015 Elsevier Ltd. All rights reserved.

No part of this publication may be reproduced, stored in a retrieval system or transmitted in any form or by any means electronic, mechanical, photocopying, recording or otherwise without the prior written permission of the publisher.

Permissions may be sought directly from Elsevier's Science & Technology Rights Department in Oxford, UK: phone (+44) (0) 1865 843830; fax (+44) (0) 1865 853333; email: permissions@elsevier.com. Alternatively, you can submit your request online by visiting the Elsevier website at http://elsevier.com/locate/permissions, and selecting Obtaining permission to use Elsevier material.

Notice
No responsibility is assumed by the publisher for any injury and/or damage to persons or property as a matter of products liability, negligence or otherwise, or from any use or operation of any methods, products, instructions or ideas contained in the material herein. Because of rapid advances in the medical sciences, in particular, independent verification of diagnoses and drug dosages should be made.

British Library Cataloguing-in-Publication Data
A catalogue record for this book is available from the British Library.

Library of Congress Control Number: 2015939555

ISBN: 978-1-78242-282-2 (print)
ISBN: 978-1-78242-294-5 (online)

For information on all Woodhead Publishing publications
visit our website at http://store.elsevier.com/

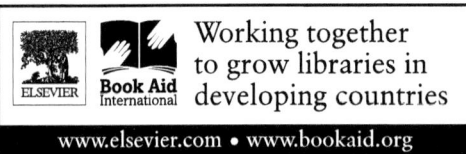

Printed and bound in the United Kingdom

Contents

Contributors	xiii
Woodhead Publishing Series in Biomaterials	xvii

1	**Advanced cardiac imaging**	**1**
	K. Nieman, O. Gaemperli, P. Lancellotti, S. Plein	
	1.1 Introduction	1
	1.2 Imaging the heart	1
	1.3 Techniques	3
	1.4 Shared themes and challenges	8
	1.5 Approach of the book	11

Part One Technological Developments in Cardiac Imaging 13

2	**Ultrasound/echocardiography**	**15**
	N.E. Hasselberg, T. Edvardsen	
	2.1 Introduction	15
	2.2 Three-dimensional echocardiography	16
	2.3 Contrast echocardiography	23
	2.4 Deformation imaging	32
	2.5 Future trends	39
	2.6 Further reading	45
	References	45
3	**Single-photon emission computed tomography**	**47**
	R.R. Buechel, P.A. Kaufmann O. Gaemperli	
	3.1 Introduction	47
	3.2 Physical principles of SPECT	47
	3.3 Camera designs	50
	3.4 Tracers	54
	3.5 Image processing and reconstruction	56
	3.6 Low-dose SPECT	62
	3.7 Dynamic SPECT	63
	3.8 Hybrid imaging	64
	References	67
4	**Positron emission tomography**	**71**
	P. Knaapen, M. Lubberink	
	4.1 Introduction	71
	4.2 Principles of PET	71

4.3	Clinical applications	78
4.4	Conclusion	90
	References	91

5 Computed tomography 97
K. Nieman, A. Coenen, M. Dijkshoorn

5.1	Development of cardiac CT	97
5.2	Technical principles and contemporary technology	97
5.3	CT performance, image quality parameters, and artifacts	106
5.4	Cardiac CT applications	111
5.5	Postprocessing, secondary reconstruction, and assisted interpretation	116
5.6	Radiation and dose reduction	117
5.7	Estimating the hemodynamic significance of CAD	120
5.8	Future perspectives	123
	References	123

6 Magnetic resonance imaging 127
V.M. Ferreira, M.D. Robson, T.D. Karamitsos, M.M. Bissell, D.J. Tyler, S. Neubauer

6.1	Introduction	127
6.2	Basic principles of NMR	127
6.3	Fast imaging	135
6.4	Perfusion, blood-oxygen-level-dependent, and late gadolinium enhancement imaging	138
6.5	Quantitative mapping techniques	141
6.6	Three-dimensional time-resolved (4D) flow	146
6.7	Magnetic resonance spectroscopy	148
6.8	Hyperpolarization	151
6.9	Latest technical developments and future trends	155
6.10	Sources of further information	156
	Acknowledgments	157
	References	158

Part Two Clinical Applications of Cardiac Imaging 171

7 Noninvasive coronary angiography 173
M. Premaratne, B.J.W. Chow

7.1	Introduction	173
7.2	Coronary artery calcium	173
7.3	CT coronary angiography	176
7.4	Limitations	189
7.5	The future	190
7.6	Coronary magnetic resonance imaging	190
	References	193

8	**Atherosclerotic plaque**	**203**
	P. Singh, A. Tawakol	
	8.1 Introduction	203
	8.2 Non-invasive imaging of atherosclerosis	204
	8.3 Computed tomography	206
	8.4 Conclusions	217
	References	217
9	**Myocardial ischemia**	**227**
	K. Goetschalckx, F.E. Rademakers	
	Abbreviations	227
	9.1 Pathophysiology of ischemia	227
	9.2 Invasive diagnosis of ischemia	234
	9.3 Noninvasive detection and quantification of ischemia	239
	9.4 Diagnostic platform	261
	9.5 Risk stratification and prognosis	261
	9.6 Noninvasive follow-up of the patient with known coronary artery disease	264
	References	264
10	**Myocardial infarction**	**271**
	A. Flotats, B.L. Gerber, S. Gurunathan, A. Mahnken, T.A. Magalhães, C.E. Rochitte, R. Senior	
	10.1 Introduction	271
	10.2 Echocardiography	280
	10.3 Nuclear imaging	288
	10.4 CMR imaging	297
	10.5 Multidetector CT	303
	10.6 Guidelines for use of imaging in AMI	312
	10.7 Conclusion	313
	References	313
11	**Myocardial viability**	**327**
	A.J. Ludman, C.D. Anagnostopoulos, P. Leeson, F. Pugliese, S.E. Petersen	
	11.1 Background, terms, and definitions	327
	11.2 Multimodality imaging for myocardial viability assessment	332
	11.3 The role of myocardial viability assessment in clinical decision-making	347
	11.4 Current research, emerging techniques, and hybrid imaging	353
	11.5 Conclusion	355
	Acknowledgements	355
	References	355
12	**Contractile function and heart failure**	**367**
	E. Donal, E. Galli, M. Lederlin, A. Manrique	
	12.1 Introduction	367
	12.2 Echocardiographic approach to the LV contractility	369

	12.3 Assessment of RV function	374
	12.4 Assessment of contractile function by CMR	383
	12.5 Assessment of ventricular function using radionuclide techniques	387
	References	392

13 Cardiomyopathy — 399
A.J. Baksi, D.J. Pennell

13.1	Introduction	399
13.2	Dilated cardiomyopathy	406
13.3	Non-compaction cardiomyopathy	411
13.4	Stress (Takotsubo) cardiomyopathy	413
13.5	Arrhythmogenic (right) ventricular cardiomyopathy	414
13.6	Hypertrophic cardiomyopathy	416
13.7	Hypertrophic phenocopies	421
13.8	Infiltrative disease/restrictive cardiomyopathy	422
13.9	Cardiac iron overload	427
13.10	Pericardial constriction	428
13.11	Limitations of imaging	428
13.12	Likely future trends	428
13.13	Conclusions and reflection	429
	Resources	430
	References	431

14 Myocarditis — 439
R. Wassmuth, J. Schulz-Menger

14.1	Clinical background	439
14.2	Biopsy as "the invasive standard"	441
14.3	Therapeutic options	443
14.4	Imaging	443
14.5	Summary	454
	References	454

15 Systemic diseases — 459
M. Lombardi, A. Gimelli, M. Galderisi

15.1	Arterial systemic hypertension	459
15.2	Diabetic cardiomyopathy	465
15.3	Inotropic reserve in diabetic patients	467
15.4	Metabolic syndrome	469
15.5	Autoimmune connective tissue disorders	472
15.6	Thyroid disease	474
15.7	Systemic vasculitis	475
	References	478

16 Acquired valvular heart disease — 489

Aortic root — 489
V. Polsani, X. Zhou, M. Vannan

16.1	Annulus size and calcification	489

16.2	Aortic valve leaflets	491
16.3	Sinus of Valsalva and sinotubular junction	493
	References	494

Aortic stenosis — 496
V. Polsani, X. Zhou, M. Vannan

16.4	Aortic valve/root morphology	496
16.5	Severity of aortic stenosis	496
16.6	Synthesis	500
	References	500

Aortic regurgitation — 503
V. Polsani, X. Zhou, M. Vannan

16.7	Aortic valve/root morphology	503
16.8	Severity of aortic regurgitation	503
	References	508

Mitral regurgitation — 510
P. Lancellotti

16.9	Introduction	510
16.10	Aetiology and mechanisms	510
16.11	2D/3D echocardiographic evaluation	511
16.12	Cardiac magnetic resonance	518
16.13	Multislice cardiac computed tomography	521
16.14	Conclusion	522
	References	523

Tricuspid and pulmonary valves — 526
D. Muraru, M.P. Marra, L.P. Badano

16.15	Tricuspid valve	526
16.16	Pulmonary valve	533
	References	540

Prosthetic valves — 541
H. Mahjoub, P. Pibarot

	Abbreviations	541
16.17	Introduction	541
16.18	Echocardiography	542
16.19	Cinefluoroscopy	557
16.20	Computed tomography	559
16.21	Nuclear imaging	562
16.22	Magnetic resonance imaging	562
16.23	Conclusion	563
	References	563

Interventional imaging for transcatheter valve procedures — 567
J. Zamorano, C. Fernández-Golfín

16.24	Transcatheter aortic valve implantation	567
16.25	Transoesophageal echocardiography approach before TAVI	567

16.26	Transoesophageal echocardiography during prosthesis implantation	568
16.27	Percutaneous transcatheter repair of paravalvular regurgitation	569
16.28	TEE before transcatheter repair of paravalvular regurgitation	569
16.29	TEE during percutaneous transcatheter repair of paravalvular regurgitation	570
16.30	Percutaneous mitral valve intervention by edge-to-edge repair	571
16.31	TEE for patients selection for edge-to-edge repair	571
16.32	TEE during edge-to-edge repair	571
16.33	Conclusion	572
	References	573

Endocarditis — 574
G. Habib, S. Camilleri, J.-Y. Gaubert

16.34	Introduction	574
16.35	Echocardiography	574
16.36	Molecular imaging	577
16.37	Multislice computed tomography	580
16.38	Magnetic resonance imaging	581
16.39	Conclusion	581
	References	581

17 Cardiac tumours — 585
J.P. Greenwood, M. Motwani, A.M. Crean

17.1	Introduction	585
17.2	Echocardiography	585
17.3	Cardiovascular magnetic resonance	588
17.4	Cardiac computed tomography	591
17.5	Nuclear imaging techniques	591
17.6	Cardiac masses	593
17.7	Conclusions	610
	References	612

18 Pericardial diseases — 617
B. Cosyns, B. Paelinck, O. Cappeliez

18.1	Introduction	617
18.2	Technical aspects	617
18.3	The pericardium: normal findings	620
18.4	Clinical scenarios	621
18.5	Cardiac masses (cysts, diverticula, hematoma, tumors)	629
18.6	Congenital absence of pericardium	632
	References	633

19 Congenital heart disease — 635
A.A. Pasquet, B.L. Gerber

	Abbreviations and acronyms	635
19.1	Introduction	635

	19.2 Imaging modalities	**636**
	19.3 Specific lesions	**641**
	19.4 Summary	**655**
	References	**655**
20	**Diseases of the thoracic aorta and pulmonary arteries**	**661**
	R. Salgado, J. Habets, R.P.J. Budde, T. Leiner	
	20.1 Introduction	**661**
	20.2 Acute aortic syndrome	**661**
	20.3 Vasculitis	**675**
	20.4 Imaging of the postoperative aorta	**681**
	20.5 Pulmonary circulation	**686**
	20.6 Aneurysmatic disease	**694**
	References	**702**
21	**Arrhythmia**	**707**
	S.C.A.M. Bekkers, B.L. Kietselaer, L. Pison	
	21.1 Introduction	**707**
	21.2 Fluoroscopy	**707**
	21.3 Ultrasound	**711**
	21.4 Computed tomography	**717**
	21.5 Cardiac magnetic resonance imaging	**720**
	21.6 Electroanatomic mapping	**724**
	21.7 Radionuclide imaging	**726**
	21.8 Image integration	**727**
	References	**729**
22	**Imaging guided interventions**	**735**
	D. Braun, B. Bischoff, J. Hausleiter	
	22.1 Introduction	**735**
	22.2 Transcatheter aortic valve implantation	**735**
	22.3 Percutaneous edge-to-edge repair of the mitral valve	**744**
	22.4 Occlusion of left atrial appendage	**751**
	22.5 Interventional closure of ASD and PFO	**758**
	22.6 Interventional closure of paravalvular leaks	**759**
	22.7 Pre-interventional imaging in coronary CTO	**761**
	References	**762**
Index		**765**

Contributors

C.D. Anagnostopoulos Biomedical Research Foundation Academy of Athens, Athens, Greece

L.P. Badano University of Padua, Padua, Italy

A.J. Baksi Royal Brompton Hospital, London, UK

S.C.A.M. Bekkers Maastricht University Medical Center, Maastricht, The Netherlands

B. Bischoff Klinikum Großhadern der Ludwig-Maximilians-Universität München, Munich, Germany

M.M. Bissell University of Oxford, Oxford, UK

D. Braun Klinikum Großhadern der Ludwig-Maximilians-Universität München, Munich, Germany

R.P.J. Budde Erasmus Medical Center, Rotterdam, The Netherlands

R.R. Buechel University Hospital Zurich, Zurich, Switzerland

S. Camilleri Hôpital de la Timone, Marseille, France

O. Cappeliez CHIREC, Brussels, Belgium

B.J.W. Chow University of Ottawa Heart Institute, Ottawa, ON, Canada

A. Coenen Erasmus MC, Rotterdam, The Netherlands

B. Cosyns Universitair Ziekenhuis Brussel, Brussels, Belgium

A.M. Crean Peter Munk Cardiac Centre, Toronto, ON, Canada

M. Dijkshoorn Erasmus MC, Rotterdam, The Netherlands

E. Donal CHU Rennes, Rennes, France; LTSI, INSERM 1099, Université Rennes-1, Rennes, France

T. Edvardsen Oslo University Hospital, Rikshospitalet, & University of Oslo, Oslo, Norway

C. Fernández-Golfín University Hospital Ramon y Cajal, Madrid, Spain

V.M. Ferreira University of Oxford, Oxford, UK

A. Flotats Hospital de la Santa Creu i Sant Pau, Universitat Autònoma de Barcelona, Barcelona, Spain

O. Gaemperli University Hospital Zurich, Zurich, Switzerland

M. Galderisi Federico II University Hospital, Naples, Italy

E. Galli CHU Rennes, Rennes, France; LTSI, INSERM 1099, Université Rennes-1, Rennes, France

J.-Y. Gaubert Hôpital de la Timone, Marseille, France

B.L. Gerber Cliniques Universitaires St. Luc Université Catholique de Louvain, Brussels, Belgium

A. Gimelli UOC Nuclear Medicine at Fondazione CNR/Regione Toscana 'G. Monasterio', Pisa, Italy

K. Goetschalckx University Hospitals Leuven, Leuven, Belgium

J.P. Greenwood University of Leeds, Leeds, UK

S. Gurunathan Royal Brompton Hospital, Imperial College, London, UK

J. Habets University Medical Center Utrecht, Utrecht, The Netherlands

G. Habib Hôpital de la Timone, Marseille, France

N.E. Hasselberg Oslo University Hospital, Rikshospitalet, & University of Oslo, Oslo, Norway

J. Hausleiter Klinikum Großhadern der Ludwig-Maximilians-Universität München, Munich, Germany

T.D. Karamitsos Aristotle University of Thessaloniki, Thessaloniki, Greece

P.A. Kaufmann University Hospital Zurich, Zurich, Switzerland

B.L. Kietselaer Maastricht University Medical Center, Maastricht, The Netherlands

P. Knaapen VU University Medical Center, Amsterdam, The Netherlands

P. Lancellotti University of Liège Hospital, CHU Sart Tilman Liège, Belgium; GVM Care and Research, E.S. Health Science Foundation, Lugo (RA), Italy

M. Lederlin CHU Rennes, Rennes, France

P. Leeson University of Oxford, Oxford, UK

T. Leiner University Medical Center Utrecht, Utrecht, The Netherlands

M. Lombardi IRCCS, Policlinico San Donato, Milan, Italy

M. Lubberink Uppsala University Hospital and Nuclear Medicine & PET, Uppsala University, Uppsala, Sweden

A.J. Ludman Royal Devon & Exeter NHS Foundation Trust, Exeter, UK

T.A. Magalhães Hospital do Coração, HCOR, University of São Paulo Medical School, São Paulo, Brazil

H. Mahjoub Université Laval/Laval University, Québec, QC, Canada

A. Mahnken Philipps University, Marburg, Germany

A. Manrique CHU de Caen, Caen, France; Université de Caen Basse-Normandie, Caen, France

M.P. Marra University of Padua, Padua, Italy

M. Motwani University of Leeds, Leeds, UK

D. Muraru University of Padua, Padua, Italy

S. Neubauer University of Oxford, Oxford, UK

K. Nieman Erasmus MC, Rotterdam, The Netherlands

B. Paelinck Antwerp University Hospital, Edegem, Belgium

A.A. Pasquet Cliniques Universitaires St. Luc Université Catholique de Louvain, Brussels, Belgium

D.J. Pennell Royal Brompton Hospital, London, UK

S.E. Petersen The London Chest Hospital, London, UK

P. Pibarot Université Laval/Laval University, Québec, QC, Canada

L. Pison Maastricht University Medical Center, Maastricht, The Netherlands

S. Plein University of Leeds, Leeds, United Kingdom

V. Polsani Marcus Heart Valve Center, Piedmont Heart Institute, Atlanta, GA, USA

M. Premaratne University of Ottawa Heart Institute, Ottawa, ON, Canada; Canberra Hospital, Garran, ACT, Australia

F. Pugliese The London Chest Hospital, London, UK

F.E. Rademakers KU Leuven, Leuven, Belgium

M.D. Robson University of Oxford, Oxford, UK

C.E. Rochitte Hospital do Coração, HCOR, University of São Paulo Medical School, São Paulo, Brazil

R. Salgado Antwerp University Hospital, Antwerp, Belgium

J. Schulz-Menger Universitätsmedizin Berlin, A Joint Institution of Charite and Max-Delbruck-Center, Berlin, Germany; HELIOS Klinikum Berlin-Buch, Berlin, Germany

R. Senior Royal Brompton Hospital, Imperial College, London, UK

P. Singh Weill Cornell Medical College, New York Presbyterian Hospital, New York, NY, USA

A. Tawakol Harvard Medical School, Massachusetts General Hospital, Boston, MA, USA

D.J. Tyler University of Oxford, Oxford, UK

M. Vannan Marcus Heart Valve Center, Piedmont Heart Institute, Atlanta, GA, USA

R. Wassmuth Oberhavel-Kliniken Hennigsdorf, Hennigsdorf, Germany; Universitätsmedizin Berlin, A Joint Institution of Charite and Max-Delbruck-Center, Berlin, Germany

J. Zamorano University Hospital Ramon y Cajal, Madrid, Spain

X. Zhou Chinese PLA General Hospital

Woodhead Publishing Series in Biomaterials

1. **Sterilisation of tissues using ionising radiations**
   Edited by J. F. Kennedy, G. O. Phillips and P. A. Williams
2. **Surfaces and interfaces for biomaterials**
   Edited by P. Vadgama
3. **Molecular interfacial phenomena of polymers and biopolymers**
   Edited by C. Chen
4. **Biomaterials, artificial organs and tissue engineering**
   Edited by L. Hench and J. Jones
5. **Medical modelling**
   R. Bibb
6. **Artificial cells, cell engineering and therapy**
   Edited by S. Prakash
7. **Biomedical polymers**
   Edited by M. Jenkins
8. **Tissue engineering using ceramics and polymers**
   Edited by A. R. Boccaccini and J. Gough
9. **Bioceramics and their clinical applications**
   Edited by T. Kokubo
10. **Dental biomaterials**
    Edited by R. V. Curtis and T. F. Watson
11. **Joint replacement technology**
    Edited by P. A. Revell
12. **Natural-based polymers for biomedical applications**
    Edited by R. L. Reiss et al
13. **Degradation rate of bioresorbable materials**
    Edited by F. J. Buchanan
14. **Orthopaedic bone cements**
    Edited by S. Deb
15. **Shape memory alloys for biomedical applications**
    Edited by T. Yoneyama and S.Miyazaki
16. **Cellular response to biomaterials**
    Edited by L. Di Silvio
17. **Biomaterials for treating skin loss**
    Edited by D. P. Orgill and C. Blanco
18. **Biomaterials and tissue engineering in urology**
    Edited by J.Denstedt and A. Atala
19. **Materials science for dentistry**
    B. W. Darvell

20 **Bone repair biomaterials**
   Edited by J. A. Planell, S. M. Best, D. Lacroix and A. Merolli
21 **Biomedical composites**
   Edited by L. Ambrosio
22 **Drug–device combination products**
   Edited by A. Lewis
23 **Biomaterials and regenerative medicine in ophthalmology**
   Edited by T. V. Chirila
24 **Regenerative medicine and biomaterials for the repair of connective tissues**
   Edited by C. Archer and J. Ralphs
25 **Metals for biomedical devices**
   Edited by M. Niinomi
26 **Biointegration of medical implant materials: Science and design**
   Edited by C. P. Sharma
27 **Biomaterials and devices for the circulatory system**
   Edited by T. Gourlay and R. Black
28 **Surface modification of biomaterials: Methods analysis and applications**
   Edited by R. Williams
29 **Biomaterials for artificial organs**
   Edited by M. Lysaght and T. Webster
30 **Injectable biomaterials: Science and applications**
   Edited by B. Vernon
31 **Biomedical hydrogels: Biochemistry, manufacture and medical applications**
   Edited by S. Rimmer
32 **Preprosthetic and maxillofacial surgery: Biomaterials, bone grafting and tissue engineering**
   Edited by J. Ferri and E. Hunziker
33 **Bioactive materials in medicine: Design and applications**
   Edited by X. Zhao, J. M. Courtney and H. Qian
34 **Advanced wound repair therapies**
   Edited by D. Farrar
35 **Electrospinning for tissue regeneration**
   Edited by L. Bosworth and S. Downes
36 **Bioactive glasses: Materials, properties and applications**
   Edited by H. O. Ylänen
37 **Coatings for biomedical applications**
   Edited by M. Driver
38 **Progenitor and stem cell technologies and therapies**
   Edited by A. Atala
39 **Biomaterials for spinal surgery**
   Edited by L. Ambrosio and E. Tanner
40 **Minimized cardiopulmonary bypass techniques and technologies**
   Edited by T. Gourlay and S. Gunaydin
41 **Wear of orthopaedic implants and artificial joints**
   Edited by S. Affatato
42 **Biomaterials in plastic surgery: Breast implants**
   Edited by W. Peters, H. Brandon, K. L. Jerina, C. Wolf and V. L. Young
43 **MEMS for biomedical applications**
   Edited by S. Bhansali and A. Vasudev

44 **Durability and reliability of medical polymers**
   Edited by M. Jenkins and A. Stamboulis
45 **Biosensors for medical applications**
   Edited by S. Higson
46 **Sterilisation of biomaterials and medical devices**
   Edited by S. Lerouge and A. Simmons
47 **The hip resurfacing handbook: A practical guide to the use and management of modern hip resurfacings**
   Edited by K. De Smet, P. Campbell and C. Van Der Straeten
48 **Developments in tissue engineered and regenerative medicine products**
   J. Basu and J. W. Ludlow
49 **Nanomedicine: Technologies and applications**
   Edited by T. J. Webster
50 **Biocompatibility and performance of medical devices**
   Edited by J-P. Boutrand
51 **Medical robotics: Minimally invasive surgery**
   Edited by P. Gomes
52 **Implantable sensor systems for medical applications**
   Edited by A. Inmann and D. Hodgins
53 **Non-metallic biomaterials for tooth repair and replacement**
   Edited by P. Vallittu
54 **Joining and assembly of medical materials and devices**
   Edited by Y. (Norman) Zhou and M. D. Breyen
55 **Diamond-based materials for biomedical applications**
   Edited by R. Narayan
56 **Nanomaterials in tissue engineering: Fabrication and applications**
   Edited by A. K. Gaharwar, S. Sant, M. J. Hancock and S. A. Hacking
57 **Biomimetic biomaterials: Structure and applications**
   Edited by A. J. Ruys
58 **Standardisation in cell and tissue engineering: Methods and protocols**
   Edited by V. Salih
59 **Inhaler devices: Fundamentals, design and drug delivery**
   Edited by P. Prokopovich
60 **Bio-tribocorrosion in biomaterials and medical implants**
   Edited by Y. Yan
61 **Microfluidic devices for biomedical applications**
   Edited by X-J. James Li and Y. Zhou
62 **Decontamination in hospitals and healthcare**
   Edited by J. T. Walker
63 **Biomedical imaging: Applications and advances**
   Edited by P. Morris
64 **Characterization of biomaterials**
   Edited by M. Jaffe, W. Hammond, P. Tolias and T. Arinzeh
65 **Biomaterials and medical tribology**
   Edited by J. Paolo Davim
66 **Biomaterials for cancer therapeutics: Diagnosis, prevention and therapy**
   Edited by K. Park
67 **New functional biomaterials for medicine and healthcare**
   E.P. Ivanova, K. Bazaka and R. J. Crawford

68 Porous silicon for biomedical applications
   Edited by H. A. Santos
69 A practical approach to spinal trauma
   Edited by H. N. Bajaj and S. Katoch
70 Rapid prototyping of biomaterials: Principles and applications
   Edited by R.Narayan
71 Cardiac regeneration and repair Volume 1: Pathology and therapies
   Edited by R-K. Li and R. D. Weisel
72 Cardiac regeneration and repair Volume 2: Biomaterials and tissue engineering
   Edited by R-K. Li and R. D. Weisel
73 Semiconducting silicon nanowires for biomedical applications
   Edited by J.L. Coffer
74 Silk biomaterials for tissue engineering and regenerative medicine
   Edited by S. Kundu
75 Biomaterials for bone regeneration: Novel techniques and applications
   Edited by P.Dubruel and S. Van Vlierberghe
76 Biomedical foams for tissue engineering applications
   Edited by P. Netti
77 Precious metals for biomedical applications
   Edited by N. Baltzer and T. Copponnex
78 Bone substitute biomaterials
   Edited by K. Mallick
79 Regulatory affairs for biomaterials and medical devices
   Edited by S. F. Amato and R. Ezzell
80 Joint replacement technology Second edition
   Edited by P. A. Revell
81 Computational modelling of biomechanics and biotribology in the musculoskeletal system: Biomaterials and tissues
   Edited by Z. Jin
82 Biophotonics for medical applications
   Edited by I. Meglinski
83 Modelling degradation of bioresorbable polymeric medical devices
   Edited by J. Pan
84 Perspectives in total hip arthroplasty: Advances in biomaterials and their tribological interactions
   S. Affatato
85 Tissue engineering using ceramics and polymers Second edition
   Edited by A. R. Boccaccini and P. X. Ma
86 Biomaterials and medical-device associated infections
   Edited by L. Barnes and I. R. Cooper
87 Surgical techniques in total knee arthroplasty (TKA) and alternative procedures
   Edited by S. Affatato
88 Lanthanide oxide nanoparticles for molecular imaging and therapeutics
   G. H. Lee
89 Surface modification of magnesium and its alloys for biomedical applications Volume 1: Biological interactions, mechanical properties and testing
   Edited by T. S. N. Sankara Narayanan, I. S. Park and M. H. Lee

90 Surface modification of magnesium and its alloys for biomedical applications Volume 2: Modification and coating techniques
   Edited by T. S. N. Sankara Narayanan, I. S. Park and M. H. Lee
91 Medical modelling: the application of advanced design and rapid prototyping techniques in medicine Second Edition
   Edited by R. Bibb, D. Eggbeer and A. Paterson
92 Switchable and responsive surfaces and materials for biomedical applications
   Edited by Z. Zhang
93 Biomedical textiles for orthopaedic and surgical applications: fundamentals, applications and tissue engineering
   Edited by T. Blair
94 Surface coating and modification of metallic biomaterials
   Edited by C. Wen
95 Hydroxyapatite (HAP) for biomedical applications
   Edited by M. Mucalo
96 Implantable neuroprostheses for restoring function
   Edited by K. Kilgore
97 Shape memory polymers for biomedical applications
   Edited by L. Yahia
98 Regenerative engineering of musculoskeletal tissues and interfaces
   Edited by S.P. Nukavarapu, J.W. Freeman and C.T. Laurencin
99 Advanced cardiac imaging
   Edited by K. Nieman, O. Gaemperli, P. Lancellotti and S. Plein
100 Functional Marine Biomaterials: Properties and Applications
   Edited by Se-Kwon Kim
101 Shoulder and elbow trauma and its complications: Volume 1: The Shoulder
   Edited by R. M. Greiwe
102 Nanotechnology-Enhanced Orthopedic Materials: Fabrications, Applications and Future Trends
   L. Yang
103 Medical devices: Regulations, standards and practices
   Seeram Ramakrishna, Lingling Tian, Charlene Wang, Susan Liao and Wee Eong Teo
104 Biomineralisation and biomaterials: fundamentals and applications
   Prof. Conrado Aparicio and Prof. Maria Pau Ginebra

Advanced cardiac imaging

K. Nieman[*], O. Gaemperli[†], P. Lancellotti[‡,§], S. Plein[¶]
[*]Erasmus MC, Rotterdam, The Netherlands; [†]University Hospital Zurich, Zurich, Switzerland; [‡]University of Liège Hospital, CHU Sart Tilman, Liège, Belgium; [§]GVM Care and Research, E.S. Health Science Foundation, Lugo (RA), Italy; [¶]University of Leeds, Leeds, United Kingdom

1.1 Introduction

One cannot cure without knowing what is wrong, which is why diagnostic techniques are essential to practice medicine. The heart is a mechanical organ, a pump consisting of moving structures, directed flow, electric controls, and an efficient oxygen and nutrient supply system. These physical phenomena can be investigated in many ways, externally by physical examination, auscultation, or electrocardiogram; invasively using catheters; and more recently by various types of noninvasive cross-sectional imaging modalities. In this book we focus on the fast-developing field of noninvasive cross-sectional imaging of the heart. There is perhaps no other organ where imaging is more important for the clinical management than the heart. While the principal purpose of cardiac imaging is the diagnosis of disease, its impact reaches further than that. Imaging provides information on the severity of disease, the prognostic consequences of abnormalities, and thereby guides imaging decisions. Nowadays, arrhythmia, coronary disease, and an increasing number of structural cardiovascular conditions can be treated by minimally invasive intervention procedures. These catheter-based procedures rely on noninvasive imaging for patient selection, preparation, and direct procedural guidance. While for most healthcare professionals imaging is most tangible in clinical care, diagnostic techniques are becoming more important in research as well. Imaging can improve our understanding of cardiovascular physiology and disease and serve as a noninvasive monitor of disease progression—for instance as a surrogate marker to assess the effect of pharmacological or mechanical interventions (Figure 1.1).

1.2 Imaging the heart

The notion that imaging of the heart is important does not imply that it is easy. As a matter of fact, the heart was rarely the first organ to be interrogated by new imaging techniques. There are several reasons why the heart is more difficult to image in comparison to other parts of the body, although the gravity of these limitations varies between modalities and applications. The most distinguishing characteristic of the heart is its perpetual movement, by contraction, but also as a result of respiration. To visualize the heart, images need to be taken very quickly (echocardiography) and the acquisition needs to be synchronized to the rhythm of the heart (CT, CMR, nuclear

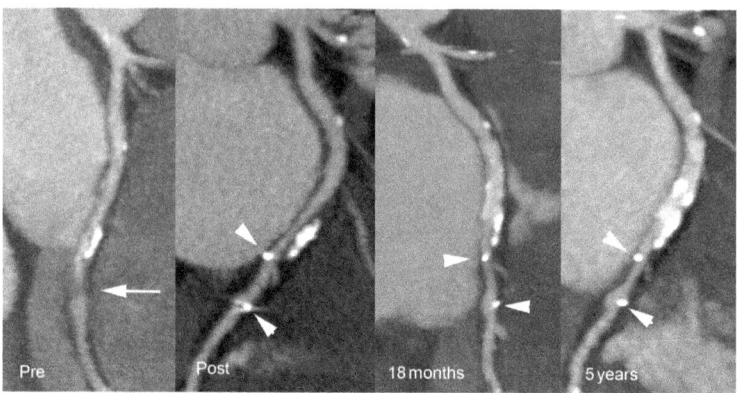

Figure 1.1 Cardiac CT as a research endpoint. Coronary CT angiography depicting a severe stenosis (arrow) in the distal left circumflex branch (PRE). CT imaging performed immediately after (POST) implantation of a bioresorbable coronary scaffold shows two markers at each end of the device (arrow heads). CT imaging confirms patency with minimal lumen loss during follow up at 18 months and 5 years. Imaging was performed as part of the ABSORB trial (see Chapter 5).

imaging), unless one is willing to accept the motion blurring when larger structures are investigated (nongated nuclear and CMR techniques). The heart's position fairly deep within the body, protected by the rib cage, poses additional challenges, limiting the acoustic windows for echocardiography, creating excessive image noise on CT, reducing the radiofrequency signal for CMR, or causing attenuation artifacts on nuclear images. Respiratory motion is relevant for longer imaging protocols involving smaller structures. Particularly for angiographic studies using arterial contrast enhancement, short scans are preferable, necessitating very fast acquisition of imaging data.

When imaging techniques are described, or perhaps compared, a number of image quality parameters are taken into account. The temporal resolution is the time needed to acquire a single image, which resembles the shutter time of an optical photo camera. Obviously fast-moving structures (valves) require a high temporal resolution. The scan time generally refers to the entire or a specific part of the examination. The spatial resolution refers to the ability to differentiate small structures, while the contrast resolution describes how well tissue types can be distinguished. Imaging of the coronary arteries or suspected endocarditis demands high spatial resolution, while myocardial infiltration benefits from high sensitivity to detect variation in tissue characteristics. Stochastic variance of the imaging signal, or irregularities arising elsewhere in the process, causes image noise. The noise level is often reported in relation to the image signal (signal-to-noise ratio) or (tissue) contrast (contrast-to-noise ratio). Performance parameters are interchangeable within a range, and trade-offs are often necessary (Figure 1.2). During echocardiography, the sector width can be narrowed to increase the frame rate. During CMR, the spatial resolution can be increased, but at the price of a longer scan time. Reconstruction of thicker CT cuts will improve the contrast-to-noise ratio, but sacrifice in-plane spatial resolution. Particularly for techniques involving radiation, image quality needs to be balanced against radiation dose, and the challenge is to provide diagnostic image quality at the lowest possible dose.

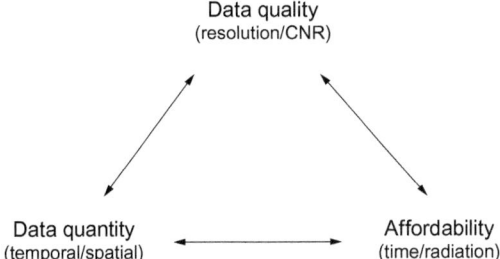

Figure 1.2 Trade-offs in cardiac imaging.

1.3 Techniques

1.3.1 Echocardiography

In the early 1950s, Edgler and Hertz described for the first time the use of cardiac ultrasound for assessing mitral valve movement. Since this landmark event, many discoveries have been made in the field of echocardiography that are presently used in daily practice. M-mode echocardiography was supplemented by 2D echocardiography in the mid 1960s, with the important additions of Doppler signals (1970s) and the combination of color Doppler (1980s) with 2D imaging. In the late 1980s, the transeosophageal approach completed the armamentarium of echocardiography. With the help of engineers, transeosophageal echocardiography quickly evolved from monoplane to biplane to present-day multiplane imaging. In parallel to the developments in transducer technology, image quality was consistently improved by using native second harmonic imaging and contrast agent. A significant step forward has been the development of 3D echocardiography and the possibility to quantitatively evaluate regional myocardial deformation by 2D/3D speckle tracking (Figure 1.3). 3D echocardiography provides surgeons planning to repair a valve with images very similar to what they see at the time of surgery. Deformation imaging allows characterization of cardiac mechanics and detection of subclinical myocardial dysfunction. Echocardiography is harmless and combines low-cost high-quality technology with easy accessibility. It provides rapid quantitative information about cardiac structure and function at the bedside. It is the first-line imaging test in the diagnostic work-up and monitoring of most cardiac diseases.

1.3.2 Nuclear cardiology

The introduction of nuclear imaging dates back to the first scintillator cameras developed by Anger in the early 1960s. Hence, besides echocardiography, nuclear imaging can be considered one of the oldest noninvasive imaging techniques in cardiology. This technology requires the injection of a mildly radioactive compound, which is distributed within the body according to the biological behavior of the carrier molecule, and decays by emission of photons, which then are picked up by the detector assembly.

The first scintigraphy devices used in clinical practice consisted of a simple flat camera allowing only planar two-dimensional image acquisition. Since then, numerous

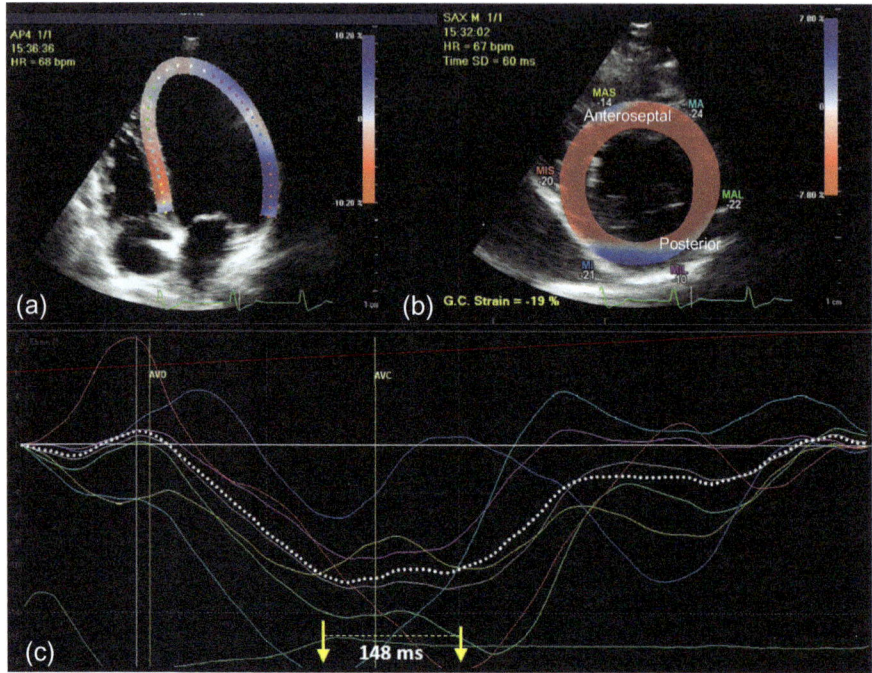

Figure 1.3 Myocardial strain imaging by echocardiography (Chapter 21).

technical developments have improved the technique to increase their utility in clinical practice. The SPECT technique (single-photon emission computed tomography) consists of rotating detector panels that allow the acquisition of 3D information from various angles and is an integral requirement for cardiac imaging. Positron emission tomography (PET) consists of a complete detector ring equipped with special detector crystals. This assembly is designed to detect coincident photons originating from positron emitters and has thereby a higher spatial resolution than SPECT. The last two decades have witnessed an increasing interest in cardiac imaging with the developments of dedicated cardiac SPECT cameras. These devices are characterized by small-footprint detector arrays, specialized collimators, and dedicated image reconstruction algorithms. By this means, they improve image resolution and patient comfort, reduce acquisition times, and lower radiation exposure for cardiac imaging.

The feature that distinguishes nuclear imaging from other techniques is the principle of radiotracer injection and photon emission as compared to transmissional cross-sectional techniques. Very low concentrations of radiolabeled compound (in the nanomolar range) in the region of interest are enough to generate a signal strong enough to be picked up by current state-of-the-art cameras. As a result, nuclear imaging is an ideal technique to detect functional aspects of normal or diseased cardiac physiology (Figure 1.4). Myocardial perfusion is the most important application; however, the technique also allows interrogation of other biological conditions (metabolism, innervation, inflammation, etc.), which have important avenues for clinical and experimental cardiology.

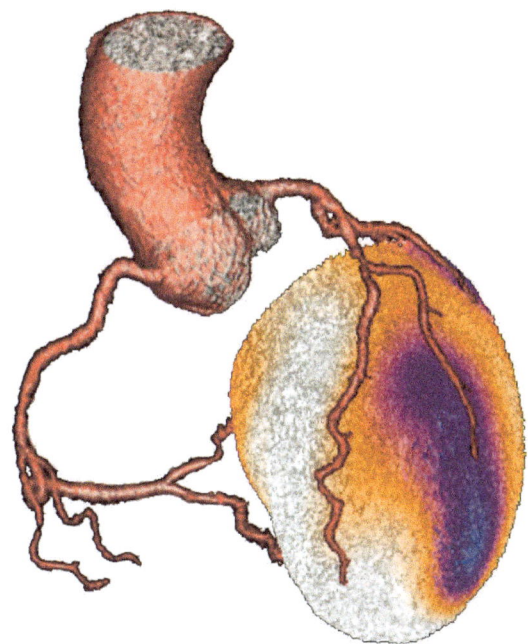

Figure 1.4 Combined SPECT-CT imaging. Hydrid SPECT-CT combining the anatomical information from coronary CT angiography and the functional imaging from SPECT myocardial perfusion imaging. Simultaneous presentation indicates that ischemia is present in the territory supplied by the diagonal branch.

1.3.3 Cardiac CT

Computed tomography was introduced in the early 1970s, although the heart remained largely off-limits until the turn of the millennium. With the introduction of multidetector scanners, fast and continuous tube rotation, ECG-synchronization and dedicated cardiac image reconstruction algorithms, cardiac CT became a clinical reality. Cardiac CT is most appreciated for its high spatial resolution and ability to depict detailed cardiovascular morphology in a very short time.

The clinically most distinguishing application of cardiac CT is noninvasive imaging of the coronary arteries to rule out coronary artery disease in a range of different situations. Also in the context of minimally invasive procedures (ablation procedures, TAVI) cardiac CT provides critical information to safely guide these interventions. Because the examination is fast and relatively easy to perform, with relative independence of patient characteristics and cooperation, cardiac CT is the most applied technique for visualizing acute cardiovascular pathology (aortic dissection) and functions as a backup to echocardiography and CMR in various situations, but also finds its utility in young patients with congenital conditions (Figure 1.5).

Over the past few years, technical innovation has focused on reducing the radiation exposure, effectively reducing doses associated with coronary CT angiography from more than 15 mSv to below 5 mSv in routine use, to even below 1 mSv with

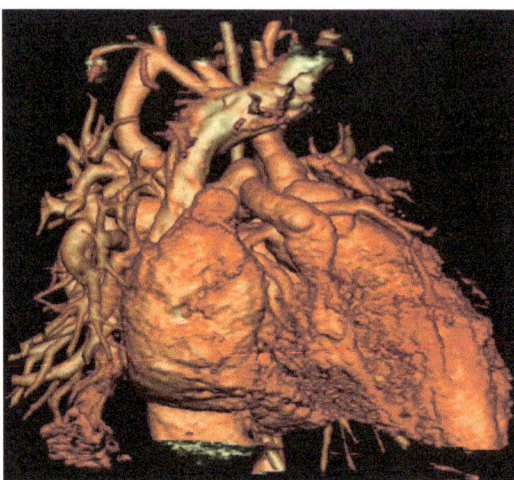

Figure 1.5 Paediatric cardiac CT. Cardiac CT scan of a young patient born with atresia of the tricuspid valve.

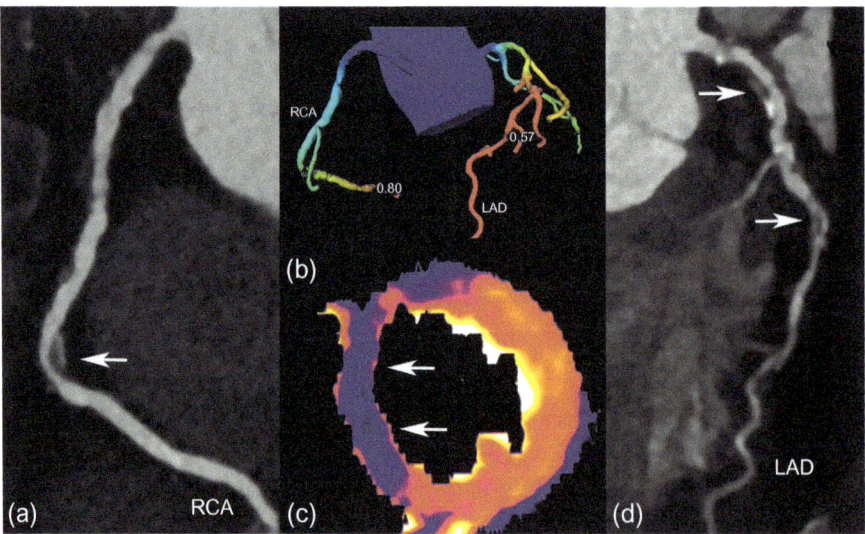

Figure 1.6 Comprehensive cardiac CT exam. Coronary CT angiography shows two-vessel disease of the RCA and LAD (a,d, arrows). CTA-derived fractional flow reserve estimation indicates that the lesion in the LAD is hemodynamically obstructed: CTA-FFR = 0.57 (b), which is confirmed by CT myocardial perfusion imaging (c).

contemporary technology in selected patients. A number of applications for functional CT assessment of ischemic heart disease have been developed recently, which include myocardial perfusion imaging and CTA based simulations of fractional flow reserve (Figure 1.6). There is ongoing research in the field of plaque characterization, valve imaging, and visualization of myocardial infarction.

1.3.4 Cardiac MR

MRI has been used in medical imaging for many decades, and the first images of the heart were obtained soon after. However, like CT, CMR only became a clinical reality in the 1990s, when fast imaging techniques and reliable ECG-synchronization were introduced. The key advantage of CMR is that it is free of ionizing radiation and it produces images with high tissue contrast in any desired plane. By varying image acquisition parameters and, in many cases, the addition of external contrast agents, both morphological and functional information can be derived and numerous tissue characteristics interrogated by CMR, making it a very versatile technique.

The clinical applications of CMR today span from congenital to acquired heart disease and include imaging of cardiac masses and the pericardium as well as the vasculature. In congenital heart disease, CMR is part of standard clinical care because of the wide-ranging information it provides and its safety as a nonionizing radiation test. In cardiomyopathies, CMR guides classification and detection of more subtle disease; in CAD, CMR now has Class 1A indication for the detection of ischemia and provides unique information on tissue viability.

Recent advances have seen the development of multidirectional flow images (Figure 1.7), quantitative measurements of tissue components such as the extracellular volume fraction and targeted imaging of inflammation and other pathological processes (Figure 1.8). Metabolic imaging with MR spectroscopy has been performed for decades; however, methods known as hyperpolarization have recently offered

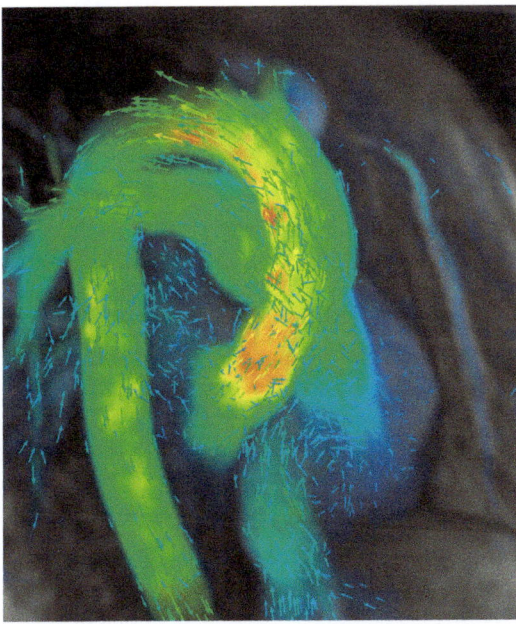

Figure 1.7 4D Flow by MRI. Blood flow in 3D through the great thoracic vessels using cardiac magnetic resonance.

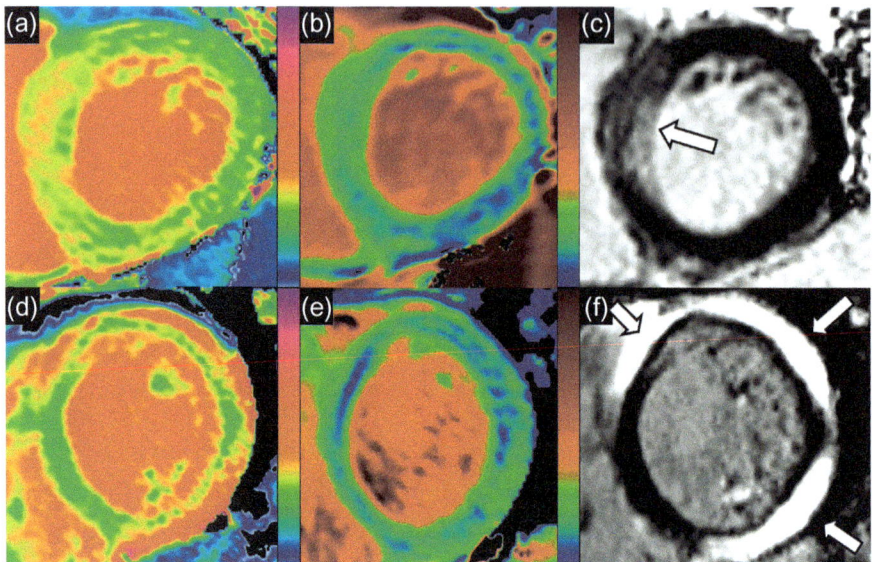

Figure 1.8 MRI tissue characterization. T1 and T2 mapping for myocardial tissue characterization (from Chapter 6).

unparalleled opportunities for signal enhancement of spectroscopic methods with many new imaging targets likely to emerge in the coming years.

1.4 Shared themes and challenges

1.4.1 Multimodality imaging

The rapid innovation of noninvasive imaging techniques, and the expanding number of applications for each modality, has enriched and generally improved the care of patients with cardiovascular disease over the past decades. Different techniques offer different perspectives and potentially better understanding of clinical cardiovascular disease processes. There are true hybrid, multimodality systems, such as SPECT-CT or PET-MRI, but the combination of CT coronary angiography with perfusion imaging on the same scanner, or a combined comprehensive CMR protocol that includes contractile function, stress perfusion, and infarct imaging can also be considered a multifaceted test (Figures 1.9 and 1.10). However, an abundance of diagnostic options can also cause confusion in daily practice. To detect and characterize ischemic heart disease, today's physician can choose between noninvasive coronary imaging by CT, vasodilator mediated perfusion imaging by CMR or nuclear techniques, or dobutamine stress imaging using echocardiography or CMR, with several more techniques and applications around the corner. While (conflicting) evidence exists to favor one test over another, individual choices turn out to be much more complicated. Individual performance depends on local expertise, available technology, patient characteristics,

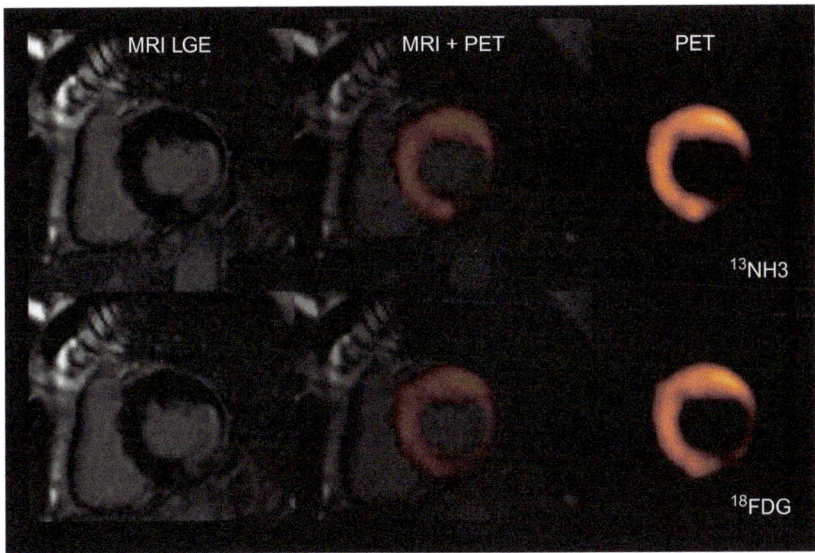

Figure 1.9 Hybrid CMR and PET imaging. Modified from *International Journal of Cardiology*, 167 (5), Anagnostopoulos et al. Assessment of myocardial perfusion and viability by Positron Emission Tomography, 2013, with permission from Elsevier (from Chapter 11).

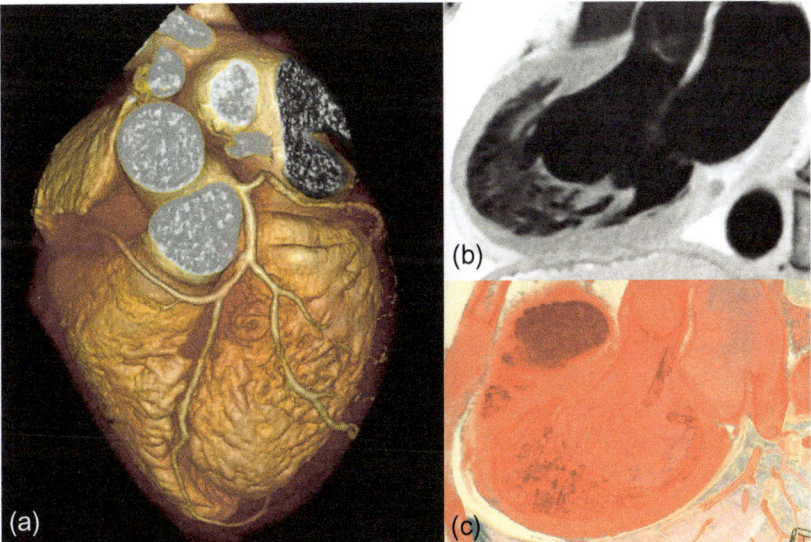

Figure 1.10 Noncompaction cardiomyopathy. Cardiac CT scan of a patient with noncompaction cardiomyopathy and a single coronary artery.

and preferences. In-depth understanding of the strengths and weaknesses of each technique is required to make the most optimal diagnostic choices. The threat of stacking tests and diagnostic overconsumption requires conscious diagnostic decisions. A multimodality mentality does not imply that multiple techniques should be employed at every opportunity, but rather that the physician can choose the most optimal technique for the right patient at the right time to guide management, without trying to solve each problem every time with the same diagnostic tool. The future requires physicians with a broad understanding of the different imaging techniques and knowledge of how these can be applied most effectively, to improve care but also to contain medical expenses.

1.4.2 Evidence-based imaging

In the future local experience, technical validations and registry data will no longer suffice to support our diagnostic choices. The fact that a specific test result predicts outcome is not evidence that performance of the test itself improves prognosis and is therefore justified. The bar has been raised for aspiring new imaging techniques, requiring demonstration of incremental value to other techniques, preferably in prospective trial designs, evaluating hard clinical or economic endpoints. Randomized controlled trials to demonstrate the efficacy of diagnostic tests are challenging because blinding is impossible and the benefit of the test can only be measured by the subsequent therapeutic decisions. Many applications are considered generic, which makes funding of large trials less attractive to manufacturers of imaging equipment. The rapid pace at which imaging techniques are introduced, improved, and adopted harbor the risk of results that run obsolete long before publication. Nevertheless, RCTs may eventually be unavoidable, and several groups have already embarked on the challenge of randomized clinical effectiveness trials [ROMICAT2, ACRIN-PA, MR INFORM PROMISE, CRESCENT, ISCHEMIA].

1.4.3 Imaging safety

An important consideration when choosing between imaging techniques is safety. Echocardiography is generally the safest option, as it requires no radiation and can be performed without the need for contrast medium in the majority of examinations. CMR does not require ionizing radiation and is generally regarded as a safe technique in competent hands and absent contra-indications. Complications related to MR contrast medium are rare. Nuclear imaging and computed tomography cannot be performed without ionizing radiation, which exposes patients to a small but non-negligible risk of malignant disease development. Over the past decade, doses used in both techniques have decreased substantially. Nevertheless, avoidance of radiation should be preferred if equivalent information can be obtained by other means. Iodine containing contrast media, as used in CT or invasive angiography, potentially harm renal function, and precautions are required in patients with kidney dysfunction. Use of medication during diagnostic examinations, including inotropic medication, vasodilators, or heart rate modulation, rarely cause complications, but examiners need to be prepared to handle complications.

1.4.4 Multidisciplinary collaboration

While echocardiography is generally established entirely within the department of cardiology, this is often not the case for the other noninvasive cardiac imaging techniques discussed in this book. In most centers, cardiac CT and CMR are performed within a variable form of collaboration between the departments of cardiology and radiology. In many parts of the world, SPECT and PET scanners are installed within the department of nuclear medicine or radiology. Advanced cardiac imaging benefits from constructive collaboration between imaging and clinical specialists. But also for cardiovascular clinicians with limited operational imaging involvement, an understanding of the possibilities and limitations of advanced cardiac imaging is essential for practicing contemporary cardiovascular medicine.

1.5 Approach of the book

This book was conceived in line with the considerations above. Instead of discussing the imaging modalities separately, we challenged the authors to discuss the relative and complementary value of different techniques within the context of specific clinical questions or situations. The first chapters focus on the general principles and latest trends in research and technical development for each of the modalities. Subsequent chapters discuss the advantages, disadvantages, and complementary value of imaging in different situations. Several chapters have been dedicated to the emerging role of imaging guided interventions of structural heart disease and electrophysiological conditions.

Part One

Technological developments in cardiac imaging

Ultrasound/echocardiography

N.E. Hasselberg[*,†], T. Edvardsen[*,†]
*Oslo University Hospital, Rikshospitalet, Oslo, Norway; †University of Oslo, Oslo, Norway

2.1 Introduction

The traditional echocardiographic techniques are widely used and form a routine complete echocardiographic examination:

- M-mode recordings, guided by two-dimensional (2D) echocardiographic images, are used for quantification of cardiac dimension and timing of rapid cardiac motions [1]. It is recommended that left ventricular (LV) internal diameters and wall thickness are measured by M-mode since they show excellent temporal resolution and may complement 2D images in separating structures such as trabeculae adjacent to the posterior wall, false tendons, or the moderator band next to the septum from the endocardium [1]. Linear measurements from M-mode have proven to be reproducible with low intra- and inter-observer variability. However, even with 2D guidance, it may not be possible to align the M-mode cursor perpendicular to the long axis of the ventricle, which is mandatory to obtain a true minor axis dimension measurement. One practical solution to this problem is to use the "anatomical" M-mode technique, which allows the user to steer the M-mode line to any angle that he or she chooses through the 2D image. The disadvantage of this technique is poorer temporal and spatial resolution compared to the real M-mode technique. Furthermore, linear measurements for size and function assessment are problematic when there are marked regional differences in function.
- 2D echocardiographic images provide detailed anatomic data in a given tomographic image. With 2D images, pathology in the cardiac cavities, myocardial walls, and valvular apparatus are visualized, as are malformations, tumours, and masses. 2D images are important for quantifying chamber volumes and myocardial mass. LV function is traditionally assessed by ejection fraction (EF). End-diastolic and end-systolic volumes are measured by using the bi-plane method of discs' summation (modified Simpson's rule). LVEF is then calculated from these respective 2D LV volumes, making EF a strictly volumetric measure of LV function. In contrast, strain by deformation imaging directly measures the intrinsic contractile properties of the myocardium. Echocardiographic strain has been shown to be a more accurate tool for quantification of myocardial function compared to EF [2].
- Doppler flow imaging, with continuous wave and pulsed wave, is analyzed by spectral analysis and assesses blood flow direction, velocity, and signal amplitude. From this, we can calculate pressure gradients over the cardiac valves and assess diastolic function by interpreting the blood flow patterns.
- Colour Doppler flow imaging (multiple sample volumes of pulsed wave Doppler along each ultrasound line) visualizes location, expansion, direction, and timing of blood flow in the cardiac chambers and through the valves or shunts.

These traditional parameters are first-line measures and provide important diagnostic and prognostic information that cannot be entirely replaced by more advanced echocardiographic techniques. In general, the traditional measures have high specificity. If they show evidence of true pathology, given acceptable image quality, there is often no further need for more advanced techniques. For example, EF has excellent diagnostic and prognostic value when myocardial function is severely depressed and EF is low (<35%). The advanced imaging techniques have their strength in having higher sensitivity for minor pathologic changes. Echocardiographic strain may show subtle reduction in LV function before symptoms appear and EF falls and contrast echocardiography may reveal early regional dysfunction in a patient with poor image quality on normal 2D images.

In this chapter of advanced echocardiography, we will describe three-dimensional echocardiography, contrast echocardiography, and deformation imaging by ultrasound. We will end the chapter with a section describing promising echocardiographic methods with the potential of obtaining clinical importance in the near future.

2.2 Three-dimensional echocardiography [3,4]

Three-dimensional (3D) echocardiography represents a large and important advancement in cardiac ultrasound. Real-time 3D acquisition and imaging of the heart from any preferable angle have become possible with advancements in transducer and computer technologies. 3D echocardiography is especially useful and applies additional information over 2D echocardiography in the assessment of:

- Cardiac volumes and mass independently of geometric assumptions
- Heart valves
- Regurgitant lesions, jets, and shunts (3D echocardiography colour Doppler)

In addition, the 3D technique has theoretical benefits compared to 2D in:

- LV regional function and dyssynchrony
- 3D stress echocardiography

2.2.1 Matrix-array transducer

Developments in hardware and software have resulted in fully sampled matrix-array transducers providing improved real-time imaging of the beating heart. 3D echocardiography matrix-array transducers are composed of about 3000 piezoelectric elements with operating frequency 2–4 MHz for transthoracic echocardiography (TTE) and 5–7 MHz for transoesophageal echocardiography (TEE). The piezoelectric elements are simultaneously active and arranged in a grid fashion. A large number of digital channels are required to connect the fully sampled elements. To avoid excessive power consumption and a wide transducer cable, several small circuits are incorporated into the transducer to allow partial beam forming in the probe. While the transducer is maintained in fixed orientation, the ultrasonic beam can steer automatically in multiple directions. This beam steering and signal processing take place automatically in the scanning probe itself. The newest generation of transducers is becoming smaller, and one single transducer can acquire both 2D and 3D studies of excellent quality. Transducers today provide better side-lobe suppression, less transducer footprint, and increased sensitivity and penetration.

2.2.2 Data acquisition—two modes

2.2.2.1 Real-time 3D echocardiographic imaging

Acquisition consists of multiple pyramidal datasets per second in one single heartbeat. The data are visualized in real-time scanning, beat after beat, while performing the examination as in conventional 2D scanning. Real-time 3D echocardiography imaging has no limitation imposed by rhythm disturbances or respiratory motion, but the temporal and spatial resolution is poorer than 2D imaging.

Real-time 3D narrow volume
Beat-by-beat view with a thicker image plane (slice) than for normal 2D imaging. The thick slice can be rotated.

Real-time 3D zoomed
A full-volume image of an enlarged area of interest. The perspective is like taking a photograph from inside the heart. Spatial and temporal resolutions are poor, and the image must be rotated to gain all anatomical information.

Real-time 3D colour Doppler
Colour Doppler acquisition at lower frame rates than for gray tone data.

2.2.2.2 ECG-triggered multi-beat 3D echocardiographic imaging

Multiple high-resolution narrow volumes of data over consecutive heartbeats are stitched together.

Full volume 3D (gated)
A single volumetric dataset is created from several smaller subvolumes not obtained simultaneously but from consecutive heart cycles. Small subvolumes provide high spatial and temporal resolution. Since the gated image is a sum of 2–7 heart cycles, it is susceptible to artifacts from body movement, respiratory motion, or irregular heart rhythms (Figure 2.1).

2.2.3 Challenges and limitations

The technical aspects of acquiring high-quality 3D echocardiography suitable for diagnostic or therapeutic purposes are similar to those for 2D echocardiography. In addition, incorrect gain settings and respiratory or ECG gating may lead to reconstruction artefacts.

2.2.3.1 Temporal versus spatial resolution

The main trade-off in 3D echocardiography is between temporal resolution and spatial resolution. Increasing spatial resolution, i.e., the number of scan lines per volume, require more time for acquisition, resulting in a falling temporal resolution. By reducing volume size, one can increase temporal resolution by simultaneously maintaining spatial resolution.

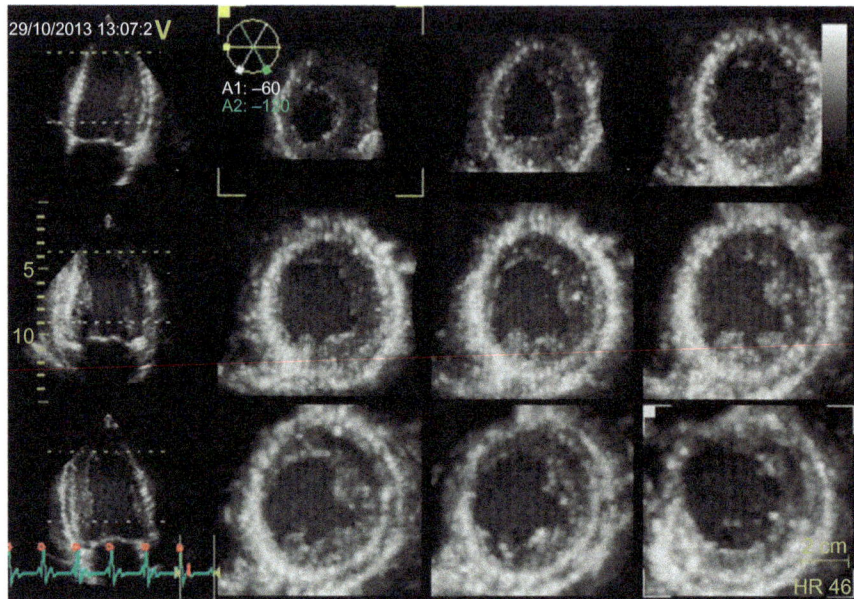

Figure 2.1 Multi-beat 3D echocardiographic imaging. Multislice image showing nine short-axis planes of the left ventricle created from six subvolumes from six consecutive heartbeats. Courtesy of Richard J. Massey, sonographer, Oslo University Hospital, Norway.

2.2.3.2 ECG gating and breath hold

Gated imaging fails when the patient is unable to perform adequate breath holding or when the heart rhythm is irregular. These situations result in stitching artifacts, which are seen as artificial lines in the image, representing interjections between neighbor subvolumes attained from different cardiac cycles. Suboptimal ECG tracings without distinct R-waves deteriorate correct gating of the subvolumes.

The gating artifacts can be minimized in different ways. One should always wait until a regular rhythm appears and be aware that full-volume gated images are not possible in patients with atrial fibrillation. For reducing respiratory artifacts, one asks the patient for breath holding, preferably during the expiration phase.

2.2.3.3 Echo dropouts

Dropouts can result from low gain settings and appear as "holes" in anatomic structures. The dropouts can falsely be identified as defects in the tissue, and they may artificially eliminate anatomic structures, making them invisible. Dropouts cannot be recovered during post processing. To avoid dropouts, it is recommended that both time gain compensation and compression settings are adjusted in the midrange and optimized with slightly higher gain control than at normal 2D acquisition. This allows the greatest flexibility during post processing. Optimizing lateral and axial resolution is just as important during 3D as in 2D acquisition.

2.2.4 Cropping

Cropping can be done in 3D zoom mode and gated full-volume mode to view the interior of the heart. Unlike 2D echocardiography, cropping is essential for 3D echocardiography to enable the visualization of the region of interest and the bypassing of structures in front of this region. Different perspectives of a structure can be obtained by alternating between rotating and recropping. For example, the aortic valve can be seen from the aorta, from the LV or in a long-axis orientation. Cropping and rotation can be done at data acquisition, with the advantage of obtaining better spatial and temporal resolution, but with the disadvantage of the inability to uncrop later. If cropping is performed as part of post processing, one will retain more information, but at a cost of lower spatial and temporal resolution.

The most frequently used cropping planes are the transverse plane, dividing the heart into superior and inferior parts; saggital plane, dividing the heart into right and left parts; and coronal plane, dividing the heart into anterior and posterior parts.

2.2.5 Post acquisition display

The 3D dataset is displayed using 3D visualization software packages:

2.2.5.1 Volume rendering

Volume rendering is a technique using different types of algorithms to preserve all 3D echocardiographic information and project it after processing onto a 2D plane for viewing. The volume-rendered 3D echocardiographic dataset can be electronically segmented and sectioned, cropped, and rotated to provide complex spatial relationships in a 3D display. It is especially useful for evaluating valves and nearby structures (Figures 2.2 and 2.5).

2.2.5.2 Surface rendering

Structures or organs are shown to the observer as either a solid or a wireframe (cage) 3D object. It is obtained by manually tracing or using semiautomatic border detection algorithms to trace the endocardium in cross-sectional images generated from the 3D dataset. These contours are combined to generate a 3D shape. Surface rendering provides quantification of chamber volumes (can be displayed graphically throughout the cardiac cycle) and function by EF but often fails to provide detailed information of cardiac structures or textures (Figures 2.3 and 2.4).

2.2.5.3 3D tomographic slices

By slicing the volumetric data, one can obtain multiple simultaneous 2D plane views. This provides the acquisition of different cutting planes from virtually any acoustic window, including 2D cutting planes which are difficult or virtually impossible to obtain with standard 2D transducer manipulation. 2D parallel tomographic slices with uniformly spaced 2D parallel slices can be obtained. The ability to "move through"

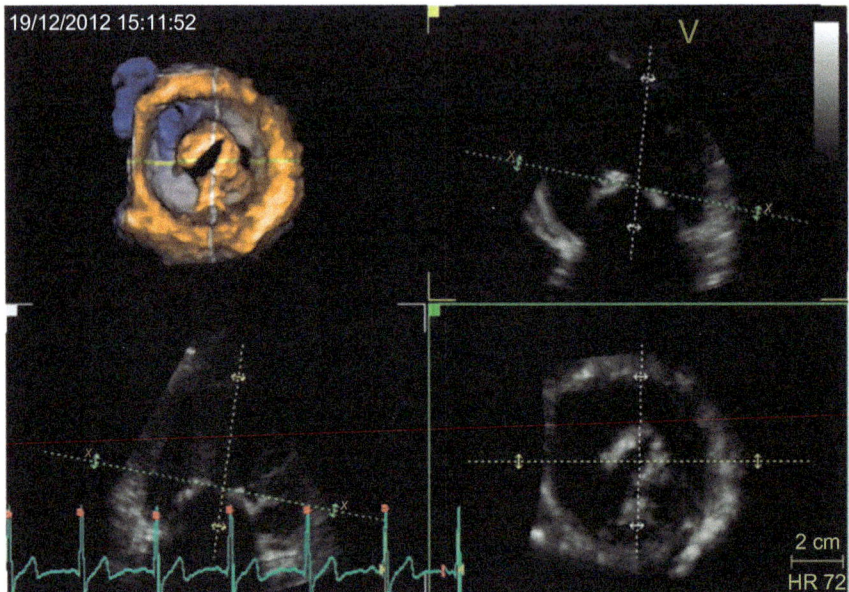

Figure 2.2 3D echocardiography of a patient with mitral stenosis. Upper left panel shows the 3D image. Upper right and lower panels show 2D slices (by flexislice method) created from the 3D dataset. The accurate mitral valve area can be traced and measured from the 2D image.
Courtesy of Richard J. Massey, sonographer, Oslo University Hospital, Norway.

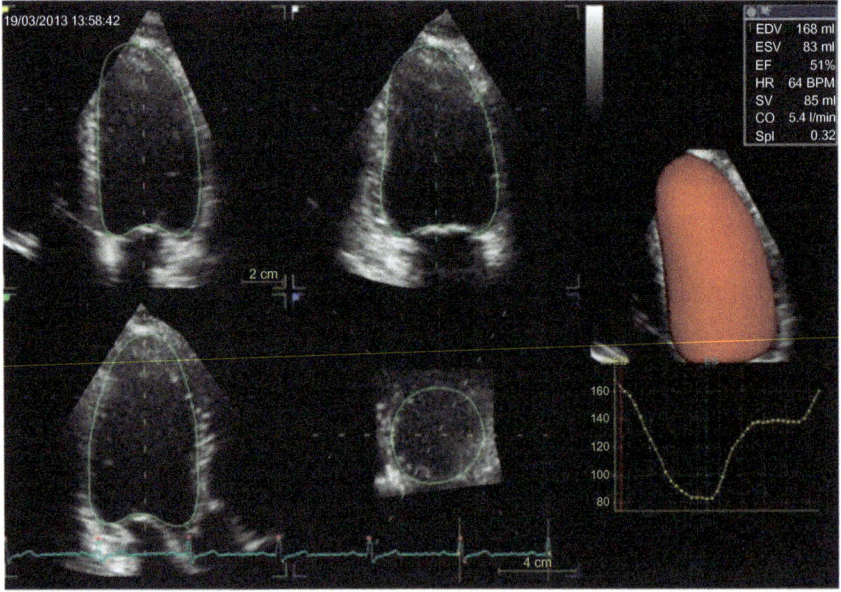

Figure 2.3 Surface rendering image. The left ventricle depicted by its surface as a solid 3D object (red) is derived from a manual correction of the semi-automated endocardial border detection in all three apical views. Left ventricular volume throughout the cardiac cycle is shown in the graph (lower right).
Courtesy of Richard J. Massey, sonographer, Oslo University Hospital, Norway.

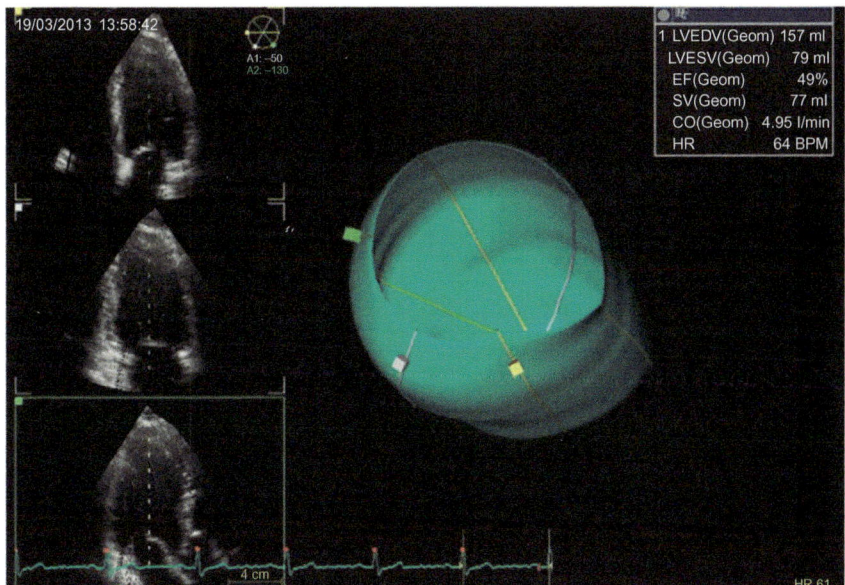

Figure 2.4 Surface rendering image. 3D image of the left ventricular cavity (blue).
Courtesy of Richard J. Massey, sonographer, Oslo University Hospital, Norway.

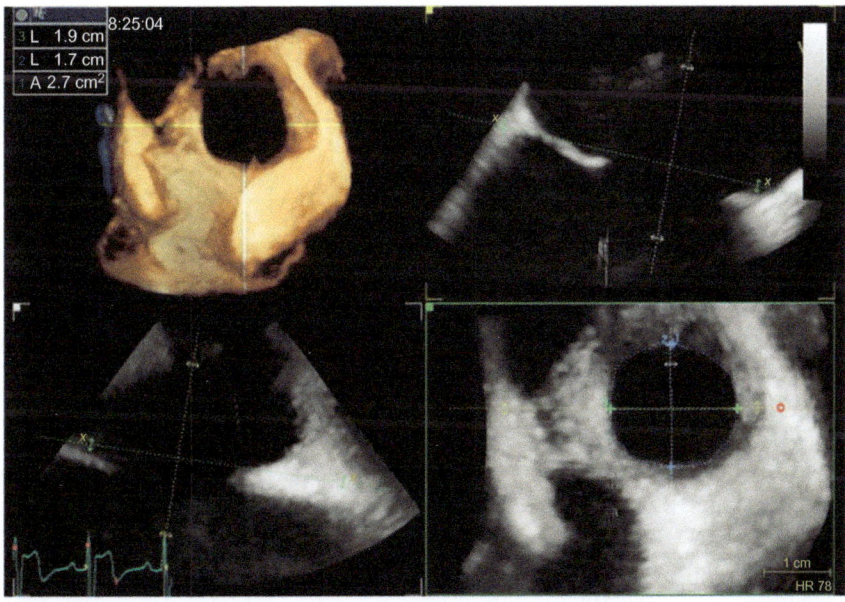

Figure 2.5 Transesophageal 3D echocardiography of a patient with an atrial septal defect. Upper left figure shows a 3D image, with the defect seen from the right atrium. By flexislice method, 2D plane images can be made from any plane preferable in the 3D dataset. Geometry and area of the defect can be accurately assessed to help choosing correct device for defect closure.
Courtesy of Richard J. Massey, sonographer, Oslo University Hospital, Norway.

the 3D dataset in any 2D plane allows accurate measurements of chamber dimensions, valve, or septal defect areas as well as improved evaluation of the morphology and function of structures. During stress echocardiography, the ability to display multiple LV planes simultaneously speeds the image acquisition.

2.2.6 3D colour Doppler

Colour Doppler adds flow information onto the 3D morphology. 3D colour Doppler acquisitions are performed using real-time 3D or multi-beat full volume acquisition.

TEE provides the best colour Doppler image quality and is recommended over TTE for detailed colour flow analysis.

3D colour Doppler analyses provide images for evaluation of distal jets, proximal flow field of valvular flow regurgitation, and flow through septal defects. 3D colour Doppler flow mapping is able to qualitatively visualize size and shape of valvular and paravalvular regurgitations as well as the underlying pathology, enabling exact definition of jet origin, size, propagation, and relationship with adjacent structures. Cropping can be performed according to the intended analysis. For example, to evaluate regurgitant jets, it is recommended that the 3D colour Doppler data be cropped to view two long-axis views (one at the narrowest and one at the broadest width of the jet) and the short-axis view at the level of the vena contracta.

Poor spatial and temporal resolutions are limitations to 3D colour Doppler acquisitions. Currently, live 3D colour Doppler is limited to small volumes with low temporal resolution. As an alternative, multi-beat full volumes deliver higher frame rates up to 40 voxels/second, but are limited by stitching artifacts with displacements between different subvolumes. New 3D colour Doppler technology is being developed to reduce these problems.

2.2.7 Stress echocardiography

The advantages of 3D over 2D stress echocardiography are better visualization of the LV apex, shorter scanning time, rapid acquisition of peak stress images before heart rate declines in recovery, and evaluation of multiple segments from different planes from a single dataset. Disadvantages are lower spatial and temporal resolution than with 2D acquisition. Most stress 3D echocardiography software allows displaying the same view at rest and different stress-stages simultaneously, side-by-side, for comparison. Both physical stress and pharmacologic stress (dobutamine, atropine, or dipyridamine) can be used. Contrast agents can be added for improved endocardial delineation or assessment of myocardial perfusion.

The main and maybe most advantageous difference between 2D and 3D stress echocardiography is the significantly shorter scanning time required at each stress level and for the complete study using 3D echocardiography. There is no need to change the transducer position during apical scanning once the optimal window is identified. Therefore, it is easier to catch the narrow time window of peak stress; this increases the sensitivity to detect ischemic mechanical changes, which is most likely to appear at the highest heart rates. Because of its ability to acquire the entire LV volume within one beat, 3D stress echocardiography is likely to be incorporated into clinical practice in the near future.

2.2.8 Implementation of 3D

Implementing 3D in clinical practice calls for a feasible workflow. So far, the 2D image quality obtained by the 3D probe has been insufficient compared to a modern 2D probe. It is too time-consuming to perform a full 3D echocardiographic examination on top of the traditional 2D examination. The newest 3D TTE and TEE probes deliver 2D echocardiographic images comparable to those delivered by dedicated 2D transducers. Ultrasound companies are developing more accurate automated chamber quantification and automated display of standard 3D and 2D cut planes from each window acquisition. What also needs to be optimized is the way 3D echocardiographic data is stored and recalled for analysis. A 2D exam requires about 300–500 MB of storage space for raw data, while a combined 2D and 3D examination requires 1.5 GB [1]. The large datasets are a challenge to the local digital systems of laboratories in regard to transmission and overall storage capacity.

2.2.9 Conclusions

3D echocardiography's full potential is far from being exploited clinically today. With advancements in 3D acquisitions techniques and software improving image quality and reducing the time it takes for image acquisition and post processing, the clinical role of 3D echocardiography will grow. Assessment of the right ventricle has failed with 2D echocardiography; hopefully, 3D imaging will improve the accuracy and reproducibility of RV volume and function assessment. Potential clinical applications where 3D echocardiography may be routinely performed are dyssynchrony assessment, strain imaging, and evaluation of prosthetic valves. Today, low spatial and temporal resolution of larger volumes remain as limitations. Obtaining a real-time single-heartbeat-full volume dataset with high spatial and temporal resolution and live 3D color Doppler of wide angle should be feasible in the future and will increase utility and efficiency of 3D echocardiography.

2.3 Contrast echocardiography [3–6]

2.3.1 Ultrasound contrast agents

The ultrasound contrast agents are acoustically active microbubbles consisting of an outer phospholipid or albumin shell encapsulating an inner high-molecular-weight gas. They are strong ultrasound reflectors, i.e., the backscatter they create results in intense echocardiographic signals that are stronger than the ultrasound waves (echoes) from the surrounding tissue and blood cells. Because the agents remain intravascular, they act as red blood cell tracers. The first-generation agents (inner gas was air) were safe but dissipated too quickly to be of clinical value. Second-generation agents consist of a gas that has high density, high molecular weight, and low solubility, making the microbubbles more stable. The bubbles do not accumulate, are biologically inert, and are considered safe.

There are three second-generation contrast agents approved for echocardiographic studies: Definity, Optison and SonoVue (not approved in the US) (Table 2.1).

2.3.2 Physics of microbubbles

The microbubbles must be able to resist destruction at normal ultrasound power outputs. Changes to both the inner gas and to a thicker outer shell confer stability and have improved the durability of the bubbles, ensuring the ability to cross the pulmonary capillary bed and reach the LV cavity intact. A microbubble's ultrasound characteristics depend on its size and the composition of the outer shell and the gas. Backscatter is proportional to the sixth power of the radius, leading to best acoustic signal from the largest bubbles being able to cross through the lung microvasculature. Also, there is a positive linear relationship between concentration and signal intensity. Ultrasound wave pressure compresses and expands the microbubbles, which start to oscillate. The volume expansion of a microbubble is maximal at a specific frequency called the natural resonant frequency and is inversely related to its size. At this resonant frequency, the microbubble scatters and absorbs ultrasound and can present nonlinear vibrations when the insonifying acoustic pressure is high enough. Consequently, the bubble oscillation contains second and higher multiples of the transmitted frequency. The backscattered signal from the microbubble therefore contains not only the fundamental frequency but also harmonic frequencies, most notably at twice the fundamental frequency (second harmonics). This nonlinear reflection is not shown by tissue, allowing the separation of response from the microbubbles from that of surrounding tissue. Finally, as the peak ultrasound wave pressure becomes more intense, many of the microbubbles are disrupted, exhibiting an irreversible, transient, and intense scattering depending on the type of gas released and its dissolution in the liquid. This scattered signal is also highly nonlinear.

2.3.3 Administration

Contrast agents are made available by mixing saline with dry powder of contrast followed by intravenously administration as bolus injection or as a continuous infusion.

Bolus injections are acceptable for studies in which the aim is to improve endocardial border delineation, perform LV opacification, or enhance Doppler signals. It is not recommended in perfusion studies.

Continuous infusion provides a steady-state concentration of microbubbles and reduces the likelihood of artefacts. It also allows calculation of myocardial blood flow, as both microbubble velocity and myocardial blood volume can be calculated if there is a steady-state concentration of contrast. Continuous infusions are mandatory for perfusion imaging and are also often recommended for endocardial border delineation and LV opacification purposes.

Table 2.1 Characteristics of three contrast agents available for echocardiography

	Gas	Bubble size	Shell composition	Side effects
SonoVue	Sulfur hexafluoride	2–8 µm	Lipid	Headache Nausea Chest pain Injection site reaction Hyperglycemia Parasthesia Vasodilation
Optison	Perfluoropropane	3.0–4.5 µm	Albumin	Headache Nausea/vomiting Warm sensation Flushing Dizziness
Luminity (definity)	Perfluoropropane	1.1–2.5 µm	Lipid	Headache Flushing Back pain Rash/uticaria Wheezing Anaphylaxis

Modified from EAE recommendation [5].

2.3.4 Safety of contrast imaging

Several clinical trials have demonstrated safety of using contrast agents with no increase in adverse events. Side effects are usually mild and transient (Table 2.1). Optison and Luminity may be used in patients with acute coronary syndrome. However, serious side effect have been seen at a low estimated incidence of 1:10 000. The Food and Drug Administration highlight the risk of serious cardiopulmonary reactions during or within 30 minutes following the administration of contrast agents and recommend that high-risk patients with pulmonary hypertension or unstable cardiopulmonary conditions should be closely monitored during and for at least 30 minutes after administration. Overall, it is concluded that contrast echocardiography is very safe in clinical practice [5]. The only absolute contraindications for contrast agent administration are in patients with large intracardial shunts or with known hypersensitivity to the agent.

2.3.5 Mechanical index and imaging modes

Mechanical index (MI) is a measure of the power generated by an ultrasound transducer within an acoustic field.

2.3.5.1 High MI (0.4–0.6) in intermittent static imaging

When microbubbles are exposed to a high MI, they are disrupted almost immediately. With each destructive pulse, high amplitude backscatter rich in harmonics is returned to the transducer, enabling static images. The burst of harmonics provides high sensitivity for contrast detection (seen as bright colour), but the bubbles are irreversibly damaged and can no longer oscillate and thus generate further harmonic signals (i.e., they cannot continue to enhance the image). High MI imaging is therefore not suitable for continuous real-time imaging. Continuous high MI imaging would result in persistent bubble destruction, which prevents detection of microbubbles in the myocardium. Intermittent imaging mode is therefore used where one imaging frame with high MI is created every 1–10 cycles triggered by the ECG. The time between destructive pulses allows the microbubbles to replenish the myocardium. High MI imaging has high sensitivity, as the harmonic signals generated by bubble destruction at high MI are rich and stronger than those emitted at a lower MI. Disadvantages is that one cannot assess wall motion and function because only static images are created at the high MI ultrasound wave and the burst of of harmonics create confounding tissue signals and impairs endocardial delineation. Also, contrast-specific imaging modalities are necessary to suppress these signals (i.e., power Doppler, ultra-harmonics, and power pulse inversion), and it is technically more challenging than low MI imaging. Another disadvantage is that the technique uses large amounts of contrast agent, as microbubbles are repeatedly destroyed and readministered.

2.3.5.2 Low to intermediate MI (<0.1–0.3) in real-time continuous imaging

Real-time imaging uses sufficiently low MI to ensure that microbubbles will oscillate and resonate but not explode from the continuous exposure to the ultrasound waves. Using low MI generates virtually no harmonic signal from non-contrast-enhanced tissue. Therefore, even low amplitude microbubble backscatter can be isolated from tissue signals for processing, and background subtraction techniques are usually not necessary. The low MI real-time imaging provides the best LV opacification with excellent LV endocardial border enhancement, as it demonstrates a sharp demarcation between the cavity with contrast and the myocardium. With an increased contrast concentration, the display of LV opacification of the myocardium shows myocardial perfusion. Continuous imaging, therefore, enables simultaneous assessment of myocardial wall motion and perfusion in real time. However, frame-rate is held low in order to reduce bubble destruction.

During real-time imaging, all the microbubbles can be intentionally totally destroyed by a "flash" of high MI ultrasound pulses and contrast replenishment from the continuous contrast infusion is then observed to allow qualitative and quantitative assessment of myocardial perfusion. There is less contrast needed than with intermittent high MI imaging. A disadvantage of low MI imaging is that the bubbles generate less acoustic signal, making the method less sensitive for contrast detection than high MI imaging.

2.3.5.3 Recommendations from the European Association of Cardiovascular Imaging (EACVI) [4]

Given the advances in contrast-specific imaging techniques, the use of low MI imaging for myocardial contrast echocardiography is recommended, as it provides simultaneous assessment of myocardial function and perfusion.

2.3.6 Contrast imaging modes

2.3.6.1 LV opacification and endocardial delineation

The myocardial vessels comprise only 7% of the myocardium. The myocardial opacification is, therefore, always much less intense than chamber opacification, reassuring excellent endocardial delineation and differentiation between LV cavity and myocardium. This provides improved accuracy for calculation of LV volumes and EF, reduced inter- and intraobserver variability, and improved detection of regional wall motion abnormalities both at rest and in stress echocardiography.

High MI imaging is not an option for LV opacification imaging, as the continuous bubble destruction would deteriorate image quality significantly. Thus, the two options are between low MI and intermediate MI. Intermediate MI (e.g., 0.1–0.3) is feasible as a real-time technique. There is more bubble destruction than with low MI imaging, but the advantage is that the stronger nonlinear oscillations generated by the microbubbles (since they resonate more with increasing MI) yield a stronger acoustic signal. Low MI imaging (<0.1) generates virtually no tissue signal, which is good in most cases; however, sometimes the returning signals are very weak and thus subtle structural abnormalities may be missed (Figure 2.6).

2.3.6.2 Tissue characterization

One can differentiate tissue according to whether it is perfused. A non-perfused apical thrombus showing no contrast signal will be differentiated from perfused tissue, as for example a vascular tumour, reflecting signals from contrast (Figure 2.7).

2.3.6.3 Myocardial perfusion

With a continuous infusion of microbubbles, the entire myocardium gets fully saturated. The contrast signal intensity represents the capillary blood volume, which makes up 90% of the myocardial blood volume. Reduced contrast signal will therefore reflect a similar reduction in myocardial capillary blood volume. Myocardial perfusion is defined as tissue blood flow at the capillary level. As microbubbles are red blood cell tracers, the product of peak microbubble intensity (representative of myocardial blood volume) and their rate of appearance (representative of blood velocity) equal myocardial blood flow. Following destruction and depletion of microbubbles in the myocardium with high MI bursts during low MI real-time imaging (i.e., destruction–replenishment imaging), the intensity, distribution, and velocity of replenishment of microbubble contrast within the myocardium reflect the global and

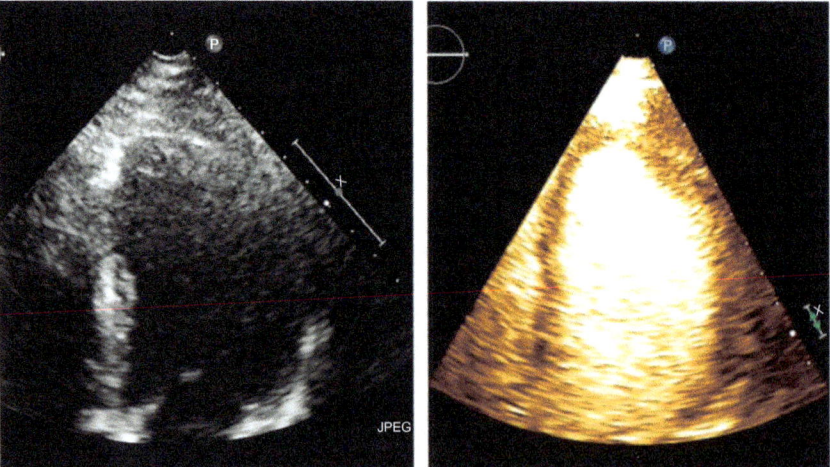

Figure 2.6 Left: Non-contrast-enhanced echocardiographic image showing poor apical and lateral endocardial delineation in a patient. Right: Contrast-enhanced image from the same patient. Continuous low mechanical index imaging with left ventricular opacification provides excellent endocardial border delineation and differentiation between left ventricular cavity and myocardium in the apical and lateral walls.
Courtesy of Mai Tone Lønnebakken, MD, PhD. Haukeland University Hospital, Bergen, Norway.

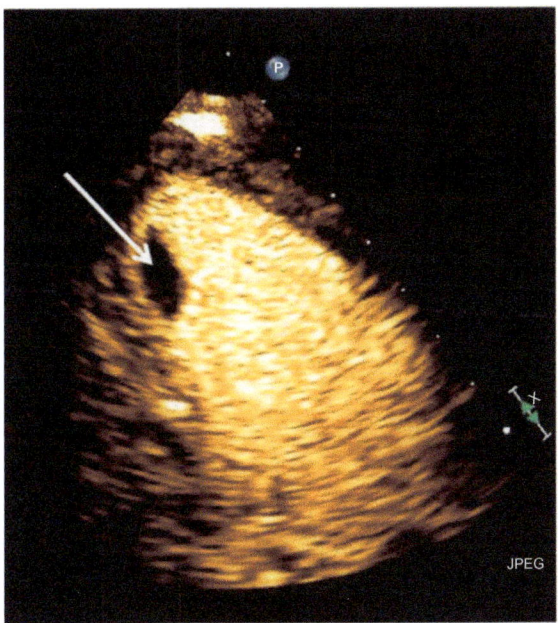

Figure 2.7 Contrast echocardiography with continuous low mechanical index imaging in apical two-chamber view showing and confirming an apical thrombus (arrow). The thrombus does not enhance contrast and can therefore be differentiated from vascularized tissue. Courtesy of Mai Tone Lønnebakken, MD, PhD. Haukeland University Hospital, Bergen, Norway.

regional myocardial perfusion. Potentially, echocardiographic perfusion imaging can improve diagnosis of coronary artery disease, assessment of myocardial viability, and monitoring after reperfusion interventions (Figure 2.8).

Ultrasound contrast agents are not yet approved for myocardial perfusion imaging even though the benefit of this application is increasingly recognized. Furthermore, routine use of contrast agents for myocardial perfusion is not appropriately reimbursed in some countries. Contrast echocardiography has been used since the 1980, but the technical aspects of performing and interpreting the destruction–replenishment imaging are difficult and need more effort to be learned than contrast echocardiography for endocardial border delineation and LV opacification. All these are limiting factors in implementing the echocardiographic perfusion imaging clinically.

2.3.7 Stress echocardiography with contrast

Contrast has been shown to improve visualization of regional wall motion abnormalities and improve study quality and diagnostic accuracy during both exercise and pharmacological stress echocardiography. It has been shown to be cost-efficient to use contrast stress echocardiography for risk stratification in patients admitted to hospital with chest pain. Inter-observer variability of image interpretation is clearly reduced using contrast. The diagnostic accuracy of contrast echocardiography in patients with

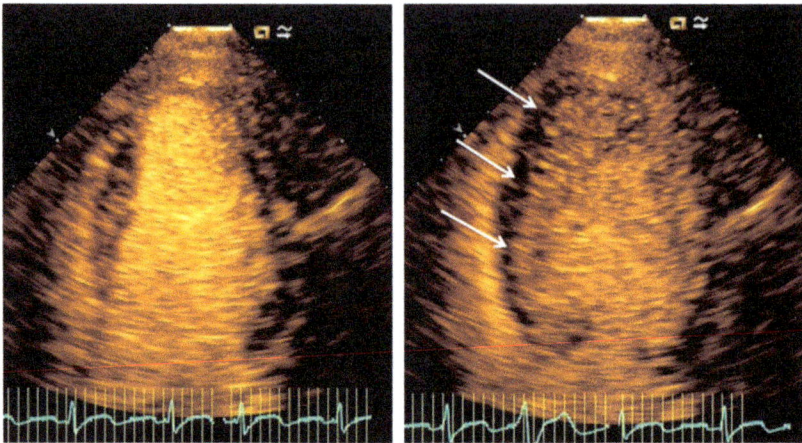

Figure 2.8 Destruction–replenishment contrast imaging for assessment of myocardial perfusion. Left: Image during continuous low mechanical index imaging with continuous contrast infusion shows hypoperfused myocardium in the interventricular septum (dark) compared to lateral wall (bright from contrast). Right: After a high mechanical index burst with resulting contrast destruction, the replenishment of contrast is delayed in the septum, seen by an even larger difference in contrast enhancement between septum (darker myocardium, arrows) and lateral wall. Both images confirm hypoperfusion in the septum, probably due to coronary artery disease.
Courtesy of Mai Tone Lønnebakken, MD, PhD. Haukeland University Hospital, Bergen, Norway.

poor image quality on conventional stress echocardiography has been shown to be equal those with optimal image quality on conventional echocardiography.

2.3.7.1 Coronary flow reserve—offline image processing

Quantification of images obtained at rest and at stress allows for the calculation of myocardial blood volume and the speed at which erythrocytes travel. The product of these two gives the myocardial blood flow as previously explained. The ratio of flow at stress compared to flow at rest then yields the coronary flow reserve (CFR).

2.3.8 EACVI recommendations for LV opacification contrast echocardiography [5]

In patients with suboptimal images

- to enable improved endocardial visualization and assessment of LV structure, function, and wall motion when two or more contiguous segments are not seen on non-contrast images.
- to have accurate and repeated measurements of LV volumes and EF on 2D echocardiography.
- to increase confidence of the interpreting physician.
- to confirm and exclude the echocardiographic diagnosis of the following LV structural abnormalities, when non-enhanced images are suboptimal for definite diagnosis:
  - apical hypertrophic cardiomyopathy
  - LV thrombus

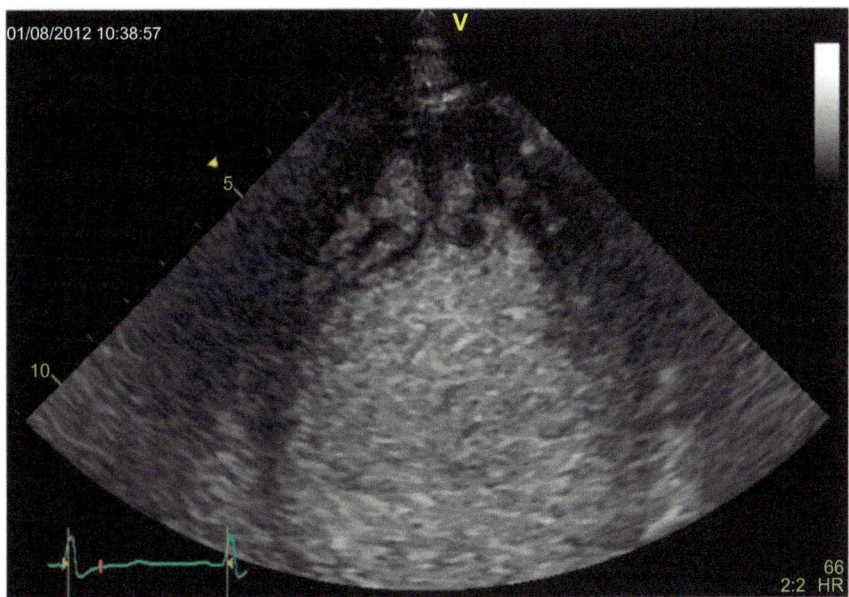

Figure 2.9 Contrast echocardiography with continous low mechanical index imaging in a patient with left ventricular non-compaction cardiomyopathy. The contrast enhancement in the left ventricular cavity helps delineate the endocardial border to show apical trabeculation. Courtesy of Trine F. Håland, MD. Oslo University Hospital, Norway.

- non-compaction cardiomyopathy (Figure 2.9)
- pseudoaneurysm of the ventricle

In stress echocardiography

- when two or more endocardial borders of contiguous segments of LV are not well visualized.

The ESC guidelines on stable angina pectoris recommends contrast during stress echocardiography, as it not only enhances image quality, but also improves reader confidence and enhances accuracy of detection of coronary artery disease.

2.3.9 Conclusions

Contrast echocardiography is a safe and practical technique with a variety of potential applications both at rest and stress. Contrast echocardiography provides assessment of cardiac structures and function in patients with suboptimal image quality and can estimate myocardial perfusion and calculate CFR. Contrast imaging can reduce the need for additional, costly, and more hazardous tests.

Despite several studies confirming the value and advantages of contrast echocardiography, implementation of the technique in clinical practice has been slower than anticipated. The price of the contrast agents is still high. Furthermore, the need of an intravenous access, an extra person to administer contrast for bolus-injections, and post processing may be considered inconvenient and too time-consuming to arrange in a busy echocardiographic laboratory.

2.4 Deformation imaging

Ventricular deformation occurs in longitudinal, circumferential, and radial direction. The apex rotates counter clockwise (seen from the apex) and the base rotates clockwise during LV ejection, with the entire process reversing during relaxation. This opposite rotation results in a twisting motion called torsion [7,8]. Traditionally, LV function is evaluated by 2D and M-mode echocardiography using subjective and semi quantitative methods. Tissue Doppler imaging (TDI) and speckle tracking echocardiography (STE) are now used as quantitative and more objective methods for assessment of global and regional systolic and diastolic function. While TDI can measure displacement, velocity, strain rate and strain, STE is used to measure myocardial strain directly and can quantify LV rotation (Table 2.2).

2.4.1 Tissue Doppler imaging

2.4.1.1 Myocardial velocity imaging

The Doppler principle, traditionally used to measure blood flow velocities, may also be used to measure myocardial velocities. Myocardium is moving much slower than blood; therefore, Doppler frequencies from myocardium are lower and signal amplitudes are higher. Signals are easily separated using filters to reject high velocity, low amplitude echoes from blood to manage only echoes from tissue.

TDI provides myocardial velocities by using colour Doppler mode or pulsed Doppler mode.

Colour Doppler

TDI uses an auto-corrector technique to calculate and display multigated points of colour-coded velocities along a series of ultrasound scan lines within the 2D sector. Myocardial velocities may be imaged as colour-coded velocities on top of

Table 2.2 **Quantitative measures of myocardial mechanics [9]**

Velocity (cm/s)	Speed of the movement of a cardiac structure
Displacement (cm)	Distance a cardiac structure moves between two consecutive frames
Strain (fraction, %)	Fractional change in length of a myocardial segment, i.e., percentage deformation
Strain rate (1/s)	Rate of change in strain
Rotation (degrees)	Circular motion of the myocardium around the longitudinal axis of the LV
Twist angle (degrees)	Absolute apex to base difference in LV rotation
Torsion (degrees/cm)	Gradient in twist angle from apex to base

a 2D grayscale image. Depending of the width and depth of the sector, the frame rate is 80–200 frames per second and usually higher than the corresponding grayscale image.

Velocity analyses are typically done as part of post processing. The most common assessed velocities are the peak systolic ejection velocity (s') and peak early diastolic lengthening velocity (e') for assessment of systolic and diastolic function respectively. Velocities can be assessed and compared between different regions of the myocardium by placing the sample volume at different locations.

One should appreciate that velocities obtained from the 2D colour mode are mean values and therefore lower than the corresponding values obtained from pulsed Doppler (Figure 2.10).

Pulsed Doppler

Velocities can be assessed by using spectral tissue Doppler with pulsed-Doppler activated. This is the main method for measuring mitral annular velocities for diastolic function assessment. The velocities obtained are peak velocities, and the comparable mean velocities obtained from colour Doppler method are typically 25% lower. Pulsed Doppler mode has disadvantages: it has limited spatial resolution, velocities can only be recorded from one region, and offline analyses of locations other than those archived are not possible (Figure 2.11).

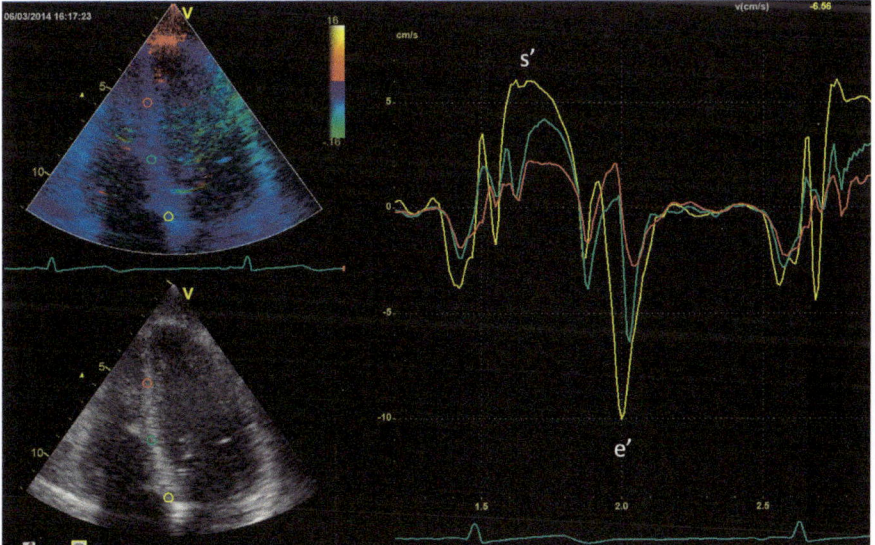

Figure 2.10 Myocardial velocity traces by colour Doppler mode derived from tissue Doppler imaging. Peak velocities decrease from base to apex shown by highest velocities in tracing from basal sample volume (yellow curve) and lowest velocities in apical tracing (red curve). s', peak systolic ejection velocity. e', peak early diastolic filling velocity.

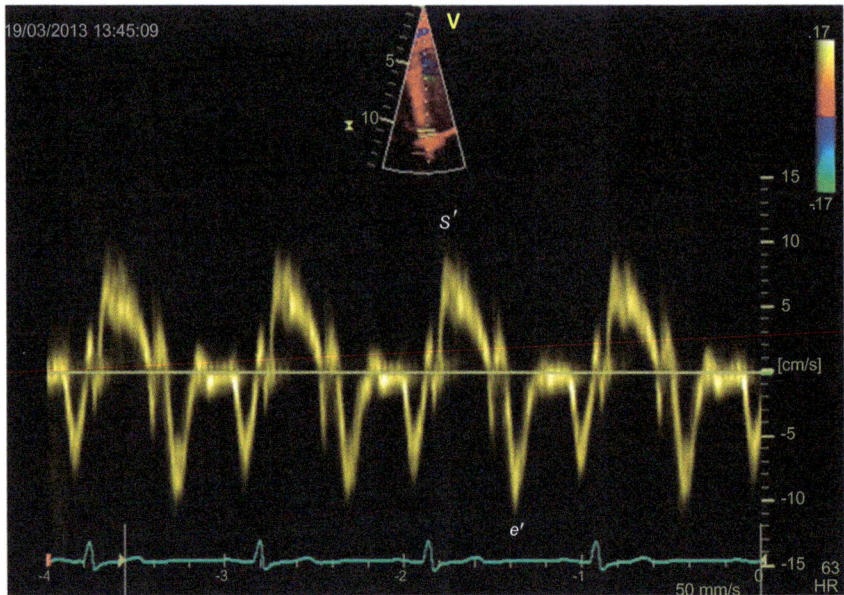

Figure 2.11 Myocardial velocity imaging by pulsed Doppler mode derived from tissue Doppler imaging. Sample volume is placed at the septal mitral annulus. s', peak systolic ejection velocity. e', peak early diastolic filling velocity.

Limitations to velocity imaging

Angle dependency Only velocity components in the beam direction are recorded; therefore, velocity imaging by Doppler is angle dependent. The ultrasound beam should be aligned parallel to the LV wall in long-axis imaging and perpendicular to the wall in short-axis imaging. Also, apical velocities are inaccurate in long-axis view because the apical curvature hinders adequate ultrasound beam alignment.

Movement of sample volume The velocities are measured within a defined sample volume. Underlying myocardium may move independently of the sample volume due to motion of the heart. This is not adjusted for, and the velocities from Doppler will be influenced not only by myocardial deformation but also on total cardiac motion.

Reverberations Reverberations lead to falsely reduced velocities.

Tethering and cardiac translation The myocardial velocities are summarized from contraction in the defined segment, motion from tethering to neighbor segments, and translation of the entire heart. This implies that velocities in one region of the myocardium may be influenced by motion in adjacent tissue since myocardium in neighbor regions is tethered together. During the cardiac cycle, the base moves toward the apex during systole and returns back in diastole. The apex remains more or less still. Due to these facts, there are normal differences in TDI velocities and displacement, with both velocity and displacement increasing from apex to base. Interpretation of regional TDI velocities is often difficult since the distinction of pathology from normal variation may be challenging.

Load dependency TDI velocities are load dependent. When TDI is used for assessment of regional function however, this limitation is less important since regional differences persists with changes in load.

2.4.1.2 Displacement imaging

With temporal integration of myocardial velocities, the displacement of one LV region is obtained. Displacement is not widely used in clinical echocardiography despite certain minor advantages to velocities. From its dependence on velocity, displacement imaging holds the same TDI limitations as described for velocity.

2.4.1.3 Strain imaging

Strain is defined as deformation and is a measure of how much an object has been deformed relative to its original length. Strain can quantify regional myocardial systolic function in comparison to EF, which is a global measure of LV function. The first available clinical method for cardiac strain assessment was magnetic resonance imaging (MRI) with tissue tagging. Limitations like costs and time consumption of MRI have led to difficulties to implement MRI for clinical strain assessment. Today, we calculate strain and strain rate (SR) more easily from echocardiographic TDI or STE.

Definition of strain and strain rate

Strain is deformation of a material, relative to its original length. Strain is in fact dimensionless; however, in cardiac mechanics, strain is most often presented as the percent change in dimension. The strain concept is complex, but linear strain is defined as Lagrangian strain, ε:

$$\varepsilon = (L - L_0) / L_0 \times 100\% \tag{2.1}$$

L_0 is baseline length of a myocardial segment, and L is the instantaneous length at the time of measurement. End-diastole is considered zero strain at length L_0 [10]. The strain rate is the rate by which the deformation occurs, i.e., deformation/strain per time unit.

Myocardial shortening or thinning is after definition assigned negative strain values and percentage lengthening, thickening, or stretching are given positive strain values. This implies that normal longitudinal and circumferential shortening function provides negative strain values while normal radial and transverse thickening function have positive strain values.

The theory behind the ability to measure strain by TDI is that myocardial velocity gradient is an estimate of SR, and therefore strain can be calculated as the temporal integral of SR. SR is calculated from the difference in velocity (V) between two sample volumes (1 and 2) relative to the distance (D) between them.

$$SR = V_1 - V_2 / D \tag{2.2}$$

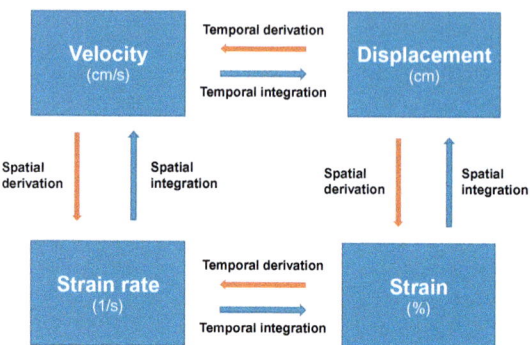

Figure 2.12 Relationship between velocity, displacement, strain rate, and strain.

Velocity difference between two adjacent regions implies compression or lengthening of the tissue in between. In long-axis view, SR measures systolic regional shortening rate while strain measures regional shortening fraction.

The four dimensions of velocity, displacement, strain rate, and strain are mathematically related, as shown in Figure 2.12.

Limitations of strain and strain rate by TDI

SR can be considered a normalized myocardial velocity, which is not influenced by motion of the heart (translation) or motion of neighbor segments. As previously explained, velocities will increase in normal hearts from apex toward the base. In contrast, strain and SR are similar in all segments between apex and base and is therefore more suitable for estimating regional systolic function.

Signal noise Random noise can potentially result in large inaccuracy of SR since errors in SR are the sum of errors of the two velocities. Strain is less susceptible to random noise than SR since integration tends to eliminate random noise.

Resolution SR and strain from TDI requires the sample volume to fit within the myocardium at an adequate distance from each other, an adequate pulse repetition frequency, and sufficient frame rate. Sufficient frame rate depends on what heart cycle event we want to assess. SR has limited lateral resolution, which limits the ability to measure strain and SR in the subendocardium or subepicardium separately. Also, if the sample volume is placed too far to either side on the myocardial wall, there is a risk that the signal partly represents velocities in the blood pool or the pericardium respectively.

Angle dependency SR and strain imaging derived from TDI are sensitive to misalignment between cardiac axis and ultrasound beam. One should align the ultrasound beam as parallel to the LV wall of interest as possible, use the smallest sector possible and record from one wall at a time.

Reverberations Reverberations cause significant errors in SR imaging. Even a small error in local velocity will create large errors in velocity gradient. Better scanning window is the only way to avoid the reverberations.

2.4.1.4 TDI in clinical use

Velocity imaging is the preferred TDI method for assessing regional function. Displacement imaging lacks validation for clinical use and is not recommended routinely. Strain and SR from TDI are neither widely used in routine clinical practice. Clinical assessment of strain is rather obtained from STE since it can be calculated offline with semiautomatic software from a routine echocardiographic exam and has fewer limitations.

2.4.2 Speckle tracking echocardiography

STE calculates strain from tracking speckles in grayscale B-mode images. The speckles are created as artifacts from constructive and destructive interference of ultrasound backscattered from structures smaller than the ultrasound wavelength. Speckles function as natural acoustic markers, which are tracked from frame to frame. The random distribution of the speckles ensures that each region of the myocardium has a unique speckle pattern, like a unique fingerprint. The speckles, i.e., the fingerprints, will follow the motion of the myocardium and move from one image frame to the next. This change in position of the speckles is registered by the software, which automatically measures the distance between speckles to calculate the myocardial strain. Since calculation of distance between speckles is not dependent on the angle of the ultrasound beam, STE is an angle-independent strain method. Measurements can be made simultaneously from different regions of the heart (Figures 2.13 and 2.14).

A meta-analysis reports on normal reference values of LV global strain by STE [11] (Table 2.3).

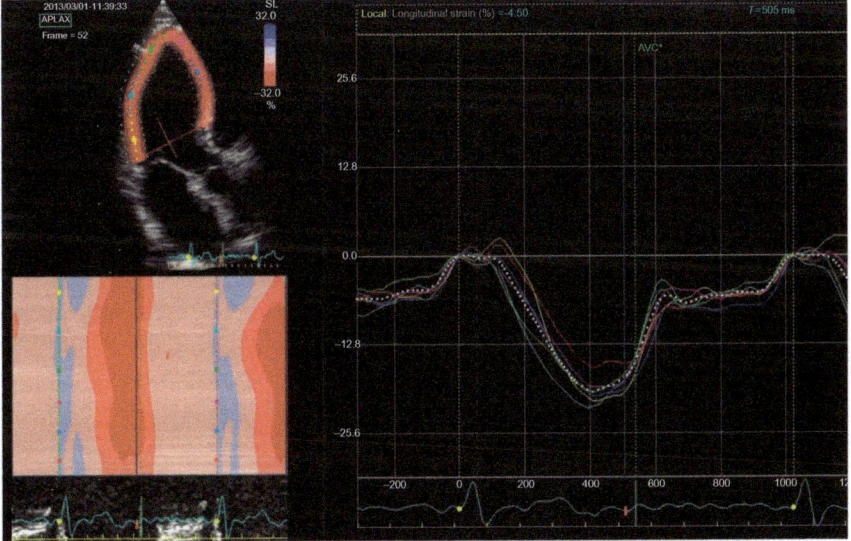

Figure 2.13 Two-dimensional speckle tracking echocardiography from apical view. Longitudinal strain traces from the six left ventricular segments in apical long-axis view show normal negative strain values in a healthy individual.

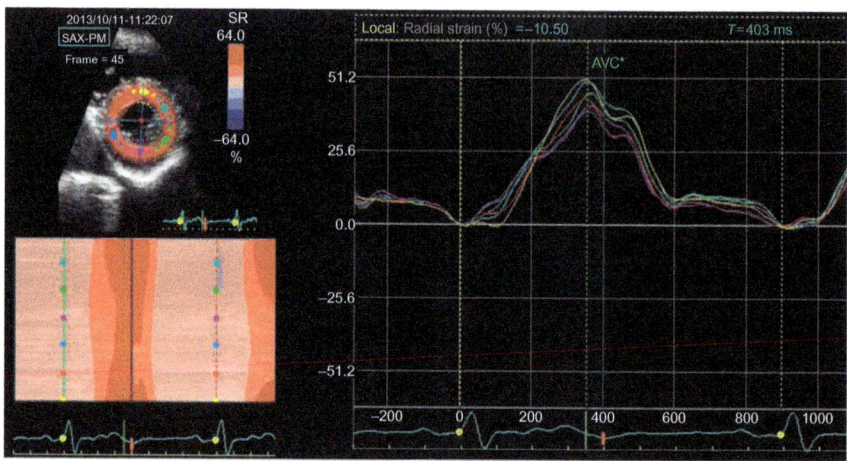

Figure 2.14 Two-dimensional speckle tracking echocardiography from parasternal short-axis view. Radial strain traces from the six left ventricular segments at the papillary level show normal positive strain values in a healthy individual.

Table 2.3 Normal reference values of LV global strain by 2D speckle tracking echocardiography (STE) [11]

LV strain by STE	Mean strain value (95% CI)	Range of mean values between the studies	Included in the meta-analysis
Global longitudinal strain (GLS)	−19.7% (−20.4% to −18.9%)	−15.9% to −22.1%	28 Studies 2597 Subjects
Global circumferential strain (GCS)	−23.3% (−24.6% to −22.1%)	−27.8% to −20.9%	14 Studies 599 Subjects
Global radial strain (GRS)	47.3% (43.6% to 51.0%)	35.1% to 59.0%	12 Studies 568 Subjects

2.4.2.1 Differences of strain from STE versus strain from TDI

STE measures strain from distance between two points within a defined piece of myocardium whereas TDI measures strain from velocities from a fixed point in space with reference to the external probe. Importantly, TDI measures strain from integrating SR, while STE measures strain directly from measuring the change in length of myocardium relative to its original length.

The most obvious advantage of STE strain is that STE strain is angle-independent and is not affected by tethering or by cardiac translation. This enables assessment of circumferential and radial strain from short-axis view and longitudinal strain from curved apical segments. STE analyses can be performed after image acquisition. Also, STE strain can be used to measure LV rotation.

2.4.2.2 Limitations of STE strain

Strain from STE shares some limitations with TDI

- Load dependency
- Low frame rate, i.e., temporal resolution, may lead to undersampling giving reduced peak values and loss of whole events, like for example the short isovolumic phases.
- Dropouts. If there are dropouts with no B-mode data, there will be no speckles to track.
- Reverberations. Motionless artifacts give falsely low strain and must be excluded from the STE analysis.

2.4.2.3 Three-dimensional (3D) STE

A limitation of 2D STE strain is the assumption that speckles move only in one plane linear along the 2D scanning sector plane. This is an unrealistic assumption since myocardium surely moves in and out of the 2D scanning sector. Therefore speckles can be lost in 2D STE analysis. 3D echocardiography allows following the speckles in the 3D space within each segmental myocardial volume, irrespective of the direction of their displacement.

Using 3D STE, the speckles are automatically identified and followed throughout the cardiac cycle. Strain values are computed as with 2D STE with frame-by-frame tracking in the 3D volume. Time-strain curves can be displayed for any single LV segment using different visualization solutions. From one single 3D dataset, all the different strain components, i.e., longitudinal, circumferential, radial, and rotation, can be quantified. An important limitation to 3D speckle tracking strain is the low spatial and temporal resolution of real-time 3D echocardiography (Figures 2.15 and 2.16) [4].

2.5 Future trends

2.5.1 Image quality

The most crucial and essential prerequisite for a successful echocardiographic examination is good image quality. Images with high spatial and temporal resolution with minimal artifacts are fundamental to assure reliability and reproducibility of evaluations of cardiac dimensions and function. Improved transducers, processing power, and computational capabilities of echocardiographic machines and software could all increase image quality and should always be a main focus in future echocardiographic developments. Easier and faster image acquisition with less operator dependence will increase the implementation of echocardiography even more in clinical practice, especially important for the interventional field where fast image acquisition is required. Reliable automated measures of cavity volumes and dimensions will probably increase.

2.5.2 Interventional echocardiography

Echocardiography is used not only for diagnosis and treatment evaluation, but also as a tool for treatment planning and guiding of device placements and electrophysiological

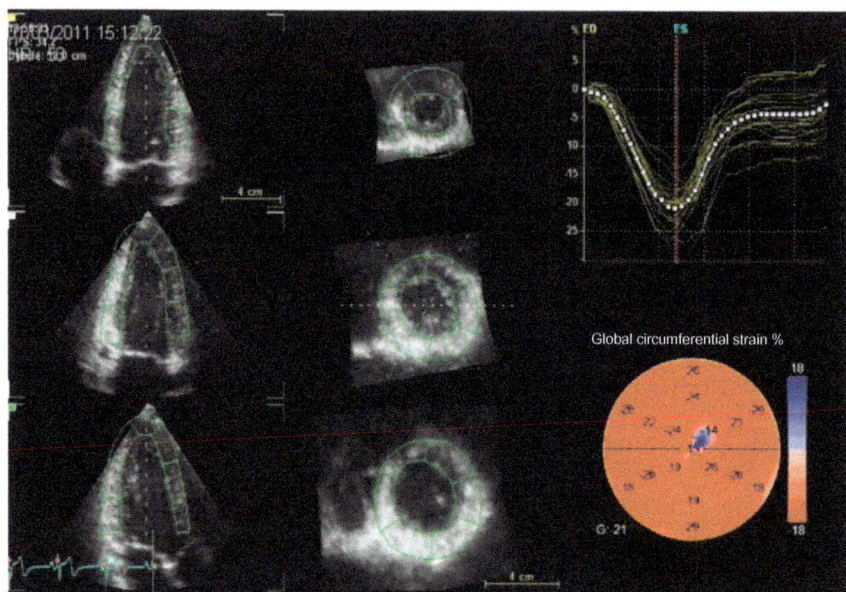

Figure 2.15 Three-dimensional speckle tracking echocardiography. Circumferential strain traces (upper right) and "bulls eye" image (lower right) show normal negative circumferential strain values in the 17 left ventricular segments.
Courtesy of Richard J. Massey, sonographer, Oslo University Hospital, Norway.

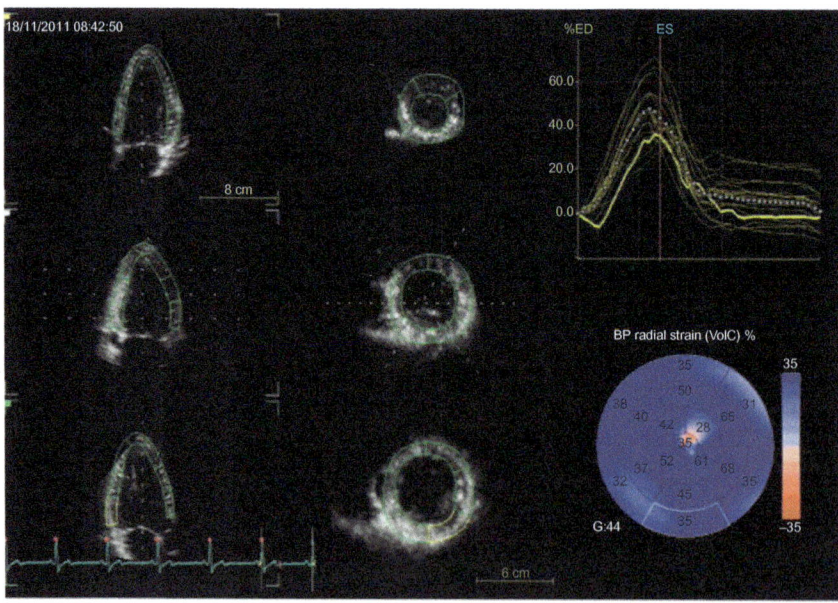

Figure 2.16 Three-dimensional speckle tracking echocardiography. Radial strain traces (upper right) and "bulls eye" image (lower right) show normal positive strain values in the 17 left ventricular segments.
Courtesy of Richard J. Massey, sonographer, Oslo University Hospital, Norway.

procedures. Advances for improving image quality in 3D echocardiography will probably lead 3D to be the modality of choice for guiding percutaneous valve procedures as TAVI and Mitraclip as well as ablation procedures and septal defect closures (see Chapter 22).

2.5.2.1 Intracardiac echocardiography

Intracardial echocardiography (ICE) has been introduced. The femoral venous access is used to place an ultrasound transducer on the tip of the catheter in the right atrium. The clinical applications of ICE today are monitoring of atrial septal defect, persistent foramen ovale and left atrial appendage closure, percutaneous mitral commisurotomy, and TAVI and Mitraclip procedures. ICE guides and monitors atrial septal puncture better than fluoroscopy by identifying the optimal place of puncture and hence minimizing the risk of complications. The benefits of ICE are better visualization of the atrial septum, septal defect rims, reduction of radiation exposure from fluoroscopy, and no need for general anesthesia (in contrast to TEE). The main disadvantage is the cost. The cable and transducer are expensive and can only be used once. So far only 2D ICE is in use. 3D ICE is needed and will probably be available in the near future.

2.5.2.2 Fusion imaging

The different cardiac imaging modalities have different and important roles and cannot entirely be replaced by one another. Multimodality evaluation of cardiac images and signals is an upcoming field in cardiac imaging presently and for the years to come. Many challenges need to be overcome, but technology is progressing fast, and indeed the new multimodality approaches have already started to reach the clinical arena. Real-time 3D echocardiographic data can be combined with live fluoroscopy for guidance of ablation and percutaneous valves procedures (EchoNavigator, Phillips). Coronary CT angiography data can be fused with echocardiographic strain data to combine morphological information of coronary stenosis with myocardial function. Myocardial viability data from MRI can be combined with myocardial function by echocardiographic strain.

Fusion of several 3D echocardiographic datasets can improve the value of the 3D imaging. For example, fused 3D echocardiographic datasets increase information about the left atrial anatomy, which will better guide ablation procedures. Multiple TEE 3D datasets from different locations of the aorta can be fused to quantify the total plaque burden in the entire length of the aorta and hence risk assessment.

2.5.3 Myocardial perfusion by contrast echocardiography

Nuclear techniques like SPECT are traditional imaging modalities, which have been in use for several decades for assessing myocardial perfusion in detection of coronary artery disease. SPECT and contrast echo do not provide similar information on myocardial perfusion, which may result in different sensitivities to detect ischemia. Cardiac MRI use has grown exponentially since its introduction approximately 20 years ago, but lack of availability in all hospitals limits its widespread use.

Myocardial perfusion with contrast echocardiography has in several clinical trials been shown to increase ischemia detection. In stress echocardiography, adding perfusion on top of wall motion abnormality-assessment has shown to increase sensitivity and accuracy of the stress test to detect coronary artery disease and improve prognostic stratification. Today, none of the contrast agents are approved for myocardial perfusion imaging anywhere in the world. Perfusion imaging by contrast echocardiography to assess ischemia and viability is widely available, fast to perform, considered safe, and does not expose the patient to radiation. It should therefore increase as a modality for myocardial perfusion imaging assessment (Figure 2.17).

2.5.4 Molecular imaging by contrast echocardiography

Molecular imaging refers to an image reflecting a molecular process like gene expression, protein synthesis, and inflammation [12]. Molecular imaging has potential for early and definite diagnosis, evaluation of treatment response, delivery of therapy, and monitoring progression. Different application fields are under research in cardiovascular molecular imaging: detection of atherosclerosis, myocardial ischemia, myocardial remodeling, angiogenesis, myocarditis, transplant rejection and thrombus, and prediction of arrhythmias and stability of plaques and aortic aneurysms.

Microbubbles are used as contrast agents in echocardiography, and they can be targeted by either alterations of shell components or conjugation of ligands to the

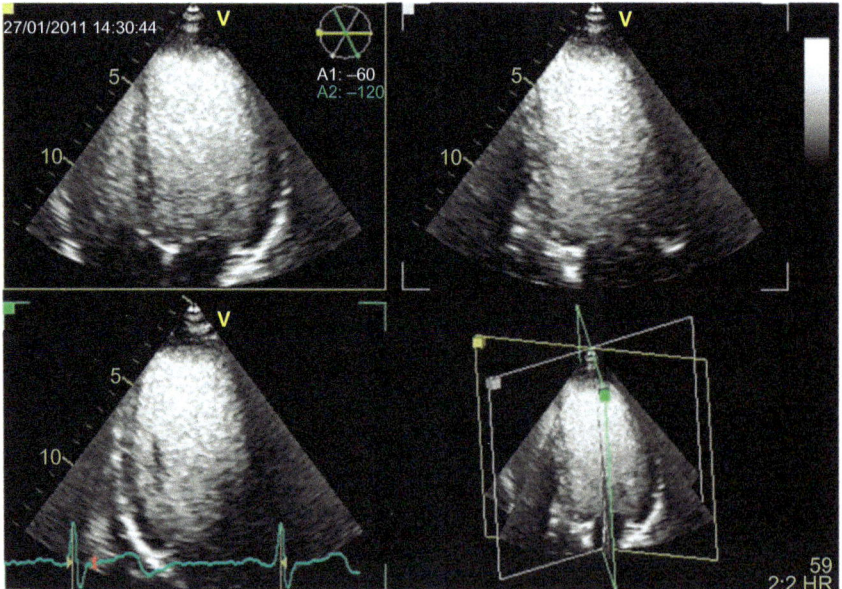

Figure 2.17 Continuous low mechanical index contrast enhanced imaging in 3D-echocardiography. Myocardial perfusion is assessed from the three apical views simultaneously. 2D planes/slices are obtained from the 3D dataset.
Courtesy of Richard J. Massey, sonographer, Oslo University Hospital, Norway.

microbubble surface using a molecular spacer "arm." Microbubbles are localized to myocardium via adhering to endothelial leukocytes that have been activated by oxygen free radicals or inflammation. Microbubbles have been shown to target the very early atherosclerotic lesions by sticking to the early exposed endothelial adhesion molecules. Research is also done to make conjugated microbubbles specifically detect plaques with high rupture risk and to target microthrombosis. Transient ischemia expose specific endothelial adhesion molecules involved in the initial rolling of leucocytes along the endothelial surface. To target these molecules with microbubbles could be exploited as "Ischemic memory" imaging and be advantageous in patients with suspected acute coronary syndrome.

The ability of microbubbles to stick to activated endothelial cells clearly indicates a potential role of contrast echocardiography to visualize tumour angiogenesis and transplant rejections. Labeled stem cells can be detected by ultrasound to assess distribution, engraftment, survival, etc.

Contrast agents have been effective in identifying the septal perforator arteries that supply the thickened septum in hypertrophic cardiomyopathy and could therefore guide alcohol ablation.

When ultrasound waves destroy microbubbles, conjugated molecules can be released. This opens for therapy where microbubbles first target the tissue with disease of interest and then deliver conjugated drugs or genes. In animal models drug delivery from conjugated microbubbles has shown to be directly related to the MI applied. Synthetic DNA can be conjugated to microbubbles and when released by high MI ultrasound in targeted tissue, DNA can block translation of mRNA into proteins. Likewise, promoter genes could be delivered by microbubbles to start translation of genes to increase synthesis of a specific protein.

High MI impulses have shown to create microspheres in the endothelium, permitting drugs conjugated to microbubbles to pass into the subendotelial space.

A disadvantage of echocardiographic molecular imaging is that microbubbles are confined to the vascular space. The technique therefore cannot assess components of plaques or myocytes. The advantages are low cost, high availability, and fast acquisition that can be performed bedside. The signal from microbubbles can be eliminated quickly by high MI ultrasound and new microbubbles can be injected directly for new assessments without interference from the previous microbubble signal.

2.5.5 Clinical indices

Echocardiographic measures today are descriptive, and no interpretation is linking the measure to a clinical condition or risk, at least not by the echocardiographic companies. In future echocardigorahic machines there might be integrated algorithms calculating clinical indices. An example is indices for myocardial mechanical dyssynchrony. Mechanical dispersion from strain echocardiography has been introduced as a novel index to predict malignant ventricular arrhythmias. An unresolved challenge in current cardiology is prediction of sudden cardiac arrest from ventricular arrhythmias. Mechanical dispersion is defined as standard deviation of time to peak longitudinal strain in 16 LV segment and is therefore of measure of how homogenous or heterogeneous the LV segments are contracting. Mechanical dispersion is thought to reflect underlying arrhythymogenic electrical dispersion, and studies have shown that mechanical dispersion predicts ventricular arrhythmias in both ischemic and non-ischemic cardiomyopathies. Mechanical dispersion is an example of a clinical index, which can be measured directly from the echocardiographic software. It is probably still far-fetched to think that we will get a change from pure descriptive information from an echocardiographic examination to receiving an automatic report with diagnostic and risk assessment interpretation. The echocardiographic companies will be reluctant to the legal responsibilities this may bring about.

2.5.6 Tissue characterization

Echocardiographic tissue characterization can use integrated backscatter signals (IBS) to visualize myocardial fibrosis [13]. The elastic property of myocardial tissue affects its acoustic impedance. Collagen deposition in myocardial fibrosis decreases tissue elasticity, and this alters the echocardiographic signal, measurable by IBS. IBS's ability to reflect fibrosis has been validated against open and percutaneous endomyocardial biopsy in aortic stenosis, dilated cardiomyopathy, and transplanted hearts. Also, IBS correlates with diastolic function in hypertrophic cardiomyopathy and with collagen biomarker in hypertension. It has not been shown if IBS relate to clinical outcomes. IBS was first described in the late 1970s. However, after 3 decades, its true clinical potential has not yet been fully clarified to justify clinical implementation of the method. The advantages of IBS in fibrosis detection over MRI are that IBS is inexpensive, easily available, and does not require a contrast agent. With further developments and knowledge, IBS may therefore be used for tissue characterization in the future.

Elastography maps the elastic properties and stiffness of soft tissue by external squeezing or compression. A variety of elastography techniques have been developed in research laboratories during the past 25 years. Elastography can be divided into strain methods and shear-wave methods, where only shear wave is able to estimate true elastic modulus. It is still early days for ultrasound elastography; it has not become a routine method in cardiology yet. So far, detection of tumors in breast, prostate, and thyroid together with measurement of liver stiffness by shear-wave elastography to stage fibrosis using the "Fibroscan" system have been the main clinical applications. Clinical evidence for echocardiographic elastography is building up, and with further developments, it has potential to become an easy, safe, and bedside method for detection of myocardial fibrosis.

The future holds increasing importance and opportunities for further implementation of echocardiography and expansion of its applications. As opposed to other imaging modalities, echocardiography is a non- or minimally invasive method without exposure to radiation. Also, since echocardiography can be performed during therapeutic procedures, it will be increasingly welcomed into the laboratories of interventionalists and electrophysiologists.

2.6 Further reading

We refer the reader to further literature on advanced echocardiography.

2.6.1 Books

"The Practice of Clinical Echocardiography". Author: Catherine Otto.
"The EAE Textbook of Echocardiography". Authors: Galiuto, Badano, Fox, Sicari, and Zamorano.

2.6.2 Journals

European Heart Journal—Cardiovascuar Imaging
Journal of the American Society of Echocardiography

2.6.3 Web-pages

European Association of Cardiovascular Imaging (EACVI)

- Guidelines, position papers and consensus documents from the EACVI
- Scientific material in educational sections in the homepage

References

[1] Lang RM, Bierig M, Devereux RB, Flachskampf FA, Foster E, Pellikka PA, et al. Recommendations for chamber quantification. Eur J Echocardiogr 2006;7(2):79–108.
[2] Gjesdal O, Helle-Valle T, Hopp E, Lunde K, Vartdal T, Aakhus S, et al. Noninvasive separation of large, medium, and small myocardial infarcts in survivors of reperfused ST-elevation myocardial infarction: a comprehensive tissue Doppler and speckle-tracking echocardiography study. Circ Cardiovasc Imaging 2008;1:3189–96.
[3] Lang RM, Badano LP, Tsang W, Adams DH, Agricola E, Buck T, et al. EAE/ASE recommendations for image acquisition and display using three-dimensional echocardiography. Eur Heart J Cardiovasc Imaging 2012;13(1):1–46.
[4] European Association of Cardiovascular Imaging (EACVI). Education: "Tool box 3D ECHO" and "Tool box CONTRAST ECHO". Available from: http://www.escardio.org/communities/EACVI/pages/welcome/aspx; 2013.
[5] Senior R, Becher H, Monaghan M, Agati L, Zamorano J, Vanoverschelde JL, et al. Contrast echocardiography: evidence-based recommendations by European Association of Echocardiography. Eur J Echocardiogr 2009;10(2):194–212.
[6] Kaul S. Myocardial contrast echocardiography: a 25-year retrospective. Circulation 2008;118(3):291–308.
[7] Otto CM. The practice of clinical echocardiography. 4th ed. Philadelphia: Elsevier/Saunders; 2012.
[8] Edvardsen T, Haugaa KH. Imaging assessment of ventricular mechanics. Heart 2011;97(16):1349–56.
[9] Otto CM. Textbook of clinical echocardiography. 5th ed. Philadelphia: Elsevier/Saunders; 2013.

[10] Støylen A. Strain rate imaging. Trondheim: Norwegian University of Science and Technology; 2013. Available from http://www.folk.ntnu.no/stoylen/strainrate.
[11] Yingchoncharoen T, Agarwall S, Popovic ZB, Marwick TH. Normal ranges of left ventricular strain: a meta-analysis. J Am Soc Echocardiogr 2013;26(2):185–91.
[12] Lindner JR, Sinusas A. Molecular imaging in cardiovascular disease: which methods, which diseases? J Nucl Cardiol 2013;20(6):990–1001.
[13] Hoskins PR, Svensson W. Current state of ultrasound elastography. Ultrasound 2012;20:3–4.

Single-photon emission computed tomography

R.R. Buechel, P.A. Kaufmann, O. Gaemperli
University Hospital Zurich, Zurich, Switzerland

3.1 Introduction

Radionuclide imaging today is an active and growing branch of medical diagnostics. Over the past decades, radionuclide imaging has advanced to become a cornerstone for the accurate diagnosis and appropriate management of a variety of medical conditions. Interestingly, however, it has its origins in the cardiovascular field: it was in the late 1920s when Herrmann L. Blumgart published his "Studies on the velocity of blood flow" in *The Journal of Clinical Investigation*, marking the birth of nuclear medicine [1]. Through the following decades, the invention of the scintillation camera by Hal Anger [2] and the commercial supply of readily available radiotracers have set the ground for its introduction in the clinical arena. The technique was further elaborated by the development of multiplane tomographic scanners, which have promoted its use for cardiac applications in daily clinical routine. Aside from ^{18}F-fluorodeoxyglucose positron emission tomography (FDG PET), the growth of nuclear medicine in the recent past has been mainly driven by the increasing use of single-photon emission computed tomography (SPECT) myocardial perfusion imaging studies. Today, over 10 million nuclear cardiology procedures are performed every year in the United States alone [3]. However, cardiac SPECT has also raised public attention as a main contributor to the growing healthcare costs and increasing individual radiation exposure from diagnostic medical procedures that has been observed over the past two decades [4]. This has prompted considerable efforts to limit radiation exposure, shorten acquisition protocols, and reduce costs, while at the same time improving diagnostic performance. The following sections provide an overview of the most important technical developments in cardiac SPECT imaging, including radionuclides, detector technology and camera design, and image reconstruction and processing. We place special emphasis on the most recent advances and developments that are currently becoming standard practice in many centers around the world or are likely to play an important role in the future.

3.2 Physical principles of SPECT

Gamma radiation refers to a form of electromagnetic radiation of very high frequency and high energy per photon, and consequently a deep penetration depth in human tissue (as opposed to relatively nonpenetrating, low-energy alpha and beta particles): the imperative necessity for all imaging purposes. The process of capturing emitted gamma

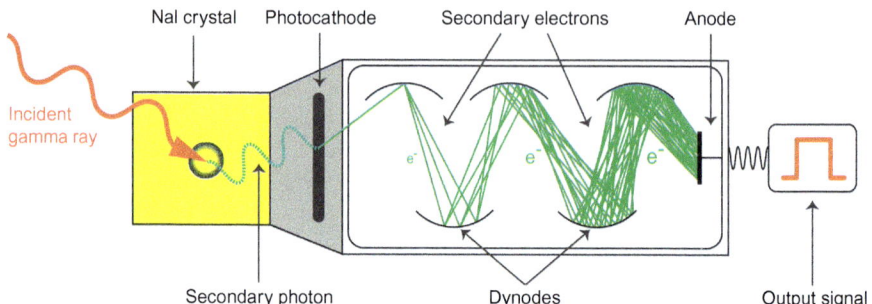

Figure 3.1 Schematic drawing illustrating the basic functionality of a conventional sodium iodide scintillation detector.

rays from a radioactive source using a gamma camera is called scintigraphy (Figure 3.1). The gamma camera contains one or multiple detectors made of an organic and optically clear crystal plane of very high density, a sensitive photomultiplier tube, and all the necessary electronics to process the photomultiplier tube output. To maximize electromagnetic interaction with the gamma rays, crystals made of elements with a high atomic number are implemented in the detectors, usually consisting of sodium iodide with thallium doping. When an emitted photon hits the crystal it causes the latter to scintillate, hence inducing an extremely short-lived (10^{-6} s) light impulse. In physical terms, the term scintillation describes the process of an electron in a crystal's atom being dislocated (excited) by a gamma ray then returning to a stable energy state shortly afterward, thereby releasing a light impulse (scintillation). As the photons of this light impulse (secondary photons) reach the photomultiplier tube's photocathode, the latter emits electrons as a result of the photoelectric effect. These electrons are then accelerated and directed by an electric potential so as to hit the first dynode of the tube. The impact of one single electron on the dynode releases a number of secondary electrons, thus creating a growing avalanche of secondary electrons that strike the next dynode: By this means, the electrical signal is being amplified to the extent of a measurable output signal representing the event of the initial photon hitting the photocathode (Figure 3.1). Importantly, the output signal also inherits information about the energy of the original incident radiation on the scintillator. Thus, both intensity and energy of the radiation is being measured.

While this outlined principle permits the measurement of incident radiation, it does not allow for spatial allocation of the origin of gamma radiation *per se* because emitted gamma rays are subject to scattering within the human body, leading to stray gamma rays. To avoid misallocation, collimators consisting of parallel holes within a block of a material impermeable for gamma rays (i.e., mostly lead) are employed. The alignment of a collimator in front of the detector ensures that only parallel incident gamma rays strike the detector, thus allowing for two-dimensional allocation of the origin of the measured radiation (Figure 3.2). The smaller and the longer the holes in the collimator, the fewer photons will get through to the scintillator, thereby increasing image resolution at the cost of lower count density and higher image noise. Conventional cardiac SPECT cameras are equipped with parallel-hole low-energy

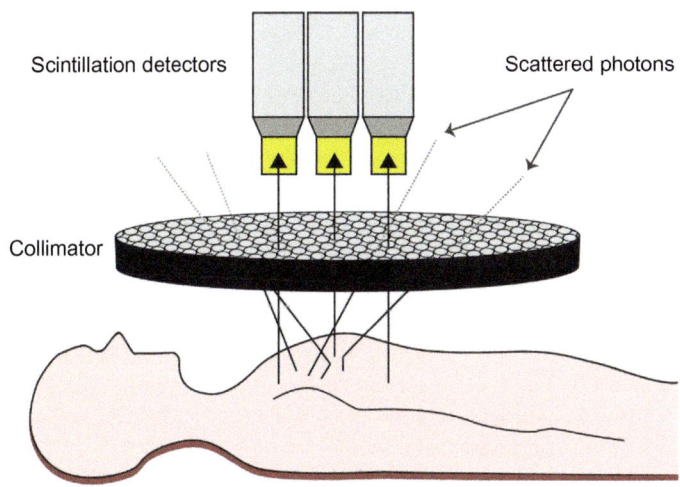

Figure 3.2 A collimator made of a high-density material prevents stray gamma rays (dotted lines) to reach the detector surface. Only parallel incident gamma rays (solid lines) pass through the holes within the detector and finally hit the detectors' crystals.

high-resolution collimators; however, some of the newer devices are mounted with pinhole collimators.

For the assessment of the heart and exact localization of myocardial perfusion defects, planar scintigraphy is not very well suited due to its two-dimensional nature. The advent of SPECT has therefore greatly improved the interpretation of myocardial perfusion scans: one or multiple scintillation detectors rotate in a step-wise fashion around the patient over an arc of at least 180°, enabling reconstruction of a tomographic data set of the heart using sophisticated reconstruction algorithms (see Section 3.5). The result is a three-dimensional image of the heart that allows the exact localization of perfusion defects within the myocardial wall (Figure 3.3).

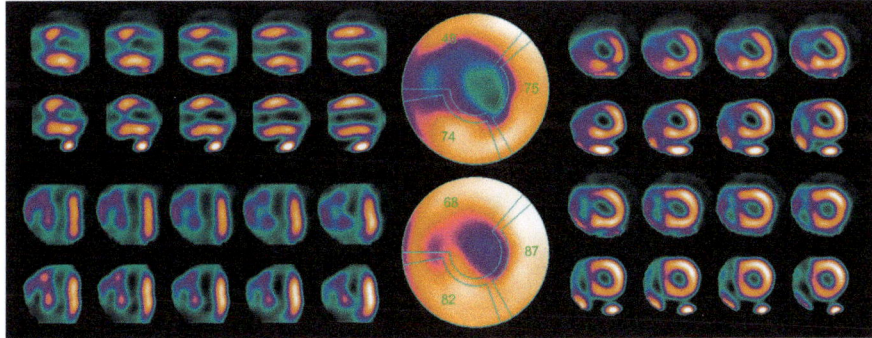

Figure 3.3 Myocardial perfusion SPECT study. Vertical (top left), horizontal (bottom left), short axis (right), and polar plots (middle) are depicted with acquisition at stress and rest aligned in the top and the bottom rows, respectively. The polar plots in the middle show a resting apical perfusion defect with partial reversibility particularly in the septal wall, indicating nontransmural apical scar with additional septal ischemia.

3.3 Camera designs

Since the introduction of the first SPECT camera, changes of camera designs were confined to optimizing the performance of sodium iodide detectors and to implementing multiple detectors in a single camera system. Furthermore, with the increasing demand for cardiac SPECT, manufacturers have released a number of devices that are specifically dedicated to cardiac imaging. These cameras are characterized by multiple small-footprint detector heads that center easily on the heart and allow imaging in supine or upright position, are compact and easy to fit in a small room, avoid claustrophobia, and improve patient comfort (Figure 3.4). Despite their common purpose, however, devices from various vendors still offer many different features with regard to detector technology, collimator design, and software solutions (see later discussion). These advances have led to a substantial reduction of the time needed for image acquisition. Due to the step-wise fashion of tomographic image acquisition by rotation around the patient's chest, the total time needed for completion of a 180° arc with a

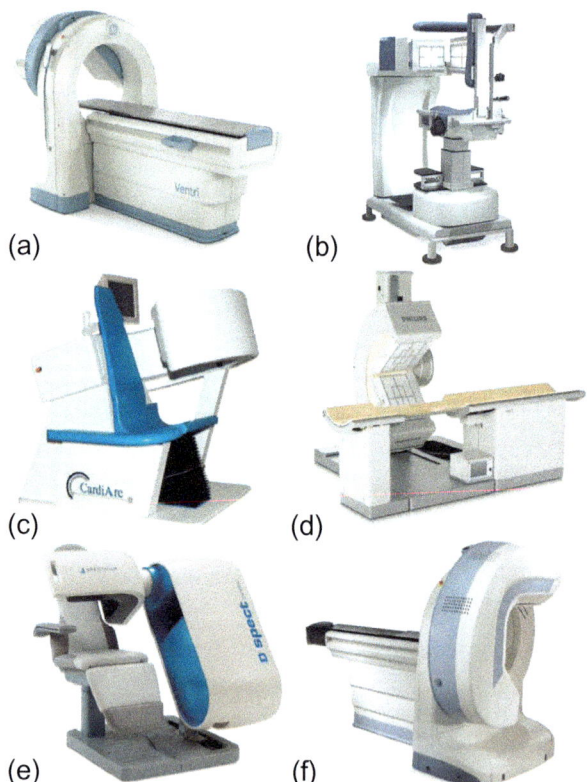

Figure 3.4 Selection of dedicated cardiac SPECT cameras: (a) Ventri, GE Healthcare. (b) Digirad Cardius 3 XPO. (c) CardiArc. (d) CardioMD, Philipps Healthcare. (e) D-SPECT, Spectrum Dynamics. (f) Discovery NM 530c, GE Healthcare.

single detector head system used to be considerable. The advent of dual-head systems and, more recently, triple-head systems, however, has enabled nuclear cardiologists to perform an examination within 10–20 min.

A recent revolutionary milestone in technical innovation for cardiac SPECT has been the introduction of semiconductor detector technology using synthetic crystals composed of cadmium-zinc-telluride (CZT). CZT is artificially grown as a single crystal; it has a very high density and effective atomic number with a higher attenuation coefficient for photons than that of conventional sodium iodide crystals, allowing the application of thinner detectors. More importantly, however, the mechanism of function of CZT detectors differs fundamentally from a conventional sodium iodide detector: CZT detectors allow direct conversion of light into an electrical signal. When a photon hits the CZT detector, the impact generates directly an anion and a cation. Through application of an electric field, the charge carriers are swept to the cathode and anode of the system, inducing a current pulse that can be recorded. Thus, contrary to conventional detectors, CZT detectors avoid the need for bulky photomultiplier tubes, thereby reducing the size of the detector head and improving the theoretical in-plane resolution.

A CZT detector consists of the crystal and multiple underlying anodes, each reflecting a pixel. If, for example, a detector consists of 16 × 16 pixels, each with an edge length of about 2.5 mm, this results in a form factor that is strikingly smaller than a conventional scintillation detector (Figure 3.5).

The intrinsic spatial resolution of current CZT detectors is approximately 4 mm, which is substantially better than the typical 10 mm achieved with conventional sodium iodide detectors [5]. One of the reasons for this increase is that due to thinner crystals in CZT detectors, the charge carriers are detected by an anode that is only millimeters away from the original photon–crystal interaction. This allows a much more accurate spatial localization of the original incident than with a conventional detector where "triangulation" to the photon's origin happens at the level of the photomultiplier several centimeters away from the crystal. Therefore, spatial resolution in a CZT detector is mostly only limited by pixel size, which in turn is restricted by how densely the electronics needed for recording power currents can be packed. Thus, as intrinsic resolution is mainly dependent on the size of a pixel, it can be expected to improve further with advancing miniaturization.

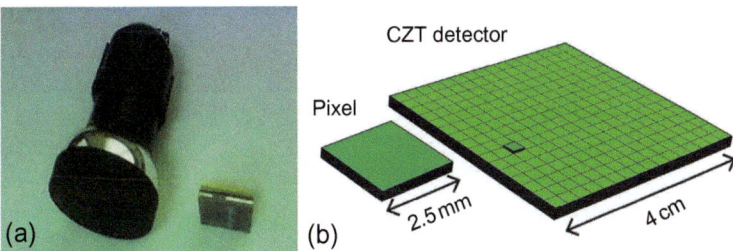

Figure 3.5 (a) A conventional sodium iodide scintillation detector with photomultiplier tube (left) in comparison with a much smaller cadmium-zinc-telluride (CZT) detector (right). (b) The latter consists of 16 × 16 pixels, resulting in an edge length of only about 4 cm.

However, it has to be taken into account that superior intrinsic properties of a detector *per se* are meaningless without similar extrinsic properties that are set by the surrounding system design. For example, the most important extrinsic factor influencing the system trade-off between sensitivity and resolution is the collimator: a high-resolution collimator depicts only a very narrow column of activity from the patient, and therefore provides excellent spatial resolution at the expense of sensitivity. By contrast, a high sensitivity collimator accepts incoming photons from a wider range of angles, therefore increasing sensitivity at the expense of resolution. In novel camera systems, the high intrinsic resolution of CZT detectors allows the use of parallel-hole or multipinhole collimators with relatively large holes focused on the heart in order to improve count sensitivity.

Moreover, CZT detectors also show better energy discrimination than sodium iodide scintillation detectors, allowing a distinction between scattered and unscattered radiation more accurately, and thereby further improving image resolution [6]. Accurate energy resolution is also a prerequisite for simultaneous imaging with more than one isotope; this is an area of ongoing research for CZT-based gamma cameras.

While all cameras have a specific limitation regarding the maximum count rates that can be measured, SPECT systems based on conventional scintillation detectors additionally show a nonlinear response with rising count rates leading to a roll-off and even to paralysis at high count rates (due to a detector "dead-time" that exceeds the rate of incoming photons). CZT detectors, by contrast show a linear count rate response up to the system maximum. The latter is limited only by computational power of the system. Hence, at present, the count rate performance of a CZT camera is twice as high as that of a conventional SPECT camera.

However, the most important advantage of CZT detectors arises from miniaturization of the detectors with inherent advantages for the geometry of the scanner. The small size of the CZT detectors allows for a detector geometry that rather resembles the design of a PET (positron emission tomography) more than a SPECT scanner. A large array of detectors is mounted on a detector arch and aligned in a curved geometry around the patient in order to face specifically the heart and thereby increase true counts from the area of interest. Instantaneous acquisition of cardiac activity from different projection angles becomes possible (Figure 3.6).

In summary, while the CZT detectors themselves constitute a milestone of technological development in terms of sensitivity, spatial and energy resolution, the true leap forward in innovation arises from the combination of such detectors with new collimator designs and modern iterative reconstruction algorithms in novel dedicated cardiac camera systems that are preferably equipped with a stationary array of multiple detectors. It is the combination of the above that has led to a 5–10-fold increase in system sensitivity and a twofold increase in image resolution and allows imaging of the heart within less than 5 min (Figure 3.7), while at the same time yielding images with substantially better image quality at higher resolutions than state-of-the-art conventional SPECT cameras (Figure 3.8).

The clinical impact of shorter acquisition time lies not only in improved patient comfort and increased patient throughput and greater scanner efficiency. As an

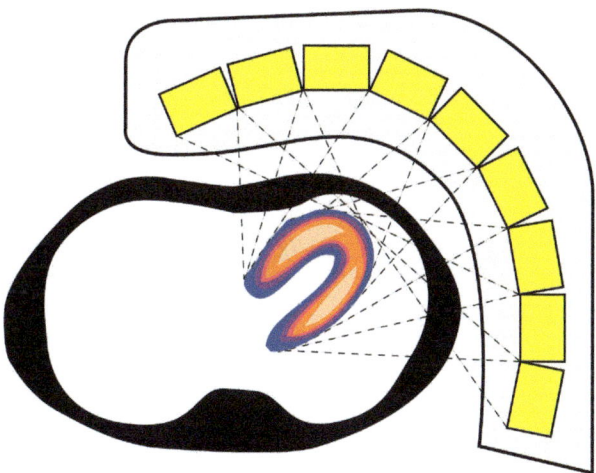

Figure 3.6 The small form factor of CZT detectors allows mounting a large array of detectors on an arch aligned around the patient and focused on the heart. Thus, rotation of the detectors around the patient is unnecessary, and instantaneous tomographic acquisition of the heart becomes possible.

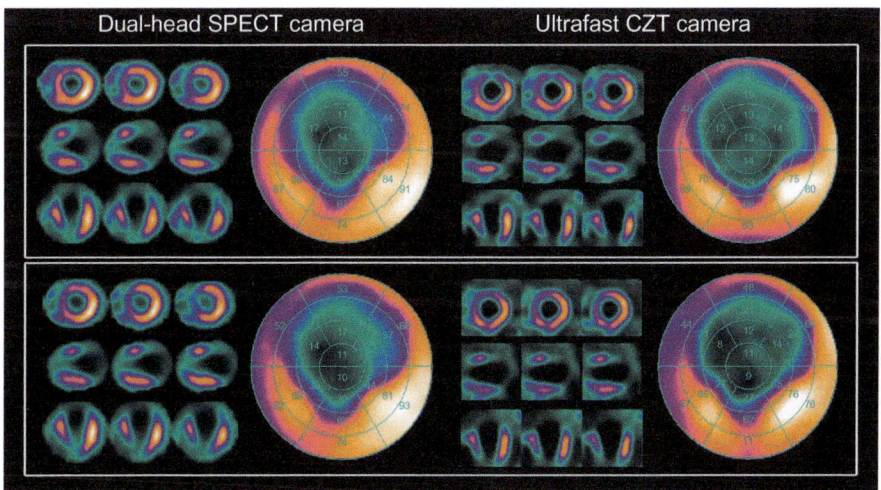

Figure 3.7 Comparison between conventional SPECT imaging with 15 min acquisition time and CZT imaging with an acquisition time of 3 min for stress (top row) and 2 min for rest (bottom rows).
Reproduced with permission of Springer from Ref. [7].

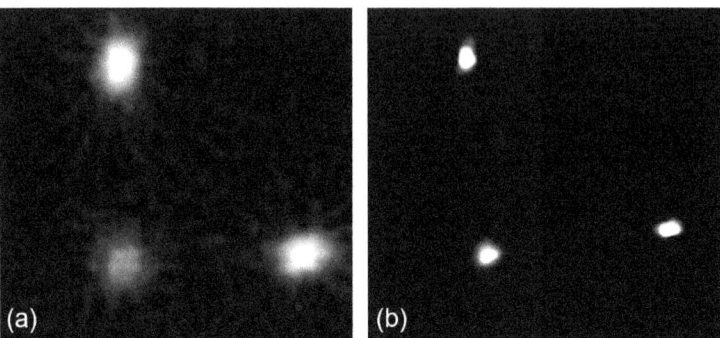

Figure 3.8 Point sources imaged on a conventional cardiac SPECT camera (a) and a CZT Camera (b) clearly demonstrating the higher resolution of the CZT system. Reproduced with permission of Springer from Ref. [6].

alternative to shortened acquisition time, this new technology can be used to reduce tracer activity and, consequently, effective radiation exposure (see also Section 3.6).

3.4 Tracers

The ideal tracer for myocardial perfusion and viability SPECT imaging should have biochemical properties that allow it to be entirely and evenly distributed solely within the myocardium after high first-pass extraction from the blood, to be biologically inert, to be retained within the myocardium until imaging is completed and to be completely extracted afterward. Regarding physical aspects, it should emit gamma rays at a high energy, have a relatively short half-life, and be able to be easily and cost-effectively manufactured. While such an ideal tracer does not exist, the available radiopharmaceuticals today offer a variety of advantages and disadvantages, demanding from the nuclear physician a profound knowledge of the tracer to distinctively utilize the respective tracer for certain clinical questions. The following section provides an overview on the most common tracers along with a brief outlook on future trends.

Radioactive tracers are synthetic chemical compounds consisting of an endogenous or exogenous carrier molecule that partakes in human metabolism and in which one or more atoms have been replaced by a radioisotope through which its natural decay allows for imaging of the compound. Today's most commonly used radioisotope for cardiac SPECT is the metastable 99m-Technetium (^{99m}Tc), which is available in different commercially available compounds such as sestamibi (Cardiolite®, Du Pont™), tetrofosmin (Myoview®, GE Healthcare™), and teboroxime (CardioTec®, Squibb Diagnostics™). By contrast, 201-Thallium (^{201}Tl) acts as a potassium analogue and can therefore be used for imaging without the need of a biochemical carrier molecule as it partakes in myocardial metabolism, mostly via Na$^+$/K$^+$—adenosine triphosphate sarcolemmal membrane transport system. Although ^{201}Tl provides certain advantages over ^{99m}Tc-labeled agents, such as lower gastrointestinal activity or redistribution properties that render additional resting injection potentially redundant, ^{99m}Tc-based tracers

Table 3.1 **Characteristics of the most commonly used myocardial SPECT imaging tracers**

	Emission energy (keV)	Radioisotope half-life (h)	First pass extraction (%)	Redistribution
^{201}Tl	75	73	82–88	Yes
^{99m}Tc-sestamibi	140	6	55–68	No
^{99m}Tc-tetrofosmin	140	6	54	No

are often preferred for their higher energy and their shorter half-life leading to higher count rates and better image quality at a lower radiation exposure. Table 3.1 provides a summary of the physical properties of the most commonly used radioisotopes.

Due to their particular biochemical properties, the time-course of uptake and clearance of the presently available ^{99m}Tc-compounds differs dramatically: sestamibi and tetrofosmin have a medium uptake rate and a very slow myocardial clearance allowing imaging for several hours after injection, whereas ^{99m}Tc-teboroxime is a boronic acid adduct of technetium dioxime complex that is highly extracted at the myocardial first-pass and shows rapid blood clearance allowing imaging immediately after injection but only within a very limited time frame (circa 10–15 min). Hence, teboroxime has been mostly replaced by sestamibi and tetrofosmin due to effectiveness considerations in daily clinical routine. However, teboroxime may experience a future revival along with the technical advances in cardiac SPECT due to its higher and—more importantly—much more linear myocardial uptake even at high myocardial blood flows, rendering it a potentially ideal tracer for quantitative assessment of myocardial blood flow in combination with the newest generation of CZT scanners [6]. The lipophilic neutral, ^{99m}Tc-labeled compound ^{99m}Tc-N-NOET shares many characteristics with teboroxime, including its high first pass extraction by the myocardium and an uptake that correlates with myocardial blood flow over a wide range of flow, but is not commercially available in Europe. Furthermore, there is ongoing research into the development of new SPECT tracers, noteworthy a group of ^{99m}Tc-labeled agents that have crown ether functional groups (e.g., ^{99m}Tc DBODC5, ^{99m}Tc-N-MPO, or ^{99m}Tc-15C5-PNP), which lead to a more rapid clearance from the liver, potentially enabling better delineation of the inferior wall of the left ventricle. Other research focuses on novel tracers with improved flow versus extraction relationship (e.g., ^{125}I-ZIROT). However, many of these tracers remain experimental and have not yet reached the clinical arena.

While the tracers mentioned above are used for myocardial perfusion and viability imaging, other tracers can be used to assess myocardial innervation. The 123-Iodine labeled meta-iodobenzylguanidine (^{123}I-MIGB) resembles the biochemical structure of noradrenaline and is thus taken up by presynaptic catecholamine transporters allowing imaging of the sympathetic innervation of the myocardium. Increased cardiac sympathetic innervation leads to reduced presynaptic uptake of the noradrenaline analogue ^{123}I-MIBG and has been associated with adverse left ventricular remodeling, progression of heart failure and increased risk of sudden cardiac death in heart failure patients [8].

3.5 Image processing and reconstruction

3.5.1 Filtered back projection (FBP)

As mentioned before, with SPECT cameras, tomography of the heart is performed by rotation of the detector heads around the patient's chest or by an array of detectors aligned around the patient. Whatever the design, however, each detector acquires a two-dimensional image of a three-dimensional object, leading to overlapping of structures that are actually separated from each other (e.g., parts of the apex are projected in front of the base in a left anterior oblique view). Reconstruction algorithms are needed to correct for this essential problem. The concept of back projection is to virtually run the projections obtained by a detector back through the source to obtain a rough approximation of the original due to constructive interaction of the projections in regions that correspond to the original source of emission (Figure 3.9a). In filtered back

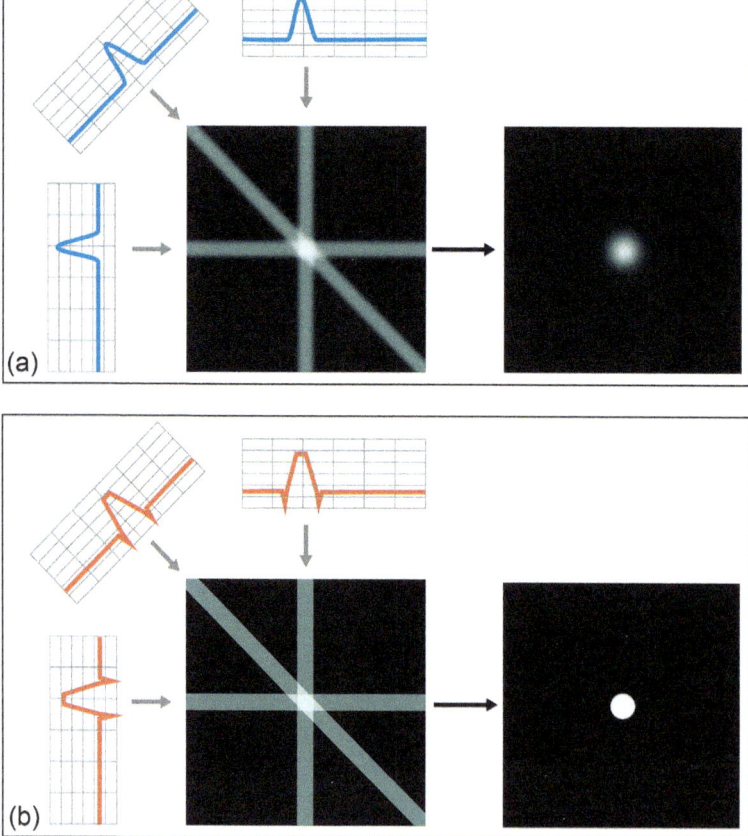

Figure 3.9 Unfiltered back projection (a) leads to smearing of the original view along the path it was originally acquired, resulting in a blurry image. During filtered back projection (b), each view is filtered before being back projected, resulting in an exact and sharp reconstruction of the original image.

Single-photon emission computed tomography

projection (FBP), a high-pass filter (a so-called ramp filter, most commonly) is applied to eliminate the blurring artifacts that result from simple back projection (Figure 3.9b).

FPB can be performed very quickly without the need for high-end CPU power and therefore quickly gained wide popularity after its introduction in the 1970s. However, there are limitations in terms of the image quality produced, particularly in low-count areas. To a large extent, this is due to the necessary filtering, which accentuates image noise and can result in streak artifacts (Figure 3.10).

3.5.2 Iterative reconstruction

Iterative reconstruction describes the process of obtaining the best possible solution for a model that depends on one or more unobserved variables (such as the true activity distribution in three-dimensional space in cardiac SPECT) by step-wise or successive approximation. In short, a virtual initial estimate of the activity distribution is made; based on this starting point, another estimate is made as to the counts that would be acquired in each projection (using "forward projection"). These projections are compared with the actual acquired measurement, and the original estimate is updated by the information of this comparison (using "back projection"). The process is repeated a given number of times (iterations) until the change between estimate and acquisition becomes minimal: the algorithm has converged to the best possible

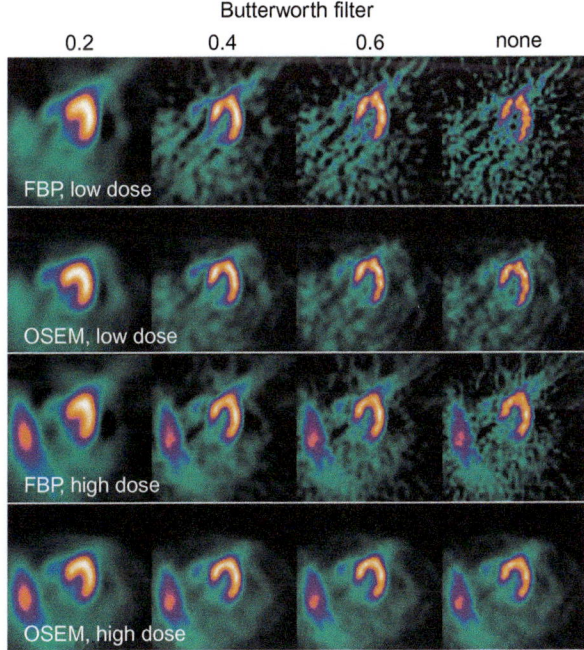

Figure 3.10 Filtered back projection (FBP) versus ordered subset expectation-maximization (OSEM) iterative reconstruction for different total counts and with a Butterworth postprocessing filter at different intensities. Low dose = 300 MBq 99mTc-tetrofosmin; high dose = 900 MBq 99mTc-tetrofosmin.

solution. Of note, unlike FBP, no filtering is necessary to reach a solution through this process but a postreconstruction smoothing filter (e.g., a Gaussian filter) is commonly used to control noise. The most commonly used iterative reconstruction algorithm relying on this basic principle is called expectation-maximization (EM). The main disadvantage of iterative reconstruction using EM is the required computational time: Depending on the number of iterations and the complexity of the model, the calculation of each projection (typically for 64 or 128 angles) may take as long as a complete FBP reconstruction. The most widely applied technique to improve the speed of iteration is called ordered subsets expectation-maximation (OSEM), where an update is based only on a few selected projections (subsets). This reduces computational time by a factor of up to 30 and has led to a widespread use of iterative reconstruction in nuclear cardiac imaging.

The latest, most refined iterative reconstruction algorithms incorporate statistically based noise suppression along with a technique called resolution recovery. The latter is achieved by taking into account the fact that the spatial resolution of a gamma camera decreases as the distance from the collimator surface to the source increases. By compensating for this effect, it has become possible to improve signal-to-noise ratio while maintaining spatial resolution. Such state-of-the-art algorithms allow for a significant reduction of scan-time or of radiation dose of up to 50% and are now integrated in various EM or OSEM iterative reconstruction software (e.g. Evolution for Cardiac™ by GE Healthcare, Astonish™ by Philips, Flash3D™ by Siemens Medical Solution, etc.). Importantly, as mentioned, variations of these algorithms have been implemented in new CZT camera designs to further improve spatial and contrast resolution while reducing image noise all at greatly reduced scan times.

3.5.3 Attenuation correction

A vast majority (>80%) of all emitted photons are deflected from their original linear path through the human body, leading to a substantially reduced count rate reaching the detector. Nonuniform photon attenuation occurs through inhomogeneous density of different structures in and around the chest and is of particular concern in SPECT imaging where additional inconsistencies arise due to changing viewing angles. Furthermore, in SPECT, photon energies are relatively low (75 keV with ^{201}Tl and 140 keV with ^{99m}Tc) and thus more susceptible to attenuation compared to PET (511 keV with positron-emitting radionuclides). In order to exactly correct for attenuation, one would have to know the exact distribution of the source activity within the object of interest during acquisition; a prerequisite that is obviously not fulfilled in SPECT imaging. Adequate correction for this phenomenon is of importance, as attenuation impairs specificity of cardiac SPECT. Commercially available correction methods, however, have only recently been made available with the basic principle of measuring the density distribution and the arising attenuation by means of a transmission scan. Various techniques with different radioactive point or line sources such as ^{241}Americium, ^{153}Gadolinium, or ^{99m}Technetium have been proposed but yielded suboptimal results. By contrast, computed tomography (CT) has shown more promising results for attenuation correction of SPECT [9], despite the fact that the energy

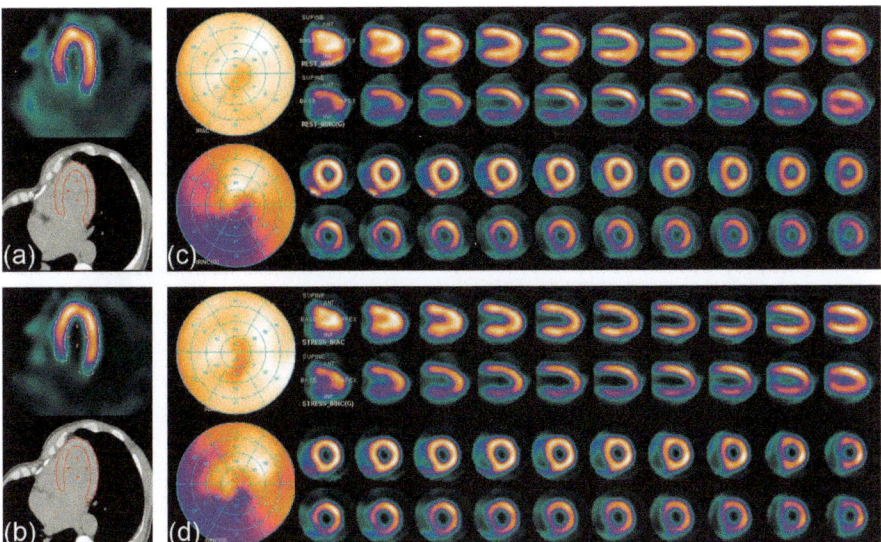

Figure 3.11 Manual registration of the low-dose CT with the SPECT from rest (a) and stress (b) acquisition. The effect of CT attenuation correction for rest (c) and stress (d) is clearly visible when uncorrected polar plots and slices (c and d, bottom rows) are compared with the corresponding corrected polar plots and slices (c and d, top rows). Thus, the inferior und septal defects are clearly unmasked as attenuation induced artifacts and this patient's perfusion scan can be reported as normal.

spectrum of the photons emitted from a CT X-ray tube is polychromatic compared to the monochromatic gamma photons from a radioactive source. Moreover, the photon flux is much higher with CT, enabling acquisition of transmission images for attenuation correction within mere seconds. However, most current dedicated SPECT scanners are not equipped with an integrated CT system for attenuation correction (Figure 3.4). This can be overcome by using a standalone CT device to create low-dose (<1 mSv) native scans of the chest, which are afterward manually co-registered with the emission scans to create accurate and reliable attenuation maps (Figure 3.11). However, manual co-registration has to be performed with due care, as misregistration creates an inaccurate attenuation map that *per se* may introduce new artifacts (Figure 3.12). Furthermore, if performed using ECG-triggering and acquired within a single breath-hold, such a native low-dose CT scan can be used to additionally assess the amount of coronary calcification by calculating the coronary artery calcium score [10].

3.5.4 Gated SPECT

The term gated SPECT commonly refers to electrocardiogram (ECG)-gated SPECT. After injection of a perfusion tracer, a set of dynamic images synchronized to the patient's ECG is obtained within multiple equal intervals (so-called "bins") during each cardiac cycle. Each bin contains the cumulated counts occurring during the predefined segment of the RR-cycle collected over the entire duration of the scan. The result is a

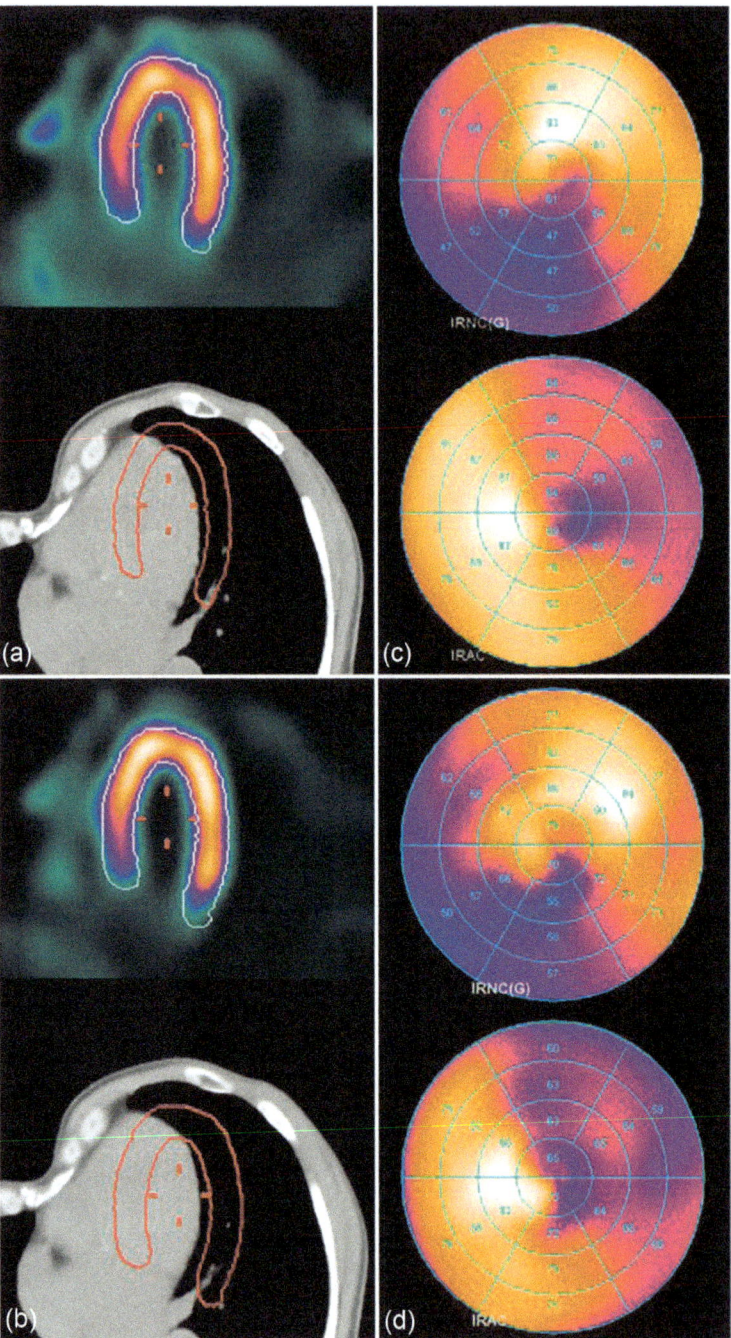

Figure 3.12 Marked misregistration of the low-dose CT with the SPECT from rest (a) and stress (b) acquisition. The soft-tissue attenuation visible in the inferior and septal myocardial wall in the uncorrected polar plots of the rest (c, top) and stress (d, top) acquisition is corrected by application of the resulting attenuation map. However, misalignment between transmission and emission scans results in a notable artifact in the anterolateral wall (c and d, bottom). The patient is the same as in Figure 3.11, where appropriate alignment of transmission and emission scans demonstrates normal perfusion of the entire left ventricle.

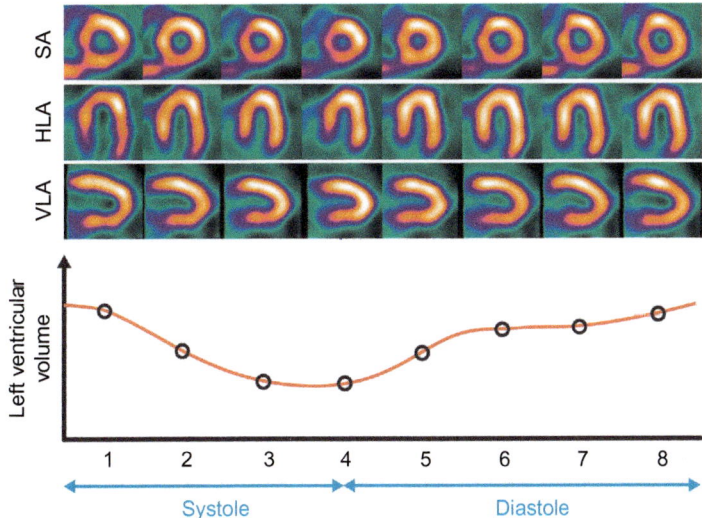

Figure 3.13 Electrocardiogram-gated SPECT using 8 bins. SA = short axis, HLA = horizontal long axis, VLA = vertical long axis.

number of images representing snapshots of the heart at different timepoints throughout systole and diastole, allowing for comprehensive analysis of the left ventricular volumes and function including assessment of regional motion, regional thickening, and left ventricular ejection fraction (Figure 3.13).

The concept of ECG gating introduced an additional set of information from myocardial perfusion SPECT. Most importantly, however, it has also improved the diagnostic accuracy of perfusion SPECT. It helps to distinguish true fixed perfusion defects with regional wall motion abnormalities from attenuation artifacts (particularly in the inferior wall), thereby reducing the false positive rates of the technique [11]. Moreover, adding resting or post-stress gated information to perfusion data adds independent prognostic information and helps to improve risk stratification [12]. The accuracy of gated SPECT to estimate volumes and ejection fraction is improved by a high number of bins (e.g., 16 versus 8 bins). However, this is counteracted by low count statistics in each bin if the number of bins is increased indefinitely, which results in poor image quality and difficulties in endo- and epicardial border delineation. Therefore, to achieve acceptable count density in each bin, gated data are acquired over many cardiac cycles. The number of bins commonly used today varies between 8 and 16—to increase the amount of bins would eventually lead to unacceptably long scan durations.

As mentioned above, gated SPECT is acquired over many cardiac cycles and substantial variations of the duration of each cardiac cycle may cause temporal blurring due to interference of counts from adjacent bins. Modern software packages correct for this by rejecting individual beats that are outliers in terms of the R-R-interval (bad beat rejection). If the acceptance window is being narrowed, more arrhythmic heartbeats are rejected at the cost of lower count statistics and noisier images. This can only be compensated by increasing scan duration unless gating is abandoned altogether or the acceptance window is expanded. Thus, gated SPECT is not always possible or may be inaccurate in patients with an irregular heart rhythm (e.g., atrial fibrillation or frequent extrasystolic beats). Other artifacts can originate from trigger failure and erroneous triggering of tall, peaky T waves. These artifacts should be recognized early into the scan.

3.5.5 List mode acquisition

List mode refers to a special scanning mode in which each event and its precise time of occurrence with regard to co-registered physiological signals (i.e., ECG, breathing) is recorded. After image acquisition, image data can be sorted retrospectively into "frames" or "bins" by grouping image data obtained from corresponding time intervals. This provides high flexibility in data processing and image reconstruction using ECG or respiratory gating, dynamic image frames for functional analysis, or simple addition of information into static images.

This feature may be of interest in reducing motion artifacts, as it allows removing certain frames along the timeline of acquisition (e.g., the time frame with patient motion) but also offers interesting new possibilities particularly in combination with CZT cameras where respiratory and ECG gating is more robust than with conventional rotating camera designs. The originally acquired raw data set can be retrospectively cut using a list mode interface tool resulting in a secondary data set that includes only certain respiratory phases. Alternatively, real-time respiratory triggering is feasible as the scanning process can be paused and resumed at any chosen moment. Intermittent inspiratory breath-hold imaging may separate gastrointestinal activity from the inferior myocardial wall and reduce artifacts from soft-tissue attenuation and/or spill-over of gastrointestinal activity [13]. Furthermore, list mode acquisition is an important prerequisite for dynamic SPECT imaging and thereby has opened up a new field of research (see Section 3.7).

3.6 Low-dose SPECT

Depending on the tracer being used, a standard one-day stress/rest protocol for cardiac SPECT imaging results in a radiation dose exposure to the patient of around 10–15 millisieverts (mSv) [14]. In all radionuclide imaging studies, image quality is dictated by a trade-off between injected dose and acquisition time. In a given set-up (same patient, tracer, camera, and reconstruction algorithm), lowering injected dose (to lower patient radiation exposure) will inevitably result in lower image quality unless acquisition times are increased. Conversely, shortening acquisition times (to improve patient throughput and patient comfort and avoid motion artifacts) mandates an increase in injected dose to maintain image quality. Thus, considerable efforts have gone into the development of new protocols, more sensitive cameras, and improved reconstruction algorithms to allow cutting down on patient dose and/or scan time. Older conventional multihead SPECT cameras had limited potential, as their reconstruction algorithms are based on FBP, which is—as mentioned above—particularly prone to degradation of image quality at low count statistics. Thus, the first attempt of dose reduction consisted of stress-only imaging: In the presence of a normal stress myocardial perfusions SPECT study (including gated information), a rest study becomes redundant and can therefore be skipped. This results in a significant reduction of radiation exposure by approximately 50–75% (for a two-day versus one-day protocol, respectively). Since the prevalence of pathological SPECT scans has declined considerably over the past 2 decades and is now lower than 10% [15], such individualized stepwise imaging strategies could be widely applied and could potentially avoid "unnecessary" rest studies in up to 90% of patients. Large longitudinal cohort studies of consecutive patients have shown identical outcomes in patients with stress only imaging compared to patients with normal stress/rest studies [16]. However, this approach requires a very dynamic institutional setup where image reading is performed after each SPECT scan and the decision to continue made immediately by an experienced reader.

Novel OSEM reconstruction algorithms with resolution recovery compensate for decreasing spatial resolution as the distance from source to collimator increases, resulting in a distinctly improved signal-to-noise ratio. It has been shown that it is possible to use half the tracer activity with no significant loss of image quality using these novel iterative reconstruction algorithms [17]. Thus, conventional SPECT cameras equipped with such state-of-the-art reconstruction algorithms allow half-dose imaging, cutting radiation dose exposure nearly in half [18].

While integration of more sophisticated reconstruction methods increases system sensitivity regardless of the camera design, the combination of such algorithms with CZT cameras has finally led to systems whose efficiency is far beyond that of a conventional SPECT resulting in a 5–10-fold increase in sensitivity [5]. This advantage may be used to substantially shorten the time needed for image acquisition down to 2 min [7]. Conversely, tracer activity may be reduced by a factor of up to twofold, resulting in a radiation dose exposure of around 5 mSv [19]. Such a reduction in radiation dose exposure addresses valid concerns about ionizing radiation from medical imaging and places SPECT at the same level with PET or invasive angiography.

3.7 Dynamic SPECT

Dynamic cardiac imaging consists of tracking the tracer kinetic properties after it is injected into the circulation and to observe its inflow and wash-out from different compartments (such as the blood pool and the myocardium) as a function of time. This yields time–activity curves (TAC) for any given region of interest. Knowing the particular radiokinetic properties of a given perfusion tracer, the TACs are used to calculate absolute myocardial blood flow using pixel-wise kinetic modeling. Absolute blood flow quantification is established with myocardial perfusion PET imaging (see Chapter 4); its reproducibility has been proven in several studies and the technique has been validated against invasive angiography and radiolabeled microspheres. However, conventional SPECT is a semiquantitative technique where regional differences in perfusion is detected by visual comparison with remote, nonaffected territory. Until recently, SPECT lacked important characteristics to be suitable for dynamic blood flow imaging: These were low-count statistics with conventional tracers and scanners, and the lack of a robust method for attenuation correction. These limitations have been overcome to a certain extent by the introduction of CZT devices and their increases system sensitivity, opening up a completely new field of research in SPECT imaging.

Nonetheless, dynamic perfusion imaging with SPECT remains challenging: the currently used ^{99m}Tc-labeled tracers are characterized by a nonlinear relationship between myocardial extraction and blood flow with an early "roll-off" phenomenon at high blood flow values. However, as quantitation of myocardial blood flow with PET has so far not been widely applied in clinical routine, due to high costs and relatively complicated procedures, including the production of PET tracers with a very short half-life (e.g., ^{13}N-labeled ammonia or ^{15}O-labeled water), a number of attempts have been made to accomplish quantitative imaging with SPECT, some of them dating back more than 10 years. Some studies have shown that calculation of coronary flow reserve (CFR) is feasible by serial dynamic imaging of the pulmonary artery or the ascending aorta during the first pass of the tracer to calculate an input curve that was then used as a reference ratio to calculate the relative increase of myocardial blood flow from rest to stress [20]. These approaches, however, yield results that represent a relative increase rather than actual absolute measurements of blood flow and have been shown to underestimate CFR when compared to PET, mostly due to the nonlinear uptake of the available SPECT tracers. Furthermore, while CFR is an important value, the integration of absolute blood flow at rest and—more importantly—hyperemic flow during stress is essential for the interpretation of the results (e.g., CFR may be underestimated in a setting with high flow at rest even though hyperemic flow is normal).

Novel CZT cameras with a stationary array of detectors aligned around the patient also overcome the scanner-inherent limitations of standard SPECT when it comes to dynamic imaging because dynamic instantaneous tomographic acquisition without the need of camera rotation becomes possible—much like in a PET scanner. Additionally, the fast imaging protocols and the high photon sensitivity of CZT cameras may finally also allow the use of tracers with better extraction over a larger range of coronary blood flow rates, such as teboroxime: A SPECT tracer that was developed in 1989 but has not been widely used in the past because of its rapid myocardial clearance, making it unsuitable for long imaging protocols with conventional SPECT cameras. Whichever tracer will proof to be most effective, it is indisputable that the introduction of novel CZT cameras has refueled this interesting field of research and that very recent feasibility studies in humans have already shown promising results using conventional ^{99m}Tc-labeled SPECT tracers (Figure 3.14) [21].

3.8 Hybrid imaging

Hybrid imaging refers to the combination and fusion of two datasets by which both modalities contribute to image information through co-localization of anatomical and functional imaging techniques [22]. Datasets suitable for fusion may be derived from various modalities such as SPECT, PET, magnetic resonance imaging (MRI), coronary computed tomography angiography (CCTA), or echocardiography. In a wider sense, the term hybrid imaging may also apply to the combination of images that *per*

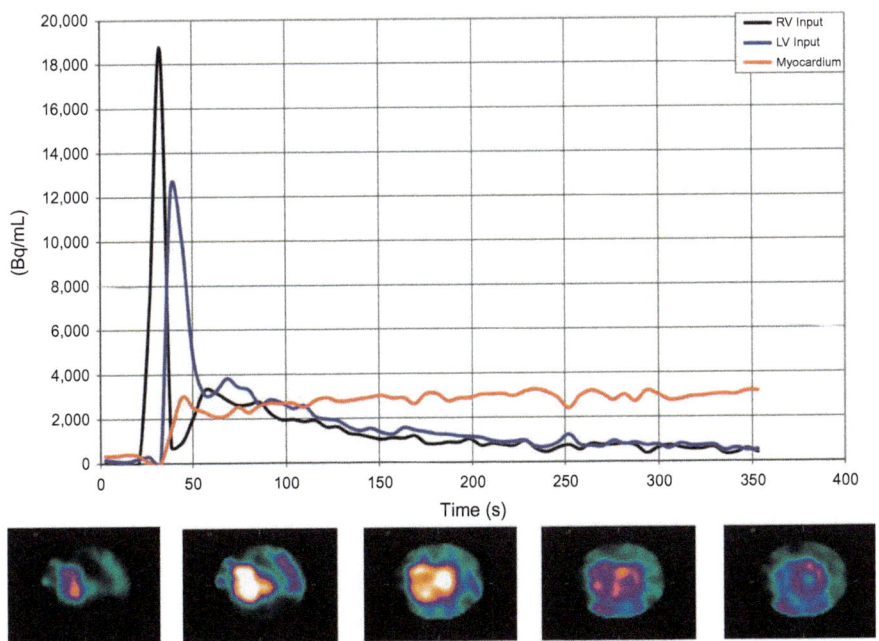

Figure 3.14 Dynamic acquisition with a CZT camera using ^{99m}Tc-sestamibi. Right and left ventricular blood pool and myocardial tissue time–activity curves are shown in the upper panel. The lower panel shows corresponding 6-second images at midventricular short axis. Reproduced with permission of the Society of Nuclear Medicine and Molecular Imaging from Ref. [21].

se do not provide neither anatomical nor functional information but are rather used to contribute to improved image quality of either modality (e.g., the combination of SPECT and a low-dose CT used for attenuation correction).

Datasets derived from SPECT and CCTA are most commonly used for hybrid imaging because both are three-dimensional datasets and the diagnostic information obtained from SPECT and CCTA is complementary: By offering information on the hemodynamic relevance of a coronary artery lesion identified by CCTA, SPECT increases the specificity of the latter. By contrast, CCTA extends the value of SPECT through diagnosis of nonobstructive atherosclerosis or the identification of multivessel disease (with possible balanced ischemia not detectable by semiquantitative perfusion imaging modalities). Importantly, however, further incremental value arises from spatial co-localization of a myocardial perfusion defect with the subtending coronary artery (Figure 3.15). Such hybrid imaging is, thus, more powerful than the sum of its parts because it provides information beyond that achievable with either data set alone [23].

Spatial co-localization may be achieved by mental synthesis through allocation of a myocardial segmentation model to one of the three main coronary arteries. However, such side-by-side analysis relies heavily on the standard distribution of myocardial perfusion territories, which is known to be inaccurate in more than half of the patients due to individual anatomical variability [24]. Therefore, true hybrid imaging, that is,

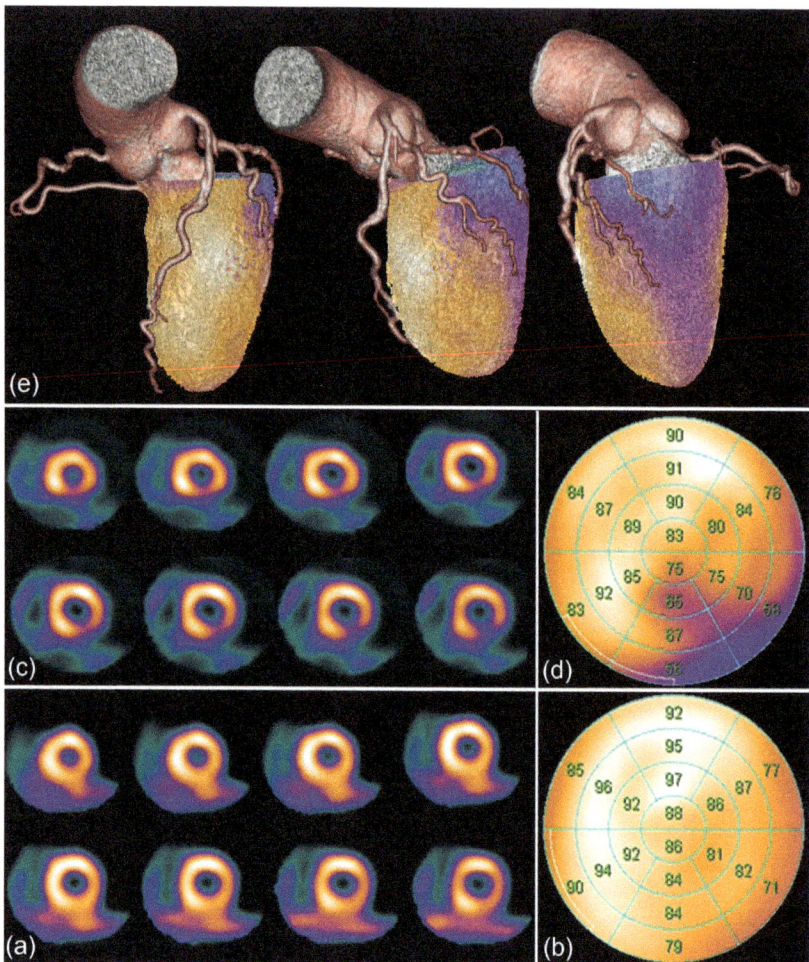

Figure 3.15 Short-axis slices and polar plots of myocardial perfusion SPECT imaging of a male patient at rest (a and b) and during pharmacologically induced stress (c and d) clearly depict a reversible infero-latero-basal perfusion defect. Volume rendered, co-registered, and fused hybrid SPECT/CCTA imaging (e; three perspectives of the same dataset are shown) clearly identifies the left circumflex artery as the subtending coronary artery, rather than the right coronary artery.

volume rendered, co-registered, and fused datasets should be preferred over sole side-by-side analysis. Accurate co-registration, however, is of utmost importance for reliable allocation of subtending coronary arteries with myocardial perfusion defects. SPECT and CCTA both are imaging modalities that provide a three-dimensional dataset of the entire heart by default that substantially facilitates the process of image fusion. Image acquisition may be performed on a hybrid scanner or obtained from separate stand-alone devices with manual, software-based co-registration of both datasets (Figure 3.16). The latter is fast and accurate [25], whereas even in automated co-registration of datasets,

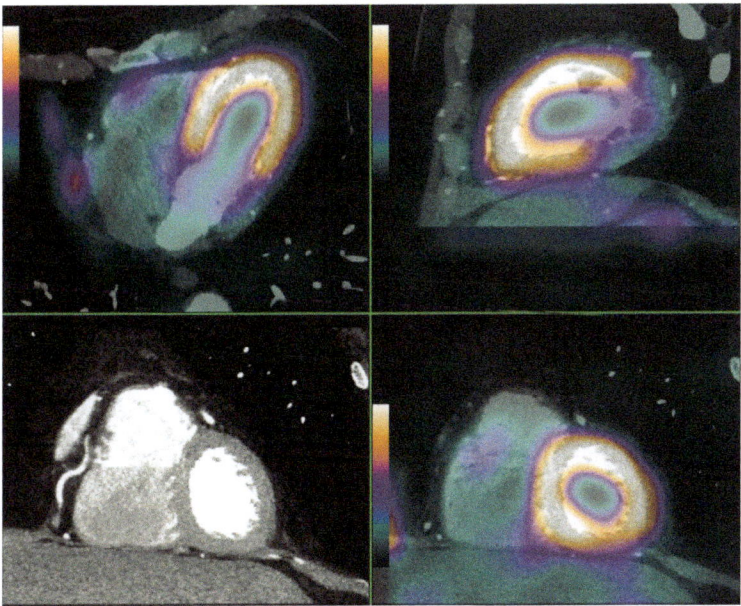

Figure 3.16 Manual software-based co-registration of SPECT and CCTA volume datasets in two-dimensional planes (same patient as in Figure 3.15).

careful review is mandatory and manual correction must be performed occasionally because errors in automatic registration may arise from breathing motion and cardiac contraction even if both datasets are acquired on a single hybrid scanner.

In summary, the integration of coronary anatomy by CCTA and documentation of myocardial perfusion through SPECT allows accurate and effective identification of (1) patients with normal coronaries who can safely be deferred from any further testing, (2) patients with nonobstructive coronary lesions where more aggressive prevention may be advisable, (3) patients with coronary artery disease who should undergo revascularization versus patients who may be benefiting more from anti-ischemic therapy, and (4) the culprit lesion in patients with multiple coronary artery lesions.

References

[1] Blumgart HL, Weiss S. Clinical studies on the velocity of blood flow: IX. The pulmonary circulation time, the velocity of venous blood flow to the heart, and related aspects of the circulation in patients with cardiovascular disease. J Clin Invest 1928;5:343–77.
[2] Anger HO. Scintillation camera with multichannel collimators. J Nucl Med 1964;5:515–31.
[3] Delbeke D, Segall GM. Status of and trends in nuclear medicine in the United States. J Nucl Med 2011;52(Suppl. 2):24S–8S.
[4] Einstein AJ, Moser KW, Thompson RC, Cerqueira MD, Henzlova MJ. Radiation dose to patients from cardiac diagnostic imaging. Circulation 2007;116:1290–305.
[5] Gambhir SS, Berman DS, Ziffer J, Nagler M, Sandler M, Patton J, et al. A novel high-sensitivity rapid-acquisition single-photon cardiac imaging camera. J Nucl Med 2009;50:635–43.

[6] Bocher M, Blevis IM, Tsukerman L, Shrem Y, Kovalski G, Volokh L. A fast cardiac gamma camera with dynamic SPECT capabilities: design, system validation and future potential. Eur J Nucl Med Mol Imaging 2010;37:1887–902.

[7] Buechel RR, Herzog BA, Husmann L, Burger IA, Pazhenkottil AP, Treyer V, et al. Ultrafast nuclear myocardial perfusion imaging on a new gamma camera with semiconductor detector technique: first clinical validation. Eur J Nucl Med Mol Imaging 2010;37:773–8.

[8] Nakata T, Nakajima K, Yamashina S, Yamada T, Momose M, Kasama S, et al. A pooled analysis of multicenter cohort studies of (123)I-mIBG imaging of sympathetic innervation for assessment of long-term prognosis in heart failure. JACC Cardiovasc Imaging 2013;6:772–84.

[9] Fricke E, Fricke H, Weise R, Kammeier A, Hagedorn R, Lotz N, et al. Attenuation correction of myocardial SPECT perfusion images with low-dose CT: evaluation of the method by comparison with perfusion PET. J Nucl Med 2005;46:736–44.

[10] Schepis T, Gaemperli O, Koepfli P, Ruegg C, Burger C, Leschka S, et al. Use of coronary calcium score scans from stand-alone multislice computed tomography for attenuation correction of myocardial perfusion SPECT. Eur J Nucl Med Mol Imaging 2007;34:11–9.

[11] DePuey EG, Rozanski A. Using gated technetium-99m-sestamibi SPECT to characterize fixed myocardial defects as infarct or artifact. J Nucl Med 1995;36:952–5.

[12] Sharir T, Germano G, Kavanagh PB, Lai S, Cohen I, Lewin HC, et al. Incremental prognostic value of post-stress left ventricular ejection fraction and volume by gated myocardial perfusion single photon emission computed tomography. Circulation 1999;100:1035–42.

[13] Buechel RR, Pazhenkottil AP, Herzog BA, Husmann L, Nkoulou RN, Burger IA, et al. Real-time breath-hold triggering of myocardial perfusion imaging with a novel cadmium-zinc-telluride detector gamma camera. Eur J Nucl Med Mol Imaging 2010;37:1903–8.

[14] Cerqueira MD, Allman KC, Ficaro EP, Hansen CL, Nichols KJ, Thompson RC, et al. Recommendations for reducing radiation exposure in myocardial perfusion imaging. J Nucl Cardiol 2010;17:709–18.

[15] Rozanski A, Gransar H, Hayes SW, Min J, Friedman JD, Thomson LE, et al. Temporal trends in the frequency of inducible myocardial ischemia during cardiac stress testing: 1991 to 2009. J Am Coll Cardiol 2013;61:1054–65.

[16] Chang SM, Nabi F, Xu J, Raza U, Mahmarian JJ. Normal stress-only versus standard stress/rest myocardial perfusion imaging: similar patient mortality with reduced radiation exposure. J Am Coll Cardiol 2010;55:221–30.

[17] Valenta I, Treyer V, Husmann L, Gaemperli O, Schindler MJ, Herzog BA, et al. New reconstruction algorithm allows shortened acquisition time for myocardial perfusion SPECT. Eur J Nucl Med Mol Imaging 2010;37:750–7.

[18] Slomka PJ, Dey D, Duvall WL, Henzlova MJ, Berman DS, Germano G. Advances in nuclear cardiac instrumentation with a view towards reduced radiation exposure. Curr Cardiol Rep 2012;14:208–16.

[19] Duvall WL, Croft LB, Ginsberg ES, Einstein AJ, Guma KA, George T, et al. Reduced isotope dose and imaging time with a high-efficiency CZT SPECT camera. J Nucl Cardiol 2011;18:847–57.

[20] Sugihara H, Yonekura Y, Kataoka K, Fukai D, Kitamura N, Taniguchi Y. Estimation of coronary flow reserve with the use of dynamic planar and SPECT images of Tc-99m tetrofosmin. J Nucl Cardiol 2001;8:575–9.

[21] Ben-Haim S, Murthy VL, Breault C, Allie R, Sitek A, Roth N, et al. Quantification of myocardial perfusion reserve using dynamic SPECT imaging in humans: a feasibility study. J Nucl Med 2013;54:873–9.

[22] Gaemperli O, Bengel FM, Kaufmann PA. Cardiac hybrid imaging. Eur Heart J 2011;32:2100–8.
[23] Sato A, Nozato T, Hikita H, Miyazaki S, Takahashi Y, Kuwahara T, et al. Incremental value of combining 64-slice computed tomography angiography with stress nuclear myocardial perfusion imaging to improve noninvasive detection of coronary artery disease. J Nucl Cardiol 2010;17:19–26.
[24] Javadi MS, Lautamaki R, Merrill J, Voicu C, Epley W, McBride G, et al. Definition of vascular territories on myocardial perfusion images by integration with true coronary anatomy: a hybrid PET/CT analysis. J Nucl Med 2010;51:198–203.
[25] Slomka PJ, Baum RP. Multimodality image registration with software: state-of-the-art. Eur J Nucl Med Mol Imaging 2009;36(Suppl. 1):S44–55.

Positron emission tomography

P. Knaapen*, M. Lubberink†
*VU University Medical Center, Amsterdam, The Netherlands; †Uppsala University Hospital and Nuclear Medicine & PET, Uppsala University, Uppsala, Sweden

4.1 Introduction

Positron emission tomography (PET) is a radionuclide imaging technique that allows for noninvasive quantification of biochemical pathways *in vivo*. Utilizing positron emitting labeled compounds of interest, a myriad of biological processes can be visualized in the human heart. As such, PET has been proven invaluable to investigate cardiovascular biology and physiology noninvasively. Due to its limited availability, methodologic complexity, and high cost, cardiac PET has long been considered to be a research tool only. In recent years, however, PET technology has been fused with computed tomography (CT) as well as magnetic resonance imaging (MRI). In a short period of time, these hybrid devices have gained great popularity, predominantly driven by their success in clinical oncology, which has led to an exponential growth of the numbers of scanners installed worldwide. This growth in hardware has been paralleled by improvements in radiotracer availability and advances in postprocessing software. Consequently, cardiac PET has witnessed more widespread use and routine implementation in the clinical arena. Assessment of myocardial perfusion and substrate metabolism are of particular value in the evaluation of patients with (suspected) coronary artery disease (CAD) to detect ischemia and myocardial viability. Moreover, PET has the potential to probe a number of complex functions like myocardial innervation, energetics, inflammation, receptor mapping, and gene reporting, some of which may ultimately prove to be of clinical value.

This chapter will outline the fundamental principles of PET and technical considerations of cardiac PET imaging. Subsequently, the available tracers for myocardial perfusion imaging (MPI) will be highlighted with special emphasis on quantification of myocardial blood flow (MBF). Also, the added value of substrate metabolism will be discussed. Finally, future directions of molecular and hybrid imaging will be explored.

4.2 Principles of PET

4.2.1 Data acquisition

PET relies on the simultaneous detection of two annihilation photons, emitted when a positron, produced in the decay of neutron-deficient nuclides, is annihilated by colliding with an atomic electron. The most commonly used nuclides in (cardiac) PET are ^{18}F, ^{11}C, ^{13}N, ^{15}O, and ^{82}Rb (Table 4.1). Since the average range traveled by positrons

Table 4.1 Selection of validated cardiac PET tracers

Isotope	Half-life	Production	Labeled compound	Biological information
^{82}Rb	76 s	Generator	^{82}Rubidium	Perfusion
^{15}O	123 s	Cyclotron	^{15}O-water	Perfusion
			^{15}O-oxygen	Oxygen consumption
			^{15}O-carbonmonoxide	Blood volume
^{13}N	9.97 min	Cyclotron	^{13}N-ammonia	Perfusion
^{11}C	20.4 min	Cyclotron	^{11}C-palmitate	Fatty acid metabolism
			^{11}C-glucose	Glucose metabolism
			^{11}C-acetate	Oxygen consumption (Krebs cycle flux)
			^{11}C-hydroxyephedrine	Sympathetic neuronal catecholamine uptake
			^{11}C-epinephrine	Sympathetic neuronal catecholamine storage
			^{11}C-CGP12177	beta-adrenergic receptor density
			^{11}C-GB67	Alpha1-adrenergic receptor density
			^{11}C-PK11195	Peripheral benzodiazepine receptor density (macrophage activity, inflammation)
^{18}F	110 min	Cyclotron	^{18}F-FDG	Glucose metabolism
			^{18}F-flurpiridaz	Perfusion
			^{18}F-fluorodopamine	Sympathetic neuronal uptake and function
			^{18}F-sodium fluoride	Vascular calcification/plaque vulnerability

is small, in the order of mm, the decay can be considered to have occurred along the straight line described by the two annihilation photons. As shown schematically in Figures 4.1 and 4.2, a PET scanner consists of a number of rings of detectors. These detectors consist of a scintillating material, typically bismuth germanate (BGO) or cerium-doped lutetium(-yttrium) oxyorthosilicate (LSO or LYSO), that converts the energy of the annihilation photons into light. This light is then converted into an electrical signal by a photomultiplier, with a pulse height proportional to the energy of the incoming photon. Two photons are considered to have been emitted simultaneously when they are detected within the coincidence-timing window of the scanner, around

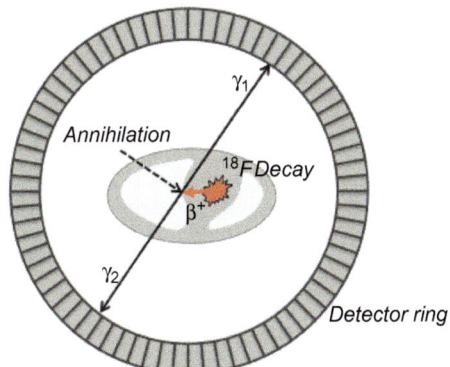

Figure 4.1 Schematic representation of an ^{18}F-decay in a PET scanner. The distance between the radioactive decay and the annihilation of the positron (β^+) is greatly exaggerated.

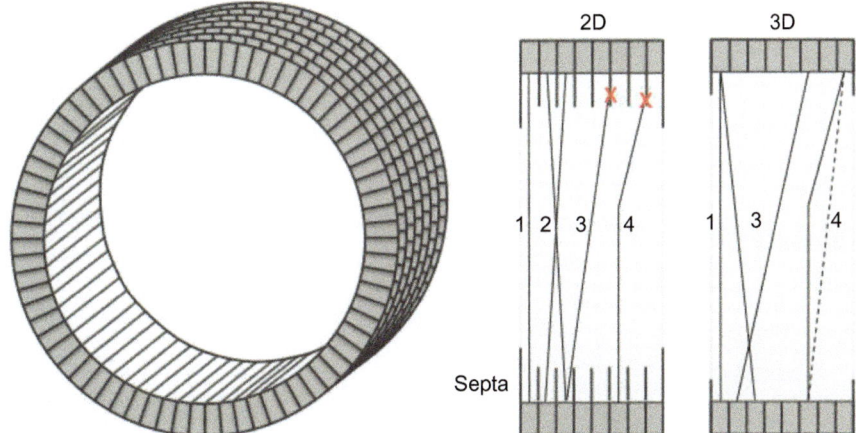

Figure 4.2 Schematic representation of a multiring PET scanner. In 2D mode, only direct coincidences (within a single ring, 1) and coincidences between adjacent rings (2) are accepted, whereas coincidences at larger axial angles (3) are not registered. The detection of scatter coincidences (4) is considerably increased in 3D mode. Typical PET(-CT, -MRI) scanners consist of several tens of these detectors rings, with a total axial FOV of 15–25 cm.

6–12 ns. Hence, all that is known when two photons are detected simultaneously is that a decay event occurred somewhere along the line between two detectors, a so-called line of response (LOR). By detection of large numbers of these annihilation photon pairs, the distribution of the positron-emitting nuclides in the part of the patient positioned within the field-of-view of the PET scanner can be reconstructed. As can be seen in Figure 4.2, acquisition can be performed either in 2D or 3D acquisition modes. To avoid confusion, the resulting images are always 3D volumes. The advantage of 2D acquisition mode, with the detector rings separated by collimating lead or tungsten septa and only accepting coincidences within a single ring or between adjacent rings, is that acquisition is done on a per-slice basis, as in CT. This reduces image reconstruction to a relatively simple 2D problem. In addition, septa reduce the fraction of random and scatter coincidences (see Section 4.2.3). 3D acquisition, accepting coincidences between all combinations of detector rings, typically result in a fivefold increase in sensitivity of several factors compared to 2D mode. This is obtained at the cost of increasing scatter and random fractions, much larger amounts of data, and more complex and computationally demanding reconstruction algorithms. Improvement in reconstruction methods and increased computer power ensure that the advantages of 3D acquisition nowadays outweigh its disadvantages, and the latest generation of scanners are no longer equipped with septa.

The implementation of faster detector materials such as LSO and LYSO has recently resulted in the emergence of time-of-flight PET (TF-PET) where the detection times of the individual photons are measured as well. In the latest generation of PET systems equipped with TF, the time difference between the arrival of both annihilation photons can be measured with a time resolution of around 500 ps, corresponding to a path length of about 17 cm (Figure 4.3). Use of TF information in image reconstruction results in a considerable improvement of signal to noise ratio, especially in large patients.

On all current PET/(-CT) scanners, image reconstruction is routinely performed using various implementations of 3D ordered subsets expectation maximization (OSEM) iterative reconstruction. Many studies have been devoted to the quantitative accuracy of OSEM reconstructions, showing results to be comparable to those obtained with analytical reconstruction methods (filtered back projection) [2].

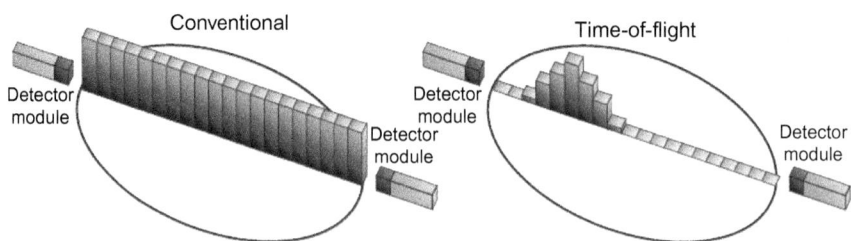

Figure 4.3 Time of flight.
Image reprinted with permission from Moses [1].

4.2.2 Attenuation

As in single-photon imaging, annihilation photons are attenuated on their way through the body, causing a reduction of the number of photons measured along a certain LOR (Figure 4.4). While the signal measured in single-photon imaging (gamma scintigraphy) is depending on the depth at which the photons are emitted, the PET signal is only dependent on the total attenuation along the LOR, which can be measured directly using a positron-emitting source rotating around the patient (Figure 4.5). This makes PET an inherently quantitative technique. As an alternative, the attenuation can be accurately estimated based on a co-registered CT image after conversion of Hounsfield units to 511 keV attenuation coefficients as implemented in all current PET–CT scanners. Especially in the thorax region, this poses a challenge compared to 511 keV transmission imaging. Since a 511 keV transmission scan typically takes several minutes to acquire, it is done during regular breathing, as is the emission PET scan itself. CT, however, provides a snapshot of the patient during a single phase of the respiratory (or cardiac) cycle. Neither 511 keV transmission scan nor CT are acquired simultaneously with the PET scan itself, which frequently results in attenuation correction misalignment artifacts in cardiac PET/CT scanning due to patient motion.

4.2.3 Corrections

In addition to attenuation correction as described in the previous section, a number of corrections have to be applied to PET data to ensure quantitatively accurate images. First, data have to be normalized, i.e., corrected for differences in detection efficiency for different LORs. This correction is usually based on a measurement with a uniform phantom that is performed on a regular basis, for example, every 3 months. Then, a correction has to be applied for dead time (the time after each event during which the

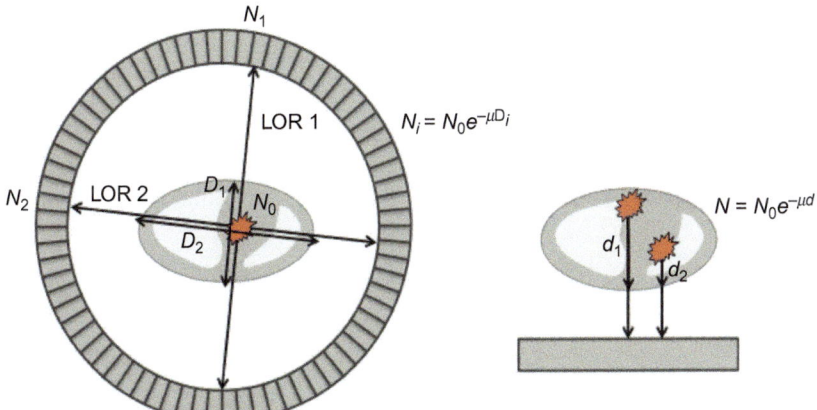

Figure 4.4 Attenuation in PET (left) compared to single-photon emission tomography (SPECT; right). In PET, attenuation is only dependent on the total path D along a line of response traversed through the patient by both annihilation photons, whereas in SPECT, attenuation is dependent on the depth at which the radioactive decay occurs.

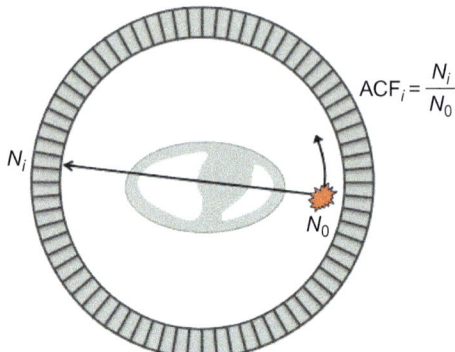

Figure 4.5 A transmission measurement using a rotating point source. In case of a positron-emitting point source (^{68}Ga), the attenuation correction for each LOR can be calculated as shown in the equation. N_0 is the number of photons emitted by the source, N_i is the number of photons detected along the LOR connecting the location of the source and detector i.

system is not able to record another event), ensuring linearity of the scanner. In this respect, dynamic cardiac studies with H$_2$^{15}O and ^{82}Rb, aimed at quantifying MBF, are the most challenging studies to be performed with PET. In these studies, count rates vary from extremely high (up to 50 million single photons per second) immediately after injection when all radioactivity is passing through the thorax, to very low after several minutes when the radioactivity has mostly decayed and has distributed throughout the body.

At high count rates, the major part of the measured coincidences can consist of random coincidences (Figure 4.6a), where two photons originating from different decays are detected within the coincidence-timing window of the scanner. The probability of random coincidences increases with the square of the single-photon count rate, and hence approximately with the square of the amount of radioactivity in the FOV of the scanner. Correction for random coincidences is based on the fact that their probability can be calculated for each LOR as the product of timing window width and the singles count rates of both detectors.

The mean attenuation length of 511 keV photons in water is about 7 cm. That implicates that after 7 cm, on average 50% of all annihilation photon pairs have undergone Compton scatter, and one of the photons has hence changed direction (Figure 4.6b).

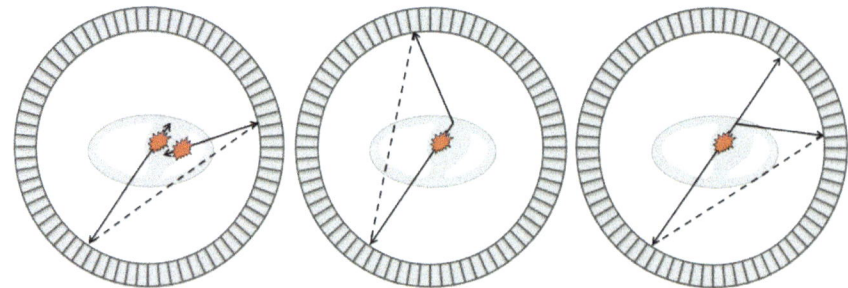

Figure 4.6 Left to right: random, scatter, and prompt gamma coincidences.

Many of these scattered photons are not detected, either because they leave the FOV of the scanner or, in 2D PET, because they do not reach the detectors due to the septa. Even if they reach the detector, Compton scatter has reduced their energy and the proportionality between photon energy and photomultiplier pulse height can be used to reject them, even though the limited energy resolution of 10–15% requires a large energy window of typically 400–600 keV. Still, depending on patient size, scatter coincidences can constitute more than 50% of the total amount of coincidences after random correction. Because of this, a lot of effort has been put into developing accurate corrections for scatter coincidences. Today, all commercial scanners utilize Monte-Carlo based correction methods, which have been extensively validated.

An additional challenge that arises with the use of ^{82}Rb is that this isotope emits gamma radiation simultaneously with positrons in about 10% of its decays. Coincidence detection of these, nonangularly correlated, photons together with one (or both) annihilation photons results in erroneous LORs, causing a quantitative bias in the resulting PET images (Figure 4.6c). This bias can be corrected for using a modification of the standard scatter correction method.

4.2.4 Image quality and accuracy

The spatial resolution of PET, that is, the minimum difference between two point sources that is needed to be able to distinguish them as separate sources in the reconstructed PET image, is mainly dependent on three factors: the size of the detector elements, the energy of the emitted positrons, and filtering applied during or post image reconstruction. The size of the detector elements is typically around 4 × 4 mm, which is the most important contribution in clinical scanners. The 2–3 cm thickness of the detectors, required to obtain a sufficient detection sensitivity, results in uncertainty on the depth of photon interaction and a corresponding degradation of the spatial resolution increasing with distance to the center of the FOV (Figure 4.7). Typical spatial resolution in images acquired with clinical scanners is around 6–7 mm.

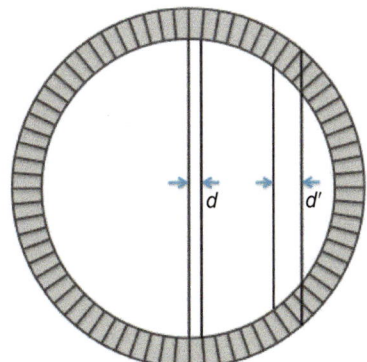

Figure 4.7 Effect of distance from the center of the FOV on spatial resolution. The effective width of a radially off-center LOR (d') is much larger than a central LOR (d) because of uncertainty of the depth at which photons interact with the detector crystal.

Since no collimation is required, the sensitivity of PET (the number of useful detected photons relative to the amount of radioactivity in the scanner) is several orders of magnitude higher than that of single-photon images. This high sensitivity allows for measurement of the radioactivity distribution not only with a high spatial resolution, but also with a temporal resolution in the order of seconds. Hence, not only the spatial distribution, but also the kinetics of molecules labeled with positron-emitting nuclides can be measured with PET.

4.3 Clinical applications

4.3.1 Myocardial perfusion

Of the available tracers, ^{82}Rb, ^{13}NH$_3$, and H$_2^{15}$O are the most commonly used for the assessment of myocardial perfusion [3]. ^{18}F-flurpiridaz is an emerging perfusion tracer not yet available for clinical use, but holds great potential and is currently being tested in phase 3 trials [4]. As will be described in this section, each of these tracers possesses unique characteristics with their individual pros and cons pertaining to (costs of) radionuclide production, physical half-life, image quality, radiation exposure, compatibility with exercise acquisition protocols, and tracer kinetics for quantification (Table 4.2). None of the perfusion tracers excels on all of these

Table 4.2 **Characteristics of cardiac perfusion tracers**

	H$_2^{15}$O	^{13}NH$_3$	^{82}Rb	^{18}F-flurpiridaz
Half-life	123 s	9.97 min	76 s	110 min
Production	Cyclotron	Cyclotron	Generator	Cyclotron
Kinetics	Freely diffusible, metabolically inert	Metabolically trapped in myocardium	Metabolically trapped in myocardium	Metabolically trapped in myocardium
Mean positron range in tissue	1.1 mm	0.4 mm	2.8 mm	0.2 mm
Scan duration	6 min	20 min	6 min	20 min
Gating/LV function	–	+	+	+
Radiation dose (3D)	~0.5 mSv	~1 mSv	~4 mSv	~5 mSv
Exercise protocol compatible	–	–	–	+
Quantification	Excellent	Good	Moderate	Very good
Image quality	Good (parametric or digital subtraction images)	Very good	Good	Excellent

features. Choice of tracer is therefore multifactorial and frequently depends on practical and logistical considerations, as well as specific requirements regarding the nature of cardiac PET program (e.g., for scientific or diagnostic purposes).

4.3.2 Perfusion tracer characteristics

$H_2^{15}O$ is characterized by fundamentally different properties as compared with ^{82}Rb, ^{13}NH$_3$, and ^{18}F-flurpiridaz [5–7]. The latter tracers are transported across the cell membrane and effectively become metabolically trapped. ^{82}Rb is a potassium analogue that is rapidly and actively taken up by myocardial cells via the Na/K ATP transporter [8], whereas ^{13}NH$_3$ is incorporated into the glutamine pool by active transport and passive diffusion processes [9]. ^{18}F-flurpiridaz is a pyridazinone derivative that avidly binds to mitochondrial complex-1 [10]. In contrast to these tracers, $H_2^{15}O$ is freely diffusible and metabolically inert. These properties have consequences for diagnostic quality of relative uptake images. Figure 4.8 displays the dynamic frame acquisition for an uptake tracer (^{82}Rb) and a freely diffusible one ($H_2^{15}O$). After intravenous bolus injection,

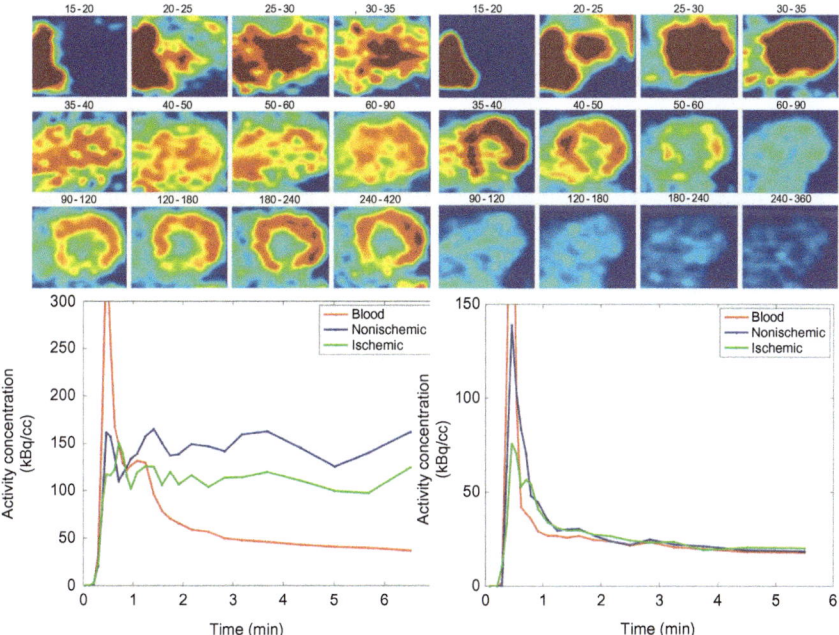

Figure 4.8 Six-minute dynamic frame sequence (short axis view) indicated in seconds for ^{82}Rb (upper left panel) and $H_2^{15}O$ (upper right panel) for the same patient with ischemia apparent by reduced tracer uptake in the inferior wall during a vasodilation study. Corresponding time–activity-curves for arterial blood, ischemic, and nonischemic myocardium are depicted in the lower panels. Note that $H_2^{15}O$ clears from myocardium after being taken up, whereas ^{82}Rb remains confined to the myocardium after initial uptake. See text for details. Image courtesy of H. Harms, PhD, and Kirstin Bouchelouche, MD, Aarhus University Hospital, Skejby.

transit of tracer through the anatomical compartments is visualized. The initial images illustrate tracer activity in the right ventricular cavity. Subsequently, the tracer bolus is dispersed into the lungs, after which it reaches the left ventricular cavity. Both ^{82}Rb and $H_2^{15}O$ are then taken up by the myocardium. As can be appreciated from the images and the matching time-activity-curves for arterial blood and myocardium, however, ^{82}Rb stays confined to the myocardium while being cleared from the intravascular compartment. Being freely diffusible, $H_2^{15}O$ promptly reaches equilibrium between blood and tissue. Consequently, "late" static uptake images of metabolically trapped compounds (^{82}Rb, ^{13}NH$_3$, and ^{18}F-flurpiridaz) have significantly higher tissue-to-background ratios as compared with $H_2^{15}O$, yielding diagnostic images of superior quality for qualitative grading of relative perfusion distribution (Figure 4.9).

The lack of diagnostic images has long prohibited the use of $H_2^{15}O$ for diagnostic imaging of CAD, and virtually all studies on qualitative imaging for CAD have been conducted with ^{82}Rb or ^{13}NH$_3$ [14]. In recent years, however, advances in scanner technology and postprocessing procedures have enabled the generation of blood volume images from the dynamic tracer acquisition through cluster image analysis (anatomical compartments are distinguished based on biological properties) [15]. Digital subtraction techniques of the blood volume from the $H_2^{15}O$ images subsequently provide high-quality radiotracer distribution images [16]. Figure 4.10 displays images highlighting this technique. These developments have enabled $H_2^{15}O$ to be utilized in clinical practice [19,20].

Image quality is further determined by the positron range in tissue. High-energy positrons have a greater tissue penetration depth before annihilation occurs and demonstrate decreased spatial resolution in comparison to low-energy positrons. In this regard, image resolution gradually increases from ^{82}Rb, $H_2^{15}O$, ^{13}NH$_3$, to ^{18}F-flurpiridaz, respectively, according to their energetic state (Figure 4.11) [4].

Moreover, the physical half-life of the radioactive compounds determines the potential acquisition duration and therefore count-statistics. The short physical half-life of ^{82}Rb and $H_2^{15}O$ allows a timeframe of only a few minutes of acquisition before the tracer is decayed to background levels, whereas ^{13}NH$_3$ and ^{18}F-flurpiridaz acquisitions can be continued till satisfactory counts-statistics are obtained, which enhances image quality. These factors result in the highest image quality of ^{18}F-flurpiridaz given its

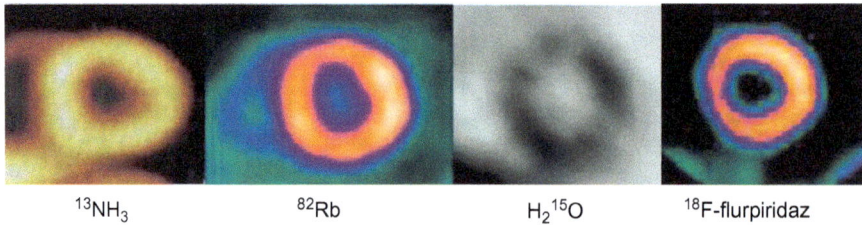

Figure 4.9 Short axis views of (late) uptake images of the different tracers used for qualitative analysis of myocardial perfusion.
Adapted from Schindler et al. [7], Yoshinaga et al. [11], Adachi et al. [12], and Bengel et al. [13].

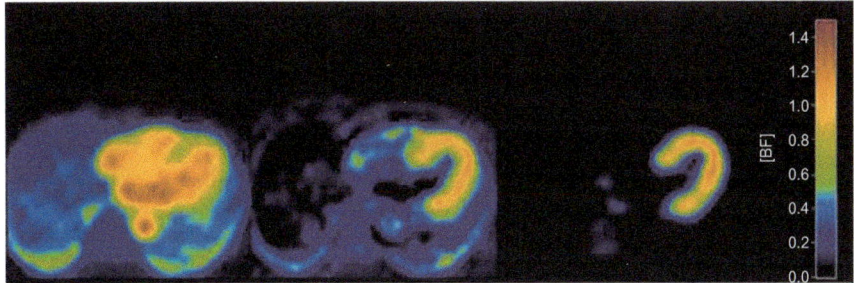

Figure 4.10 Left panel: transaxial image at the thoracic level obtained a few minutes after injection of $H_2^{15}O$. Note that the myocardium cannot be distinguished from the ventricular blood pool cavities as a result of free diffusion of tracer between blood and myocardial tissue, rendering the images unsuitable for diagnostic purposes. Middle panel: through a mathematical process (i.e., factor or cluster analysis) the blood pool can be identified and subtracted from the $H_2^{15}O$ image, yielding an image of tracer activity distribution in the myocardial wall. These images can be used to qualitatively grade tracer uptake. Right panel: parametric image of the same patient as in other panels. Perfusion is calculated at the voxel level through a modeling procedure based on the dynamic flux of tracer between arterial blood and myocardial tissue. The parametric image perfusion is given in absolute terms (mL min^{-1} g^{-1}) in the accompanying color-coded legend [17]; see text for details.
Adapted from Knaapen et al. [18].

long half-life and low positron range as opposed to relatively poor image quality of ^{82}Rb with its ultra-short half-life and high positron range.

As already alluded to, PET measures absolute levels of tracer concentration. Acquisition of PET in a dynamic fashion (i.e., multiple frames initiated upon administration of the tracer) generates time–activity curves of tracer flux between arterial blood and tissues [6]. This information allows the mathematical computation of MBF in absolute terms. The ideal tracer accumulates in/or clears from myocardium

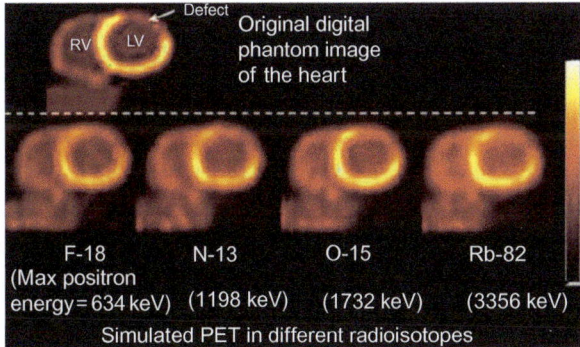

Figure 4.11 Simulated cardiac images of different positron ranges (F-18, N-13, O-15, and Rb-82) using same digital cardio-torso phantom. Blurring effect by positron range increases for higher kinetic energy of the positron.
Reprinted with permission from Rischpler et al. [4].

proportionally linear to perfusion, irrespective of flow rate or metabolic state [21]. $H_2^{15}O$ is the only tracer that meets these criteria and is therefore considered the gold standard for quantification of MBF [22]. An important limitation of the other aforementioned tracers is that myocardial extraction from arterial blood is incomplete and curvilinear with increasing flow rates, frequently referred to as the "roll-off" phenomenon (Figure 4.12) [24]. This results in progressive underestimation of MBF measurements as actual flow increases. Correction models based on animal experiments can be employed yet induce noise, particularly when large correction factors are required with severely blunted extraction at high perfusion levels. Nonetheless, based on the time-activity-curves of the arterial input (defined by a volume of interest in the left ventricular cavity or aorta) and the myocardium (by regional volume of interest selection of the myocardium) as depicted in Figure 4.8, compartment modeling procedures can be performed to calculate MBF in absolute terms (i.e., $mL\,min^{-1}\,g^{-1}$). A compartment represents a unique biochemical state of a certain type of tissue. Depending on the biological behavior of the tracer, single or multiple tissue compartment models can be used to quantify MBF (Figure 4.13) [25].

$H_2^{15}O$ and ^{82}Rb can best be described by a single compartment model [5,22,26], while metabolites of $^{13}NH_3$ and ^{18}F-flurpiridaz stay confined to a bound space in the myocardium and therefore generally a two-compartment model for these tracers is employed [27–29]. Appropriate corrections for spillover and partial volume effects are also included in these models. Each of these tracers has been tested in animal experiments against microsphere-quantified perfusion; the invasive reference standard. $H_2^{15}O$ and $^{13}NH_3$ in particular have been well validated and display close agreement with microsphere flow and demonstrate low test-retest variability (10–15%) [5,22,28,30,31]. As already mentioned, quantification of ^{82}Rb is less reliable as this tracer harbors intrinsic limitations. Nonetheless, recent studies have shown MBF measurements of ^{82}Rb to be feasible [32]. Limited data are available pertaining the quantification of ^{18}F-flurpiridaz, but its characteristics and kinetics should allow for highly reliable perfusion measurements [4,21,27]. In recent years, automated software packages have been developed, applying these validated models. Postprocessing is in the order of minutes, and these

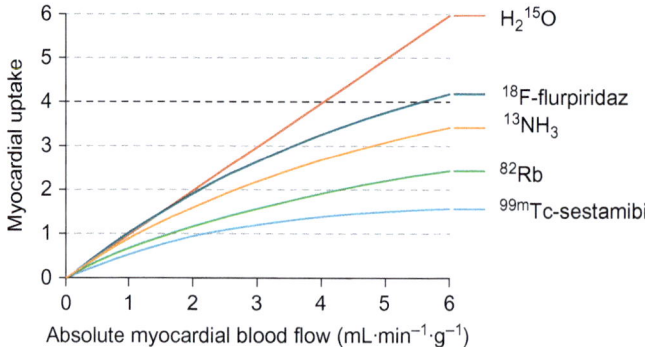

Figure 4.12 Kinetics of MPI perfusion tracers. Graphical presentation of the relationship between absolute MBF of the several PET radiotracers and actual tracer uptake. Adapted from Danad et al. [23].

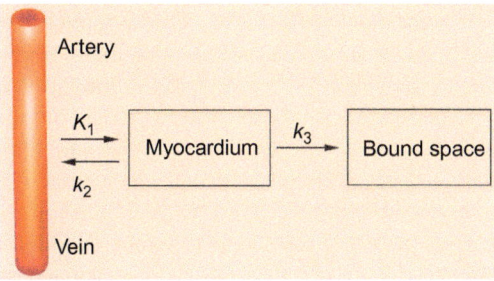

Figure 4.13 Schematic diagram of a compartment model used for quantification of MBF. For $H_2^{15}O$ and ^{82}Rb, only K_1 and k_2 are used, while for ^{18}F-flurpiridaz and $^{13}NH_3$, k_3 must be included [24].

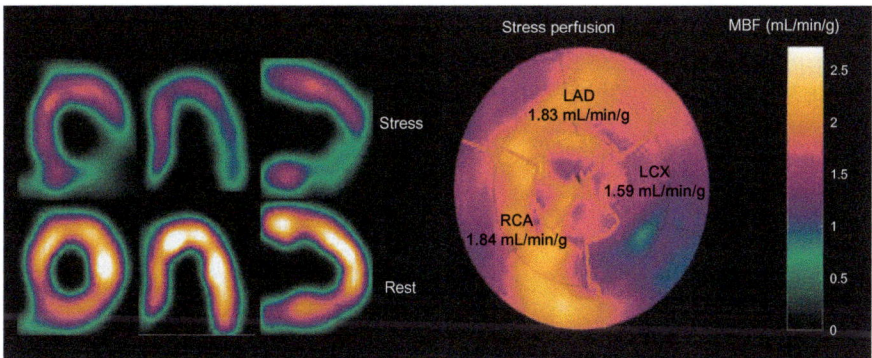

Figure 4.14 Parametric $H_2^{15}O$ images in short and long axis views as well as a parametric polar map of the left ventricle during hyperaemia [17]. These images display perfusion in absolute quantities at the voxel level and can be interpreted both qualitatively for relative perfusion defects as well as in a quantitative manner. Quantitative parametric imaging aids to unmask e.g., balanced ischemia in case of multivessel disease and/or coronary microvascular dysfunction.

packages display high reproducibility [33–35]. Moreover, parametric images can be generated that display perfusion at the voxel level, based on evaluation of the tracer kinetic model for each voxel [16,17]. These images are distinctly different from actual radiotracer uptake images as they represent a graphical illustration of quantitative MBF (Figure 4.14). This has proven to be specifically useful for $H_2^{15}O$ PET, as this tracer principally lacks visual interpretable distribution images (*vide supra*).

4.3.3 Imaging protocols

Given the short physical half of ^{82}Rb, $H_2^{15}O$, and $^{13}NH_3$, multiple acquisitions can be conducted in a single session. The half-life of ^{18}F-flurpiridaz does not allow for serial acquisitions in a single session. Administration dosage should be adjusted for the scanner hardware in order to avoid saturation and retain linearity between radionuclide concentration and PET signal. Bolus injections have proven to provide the most accurate results to quantify MBF [36]. As a rule of thumb, radionuclide activity is considered to be sufficiently decayed five half-lives after administration to commence a new scan sequence. Perfusion protocols generally consist of a rest and vasodilator stress study, although sometimes an alternative stressor like cold pressor testing is used to assess coronary endothelial function (usually by immersing the subject's hand in ice water to provoke a pain-stimulus and adrenergic response) [37]. Maximal vasodilation is achieved by intravenous administration of adenosine, dypiridamole, or regadenoson. Alternatively, inotropic stimulation (e.g., dobutamine) is used in case of contraindications for vasodilator agents (obstructive pulmonary disease or cardiac electrical conduction abnormalities). As already mentioned, attenuation correction is achieved by use of a transmission image. Traditionally, this was obtained through a rotating positron-emitting source located within in the PET gantry (e.g., ^{68}Ge). With contemporary PET/CT systems, however, tissue density maps are acquired with the CT equipment. This is usually a nongated, low-resolution CT scan obtained during tidal expiration, breath hold, or shallow breathing [38]. Some centers perform separate attenuation scans for resting and stress conditions as the stressor agent influences the anatomical position of the heart due to tachycardia and/or tachypnoe, causing misalignment between the rest attenuation map and stress emission data. During postprocessing, alignment between transmission and emission images can be verified and manually adjusted when required (Figure 4.15) [39,40]. Such a procedure is important

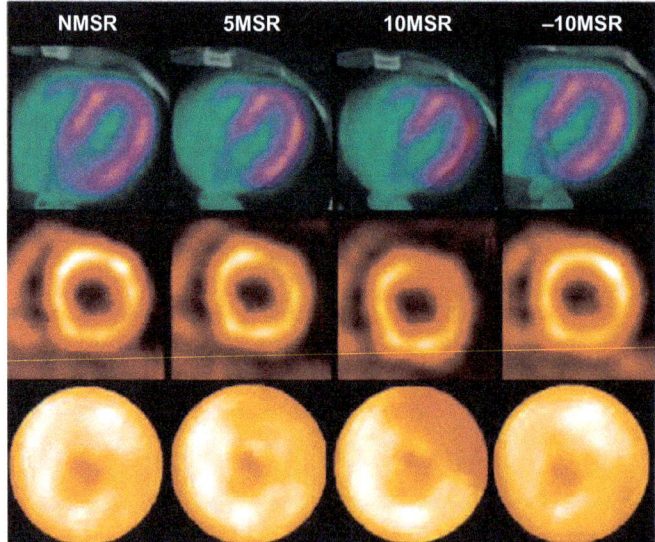

Figure 4.15 Myocardial perfusion stress ^{82}Rb PET images and polar maps demonstrate effects of no misregistration (NMSR) and effects of 5-mm misregistration (5MSR), 10-mm misregistration (10MSR), and reverse 10-mm misregistration (−10MSR) between PET and CT images. Artifactual defects are prominent in anterior and lateral walls of heart, although this patient had no disease.
Adapted from Rajaram et al. [39].

to minimize motion artifacts that may affect uptake images as well as MBF quantification. It is of interest to note that $H_2^{15}O$ does not necessarily require attenuation correction as quantification of perfusion is derived from the wash-out curve. As the image derived arterial input curve and tissue response are affected to a similar extent by attenuation, correction for attenuation does not appreciably affect flow values and can thus be omitted [41].

Most systems support list-mode acquisition, which enables additional collection of ECG and/or respiratory signals [42]. During postprocessing, these data can be utilized to retrieve information on cardiac function (left ventricular end-diastolic and end-systolic volumes, ejection fraction, and regional wall motion) [43]. New developments also enable to generate "motion frozen" images to enhance resolution, whereby only emission data from the end-diastolic and/or expiration phase are utilized to minimize the blurring effects of cardiac and respiratory motion [44]. These techniques require longer acquisition times to gather sufficient count-statistics as much of the collected data outside of these prespecified cardiac or respiratory phases are disregarded, and are therefore less suitable for very short-lived tracers [45,46].

4.3.4 Tracer production and availability

A pivotal issue that has proven to be the major obstacle for cardiac PET perfusion imaging is the necessity to produce the utilized tracers onsite. Of the currently available tracers, $H_2^{15}O$ and $^{13}NH_3$ require a cyclotron in the near proximity of the scanning facilities. ^{82}Rb is produced by a $^{82}Sr/^{82}Rb$ generator, obviating the need for a cyclotron, and is therefore more convenient to implement in clinical practice. The parent isotope ^{82}Sr, however, needs to be replenished every 28 days at relatively high costs ($20,000). Therefore, high-volume patient throughput is needed to be cost-effective. These issues of local tracer production have clearly limited the widespread use of cardiac perfusion PET. This may soon be overcome by the dawning perspective of fluorine labeled tracers such as ^{18}F-flurpiridaz [4]. Its longer physical half-life of 110 min allows for off-site production and could be as successful for cardiology as ^{18}F-FDG PET has been for clinical oncology. Another advantage of ^{18}F-labeled flow tracers is the fact that they allow to be used in physical exercise protocols whereby the radioisotope is administered during maximal exertion. ^{82}Rb, $H_2^{15}O$, and $^{13}NH_3$ require injection while the patient is lying within the scanner, as tracer decay is too rapid to transport the patient from the treadmill or stationary bike to the scanner. Furthermore, prescanning physical exercise and injection is not an option for $H_2^{15}O$ since this tracer does not accumulate in tissue. These tracers can therefore only be utilized in conjunction with pharmacological stressor agents. A disadvantage of exercise PET imaging is that quantification is lost as no arterial input function is obtained. Moreover, as with technetium labeled SPECT imaging, rest and stress images are generally acquired on separate occasions due to the relative long physical half-life of ^{18}F-labeled compounds. One-day protocols are feasible, but necessitate the second image acquisition at high tracer dosage administration (and radiation exposure) to minimize the influence of residual radioactivity [47].

4.3.5 Image interpretation

Most commonly, images are graded in a qualitative manner. Radiotracer distribution is evaluated both during rest and stress conditions. Myocardial perfusion defects are graded by their extent, severity, and location. Guidelines recommend a semiquantitative analysis using a 5 point scale system (normal=0, mild defect=1, moderate defect=2, severe defect=3, and absent uptake=4) on a 17 segment model of the left ventricle [48]. The summed scores are calculated for rest (SRS) and stress (SSS), and their difference (SDS) to identify reversibility [49]. Fixed defects are compatible with myocardial scarring or hibernating myocardium, whereas reversibility of stress induced hypoperfusion is compatible with ischemia. As already mentioned, PET acquisitions are nowadays generally acquired with a dynamic frame sequence and, next to qualitative grading, absolute quantitative MBF values are routinely provided. Normal databases display a broad base of hyperemic MBF between 2 and $5\,\text{mL}\,\text{min}^{-1}\,\text{g}^{-1}$, which is attributable to variability in minimal microvascular resistance and is dependent on age, sex, and traditional cardiovascular risk factors [50,51]. Currently, limited data are available with regard to an optimal threshold to distinguish pathological from normal hyperemic MBF and myocardial flow reserve [52]. In general, a myocardial flow reserve below two is considered abnormal whereas beyond 2.5 is deemed normal, with an ambiguous transition zone between 2.0 and 2.5 [7]. Ongoing studies are targeted to further define the normal limits of (hyperemic) perfusion.

4.3.6 Substrate metabolism

The heart is omnivorous, and its substrate metabolism includes the use of glucose, free fatty acids, lactate, and ketones [53,54]. The relative contribution of each of these given fuels is, among others, dependent on their concentration in plasma and the hormonal milieu. In general, it can be stated that in the fasting state, the heart feeds predominantly on free fatty acids, whereas after a meal, glucose becomes the major fuel substrate. Both metabolic pathways can be (quantitatively) visualized with cardiac PET in conjunction with some of the tracers listed in Table 4.1. As with myocardial perfusion, quantitative compartment models have been developed and validated for glucose and fatty acid metabolism [55,56]. This type of metabolic imaging has provided important insight in the pathophysiology of altered substrate metabolism in conditions such as diabetic and dilated cardiomyopathy [57,58], as well as allowing the monitoring of the effects of pharmacological interventions over time [59–61]. The most experience for myocardial substrate metabolism has been obtained with the glucose analogue ^{18}F-deoxyglucose (^{18}F-FDG). After intravenous injection, ^{18}F-FDG is transported across the capillary and sarcolemmal membranes by the same carrier as glucose and is then phosphorylated to ^{18}F-FDG-6-phospate by the enzyme hexokinase. For ^{18}F-FDG, this is a unidirectional pathway, and radioactivity accumulates in the myocardium in proportion to the overall rate of transsarcolemmal transport and phosphorylation of exogenous glucose [62]. The main indication for the assessment of myocardial metabolism in clinical cardiology is the evaluation of myocardial viability in ischemic heart failure [63]. An irreversible defect as documented by MPI does not distinguish myocardial scarring from viable hibernating myocardium, a condition characterized by resting hypoperfusion with preserved or even augmented glucose metabolism. Figure 4.16 shows the imaging patterns of resting MBF and glucose metabolism in a patient with (mismatch) and without myocardial viability (match) [13]. This distinction is of clinical relevance as patients with documented myocardial viability are eligible for coronary revascularization, which allows for recovery of cardiac function, whereas such a procedure is futile in patients with myocardial scarring. Although nowadays there are many alternatives for myocardial viability testing, the combination of cardiac perfusion/metabolism PET is still considered the gold standard [64].

4.3.7 Hybrid PET/CT and PET/MRI imaging

Driven by their success in clinical oncology, all currently produced PET systems are fused with CT hardware. As already discussed, low-dose CT based density mapping is now routinely used to correct for attenuation correction of the PET data. Next to attenuation correction, however, the CT hardware provides the possibility to additionally

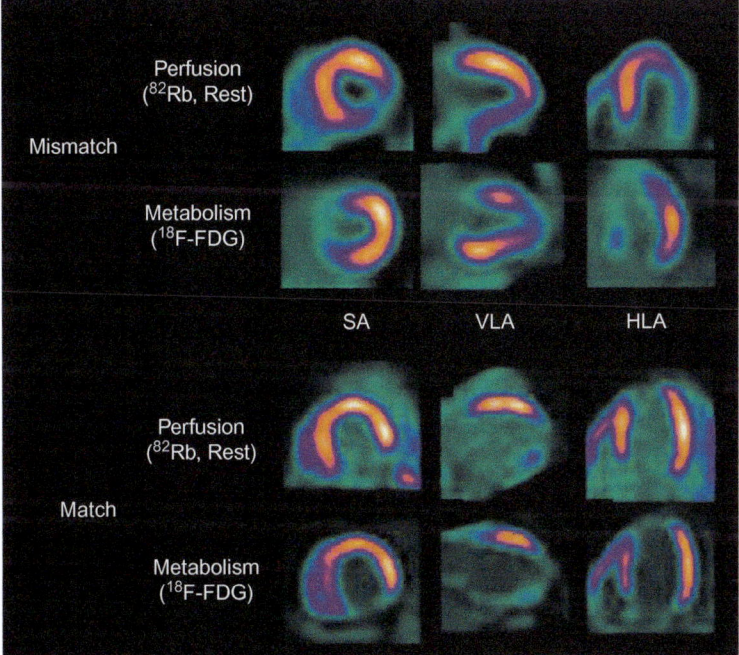

Figure 4.16 PET perfusion/metabolism imaging for assessment of myocardial viability. (Top) A mismatch with reduced rest perfusion (measured by ^{82}Rb) and preserved/increased metabolism (measured by ^{18}F-FDG) is shown in the inferolateral wall, indicating ischemically compromised but viable "hibernating" myocardium. (Bottom) A matched perfusion/metabolism defect is shown in the inferior wall, indicating nonviable scar. SA = short axis; VLA = vertical long axis; HLA = horizontal long axis.
Reprinted with permission from Bengel et al. [13].

study the coronary anatomy through calcium scoring and coronary CT angiography (CCTA) [65]. State-of-the-art PET/CT systems are currently equipped with up to 128-slices, and CCTA can be conducted at relatively low radiation burden utilizing modern scanning sequences (<3 mSv), such as prospective ECG-gating. This hybrid approach now enables the near simultaneous evaluation of coronary anatomy and function, and produces high-quality fusion images. Figure 4.17 displays such an image whereby the coronary tree is fused with a hyperemic perfusion map. Recent studies have demonstrated that this type of hybrid imaging has a higher diagnostic value than each imaging modality alone [19,20,23,67]. Particularly in case of an abnormal or equivocal CT scan, myocardial perfusion allows the evaluation of the hemodynamic consequences of the coronary lesion. As such, a more judicious referral pattern for invasive coronary angiography can be achieved [66].

Most recent attempts have been aimed at targeting not lesion severity, but vulnerability. Certain plaques are prone to rupture, provoking thrombosis and leading to unheralded events such as unstable angina and myocardial infarction. Anatomical plaque morphology can be obtained with CCTA, and vulnerable plaques are characterized by low attenuation positive remodeling, and spotty calcification [68]. Molecular imaging of such plaques with PET could further contribute to assess plaque inflammation. Initial studies to visualize coronary plaques with ^{18}F-FDG have shown this approach to be feasible [69]. Myocardial utilization of ^{18}F-FDG, however, results in poor target-to-background ratios, and the plaque signal often gets swamped by the myocardial signal, even with proper dietary preparations to minimize myocardial

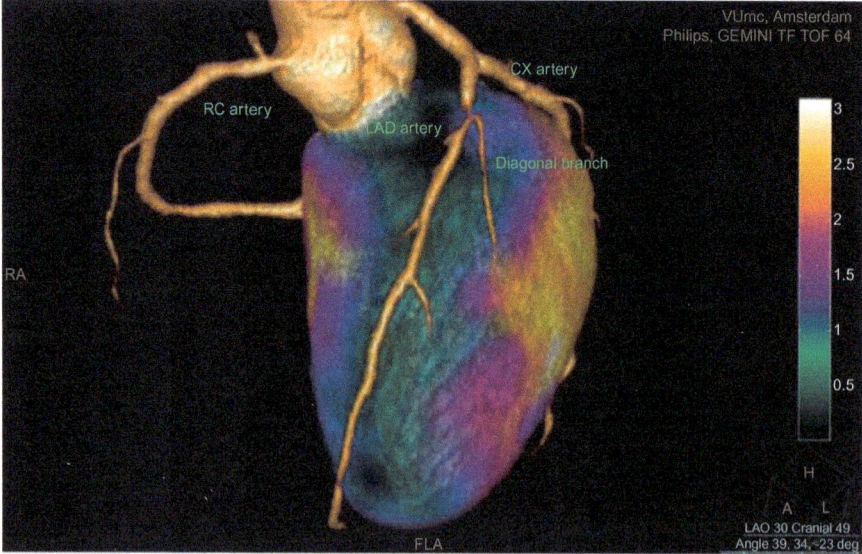

Figure 4.17 A 52-year-old male with atypical angina. Hybrid $H_2^{15}O$ PET/CTCA imaging reveals a severely reduced hyperaemic perfusion (1.25 mL min^{-1} g^{-1}) in the area supplied by the LAD artery.
Reprinted with permission from Danad et al. [66].

glucose utilization at the time of acquisition. More recently, hybrid PET/CCTA studies using ^{18}F-NaF have linked tracer uptake to active coronary calcification and plaque stability (Figure 4.18), although overlap between patients with stable CAD was still substantial [70,71]. Nonetheless, these studies illustrate that combining anatomical plaque features and vascular biology with hybrid PET/CCTA may have the potential to identify those patients at risk for acute coronary syndromes. Results from pilot trials that examine novel inflammatory plaque tracers that may visualize coronary macrophage activity (^{11}C-PK11195), matrix-metalloptroteinase (^{18}F-AS101), or integrins (^{18}F-galacto-RGD) are eagerly awaited [72,73].

Another hybrid imaging device that has been introduced is the PET/MRI system. The imaging capabilities of MRI are fundamentally different from CT; therefore, this hybrid approach offers new potential cardiac applications as compared with PET/CT. Cardiac MRI excels in imaging of myocardial function, structure, and myocardial tissue morphology, whereas coronary arteries are poorly visualized. Therefore, the strength of hybrid PET/CT lies in imaging the anatomy and function/biology of the coronary tree, whereas hybrid PET/MRI is more equipped in examining morphology and biology of the myocardium itself [74]. As opposed to PET/CT, the development of PET/MRI had to overcome some major obstacles. Conventional PET photomultiplier tubes to detect the annihilating photons are very sensitive to interference by a magnetic field. On the other hand, MRI image quality can be impaired by PET electronics–generated radiofrequency noise and magnetic field inhomogeneity. Advances in hardware, e.g., by implementation of magnetic-field–compatible solid-state PET light detectors, have enabled the commercial production of clinical PET/MRI systems [75]. Another practical limitation is the lack of accurate attenuation correction for the PET data, as MRI data cannot be used directly for attenuation correction because the MR signal is not related to the radiodensity of biologic tissue [76]. Segmentation models with standardized density values for different types of structures/organs (background, lungs, fat, bone, and soft tissue), however, have been shown to produce robust and reproducible attenuation correction for PET in such hybrid systems [77].

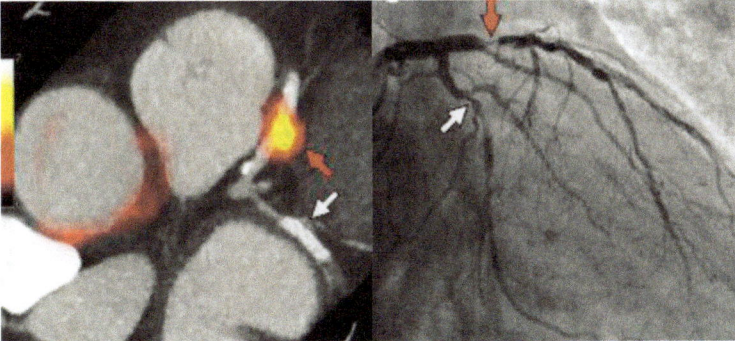

Figure 4.18 Active calcification of the LAD in a hybrid PET/CCTA image using ^{18}F-NaF. Note that the circumflex lesion is metabolically inactive.
Adapted from Joshi et al. [70].

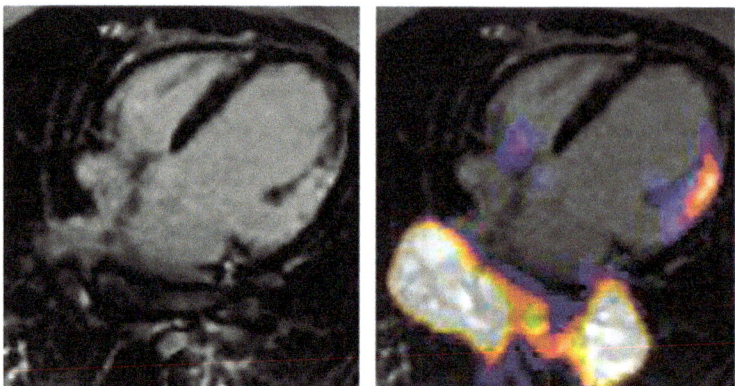

Figure 4.19 PET/MR images of patient with cardiac sarcoidosis. On four-chamber view, patchy late gadolinium enhancement can be observed in basal lateral wall (left). In this region, upregulated glucose metabolism (right) can be observed, indicating active inflammation. Also, increased ^{18}F-FDG uptake can be seen bilaterally in hilar lymph nodes.
Adapted from Rischpler et al. [74].

Although experience with PET/MRI for cardiac applications is still very limited, some indications appear to be promising. In chronic ischemic heart failure, combined viability testing with late gadolinium enhanced (LGE) MRI and ^{18}F-FDG PET could provide a more accurate assessment of the extent of morphological and metabolic viable myocardium [78]. Also, this approach may prove to be useful in the study of the inflammatory response of jeopardized myocardium after acute myocardial infarction, the extent of which appears to predict LV remodeling and may therefore guide therapy. Another potential application could be to examine patients with a reduced LV ejection fraction who are at risk for sudden cardiac death. Both myocardial scarring as documented with LGE MRI as well as myocardial innervation defects in residual viable myocardium as documented with ^{11}C-HED PET are associated with the occurrence of lethal ventricular arrhythmias in these patients. Future studies will evaluate whether a combined PET/MRI imaging strategy will be able to optimize selection criteria to guide implantable cardioverter device therapy [79]. Finally, infiltrative cardiomyopathy due, for example, to cardiac involvement of sarcoidosis could benefit from this hybrid approach (Figure 4.19). The diagnosis of cardiac sarcoidosis through noninvasive imaging is not trivial. LGE-MRI with a patchy distribution pattern is a nonspecific feature of cardiac sarcoidosis. On the other hand, ^{18}F-FDG PET imaging can reveal myocardial inflammation, although images can at times be difficult to interpret due to physiological myocardial uptake. The combination of ^{18}F-FDG PET with MRI could therefore act in a complementary way and provide a more comprehensive analysis of the disease process [74].

4.4 Conclusion

Over the past years, cardiac PET has evolved from solely a scientific research tool that enables the tracking of biochemical pathways *in vivo* in a quantitative manner, to a valuable clinical imaging modality that routinely quantifies myocardial perfusion and substrate metabolism in patients with ischemic heart disease. The fusion of PET with CT and MRI has further expedited the implementation of cardiac PET in clinical practice. These new hybrid imaging techniques allow both anatomical and biological information to be gathered within a single scanning session. Development and validation of novel tracers expand the field of molecular imaging, which may hold great potential for future clinical applications and contribute to personalization of cardiovascular medicine.

References

[1] Moses WW. Recent advances and future advances in Time-of-Flight PET. IEEE Trans Nucl Sci 2002;3:1670–5.
[2] Lubberink M, Boellaard R, van der Weerdt AP, Visser FC, Lammertsma AA. Quantitative comparison of analytic and iterative reconstruction methods in 2- and 3-dimensional dynamic cardiac 18F-FDG PET. J Nucl Med 2004;45(12):2008–15.
[3] Knaapen P, Lubberink M. Cardiac positron emission tomography: myocardial perfusion and metabolism in clinical practice. Clin Res Cardiol 2008;97(11):791–6. http://dx.doi.org/10.1007/s00392-008-0662-9.
[4] Rischpler C, Park M-J, Fung GSK, Javadi M, Tsui BMW, Higuchi T. Advances in PET myocardial perfusion imaging: F-18 labeled tracers. Ann Nucl Med 2012;26(1):1–6. http://dx.doi.org/10.1007/s12149-011-0552-5.
[5] Iida H, Kanno I, Takahashi A, et al. Measurement of absolute myocardial blood flow with $H_2^{15}O$ and dynamic positron-emission tomography. Strategy for quantification in relation to the partial-volume effect. Circulation 1988;78(1):104–15.
[6] Knaapen P, Camici PG, Marques KM, et al. Coronary microvascular resistance: methods for its quantification in humans. Basic Res Cardiol 2009;104(5):485–98. http://dx.doi.org/10.1007/s00395-009-0037-z.
[7] Schindler TH, Schelbert HR, Quercioli A, Dilsizian V. Cardiac PET imaging for the detection and monitoring of coronary artery disease and microvascular health. JACC Cardiovasc Imaging 2010;3(6):623–40. http://dx.doi.org/10.1016/j.jcmg.2010.04.007.
[8] Huang SC, Williams BA, Krivokapich J, Araujo L, Phelps ME, Schelbert HR. Rabbit myocardial 82Rb kinetics and a compartmental model for blood flow estimation. Am J Physiol 1989;256(4 Pt 2):H1156–64.
[9] Schelbert HR, Phelps ME, Huang SC, et al. N-13 ammonia as an indicator of myocardial blood flow. Circulation 1981;63(6):1259–72.
[10] Yalamanchili P, Wexler E, Hayes M, et al. Mechanism of uptake and retention of F-18 BMS-747158-02 in cardiomyocytes: a novel PET myocardial imaging agent. J Nucl Cardiol 2007;14(6):782–8. http://dx.doi.org/10.1016/j.nuclcard.2007.07.009.
[11] Yoshinaga K, Klein R, Tamaki N. Generator-produced rubidium-82 positron emission tomography myocardial perfusion imaging-from basic aspects to clinical applications. J Cardiol 2010;55(2):163–73. http://dx.doi.org/10.1016/j.jjcc.2010.01.001.
[12] Adachi I, Gaemperli O, Valenta I, et al. Assessment of myocardial perfusion by dynamic O-15-labeled water PET imaging: validation of a new fast factor analysis. J Nucl Cardiol 2007;14(5):698–705. http://dx.doi.org/10.1016/j.nuclcard.2007.05.012.
[13] Bengel FM, Higuchi T, Javadi MS, Lautamäki R. Cardiac positron emission tomography. J Am Coll Cardiol 2009;54(1):1–15. http://dx.doi.org/10.1016/j.jacc.2009.02.065.
[14] Di Carli MF, Hachamovitch R. New technology for noninvasive evaluation of coronary artery disease. Circulation 2007;115(11):1464–80. http://dx.doi.org/10.1161/CIRCULATIONAHA.106.629808.

[15] Hermansen F, Ashburner J, Spinks TJ, Kooner JS, Camici PG, Lammertsma AA. Generation of myocardial factor images directly from the dynamic oxygen-15-water scan without use of an oxygen-15-carbon monoxide blood-pool scan. J Nucl Med 1998;39(10):1696–702.
[16] Nesterov SV, Han C, Mäki M, et al. Myocardial perfusion quantitation with 15O-labelled water PET: high reproducibility of the new cardiac analysis software (Carimas). Eur J Nucl Med Mol Imaging 2009;36(10):1594–602. http://dx.doi.org/10.1007/s00259-009-1143-8.
[17] Harms HJ, Knaapen P, de Haan S, Halbmeijer R, Lammertsma AA, Lubberink M. Automatic generation of absolute myocardial blood flow images using [15O]H2O and a clinical PET/CT scanner. Eur J Nucl Med Mol Imaging 2011;38(5):930–9. http://dx.doi.org/10.1007/s00259-011-1730-3.
[18] Knaapen P, de Haan S, Hoekstra OS, et al. Cardiac PET-CT: advanced hybrid imaging for the detection of coronary artery disease. Neth Hear J 2010;18(2):90–8.
[19] Danad I, Raijmakers PG, Appelman YE, et al. Hybrid imaging using quantitative $H_2^{15}O$ PET and CT-based coronary angiography for the detection of coronary artery disease. J Nucl Med 2013;54(1):55–63. http://dx.doi.org/10.2967/jnumed.112.104687.
[20] Kajander S, Joutsiniemi E, Saraste M, et al. Cardiac positron emission tomography/computed tomography imaging accurately detects anatomically and functionally significant coronary artery disease. Circulation 2010;122(6):603–13. http://dx.doi.org/10.1161/CIRCULATIONAHA.109.915009.
[21] Maddahi J. Properties of an ideal PET perfusion tracer: new PET tracer cases and data. J Nucl Cardiol 2012;19(Suppl. 1(S1)):S30–7. http://dx.doi.org/10.1007/s12350-011-9491-8.
[22] Bergmann SR, Fox KA, Rand AL, et al. Quantification of regional myocardial blood flow in vivo with $H_2^{15}O$. Circulation 1984;70(4):724–33.
[23] Danad I, Raijmakers PG, Knaapen P. Diagnosing coronary artery disease with hybrid PET/CT: it takes two to tango. J Nucl Cardiol 2013;20(5):874–90. http://dx.doi.org/10.1007/s12350-013-9753-8.
[24] Saraste A, Kajander S, Han C, Nesterov SV, Knuuti J. PET: Is myocardial flow quantification a clinical reality? J Nucl Cardiol 2012;19(5):1044–59. http://dx.doi.org/10.1007/s12350-012-9588-8.
[25] Schmidt KC, Turkheimer FE. Kinetic modeling in positron emission tomography. Q J Nucl Med 2002;46(1):70–85.
[26] Lortie M, Beanlands RSB, Yoshinaga K, Klein R, Dasilva JN, DeKemp RA. Quantification of myocardial blood flow with 82Rb dynamic PET imaging. Eur J Nucl Med Mol Imaging 2007;34(11):1765–74. http://dx.doi.org/10.1007/s00259-007-0478-2.
[27] Nekolla SG, Reder S, Saraste A, et al. Evaluation of the novel myocardial perfusion positron-emission tomography tracer 18F-BMS-747158-02: comparison to 13N-ammonia and validation with microspheres in a pig model. Circulation 2009;119(17):2333–42. http://dx.doi.org/10.1161/CIRCULATIONAHA.108.797761.
[28] Hutchins GD, Schwaiger M, Rosenspire KC, Krivokapich J, Schelbert H, Kuhl DE. Noninvasive quantification of regional blood flow in the human heart using N-13 ammonia and dynamic positron emission tomographic imaging. J Am Coll Cardiol 1990;15(5):1032–42.
[29] Muzik O, Beanlands RS, Hutchins GD, Mangner TJ, Nguyen N, Schwaiger M. Validation of nitrogen-13-ammonia tracer kinetic model for quantification of myocardial blood flow using PET. J Nucl Med 1993;34(1):83–91.
[30] Bol A, Melin JA, Vanoverschelde JL, et al. Direct comparison of [13N]ammonia and [15O] water estimates of perfusion with quantification of regional myocardial blood flow by microspheres. Circulation 1993;87(2):512–25.
[31] Kaufmann PA, Gnecchi-Ruscone T, Yap JT, Rimoldi O, Camici PG. Assessment of the reproducibility of baseline and hyperemic myocardial blood flow measurements with 15O-labeled water and PET. J Nucl Med 1999;40(11):1848–56.

[32] Lautamäki R, George RT, Kitagawa K, et al. Rubidium-82 PET-CT for quantitative assessment of myocardial blood flow: validation in a canine model of coronary artery stenosis. Eur J Nucl Med Mol Imaging 2009;36(4):576–86. http://dx.doi.org/10.1007/s00259-008-0972-1.
[33] Harms HJ, Nesterov SV, Han C, et al. Comparison of clinical non-commercial tools for automated quantification of myocardial blood flow using oxygen-15-labelled water PET/CT. Eur Heart J Cardiovasc Imaging 2013; et177.
[34] Slomka PJ, Alexanderson E, Jácome R, et al. Comparison of clinical tools for measurements of regional stress and rest myocardial blood flow assessed with 13N-ammonia PET/CT. J Nucl Med 2012;53(2):171–81. http://dx.doi.org/10.2967/jnumed.111.095398.
[35] DeKemp RA, Declerck J, Klein R, et al. Multisoftware reproducibility study of stress and rest myocardial blood flow assessed with 3D dynamic PET/CT and a 1-tissue-compartment model of 82Rb kinetics. J Nucl Med 2013;54(4):571–7. http://dx.doi.org/10.2967/jnumed.112.112219.
[36] Hermansen F, Rosen SD, Fath-Ordoubadi F, et al. Measurement of myocardial blood flow with oxygen-15 labelled water: comparison of different administration protocols. Eur J Nucl Med 1998;25(7):751–9.
[37] Schindler TH, Zhang X-L, Prior JO, et al. Assessment of intra- and interobserver reproducibility of rest and cold pressor test-stimulated myocardial blood flow with (13)N-ammonia and PET. Eur J Nucl Med Mol Imaging 2007;34(8):1178–88. http://dx.doi.org/10.1007/s00259-007-0378-5.
[38] Souvatzoglou M, Bengel F, Busch R, et al. Attenuation correction in cardiac PET/CT with three different CT protocols: a comparison with conventional PET. Eur J Nucl Med Mol Imaging 2007;34(12):1991–2000. http://dx.doi.org/10.1007/s00259-007-0492-4.
[39] Rajaram M, Tahari AK, Lee AH, et al. Cardiac PET/CT misregistration causes significant changes in estimated myocardial blood flow. J Nucl Med 2013;54(1):50–4. http://dx.doi.org/10.2967/jnumed.112.108183.
[40] Martinez-Möller A, Souvatzoglou M, Navab N, Schwaiger M, Nekolla SG. Artifacts from misaligned CT in cardiac perfusion PET/CT studies: frequency, effects, and potential solutions. J Nucl Med 2007;48(2):188–93.
[41] Lubberink M, Harms HJ, Halbmeijer R, de Haan S, Knaapen P, Lammertsma AA. Low-dose quantitative myocardial blood flow imaging using 15O-water and PET without attenuation correction. J Nucl Med 2010;51(4):575–80. http://dx.doi.org/10.2967/jnumed.109.070748.
[42] Martinez-Möller A, Zikic D, Botnar RM, et al. Dual cardiac-respiratory gated PET: implementation and results from a feasibility study. Eur J Nucl Med Mol Imaging 2007;34(9):1447–54. http://dx.doi.org/10.1007/s00259-007-0374-9.
[43] Di Carli MF, Dorbala S, Meserve J, Fakhri El G, Sitek A, Moore SC. Clinical myocardial perfusion PET/CT. J Nucl Med 2007;48(5):783–93. http://dx.doi.org/10.2967/jnumed.106.032789.
[44] Slomka PJ, Nishina H, Berman DS, et al. "Motion-frozen" display and quantification of myocardial perfusion. J Nucl Med 2004;45(7):1128–34.
[45] Le Meunier L, Slomka PJ, Dey D, et al. Motion frozen (18)F-FDG cardiac PET. J Nucl Cardiol 2011;18(2):259–66. http://dx.doi.org/10.1007/s12350-010-9322-3.
[46] Berman DS, Germano G, Slomka PJ. Improvement in PET myocardial perfusion image quality and quantification with flurpiridaz F 18. J Nucl Cardiol 2012;19(Suppl 1(S1)):S38–45. http://dx.doi.org/10.1007/s12350-011-9487-4.
[47] Berman DS, Maddahi J, Tamarappoo BK, et al. Phase II safety and clinical comparison with single-photon emission computed tomography myocardial perfusion imaging for detection of coronary artery disease: flurpiridaz F 18 positron emission tomography. J Am Coll Cardiol 2013;61(4):469–77. http://dx.doi.org/10.1016/j.jacc.2012.11.022.

[48] Klocke FJ, Baird MG, Lorell BH, et al. ACC/AHA/ASNC guidelines for the clinical use of cardiac radionuclide imaging–executive summary: a report of the American College of Cardiology/American Heart Association Task Force on Practice Guidelines (ACC/AHA/ASNC Committee to Revise the 1995 Guidelines for the Clinical Use of Cardiac Radionuclide Imaging). Circulation 2003;108(11):1404–18. http://dx.doi.org/10.1161/01.CIR.0000080946.42225.4D.

[49] Anagnostopoulos C, Georgakopoulos A, Pianou N, Nekolla SG. Assessment of myocardial perfusion and viability by positron emission tomography. Int J Cardiol 2013;167(5):1737–49. http://dx.doi.org/10.1016/j.ijcard.2012.12.009.

[50] Danad I, Raijmakers PG, Appelman YE, et al. Coronary risk factors and myocardial blood flow in patients evaluated for coronary artery disease: a quantitative [15O]H2O PET/CT study. Eur J Nucl Med Mol Imaging 2012;39(1):102–12. http://dx.doi.org/10.1007/s00259-011-1956-0.

[51] Chareonthaitawee P, Kaufmann PA, Rimoldi O, Camici PG. Heterogeneity of resting and hyperemic myocardial blood flow in healthy humans. Cardiovasc Res 2001;50(1):151–61.

[52] Gould KL, Johnson NP, Bateman TM, et al. Anatomic versus physiologic assessment of coronary artery disease. Role of coronary flow reserve, fractional flow reserve, and positron emission tomography imaging in revascularization decision-making. J Am Coll Cardiol 2013;62(18):1639–53. http://dx.doi.org/10.1016/j.jacc.2013.07.076.

[53] Opie LH. Cardiac metabolism–emergence, decline, and resurgence. Part I. Cardiovasc Res 1992;26(8):721–33.

[54] Opie LH. Cardiac metabolism–emergence, decline, and resurgence. Part II. Cardiovasc Res 1992;26(9):817–30.

[55] de Jong HWAM, Rijzewijk LJ, Lubberink M, et al. Kinetic models for analysing myocardial [(11)C]palmitate data. Eur J Nucl Med Mol Imaging 2009;36(6):966–78. http://dx.doi.org/10.1007/s00259-008-1035-3.

[56] Ratib O, Phelps ME, Huang SC, Henze E, Selin CE, Schelbert HR. Positron tomography with deoxyglucose for estimating local myocardial glucose metabolism. J Nucl Med 1982;23(7):577–86.

[57] Rijzewijk LJ, van der Meer RW, Lamb HJ, et al. Altered myocardial substrate metabolism and decreased diastolic function in nonischemic human diabetic cardiomyopathy: studies with cardiac positron emission tomography and magnetic resonance imaging. J Am Coll Cardiol 2009;54(16):1524–32. http://dx.doi.org/10.1016/j.jacc.2009.04.074.

[58] Tuunanen H, Engblom E, Naum A, et al. Decreased myocardial free fatty acid uptake in patients with idiopathic dilated cardiomyopathy: evidence of relationship with insulin resistance and left ventricular dysfunction. J Card Fail 2006;12(8):644–52. http://dx.doi.org/10.1016/j.cardfail.2006.06.005.

[59] Tuunanen H, Engblom E, Naum A, et al. Free fatty acid depletion acutely decreases cardiac work and efficiency in cardiomyopathic heart failure. Circulation 2006;114(20):2130–7. http://dx.doi.org/10.1161/CIRCULATIONAHA.106.645184.

[60] Tuunanen H, Engblom E, Naum A, et al. Trimetazidine, a metabolic modulator, has cardiac and extracardiac benefits in idiopathic dilated cardiomyopathy. Circulation 2008;118(12):1250–8. http://dx.doi.org/10.1161/CIRCULATIONAHA.108.778019.

[61] van der Meer RW, Rijzewijk LJ, de Jong HWAM, et al. Pioglitazone improves cardiac function and alters myocardial substrate metabolism without affecting cardiac triglyceride accumulation and high-energy phosphate metabolism in patients with well-controlled type 2 diabetes mellitus. Circulation 2009;119(15):2069–77. http://dx.doi.org/10.1161/CIRCULATIONAHA.108.803916.

[62] Camici PG. Positron emission tomography and myocardial imaging. Heart 2000;83(4):475–80.

[63] Tillisch J, Brunken R, Marshall R, et al. Reversibility of cardiac wall-motion abnormalities predicted by positron tomography. N Engl J Med 1986;314(14):884–8. http://dx.doi.org/10.1056/NEJM198604033141405.
[64] Schinkel AFL, Bax JJ, Poldermans D, Elhendy A, Ferrari R, Rahimtoola SH. Hibernating myocardium: diagnosis and patient outcomes. Curr Probl Cardiol 2007;32(7):375–410. http://dx.doi.org/10.1016/j.cpcardiol.2007.04.001.
[65] Schroeder S, Achenbach S, Bengel F, et al. Cardiac computed tomography: indications, applications, limitations, and training requirements: report of a Writing Group deployed by the Working Group Nuclear Cardiology and Cardiac CT of the European Society of Cardiology and the European Council of Nuclear Cardiology. Eur Heart J 2008;29(4):531–56. http://dx.doi.org/10.1093/eurheartj/ehm544.
[66] Danad I, Raijmakers PG, Harms HJ, et al. Effect of cardiac hybrid 15O-water PET/CT imaging on downstream referral for invasive coronary angiography and revascularization rate. Eur Heart J Cardiovasc Imaging 2014;15(2):170–9. http://dx.doi.org/10.1093/ehjci/jet125.
[67] Gaemperli O, Bengel FM, Kaufmann PA. Cardiac hybrid imaging. Eur Heart J 2011;32(17):2100–8. http://dx.doi.org/10.1093/eurheartj/ehr057.
[68] Camici PG, Rimoldi OE, Gaemperli O, Libby P. Non-invasive anatomic and functional imaging of vascular inflammation and unstable plaque. Eur Heart J 2012;33(11):1309–17. http://dx.doi.org/10.1093/eurheartj/ehs067.
[69] Teräs M, Kokki T, Durand-Schaefer N, et al. Dual-gated cardiac PET-clinical feasibility study. Eur J Nucl Med Mol Imaging 2010;37(3):505–16. http://dx.doi.org/10.1007/s00259-009-1252-4.
[70] Joshi NV, Vesey AT, Williams MC, et al. (18)F-fluoride positron emission tomography for identification of ruptured and high-risk coronary atherosclerotic plaques: a prospective clinical trial. Lancet 2013;http://dx.doi.org/10.1016/S0140-6736(13)61754-7.
[71] Dweck MR, Chow MWL, Joshi NV, et al. Coronary arterial 18F-sodium fluoride uptake: a novel marker of plaque biology. J Am Coll Cardiol 2012;59(17):1539–48. http://dx.doi.org/10.1016/j.jacc.2011.12.037.
[72] Davies JR, Rudd JHF, Weissberg PL, Narula J. Radionuclide imaging for the detection of inflammation in vulnerable plaques. J Am Coll Cardiol 2006;47(8 Suppl.):C57–68. http://dx.doi.org/10.1016/j.jacc.2005.11.049.
[73] Bengel FM. Atherosclerosis imaging on the molecular level. J Nucl Cardiol 2006;13(1):111–8. http://dx.doi.org/10.1016/j.nuclcard.2005.11.003.
[74] Rischpler C, Nekolla SG, Dregely I, Schwaiger M. Hybrid PET/MR imaging of the heart: potential, initial experiences, and future prospects. J Nucl Med 2013;54(3):402–15. http://dx.doi.org/10.2967/jnumed.112.105353.
[75] Pichler BJ, Wehrl HF, Judenhofer MS. Latest advances in molecular imaging instrumentation. J Nucl Med 2008;49(Suppl 2(Suppl.2)):5S–23S. http://dx.doi.org/10.2967/jnumed.108.045880.
[76] Pichler BJ, Judenhofer MS, Wehrl HF. PET/MRI hybrid imaging: devices and initial results. Eur Radiol 2008;18(6):1077–86. http://dx.doi.org/10.1007/s00330-008-0857-5.
[77] Wagenknecht G, Kaiser H-J, Mottaghy FM, Herzog H. MRI for attenuation correction in PET: methods and challenges. MAGMA 2013;26(1):99–113. http://dx.doi.org/10.1007/s10334-012-0353-4.
[78] Adenaw N, Salerno M. PET/MRI: current state of the art and future potential for cardiovascular applications. J Nucl Cardiol 2013;20(6):976–89. http://dx.doi.org/10.1007/s12350-013-9780-5.
[79] de Haan S, Knaapen P, Beek AM, et al. Risk stratification for ventricular arrhythmias in ischaemic cardiomyopathy: the value of non-invasive imaging. Europace 2010;12(4):468–74. http://dx.doi.org/10.1093/europace/euq064.

Computed tomography

K. Nieman, A. Coenen, M. Dijkshoorn
Erasmus MC, Rotterdam, The Netherlands

5.1 Development of cardiac CT

In 1972, the first CT scanner was designed by the engineer Geoffrey N. Hounsfield at an English company named EMI Ltd. Together with Allan C. Cormack, a physicist from Cape Town who developed the mathematical foundation for the reconstruction of cross-sectional images from transmission measurements, Hounsfield was honored with the Nobel Prize for Physiology or Medicine in 1979. The first CT scanners, at this time known as a computerized axial tomography (CAT) scanner, were limited to cranial imaging, until whole-body scanners were released in 1975. The rotation speed of these first mechanical CT scanners was insufficient to image moving organs. Therefore, in the late 1970s, a very fast CT system without rotating parts was developed, dedicated to imaging the heart. The electron-beam CT scanner (cine CT; ultrafast CT) has a static anode and detector rings on opposite sides of the gantry. By electromagnetically directing an electron beam along the tungsten anode ring, images can be acquired in a very short time (50 ms or less). EBCT has been used for different cardiovascular applications, including calcium imaging, CT coronary angiography, and myocardial perfusion imaging. Because of high operating costs and technical obstacles for further (multislice) development, the EBCT technology has largely disappeared from clinical use. Introduced in the early 1990s spiral CT permitted fast coverage of large body sections, which was particularly useful for angiographic CT applications. Spiral CT requires continuous tube-detector rotation, which could only be accomplished by removing the physical connections (wires) between the stationary and rotating scanner elements. As for all CT scanners today, the cables have been replaced by slip-ring and wireless technology that allows for energy and data exchange via nonfixed connections. Since the end of the 1990s, CT scanners have been equipped with an ever-increasing number of detector rows. The combination of spiral imaging, faster rotation speeds, more efficient reconstruction algorithms (half-scan algorithms), and multiple detectors allowed for detailed imaging of the moving heart and coronary arteries in the early 2000s (Figure 5.1).

5.2 Technical principles and contemporary technology

5.2.1 Computed tomography

5.2.1.1 Roentgen generation

The goal of computed tomography is to differentiate tissues and structures within the human body in a cross-sectional manner. What CT measures is the degree by which material affects roentgen radiation as it passes through. Conventional X-ray images

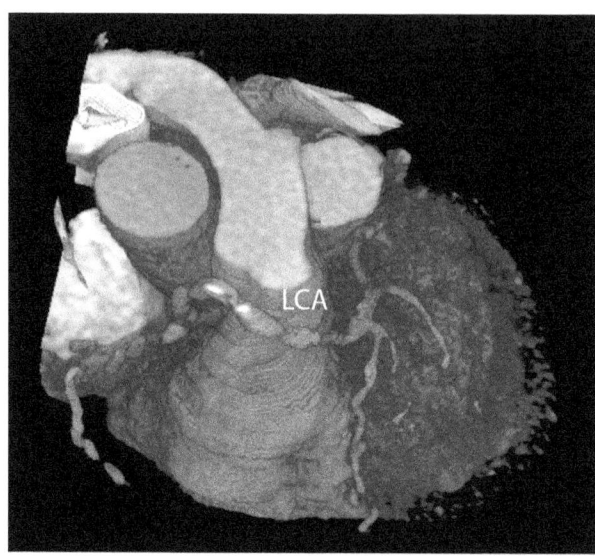

Figure 5.1 Four-slice cardiac CT. Four-slice CT coronary angiography of a patient with an aberrant left coronary artery originating from the right coronary sinus and coursing around the right ventricular outflow tract.

are projection images that display the cumulative roentgen attenuation of an entire object. Computed tomography is a technique that acquires a large number of projection images from different rotational angles and uses the cumulative attenuation profiles to calculate the spatial distribution of the roentgen attenuation throughout the interrogated cross-sectional plane. In cardiac imaging, where temporal resolution is essential, projections acquired during half of a full system rotation are sufficient for image reconstruction.

The core components of a CT system are the X-ray tube and the roentgen detectors, which are positioned at opposing sides of the scanner gantry. The high-power roentgen generator produces X-rays with a variable energy level; the maximum kV level is selectable, generally between 70 and 150 kV. The tube potential (kV) relates to the energy level of the photons, where X-ray with a higher kV are more penetrating than the weaker low kV photons. The X-ray beam is not a monochromatic source at a single kV level, but will include a spectrum of energy levels. The lowest energy levels, which do not contribute to the image generation, are filtered out before they enter the gantry. The number of photons per time unit (flux) is expressed in milli-Ampere. The point where electrons from the cathode collide with the anode to generate roentgen photons is called the focal spot. A small focal spot improves spatial resolution, but creates more heat at a constant flux. The anode rotates to better disperse the heat. Repetitive alternation of the focal spot (or more accurately focal ring) by electromagnetically changing the direction of the electrons allows for double-image sampling. Acquisition of slightly overlapping images using the "flying focal spot" improves the image quality in the longitudinal direction. Collimators are used to shape the X-ray beam to fit the detectors on the opposite side of the gantry.

5.2.1.2 Roentgen detection

The purpose of the detectors on the opposite side is to detect and quantify photons, augment the signal, and convert it to digital form. The requirements for the detectors are high. They need to be small, with minimal dead space separating them in the interest of spatial resolution; the reaction to exposure needs to be fast and proportional; and after exposure the detectors need to return to standby immediately to receive the following exposure. Sensitivity needs to be high, and (electronic) noise as low as possible. In order to accommodate faster scanning and multidetector row configuration, detectors with xenon ionization chambers have been replaced by solid-state scintillating ceramic detectors, which have shorter decay times. The ceramics convert the X-ray photons into light, which is then detected and converted to a proportional electrical signal. These electric signals are then collected for further processing and image reconstruction (Figure 5.2). New integrated and miniaturized electronics designs can reduce electronic noise.

Originally, CT scanners were equipped with a single row of detectors, exposed by a narrow fan-shaped X-ray beam. The number of parallel rows of detectors has increased dramatically over the past 15 years. Contemporary scanners have between 64 and 320 rows of detectors, each measuring 0.5–0.625 mm in width, as measured in the center of rotation. Per rotation, current scanners can cover a longitudinal distance between 38 and 160 mm. The number and width of the detector system is referred to as the detector collimation, for instance $128 \times 0.625 \, mm = 80 \, mm$.

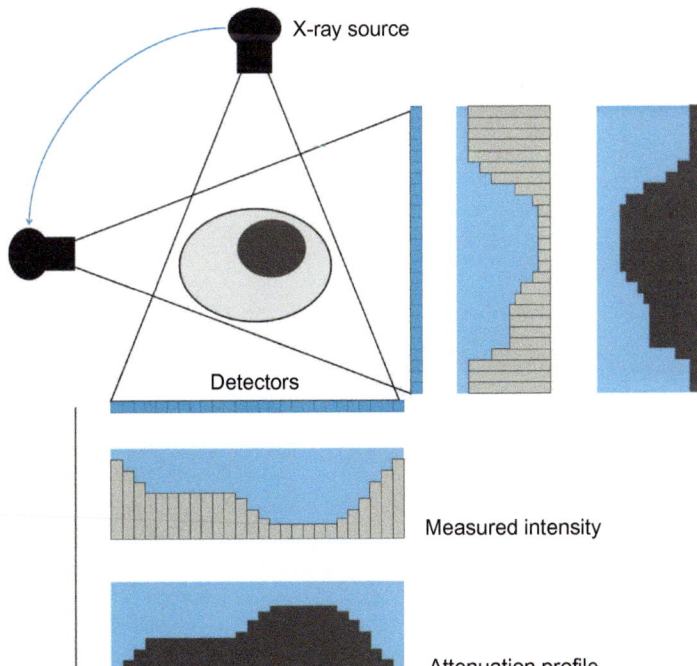

Figure 5.2 Attenuation profiles.

5.2.1.3 Dual-source CT

Dual-source CT systems are equipped with a double tube-detector system. The two systems are mounted on the scanner by a rotational offset of 90–95°. The main purpose of the system is to improve temporal resolution, which is the time needed to acquire data for a single image. Instead of needing a half rotation to acquire the images, all required projections can be gathered using in a 90° rotation using the dual-source system. Additional applications are double-output imaging in very obese patients, ultra-fast z-axis coverage scan modes to avoid motion in uncooperative (pediatric) patients, and improved tissue differentiation by imaging at nonidentical tube voltages (dual-energy CT).

5.2.1.4 Scan modes

CT scanners can operate in different acquisition modes, which become evident from the movement of the table (Figure 5.3). Of the available scan modes in use today, the axial mode has been in operation from the beginning. In this mode, one set of axial

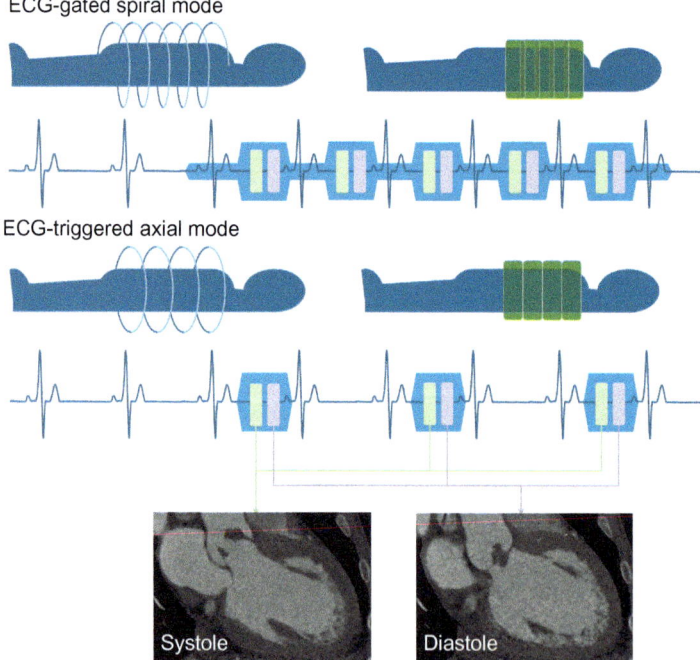

Figure 5.3 Scan modes. The spiral scan mode (helical mode) continuously exposes the patient, and images are reconstructed afterward using the recorded ECG (ECG-gated image reconstruction). The exposure can be reduced by applying ECG-triggered tube modulation ("pulsing"). Nominal exposure is only applied during a selected phase, while the tube power is lowered during the remainder of the heart cycle. The ECG-triggered axial scan mode ("step-and-shoot" or "prospective mode") acquires images with the table in a stationary position during the desired phase. To have the availability of multiple phases for reconstruction, the exposure time can be extended ("padding").

images is acquired while the table remains stationary. After each acquisition, the table moves to the next consecutive position. In cardiac CT, this is also referred to as the sequential, step-and-shoot, or prospective mode. After the physical connections (cables) between the rotating and stationary parts of the scanner had been removed, continuous rotation of the tube-detector system combined with uninterrupted table propagation became possible. This scan mode, referred to as spiral or helical scanning, allows much faster longitudinal coverage, which was essential to the development of CT angiography. Because projections are acquired at slightly incremental table positions, a form of longitudinal interpolation is necessary before axial images can be reconstructed. If the width of the detectors rows completely cover the organ of interest, such as is the case with 320-row imaging of the heart, no table movement is required anymore. If the same section is imaged repetitively, structural motion or dynamic contrast enhancement may be visualized. Serial imaging may be accomplished by repeating a complete volumetric scan, repeating acquisitions at the same table location, or a combination of the two (shuttle mode).

5.2.2 ECG-synchronized CT of the heart

The most important aspect of cardiac imaging, which separates it from most other applications, is the need for ECG synchronization. This includes two aspects. First, if all images cannot be acquired by a single acquisition during a single heart cycle, then each partition of the total scan needs to be acquired during the exact same phase of contraction over several heart cycles. Imaging with neglect of cardiac phases will cause blurring, nonalignment, or even loss of entire structures. Secondly, the temporal resolution of cardiac CT is limited. This means that the heart cannot be imaged well without blurring during phases of rapid displacement. The preferential phases to image the heart are during mid-diastole, just before atrial contraction, or at the end of systole. To create images during the same phase of relative cardiac immobility, either the data acquisition or the image reconstruction needs to be synchronized to the rhythm of the heart. Several cardiac scan modes, with modifications, can accomplish this: the ECG-gated conventional-pitch spiral mode, the ECG-triggered axial mode, the ECG-triggered stationary mode, and the ECG-triggered high-pitch spiral mode.

5.2.2.1 ECG-gated spiral CT

While not the earliest cardiac scan mode, it was the ECG-gated spiral CT that propelled the development of noninvasive CT coronary angiography. The principle of the ECG-gated spiral mode is the acquisition of a continuous, spatially overlapping spiral CT scan, with a simultaneous recording of an ECG trace (Table 5.1). Using the ECG trace, CT data acquired during the same phase of contraction is gathered to reconstruct a complete data set. The advantage of ECG-gated spiral CT is that the technique is very robust and flexible. Images can be reconstructed during any cardiac phase, allowing selection of the optimal dataset with the fewest motion artifacts. The moment of reconstruction (reconstruction window) can be placed anywhere within the heart cycle. It can be positioned at an absolute time interval after the previous R-wave

Table 5.1 **Spiral and axial scan modes**

	ECG-gated spiral CT	ECG-triggered axial CT
Synonyms	Helical mode Spiral mode	Prospective mode Sequential mode Step-and-shoot mode
ECG synchronization	Retrospectively, from recorded ECG trace	Prospectively, from online ECG signal
Table motion	Continuous	Interrupted
Exposure	Continuous	Interrupted
Scan duration	Predictable, based on selected table speed (based on expected heart rate)	Less predictable, depending on actual heart rate and rhythm regularity
Modifications	Prospectively ECG-triggered tube current modulation (*pulsing*) to reduce tube output during low-priority phases	Prolonged exposure to increase available cardiac phases (*padding*)
Advantages	Robust, arrhythmia resistant	Lower radiation exposure

or before the next R-wave. Alternatively, it can be placed at a relative position, for instance at 70% of the R-to-R interval. After the scan has been performed, the ECG synchronization may be manually corrected, for each individual beat, if necessary. Spiral CT acquisition allows for overlapping image reconstruction at smaller increments to improve perceived longitudinal image quality. The major drawback of ECG-gated spiral CT is the high radiation exposure caused by oversampling. The pitch is a term used in spiral CT to quantify the scan speed and is defined as the distance the table moves per tube-detector rotation. For nongated spiral CT scans, the table could advance by as much as twice the detector collimation width per rotation. In that case, the pitch is 2 (without unit). This is different for cardiac CT. To be able to reconstruct every cardiac phase, each table position needs to be sampled during an entire heart cycle. To anticipate changes in heart rate, the exposure per table position is generally more than a single heart cycle. Depending on the heart rate, the pitch varies from 0.15 to 0.5 for ECG-gated spiral CT. The amount of radiation used per longitudinal distance is relatively high for the conventional ECG-gated spiral CT. One can calculate that when the temporal resolution of a 4-slice scanner is 250 ms (at a rotations time of 500 ms), and each position is scanned for 1.5 heart cycles at a heart of 60/min, then the ratio of minimal needed exposure is 1/6th of the actual exposure. Modifications of the ECG-gated spiral mode have been designed to reduce the overall exposure. Using the prospective ECG-triggered tube current modulation, it is possible to reduce the tube output to 4–20% of the nominal output during the phases that are less likely to be needed for evaluation. The ECG-triggered tube output modulation, also known as ECG pulsing, can significantly reduce the overall exposure. While these algorithms are more vulnerable to arrhythmia than conventional ECG-gated spiral algorithms, advantages in terms of ECG editing are still retained. However, in patients with a stable heart rate, axial scan protocols have largely replaced spiral protocols as the default scan mode.

5.2.2.2 ECG-triggered axial CT

The axial scan mode implies that images are acquired with a stationary table position. Timing of the scan within the heart cycle is planned in advance, and the online ECG trace is used to trigger the image acquisition. Based on the previous heart cycles, the scanner estimates when the desired cardiac phase will take place. After the acquisition of a single set of images, the table will move to the next consecutive position and wait for a trigger. The advantage of the axial mode (also known as sequential, prospectively triggered, or step-and-shoot mode) is that exposure only occurs during the phase that is intended for reconstruction, thereby minimizing the overall radiation dose. The drawback of a prospectively triggered acquisition is that it relies on the regularity of the heart rhythm and that no alternative cardiac phases can be reconstructed in case of suboptimal image quality. Because advancement of the table takes time, acquisition generally occurs every second heartbeat, or every third heartbeat in case of a fast heart rate. Using earlier generations multislice CT with slower rotation speeds, this acquisition mode was considered unacceptably vulnerable to arrhythmia. Then, interpretation often required comparison of datasets reconstructed during different phases of contraction. Contemporary faster scanners, aided by betablockers, have made image quality more reliable. In addition, the ECG-triggering algorithms have become smarter. In case of a premature beat, the acquisition at a given location can be stopped and repeated once regularity is restored. In addition, the duration of exposure at each location can be extended beyond the minimum required for a single-phase reconstruction, sometimes called "padding", to allow for reconstruction of several cardiac phases while still avoiding exposure during other phases.

5.2.2.3 ECG-triggered stationary mode

If the number of detector rows allows for complete coverage of the organ of interest, then no table movement is necessary. Some of the recently released scanners have a detector collimation of 16 cm, which covers the entire heart. Without the need for table movement, images can be acquired in a single heart cycle, or exposure at the same location can be extended to several heart cycles to improve temporal resolution (discussed elsewhere), using ECG-triggering to image the desired cardiac phase.

5.2.2.4 ECG-triggered high-pitch mode

Second- and third-generation dual-source CT scanners have the option of an ECG-triggered high-pitch spiral scan protocol. Operating at a high table speed, the entire heart can be covered during a single cardiac cycle. Although the entire acquisition takes 150–250 ms, individual images are acquired with a temporal resolution of 66–75 ms. The advantage of the ECG-triggered high-pitch protocol (also referred to as Flash®) is that the entire heart is acquired during a single cycle, although there is a small phase shift from the first to the last image, at a very low exposure. The drawback is that only a single cardiac phase is available, and that the prolonged exposure within the heart cycle requires a low and regular heart rate.

5.2.3 Image reconstruction

While the concepts of computed tomography were developed a long time ago, the rate of development was largely driven by progress in computer technology. The quantity of information created by a CT scanner is immense, and reconstruction of images out of the attenuation profiles requires substantial processing power. The objective of image reconstruction is to display the distribution of a specific tissue characteristic throughout a cross-section or volume. In case of CT, this property is the tissue-specific roentgen attenuation coefficient (μ). To calculate this, we have at our disposal a large number of attenuation profiles obtained from a series of rotational angles, which are summations of the attenuation of X-ray through an object consisting of tissues with varying attenuation coefficients. The challenge of CT imaging is to estimate the attenuation distribution based on these samples. From the calculated, spatially distributed attenuation values, a so-called CT number is calculated. The CT number, expressed in Hounsfield units (HU), represents the relative attenuation compared to water and is calculated as:

$$\text{CT Number}(\text{HU}) : \left[(\mu_{\text{tissue}} - \mu_{\text{water}}) / \mu_{\text{water}} \right] * 1000 \tag{5.1}$$

By default, the CT number of water is 0 HU. Air has a CT number close to -1000 HU, while metal ranges up to 3000 HU. While a detailed mathematical discussion of CT image reconstruction techniques is beyond the scope of this chapter, general principles and characteristics will be discussed for two reconstruction techniques in practice today.

5.2.3.1 Filtered back-projection

Filtered back-projection (FBP) is an analytical reconstruction technique that dominated the field during the past decades. Images are created by back-projecting individual attenuation measurement for each point in space. Over time, these algorithms have been adapted from relatively simple 2D axial fan beam projections to multislice, spiral, and eventually cone-beam reconstruction algorithms. The advantage of FBP is their computational efficiency, which is accomplished by several simplifications with regard to the acquisition geometry.

5.2.3.2 Iterative reconstruction

Over the past few years, iterative reconstruction techniques were reintroduced—Hounsfield used iterative reconstruction in the first CT scanners—to improve image quality (Figure 5.4). These more calculation-intensive algorithms are still in a phase of development, and new improved algorithms are introduced on a regular basis [1]. Instead of a single reconstruction by analytical reconstruction algorithms, iterative reconstruction requires a repetitive sequence of reconstructions to arrive at a more accurate image, ideally taking into account the X-ray behavior and scanner geometry. Various iterative reconstruction techniques, of which the complexity has only partially been disclosed, have been introduced by different vendors. The basic principle is that

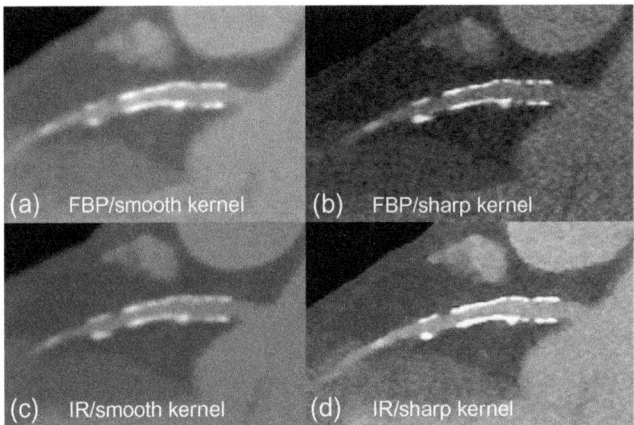

Figure 5.4 Filtered back-projection, iterative reconstruction, and selective kernels. Four examples of the same CT scan of a patient with a stent in the left main coronary artery reconstructed with filtered back-projection (FBP) or an iterative reconstruction algorithm (IR), and a smooth kernel or a sharp convolution kernel.

the measured raw data is compared to artificial raw data from a forward projection of a volumetric object estimate (which can be a regular FBP reconstruction). The correction term determined from this comparison serves to improve the reconstruction of the scanned data, after which the process is repeated several times. Statistical methods for iterative reconstruction incorporate the photon counting statistics into the reconstruction process, mainly to reduce noise, which can be applied in the raw data domain (preprocessing), the image domain (postprocessing), or during the iterative reconstruction process.

The principle of model-based iterative reconstruction techniques is that they take into account and try to model the data acquisition process. Correction models include the system optics and geometry, SNR-dependent prioritization of scan data, and spatially optimized noise regularization with edge preservation. Using these models, the synthesized images are compared to the projection data and modified accordingly in several steps. The result of these iterative reconstruction processes is improved image quality, in terms of spatial resolution and reduction of noise and reconstruction artifacts. The process is more computationally demanding, and requires more computer power and time to obtain the images. Apart from improved image quality, iterative reconstruction techniques have further propelled the potential for low-dose cardiac CT imaging.

5.2.3.3 Selectable reconstruction algorithms

Computational reconstruction algorithms, also known as kernels, can modify image impression. The operator can adjust the smoothness or sharpness of the images according to his diagnostic needs in trade-off with more or less noise. In general, smooth kernels are selected to depict subtle contrast differences between larger structures (myocardial perfusion defects), while sharper kernels are preferred to for detailed structural inspection and to reduce blooming from high-density structures (coronary stents).

5.2.4 Multienergy imaging

Absorption of roentgen by matter is the result of photoelectric absorption and Compton scattering. The proportion of each depends on the type of material (atomic number and electron density) and the energy of the roentgen. The degree by which attenuation changes within a tissue at different energy levels reflects differences in the atomic number. By resolving energy-dependent changes in attenuation, improved tissue characterization can be achieved. CT vendors have taken different approaches toward the development of multienergy, or spectral CT. Using a dual-source CT system, the two roentgen tubes can each be operated at a different tube voltage. Using a single-source CT system, rapid switching of the tube current can be performed to acquire dual-energy datasets. Alternatively, switching between high and low kV can take place for subsequent rotations. Finally, separation of different energy levels can be achieved using multilayered detectors. None of these approaches is ideal, and each has specific drawbacks [2]. Radiation exposure of a dual-energy scan is generally higher compared to a single-low energy scan.

The most promising spectral imaging application in cardiac CT is in myocardial perfusion and infarct imaging. Selective visualization of iodine (iodine mapping) could benefit differentiation and perhaps quantification of myocardial perfusion. Also for delayed-enhancement imaging, selective iodine mapping and suppression of the myocardial attenuation could improve differentiation of infracted myocardium.

5.3 CT performance, image quality parameters, and artifacts

The quality of a CT scan depends on many parameters (Table 5.2). Some of these are dependent on given limitations of roentgen physics, scanner design, and reconstruction algorithms. Others can be modified by the team performing the examination, such as heart rate, reconstruction parameters, postprocessing, and display. Taking a practical approach, the most relevant image quality parameters are discussed below. Image quality includes spatial resolution, temporal resolution, contrast resolution, and noise, although they are interdependent. The ability to differentiate small structures is affected by contrast gradients and motion blurring. Unfortunately, optimization in image quality in terms of scanner design and scan protocols are limited by increases in radiation use. In the spirit of the ALARA principle (as low as reasonably achievable), the image quality should be sufficient to make a confident diagnosis, without unnecessarily increasing radiation exposure to the patient.

5.3.1 Temporal resolution and heart rhythm

When imaging a (continuously) moving object, temporal resolution is crucial. In fundamental terms, temporal resolution is the time needed to acquire an image. In practical terms, the occurrence of motion blurring depends on the speed of the camera as well as the motion intensity of the object (Figure 5.5).

Table 5.2 **Image quality parameters**

	Temporal resolution and ECG synchronization	Spatial resolution	Tissue contrast and image noise
Scanner hardware	Rotation speed Number of roentgen tube-detector systems	Focal spot size Tube-detector distance Detector size[a]/characteristics Profiles per rotation	Detector design Detector size
Scan protocol	Exposure timing Exposure duration per cycle[a]	Tube current (mA)[a] Pitch[a] (spiral) Rotation speed	Tube current (mA)[a] Tube voltage (kV) X-ray filtering
Contrast protocol			Contrast medium (iodine concentration) Injection protocol
Image reconstruction	Multicycle reconstruction[a] ECG editing	Reconstruction algorithm Slice thickness Field of view size Slice increment Reconstruction matrix Filtering kernels	Reconstruction algorithm Slice thickness Field of view size Increment Filtering kernels
Post-processing and display		Magnification Slice/slab thickness Axial versus oblique cross-sections	Maximum intensity projections Window display settings
Patient characteristics	Heart rate and modulation Arrhythmia		Body size

[a]Optimization likely to increase radiation exposure directly or indirectly.

As discussed previously, a CT scanner requires a minimum of 180° of projections to reconstruct an image. Contemporary scanners have rotation times between 250 and 350 ms. Compared to the exponential steps made in the number of detector rows and image computation speed, a merely twofold improvement of tube-detector rotation speed over the past decade may seem only modest. However, the centrifugal forces created by the massive tube-detector system increase exponentially with each acceleration and therefore physically limit further acceleration. Using a conventional half-scan reconstruction algorithm, the temporal resolution of contemporary scanners ranges between 125 and 175 ms. All structural displacement taking place during this interval negatively affects image quality.

Despite the admirable engineering accomplishment of the currently available rotation speed, this is still insufficient to image the heart free of motion throughout the

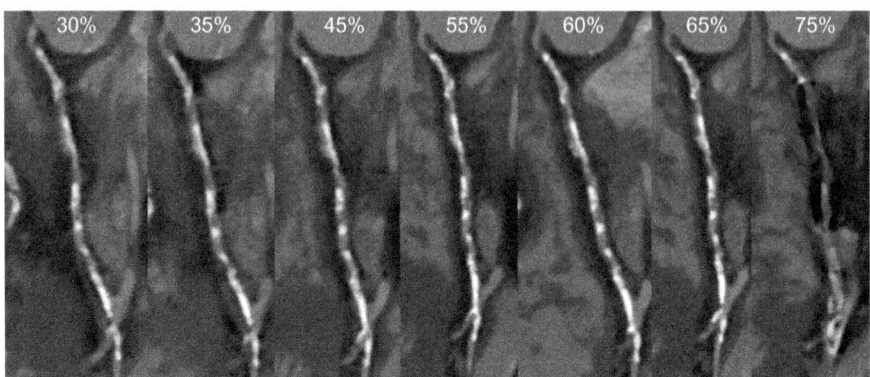

Figure 5.5 Cardiac motion artifacts. Cardiac CT with a dual-source CT scanner with exposure between 30% and 75%. In terms of motion, 60–70% bares the best intervals to assess the right coronary artery in this case.

cardiac cycle. Within a heart cycle, there are two periods where cardiac motion is relatively slow, mid-diastole and end-systole, which is when the best quality images can be collected. Accurate and reproducible timing depends on the quality of the ECG signal, robustness of the ECG interpretation algorithm, handling of arrhythmia, selection of the best phase for image acquisition/reconstruction, and regularity of the heart rhythm.

Even if timed perfectly, the fundamental temporal resolution of CT remains a challenge. This is particularly relevant in patients with a fast heart rate. While the heart cycle shortens, with relatively most shortening occurring in the preferred mid-diastolic phase, the relative proportion needed for image acquisition/reconstruction (150 ms) doubles from 12.5% at 50 beats per minute, to 25% at a heart rate of 100 per minute. In terms of hardware and reconstruction techniques, several approaches have been taken to improve the temporal resolution and improve image quality at higher heart rates.

Multisegmental reconstruction algorithms combine data from different heart cycles to reconstruct images. If at the same moment within two consecutive heart cycles, different projections were collected, then the effective temporal resolution can be improved by combining these data. The efficiency of this approach depends on the heart rate in relation to the rotation speed of the scanner, and varies between 0 and 50% for a bi-segmental reconstruction algorithm (Figure 5.6). A drawback of this approach is that each position needs to be scanned two or more times to combine a corresponding number of heart cycles, which translates into increased radiation exposure.

Dual-source CT was designed to improve the temporal resolution of CT by combining the data from two tube-detector system, that each acquire data at an angular offset of 90°, thereby collecting 180° of projections during a 90° scanner rotation. The third generation dual-source scanners rotate at 250 ms, resulting in a 66-ms temporal resolution.

Within the technical boundaries of the available technology, effective temporal resolution can be improved by reducing the heart rate, through administration of betablockers, calcium channel antagonists, sinus node blockers, or anxiolytic medication.

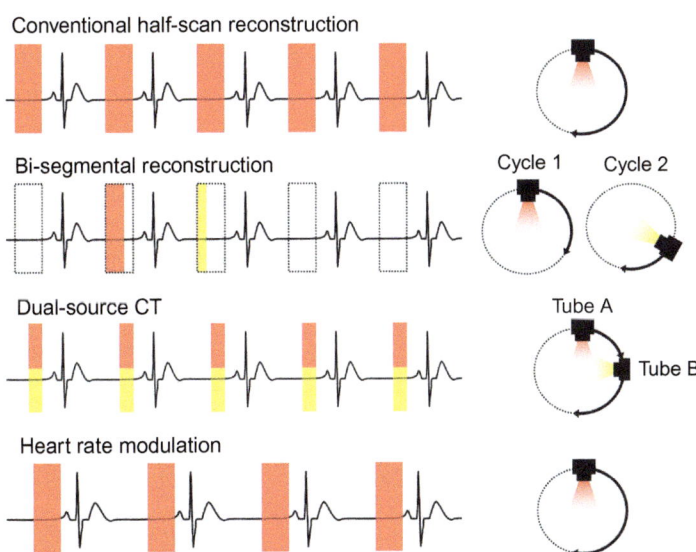

Figure 5.6 Temporal resolution. The absolute temporal resolution can be improved by increasing the rotation speed of the system, multisegmental reconstruction algorithms, or dual-source scanning. The relative temporal resolution can be improved by slowing down the heart rate.

One of the basic assumptions in CT reconstruction is that the structures in the image are stationary. Unfortunately, that is not the case for cardiac imaging, which is one of the limitations in coronary imaging. Motion-correcting algorithms are currently under development to reduce motion blurring. By assessing the position of the coronary arteries over time from images derived at different phases during the cycle, reconstruction can be optimized taking into account the displacement of the structure of interest.

5.3.2 Spatial resolution

Spatial resolution refers to the ability to differentiate small structures. The fundamental spatial resolution of a CT scanner is largely hardware dependent, and quantified in experiments with stationary phantoms with sharp contrast differences under ideal conditions. If we consider the spatial resolution the ability to identify small structures on cardiac CT images, then in practical terms spatial resolution is the result of patient characteristics, roentgen characteristics, scanner design, scan protocol, reconstruction algorithms, postprocessing, and methods of display. Some of these factors are nonmodifiable, while others are susceptible to optimization. We can distinguish between in-plane (or axial, or XY) resolution within a single cross-sectional image, or the through-plane (or longitudinal, or Z) resolution that refers to the coronal/sagittal planes. In terms of hardware, the fundamental spatial resolution improves with a smaller focal spot. The size and quality of the detectors directly affect the spatial resolution. Miniaturization of the detectors is limited by the necessity of much higher tube currents to compensate increased image noise. Other relevant detector characteristics are the dead space versus the need to limit "cross talk" between detectors elements. The number of projections per rotation is directly related to image quality and spatial resolution, but limited by the rotation speed and the time the detectors need to "recover" and get ready for the next measurement (afterglow). Contemporary CT scanners have a fundamental, in vitro spatial resolution ranging between 0.3 and 0.6 mm in all three dimensions.

The type of reconstruction and the use of filtering kernels also affect the spatial resolution. A sharp kernel with edge enhancement will make differentiation of structures better (as long as noise is within limits), while smoother kernels will reduce spatial resolution to some extent. Because the matrix dimensions are usually fixed (at 512×512 for cardiac imaging), selecting a small area for image reconstruction (field of view) will reduce the size of the in-plane image elements (pixels). By reconstructing thin slices, at an even shorter longitudinal interval (overlapping), the thickness of the image elements (voxels) can be reduced. While it is technically possible to create very small voxels ($0.1 \times 0.1 \times 0.1$ mm), it generally does not benefit image quality to reduce the voxel size below the fundamental resolution of the scanner. A comparison has been made with the zoom function on digital cameras, where the optical zoom refers to the fundamental spatial resolution, and the voxel size refers to the digital zoom. The latter enlarges the image through interpolation, but without adding information data that would reveal further detail.

5.3.3 Contrast resolution versus image noise

The contrast resolution is the difference in measured signal between two materials (tissues). In cardiac imaging, it may refer to the difference between the coronary lumen and the surrounding tissues, or the contrast between infarcted and healthy myocardium. Often the contrast level is expressed relative to the random image noise on CT images (Figure 5.7). Noise negatively affects the ability to see signal intensity differences between tissues, and hence the ability to identify small structures (spatial resolution).

The ability to separate tissues depends on differences in roentgen attenuation characteristics. If these differences are too small, contrast may be improved using contrast media. Taking iodine-based contrast media for coronary angiography as an example, the improvement in contrast is directly related to the achieved concentration of iodine atoms within the coronary arteries. However, the tissue-specific attenuation characteristics (attenuation coefficient) vary with the energy level of the roentgen. Using dual-energy CT, these differences can be exploited to improve the contrast between tissues (atoms).

In general terms, statistical (image) noise decreases with a higher sampling rate. If per measurement more photons are collected per detector element, then the measured attenuation coefficient is more likely to approximate the truth. Therefore, on a detector level, noise will decrease at higher tube currents (higher mA) and larger detector sizes. Also the detector technology, including electronic noise, will affect the image quality. Because random photons scatter occurs easier at lower energy levels, decreasing

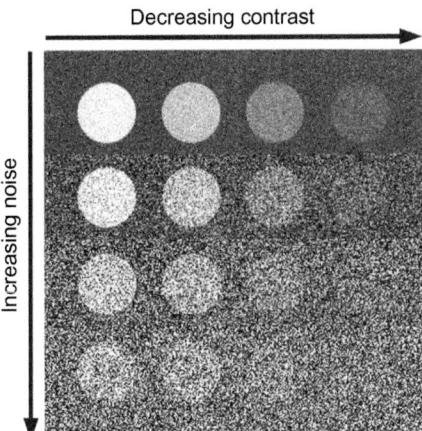

Figure 5.7 Image contrast versus noise. The ability to differentiate structures is affected both by contrast and noise. The same shapes with decreasing contrast to the surrounding are subjected to an increasing degree of image noise. Noise is better tolerated when contrast is sufficient, and vice versa.

the tube potential (kV) will generally increase image noise. In terms of reconstruction parameters, levels of noise will decrease with iterative reconstruction algorithms, smoother kernels, thicker slices, and larger fields of view. To improve appreciation of small differences in attenuation between tissues, one can increase the slice thickness (data averaging to decrease noise) or adjust the window display settings.

5.4 Cardiac CT applications

5.4.1 Coronary CT angiography

CT angiography of the coronary arteries (CCTA) is generally performed to exclude (or confirm) obstructive coronary artery disease (CAD). Besides the coronary lumen, and in contrast to invasive coronary angiography, CCTA allows assessment of the atherosclerotic artery wall. The diagnostic accuracy and clinical use of CCTA will be discussed in separate chapters (Figure 5.8).

Today, the default CCTA scan protocol at many centers is an ECG-triggered axial scan mode, with limited exposure duration (depending on the heart rate). The tube voltage is maintained as low as patient size, image requirement, and roentgen tube current limits allow.

Contrast is injected through a peripheral IV access, generally followed by a saline bolus to push forward the contrast medium. The contrast injection protocol depends on the indication and structure of interest, iodine concentration, patient size, scan duration, and roentgen tube settings, as well as institutional preferences. Timing of the scan during optimal contrast enhancement can be achieved by performing a test bolus to determine the circulation time, or by bolus tracking, in which case the arrival of the

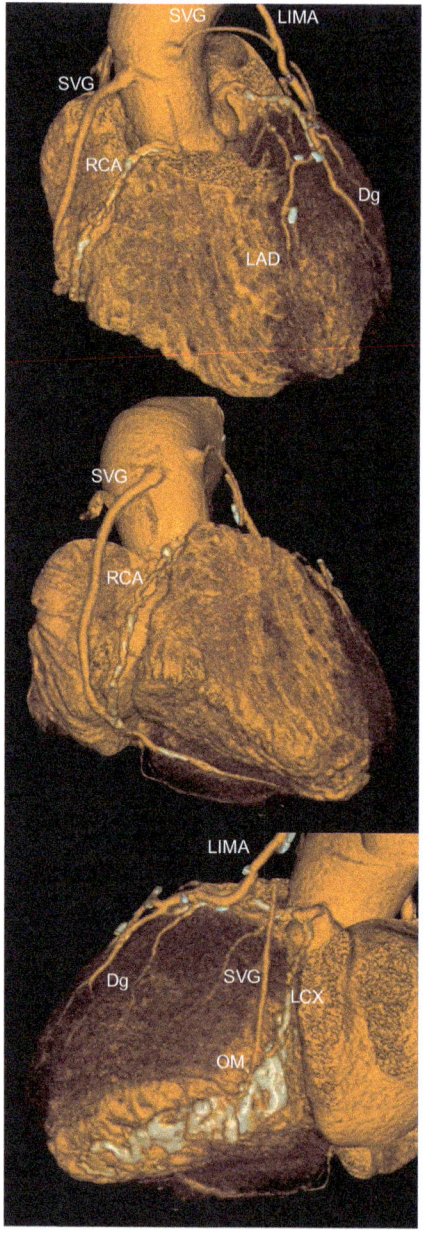

Figure 5.8 CT angiography after bypass graft surgery. Volumetric reconstructions of a CT angiogram in a patient with a history of bypass graft surgery and a lateral myocardial infarction. A left internal mammary artery graft is anastomosed side-to-side to a diagonal branch (Dg) and end-to-side to the left anterior descending coronary artery (LAD). One venous graft (SVG) is anastomosed to the distal right coronary artery (RCA), another to a small obtuse marginal branch (OM) from the left circumflex coronary artery (LCX). The small marginal branch supplies a nonvital, calcified myocardial scar.

contrast bolus is monitored online. Because of the small vessel size and detailed pathology, high image quality is essential for CCTA, which can be improved with proper patient preparation. This includes, information about the test, practice of the breath hold, (pharmacological) lowering of the heart rate, and vasodilation by sublingual nitrates.

Generally, thin slices are reconstructed for coronary CT angiograms, with the reconstructed field of view centered around the heart. Depending on the duration of exposure, images will be reconstructed during one or several cardiac phases. Contemporary scanners may automatically select the least motion-affected phase for reconstruction. For patients with extensive calcification or stents, sharper filtering kernels can be selected to limit blooming artifacts.

Images are interpreted on dedicated 3D workstations with the use of various applications for secondary reconstruction. CT guidelines recommend a systematic evaluation of the plaque burden and categorical classification of lumen obstruction severity.

5.4.2 Calcium scan

The calcium scan is an ECG-synchronized CT scan of the heart without injection of contrast medium (Figure 5.9). It is performed to semiquantify the amount of calcium in the coronary arteries, generally with the purpose of risk stratification in the preventive setting, or to exclude obstructive CAD in (symptomatic) patients. Particularly in case of nonsymptomatic individuals, radiation reduction is important, which is why the scan is generally performed using an ECG-triggered axial scan mode and short (single-phase) exposure. By convention, 3-mm thick slices are reconstructed for analysis. Structures with an attenuation value above 130HU, assumed calcified tissue, will be presented for semi-automatic selection by the reader, after which the total calcium amount will be semiquantified using the Agatston score or a measure of volume or mass. New iterative algorithms and lower kV settings can reduce the radiation exposure of calcium imaging, but will modify the measured calcium density and result in nonstandard calcium scores. Therefore calcium score is by default performed with 120 kV and FBP unless dedicated conversion factors become available.

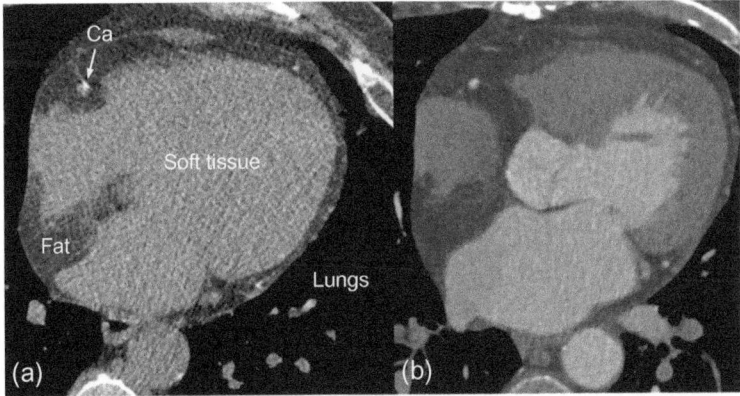

Figure 5.9 Native and contrast-enhanced cardiac CT.

5.4.3 Dynamic reconstructions for contractile function analysis

If the heart is exposed during the entire heart cycle, images can be reconstructed at any temporal point within the cardiac cycle. By comparing the end-diastolic and end-systolic datasets, an accurate assessment can be made of the global ventricular function (Figure 5.10). The high spatial resolution and clear contrast between the myocardium and cavity allow for accurate (automatic) segmentation and measurement of the cavity size and myocardial mass [3]. From these measurements, stroke volume, ejection fraction, and cardiac output can be calculated.

If a temporal series of CT reconstructions are displayed in rapid sequence, the impression of a contracting heart can be created. Contrary to real-time cardiac imaging techniques, the moving CT images merely display the heart during a single heart cycle, which is generally a different heart cycle for the different parts of the scan. From these images, regional myocardial contractility or valvular mobility can be assessed.

Because of the relatively high radiation exposure, and availability of other lower-risk modalities, cardiac CT is rarely requested for functional investigations. Exceptions

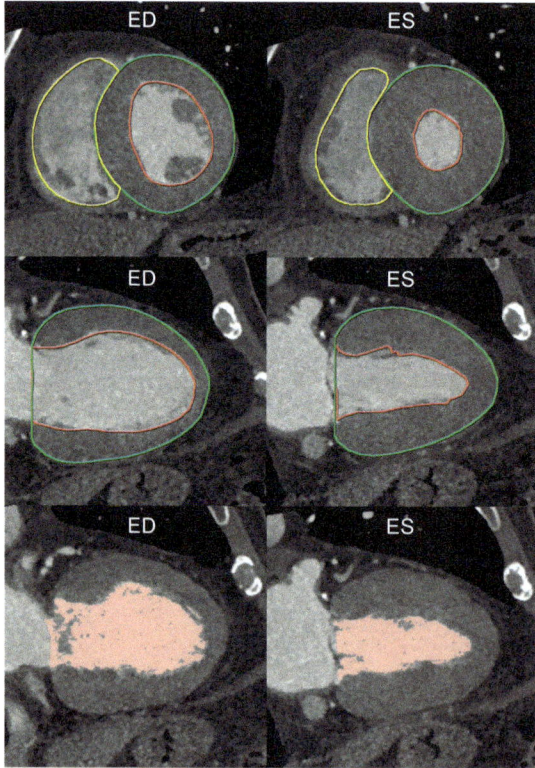

Figure 5.10 Left ventricular function. End-diastolic (ED) and end-systolic (ES) cross-sections of the heart. Endo- and epicardial wall segmentation can be performed of the left and right ventricle to measure the ventricular dimensions and assess the global left ventricular function. Alternatively, the volume of the left ventricular cavity can be determined by "blood-pool" method, in which case all volume elements with an attenuation corresponding to enhanced blood are identified and summed.

include the interpretation of prosthetic valves (endocarditis/thrombosis), or those with contraindications to both echocardiography and MRI [4,5]. This may change in the future with the development of low-dose functional scan protocols. Because assessment of the left ventricle does not require similarly high image quality, the tube current can be reduced to 4–20% of the nominal tube output during the systolic phase.

5.4.4 Infarct imaging

A decade before delayed-enhancement imaging became a trademark investigation for cardiac MRI, investigators reported similar infarct enhancement by CT [6]. Acute myocardial infarction changes the contrast medium kinetics of the myocardium. It results in reduced contrast wash-in because of vascular obstruction and delayed washout of accumulated contrast medium as a result of myocyte damage and oedema. In chronic myocardial infarction, contrast medium accumulates in the increased interstitial space of fibrous tissue. Lingering contrast medium can be visualized by CT (or MRI) and differentiates necrotic/fibrotic myocardium from healthy myocardium, which is characterized by fast washout of contrast medium [7]. In acute infarction, the enhanced myocardium may show dark hypo-enhanced core, referred to as microvascular obstruction [8]. These regions of very poor perfusion are associated with adverse clinical outcome. In chronic infarction, muscle and scar tissue may eventually be replaced by fat tissue. Fat tissue is readily detected by CT, even on nonenhanced images [9].

Delayed-enhancement imaging by CT is more challenging in comparison to MRI (Figure 5.11). Contrast between healthy and abnormal myocardium requires sufficient

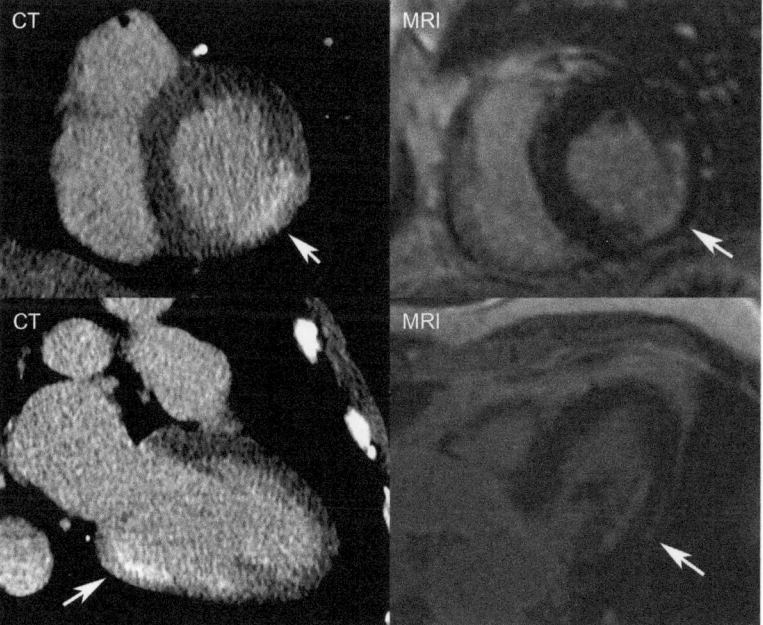

Figure 5.11 Delayed-enhancement imaging. Patient with an old infero-lateral myocardial infarction (arrows) imaged by delayed-enhancement CT and MRI.

contrast medium injection and tube current (preferably at a low kV level). Images are generally acquired between 5 and 15 min after contrast injection. Reconstruction of thicker slices, displayed at narrow display settings, improves interpretation.

CT infarct imaging is generally reserved for patients with contraindications to MRI.

5.5 Postprocessing, secondary reconstruction, and assisted interpretation

The quantity of detailed data created during a CT scan is enormous. Accurate, quantitative, and efficient interpretation and comprehensive reporting to referring physicians requires the use of secondary post-processing tools (Figure 5.12). Use of oblique

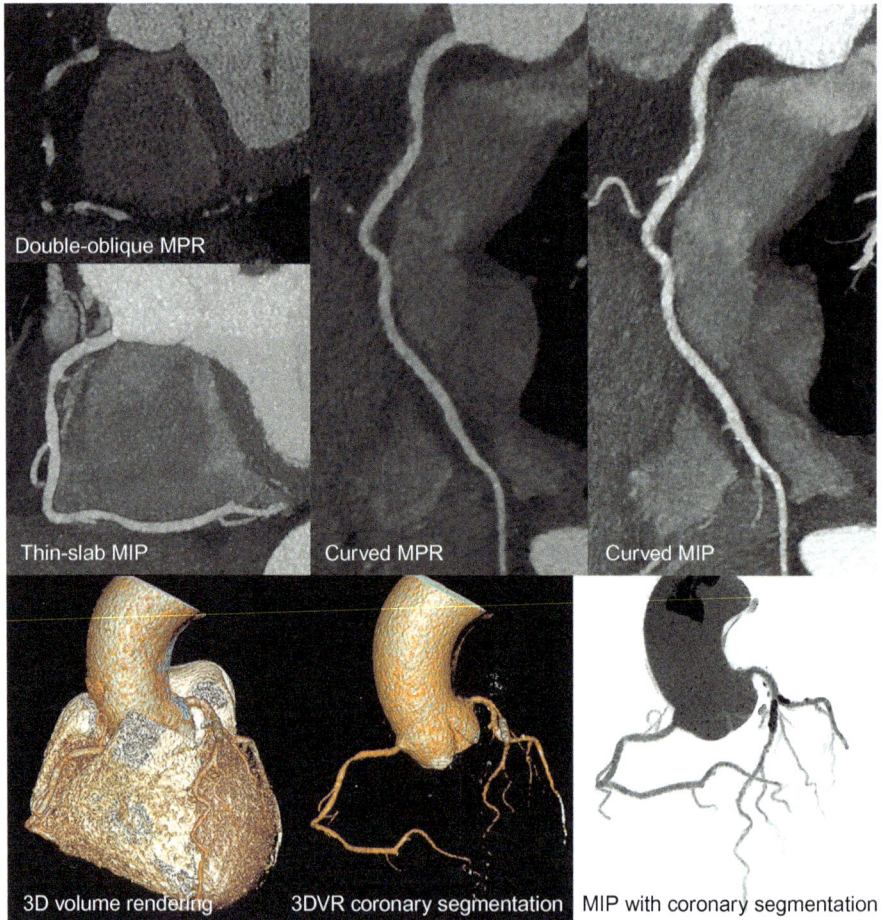

Figure 5.12 Qualitative postprocessing tools. Multiplanar reformation (MPR); maximum intensity projection (MIP); three-dimensional volume rendering (3DVR).

cross-section (multiplanar reformations, MPR) and maximum intensity projections (MIPs) allow for assessment of longer segments of the coronary arteries and compare luminal dimensions. Quantitative tools are available to assess attenuation, dimensions, angles, etc., as well as more complex assessment such as stenosis severity and contractile function. The use, for instance, of curved reconstruction along vessel and three-dimensional reconstructions are effective means to summarize and communicate findings with others. Because of various reasons related to image quality, digital CT images are very suitable for automated post-processing and quantification tools, in comparison to for instance echocardiography and magnetic resonance imaging.

5.6 Radiation and dose reduction

Roentgen is an ionizing form of electromagnetic radiation associated with various health risks, of which the development of malignant cancer is the most relevant in cardiac CT. The potential hazards of medical radiation are heavily debated. Given the high background incidence of malignancies, the varying natural exposure to radiation, the delay in the occurrence of radiation induced disease, selection bias toward those requiring CT scans, and various other aspects, it is difficult to determine the risk of medical radiation exposure. While it is difficult to quantify the exact risks, there is no reason to assume they are nonexistent. As for any diagnostic or therapeutic procedure, the risks and benefits need to be assessed and compared to alternative diagnostic approaches. If the CT scan is needed, efforts should be made to keep radiation as low as reasonably possible.

5.6.1 Measurement and reporting of dose

The radiation dose from CT is reported using different parameters. The CT dose index (CTDI) is the energy/dose absorbed from the acquisition slice, as measured by an ionization chamber in a standardized 32 cm cylindrical body phantom. Accounting for the different absorption characteristics between the center and the periphery of the weighted CTDI ($CTDI_w$) can be calculated. To account for the overlapping exposure with spiral scan modes, the volumetric CTDI ($CTDI_{vol}$) can be calculated. Because the absorbed dose of a patient depends on the longitudinal range of the scan, the $CTDI_{vol}$ is multiplied with the scan length to obtain the dose-length product (DLP). As some tissues are more sensitive to radiation than others, the DLP can be multiplied with body-region specific coefficient to estimate the effective dose of the CT scan. The coefficient (k) for a CT scan of the adult thorax is 0.0017, for adult cardiac CT scans often 0.0014 is used. Despite limitations of this approximation, this number best represents the risk of the scan to the patients. Since patients do not have the same habitus as the standardized 32 cm CTDI phantom the calculated dose represents only an estimation. Particularly in slim and pediatric patients, the true effective dose may be (severely) underestimated. In addition to the tissue coefficient, a correction factor for low kV should be applied.

5.6.2 Radiation exposure and dose reductions in cardiac CT

Why has there been so much attention given to the radiation exposure of cardiac CT? While the diagnostic performance of cardiac CT improved dramatically from 4- to 64-slice CT, this came at the expense of increasing exposure to radiation. Using standard ECG-gated spiral CT protocols, the radiation exposure of 64-slice scanners exceeded that of single-photon emission tomography (SPECT, 15–20 mSv). Why is the dose of a cardiac CT so high in comparison to CT examinations of other body regions? Because the coronaries and their pathology are small, sufficient contrast and spatial resolution require a high photon flux. But most important, or most avoidable, earlier CT technology with spiral CT scan protocols obtained images throughout the cardiac cycle. Continuous scanning at a slow table feed (pitch) results in a high radiation dose.

Since then, various innovations have been introduced, with regard to hardware, scan protocols, and reconstruction techniques (Table 5.3). Also, increased radiation awareness within the cardiac imaging community was important to adopt these new techniques and implement further measures to reduce radiation exposure [10].

In terms of hardware, many components directly or indirectly affect the exposure to radiation. These include tube shielding, filters, and collimation, as well as collimation and efficiency of the detector system. Over the past years, there has been a trend toward the use of lower tube voltages, in part facilitated by the use of more powerful roentgen generators and iterative reconstruction algorithms. Radiation can be reduced for ECG-gated spiral mode CT using ECG-triggered tube current modulation. During phases that are unlikely to be involved in the evaluation, the tube current is turned lower. Using ECG-triggered axial scan modes, exposure can be completely restricted to the phase of interest [11]. Efficiency of tube modulation (pulsing) and axial scanning depends on the duration of full exposure during each cycle.

Table 5.3 **Reduction of radiation exposure in cardiac CT**

Hardware	Roentgen generator and tube power to allow low kV protocols
	Collimation and filtering
	Detector efficiency
Scan mode and ECG-based modulations	Prospective ECG-gated tube modulation for spiral CT
	ECG-triggered axial scan protocols with narrow exposure windows
	ECG-triggered high-pitch spiral scan protocols
Scan settings	Minimizing tube potential and current
	Minimal scan range
Reconstruction	Iterative reconstruction algorithms
Patient preparation	Heart rate reduction

Acceptance of lower (but diagnostic) image quality, shorter scan ranges, heart rate modulation, and readiness to use narrower ECG-modulated exposure have all contributed to lower reported patient doses over the past years. Since the peak in exposure with first generation 64-slice CT, radiation exposure has decreased at a consistent pace. The average radiation dose of a standard ECG-triggered axial CT scan with narrow exposure window and a 100-kV tube voltage, the effective dose does not need to exceed 3–4 mSv, while in selected (and prepared) patients further customized scan protocols will achieve doses well below 1 mSv [12] (Figure 5.13).

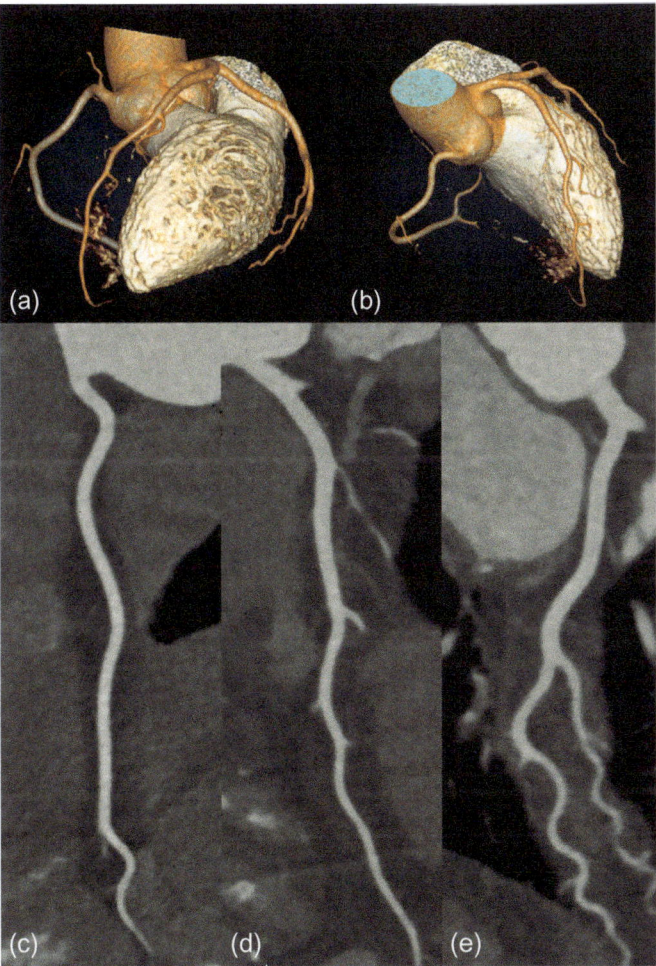

Figure 5.13 Low-dose coronary CT angiography. Coronary CT angiography using a third generation dual-source CT scanner, an ECG-triggered high-pitch spiral scan mode and a 80-kV tube current. The dose-length product was 32 mGy-cm, corresponding to an effective dose of approximately 0.5 mSv.

5.7 Estimating the hemodynamic significance of CAD

5.7.1 Myocardial perfusion imaging

CCTA is a reliable technique to rule out CAD with a negative predictive value approaching 100%. However, CCTA tends to overestimate angiographic severity, particularly in the presence of calcified atherosclerosis. Nowadays, management decisions are largely based on the functional severity of CAD, which only diffusely correlates with the angiographic severity. As a consequence, patients with angiographic stenosis of unknown functional severity will require additional testing to determine the need for myocardial revascularization. Similar to other noninvasive imaging techniques (SPECT, PET, MRI, echocardiography), cardiac CT is capable of visualizing vasodilator-mediated myocardial hypo-perfusion, indicating reversible myocardial ischemia.

5.7.1.1 Static MPI

Most myocardial perfusion imaging experience has been obtained with the so-called static perfusion technique [13,14]. During pharmacological vasodilation, a single CT angiogram is acquired during the early phase of myocardial contrast passage. Ischemic myocardium is identified by a relative decrease in myocardial enhancement. Demonstration of enhancement differences requires careful timing of the scan. Image interpretation is affected by contrast-related beam-hardening artifacts. Images may be compared to resting images (for instance the CCTA) to assess reversibility and differentiation from myocardial scar [15].

5.7.1.2 Dynamic MPI

Similarly to MRI or PET, myocardial enhancement can be imaged in a dynamic fashion. While the contrast flows in and out of the myocardium, a series of images are acquired to show temporal changes in myocardial enhancement. From the time-attenuation curves, the absolute myocardial perfusion can be estimated using a variety of physiological models [16] (Figure 5.14). The advantage of dynamic MPI and quantification of myocardial blood flow is that assessment of disease does not require a normal reference. There may be less susceptibility to beam-hardening artifacts. A drawback is the complexity and higher exposure to radiation to the patient [17]. Performance of dynamic MPI requires complete cardiac coverage, which can be achieved with wide-detector scanners or by repeatedly alternating the table position. The latter approach is characterized by a lower radiation exposure but also lower maximum sample rate.

5.7.2 Coronary contrast opacification patterns

Contrast enhancement of the coronary artery is not homogenous and generally decreases toward the periphery. Obstructive CAD may further affect contrast enhancement. This is most evident in complete coronary occlusion, in which case enhancement is often significantly lower distal to the lesion. There may in fact even be a reversed

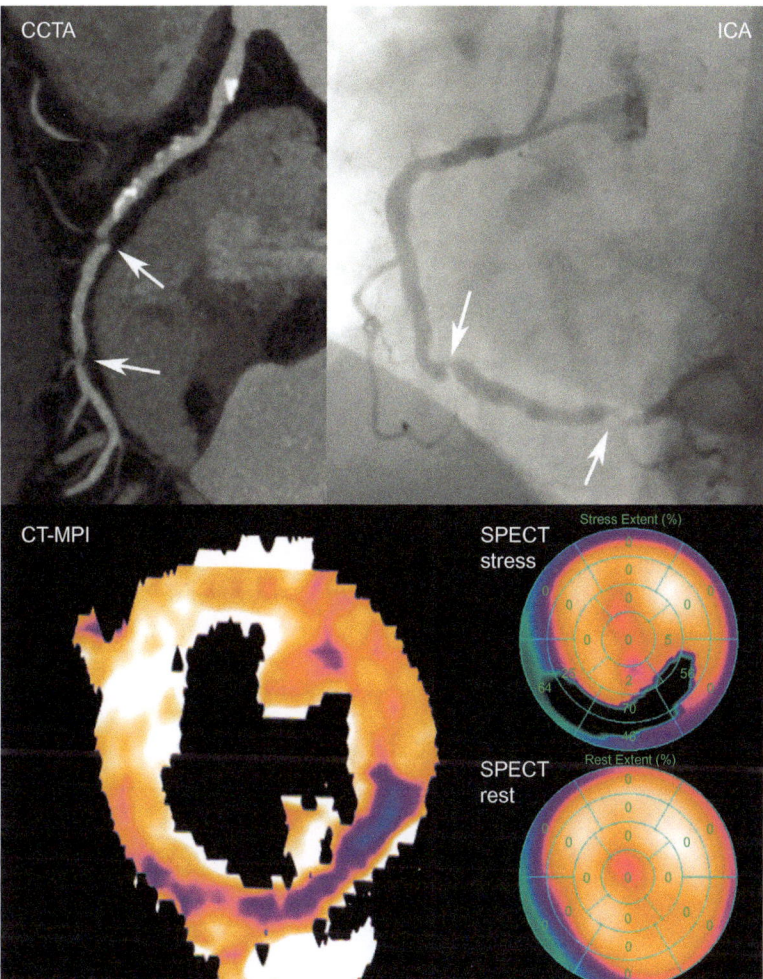

Figure 5.14 Stress myocardial perfusion imaging. Patient with obstructive disease of the right coronary artery by CT and invasive angiography. Dynamic stress CT myocardial perfusion imaging shows an area of low myocardial blood flow in the infero-lateral wall (40–60 ml/100 g/min), in comparison to normally perfused myocardium (120–170 ml/100 g/min). SPECT myocardial perfusion imaging shows a corresponding area of reversible ischemia.

opacification gradient as a result of collateral filling, which allows differentiation of total occlusion from subtotal stenosis with maintained anterograde flow. Several investigators have demonstrated that in hemodynamically significant disease, proximal to distal coronary opacification decreased more than in patients without obstruction of the coronary lumen. Either the ratio between the proximal and distal coronary artery is calculated with correction for the aortic attenuation changes, or the trans-coronary attenuation gradient (TAG) is calculated throughout the coronary artery tree [18–20]. Failure to reproduce these results has been reported by others [21]. Effectiveness of the approach may be dependent on scanner technology (single beat scan preferable) as well as the scan methodology. Bolus tracking and a relative late scan start may attenuate the coronary attenuation gradient, in comparison to an earlier test bolus mediated scan initiation.

5.7.3 CT-based fractional flow reserve

An alternative approach to estimating the functional severity of angiographic CAD is by model-based calculation of the fractional flow reserve using computational fluid dynamics (Figure 5.15). The shape and size of the coronary arteries and the myocardium are derived from the cardiac CT scan. Using a physiological model, with input of the myocardial mass from CT, and several physiological parameters (blood pressure, heart rate) the resting coronary flow and peripheral resistance can be calculated. Numerical computation of Navier-Stoke equations by applying computational fluid dynamics allows for the calculation of coronary blood flow and pressure throughout the coronary artery tree. By simulation, the effect of vasodilation, and lowered peripheral resistance, the blood pressure can be determined and compared to the aortic pressure to compute a fractional flow reserve [22].

The first CT-FFR approach by HeartFlow, Inc., has been the most validated algorithm to date [23,24]. While correlation with invasive FFR is modest, CTA-FFR does improve the performance of CCTA to identify hemodynamically significant CAD by correctly reclassifying a substantial proportion of overestimations. Contrary

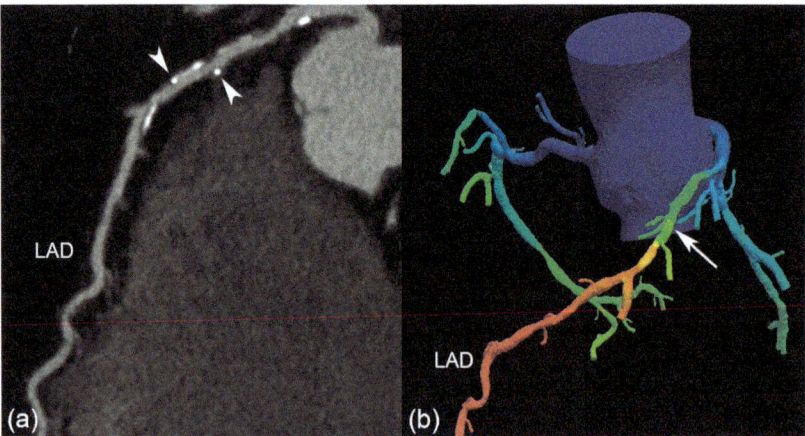

Figure 5.15 CT-based fractional flow reserve. Coronary CT angiogram (a) of a patient who underwent percutaneous intervention with a bio-resorbable scaffold 5 years prior. Only the platinum markers of the scaffold are visible (arrows) on CT. On the three-dimensional reconstruction of the coronary arteries, the FFR_{CT} is displayed in color (b). Green-blue represent normal values, orange to red indicates an FFR_{CT} value below 0.80. Despite the absence of a single lesion exceeding 50% diameter reduction, diffuse atherosclerotic disease results in a significant gradient over the LAD, which was confirmed by invasive fractional flow reserve (FFR).

to alternative functional testing by CT or other modalities, CTA-FFR does not require additional testing or exposure to contrast and/or radiation. Accurate CTA-FFR calculations require high-quality CT data and are negatively affected by calcification, ECG synchronization inaccuracies, and motion artifacts. Certain generalizations concerning the form–function relations and the expected response to adenosine may not apply in all situations and individual cases. Recently, computationally less demanding CTA-FFR algorithms have been introduced, which allow local processing by the clinicians with immediate availability of the CTA-FFR results [25].

5.8 Future perspectives

In terms of technology, cardiac CT is still developing at a rapid pace. Scanners continue to improve on rotation speed, X-ray power, longitudinal coverage, and detector efficiency. Reconstruction techniques will further evolve to improve image quality, reduce radiation exposure, and even reduce cardiac motion artifacts. CT will advance from a single-parameter technique to a more diverse interrogation of tissue properties with the use of spectral imaging. Adaptation of cardiac CT will continue as the reliability of the technique is now associated with ever-decreasing radiation exposures. The introduction of applications such as myocardial perfusion imaging and CT-based fractional flow reserve simulations, to assess the functional severity of obstructive coronary disease will allow CT to complement the anatomical information derived for the CT angiogram.

References

[1] Beister M, Kolditz D, Kalender WA. Iterative reconstruction methods in X-ray CT. Phys Med 2012;28(2):94–108.

[2] So A, Hsieh J, Narayanan S, Thibault JB, Imai Y, Dutta S, et al. Dual-energy CT and its potential use for quantitative myocardial CT perfusion. J Cardiovasc Comput Tomogr 2012;6(5):308–17.

[3] Mahnken AH, Koos R, Katoh M, Spuentrup E, Busch P, Wildberger JE, et al. Sixteen-slice spiral CT versus MR imaging for the assessment of left ventricular function in acute myocardial infarction. Eur Radiol 2005;15(4):714–20.

[4] Fagman E, Perrotta S, Bech-Hanssen O, Flinck A, Lamm C, Olaison L, et al. ECG-gated computed tomography: a new role for patients with suspected aortic prosthetic valve endocarditis. Eur Radiol 2012;22(11):2407–14.

[5] Symersky P, Budde RP, de Mol BA, Prokop M. Comparison of multidetector-row computed tomography to echocardiography and fluoroscopy for evaluation of patients with mechanical prosthetic valve obstruction. Am J Cardiol 2009;104(8):1128–34.

[6] Siemers PT, Higgins CB, Schmidt W, Ashburn W, Hagan P. Detection, quantitation and contrast enhancement of myocardial infarction utilizing computerized axial tomography: comparison with histochemical staining and 99mTc-pyrophosphate imaging. Invest Radiol 1978;13(2):103–9.

[7] Gerber BL, Belge B, Legros GJ, Lim P, Poncelet A, Pasquet A, et al. Characterization of acute and chronic myocardial infarcts by multidetector computed tomography: comparison with contrast-enhanced magnetic resonance. Circulation 2006;113(6):823–33.

[8] Lardo AC, Cordeiro MA, Silva C, Amado LC, George RT, Saliaris AP, et al. Contrast-enhanced multidetector computed tomography viability imaging after myocardial infarction: characterization of myocyte death, microvascular obstruction, and chronic scar. Circulation 2006;113(3):394–404.

[9] Nieman K, Cury RC, Ferencik M, Nomura CH, Abbara S, Hoffmann U, et al. Differentiation of recent and chronic myocardial infarction by cardiac computed tomography. Am J Cardiol 2006;98(3):303–8.

[10] Halliburton SS, Abbara S, Chen MY, Gentry R, Mahesh M, Raff GL, et al. Society of Cardiovascular Computed Tomography. SCCT guidelines on radiation dose and dose-optimization strategies in cardiovascular CT. J Cardiovasc Comput Tomogr 2011;4(5):198–224.

[11] Neefjes LA, Rossi A, Genders TS, Nieman K, Papadopoulou SL, Dharampal AS, et al. Diagnostic accuracy of 128-slice dual-source CT coronary angiography: a randomized comparison of different acquisition protocols. Eur Radiol 2013;23(3):614–22.

[12] Marwan M, Mettin C, Pflederer T, Seltmann M, Schuhbäck A, Muschiol G, et al. Very low-dose coronary artery calcium scanning with high-pitch spiral acquisition mode: comparison between 120-kV and 100-kV tube voltage protocols. J Cardiovasc Comput Tomogr 2013;7(1):32–8.

[13] George RT, Silva C, Cordeiro MA, DiPaula A, Thompson DR, McCarthy WF, et al. Multidetector computed tomography myocardial perfusion imaging during adenosine stress. J Am Coll Cardiol 2006;48(1):153–60.

[14] Kurata A, Mochizuki T, Koyama Y, Haraikawa T, Suzuki J, Shigematsu Y, et al. Myocardial perfusion imaging using adenosine triphosphate stress multi-slice spiral computed tomography: alternative to stress myocardial perfusion scintigraphy. Circ J 2005;69(5):550–7.

[15] Mehra VC, Ambrose M, Valdiviezo-Schlomp C, Schuleri KH, Lardo AC, Lima JA, et al. CT-based myocardial perfusion imaging-practical considerations: acquisition, image analysis, interpretation, and challenges. J Cardiovasc Transl Res 2011;4(4):437–48.

[16] Rossi A, Uitterdijk A, Dijkshoorn M, Klotz E, Dharampal A, van Straten M, et al. Quantification of myocardial blood flow by adenosine-stress CT perfusion imaging in pigs during various degrees of stenosis correlates well with coronary artery blood flow and fractional flow reserve. Eur Heart J Cardiovasc Imaging 2013;14(4):331–8.

[17] Bamberg F, Becker A, Schwarz F, Marcus RP, Greif M, von Ziegler F, et al. Detection of hemodynamically significant coronary artery stenosis: incremental diagnostic value of dynamic CT-based myocardial perfusion imaging. Radiology 2011;260(3):689–98.

[18] Choi JH, Koo BK, Yoon YE, Min JK, Song YB, Hahn JY, et al. Diagnostic performance of intracoronary gradient-based methods by coronary computed tomography angiography for the evaluation of physiologically significant coronary artery stenoses: a validation study with fractional flow reserve. Eur Heart J Cardiovasc Imaging 2012;13(12):1001–7.

[19] Chow BJ, Kass M, Gagné O, Chen L, Yam Y, Dick A, et al. Can differences in corrected coronary opacification measured with computed tomography predict resting coronary artery flow? J Am Coll Cardiol 2011;57(11):1280–8.

[20] Wong DT, Ko BS, Cameron JD, Leong DP, Leung MC, Malaiapan Y, et al. Comparison of diagnostic accuracy of combined assessment using adenosine stress CT perfusion (CTP) + computed tomography angiography (CTA) with transluminal attenuation gradient (TAG320) + CTA against invasive fractional flow reserve (FFR). J Am Coll Cardiol 2014;10.

[21] Stuijfzand WJ, Danad I, Raijmakers PG, Marcu CB, Heymans MW, van Kuijk CC, et al. Additional value of transluminal attenuation gradient in CT angiography to predict hemodynamic significance of coronary artery stenosis. JACC Cardiovasc Imaging 2014; 7(4):374–86.
[22] Taylor CA, Fonte TA, Min JK. Computational fluid dynamics applied to cardiac computed tomography for noninvasive quantification of fractional flow reserve: scientific basis. J Am Coll Cardiol 2013;61(22):2233–41.
[23] Min JK, Leipsic J, Pencina MJ, Berman DS, Koo BK, van Mieghem C, et al. Diagnostic accuracy of fractional flow reserve from anatomic CT angiography. JAMA 2012;308(12):1237–45.
[24] Nørgaard BL, Leipsic J, Gaur S, Seneviratne S, Ko BS, Ito H, et al. NXT trial study group. Diagnostic performance of noninvasive fractional flow reserve derived from coronary computed tomography angiography in suspected coronary artery disease: the NXT trial (analysis of coronary blood flow using CT angiography: next steps). J Am Coll Cardiol 2014;63(12):1145–55.
[25] Coenen A, Lubbers MM, Kurata A, Kono A, Dedic A, Chelu RG, et al. Fractional flow reserve computed from noninvasive CT angiography data: diagnostic performance of an on-site clinician-operated computational fluid dynamics algorithm. Radiology 2015;274(3):674–83.

Magnetic resonance imaging

V.M. Ferreira*, M.D. Robson*, T.D. Karamitsos[†], M.M. Bissell*,
D.J. Tyler*, S. Neubauer*
*University of Oxford, Oxford, UK; [†]Aristotle University of Thessaloniki, Thessaloniki, Greece

6.1 Introduction

The nuclear magnetic resonance (NMR) phenomenon was first demonstrated in 1938 and applied to imaging in the early 1970s, with the first clinical scanners available from the late 1980s. Owing to the challenges of imaging the moving heart, cardiovascular magnetic resonance (CMR) only emerged as a clinical tool in the 1990s when high-performance gradient systems and advances in pulse sequence design allowed for the acquisition of high-quality static and cine images of the heart. A key property of CMR is its unique ability to perform multiparametric tissue characterization, including edema, scar, viability, perfusion, and blood flow. Thus, CMR has the capability to distinguish among acute, chronic, ischemic, and nonischemic etiologies, making it an attractive clinical tool to evaluate the cardiac patient.

In this chapter, we will review the basic principles of NMR and expand on some of the developing techniques that hold promise for clinical applications as the field continues to advance. Clinical applications will continue to stipulate shorter examination times for efficient workflow, so the section on fast imaging techniques will explore technical advances that aim toward this goal. Assessment for coronary artery disease (CAD) and ischemia is currently the top indication for CMR, and we shall discuss how combining perfusion imaging with tissue characterization techniques provides comprehensive information in aiding decision making for the patient with CAD. Novel techniques such as T1- and T2-mapping allow direct quantification of myocardial characteristics and comparisons within and between individuals and are sensitive to a wide range of myocardial pathologies, promising to provide additional disease detection beyond conventional CMR techniques. Four-dimensional flow imaging can assess flow patterns and hemodynamics within cardiac chambers and great vessels, which may be useful in the evaluation of congenital heart disease and diseases of the aorta. Finally, we will review how CMR may assess cardiac metabolism without the need for radioactive tracers using magnetic resonance spectroscopy (MRS) and hyperpolarized carbon-13 (^{13}C) imaging.

6.2 Basic principles of NMR

The principle of NMR is that when subjected to a magnetic field, nuclei with different spin states are split into different energy levels, allowing them to absorb and re-transmit electromagnetic radiation [1]. The frequency of the electromagnetic radiation and the amplitude of the signal both increase with the applied field strength. At the field-strengths used in clinical imaging, this electromagnetic radiation is in the radiofrequency (RF) range (e.g., approximately 63 MHz at 1.5 tesla (T) for the protons of hydrogen in water). Because of their biological abundance, hydrogen nuclei (^{1}H or protons) are the dominant nuclei used in CMR.

Other than ^{1}H, all nuclei with an odd number of protons or neutrons have net nuclear spin and can be used to generate NMR signal. For human cardiac applications, these are typically limited to phosphorus (^{31}P) [2], carbon (via its low natural abundance isotope ^{13}C), and sodium (^{23}Na). The NMR phenomenon is also sensitive to air and the elements, gadolinium, dysprosium, iron, and manganese, for example, but this is by their influence on the NMR visible nuclei.

The fundamentals of NMR and, hence, MRI are the large magnetic field that generates different energy levels for the nucleus. The term "spin state" is used to describe the magnetization of the nuclei. The natural spin state for the magnetization is for it to be aligned with the applied magnetic field of the magnet. It is possible to excite this spin system using RF pulses that rotate the spin state so that the spins no longer point along the direction of the magnetic field, but will precess (spin) about that direction. After excitation, the spin system will continue to transmit an RF signal, which is due to the components of the spin in the plane perpendicular to that of the magnet (the transverse plane). This transverse component of the spin system (also known as transverse magnetization) will decay with the characteristic decay time of T2, simultaneously the spin system (magnetization) will recover back to its natural (thermal equilibrium) state with the characteristic decay time of T1.

After excitation by an RF pulse, the behavior of the protons is governed by the relaxation parameters T1, T2, and T2* (Figures 6.1 and 6.2) and described later on. These depend on the microscopic environment of water and fat within the tissues. The signal also depends on the number of nuclei present, their motion, and the pulse sequence. Signals are encoded and located through the use of magnetic field gradients that alter the frequency of the nuclei's precession. The principle of spatial encoding involves the use of magnetic field gradient, which results in the resonant frequency of precession varying from one side of the patient to the other. This variation in frequency means that we can excite a single position in space if we apply a pulse of a specific RF frequency. Further, we can then change the orientation of the field gradient and collect the re-transmitted RF signal from the sample. This signal contains frequency components that are proportional to the amount of material along the direction of the field gradient. By using magnetic field gradients and these types of approaches, it is possible to fill a complete grid with the frequency components of the image. This grid is known as k-space. Fourier transformation of the k-space data yields an image of the patient. The pulse sequence defines the types and timing of the RF and gradient pulses used to encode an image. Manipulation of pulse sequence parameters allows emphasis on different characteristics of the nuclei, enabling the tailoring of diagnostic images that is the powerful feature of MRI [1].

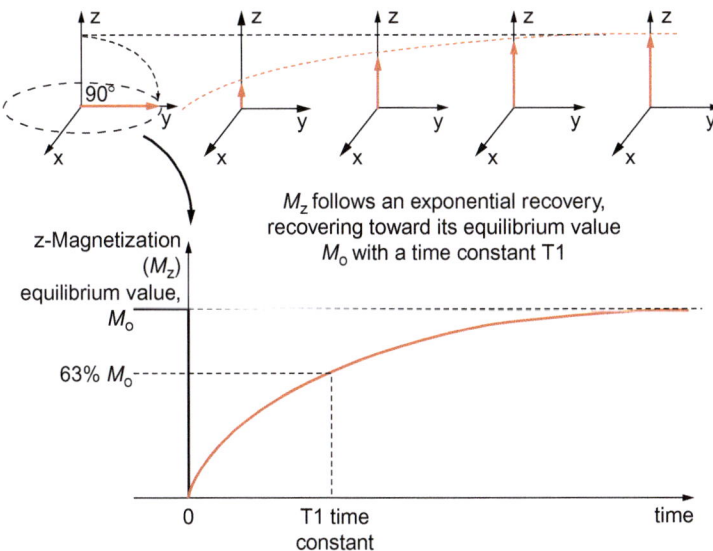

Figure 6.1 T1 relaxation process. Diagram showing the process of T1 relaxation after a 90° rf pulse is applied at equilibrium. The z component of the net magnetization, M_z is reduced to zero, but then recovers gradually back to its equilibrium value if no further rf pulses are applied. The recovery of M_z is an exponential process with a time constant T1. This is the time at which the magnetization has recovered to 63% of its value at equilibrium. As originally published by Biomed Central in [3].

6.2.1 Intrinsic MR contrast

Intrinsic MR contrast refers to the use of the natural differences in NMR parameters of tissue, and these tend to describe the relaxation parameters T1, T2, T2*, the amount of fat, and the proton density of water. At a deeper level, intrinsic contrast is more subtle, as any single pixel of an MRI image includes many millions of protons in many thousands of different environments, which flow, perfuse, diffuse, interact, and react in a manner that all can influence the MRI signal. To deal with this complexity/elegance, we generally ignore the details and (pragmatically) simplify describing each image pixel as having a single T1, T2, T2* and amounts of fat and water, and call that intrinsic contrast.

The T1 (or spin-lattice) relaxation time of the protons depends on the way the protons can reorganize back their thermal equilibrium state after an RF pulse excitation. Pure water free of other constituents has a long T1 (many seconds), but T1 is shortened by interaction with cell membranes. Protons in fat molecules have short T1. By imaging quickly with large RF pulses, it is possible to suppress protons with long T1, which emphasizes protons with short T1, a technique known as T1-weighting.

The T2 (or spin-spin) relaxation time is affected by similar factors as T1 so free water has long T2 but water bound to proteins has very short T2. The T2 relates to the time for which a nucleus will transmit its RF signal after it has been excited by an excitation pulse in a spin-echo acquisition. T2 decay is not simply caused by local

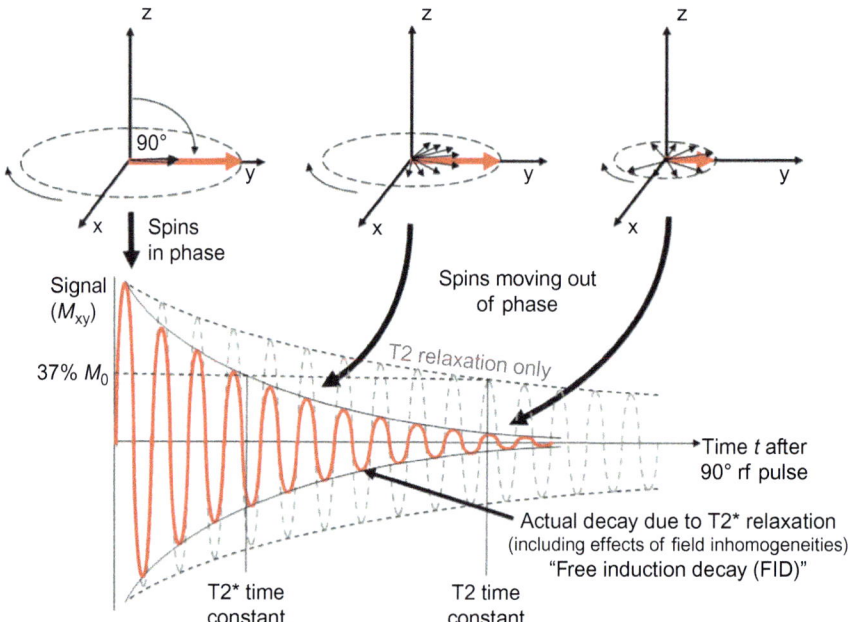

Figure 6.2 Transverse (T2 and T2*) relaxation processes. A diagram showing the process of transverse relaxation after a 90° rf pulse is applied at equilibrium. Initially the transverse magnetization (red arrow) has a maximum amplitude as the population of proton magnetic moments (spins) rotate in phase. The amplitude of the net transverse magnetization (and therefore the detected signal) decays as the proton magnetic moments move out of phase with one another (shown by the small black arrows). The resultant decaying signal is known as the free induction decay (FID). The overall term for the observed loss of phase coherence (de-phasing) is T2* relaxation, which combines the effect of T2 relaxation and additional de-phasing caused by local variations (inhomogeneities) in the applied magnetic field. T2 relaxation is the result of spin-spin interactions, and due to the random nature of molecular motion, this process is irreversible. T2* relaxation accounts for the more rapid decay of the FID signal, however the additional decay caused by field inhomogeneities can be reversed by the application of a 180° refocusing pulse. Both T2 and T2* are exponential processes with times constants T2 and T2*, respectively. This is the time at which the magnetization has decayed to 37% of its initial value immediately after the 90° rf pulse.
As originally published by Biomed Central in [3].

dephasing of the spin state in a nonuniform magnetic field (like T2* below) but is due to the component of this dephasing that cannot be refocused. Mechanistically, T2 decay is explained as being due to the random motion of spins in a nonuniform magnetic field, although in practice, T2 has many varied stochastic sources such as magnetization exchange, dipolar couplings, and chemical reactions. Delaying the time of acquisition after the spin system has been excited attenuates tissues with short T2, emphasizing nuclei with long T2 (e.g., free water). A classic application of T2-weighted imaging is in the detection of edema.

T2* relaxation is similar to T2, but requires the use of a gradient echo acquisition. T2* decay is caused by the individual spins precessing at different frequencies and, thus, moving out of phase with each other, which results in signal cancelation. T2* is extremely sensitive to iron, and is also affected by the oxygenation level of the tissue. These sources of microscopic magnetic field inhomogeneity result in dephasing of the spins and cause rapid signal decay, hence, shortening T2*. Large-scale magnetic field inhomogeneity will also influence the T2* and so care must be taken to ensure that this source does not confound T2* measurements.

6.2.2 MR contrast agents

Injectable contrast agents have multiple uses. Gadolinium-based agents shorten the T1 of protons that can exchange spin with the complexed paramagnetic ion. This increases the signal of those protons with appropriate T1-weighted pulse sequences. This approach finds application in perfusion imaging, where the blood labeled with gadolinium increases the signal where that blood perfuses, hence, providing differential contrast agents that have not yet been visited by the gadolinium [4]. The signal increase is also valuable when performing angiography to yield images that are of adequate signal to noise and high resolution. A second feature of gadolinium-based contrast agents is that they do not enter intracellular space such that in regions of extracellular space expansion the average gadolinium concentration is higher and the T1 will be shortened. This property of contrast agents is exploited in scar imaging by CMR. Iron-based particles also shorten the T1 but their dominant effect is shortening the T2* with a lesser effect on T2. Complex molecules incorporating iron or gadolinium may be used as novel targeted contrast agents but no clinically approved agent is yet available.

6.2.3 Morphological imaging

The simplest form of cardiac imaging is morphological imaging in which the goal is to determine the basic structure of the anatomy. In this case, it is desirable to differentiate the blood from the tissue. One way to achieve this is to suppress the signal from blood using a "black-blood" imaging method. Blood can be suppressed in a number of ways, but the classic approach is through the use of two inversion RF pulses: one that is slice selective to the slice of interest and the other which inverts the magnetization in the whole sample. This is followed by imaging when the magnetization of the blood is at the null point, just as the recovering magnetization crosses zero. The blood, owing to its motion, observes only one of these pulses, while the static tissue is exposed to both pulses and is thus unaffected. Careful selection of the time delay after the second inversion pulse allows images devoid of blood to be obtained, hence, the major vessels can be depicted with high quality in a fast-spin-echo or HASTE acquisition (Figure 6.3). In each case, ECG gating is used to freeze the cardiac motion in a single frame and only a single phase of the cardiac cycle is imaged.

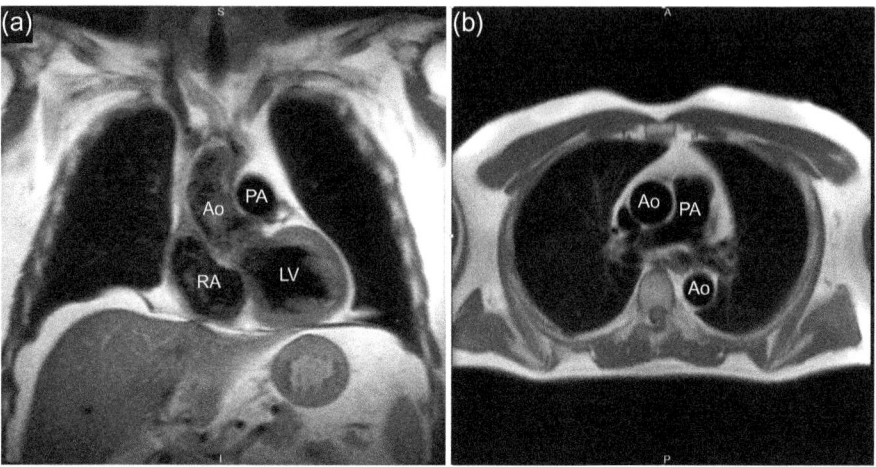

Figure 6.3 Black-blood half-Fourier acquisition single-shot turbo spin-echo (HASTE) magnetic resonance imaging. (a) Coronal MR image through the thorax. (b) Transverse MR image at the level of the pulmonary artery (PA). Ao, aorta; LV, left ventricle; RA, right atrium.

6.2.4 Cine imaging

Cine imaging generates a frame-by-frame movie of the heart, usually based on a composite of acquisition over multiple heartbeats and using ECG gating. Typically, images are acquired during a breath-hold lasting between 1 and 10 heartbeats. In this interval it is possible to collect anything between a single high-resolution ($1\,\text{mm} \times 1\,\text{mm} \times 3\,\text{mm}$) image or lower-resolution images encompassing the whole heart. The other parameter of the acquisition that is easily adjusted is the frame-rate of the resultant movie. Typically, this needs to exceed 14 frames to ensure an accurate depiction of the cardiac motion. Increased frame-rate, smaller voxel dimensions, and larger numbers of slices all increase the time required for image acquisition, hence, there is an inevitable trade-off. Frequently, a complete 3D depiction of the myocardium is obtained through collecting multiple parallel images that slice through the short-axis of the heart, which are often collected in a number of serial breath-holds (Figure 6.4).

6.2.5 Perfusion imaging

Rest perfusion imaging using gadolinium contrast agents can be used to characterize masses and tumors, while first-pass perfusion imaging under rest and stress conditions is widely used to assess for myocardial ischemia (Figure 6.5). The passage of the contrast agent through the myocardium is monitored by acquiring T1 weighted images at every heartbeat. With current methods, at least three myocardial slices can be imaged at every heart beat with an in-plane spatial resolution of less than 3 mm. Pharmacologic stress can be induced using vasodilators, such as adenosine, regadenoson, and dipyridamole, or inotropic agents such as dobutamine. Adenosine is a nonselective adenosine receptor agonist with potent vasodilator properties and is the most commonly used vasodilator for stress perfusion CMR imaging. The coronary

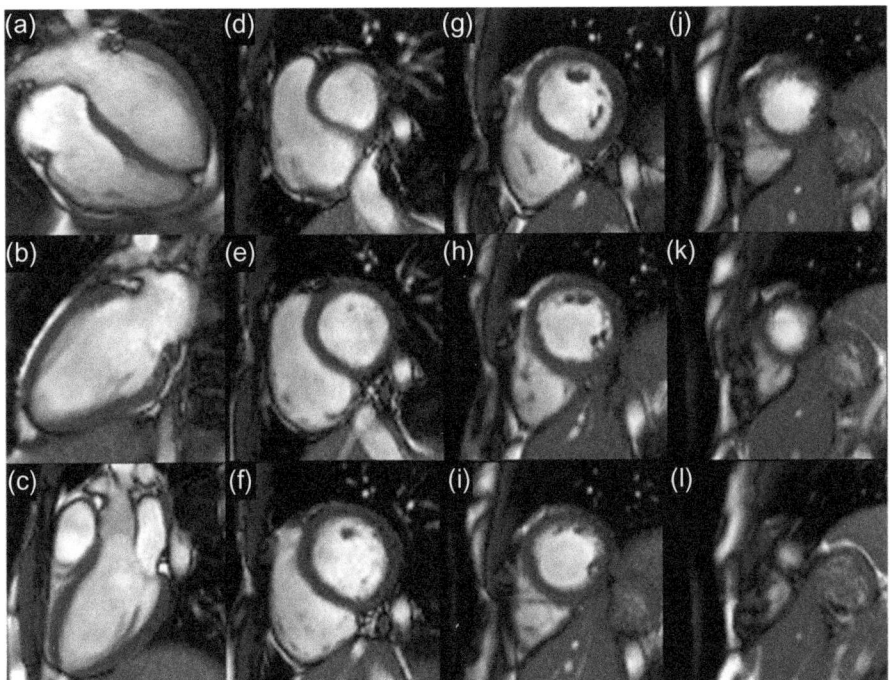

Figure 6.4 Steady-state free precession (SSFP) cine cardiac MR imaging acquired using retrospective ECG gating during breath-hold at end-expiration. (a) Horizontal long-axis view; (b) vertical long-axis view; (c) left-ventricular outflow tract view; (d–l) short-axis stack covering the ventricles from the base of the heart (d) through the atrioventricular groove to the apex (l).

vasculature downstream a stenosed artery is nearly maximally dilated at rest, with little further response under vasodilator stress in contrast to normal coronary vasculature, resulting in a relative hypoperfusion in the area subtended by the stenosed artery. Regadenosine is a newer, selective adenosine (A2A) receptor agonist, which can be administered as a bolus, while dipyridamole blocks endogenous adenosine reuptake to induce vasodilation indirectly. Dobutamine is a selective beta-1 adrenergic agonist that directly increases heart rate and contractility, typically used for the detection of ischemia-induced wall motion abnormalities, rather than first-pass perfusion imaging due to the tachycardia induced.

6.2.6 Flow imaging

Flow imaging can be used to measure the velocity of moving blood to assess for valvular lesions (stenotic or regurgitant) or blood flow within vessels and conduits. Phase-velocity imaging works by encoding the position of the blood, waiting a short amount of time and then un-encoding the position. The change in position will result in imperfect un-encoding of the position, which appears as a phase change of the signal that is proportional to the distance the blood has moved (and hence its velocity). In-plane

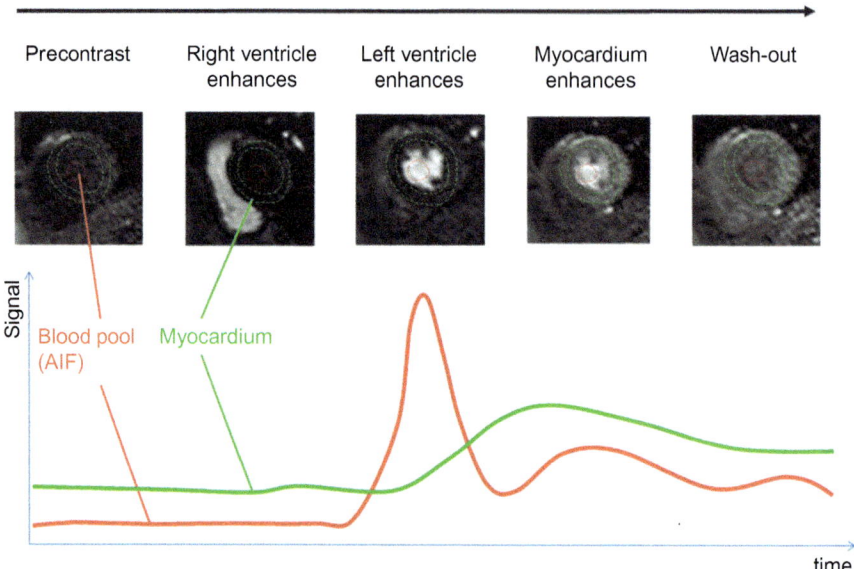

Figure 6.5 Quantitative perfusion data. For every image in the dynamic sequence, region-of interest contours describing the myocardium and a region in the blood pool are drawn. The mean signal intensity from within each region is plotted for each time point to generate plots of signal intensity versus time to show the increase in signal intensity in both the myocardium (green) and the blood pool (red). The blood pool curve is also often referred to as the arterial input function (AIF). These curves can be analyzed together to give an estimate of myocardial blood flow (MBF). As originally published by Biomed Central in [5].

flow imaging allows visual assessment of a jet along its course but does not permit flow quantification and may underestimate the velocity of narrow jets due to partial volume effects from the slice thickness. Through-plane flow has higher in-plane spatial resolution and allows for flow quantification as there is full, cross-sectional coverage of the jet. For very high velocity or turbulent flow, quantification can suffer from phase-shift errors and underestimation of the peak velocity due to its temporal resolution (25–45 ms), but CMR has the advantage of aligning velocity jets in any plane. Highly irregular rhythms will lead to inaccuracies in flow measurements, but dedicated arrhythmia sequences may improve accuracy at the cost of longer scan times.

6.2.7 MR angiography

In addition to quantifying flow, it is also possible to design pulse sequences that maximize the signal from blood to enable angiographic images. Typically these acquisitions are performed in 3D to generate a complete image of the vascular tree, which can be reconstructed on viewing workstations to allow these data to be examined carefully after acquisition. Several mechanisms can be employed to generate contrast, including intrinsic T2 contrast, in-flow or, with the use of contrast agents, T1 shortening to provide extremely rapid angiographic imaging.

6.2.8 Strengths and weaknesses of CMR

CMR has many strengths as a clinical and research tool. It does not use ionizing radiation and permits imaging in any plane. Another key advantage of CMR lies in the ability to accurately assess cardiac structures, function, and to perform tissue characterization, distinguishing ischemic from nonischemic pathologies. The quality of images can be affected by motion (cardiac, respiratory, or patient), so that image quality in patients with significant tachyarrhythmia or difficulty in breath-holding or remaining stationary can be impaired. Contraindications to CMR include claustrophobia, very large patient size and having an MRI-incompatible implant. Additionally, significant renal failure with an estimated glomerular filtration rate (eGFR) of less than 30 ml/min is a relative contraindication to contrast-enhanced CMR due to the inability to clear the gadolinium-based contrast agents with a risk of nephrogenic systemic fibrosis (NSF), although measures such as using the lower-risk macrocyclic chelates and arranging for dialysis after the CMR scan may help reduce the risk of NSF.

6.3 Fast imaging

6.3.1 Introduction: the challenge of imaging quickly

6.3.1.1 Image space versus k-space

CMR is based on techniques developed within the more general field of magnetic resonance imaging (MRI). In MRI, the image can only be collected over a period of time, as the data that constitute the final image must be collected sequentially. This signal data is then stored in a matrix known as k-space, and undergoes a mathematical transformation (the Fourier transform) to generate an image. Patient motion during acquisition will result in failure of the Fourier transform to properly reconstruct the image; resulting errors can be considerable and extremely difficult to disentangle. Therefore, over the period of image collection, it is essential for that body part to be stationary. Clearly this represents a significant challenge in the case of the human heart, owing both to the beating, but also to the asynchronous and variable breathing patterns.

6.3.1.2 The need for speed

Typical image acquisition times for MRI of noncardiac organs are one to two minutes, and even with advanced cardiac MRI it is difficult to obtain good image quality unless at least 200 ms of data are collected. This permits three basic methods for data collection:

1) Collect data over approximately 200 ms during a phase of the cardiac cycle where cardiac motion is minimal
2) Freeze the breathing motion (breath-hold or some form of respiratory triggering) and collect some of the data over several heartbeats (e.g., acquire for 20 ms on each of 10 heartbeats)
3) Collect the data faster than 200 ms (e.g., 60 ms), accepting the resultant lower image quality

Over these shorter intervals, the heart is sufficiently still to be captured accurately by the imaging sequence. ECG gating is used to synchronize the scanner acquisition to the cardiac cycle and breath-hold instructions are typically issued through headphones to the subject.

6.3.1.3 Technical restrictions (SAR, SNR, and gradient stimulation issues)

Traditionally, MR image quality was limited by the MR scanner hardware capabilities; however, with commercial improvement of scanner performance, it is now limited mainly by subject characteristics [6]. The excitation RF pulses used to stimulate the sample benefit from being short and of high amplitude, but the high-power RF pulses deliver heat into the subject. The specific absorption rate (SAR) defines how much RF power can be safely deposited into the patient and is restricted for MRI scans to limit patient heating effects. To sample k-space rapidly, magnetic field gradients are switched on and off rapidly. These changes in magnetic fields induce small currents into the subject, which can stimulate the peripheral nerves. This can be perceived as tactile stimulation or vibration on the skin; if the gradient field switching were faster, this sensation could become painful, and so gradient field switching rates are limited by the scanner hardware to prevent this. Finally, the image quality is limited by the signal-to-noise ratio (SNR) in the images; the NMR phenomenon exerts a weak effect so only a small fraction of the protons in the body is observed in an MRI scan, which limits the sensitivity and spatial resolution of images.

6.3.2 Real time versus segmentation

6.3.2.1 The benefits of real-time imaging

Imaging in real time has several benefits, as the acquisition is very fast (as short as one heartbeat), does not require breath-holding, and ECG gating is not absolutely required (although it is desirable). Further, for irregular heart rhythms, it is possible to obtain images of the variable patterns of ventricular filling and contraction. Real-time imaging is especially useful for cine and flow imaging in patients with irregular tachyarrhythmia such as rapid atrial fibrillation or frequent ectopic heartbeats.

6.3.2.2 The benefit of collecting over multiple heartbeats

In practice, collecting images in real time is difficult due to the limited amount of time available to collect the data, which compromises image quality. Image quality may be improved by collecting parts of the image (in k-space) during separate cardiac cycles. This segmentation of k-space requires good quality ECG gating and breath-holding but results in higher resolution and better image quality.

6.3.2.3 Issues with real-time data

Real-time imaging may appear to be the holy grail for cardiac function assessment, but there are deeper considerations [7]. Care must be taken to analyze data that were acquired without ECG gating, breath-holding, or assumptions of regular periodicity. For instance, in calculating the left ventricular ejection fraction, the volume of the heart is determined by adding the volume of a series of slices; if these data (from real time) cannot be aligned due to the mismatch of breathing phases, if the position of the imaging slice is not known, or if data from irregular heartbeats were combined, significant errors will arise. For these reasons, most data are presently collected in a segmented fashion using ECG-gating and breath-holding. It is likely that future work will move toward real-time imaging and address the aforementioned challenges, but at present these systems are not yet in place.

6.3.3 Sampling the data faster

6.3.3.1 Use of echo planar imaging (EPI) and spiral methods

Up until now, the methods of acquisition have focused on Cartesian acquisition schemes based primarily on balanced SSFP techniques. This approach is the stalwart of cardiac MR imaging and has driven its transformation from an interesting research tool to clinical workhorse. Data may be collected more quickly using echo planar imaging (EPI) [8–10], or spiral imaging methods [11,12]. Both of these methods use complex magnetic gradient field waveforms to contiguously sample large sections or even the whole of k-space in a short time (~20 ms). The approaches have found utility for methods such as perfusion imaging, where rapid sampling is essential.

6.3.3.2 Use of higher gradient performance

If k-space can be sampled faster, then it is possible to either improve imaging speed or quality. The simplest way to image faster would be to apply stronger imaging gradients that switch more quickly. However, as discussed earlier, with linear gradient systems, there is a limit to avoid problematic electrical currents being induced and peripheral nerve stimulation in the subject. Alternative approaches are being developed with gradient field systems that incorporate nonlinear gradients. These allow much higher gradient fields and switching rates with their associated benefits, but have much less of an issue with induced electrical currents and peripheral nerve stimulation. These technologies are not yet available on standard clinical scanners but are an active area of research.

6.3.4 Less is more: sampling smarter

6.3.4.1 Use of parallel imaging techniques

To make an MR image, it is necessary to sample k-space. A higher-resolution image requires more k-space to be acquired and hence a longer acquisition time (longer breath-holds or lower temporal resolution in a segmented acquisition). Parallel imaging is one of a series of methods that exploits MRI capabilities to collect less data and still create an image [13]. Parallel imaging simultaneously takes advantage of the additional spatial localization that is available when collecting images simultaneously from more than one receive RF coil. It is then possible to collect less of the k-space and use the fact that each coil "sees" a different region of the patient to generate the k-space that was not sampled. Presently, it is possible to accelerate 2D MRI by factors of 2 or 3 and 3D MRI by larger factors up to 10-fold or more. These approaches can also be used to collect multiple (typically 3) image slices in the time required to collect one slice. In addition to parallel imaging it is possible to use methods such as Partial

Fourier to accelerate data acquisition by factors approaching 2× speed-up, which takes advantages of fundamental symmetries in k-space.

6.3.4.2 Use of time acceleration approaches

When collecting a time series of images (e.g., in a cine or perfusion acquisition), most of the image changes vary little from one image frame to the next, which suggests a mechanism of acceleration. If it were possible to only image the changes between one image and the next, then the number of nonzero pixels in this difference image would be very small. Information theory therefore suggests that it should be possible to acquire the data associated with the difference image very quickly. These methods have been pioneered in digital imagery, such as the mpeg formats, and are very successful in that arena, achieving compression ratios of better than 200:1. In MRI, the data are collected in the k-space domain rather than the image domain, which hampers compression; however, even with this limitation, these approaches have proven effective at providing acceleration. This family of approaches is known as $k-t$ acceleration [14] and is seen to have applicability to cine and perfusion and any other acquisition that acquires a time course of images. A further current issue lies in the rapid reconstruction of images acquired in this fashion; however, further advances in the reconstruction algorithms and of the reconstruction hardware platforms address this issue.

6.3.5 Do we really need to go faster?

6.3.5.1 Navigated methods

So far, the discussion has focused on controlling the breathing motion through breath-holding. Breath-holding is a crude approach but is clinically well-tolerated and provides good-quality images. An alternative approach is to monitor the breathing cycle and only collect data when the patient is at a certain breathing position. This idea mimics the approach used for cardiac gating in which data are acquired at the same phase of the movement, whether it is the beating heart or respiration. Several ways have been used for monitoring breathing, including measuring chest expansion with a sensor and with MRI methods. MRI methods can be used to measure directly the diaphragm position to control how the imaging sequence operates in real time, either by selecting whether image data is collected, or what to do with the collected data. Simple "pencil beam" one-dimensional navigators have been commonly used for some time, but higher dimensional navigators are emerging that provide more information to the algorithms in managing breathing motion.

6.4 Perfusion, blood-oxygen-level-dependent, and late gadolinium enhancement imaging

6.4.1 Introduction

The assessment of patients with known or suspected ischemic heart disease is a major application of CMR. In the EuroCMR registry, risk stratification in suspected CAD or ischemia is the number one indication for CMR (34.2%) followed by workup of myocarditis or cardiomyopathies (32.2%) and assessment of viability (14.6%) [15]. New CMR techniques that assess myocardial oxygenation may be useful adjuncts to perfusion CMR by providing a more direct assessment of myocardial ischemia [16]. Important prognostic indices can also be derived from CMR imaging in patients with ischemic heart disease [17].

6.4.2 Viability assessment by CMR

The development of late gadolinium enhancement (LGE)-CMR in the late 1990s and extensive preclinical and clinical validation studies established CMR as a reference standard method for imaging myocardial infarction and thus indirectly assessing viability [18–20]. Using T1-weighted segmented inversion-recovery LGE sequences, high spatial resolution images of irreversible myocardial injury both in the acute and chronic setting can be acquired (Figure 6.6). This *in vivo* demonstration of the spatial extent of myocardial necrosis allows the identification of even small subendocardial infarcts previously undetectable by lower-resolution techniques such as single photon emission cardiac tomography (SPECT) [21].

Several studies have shown that the transmural extent of infarction predicts the recovery of contractile function after revascularization [22,23].

LGE-CMR not only defines the location and extent of infarction, but in acute MI also shows areas with poor tissue perfusion following primary PCI due to the "no-reflow phenomenon." Such microvascular obstruction detected by CMR has been linked to adverse ventricular remodeling and cardiovascular events after acute myocardial infarction [24,25].

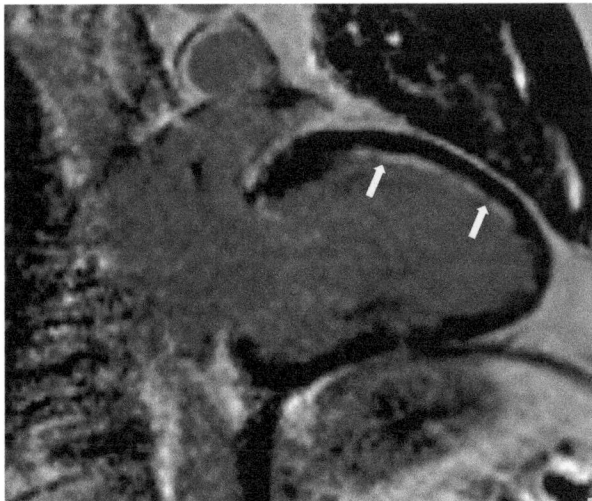

Figure 6.6 Late gadolinium enhancement image (two-chamber view) of a patient with previous subendocardial anterior myocardial infarction. The infarct appears as a white rim of enhancement (white arrows). The transmural extent of enhancement in ~25%, indicating that the majority of the anterior wall is viable.

6.4.3 Ischemia assessment by CMR

Perfusion imaging is an excellent method to assess myocardial ischemia and can be performed as part of a comprehensive CMR study in patients with acute or chronic ischemic heart disease [26]. Perfusion defects appear hypointense (dark) compared to adjacent normal myocardium during the first pass of a gadolinium-based contrast agent at maximal vasodilatation usually achieved using adenosine i.v. infusion (Figure 6.7). With the application of parallel imaging techniques and the higher field strength of 3 T, the spatial and temporal resolution of the technique is further improved, and near whole heart coverage is now possible [27,28]. The difference in spatial resolution compared to nuclear techniques is several times higher for CMR, allowing clear visualization of the subendocardial and subepicardial layers. Multiple studies have proven the clinical feasibility, safety, and high diagnostic accuracy of first-pass perfusion CMR with vasodilator stress for the detection of CAD [29–33]. In patients with contraindications to adenosine such as asthma or atrioventricular block and poor acoustic windows, dobutamine stress CMR is a reliable alternative to perfusion CMR.

Oxygenation-sensitive, or blood-oxygen-level-dependent (BOLD), CMR is a gadolinium-contrast-free technique that allows the noninvasive assessment of myocardial oxygenation [16]. Deoxygenated hemoglobin in blood can act as an intrinsic contrast agent, changing proton signals in a fashion that can be imaged to reflect the level of blood oxygenation [34]. Importantly, situations can exist where myocardial perfusion can be dissociated from oxygenation. The oxygen demand of the heart muscle may vary in different states, e.g., reduced in hibernating myocardium in line with the down-regulated contractility or increased in hypertrophic cardiomyopathy (HCM) due to the increased energy cost of contraction [35]. Even in patients with significant

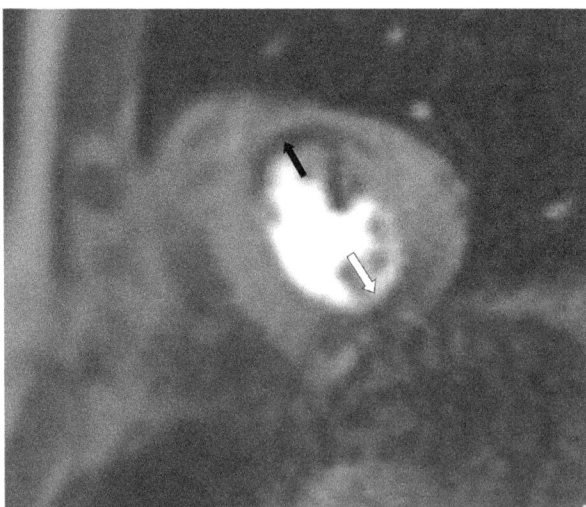

Figure 6.7 Mid short-axis view of stress perfusion scan in a patient with exertional angina. Note the areas of hypoenhancement (perfusion defects) in the anterior wall (black arrow) and the inferior wall (white arrow) compared to adjacent normal myocardium.

Magnetic resonance imaging

coronary stenoses, some degree of dissociation can occur between segmental perfusion and oxygenation [36]. Thus, compared to perfusion, regional myocardial oxygenation may be a superior parameter that more directly reflects the imbalance between oxygen demand and supply that characterizes ischemia.

6.4.4 Future directions

Further improvements in image quality with high spatial and temporal resolution can be expected for perfusion and viability CMR in the coming years [37–39]. The development of robust 3D techniques will increase the speed of data acquisition, further shortening scan time. Oxygenation imaging techniques are also expected to improve and become robust clinical tools in addition to perfusion. Finally, the cost effectiveness of a comprehensive CMR scan in patients with known or suspected ischemic heart disease compared to other imaging modalities and management strategies needs to be determined.

6.5 Quantitative mapping techniques

6.5.1 T1 mapping

Each tissue type exhibits a characteristic range of normal T1 relaxation times, deviation from which may indicate disease. Normal myocardial T1 values can be influenced by physiologic and technical factors, including temperature, age, gender, heart rate, magnetic field strength, and the pulse sequence used [40–42].

The most widely used approaches to estimate *in vivo* human myocardial T1 values are inversion-recovery and saturation-recovery based sequences. The Modified Look-Locker Inversion Recovery (MOLLI) method (2004) brought T1-mapping closer toward cardiac applications [43], and recent efforts using abbreviated variants concentrated on shortening acquisition times and minimizing heart-rate dependency [44]. Currently, MOLLI-based sequences are the most commonly used and validated [42,45,46] although saturation-recovery single-shot acquisition (SASHA) sequences are promising approaches in achieving very short imaging times without heart rate dependency [47]. Saturation recovery-based techniques may have a higher accuracy in estimating myocardial T1 times [47], while MOLLI-based methods may be more sensitive to detecting changes in disease due to additional magnetization transfer (MT) contrast [48]. Myocardial T1-mapping methods can be used for native (or precontrast) T1-mapping, postcontrast T1-mapping and extracellular volume (ECV) mapping.

6.5.1.1 Native T1 mapping

Native T1-mapping estimates myocardial T1 values before the administration of any contrast agents. MOLLI-based native T1-mapping has been extensively validated using simulations, phantoms, animal, and multicenter normal human population studies

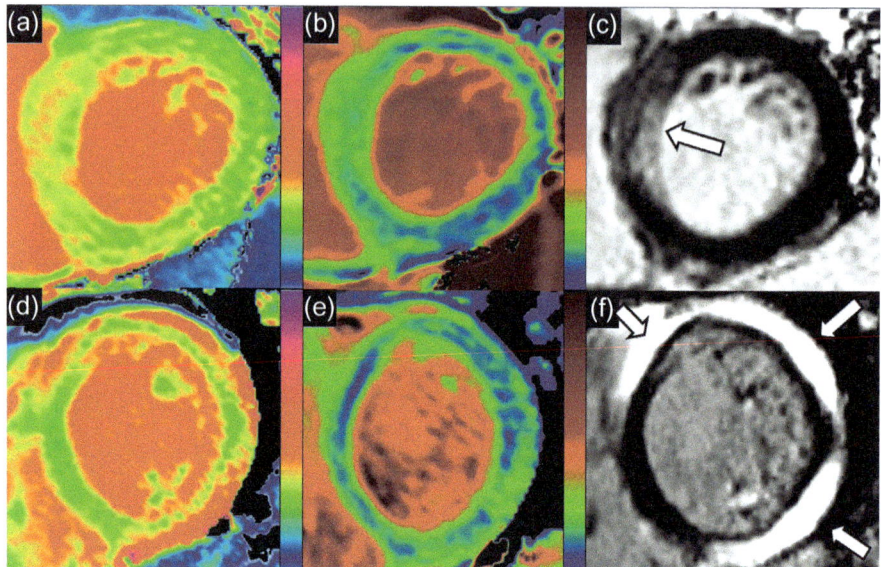

Figure 6.8 (From left to right) T1-mapping, T2-mapping and late gadolinium enhancement (LGE) imaging . (Top row) In a patient with acute myocardial infarction, LGE imaging showed subendocardial enhancement with near-transmurality in the septum (c, arrow). T1-mapping (a) showed significantly increased T1 values in the area of acute myocardial injury compared to remote myocardium with a step-down in T1 values (green) in the subendocardial infarct core. T2-mapping (b) demonstrated increased T2 in the area of infarction compared to remote myocardium. (Bottom row) In a patient with severe acute myocarditis, LGE imaging showed extensive, global subepicardial enhancement (f, arrows), sparing only the inferior septum. T1-mapping (d) showed significantly increased T1 values (red) in the areas of LGE enhancement, and T2-mapping (e) showed increased T2 in those areas.

[42–46] and was shown to be highly reproducible with a tight and stable normal range [42]. T1 values are sensitive to increased free water content [49–51], whether due to acute edema or pooling within an expanded interstitial space, and increased T1 times are observed in a number of common cardiac conditions (Figure 6.8), including acute myocardial edema [52], myocardial infarction [51,53–55], myocarditis [56,57], hypertrophic and dilated cardiomyopathy [58–60], cardiac amyloidosis [61,62], cardiac involvement in systemic diseases [59,60,63–66], and diffuse fibrosis, with histopathologic correlation in the latter [67]. Native myocardial T1 values may be lowered by fat or iron content and thus are also useful in characterizing Anderson-Fabry disease [68,69], fat in cardiac masses [70], and myocardial iron overload [71,72]. The main advantage of native T1-mapping is that it does not require intravenous administration of contrast agents, saving time, cost, and improving patient comfort. This is particularly useful in patients with contraindication to gadolinium-based contrast agents. Native T1-mapping can display nonischemic patterns of myocardial injury previously only possible using late gadolinium enhanced imaging [73] and can potentially be used in the future for gadolinium-free CMR protocols.

6.5.1.2 Postcontrast T1 mapping

Postcontrast T1-mapping estimates myocardial T1 values at a fixed time point after the injection of gadolinium contrast agents, which shorten T1 times. Postcontrast T1 values depend on a number of factors, including the type and dosage of gadolinium contrast used, the postcontrast acquisition time, body fat percentage, hematocrit, and renal function [74–76]. Isolated (single time-point) postcontrast T1-mapping has been shown to detect significantly lower T1 values in myocardial infarction [55,77], cardiomyopathy [59,60,78], amyloidosis [79], and diffuse myocardial fibrosis [80–83], but is insufficient to measure ECV when compared against histology and ECV mapping [75]. These, together with the difficulty in directly comparing isolated postcontrast T1 values between subjects, may limit its reproducibility and clinical applicability as a quantitative technique [84].

6.5.1.3 Extracellular volume (ECV) estimation and mapping

Expansion of the myocardial interstitial space may serve as a marker for myocardial fibrosis in a number of myocardial diseases [67,75,76,85–87]. It is possible to quantify the myocardial interstitial space in the human myocardium, as demonstrated *in vitro* using gadolinium-enhanced MRI [88], and *in vivo* using equilibrium contrast cardiovascular magnetic resonance (EQ-CMR) [89], both with good correlation to collagen volume fraction (CVF) [88–90]. ECV can be estimated using the formula:

$$\text{Extracellular volume fraction}(\text{ECV}) = \lambda \times (1 - \text{hematocrit}) \tag{6.1}$$

where the partition coefficient $\lambda = \dfrac{(1/T1)_{\text{postcontrast myocardium}} - (1/T1)_{\text{precontrast myocardium}}}{(1/T1)_{\text{postcontrast blood}} - (1/T1)_{\text{precontrast blood}}}$

and requires a constant infusion of contrast, which can be time-consuming for practical applications. This state of equilibrium can be closely approximated by the bolus contrast technique with delayed (15 min) postcontrast measurement, known as dynamic-equilibrium (DynEq) CMR [76]. ECV appears to be slightly higher in women [45,91] and to increase with age, both in healthy human cohorts [45,92] and in mice, with strong correlation to the extent of myocardial fibrosis [92]. Increased myocardial ECV has been shown in myocardial infarction, myocarditis, hypertrophic, and dilated cardiomyopathy, cardiac amyloidosis, diabetes, obesity, and other cardiac conditions with diffuse myocardial fibrosis (Figure 6.9) [65,66,88,93–99]. ECV calculation can correct for some of the variables confounding isolated postcontrast T1-mapping, and is less dependent on magnetic field strength than T1 values. However, the number of variables required can magnify noise and variability within the technique. Its accuracy also relies on the assumption that contrast concentration is equal in a strict two-compartment model, but can be affected by incomplete dynamic equilibrium, contrast transfer into other compartments, and a faster renal clearance than exchange rate between compartments [75]. Like native T1 times, expansion of ECV is nonspecific and can be due to reasons other than myocardial fibrosis, such as edema or infiltrative diseases.

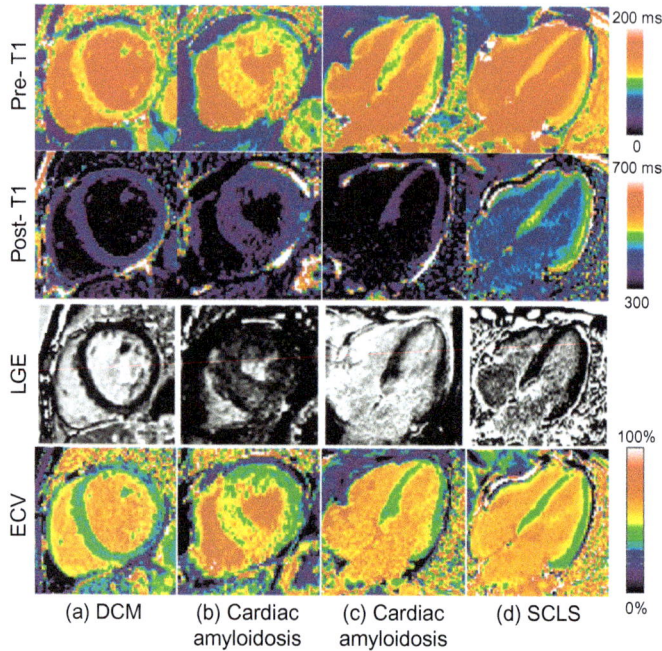

Figure 6.9 Examples illustrating cases with diffuse abnormalities in myocardial ECV, which are challenging to assess with conventional LGE. Precontrast T1-maps (top row), postcontrast T1-maps (second row), late gadolinium enhancement (third row), and ECV maps (bottom row) for patients with various cardiomyopathies: (a) nonischemic DCM with diffusely elevated ECV and normal appearing LGE, (b) cardiac amyloidosis with "patchy" LGE enhancement, (c) cardiac amyloidosis with diffusely elevated ECV and globally nulled LGE, and (d) systemic capillary leak syndrome (SCLS) with globally elevated ECV due to edema and normal LGE.
As originally published by Biomed Central in [93].

6.5.2 T2 mapping

Myocardial T2 (spin-spin) time is strongly correlated to myocardial water content and edema in animal studies [49,100]. T2-mapping is sensitive to detecting changes in acute myocardial infarction, myocarditis (Figure 6.8), and heart transplant rejection [101–106]. T2-mapping [107], as well as native T1-mapping [52], can circumvent many of the technical limitations of conventional T2-weighted imaging for edema [108], which rely on comparisons of relative signal intensities and reference regions of interest to detect changes within the myocardium. However, at high heart rates, incomplete T1 recovery may result in T1-weighting and underestimation of T2 relaxation times on SSFP-based T2-maps, although increasing the TR may circumvent this issue [101]. T2-mapping is found to be reproducible and feasible in differentiating edematous from normal myocardium; like other quantitative mapping techniques, it is susceptible to partial volume affects and motion, which can result in false positive findings [101,107,109].

6.5.3 T2* mapping

T2* relaxation time is shortened by paramagnetic molecules, such as iron and oxygen, which induce local magnetic field inhomogeneity. T2* imaging (Figure 6.10) has applications in detecting myocardial iron overload, intramyocardial hemorrhage, reperfusion injury in acute myocardial infarction [111–113] or, in conjunction with BOLD imaging, assessment of tissue oxygenation, myocardial perfusion reserve, or vasodilatory function [114]. Conventional myocardial T2* mapping can be challenging due to relatively long breath-holds, artifacts due to fast-flowing blood, and susceptibility artifacts in areas of B_0 field inhomogeneity, resulting in image distortion and signal loss [115,116]. As T1 relaxation times are also shortened by paramagnetic molecules with fewer technical limitations, native T1-mapping has been proven superior to T2* imaging in detecting myocardial iron overload [71,72] and may have a role where T2* imaging has proven useful.

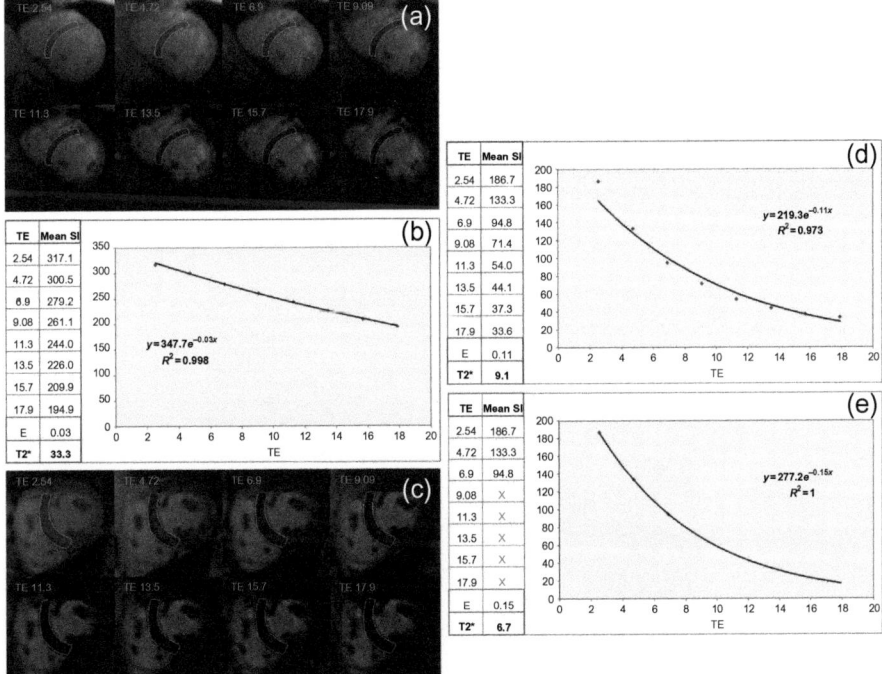

Figure 6.10 T2* imaging to assess myocardial iron overload. (a) T2* scan of a normal heart showing slow signal loss with increasing TE. (b) Decay curve for normal heart. T2*=33.3 ms. (c) Heavily iron overloaded heart. Note there is substantial signal loss at TE=9.09. (d) Decay curve for heavily iron overloaded heart showing rapid signal loss with increasing TE. The curve plateaus as myocardial SI falls below background noise. (e) Values for higher TEs are removed (truncation method) resulting in a better curve fit and a lower T2* value. As originally published by BioMed Central in [110].

6.5.4 Future directions

One of the challenges of current mapping techniques is the limited resolution and the resulting partial volume effect, leading to difficulty in characterizing the apex, right ventricle, and atrial walls. The establishment of comparable reference normal ranges and thresholds for detecting disease across different platforms is important for general clinical application [84]. Further validation of mapping techniques against histopathology is much needed to elucidate the exact mechanisms for the detected signal changes. Ongoing efforts to render mapping techniques more applicable in the clinical setting may include even faster imaging times, immunity to tachyarrhythmia, free-breathing methods, and immediate visual diagnostic maps with minimal postprocessing steps. Ultra high-field (e.g., 7 T) CMR for human applications provide further opportunities to explore the diagnostic capabilities of mapping techniques [117,118].

6.6 Three-dimensional time-resolved (4D) flow

6.6.1 Introduction

To image the blood flow within the heart and great vessels (Figure 6.11), 3-dimensional time-resolved flow (4D flow) acquires magnitude (anatomical) and velocity encoded (flow) images in one sequence acquisition. Currently, the average acquisition time is 10–25 min for a 4D flow assessment of the aorta and 20–40 min for an assessment of the whole heart. To reduce breathing artifacts, the 4D flow sequence is respiratory

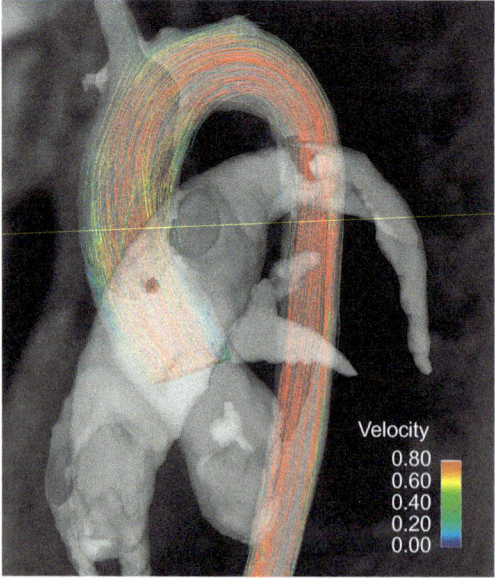

Figure 6.11 4D flow MRI in the aorta of a healthy volunteer.

gated, using only the images acquired in end-expiration. Data quality can be improved by using intra-vascular gadolinium based contrast agents or a higher magnetic field strength. Once the data acquisition is complete, the dataset can be visualized off-line using a variety of postprocessing tools, some of which are commercially available. Additionally, a number of quantifications can be made using the 4D flow dataset. For aortic flow, these include parameters such as wall shear stress (a measure to estimate the friction of the blood volume against the vessel wall), pulse wave velocity (a measure of arterial stiffness), the flow angle at which the blood jets leave the aortic valve, and the amount of helical, rotational, and turbulent blood flow. Quantification within the heart often also requires separate anatomical images to be acquired in the same CMR scan for co-localization with the 4D flow dataset to aid anatomical orientation. This then allows quantification of intra-cardiac kinetic energy, flow volumes, and assessment of ventricular efficiency.

6.6.2 Flow in the aorta—clinical applications

Advanced flow assessment in the aorta using 4D flow MRI has been used in a variety of pathologies, the most intensively studied being bicuspid aortic valve disease. Visualization of the ascending aortic blood flow has revealed a marked helical (anterograde rotational movement) blood flow pattern [119] with an increased wall shear stress [120], which have shown an association with aortic dilation [121]. In the future, these 4D flow measurements might form new imaging biomarkers for risk stratification of aortic dilation in bicuspid aortic valve disease. In contrast, aortic aneurysms with a tricuspid aortic valve have shown a decrease in wall shear stress and an increase in vortical flow pattern [122]. As an increase in wall shear stress is thought to be a risk factor, 4D flow assessment for risk stratification may prove less useful in this patient group. Marfan syndrome also showed a marked increase in vortical flow in the sinuses and an increase in helical flow in the proximal descending aorta [123], which may explain the increased risk for aortic dissection in these areas in Marfan syndrome. 4D flow MRI has also been used to assess the effectiveness of different surgical methods, such as the preservation of vortical flow in the sinuses of Valsalva in different aortic root replacement techniques with valve-sparing surgery [124]. Furthermore, aortic and pulmonary blood flow has been assessed in different surgical approaches of the arterial switch procedure in transposition of the great arteries [125]. 4D flow MRI has also been used in congenital heart disease to assess collaterals in aortic coarctation, as well as remaining flow disturbances within the aortic lumen after coarctation repair [126].

6.6.3 Flow in the heart—clinical applications

Clinical applications for intra-cardiac flow visualization and quantification are still in the early stages and are likely to expand in the coming years. Flow quantification has been proven useful in heart failure [127]. In patients with clinically compensated dilated cardiomyopathy and mild LV remodeling, 4D flow analysis already revealed marked changes in kinetic energy, flow volumes, and reduced ventricular efficiency [128]. Changes have also been shown in atrial fibrillation where intra-atrial hemodynamics were improved in patients who have undergone cardioversion compared to those that suffered from persistent atrial fibrillation [129]. In congenital heart disease, 4D flow MRI now allows a more detailed assessment of the extra-cardiac conduit in the Fontan circulation. Differential flow assessment can now quantify the amount of inferior and superior vena cava flow that enters the right and left pulmonary artery, respectively [130].

6.6.4 Challenges and future directions

The main challenges in 4D flow MRI are the currently long acquisition time with a relatively low temporal resolution (40 ms) and the complex analysis process. Commercially developed software is becoming available that allows easy visualization, and research groups are working on automating the data analysis process for quantification. Further sequence development is aimed at reducing the acquisition time. All of these developments are essential to enable integration of 4D flow MRI into clinical practice. This will allow comprehensive flow assessment in, for example, complex congenital heart disease in a single acquisition sequence. In time, it might also be used as a more sensitive imaging biomarker for risk stratification of patients who are susceptible to aortic dissection, and in planning surgical and catheter interventions. 4D flow MRI may also prove useful in monitoring treatment effects.

6.7 Magnetic resonance spectroscopy

6.7.1 Background

MRS is the only noninvasive imaging technique that allows measurements of cardiac metabolism *in vivo* without relying on external radioactive tracers (see [131] for a review). Many nuclei can be investigated with MRS: the most relevant ones for cardiac spectroscopy are ^{1}H, ^{31}P, and ^{13}C. In addition to H_2O, ^{1}H MRS detects a large number of other metabolites, such as total creatine, lactate, deoxymyoglobin, and, most importantly, myocardial triglyceride (fat) content. ^{31}P MRS provides a window into cardiac energy metabolism, in particular adenosine triphosphate (ATP) and phosphocreatine (PCr). ^{13}C MRS allows assessment of various metabolic pathways of intermediary metabolism such as glycolysis, Krebs cycle flux, or beta-oxidation. The great limitation of MRS is that its signals are about 100,000 times weaker than the signals interrogated in standard MR imaging. For that reason, temporal and spatial resolution of MRS is poor, and the method is currently limited to research studies.

6.7.1.1 Technical considerations (see [132] for a review)

Most human cardiac MRS studies have employed the ^{31}P nucleus. The only hardware requirement on top of the standard MRI equipment is a nucleus-specific MR coil (e.g., ^{31}P-coil) and, secondly, a broadband RF transmitter. To excite nonproton nuclei, specific spectroscopy acquisition sequences and postprocessing techniques are required. Before acquiring spectroscopy data, the magnetic field has to be homogenized by careful shimming. Using one of several available localization sequences, we obtain a spectroscopy signal limited to one or several voxels in the heart. For an MR spectrum, many RF pulses have to be applied and their resulting signals, the free induction decays (FIDs), have to be signal averaged to obtain a ^{31}P spectrum with sufficient SNR. Correction factors have to be applied for the effects of saturation and blood contamination. The resulting ^{31}P MR spectrum (Figure 6.12) then allows quantification of the relative concentrations of each metabolite. Absolute quantification in mmol/l is more difficult and has only been done in a few pilot studies. A typical ^{31}P spectrum shows six resonances: three peaks for the three ^{31}P-atoms of ATP (alpha, beta and gamma), PCr, 2,3-diphosphoglycerate (from erythrocytes), and phosphodiesters (signal from membrane phospholipids). The ratio of PCr to ATP (PCr/ATP ratio) provides a powerful index of the energetic state of the heart. Whenever ATP demand outstrips supply, phosphocreatine levels fall, lowering the PCr/ATP ratio. The PCr/ATP ratio is also sensitive to changes in the total creatine pool, which can occur in

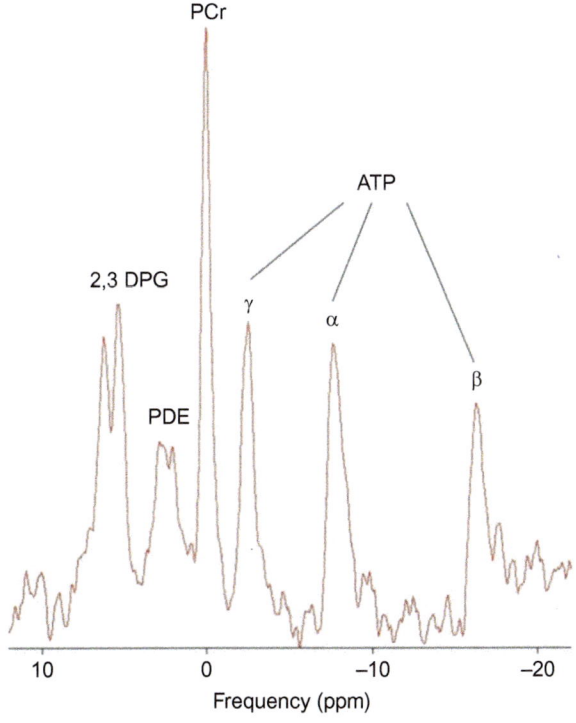

Figure 6.12 A typical ^{31}P spectrum shows six resonances: three peaks for the three ^{31}P-atoms of ATP (alpha, beta, and gamma), PCr, 2,3-diphosphoglycerate (from erythrocytes), and phosphodiesters (signal from membrane phospholipids). The ratio of PCr to ATP (PCr/ATP ratio) provides a powerful index of the energetic state of the heart.

hypertrophy and heart failure [133]. Typically, at 1.5 T, ^{31}P spectra are obtained from 20 to 70 ml voxels in 20–40 min, with a measurement variability for PCr/ATP of 15%. At higher fields strengths (3 T, 7 T) substantial SNR gains can be achieved.

The ^{1}H nucleus has great potential for spectroscopy, as a large number of resonances can theoretically be quantified [134–136]. However, many of those are not yet identified and, in addition, many are overlapping. Most important is the measurement of myocardial lipid (triglyceride) content. For ^{1}H MRS, the strong water signal needs to be suppressed with an additional MR pulse. ^{13}C MRS studies are currently severely limited by its very low SNR, but, as will be explained in the following section, ^{13}C hyperpolarization offers an exciting new technology, increasing spectroscopy signal by five orders of magnitude [137].

6.7.2 Clinical applications of MRS

6.7.2.1 Ischemic heart disease

With the PCr/ATP ratio exquisitely sensitive to any imbalance between oxygen demand and supply, ^{31}P MRS is in principle a powerful technique to detect the presence of myocardial ischemia [138]. Secondly, ^{31}P MRS can in principle be used to identify viable versus nonviable myocardium, as viable myocardium contains normal levels of ATP and PCr, while nonviable myocardium contains negligible amounts. Although in principle highly promising as an intrinsic contrast method, currently clinical ^{31}P MRS is practically limited by its low spatial and temporal resolution and therefore remains a research tool.

6.7.2.2 Heart failure

The failing heart is "an engine out of fuel," and deranged cardiac energetics are thought to be a major player in the development of chronic heart failure [133]. Accordingly, clinical ^{31}P MRS studies have demonstrated a reduction of the PCr/ATP ratio in heart failure [139,140]. Furthermore, the PCr/ATP ratio is a powerful indicator of prognosis [141]. Newer developments in heart failure are the measurement of absolute concentrations of high-energy phosphates [142] and the measurement of ATP turnover (creatine kinase flux) with MRS saturation transfer methods.

MRS is highly suited to monitor the response of the failing myocardium to therapy [140].

More recently, improvements in the PCr/ATP ratio have been demonstrated by novel metabolic agents such as trimetazidine or allopurinol [143,144]. In the future, it is possible that assessment of the energetic response of the myocardium to novel heart failure drugs may emerge as a surrogate imaging biomarker for their long-term prognostic effects.

6.7.2.3 Other pathologies

Reduced PCr/ATP ratios and steatosis have also been shown in patients with aortic stenosis [145,146]. HCM shows derangement of cardiac energetics independent of the degree of hypertrophy [147]. Diabetes [148] and obesity [149] also lead to impairment in myocardial energetics as demonstrated by ^{31}P MRS and weight loss can normalize energetic abnormalities [150].

6.7.3 Future developments

Cardiac MR spectroscopy has been around for several decades and, while providing many important scientific insights into cardiac metabolism, has not yet been established as a routine clinical method. However, two recent developments give reason for optimism. Firstly, very high field magnets, such as 7 T, have now become a realistic possibility, and we have recently shown that ^{31}P MRS at 7T shows very substantial gains in signal to noise [151]. Secondly, the innovative technique of hyperpolarized ^{13}C MRS allows us to bring the spectroscopy signal almost up to the level of the standard MRI signal, thus opening the possibility of rapid, high-resolution metabolic studies in patients with heart disease. These opportunities will be explained in the subsequent section.

6.8 Hyperpolarization

6.8.1 Introduction

As described in the previous section, one of the major limitations of magnetic resonance (MR) spectroscopy is the low SNR. This limitation results from a combination of factors, including the low concentration of metabolites under study, the inherently low sensitivity of nuclei other than protons (e.g., ^{31}P, ^{23}Na, ^{19}F), and the low natural abundance of certain nuclei (e.g., ^{13}C).

The recent development of a novel technique referred to as "hyperpolarization" based on a process called dynamic nuclear polarization (DNP), has provided a means to overcome this fundamental limitation of MR spectroscopy [152]. Hyperpolarization aims to generate an injectable compound whose signal is temporarily enhanced by several orders of magnitude, enabling enzyme-controlled reactions to be monitored *in vivo* in real time.

While several other hyperpolarization techniques have also been developed, including the optical pumping of noble gasses, parahydrogen-induced polarization (PHIP), and brute force polarization, the aim of this section is to describe the development and application of hyperpolarization via the DNP process for the assessment of metabolism in the normal and diseased heart [137].

6.8.2 Hyperpolarization theory

When a sample is placed in a magnetic field, the nuclei inside act like small bar magnets, aligning either in the same direction as the magnetic field or in the opposite direction. This generates two different populations with slightly different energy levels. At room temperatures, the difference between these two populations is very small, leading to a very low signal (low polarization, Figure 6.13a). The process of

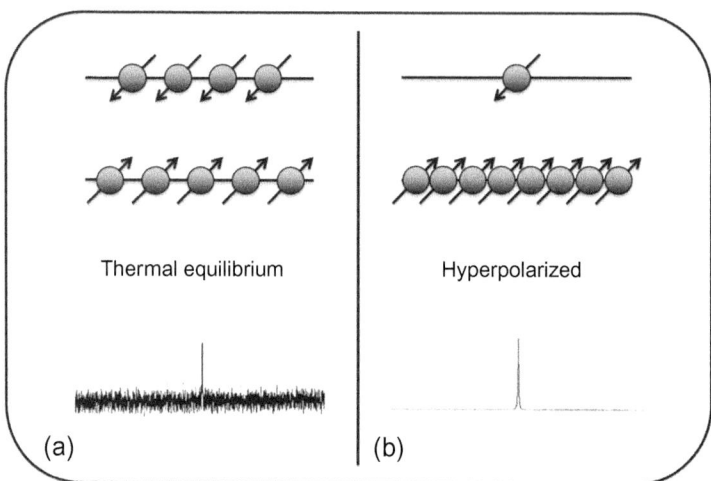

Figure 6.13 Polarization enhancement through hyperpolarization. (a) At thermal equilibrium there are a similar number of spins in the two energy states leading to a low polarization and an inherently low signal-to-noise ratio. (b) Following the process of hyperpolarization, there is an excess of spins in the lower energy level leading to an enhanced polarization and increased signal-to-noise ratio.

hyperpolarization forces the nuclei from the higher energy state (aligned against the magnetic field) into the lower energy state (aligned with the magnetic field), generating a large difference in the population of the two energy levels (high polarization) and therefore a dramatically enhanced signal (Figure 6.13b) [153].

6.8.3 Methodological considerations

To achieve this large enhancement in sensitivity, it is necessary to mix the sample to be hyperpolarized (which is enriched with ^{13}C) with a source of free electrons (called a radical). This mixture is then cooled to very low temperatures (~1 K) inside a high magnetic field (3–5 T) and irradiated with microwaves at a frequency defined by the properties of the sample, the radical, and the strength of the magnetic field. The polarization of the sample enhances slowly over a period of 1–2 h [153]. When a steady-state level of polarization has been achieved, the sample is rapidly dissolved using a bolus of superheated liquid to generate a tracer, which is suitable for injection [152]. The enhanced polarization then decays over a period of several minutes, depending on the sample under study.

6.8.4 Review of preclinical literature

There has been great interest in the application of hyperpolarization in the fields of both oncology [154] and cardiology [137], with most interest focusing on the metabolism of hyperpolarized pyruvate. Pyruvate has been extensively studied as it hyperpolarizes well (polarization levels of 30–50%), has a relatively long decay time (3–5 min) and holds a key position in the metabolic breakdown of carbohydrates.

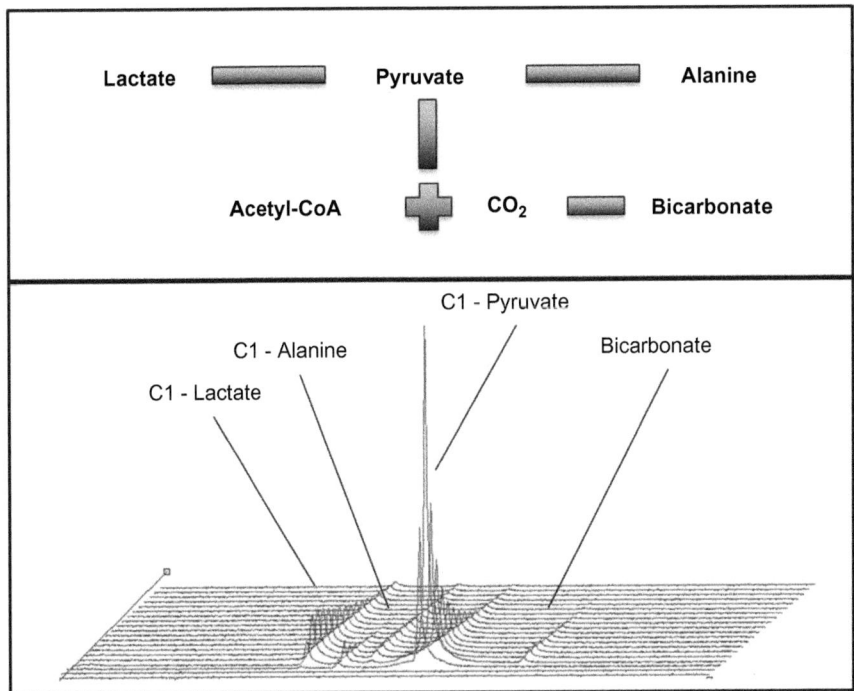

Figure 6.14 Metabolism of hyperpolarized [1-^{13}C]pyruvate. Conversion of the hyperpolarized pyruvate into lactate (via lactate dehydrogenase), alanine (via alanine aminotransferase), and bicarbonate (via pyruvate dehydrogenase and carbonic anhydrase) can be observed.

Initial studies with pyruvate labeled with ^{13}C at the first carbon position ([1-^{13}C] pyruvate) were undertaken in the remotely perfused rat heart and demonstrated that conversion of pyruvate into lactate (via lactate dehydrogenase), alanine (via alanine aminotransferase), and CO_2/bicarbonate (via pyruvate dehydrogenase and carbonic anhydrase) could be observed with high temporal resolution (Figure 6.14) [155]. This work was rapidly transferred to the *in vivo* heart, where Schroeder and colleagues demonstrated that the flux of ^{13}C pyruvate through pyruvate dehydrogenase (PDH) offered a sensitive measure of disease severity in the type 1 diabetic rat heart [156].

In addition to pyruvate labeled with ^{13}C at the first carbon position, work has also been undertaken with pyruvate labeled with ^{13}C at the second carbon position ([2-^{13}C] pyruvate). Schroeder and colleagues have shown, in both the perfused [157] and *in vivo* rat heart [158], that the conversion of hyperpolarized pyruvate, via acetyl-CoA, into intermediates of the TCA cycle can be monitored in real time (Figure 6.15).

In addition to monitoring enzymatic fluxes, the utility of hyperpolarized pyruvate to monitor treatment response has been demonstrated in a rat model of cardiac hypertrophy [159]. Atherton and colleagues demonstrated that following treatment with the PDH activator, dichloroacetate, the level of hypertrophy was reduced as PDH flux was restored.

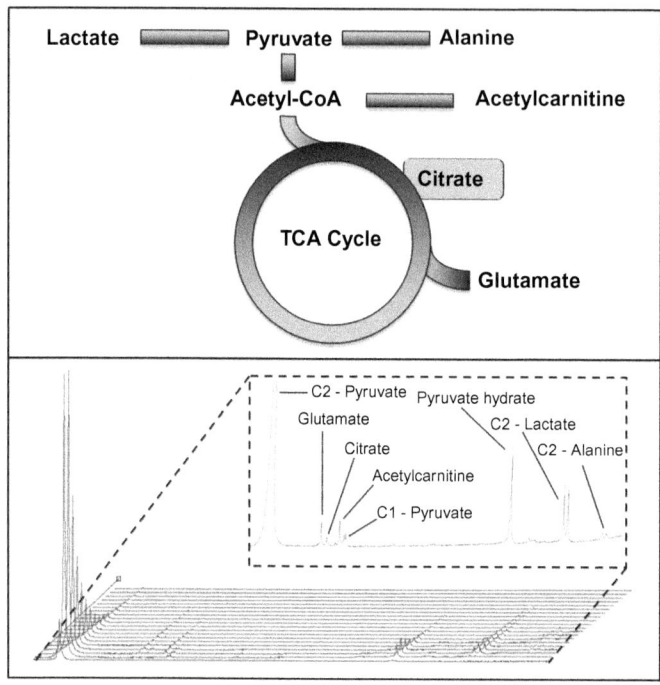

Figure 6.15 Metabolism of hyperpolarized [2-^{13}C]pyruvate. Conversion of the hyperpolarized pyruvate into the TCA cycle intermediates citrate and glutamate can be observed along with the production of acetylcarnitine via carnitine acetyltransferase.

A great deal of developmental work has also been undertaken to extend these spectroscopic studies into imaging studies, whereby the spatial distribution of metabolism can be mapped. Lau et al. have demonstrated a rapid imaging technique, which can map the distribution of pyruvate, lactate, and bicarbonate in a single breath-hold [160]. Such sequences have been applied in the setting of myocardial infarction [161] and dilated cardiomyopathy (Figure 6.16) [162] to explore the spatial variation of pathological metabolism.

6.8.5 Future clinical perspectives

The success of these preclinical studies, alongside similar studies in the field of oncology, has led to the first clinical trial of this novel technique at the University of California in San Francisco. With approval from the FDA, a phase 1 ascending-dose study was undertaken to assess the safety, tolerability, and imaging potential of hyperpolarized pyruvate in subjects with prostate cancer (http://clinicaltrials.gov/show/NCT01229618). Initial results indicate that the conversion of hyperpolarized pyruvate into hyperpolarized lactate may prove to be a useful marker of malignancy [163]. Whilst the accumulation of lactate in tumors is well known, hyperpolarization is currently the only technique to be able to assess the level of lactate noninvasively in humans. The development of a

Magnetic resonance imaging 155

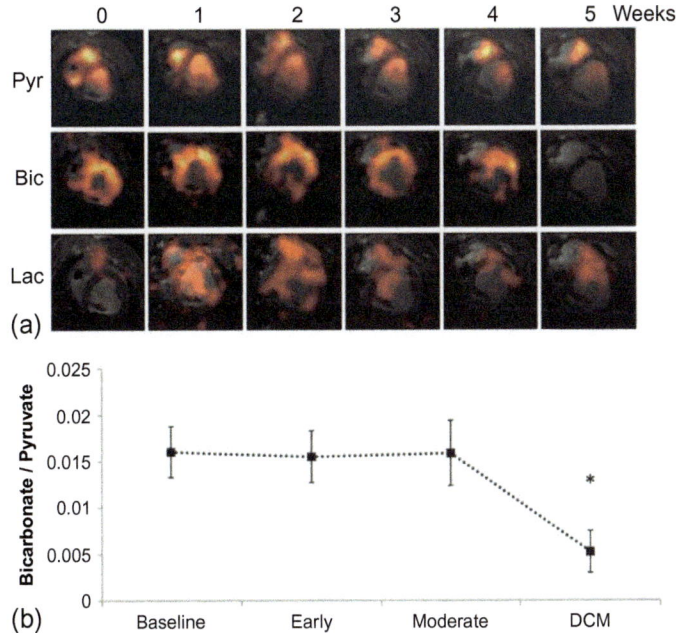

Figure 6.16 Imaging the metabolism of hyperpolarized [1-^{13}C]pyruvate in the failing pig heart. (a) Imaging the spatial distribution of pyruvate, bicarbonate, and lactate in the pig heart during the progression into heart failure. (b) Quantification of the images in (a) shows that the production of bicarbonate from hyperpolarized pyruvate is only reduced in the later stages of heart failure. Figure reproduced with permission from Schroeder et al. Hyperpolarized C-13 magnetic resonance reveals early and late-onset changes to *in vivo* pyruvate metabolism in the failing heart. Schroeder et al. [162]

commercial hyperpolarizer system capable of generating sterile tracers suitable for human injection [164] means that the translation of cardiac hyperpolarization studies from animals into humans is just around the corner [137].

6.9 Latest technical developments and future trends

Technical developments will continue to push the boundaries in making CMR faster and easier with expanding diagnostic capabilities that could assess even more aspects of the human cardiovascular system, myocardial tissue characteristics and metabolism. Hardware advances such as high-field (3 T) and ultra-high-field (7 T) MR systems [165–168] promise to deliver higher SNRs, image spatial resolution, and contrast. Phased array coils, multiple receiver channel systems, and parallel transmit technology work toward improving sensitivity and speed. Methods such as undersampling of k-space, noncartesian acquisitions, and compressed sensing all contribute toward decreasing imaging times, while single heartbeat acquisition in real time will facilitate acute cardiac imaging and CMR-guided interventions. Rapid whole-heart single breath-hold methods [169,170] and automated acquisition and image postprocessing [171] may provide cost-effective and high through-put strategies to help transition CMR into widespread clinical practice.

MR angiography (MRA) of the coronary arteries will benefit from high-field CMR with higher SNR, improved spatial resolution, and shorter acquisition times to better visualize distal and branch coronary segments [172,173]. Imaging of the vessel wall to assess plaque characteristics is also important to the evaluation of atherosclerotic CAD [174]; intravascular CMR at high field-strength using loopless CMR detectors has been shown to provide high-resolution images of atherosclerotic plaques including fibrous cap thickness over a range of about 100–1000 µm [175]. As discussed, 4D flow assessments may improve care in congenital heart disease, valvular and aortic diseases, and possibly in planning interventions tailored to flow dynamics unique to the individual.

Nongadolinium contrast techniques may be desirable to achieve wider clinical applicability and cost savings. Stress perfusion imaging may also be combined with arterial spin labeling (ASL), or mapping techniques in addition to BOLD imaging to avoid gadolinium administration. Mapping techniques appear to be highly sensitive to myocardial water, and may open the field to quantitative, gadolinium-free CMR imaging. Ultrashort echo time (UTE) imaging of very short T2 components in tissues may allow detection of fibrosis and calcification in the myocardium and atherosclerotic plaques [176–178]. Molecular imaging [174,179–181], by linking MR contrast agents to a ligand that targets specific molecules, receptors, or cell surface markers, may shed insights into disease mechanisms, improve diagnosis, drug delivery, targeted treatment, and monitoring of disease course.

Myocyte structure and metabolism may also be imaged using CMR. Diffusion tensor imaging (DTI) [182] allows the examination of myocyte orientation and disarray, which is especially of interest in the study of HCM [183] and adverse cardiac remodeling. As discussed, MRS allows the noninvasive study of myocardial metabolism using nonproton nuclei like ^{13}C, ^{23}Na, ^{31}P without the need for radioactive tracers. Ultra high-field (7 T) imaging holds significant promise for improving the low SNR that has traditionally plagued MRS [151] while dynamic nuclear polarization (DNP) of ^{13}C allows the examination of metabolic pathways (^{13}C-pyruvate) and tissue pH (^{13}C-bicarbonate).

To summarize, CMR will become more integrated into widespread clinical practice as technical advances facilitate better diagnostic image quality and ease of application both for health care professionals and patients. CMR holds the most promise to become the "one-stop shop" cardiac imaging modality able to assess the whole heart noninvasively without the need for radiation or exogenous contrast agents.

6.10 Sources of further information

6.10.1 Selected reference texts

- Cardiovascular magnetic resonance, 2nd ed. by Manning WJ, Pennell DJ (April 19, 2010).
- MRI and CT of the cardiovascular system by Higgins CB, Albert de Roos MD (August 12, 2013).
- Cardiovascular magnetic resonance imaging: textbook and atlas by Hombach V, Merkle N, Rasche V (November 1, 2012).

- Cardiovascular magnetic resonance spectroscopy by Schaefer S. Balaban RS (December 21, 2012).
- Magnetic resonance angiography: principles and applications by Carr JC, Carroll TJ (January 17, 2012).
- Magnetic resonance imaging of congenital heart disease by Syed MA, Mohiaddin RH (December 18, 2012)
- Cardiovascular magnetic resonance (Oxford Specialist Handbooks in Cardiology) by Myerson S, Francis JM, Neubauer S (April 19, 2010).
- Cardiovascular MR manual by Plein S, Greenwood J, Ridgway JP (December 27, 2010)
- Atlas of cardiovascular magnetic resonance (Current Medicine) by Manning WJ, Braunwald E (January 30, 2009).

6.10.2 Professional bodies

- European Association of Cardiovascular Imaging (EACVI) (www.escardio.org)
- European Society of Cardiology (www.escardio.org)
- The Society for Cardiovascular Magnetic Resonance (www.scmr.org)
- British Society of Cardiovascular Magnetic Resonance (www.bscmr.org)
- Canadian Society for CMR (www.canscmr.org)
- International Society for Magnetic Resonance in Medicine (www.ismrm.org)
- British Society of Cardiovascular Imaging (www.bsci.org.uk)
- The North American Society for Cardiac Imaging (www.nasci.org)
- Radiological Society of North America (www.rsna.org)
- American College of Cardiology (www.acc.org)
- American College of Radiology (www.acr.org)
- American Heart Association (www.heart.org)
- British Cardiac Society (www.bcs.com)

6.10.3 MRI safety

- www.mrisafety.com
- www.FDA.gov/cdrh/safety/mrisafety.html
- www.magneticresonancesafetytesting.com
- www.imrser.org

Acknowledgments

The authors of this chapter acknowledge BioMed Central as the original publisher of selected figures in this chapter as indicated by references to the original authors and publications. The authors also acknowledge Oxford University Press as the original publisher of Figure 6.16 reproduced with permission from Schroeder et al., hyperpolarized C-13 magnetic resonance reveals early- and late-onset changes to *in vivo* pyruvate metabolism in the failing heart [162].

VMF is funded by the National Institute for Health Research (NIHR) Oxford Biomedical Research Centre based at The Oxford University Hospitals NHS Trust and the University of Oxford. MDR is funded by the Medical Research Council. DT is funded by a British Heart Foundation Senior Research Fellowship (FS/14/17/30634). SN acknowledges support from the British Heart Foundation Centre of Research Excellence, Oxford, and from the Oxford NIHR Biomedical Research Centre.

References

[1] Hashemi RH, Bradley WG, Lisanti CJ. MRI: the basics. Philadelphia, PA: Lippincott Williams & Wilkins; 2010.
[2] Neubauer S. The failing heart–an engine out of fuel. N Engl J Med 2007;356:1140–51.
[3] Ridgway JP. Cardiovascular magnetic resonance physics for clinicians: part I. J Cardiovasc Magn Reson 2010;12:71.
[4] Coelho-Filho OR, Rickers C, Kwong RY, Jerosch-Herold M. MR myocardial perfusion imaging. Radiology 2013;266:701–15.
[5] Biglands JD, Radjenovic A, Ridway JP. Cardiovascular magnetic resonance physics for clinicians: part II. J Cardiovasc Magn Reson 2012;14:66.
[6] Shellock FG, Kanal E. Magnetic resonance: bioeffects, safety, and patient management. Philadelphia: Lippincott-Raven; 1996.
[7] Nayak KS, Hu BS. The future of real-time cardiac magnetic resonance imaging. Curr Cardiol Rep 2005;7:45–51.
[8] Chrispin A, Small P, Rutter N, Coupland RE, Doyle M, Chapman B, et al. Echo planar imaging of normal and abnormal connections of the heart and great arteries. Pediatr Radiol 1986;16:289–92.
[9] Sakuma H, Takeda K, Higgins CB. Fast magnetic resonance imaging of the heart. Eur J Radiol 1999;29:101–13.
[10] Stehling MK, Turner R, Mansfield P. Echo-planar imaging: magnetic resonance imaging in a fraction of a second. Science 1991;254:43–50.
[11] Delattre BM, Heidemann RM, Crowe LA, Vallee JP, Hyacinthe JN. Spiral demystified. Magn Reson Imaging 2010;28:862–81.
[12] Meyer CH, Hu BS, Nishimura DG, Macovski A. Fast spiral coronary artery imaging. Magn Reson Med 1992;28:202–13.
[13] Larkman DJ, Nunes RG. Parallel magnetic resonance imaging. Phys Med Biol 2007;52:R15–55.
[14] Tsao J, Boesiger P, Pruessmann KP. k-t BLAST and k-t SENSE: dynamic MRI with high frame rate exploiting spatiotemporal correlations. Magn Reson Med 2003;50:1031–42.
[15] Bruder O, Wagner A, Lombardi M, Schwitter J, Van Rossum A, Pilz G, et al. European cardiovascular magnetic resonance (EuroCMR) registry–multi national results from 57 centers in 15 countries. J Cardiovasc Magn Reson 2013;15:9.
[16] Friedrich MG, Karamitsos TD. Oxygenation-sensitive cardiovascular magnetic resonance. J Cardiovasc Magn Reson 2013;15:43.
[17] Lipinski MJ, Mcvey CM, Berger JS, Kramer CM, Salerno M. Prognostic value of stress cardiac magnetic resonance imaging in patients with known or suspected coronary artery disease: a systematic review and meta-analysis. J Am Coll Cardiol; 2013.
[18] Arai AE. Magnetic resonance imaging for area at risk, myocardial infarction, and myocardial salvage. J Cardiovasc Pharmacol Ther 2011;16:313–20.
[19] Kim RJ, Fieno DS, Parrish TB, Harris K, Chen EL, Simonetti O, et al. Relationship of MRI delayed contrast enhancement to irreversible injury, infarct age, and contractile function. Circulation 1999;100:1992–2002.
[20] Simonetti OP, Kim RJ, Fieno DS, Hillenbrand HB, Wu E, Bundy JM, et al. An improved MR imaging technique for the visualization of myocardial infarction. Radiology 2001;218:215–23.
[21] Wagner A, Mahrholdt H, Holly TA, Elliott MD, Regenfus M, Parker M, et al. Contrast-enhanced MRI and routine single photon emission computed tomography (SPECT) per-

fusion imaging for detection of subendocardial myocardial infarcts: an imaging study. Lancet 2003;361:374–9.
[22] Kim RJ, Wu E, Rafael A, Chen EL, Parker MA, Simonetti O, et al. The use of contrast-enhanced magnetic resonance imaging to identify reversible myocardial dysfunction. N Engl J Med 2000;343:1445–53.
[23] Selvanayagam JB, Kardos A, Francis JM, Wiesmann F, Petersen SE, Taggart DP, et al. Value of delayed-enhancement cardiovascular magnetic resonance imaging in predicting myocardial viability after surgical revascularization. Circulation 2004;110:1535–41.
[24] Larose E, Rodes-Cabau J, Pibarot P, Rinfret S, Proulx G, Nguyen CM, et al. Predicting late myocardial recovery and outcomes in the early hours of ST-segment elevation myocardial infarction traditional measures compared with microvascular obstruction, salvaged myocardium, and necrosis characteristics by cardiovascular magnetic resonance. J Am Coll Cardiol 2010;55:2459–69.
[25] Wu KC, Zerhouni EA, Judd RM, Lugo-Olivieri CH, Barouch LA, Schulman SP, et al. Prognostic significance of microvascular obstruction by magnetic resonance imaging in patients with acute myocardial infarction. Circulation 1998;97:765–72.
[26] Karamitsos TD, Dall'armellina, E, Choudhury RP, Neubauer S. Ischemic heart disease: comprehensive evaluation by cardiovascular magnetic resonance. Am Heart J 2011;162:16–30.
[27] Cheng AS, Pegg TJ, Karamitsos TD, Searle N, Jerosch-Herold M, Choudhury RP, et al. Cardiovascular magnetic resonance perfusion imaging at 3-tesla for the detection of coronary artery disease: a comparison with 1.5-tesla. J Am Coll Cardiol 2007;49:2440–9.
[28] Lockie T, Ishida M, Perera D, Chiribiri A, De Silva K, Kozerke S, et al. High-resolution magnetic resonance myocardial perfusion imaging at 3.0-Tesla to detect hemodynamically significant coronary stenoses as determined by fractional flow reserve. J Am Coll Cardiol 2011;57:70–5.
[29] Greenwood JP, Maredia N, Younger JF, Brown JM, Nixon J, Everett CC, et al. Cardiovascular magnetic resonance and single-photon emission computed tomography for diagnosis of coronary heart disease (CE-MARC): a prospective trial. Lancet 2012;379:453–60.
[30] Hamon M, Fau G, Nee G, Ehtisham J, Morello R. Meta-analysis of the diagnostic performance of stress perfusion cardiovascular magnetic resonance for detection of coronary artery disease. J Cardiovasc Magn Reson 2010;12:29.
[31] Karamitsos TD, Arnold JR, Pegg TJ, Cheng AS, Van Gaal WJ, Francis JM, et al. Tolerance and safety of adenosine stress perfusion cardiovascular magnetic resonance imaging in patients with severe coronary artery disease. Int J Cardiovasc Imaging 2009;25:277–83.
[32] Klem I, Heitner JF, Shah DJ, Sketch Jr MH, Behar V, Weinsaft J, et al. Improved detection of coronary artery disease by stress perfusion cardiovascular magnetic resonance with the use of delayed enhancement infarction imaging. J Am Coll Cardiol 2006;47:1630–8.
[33] Nagel E, Klein C, Paetsch I, Hettwer S, Schnackenburg B, Wegscheider K, et al. Magnetic resonance perfusion measurements for the noninvasive detection of coronary artery disease. Circulation 2003;108:432–7.
[34] Wacker CM, Hartlep AW, Pfleger S, Schad LR, Ertl G, Bauer WR. Susceptibility-sensitive magnetic resonance imaging detects human myocardium supplied by a stenotic coronary artery without a contrast agent. J Am Coll Cardiol 2003;41:834–40.
[35] Karamitsos TD, Dass S, Suttie J, Sever E, Birks J, Holloway CJ, et al. Blunted myocardial oxygenation response during vasodilator stress in patients with hypertrophic cardiomyopathy. J Am Coll Cardiol 2013;61:1169–76.

[36] Karamitsos TD, Leccisotti L, Arnold JR, Recio-Mayoral A, Bhamra-Ariza P, Howells RK, et al. Relationship between regional myocardial oxygenation and perfusion in patients with coronary artery disease: insights from cardiovascular magnetic resonance and positron emission tomography. Circ Cardiovasc Imaging 2010;3:32–40.

[37] Jogiya R, Kozerke S, Morton G, De Silva K, Redwood S, Perera D, et al. Validation of dynamic 3-dimensional whole heart magnetic resonance myocardial perfusion imaging against fractional flow reserve for the detection of significant coronary artery disease. J Am Coll Cardiol 2012;60:756–65.

[38] Manka R, Paetsch I, Kozerke S, Moccetti M, Hoffmann R, Schroeder J, et al. Whole-heart dynamic three-dimensional magnetic resonance perfusion imaging for the detection of coronary artery disease defined by fractional flow reserve: determination of volumetric myocardial ischaemic burden and coronary lesion location. Eur Heart J 2012;33:2016–24.

[39] Yorimitsu M, Yokoyama K, Nitatori T, Yoshino H, Isono S, Kuhara S. Whole-heart 3D late gadolinium-enhanced MR imaging: investigation of optimal scan parameters and clinical usefulness. Magn Reson Med Sci 2012;11:9–16.

[40] Bottomley PA, Foster TH, Argersinger RE, Pfeifer LM. A review of normal tissue hydrogen NMR relaxation times and relaxation mechanisms from 1-100 MHz: dependence on tissue type, NMR frequency, temperature, species, excision, and age. Med Phys 1984;11:425–48.

[41] Messroghli DR, Plein S, Higgins DM, Walters K, Jones TR, Ridgway JP, et al. Human myocardium: single-breath-hold MR T1 mapping with high spatial resolution—reproducibility study. Radiology 2006;238:1004–12.

[42] Piechnik S, Ferreira V, Lewandowski A, Ntusi N, Banerjee R, Holloway C, et al. Normal variation of magnetic resonance T1 relaxation times in the human population at 1.5T using ShMOLLI. J Cardiovasc Magn Reson 2013;15:13.

[43] Messroghli DR, Radjenovic A, Kozerke S, Higgins DM, Sivananthan MU, Ridgway JP. Modified look-locker inversion recovery (MOLLI) for high-resolution T 1 mapping of the heart. Magn Reson Med 2004;52:141–6.

[44] Piechnik SK, Ferreira VM, Dall'armellina E, Cochlin LE, Greiser A, Neubauer S, et al. Shortened modified look-locker inversion recovery (ShMOLLI) for clinical myocardial T1-mapping at 1.5 and 3 T within a 9 heartbeat breathhold. J Cardiovasc Magn Reson 2010;12:69.

[45] Liu C-Y, Chang Liu Y, Wu C, Armstrong A, Volpe GJ, Van Der Geest RJ, et al. Evaluation of age related interstitial myocardial fibrosis with cardiac magnetic resonance contrast-enhanced t1 mapping in the multi-ethnic study of atherosclerosis (MESA). J Am Coll Cardiol 2013;62(14):1280–7.

[46] Messroghli DR, Greiser A, Frählich M, Dietz R, Schulz-Menger J. Optimization and validation of a fully-integrated pulse sequence for modified look-locker inversion-recovery (MOLLI) T1 mapping of the heart. J Magn Reson Imaging 2007;26:1081–6.

[47] Chow K, Flewitt JA, Green JD, Pagano JJ, Friedrich MG, Thompson RB. Saturation recovery single-shot acquisition (SASHA) for myocardial T1 mapping. Magn Reson Med 2014;71(June (6)):2082–95.

[48] Robson MD, Piechnik SK, Tunnicliffe EM, Neubauer S. T1 measurements in the human myocardium: The effects of magnetization transfer on the SASHA and MOLLI sequences. Magn Reson Med 2013, [Epub ahead of print].

[49] Higgins CB, Herfkens R, Lipton MJ. Nuclear magnetic resonance imaging of acute myocardial infarction in dogs: alterations in magnetic relaxation times. Am J Cardiol 1983;52:184–8.

[50] Scholz TD, Martins JB, Skorton DJ. NMR relaxation times in acute myocardial infarction: relative influence of changes in tissue water and fat content. Magn Reson Med 1992;23:89–95.
[51] Williams ES, Kaplan JI, Thatcher F. Prolongation of proton spin lattice relaxation times in regionally ischemic tissue from dog hearts. J Nucl Med 1980;21:449–53.
[52] Ferreira V, Piechnik S, Dall'armellina, E, Karamitsos T, Francis J, Choudhury R, et al. Non-contrast T1-mapping detects acute myocardial edema with high diagnostic accuracy: a comparison to T2-weighted cardiovascular magnetic resonance. J Cardiovasc Magn Reson 2012;14:42.
[53] Dall'armellina, E, Ferreira VM, Kharbanda RK, Prendergast B, Piechnik SK, Robson MD, et al. Diagnostic value of pre-contrast T1 mapping in acute and chronic myocardial infarction. JACC Cardiovasc Imaging 2013;6:739–42.
[54] Dall'armellina E, Piechnik S, Ferreira V, Si QL, Robson M, Francis J, et al. Cardiovascular magnetic resonance by non contrast T1 mapping allows assessment of severity of injury in acute myocardial infarction. J Cardiovasc Magn Reson 2012;14:15.
[55] Messroghli DR, Walters K, Plein S, Sparrow P, Friedrich MG, Ridgway JP, et al. Myocardial T1 mapping: application to patients with acute and chronic myocardial infarction. Magn Reson Med 2007;58:34–40.
[56] Ferreira V, Piechnik S, Dall'armellina E, Karamitsos T, Francis J, Ntusi N. T1-mapping for the diagnosis of acute myocarditis using cardiovascular magnetic resonance - comparison to T2-weighted and late gadolinium enhanced imaging. JACC Cardiovasc Imaging 2013; http://dx.doi.org/10.1016/j.jcmg.2013.03.008, Online before print.
[57] Luetkens JA, Doerner J, Thomas DK, Dabir D, Gieseke J, Sprinkart AM, et al. Acute myocarditis: multiparametric cardiac MR imaging. Radiology 2014;132540.
[58] Dass S, Suttie JJ, Piechnik SK, Ferreira VM, Holloway CJ, Banerjee R, et al. Myocardial tissue characterization using magnetic resonance noncontrast T1 mapping in hypertrophic and dilated cardiomyopathy. Circ Cardiovasc Imaging 2012;5:726–33.
[59] Puntmann VO, D'Cruz D, Smith Z, Pastor A, Choong P, Voigt T, et al. Native myocardial T1 mapping by cardiovascular magnetic resonance imaging in subclinical cardiomyopathy in patients with systemic lupus erythematosus. Circ Cardiovasc Imaging 2013;6:295–301.
[60] Puntmann VO, Voigt T, Chen Z, Mayr M, Karim R, Rhode K, et al. Native T1 mapping in differentiation of normal myocardium from diffuse disease in hypertrophic and dilated cardiomyopathy. JACC Cardiovasc Imaging 2013;6:475–84.
[61] Fontana M, Banypersad SM, Treibel TA, Maestrini V, Sado DM, White SK, et al. Native T1 mapping in transthyretin amyloidosis. JACC Cardiovasc Imaging 2014;7:157–65.
[62] Karamitsos TD, Piechnik SK, Banypersad S, Fontana M, Ntusi N, Ferreira VM, et al. Non-contrast T1 mapping for the diagnosis of cardiac amyloidosis. JACC Cardiovasc Imaging 2012; http://dx.doi.org/10.1016/j.jcmg.2012.11.013 published online before print.
[63] Holloway CJ, Ntusi N, Suttie J, Mahmod M, Wainwright E, Clutton G, et al. Comprehensive cardiac magnetic resonance imaging and spectroscopy reveal a high burden of myocardial disease in HIV patients. Circulation 2013;128:814–22.
[64] Been M, Thomson BJ, Smith MA, Ridgway JP, Douglas RHB, Been M, et al. Myocardial involvement in systemic lupus erythematosus detected by magnetic resonance imaging. Eur Heart J 1988;9:1250–6.
[65] Ntusi N, Piechnik S, Francis J, Ferreira V, Matthews P, Robson M, et al. Diffuse myocardial fibrosis and inflammation in rheumatoid arthritis: insights from cardiovascular magnetic resonance T1 mapping. JACC Cardiovasc Imaging 2015;8(5):526–36.

[66] Ntusi N, Piechnik S, Francis J, Ferreira V, Rai A, Matthews P, et al. Subclinical myocardial inflammation and diffuse fibrosis are common in systemic sclerosis—a clinical study using myocardial T1-mapping and extracellular volume quantification. J Cardiovasc Magn Reson 2014;16:21.

[67] Bull S, White SK, Piechnik SK, Flett AS, Ferreira VM, Loudon M, et al. Human noncontrast T1 values and correlation with histology in diffuse fibrosis. Heart 2013;99:932–7.

[68] Sado DM, White SK, Piechnik SK, Banypersad SM, Treibel T, Captur G, et al. Identification and assessment of anderson-fabry disease by cardiovascular magnetic resonance noncontrast myocardial T1 mapping. Circ Cardiovasc Imaging 2013;6:392–8.

[69] Thompson RB, Chow K, Khan A, Chan A, Shanks M, Paterson I, et al. T1 mapping with CMR is highly sensitive for Fabry disease independent of hypertrophy and gender. Circ Cardiovasc Imaging 2013;6:637–45.

[70] Ferreira VM, Holloway CJ, Piechnik SK, Karamitsos TD, Neubauer S. Is it really fat? Ask a T1-map. Eur Heart J Cardiovasc Imaging 2013;14(11):1060.

[71] Sado DM, Maestrini V, Piechnik SK, Banypersad SM, White SK, Flett AS, et al. Noncontrast myocardial T1 mapping using cardiovascular magnetic resonance for iron overload. J Magn Reson Imaging 2014 Aug 8. http://dx.doi.org/10.1002/jmri.24727. [Epub ahead of print].

[72] Feng Y, He T, Carpenter J-P, Jabbour A, Alam MH, Gatehouse PD, et al. In vivo comparison of myocardial T1 with T2 and T2* in thalassaemia major. J Magn Reson Imaging 2013;38:588–93.

[73] Ferreira V, Piechnik S, Dall'armellina, E, Karamitsos T, Francis J, Ntusi N, et al. Native T1-mapping detects the location, extent and patterns of acute myocarditis without the need for gadolinium contrast agents. J Cardiovasc Magn Reson 2014;16:36.

[74] Kawel N, Nacif M, Zavodni A, Jones J, Liu S, Sibley C, et al. T1 mapping of the myocardium: intra-individual assessment of post-contrast T1 time evolution and extracellular volume fraction at 3T for Gd-DTPA and Gd-BOPTA. J Cardiovasc Magn Reson 2012;14:26.

[75] Miller CA, Naish JH, Bishop P, Coutts G, Clark D, Zhao S, et al. Comprehensive validation of cardiovascular magnetic resonance techniques for the assessment of myocardial extracellular volume. Circ Cardiovasc Imaging 2013;6:373–83.

[76] White SK, Sado DM, Fontana M, Banypersad SM, Maestrini V, Flett AS, et al. T1 Mapping for myocardial extracellular volume measurement by CMR: bolus only versus primed infusion technique. JACC Cardiovasc Imaging 2013;6:955–62.

[77] Chan W, Duffy SJ, White DA, Gao X-M, Du X-J, Ellims A-H, et al. Acute left ventricular remodeling following myocardial infarction: coupling of regional healing with remote extracellular matrix expansion. JACC Cardiovasc Imaging 2012;5:884–93.

[78] Ellims A, Iles L, Ling L-H, Hare J, Kaye D, Taylor A. Diffuse myocardial fibrosis in hypertrophic cardiomyopathy can be identified by cardiovascular magnetic resonance, and is associated with left ventricular diastolic dysfunction. J Cardiovasc Magn Reson 2012;14:76.

[79] Maceira AM, Prasad SK, Hawkins PN, Roughton M, Pennell DJ. Cardiovascular magnetic resonance and prognosis in cardiac amyloidosis. J Cardiovasc Magn Reson 2008;10:54.

[80] Iles L, Pfluger H, Phrommintikul A, Cherayath J, Aksit P, Gupta SN, et al. Evaluation of diffuse myocardial fibrosis in heart failure with cardiac magnetic resonance contrast-enhanced T1 mapping. J Am Coll Cardiol 2008;52:1574–80.

[81] Sparrow P, Messroghli DR, Reid S, Ridgway JP, Bainbridge G, Sivananthan MU. Myocardial T1 mapping for detection of left ventricular myocardial fibrosis in chronic aortic regurgitation: pilot study. AJR Am J Roentgenol 2006;187.

[82] Ling L-H, Kalman JM, Ellims AH, Iles LM, Medi C, Sherratt C, et al. Diffuse ventricular fibrosis is a late outcome of tachycardia-mediated cardiomyopathy after successful ablation. Circ Arrhythm Electrophysiol 2013;6:697–704.

[83] Ling L-H, Kistler PM, Ellims AH, Iles LM, Lee G, Hughes GL, et al. Diffuse ventricular fibrosis in atrial fibrillation: noninvasive evaluation and relationships with aging and systolic dysfunction. J Am Coll Cardiol 2012;60:2402–8.

[84] Moon J, Messroghli D, Kellman P, Piechnik S, Robson M, Ugander M, et al. Myocardial T1 mapping and extracellular volume quantification: a Society for Cardiovascular Magnetic Resonance (SCMR) and CMR Working Group of the European Society of Cardiology consensus statement. J Cardiovasc Magn Reson 2013;15:92.

[85] Jerosch-Herold M, Sheridan DC, Kushner JD, Nauman D, Burgess D, Dutton D, et al. Cardiac magnetic resonance imaging of myocardial contrast uptake and blood flow in patients affected with idiopathic or familial dilated cardiomyopathy. Am J Physiol Heart Circ Physiol 2008;295:H1234–42.

[86] White SK, Sado DM, Flett AS, Moon JC. Characterising the myocardial interstitial space: the clinical relevance of non-invasive imaging. Heart 2012;98:773–9.

[87] Won S, Davies-Venn C, Liu S, Bluemke DA. Noninvasive imaging of myocardial extracellular matrix for assessment of fibrosis. Curr Opin Cardiol 2013;28:282–9. http://dx.doi.org/10.1097/HCO.0b013e32835f5a2b.

[88] Kehr E, Sono M, Chugh SS, Jerosch-Herold M. Gadolinium-enhanced magnetic resonance imaging for detection and quantification of fibrosis in human myocardium *in vitro*. Int J Cardiovasc Imaging 2008;24:61–8.

[89] Flett AS, Hayward MP, Ashworth MT, Hansen MS, Taylor AM, Elliott PM, et al. Equilibrium contrast cardiovascular magnetic resonance for the measurement of diffuse myocardial fibrosis: preliminary validation in humans. Circulation 2010;122:138–44.

[90] Fontana M, White S, Banypersad S, Sado D, Maestrini V, Flett A, et al. Comparison of T1 mapping techniques for ECV quantification. Histological validation and reproducibility of ShMOLLI versus multibreath-hold T1 quantification equilibrium contrast CMR. J Cardiovasc Magn Reson 2012;14:88.

[91] Sado DM, Flett AS, Banypersad SM, White SK, Maestrini V, Quarta G, et al. Cardiovascular magnetic resonance measurement of myocardial extracellular volume in health and disease. Heart 2012;98:1436–41.

[92] Neilan TG, Coelho-Filho OR, Shah RV, Abbasi SA, Heydari B, Watanabe E, et al. Myocardial extracellular volume fraction from T1 measurements in healthy volunteers and mice: relationship to aging and cardiac dimensions. JACC Cardiovasc Imaging 2013;6:672–83.

[93] Kellman P, Wilson J, Xue H, Bandettini W, Shanbhag S, Druey K, et al. Extracellular volume fraction mapping in the myocardium, part 2: initial clinical experience. J Cardiovasc Magn Reson 2012;14:64.

[94] Shah RV, Abbasi SA, Neilan TG, Hulten E, Coelho-Filho O, Hoppin A, et al. Myocardial tissue remodeling in adolescent obesity. J Am Heart Assoc 2013;2(4):e000279.

[95] Banypersad SM, Sado DM, Flett AS, Gibbs SDJ, Pinney JH, Maestrini V, et al. Quantification of myocardial extracellular volume fraction in systemic AL amyloidosis: an equilibrium contrast cardiovascular magnetic resonance study. Circ Cardiovasc Imaging 2012;6:34–9.

[96] Plymen CM, Sado DM, Taylor AM, Bolger AP, Lambiase PD, Hughes M, et al. Diffuse myocardial fibrosis in the systemic right ventricle of patients late after Mustard or Senning surgery: an equilibrium contrast cardiovascular magnetic resonance study. Eur Heart J Cardiovasc Imaging 2013;14(10):963–8.

[97] Tham E, Haykowsky M, Chow K, Spavor M, Kaneko S, Khoo N, et al. Diffuse myocardial fibrosis by T1-mapping in children with subclinical anthracycline cardiotoxicity: relationship to exercise capacity, cumulative dose and remodeling. J Cardiovasc Magn Reson 2013;15:48.

[98] Ugander M, Oki AJ, Hsu LY, Kellman P, Greiser A, Aletras AH, et al. Extracellular volume imaging by magnetic resonance imaging provides insights into overt and subclinical myocardial pathology. Eur Heart J 2012;33:1268–78.

[99] Wong TC, Piehler KM, Kang IA, Kadakkal A, Kellman P, Schwartzman DS, et al. Myocardial extracellular volume fraction quantified by cardiovascular magnetic resonance is increased in diabetes and associated with mortality and incident heart failure admission. Eur Heart J; 2013.

[100] Ugander M, Bagi PS, Oki AJ, Chen B, Hsu LY, Aletras AH, et al. Myocardial edema as detected by pre-contrast T1 and T2 CMR delineates area at risk associated with acute myocardial infarction. JACC Cardiovasc Imaging 2012;5:596–603.

[101] Thavendiranathan P, Walls M, Giri S, Verhaert D, Rajagopalan S, Moore S, et al. Improved detection of myocardial involvement in acute inflammatory cardiomyopathies using T2 mapping. Circ Cardiovasc Imaging 2011;5:102–10.

[102] Usman AA, Taimen K, Wasielewski M, McDonald J, Shah S, Giri S, et al. Cardiac magnetic resonance T2 mapping in the monitoring and follow-up of acute cardiac transplant rejection: a pilot study. Circ Cardiovasc Imaging 2012;5:782–90.

[103] Wassmuth R, Prothmann M, Utz W, Dieringer M, Von Knobelsdorff-Brenkenhoff F, Greiser A, et al. Variability and homogeneity of cardiovascular magnetic resonance myocardial T2-mapping in volunteers compared to patients with edema. J Cardiovasc Magn Reson 2013;15:27.

[104] Van Heeswijk RB, Feliciano HLN, Bongard CD, Bonanno G, Coppo S, Lauriers N, et al. Free-breathing 3 T magnetic resonance T2-mapping of the heart. JACC Cardiovasc Imaging 2012;5:1231–9.

[105] Lund G, Morin RL, Olivari MT, Ring WS. Serial myocardial T2 relaxation time measurements in normal subjects and heart transplant recipients. J Heart Transplant 1988;7:274–9.

[106] Verhaert D, Thavendiranathan P, Giri S, Mihai G, Rajagopalan S, Simonetti OP, et al. Direct T2 quantification of myocardial edema in acute ischemic injury. JACC Cardiovasc Imaging 2011;4:269–78.

[107] Giri S, Chung YC, Merchant A, Mihai G, Rajagopalan S, Raman SV, et al. T2 quantification for improved detection of myocardial edema. J Cardiovasc Magn Reson 2009;11:56.

[108] Abdel-Aty H, Simonetti O, Friedrich MG. T2-weighted cardiovascular magnetic resonance imaging. J Magn Reson Imaging 2007;26:452–9.

[109] Von Knobelsdorff-Brenkenhoff F, Prothmann M, Dieringer M, Wassmuth R, Greiser A, Schwenke C, et al. Myocardial T1 and T2 mapping at 3T: reference values, influencing factors and implications. J Cardiovasc Magn Reson 2013;15:53.

[110] Schulz-Menger, et al. J Cardiovasc Magn Reson 2013;15:35.

[111] Ghugre NR, Pop M, Barry J, Connelly KA, Wright GA. Quantitative magnetic resonance imaging can distinguish remodeling mechanisms after acute myocardial infarction based on the severity of ischemic insult. Magn Reson Med 2013;70(4):1095–105.

[112] Ghugre NR, Ramanan V, Pop M, Yang Y, Barry J, Qiang B, et al. Quantitative tracking of edema, hemorrhage, and microvascular obstruction in subacute myocardial infarction in a porcine model by MRI. Magn Reson Med 2011;66:1129–41.

[113] Zia MI, Ghugre NR, Connelly KA, Strauss BH, Sparkes JD, Dick AJ, et al. Characterizing myocardial edema and hemorrhage using quantitative T2 and T2* mapping at multiple time intervals post ST-segment elevation myocardial infarction. Circ Cardiovasc Imaging 2012;5:566–72.

[114] Ghugre NR, Ramanan V, Pop M, Yang Y, Barry J, Qiang B, et al. Myocardial BOLD imaging at 3 T using quantitative T2: application in a myocardial infarct model. Magn Reson Med 2011;66:1739–47.

[115] Heinrichs U, Utting JF, Frauenrath T, Hezel F, Krombach GA, Hodenius MAJ, et al. Myocardial T2* mapping free of distortion using susceptibility-weighted fast spin-echo imaging: a feasibility study at 1.5 T and 3.0 T. Magn Reson Med 2009;62:822–8.

[116] Positano V, Pepe A, Santarelli MF, Scattini B, De Marchi D, Ramazzotti A, et al. Standardized T2* map of normal human heart in vivo to correct T2* segmental artefacts. NMR Biomed 2007;20:578–90.

[117] Hezel F, Thalhammer C, Waiczies S, Schulz-Menger J, Niendorf T. High spatial resolution and temporally resolved T2* mapping of normal human myocardium at 7.0 tesla: an ultrahigh field magnetic resonance feasibility study. PLoS One 2012;7, e52324.

[118] Rodgers CT, Piechnik SK, Delabarre LJ, Van De Moortele PF, Snyder CJ, Neubauer S, et al. Inversion recovery at 7 T in the human myocardium: measurement of T 1, inversion efficiency and B 1 +. Magn Reson Med 2013;70(4):1038–46.

[119] Hope MD, Hope TA, Meadows AK, Ordovas KG, Urbania TH, Alley MT, et al. Bicuspid aortic valve: four-dimensional MR evaluation of ascending aortic systolic flow patterns. Radiology 2010;255:53–61.

[120] Barker AJ, Markl M, Bürk J, Lorenz R, Bock J, Bauer S, et al. Bicuspid aortic valve is associated with altered wall shear stress in the ascending aorta. Circ Cardiovasc Imaging 2012;5:457–66.

[121] Bissell MM, Hess AT, Biasiolli L, Glaze SJ, Loudon M, Pitcher A, et al. Aortic dilation in bicuspid aortic valve disease: flow pattern is a major contributor and differs with valve fusion type. Circ Cardiovasc Imaging 2013;6:499–507.

[122] Burk J, Blanke P, Stankovic Z, Barker A, Russe M, Geiger J, et al. Evaluation of 3D blood flow patterns and wall shear stress in the normal and dilated thoracic aorta using flow-sensitive 4D CMR. J Cardiovasc Magn Reson 2012;14.

[123] Geiger J, Markl M, Herzer L, Hirtler D, Loeffelbein F, Stiller B, et al. Aortic flow patterns in patients with Marfan syndrome assessed by flow-sensitive four-dimensional MRI. J Magn Reson Imaging 2012;35:594–600.

[124] Markl M, Draney MT, Miller DC, Levin JM, Williamson EE, Pelc NJ, et al. Time-resolved three-dimensional magnetic resonance velocity mapping of aortic flow in healthy volunteers and patients after valve-sparing aortic root replacement. J Thorac Cardiovasc Surg 2005;130:456–63.

[125] Geiger J, Hirtler D, Burk J, Stiller B, Arnold R, Jung B, et al. Postoperative pulmonary and aortic 3D haemodynamics in patients after repair of transposition of the great arteries. Eur Radiol 2013;24:200–8.

[126] Hope MD, Meadows AK, Hope TA, Ordovas KG, Saloner D, Reddy GP, et al. Clinical evaluation of aortic coarctation with 4D flow MR imaging. J Magn Reson Imaging 2010;31:711–8.

[127] Carlhall CJ, Bolger A. Passing strange flow in the failing ventricle. Circ Heart Fail 2010;3:326–31.

[128] Eriksson J, Bolger AF, Ebbers T, CarlhäLl CJ. Four-dimensional blood flow-specific markers of LV dysfunction in dilated cardiomyopathy. Eur Heart J Cardiovasc Imaging 2013;14:417–24.

[129] Fluckiger JU, Goldberger JJ, Lee DC, Ng J, Lee R, Goyal A, et al. Left atrial flow velocity distribution and flow coherence using four-dimensional FLOW MRI: a pilot study investigating the impact of age and pre- and postintervention atrial fibrillation on atrial hemodynamics. J Magn Reson Imaging 2013;38:580–7.

[130] Bachler P, Valverde I, Pinochet N, Nordmeyer S, Kuehne T, Crelier G, et al. Caval blood flow distribution in patients with Fontan circulation: quantification by using particle traces from 4D flow MR imaging. Radiology 2013;267:67–75.

[131] Hudsmith LE, Neubauer S. Magnetic resonance spectroscopy in myocardial disease. JACC Cardiovasc Imaging 2009;2:87–96.

[132] Bottomley PA. MR spectroscopy of the human heart: the status and the challenges. Radiology 1994;191:593–612.

[133] Neubauer S. The failing heart—an engine out of fuel. New Engl J Med 2007;356:1140–51.

[134] Bottomley PA, Weiss RG. Noninvasive localized MR quantification of creatine kinase metabolites in normal and infarcted canine myocardium. Radiology 2001;219:411–8.

[135] Kreutzer U, Mekhamer Y, Chung Y, Jue T. Oxygen supply and oxidative phosphorylation limitation in rat myocardium in situ. Am J Physiol Heart Circ Physiol 2001;280:H2030–7.

[136] Schneider JE, Tyler DJ, Ten Hove M, Sang AE, Cassidy PJ, Fischer A, et al. In vivo cardiac 1H-MRS in the mouse. Magn Reson Med 2004;52:1029–35.

[137] Schroeder MA, Clarke K, Neubauer S, Tyler DJ. Hyperpolarized magnetic resonance: a novel technique for the in vivo assessment of cardiovascular disease. Circulation 2011;124:1580–94.

[138] Weiss RG, Bottomley PA, Hardy CJ, Gerstenblith G. Regional myocardial metabolism of high-energy phosphates during isometric exercise in patients with coronary artery disease. N Engl J Med 1990;323:1593–600.

[139] Neubauer S, Horn M, Pabst T, Godde M, Lubke D, Jilling B, et al. Contributions of 31P-magnetic resonance spectroscopy to the understanding of dilated heart muscle disease. Eur Heart J 1995;16:115–8.

[140] Neubauer S, Krahe T, Schindler R, Horn M, Hillenbrand H, Entzeroth C, et al. 31P magnetic resonance spectroscopy in dilated cardiomyopathy and coronary artery disease: altered cardiac high-energy phosphate metabolism in heart failure. Circulation 1992;86:1810–8.

[141] Neubauer S, Horn M, Cramer M, Harre K, Newell JB, Peters W, et al. Myocardial phosphocreatine-to-ATP ratio is a predictor of mortality in patients with dilated cardiomyopathy. Circulation 1997;96:2190–6.

[142] Beer M, Seyfarth T, Sandstede J, Landschütz W, Lipke C, Köstler H, et al. Absolute concentrations of high-energy phosphate metabolites in normal, hypertrophied, and failing human myocardium measured noninvasively with 31P-SLOOP magnetic resonance spectroscopy. J Am Coll Cardiol 2002;40:1267–74.

[143] Fragasso G, Perseghin G, De Cobelli F, Esposito A, Palloshi A, Lattuada G, et al. Effects of metabolic modulation by trimetazidine on left ventricular function and phosphocreatine/adenosine triphosphate ratio in patients with heart failure. Eur Heart J 2006;27:942–8.

[144] Hirsch GA, Bottomley PA, Gerstenblith G, Weiss RG. Allopurinol acutely increases adenosine triphospate energy delivery in failing human hearts. J Am Coll Cardiol 2012;59:802–8.

[145] Beyerbacht HP, Lamb HJ, Van Der Laarse A, Vliegen HW, Leujes F, Hazekamp MG, et al. Aortic valve replacement in patients with aortic valve stenosis improves myocardial metabolism and diastolic function. Radiology 2001;219:637–43.

[146] Mahmod M, Bull S, Suttie JJ, Pal N, Holloway C, Dass S, et al. Myocardial steatosis and left ventricular contractile dysfunction in patients with severe aortic stenosis. Circ Cardiovasc Imaging; 2013.

[147] Crilley JG, Boehm EA, Blair E, Rajagopalan B, Blamire AM, Styles P, et al. Hypertrophic cardiomyopathy due to sarcomeric gene mutations is characterized by impaired energy metabolism irrespective of the degree of hypertrophy. J Am Coll Cardiol 2003;41:1776–82.

[148] Scheuermann-Freestone M, Madsen PL, Manners D, Blamire AM, Buckingham RE, Styles P, et al. Abnormal cardiac and skeletal muscle energy metabolism in patients with type 2 diabetes. Circulation 2003;107:3040–6.

[149] Rider OJ, Francis JM, Ali MK, Holloway C, Pegg T, Robson MD, et al. Effects of catecholamine stress on diastolic function and myocardial energetics in obesity. Circulation 2012;125:1511–9.

[150] Rider OJ, Francis JM, Tyler D, Byrne J, Clarke K, Neubauer S. Effects of weight loss on myocardial energetics and diastolic function in obesity. Int J Cardiovasc Imaging 2013;29:1043–50.

[151] Rodgers CT, Clarke WT, Snyder C, Vaughan JT, Neubauer S, Robson MD. Human cardiac P magnetic resonance spectroscopy at 7 tesla. Magn Reson Med; 2013.

[152] Ardenkjaer-Larsen JH, Fridlund B, Gram A, Hansson G, Hansson L, Lerche MH, et al. Increase in signal-to-noise ratio of > 10,000 times in liquid-state NMR. Proc Natl Acad Sci U S A 2003;100:10158–63.

[153] Comment A, Van Den Brandt B, Uffmann K, Kurdzesau F, Jannin S, Konter JA, et al. Principles of operation of a DNP prepolarizer coupled to a rodent MRI scanner. Appl Magn Reson 2008;34:313–9.

[154] Kurhanewicz J, Vigneron DB, Brindle K, Chekmenev EY, Comment A, Cunningham CH, et al. Analysis of cancer metabolism by imaging hyperpolarized nuclei: prospects for translation to clinical research. Neoplasia 2011;13:81–97.

[155] Merritt ME, Harrison C, Storey C, Jeffrey FM, Sherry AD, Malloy CR. Hyperpolarized C-13 allows a direct measure of flux through a single enzyme-catalyzed step by NMR. Proc Natl Acad Sci U S A 2007;104:19773–7.

[156] Schroeder MA, Cochlin LE, Heather LC, Clarke K, Radda GK, Tyler DJ, et al. In vivo assessment of pyruvate dehydrogenase flux in the heart using hyperpolarized carbon-13 magnetic resonance. Proc Natl Acad Sci U S A 2008;105:12051–6.

[157] Schroeder MA, Atherton HJ, Dodd MS, Lee P, Cochlin LE, Radda GK, et al. The cycling of acetyl-coenzyme a through acetylcarnitine buffers cardiac substrate supply a hyperpolarized C-13 magnetic resonance study. Circ Cardiovasc Imaging 2012;5(2):201–9.

[158] Schroeder MA, Atherton HJ, Ball DR, Cole MA, Heather LC, Griffin JL, et al. Real-time assessment of Krebs cycle metabolism using hyperpolarized C-13 magnetic resonance spectroscopy. Faseb J 2009;23:2529–38.

[159] Atherton HJ, Dodd MS, Heather LC, Schroeder MA, Griffin JL, Radda GK, et al. Role of pyruvate dehydrogenase inhibition in the development of hypertrophy in the hyperthyroid rat heart a combined magnetic resonance imaging and hyperpolarized magnetic resonance spectroscopy study. Circulation 2011;123(22):2552–61.

[160] Lau AZ, Chen AP, Ghugre NR, Ramanan V, Lam WW, Connelly KA, et al. Rapid multislice imaging of hyperpolarized C-13 pyruvate and bicarbonate in the heart. Magn Reson Med 2010;64:1323–31.

[161] Lau AZ, Chen AP, Barry J, Graham JJ, Dominguez-Viqueira W, Ghugre NR, et al. Reproducibility study for free-breathing measurements of pyruvate metabolism using hyperpolarized (13) C in the heart. Magn Reson Med 2013;69:1063–71.

[162] Schroeder MA, Lau AZ, Chen AP, Gu YP, Nagendran J, Barry J, et al. Hyperpolarized C-13 magnetic resonance reveals early- and late-onset changes to in vivo pyruvate metabolism in the failing heart. Eur J Heart Fail 2013;15:130–40.

[163] Nelson SJ, Ozhinsky E, Li Y, Park I, Crane J. Strategies for rapid in vivo 1H and hyperpolarized 13C MR spectroscopic imaging. J Magn Reson 2013;229:187–97.

[164] Ardenkjaer-Larsen JH, Leach AM, Clarke N, Urbahn J, Anderson D, Skloss TW. Dynamic nuclear polarization polarizer for sterile use intent. NMR Biomed 2011;24:927–32.

[165] Suttie JJ, Delabarre L, Pitcher A, Van De Moortele PF, Dass S, Snyder CJ, et al. 7 Tesla (T) human cardiovascular magnetic resonance imaging using FLASH and SSFP to assess cardiac function: validation against 1.5 T and 3 T. NMR Biomed 2012;25:27–34.

[166] Thalhammer C, Renz W, Winter L, Hezel F, Rieger J, Pfeiffer H, et al. Two-dimensional sixteen channel transmit/receive coil array for cardiac MRI at 7.0 T: design, evaluation, and application. J Magn Reson Imaging 2012;36:847–57.

[167] Von Knobelsdorff-Brenkenhoff F, Frauenrath T, Prothmann M, Dieringer M, Hezel F, Renz W, et al. Cardiac chamber quantification using magnetic resonance imaging at 7 Tesla—a pilot study. Eur Radiol 2010;20:2844–52.

[168] Von Knobelsdorff-Brenkenhoff F, Tkachenko V, Winter L, Rieger J, Thalhammer C, Hezel F, et al. Assessment of the right ventricle with cardiovascular magnetic resonance at 7 Tesla. J Cardiovasc Magn Reson 2013;15:23.

[169] Makowski M, Wiethoff A, Jansen C, Uribe S, Parish V, Schuster A, et al. Single breath-hold assessment of cardiac function using an accelerated 3D single breath-hold acquisition technique - comparison of an intravascular and extravascular contrast agent. J Cardiovasc Magn Reson 2012;14:53.

[170] Niendorf T, Hardy CJ, Giaquinto RO, Gross P, Cline HE, Zhu Y, et al. Toward single breath-hold whole-heart coverage coronary MRA using highly accelerated parallel imaging with a 32-channel MR system. Magn Reson Med 2006;56:167–76.

[171] Attili A, Schuster A, Nagel E, Reiber JC, Geest R. Quantification in cardiac MRI: advances in image acquisition and processing. Int J Cardiovasc Imaging 2010;26:27–40.

[172] Stuber M, Botnar RM, Fischer SE, Lamerichs R, Smink J, Harvey P, et al. Preliminary report on in vivo coronary MRA at 3 Tesla in humans. Magn Reson Med 2002;48:425–9.

[173] Van Elderen SGC, Versluis MJ, Webb AG, Westenberg JJM, Doornbos J, Smith NB, et al. Initial results on in vivo human coronary MR angiography at 7 T. Magn Reson Med 2009;62:1379–84.

[174] Lipinski MJ, Frias JC, Amirbekian V, Briley-Saebo KC, Mani V, Samber D, et al. Macrophage-specific lipid-based nanoparticles improve cardiac magnetic resonance detection and characterization of human atherosclerosis. JACC Cardiovasc Imaging 2009;2:637–47.

[175] Qian D, Bottomley PA. High-resolution intravascular magnetic resonance quantification of atherosclerotic plaque at 3T. J Cardiovasc Magn Reson 2012;14.

[176] Robson MD, Tyler DJ, Neubauer S. Ultrashort TE chemical shift imaging (UTE-CSI). Magn Reson Med 2005;53:267–74.

[177] Hoerr V, Nagelmann N, Nauerth A, Kuhlmann MT, Stypmann J, Faber C. Cardiac-respiratory self-gated cine ultra-short echo time (UTE) cardiovascular magnetic resonance for assessment of functional cardiac parameters at high magnetic fields. J Cardiovasc Magn Reson 2013;15:59.

[178] Robson MD, Gatehouse PD, Bydder M, Bydder GM. Magnetic resonance: an introduction to ultrashort TE (UTE) imaging. J Comput Assist Tomog 2003;27:825–46.
[179] Liu W, Frank JA. Detection and quantification of magnetically labeled cells by cellular MRI. Eur J Radiol 2009;70:258–64.
[180] Mcateer MA, Sibson NR, Von Zur Muhlen C, Schneider JE, Lowe AS, Warrick N, et al. In vivo magnetic resonance imaging of acute brain inflammation using microparticles of iron oxide. Nat Med 2007;13:1253–8.
[181] Zhou R, Idiyatullin D, Moeller S, Corum C, Zhang H, Qiao H, et al. SWIFT detection of SPIO-labeled stem cells grafted in the myocardium. Magn Reson Med 2010;63:1154–61.
[182] Nielles-Vallespin S, Mekkaoui C, Gatehouse P, Reese TG, Keegan J, Ferreira PF, et al. In vivo diffusion tensor MRI of the human heart: reproducibility of breath-hold and navigator-based approaches. Magn Reson Med 2013;70:454–65.
[183] Mcgill L-A, Ismail T, Nielles-Vallespin S, Ferreira P, Scott A, Roughton M, et al. Reproducibility of *in-vivo* diffusion tensor cardiovascular magnetic resonance in hypertrophic cardiomyopathy. J Cardiovasc Magn Reson 2012;14:86.

Part Two

Clinical applications of cardiac imaging

Noninvasive coronary angiography

M. Premaratne*,†, B.J.W. Chow*
*University of Ottawa Heart Institute, Ottawa, ON, Canada; †Canberra Hospital, Garran, ACT, Australia

7.1 Introduction

Invasive coronary angiography (ICA) is the gold standard for the identification of anatomically obstructive coronary artery disease (CAD). However at many centers, ICA is a limited resource that is expensive and has periprocedural risks (death, cerebrovascular accident, myocardial infarction, and vascular complications). Thus, ICA may not be appropriate for all patients and best reserved for those at highest risk and who likely require coronary revascularization. A noninvasive method that can accurately diagnose and risk stratify patients could function as a gatekeeper for ICA. Technological improvements in computed tomography (CT) and cardiovascular magnetic resonance (CMR) imaging have made non-invasive coronary angiography feasible.

7.2 Coronary artery calcium

Atherosclerosis is a complex pathophysiologic process that begins with endothelial injury. Disruption of the protective endothelial layer increases its permeability and impairs its regulatory system and its ability to respond to stressors. The subsequent deposition of oxidized low-density lipid proteins results in the overexpression of cell adhesion molecules, recruitment of inflammatory cells, accumulation of lipid laden foam cells in the subendothelium, smooth muscle proliferation, and positive remodeling. As part of this process, calcium phosphate hydroxyapatite deposition occurs. Therefore, coronary calcification is a specific marker of coronary atherosclerosis.

Noncontrast enhanced cardiac CT can be used to detect and measure coronary artery calcification (CAC). It is recognized that the composition of coronary atherosclerotic plaque is variable and that calcification is a later process. Therefore, CAC is an indirect measure of total plaque burden and volume. Although noncontrast enhanced CT cannot assess the coronary lumen, there is a relationship between CAC and coronary artery stenosis (Figure 7.1). Patients with high CAC scores have a higher likelihood of having obstructive CAD and major adverse cardiovascular events (MACEs) [2–5] (Figure 7.2). However, it is important to recognize that the relationship between CAC and coronary stenosis is not linear (Figure 7.1) [7–10].

Several methods of quantifying CAC (mass score, calcium volume method, and Agatston score) have been studied [11]. The Agatston method has been the most frequently used and best validated method for quantifying CAC. Using the Agatston method, calcific coronary plaque is defined as a perivascular lesion ≥130 Hounsfield

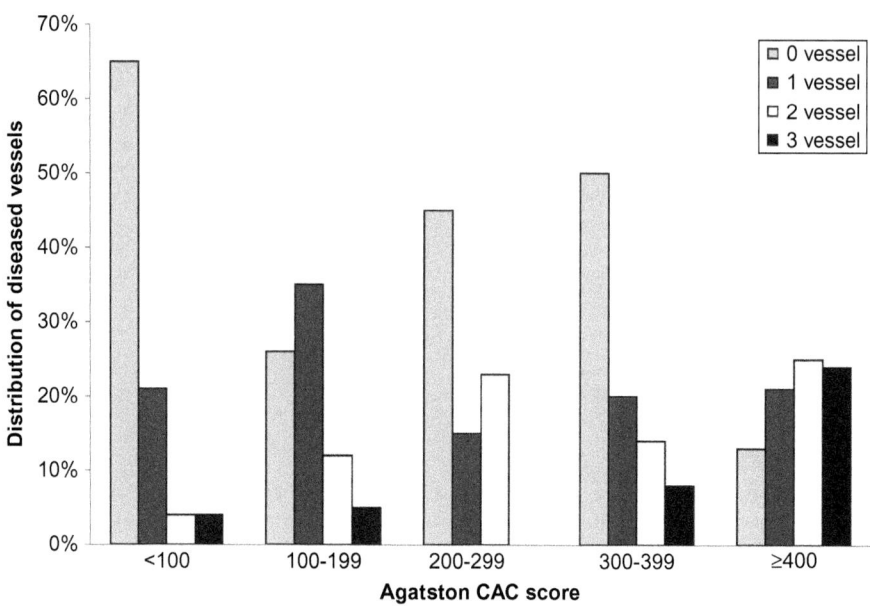

Figure 7.1 Relationship of calcium score to severity of coronary artery disease. The relationship between the severity of coronary artery calcification and severity of coronary artery disease and diseased vessels is not linear.
Adapted from Rosen et al. [1].

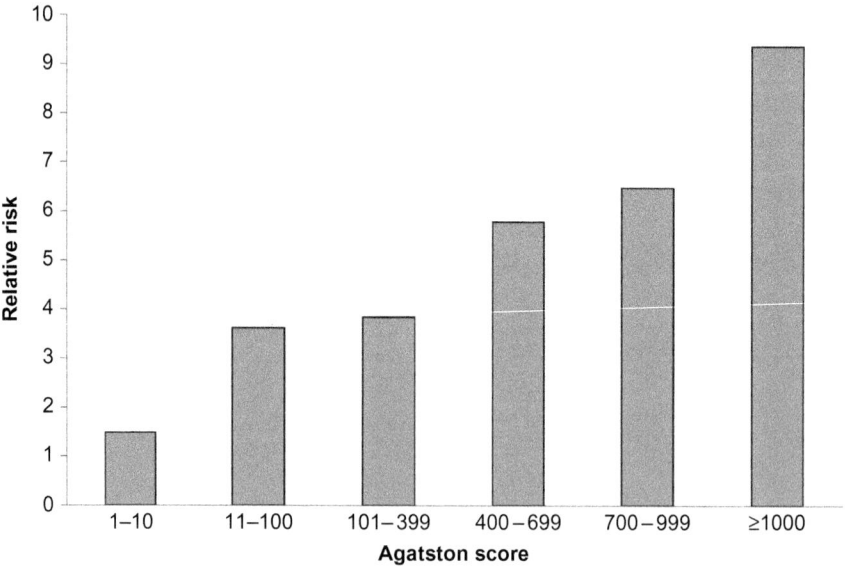

Figure 7.2 Agatston score and future adverse outcomes. The Agatston score has prognostic value. The severity of calcium score is directly related to the risk of future adverse outcomes (all-cause death).
Adapted from Budoff et al. [6].

Units (HU) with an area of ≥1 mm² (three pixels) [11]. The Agatston score is a unitless score that is calculated as the product of the area of calcium and a multiplication factor representing the maximum attenuation of each lesion (Table 7.1). The Agatston score is considered useful for refining cardiovascular risk of asymptomatic patients and has incremental prognostic value over conventional clinical risk prediction models (such as age, sex, cardiac risk factors) (Figure 7.3).

Acknowledging that the correlation between the Agatston score and obstructive CAD is fair, the absence of CAC is associated with a low risk of future adverse events [11]. In asymptomatic patients, a zero calcium score has a very low prevalence of obstructive CAD (2%) [13,14]. An important distinction is that the data from these studies was derived from patient cohorts referred for coronary

Table 7.1 Weighting factor used to calculate the Agatston score

CT hounsfield unit no.	Weighting factor[a]
0–129	0
130–199	1
200–299	2
300–399	3
>400	4

Agatston score = area of calcification (mm²) × weighting factor of the calcification.
[a] Brightest pixel in lesion.
Adapted from Agatston et al. [12].

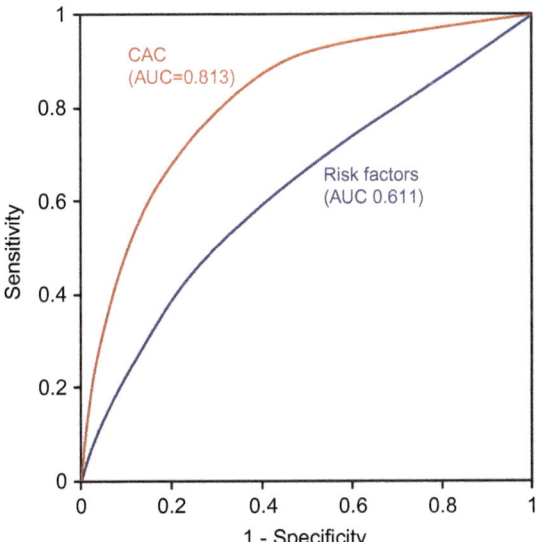

Figure 7.3 Incremental prognostic value of coronary artery calcium scoring. The Agatston score has incremental value over conventional cardiac risk factors for all-cause death. Adapted from Budoff et al. [6].

angiography, with an inherent higher prevalence of obstructive CAD compared to the group of patients subjected to cardiac CT in clinical practice. Thus, in the asymptomatic population, a zero calcium score effectively rules out obstructive CAD. Currently, according to the AHA/ACCF taskforce guidelines, calcium imaging has a Class IIa recommendation for cardiovascular risk assessment in asymptomatic adults at intermediate risk and a IIb recommendation for low to intermediate risk.

Although a zero calcium score in the asymptomatic population is reassuring, the ability to absolutely rule out obstructive CAD in the symptomatic population is more difficult. Although it may effectively rule out high-risk coronary anatomy (three vessel disease $\geq 70\%$, two vessel disease involving proximal left anterior descending artery $\geq 70\%$ or left main stenosis $\geq 50\%$), a zero calcium score cannot be used to exclude CAD as a cause of symptoms [13,15]. In the symptomatic population with a zero calcium score, the prevalence of obstructive CAD (diameter stenosis $\geq 50\%$ by CT or invasive angiography) is still 7%. It is reassuring that in clinical practice, the proportion of patients with obstructive disease is very low (0–2%) after a negative calcium scan [16,17]. The CONFIRM registry reported that less than 1% of patients with a negative calcium scan eventually required revascularization (Figure 7.5) [18].

7.3 CT coronary angiography

With the arrival of 64-slice CT scanners came significant advances in both temporal and spatial resolution, which led to the feasibility and the rapid adoption of CT coronary angiography (CTCA) for the assessment of CAD.

Luminal stenosis has been traditionally used as the measure of obstructive CAD severity. Early studies suggested that a threshold of 50% was associated with an abnormal coronary blood flow reserve and 80% threshold was associated with decreased resting coronary flow [19,20]. The Fractional Flow Reserve Vs Angiography in Multi-vessel Evaluation (FAME) trial subsequently showed that the relationship between anatomy and its hemodynamic consequences can be unpredictable [21] (Figure 7.6). The importance of calcification affecting Cardiac CT interpretation is shown in Figures 7.4 and 7.5. The increasing extent makes interpretation difficult. Patients with mild lesions (<50%) remain at risk of cardiovascular events [23], as studies have reported that >66% of infarct-related lesions arise from sites with subclinical atherosclerosis [24].

7.3.1 Accuracy

Early single-center studies demonstrated that CTCA has a high sensitivity and specificity for the detection of coronary stenosis $\geq 50\%$ [25–28]. Recent meta-analyses have confirmed that the sensitivity (91–99%) and specificity (74–96%) of CTCA is very good [29]. Not unexpectedly, the diagnostic performance improved as technology evolved with a concomitant reduction in the number of nonassessable segments [30].

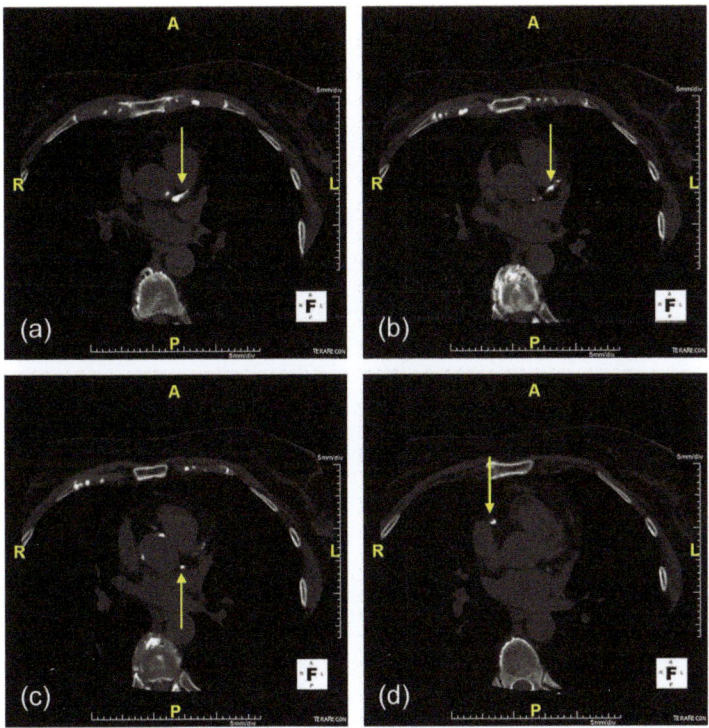

Figure 7.4 Coronary calcification and lumen evaluability. Noncontrast enhanced ECG-gated Cardiac CT, which demonstrates severe coronary artery calcification (arrows) of the left main (a), LAD (b), LCx (c), and RCA (d). In cases of severe coronary artery calcification, there is increased likelihood of nonevaluable coronary segments.

For 64-slice CTCA, a per-segment sensitivity, specificity, positive predictive value and negative predictive value of 86%, 96%, 83%, and 97%, respectively, and 98%, 91%, 93%, and 96%, respectively, has been reported on a per-patient basis [31]. It is anticipated that the operating characteristics of CTCA will improve in parallel with advancements in software (iterative reconstruction) and hardware (gantry rotation speed, detectors, dual energy acquisition).

When interpreting accuracy studies, one has to be mindful that early single-center studies were subject to multiple biases, such as referral, population, verification, and publication biases. To address this, several multicenter trials have examined the diagnostic accuracy of CTCA compared to ICA (Table 7.2). Although their results confirm those found in single-center studies, these studies were still subject to a population bias since study patients were awaiting ICA [33–35,37].

The "Coronary Artery Evaluation Using 64-Row multidetector computed tomography angiography" (CORE 64) trial studied 291 patients with and without a history of CAD, but excluded patients with Agatston score ≥600 [34]. This vendor specific study had lower sensitivity (85%) and negative predictive value (83%) than previous single center studies (Table 7.2).

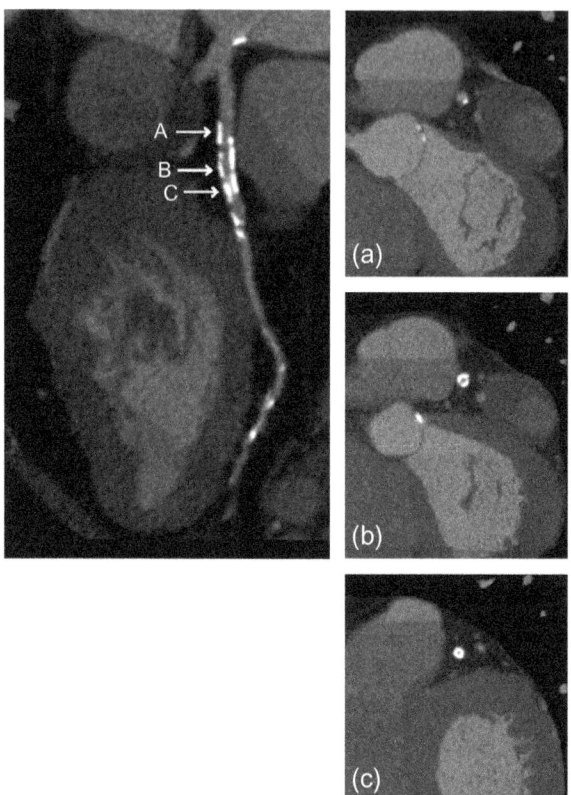

Figure 7.5 Coronary calcification and lumen evaluability. Curved multiplanar reformation (cMPR) of the left anterior descending (LAD) artery showing severe concentric calcification with blooming artifact and unevaluable lumen.

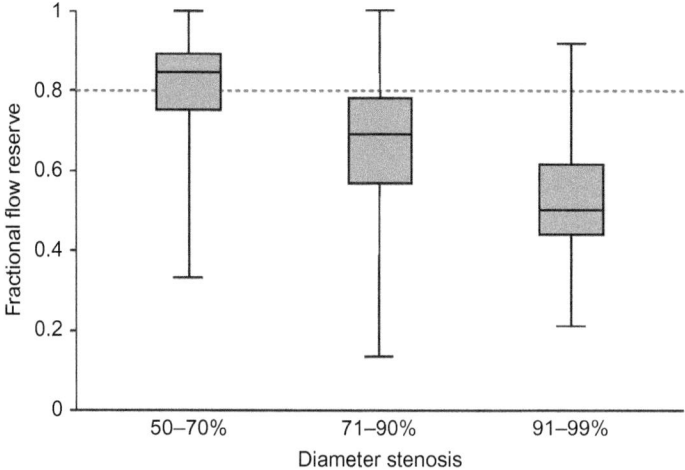

Figure 7.6 Relationship between fractional flow reserve and coronary artery stenosis. Severity of visually assessed luminal stenosis does not predict its hemodynamic significance. Adapted from Tonino et al. [22].

Table 7.2 **Multicenter studies on accuracy of CT coronary angiography**

	N	CAD (%)	Sensitivity (%)	Specificity (%)	PPV (%)	NPV (%)
ACCURACY [33]	230	25	95	83	64	99
CORE 64 [34]	291	56	85	90	91	83
Meijboom et al. [35]	360	68	99	64	86	97
OMCAS [36]	117	59	89	99	99	87

The "Assessment by Coronary Computer Tomography Individuals UndeRgoing InvAsive Coronary AngiographY" (ACCURACY) was a prospective multicenter trial that examined 230 patients without a prior history of CAD with stable anginal symptoms [33]. In a population with a low (25%) prevalence of CAD, the core lab evaluated all consecutive patients irrespective of CAC, body size, or heart rate. The sensitivity, specificity, positive predictive, and negative predictive values of the ACCURACY trial were 94%, 83%, 48%, and 99%, respectively, with an area under the curve (AUC) of 0.95.

The largest study (360 patients) was performed by Meijboom et al., and included patients with both acute and stable chest pain. This multicenter and multivendor study showed that CTCA had very high sensitivity (99%) and negative predictive value (97%) in a population with a CAD prevalence of 68% [35]. The "Ontario Multicenter CT Angiography Study" (OMCAS) was a field evaluation of CTCA accuracy in patients awaiting ICA [36]. In this study, CTCA interpretation was not performed by a core lab and was left to local centers. The results of this study are thought to reflect accuracy if CTCA were to be widely adopted into clinical practice. Not unexpectedly, there were significant variations in operating characteristics across the different centers, which may be related to patient pretest probability or local experience. Most importantly, the results support the need for identifying appropriate indications that exploit the strengths of CTCA, as well as training guidelines for both technologists and imagers.

The accuracy and applicability of CTCA will grow, as limitations relating to heart rate, arrhythmia, and calcification are overcome.

7.3.2 Plaque characterization

Although intravascular ultrasound (IVUS) is the clinically accepted tool for imaging the arterial lumen and wall, CTCA has the potential ability to visualize and characterize coronary plaque [38–40]. The potential importance of identifying vulnerable plaque is underlied by pathology studies that demonstrated that plaque rupture is the most common (60%) cause of acute coronary syndrome (ACS), with plaque erosion and calcified nodules making up the remainder [41,42]. Early studies showed that CT has the ability to distinguish noncalcified, mixed, and calcified plaques [40], and automated CTCA software have been validated against IVUS and virtual histology

IVUS [43]. The accuracy of CTCA (using IVUS as the gold standard) showed that it has a high sensitivity and specificity (90% and 92%, respectively, with an area under the curve of 0.94 to detect coronary plaque [43].

Known features of vulnerable plaque, confirmed by histology, IVUS, and CT, are outward vessel remodeling, a large necrotic core (>25% of plaque volume), vasa vasorum in the plaque, fibrous cap <65 microns thickness, macrophage infiltration of the fibrous cap, and elevated matrix metalloproteinase expression [44].

Since the majority of plaque ruptures in ACS occur in coronary plaques that do not cause luminal stenosis, routine stress testing cannot identify vulnerable plaque [45]. CTCA can visualize and differentiate several plaque components, which have been associated with future adverse cardiac events [46]. Motoyama et al., comparing patients with stable CAD and patients with ACS, showed that culprit lesions were more likely to occur in plaques with spotty calcification, outward vessel remodeling (remodeling index > 1.1), and presence of low attenuation plaque (<30 HU) (Figure 7.8). Patients with evidence of outward vessel remodeling and low attenuation plaque had a greater probability (22.2%) of experiencing ACS at two years [47], while others have shown that ring-like plaque represents thin cap fibrous atheroma [48]. The pathologic basis of ring-like plaque (the napkin ring sign) is not fully known but could represent revascularization with intraplaque hemorrhage, deep microcalcification, liponecrotic core, or completed rupture with surrounding contrast agent [38].

Thin cap fibrous atheroma are predominantly found in the proximal segments of the coronary arteries [49] with LAD predominance. In a study of 4870 CTCA patients, 474 (65%) of all lesions were subclinical and nonobstructive, with 7% exhibiting high risk features of low attenuation with outward remodeling [38].

Although CAC has been used as indirect measure of total atherosclerotic burden, it may not accurately identify individual plaque at greatest risk of rupture [41,42]. Since noncalcified plaque appears to be more commonly associated with ACS, noncontrast enhanced CT cannot identify noncalcific plaque with the highest risk features. Similarly, noncontrast enhanced CT may not reliably identify spotty calcification due to the partial volume effect when reconstructing using 2.5 and 3 mm slice thickness. Morita et al. studied 1019 patients with zero calcium score and showed that 4.6% of patients had plaque with ≥2 high-risk CT features [50]. The "Coronary CT Angiography EvaluatioN for Clinical Outcomes: An InteRnational Multicenter" (CONFIRM) registry of 23,854 patients without documented CAD, showed that all-cause mortality was associated with nonobstructive plaque [51]. Although coronary obstruction remains the most predictive CTCA feature, several studies have demonstrated that the prognostic value of nonobstructive plaque is incremental to clinical risk factors, CAD severity and LVEF [52–54].

Although the Framingham risk score (FRS) and the atherosclerotic burden on CT both predict cardiovascular outcome, Pen et al. observed in a large cohort of patients who underwent CTCA that the correlation between FRS and plaque burden was only modest ($r=0.48$) [52,53,55,56]. A significant proportion of low and intermediate FRS patients had evidence of subclinical coronary atherosclerosis and a small percentage of patients with high FRS had no visible atherosclerosis [56]. These findings demonstrate the limitations of population-generated clinical risk prediction models and the potential value of imaging to further refine individual patient risk and develop personalized treatment strategies.

While the data supporting CT features that identify plaque at risk of future rupture is quite promising, the ability to detect plaque erosions (which account for approximately 30% of ACS cases) is limited [57]. Additionally, CT alone cannot be used to detect inflammation, which has been associated with plaque rupture. Currently, there is a paucity of data that links high-risk plaque features with adverse outcomes, and therefore routine plaque screening with CTCA cannot be advocated.

7.3.3 Prognosis by CTCA

The first large prognostic study evaluating 16-slice CTCA in 1127 patients with suspected CAD with a mean follow-up of 15 months [53] showed that the presence of obstructive CAD, number of vessels with obstructive CAD, plaque distribution, and plaque burden provided independent and incremental value in predicting all-cause mortality. The prognostic value of CTCA in symptomatic patients was independent of age, gender, conventional risk factors, and coronary calcium.

The large multinational, multicenter CONFIRM registry has validated many of the observations made by single centers. The absence of disease on CTCA confers an excellent prognosis with an annualized death rate of 0.6% [52]. It appears that this excellent prognosis is sustained over time; Ostrom et al. followed patients for over seven years, and the event rate remained very low (0.3%) [54].

The CONFIRM registry evaluated the incremental contribution of CTCA-defined CAD compared with CACS and conventional risk factors in asymptomatic patients [52], which showed no improvement in risk stratification observed from information provided beyond CACS. Therefore, CTCA is currently not recommended in the general asymptomatic population.

7.3.4 Percutaneous coronary intervention

With the increasing prevalence of percutaneous coronary intervention (PCI), there is commonly a need to re-evaluate symptomatic revascularized patients. The utility of CTCA in post-PCI patients has been evaluated using EBCT, but without the ability to directly assess the stent lumen. This necessitated the assessment of luminal contrast enhancement distal to the stent as an indirect marker of stent patency. However, the accuracy of this method is unreliable in the presence of retrograde filling by collaterals. The absence of contrast distal to a stent is specific for flow limiting disease but is unlikely to be sensitive and cannot be used to exclude in-stent restenosis.

Factors that have limited stent evaluability include stent composition, luminal size, strut size, and high attenuation seen with overlapping stents. Artifacts, such as partial volume effect and beam hardening artifact, make stent struts appear larger and consequently limit the visibility of the stent lumen. Maintz studied the accessibility of stent lumen and demonstrated that *exvivo*, in the absence of cardiac motion or patient attenuation, only 50–59% of the lumen was accessible [58,59].

Stent evaluability may be improved by using a sharper kernel image reconstruction by reducing blooming artifact, but it is offset with an increase in image noise. There have been recent improvements in CTCA operating characteristics in post-PCI patients with a reduction in the frequency of nonevaluable coronary stents. Meta-analyses have examined the utility of CTCA for the assessment of coronary artery stents. In 1286 PCI patients, CTCA had a sensitivity, specificity, positive predictive value and negative predictive value of 99%, 89%, 93%, and 100%, respectively (per-patient analysis) [29,60]. Using a segment-based analysis, the sensitivity, specificity, positive predictive value, and negative predictive value were 90%, 97%, 76%, and 99%, respectively. While the sensitivity and specificity appear to be very good, these results may not be generalizable to all stents nor all centers. Stent evaluability is related to stent size with a high proportion of stents <3.0 mm being unevaluable [61–64]. Acknowledging the current limitations to stent evaluation, many centers recommend the use of stress imaging rather than CTCA in stented patients [65]. ACCF/AHA/ASE/ASNC/HFSA/HRS/SCAI/SCCT/SCMR/STS 2013 Multimodality Appropriate Use Criteria for the Detection and Risk Assessment of Stable Ischemic Heart Disease assigns the designation "maybe appropriate" for the evaluation of symptomatic patients with prior revascularization and "maybe appropriate" in asymptomatic patients with left main stent [66]. In either situation, evaluation of stents with CTCA may be best left to centers of expertise. Although the role of CTCA in the evaluation of patients with bioabsorbable coronary stents has not been well studied, we would anticipate that diagnostic accuracy be similar prior to stent absorption and superior after reabsorption (Figure 7.9).

7.3.5 Coronary artery bypass grafts

Imaging coronary artery bypass grafts (CABGs) is feasible due to the fact that grafts are large and less prone to motion artifact (Figure 7.10). Although arterial grafts are smaller than venous grafts and often have surrounding metallic clips, they are usually easily assessed. However, important to the assessment of grafts is the anastomotic site and distal run-off. The anastomotic site can still be affected by cardiac motion and native coronary disease can often be difficult to assess due to diffuse atherosclerosis, coronary calcification, and obstructive CAD. This can limit the utility of CTCA in the CABG population, especially when bypass grafts are occluded and decisions regarding revascularization of the native coronaries are needed. In many cases, ICA is still needed to guide revascularization.

7.3.6 Accuracy

Analyzing 2023 grafts in 723 patients, the accuracy of CTCA in grafts appears to be excellent (sensitivity=98%, specificity=97%, positive predictive value=93%, and negative predictive value=99%) [60] and the diagnostic accuracy of CTCA was similar in arterial and venous grafts [67]. However, many analyses focused on grafts alone and did not include distal run-off, nongrafted vessels, and segments proximal to graft anastomoses. More recent studies have examined the accuracy of CTCA grafts in addition to distal run-offs and native coronaries [68,69]. Nazeri et al. showed that sensitivity and specificity decreased from 98% and 97% (when restricted to analysis of grafts) to 89% and 94% when studying nongrafted and distal runoff segments [69]. Another study, using a per-segment detection of graft disease, showed sensitivity and specificity of 99% and 96%, respectively, while in the native vessels, sensitivity and specificity were 97% and 86%, respectively [68]. Acknowledging the potential limitations of CTCA in the CABG population, ACCF/AHA/ASE/ASNC/HFSA/HRS/SCAI/SCCT/SCMR/STS 2013 Multimodality Appropriate Use Criteria for the Detection and Risk Assessment of Stable Ischemic Heart Disease have recommended that evaluation of symptomatic patients is "maybe appropriate" but evaluation of asymptomatic patients "rarely appropriate" [66].

7.3.7 Prognosis

Acknowledging the potential limitations of diagnostic accuracy in CABG patients, the prognostic value of CTCA in this population has been examined. Using the CONFIRM registry, Small et al. studied 657 CABG patients and demonstrated the incremental value of measures of revascularized and unrevascularized territories, unprotected coronary territories (UCT) and the coronary artery protective score (CAPS) [70]. The CAPS score appeared to have independent and incremental prognostic value with the ability to appropriately reclassify 27.2% of CABG patients into high and low risk for future all-cause death.

7.3.8 Transluminal arterial gradient and corrected coronary opacification

Transluminal arterial gradient (TAG) and corrected coronary opacification (CCO) have been explored in the efforts to provide functional information that may be incremental to anatomical information. Figure 7.7 shows studies illustrating the discrepancy between the anatomical lesions and their functional significance. TAG uses attenuation samples at 1 mm intervals within the coronary lumen to assess the attenuation change over the coronary artery [71]. Patients with flow limiting lesions had a more negative slope (Figure 7.11). CCO is a similar method but uses luminal attenuation value normalized to the descending aorta, which is potentially relevant when full coverage of the heart is not possible [73]. Using this method, patients with abnormal coronary flow (TIMI < 3) had greater CCO differences between pre- and post-stenosis measurements [73].

Recognizing that multiple beat acquisitions and dense mural calcifications hamper interpretation [74], correction algorithms with dephasing of contrast delivery by relating coronary density to corresponding descending aortic opacification (TAG-CCO) or exclusion of dense calcified coronary segments (TAG-ExC) have been devised. It was shown that while CCO in arteries with lesions was lower, there was no significant difference between arteries with and without hemodynamically significant lesions.

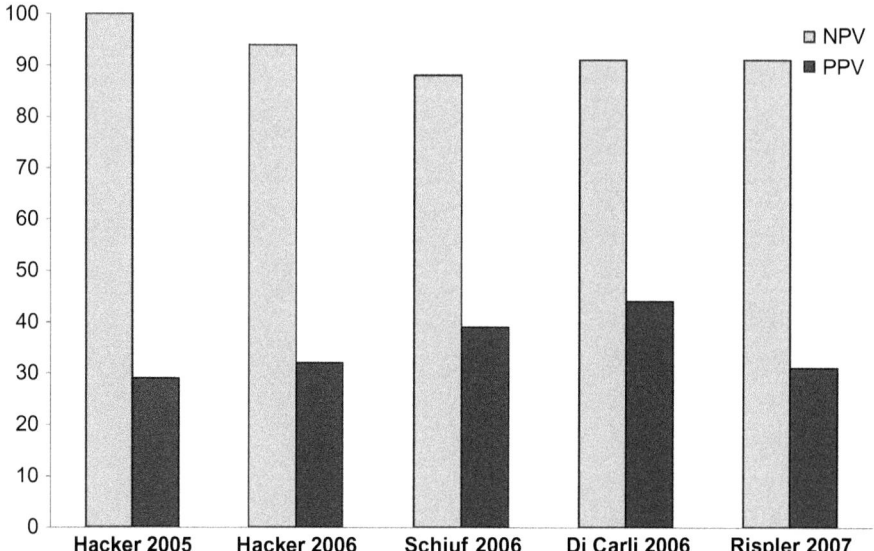

Figure 7.7 Negative and positive predictive value of CTCA stenosis. Predictive value of CTCA for myocardial ischemia.
Adapted from Hachamovitch et al. [32].

Wong et al. studied an integrated approach using TAG, CT-Perfusion, and CTA compared to invasive FFR ≤0.80 as the gold standard [75]. TAG significantly improved both sensitivity and specificity over degree of stenosis alone. Although TAG was shown to be highly reproducible and was better than CCO across a stenosis, however weaknesses of this study and other TAG studies include: small sample sizes, the need for artifact-free images along the arterial course, and the lack of information regarding individual lesions [76].

7.3.9 Fractional flow reserve with CT

Clinicians have begun to recognize the importance of ischemia testing for guiding revascularization strategies. Although this has been well studied with noninvasive methods, recent studies have supported the use of invasive measures of fractional flow reserve (FFR) [21,77]. Practice guidelines support the use of FFR for the assessment of functional significance of moderate coronary stenoses when noninvasive functional information is not available [78]. Initial analysis demonstrated that FFR detected ischemic lesions with sensitivity of 88%, specificity of 88%, and diagnostic accuracy of 93% [79,80]. The incorporation of FFR measures with ICA hopes to remove much of the oculostenotic reflex commonly observed with PCI.

While CTCA can detect and characterize anatomic stenoses, its ability to predict ischemia is modest (Figure 7.7) [17–19]. Recognizing the limitations of CTCA and anatomical imaging, several groups have examined the potential of CTCA to assess for ischemia [73,81–83].

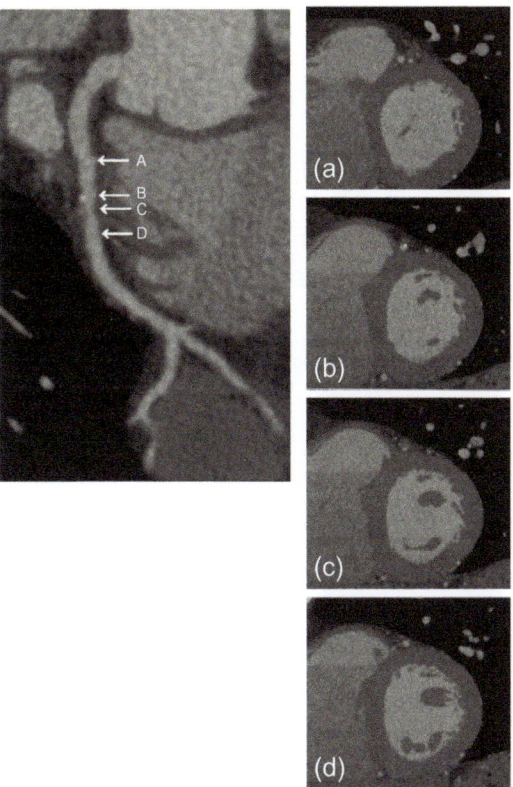

Figure 7.8 CTCA plaque imaging. Curved multiplanar reformation (cMPR) of the left anterior descending artery with a mixed plaque. (a)–(d) show cross sections: proximal to the plaque (a), inside the plaque lumen but proximal to its narrowest (b), plaque at its narrowest (c), and distal to the plaque (d).

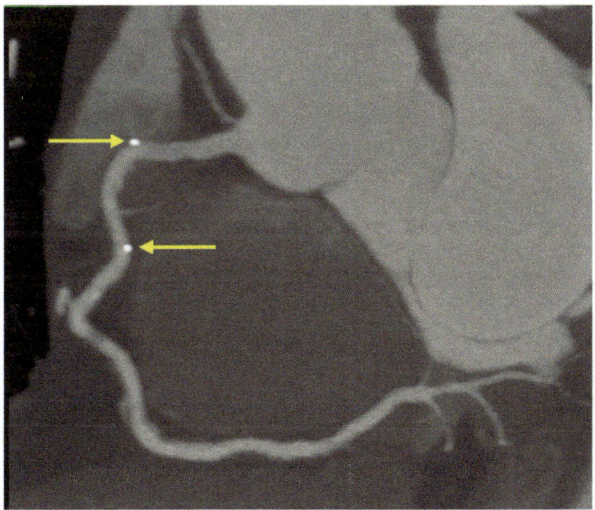

Figure 7.9 Bioresorbable scaffold imaged with CTCA. Curved multiplanar reformation (cMPR) of the right coronary artery containing a bioresorbable scaffold. Arrows illustrate the platinum markers of the device.

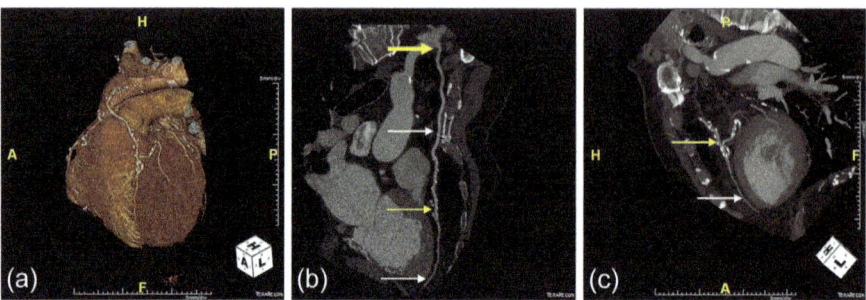

Figure 7.10 Coronary artery bypass graft imaging with CTCA. Image a: 3D Volume rendered image of the left internal thoracic artery (LITA) graft to left anterior descending (LAD). Graft evaluation included assessment of the graft origin (yellow thick arrow; Image b), graft body (white thin arrow; Image b), anastomotic site (yellow thin arrows; Images b and c), and distal run off (native distal LAD, images b and c, white thin arrow).

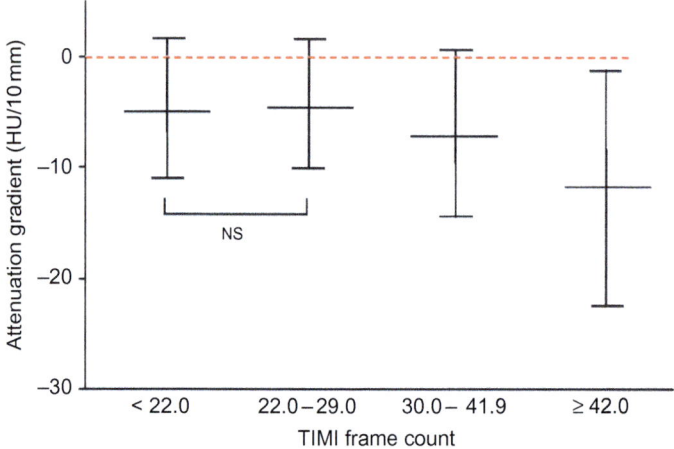

Figure 7.11 CT transluminal attenuation gradients and their relationship to TIMI flow. Adapted from Choi et al. [72].

A proprietary model using computational fluid dynamics has been used to estimate FFR with CT (FFR-CT) [84–86]. "Diagnosis of Ischemia-causing Coronary Stenoses Obtained via Non-Invasive Fractional Flow Reserve" (DISCOVER FLOW) was a prospective trial where 103 CTCA patients were assessed with FFR-CT and compared to invasive FFR [87]. Using invasive FFR < 0.8 as the gold standard, the per-vessel operating characteristics of FFR-CT were very good with an area under the curve of 0.9 for FFR-CT and 0.75 for CTCA. These results have since been confirmed in subsequent studies (Table 7.3) [51,83,84,86]. The most recent study was performed with updated software and stricter adherence to imaging protocols and had promising results [83]. Although encouraging, FFR-CT has limitations that include long processing times

Table 7.3 **The operating characteristics of FFR-CT**

	Sensitivity (%)	Specificity (%)	PPV (%)	NPV (%)	Accuracy (%)
DISCOVER-FLOW [82]	93	82	85	91	81
DeFACTO [86]	90	54	67	84	73
NXT [88]	86	79	65	93	81

For the detection of invasive FFR ≤ 0.80.

(approximately 5 h), and the need for CTCA images that are free of motion and artifact. The utility of FFR-CT in other populations, such as CABG and PCI patients, has not been studied.

7.3.10 CT myocardial perfusion imaging

Another strategy for assessing the functional significance of CTCA stenosis is the assessment of CT perfusion (CTP). With contrast administration, the subsequent myocardial enhancement is dependent on coronary flow. Similar to other methods of assessing myocardial perfusion imaging, images are acquired at rest and with pharmacologic stress (vasodilators such as Adenosine, Regadenoson, and Dipyridamole). In the absence of artifact, reduction in myocardial enhancement represents abnormal perfusion.

Dynamic myocardial perfusion imaging is another method of assessing myocardial perfusion, by examining the rates of myocardial enhancement (Table 7.4). Dynamic imaging serially records kinetics of iodinated contrast in arterial blood pool and myocardium. Time attenuation density curves are collected for the myocardium, left ventricle, and aorta, and myocardial blood flow is derived by mathematical modeling [90]. George et al. showed in early studies that MDCT-derived MBF strongly correlated with MBF measured with microspheres [91].

Potential pitfalls of stress/rest or rest/stress CTP is that the enhancement from first acquisition may still be present at the time of the second acquisition (late enhancement). Washout of contrast can be delayed in areas of scar (similar to the concept of delayed gadolinium enhancement on MRI) and depending on the sequence of rest and

Table 7.4 **Diagnostic performance of CT and SPECT myocardial perfusion imaging for the diagnosis of stenosis ≥50%**

	Sensitivity (%)	Specificity (%)	PPV (%)	NPV (%)
CT perfusion	88	55	75	75
SPECT	62	67	74	54

Adapted from [89].

stress could underestimate or overestimate myocardial ischemia or size of scar [92]. Also, the absence of software that corrects for beam-hardening artifact could lead to artifacts that appear as "hypoperfusion."

The per-vascular territory sensitivity has ranged from 76% to 96% with a specificity of 72–98% [91,92]. Some centers have proposed an algorithm of incorporating CTP into the clinical work-up of patients. In a study, 91 patients underwent CTCA and CTP if the CTCA was nondiagnostic and showed that the combination of CTCA and CTP reduced the nondiagnostic rate from 22% to 1% [92].

7.3.11 Downstream resource utilization and cost-effectiveness

When a new modality is adopted into clinical practice, it is important to demonstrate that it does not impact adversely upon cost or resource utilization. Tandon et al. studied the rate of downstream utilization of ICA and revascularization after CTCA and MPI [93]. Using a prospective matched cohort of 2442 CTCA and SPECT patients, 129 (10.7%) patients from the CTCA group and 125 (10.2%) patients were referred for ICA. When compared to SPECT, CTCA did not result in increased ICA referrals and both groups had similar rates of revascularization. There was a significantly lower rate of false positive test results in the CTCA group.

The "Study of myocardial Perfusion and coronary Anatomy imaging Roles in Coronary artery disease" (SPARC) [94] examined 1703 patients with intermediate and high pretest likelihood for CAD who underwent SPECT, PET, or CTCA. Patients were followed for rates of catheterization and medication changes. There was only a modest impact on clinical management in terms of the medication changes but CTCA patients were more likely to undergo ICA. This may be explained by the greater sensitivity of CTCA or the "oculostenotic reflex" whereby a visual anatomic lesions biases a physician toward revascularization.

Other groups have examined the cost of a CTCA strategy. Min et al. looked at two matched cohorts who underwent MPI or CTCA and evaluated their nine-month expenditures and their clinical outcomes. Downstream and total CAD costs were lower in patients undergoing CTCA and resulted in a cost savings of ($445) beyond the baseline test cost and with no differences in rates of adverse cardiac events [95]. Conversely, in a follow-up analysis of the SPARC study, the economic outcomes of PET, CTCA, and SPECT were compared. At two years, there was no significant difference in outcomes between CTCA and SPECT patients, but CTCA costs were 15% higher and were primarily driven by higher rates of referral to ICA. Since these studies are not randomized controlled trials, there is the issue of referral and selection bias [96]. Further studies examining downstream resource utilization and cost-effectiveness of CTCA are needed to better understand which tests are most likely to yield the greatest diagnostic and prognostic information without increasing the cost of healthcare [97]. An example of studies needed is the "Computed Tomographic coronary Angiography for patients with Heart Failure" (CTA-HF) [98]. This randomized, controlled trial that will examine the utility of CTCA in heart failure patients and its impact on downstream resource utilization and patient health care costs [98].

7.3.12 CTCA in the emergency department

Chest pain leads to millions of visits to the emergency department (ED) each year [99]. CTCA is an attractive modality for triaging patients because it is readily available and has the ability to image patients rapidly without the need for a stressor agent.

Groups have compared the strategy of CTCA to the "standard of care" in ED patients present with acute chest pain syndromes. The diagnostic accuracy of CTCA and SPECT was similar, but the CT strategy reduced the "time to diagnosis" [99]. Although very good at excluding obstructive CAD, 12% of CTCA patients required MPI to further evaluate patients with intermediate stenoses or unevaluable studies. The findings were confirmed in the multicenter "Coronary Computer Tomographic Angiography for Systematic triage of Acute chest pain patients to Treatment trial" (CT-STAT) [100]. This trial showed that CTCA resulted in a 50% reduction in "time to diagnosis" and patients received lower radiation doses than SPECT patients. In 1000 patients, the 'Rule Out Myocardial Infarction/Ischemia Using Computer Assisted Tomography' trial (ROMICAT-II) showed that the length-of-stay in CTCA arm was reduced by 7.6 h with no significant differences in MACE or missed ACS [101]. Similar findings were observed in the CT Angiography for Safe Discharge of Patients with Possible Acute Coronary Syndromes study with higher discharge rates and shorter hospital admissions [102]. These studies suggest that CTCA can be used effectively to triage patients with low-risk acute chest pain syndromes, facilitating early discharge.

In the "Coronary Computed Tomographic Angiography for Systematic Triage of Acute Chest Pain Patients to Treatment" (CT-STAT) trial, discharged patients were followed to ensure the safety of triaging with CTCA. At six months, normal results conferred a very low rate of MACE in both groups (myocardial perfusion imaging = 0.4% versus CTCA = 0.8%) [100]. In the 'Rule Out Myocardial Infarction/Ischemia Using Computer Assisted Tomography' (ROMICAT) trial, patients with normal or nonobstructive CTCA had very high NPV (98%) and patients with a normal CTCA had no adverse events at six months [103]. A large meta-analysis of CTA in patients with acute chest pain confirmed that the annual event rate of a negative CTCA was very low (0.16%) [104]. A meta-analysis of randomized controlled trials in the emergency department confirmed that CTCA decreased patient length of stay and cost [105]. These studies suggest that CTCA can be used in lower-risk acute chest pain syndrome patients to facilitate early diagnosis at a lower cost than current standard of care, and is unlikely to miss prognostically significant CAD.

7.4 Limitations

CTCA still has limited ability to assess areas of severe coronary calcification, which results in blooming and beam-hardening artifact (Figure 7.4). However, these may be minimized in the future with dual-energy image acquisition with mono-energetic reconstruction. Improvements in both spatial and temporal resolution are needed to further improve diagnostic accuracy of CTCA. Radiation dose continues to decline and will lead wider CTCA acceptance and applicability. Iodine contrast medium is still required to opacify coronary lumen; however, greater detector coverage has reduced contrast volumes, thereby reducing the risk of contrast induced acute kidney injury.

7.4.1 Clinical use

As evidenced by the increasing number of appropriate indications for cardiac CT, the clinical use of cardiac CT is expanding [106]. However, test selection is still complex because multiple tests are available and considered "appropriate" for the same indication [66]. Test selection is best tailored based upon local availability and expertise. At our institution, patients with low-intermediate ($\leq 60\%$) pretest probability for CAD who require noninvasive imaging are preferentially investigated with cardiac CT, while patients with >60% pretest probability for CAD or those with documented CAD are investigated with other noninvasive modalities. However, we acknowledge that other guidelines have also proposed different strategies. NICE has recommended that patients presenting with stable chest pain be stratified with the Diamond-Forrester criteria [107]. If the likelihood of disease is 10–29% then CT scanning is recommended, versus 61–90% for coronary angiography and 30–60% for SPECT, stress echocardiography, and magnetic resonance imaging. The NICE guidelines also outline that patients with a calcium score of zero can forego the CTCA portion of the examination on the basis that significant CAD has been ruled out. The absence of consensus highlights the need for further research.

7.5 The future

The simultaneous assessment of coronary anatomy and function with CT appears to be attainable and may eventually lead to the "one-stop shop." With further advancements of CTCA (improved diagnostic accuracy, radiation reduction, artifact reduction, reduced susceptibility to motion artifact), a wider acceptance of CTCA will occur. In the future, the ability to assess for ischemia and/or FFR may allow CTCA to guide revascularization strategies, thereby reducing downstream ischemia testing and the need for invasive diagnostic angiograms. Although its current function is as a "gatekeeper" by ruling-out obstructive CAD, in the future it could serve to triage patients to specific revascularization strategies (PCI or CABG).

7.6 Coronary magnetic resonance imaging

7.6.1 Introduction

CMR imaging of the coronary arteries allows assessment of the coronary arterial lumen as well as atherosclerotic plaque. Compared with CT, CMR is less commonly used, but offers several potential advantages including the absence of radiation and contrast, little limitation posed by the patient's body habitus, and the ability to combine coronary imaging with acquisition of multiple anatomic and functional parameters [108]. In experienced centers and in compliant patients, the image quality and diagnostic performance of CMR can be similar to that of cardiac CT.

However, as in all MR imaging, the acquired spatial resolution in coronary CMR is proportional to image acquisition time. Because coronary imaging requires high spatial resolution of around 1 mm to resolve coronary anatomy and less than 1 mm to identify coronary plaque and stenosis, acquisition of a coronary CMR data set typically requires several minutes. As a consequence, image quality is more variable than in CTA due to the effects of motion and registration artifacts. The anatomical course of coronary arteries can therefore generally determined reliably, but tortuous and small vessels and those running posteriorly are less reliably imaged [109].

The stationary position, straighter course, and size of bypass grafts permit more accurate evaluation with CMR [109–112]. However, like CTCA, anastomotic sites and distal run-off vessels can be problematic to image reliably. Several studies have demonstrated that the proximal graft segments are less susceptible to cardiac motion compared to the distal segments and native coronaries and can impact upon the accuracy of MRA [113]. Other potential limitations in graft patients are artifacts associated with metallic clips; proximity of sternal wires to the grafts; and severe, diffusely diseased native arteries.

Taking into the account the considerations above, and the current evidence for coronary CMR, ACCF/ACR/AHA/NASCI/SCMR 2010 Expert Consensus Document on Cardiovascular Magnetic Resonance document rated the method appropriate for the identification of coronary artery aneurysms and anomalies (Class I) and aortocoronary bypass grafts (Class II) [108].

7.6.1.1 Methods for coronary CMR

Numerous and different acquisition protocols have been described to meet the challenges of coronary CMR, including targeted and whole-heart acquisition, contrast-enhanced and noncontrast methods, and various acquisition pulse sequence designs [114].

In order to compensate for cardiac motion, acquisition is generally limited to the diastolic coronary rest period with acquisition windows of 100–150 ms, depending on the heart rate of the patient and the vessel imaged. In some patients, the systolic phase can deliver better image quality. Respiratory navigator methods are now widely used to compensate for respiratory motion. They usually track the position of the diaphragm (although cardiac or multiple navigators can also be used) and restrict acquisition to the end-expiratory phase. Navigators signals are also used to adjust for residual respiratory motion, either using fixed conversion factors (most commonly 0.6 for the ratio of diaphragmatic to cardiac motion) or more sophisticated conversion models.

The number of different pulse sequences used for coronary CMR acquisition pulse is vast. In general, methods include fat saturation and other preparation schemes to improve vessel edge detection within the surrounding tissue. Signal read out with spoiled or balanced gradient echo methods has been used, and both Cartesian and spiral k-space filling have been proposed. Comparative studies of all these parameters are sparse, with one small study suggesting that spiral and balanced fast field echo imaging offer the best signal:noise ratio, contrast:noise ratio, vessel sharpness, and qualitative results [114]. Acquiring coronary CMR images during or after the administration of contrast agents may also improve image contrast, but is not mandatory as it is in CTA. However, the effect of different imaging parameters on diagnostic performance is largely unknown.

While in the past, targeted acquisition on individual coronary arteries was mostly used to limit acquisition time; with current methods, whole-heart acquisition is feasible within a few minutes and has become the clinical standard.

7.6.1.2 Accuracy

The diagnostic accuracy of coronary CMR to detect significant coronary stenosis is best for the proximal segments of the coronary arteries [126]. In an early study, Manning and Edelman [127] showed excellent sensitivity (90%) and specificity (92%) using 2-D segmented gradient echo (2D GRE) acquisition. The introduction of whole-heart imaging with a free breathing navigator has increased the feasibility and acceptance of coronary CMR [115]. In a multicenter trial, Kim et al. analyzed this technique in 109 patients [116]. A total of 84% of coronary segments were evaluable with excellent sensitivity but relatively poor specificity. Triple vessel disease and left main disease detection was excellent with a sensitivity of 100% and a specificity of 85%. However, only the proximal coronary segments were analyzed in this study.

In a more recent multicenter study of seven Japanese hospitals, whole-heart coronary CMR was assessed against ICA for the detection of significant obstructive CAD [117] and yielded a sensitivity specificity and NPV of 88%, 72%, and 88%, respectively. This NPV was comparable to that of the CORE-64 study, suggesting that in a population with a pretest probability of <20%, coronary CMR may be comparable to CTA. However, a meta-analysis of noninvasive imaging included 89 CTCA and 20 CMR studies, and 5 of these studies directly compared the two modalities [118]. In the five studies, both sensitivity (97.2% vs. 87.4%) and specificity (87.1% vs. 70.3%) were higher for CTA than for coronary CMR. Where ionizing radiation is no concern, CTA is therefore widely considered the preferred method for noninvasive coronary imaging. CMR may be favored in patients with a very low pretest probability of CAD, especially children and young women in whom radiation exposure is associated with higher risks.

7.6.1.3 Prognosis

Prognostic CMR studies are limited, and coronary CMR has been mostly evaluated in the context of multiparametric CMR assessment [119]. In a small study, 207 patients were followed for a median of 25 months for major adverse cardiac events [120]. A total of five cardiac events were observed in the 84 patients with coronary stenosis ≥50%. No fatal cardiac events were observed in the 123 patients without significant stenosis. Albeit preliminary, these data support the potential prognostic value of a normal coronary CMR study.

7.6.1.4 Multiparametric imaging

An advantage of CMR over other noninvasive modalities is that multiple parameters can be assessed from a single study: ventricular function, myocardial perfusion, viability, and coronary artery anatomy. The inclusion of coronary CMR in such multiparametric imaging protocols has been investigated in several studies, giving inconsistent results. Most prominently, the "Cardiovascular Magnetic Resonance and Single Photon emission computed tomography for diagnosis of coronary heart disease" (CE-MARC) study was a large prospective trial assessing the diagnostic accuracy of CMR [121]. While the trial showed excellent sensitivity and specificity for multiparametric CMR compared to SPECT, the results of the coronary CMR component were less favorable. Only 55% of the 10,140 segments were of analyzable quality and the exclusion of the coronary analysis resulted in no significant decrease in sensitivity and overall accuracy. In non-ST elevation MI patients, multiparametric CMR had excellent sensitivity; however, when the accuracy of MRA for the coronaries was examined, the results were weak [122]. However, in another small study of 43 patients by Klein et al., adding coronary CMR to perfusion and LGE analysis increased the sensitivity from 79% to 96% and NPV from 78% to 94% [123]. From the available data, it is therefore uncertain if coronary CMR performed as part of a comprehensive multiparametric CMR study has incremental value over perfusion and LGE imaging. This issue is further complicated by the fact that within a multiparametric study, coronary MRA protocols cannot be optimized in the same way as in a focused coronary study, and larger future studies may need to consider protocol designs that optimize coronary CMR acquisition.

7.6.1.5 Ongoing and future developments

As for other applications, coronary CMR may benefit from imaging at higher field strength. In one comparative study, 3 T imaging yielded significant increases in signal-to-noise ratios and contrast-to-noise ratios compared to 1.5 T acquisition, but no significant improvement in image quality or diagnostic accuracy [124]. In a second study, coronary CMR at 3 T was comparable to 64-slice CTCA, with AUC for CMR 0.78 (95% CI: 0.69–0.87) and CTCA 0.82 (95% CI: 0.74–0.90) [125].

CMR has also been used for the evaluation of the coronary arterial wall. Noncontrast methods can characterize components of atherosclerotic plaques, providing images are acquired with sufficient spatial resolution. Contrast-enhanced methods in particular, with contrast agents targeting specific molecules or cells, allow visualization of pathological processes within the plaque.

References

[1] Rosen BD, Fernandes V, McClelland RL, Carr JJ, Detrano R, Bluemke DA, et al. Relationship between baseline coronary calcium score and demonstration of coronary artery stenoses during follow-up MESA (multi-ethnic study of atherosclerosis). JACC Cardiovasc Imaging 2009;2(10):1175–83.

[2] Goel R, Garg P, Achenbach S, Gupta A, Song JJ, Wong ND, et al. Coronary artery calcification and coronary atherosclerotic disease. Cardiol Clin 2012;30(1):19–47.

[3] Budoff MJ, Diamond GA, Raggi P, Arad Y, Guerci AD, Callister TQ, et al. Continuous probabilistic prediction of angiographically significant coronary artery disease using electron beam tomography. Circulation 2002;105(15):1791–6.
[4] Breen JF, Sheedy 2nd PF, Schwartz RS, Stanson AW, Kaufmann RB, Moll PP, et al. Coronary artery calcification detected with ultrafast CT as an indication of coronary artery disease. Radiology 1992;185(2):435–9.
[5] Haberl R, Becker A, Leber A, Knez A, Becker C, Lang C, et al. Correlation of coronary calcification and angiographically documented stenoses in patients with suspected coronary artery disease: results of 1,764 patients. J Am Coll Cardiol 2001;37(2):451–7.
[6] Budoff MJ, Shaw LJ, Liu ST, Weinstein SR, Mosler TP, Tseng PH, et al. Long-term prognosis associated with coronary calcification: observations from a registry of 25,253 patients. J Am Coll Cardiol 2007;49(18):1860–70.
[7] Marwan M, Ropers D, Pflederer T, Daniel WG, Achenbach S. Clinical characteristics of patients with obstructive coronary lesions in the absence of coronary calcification: an evaluation by coronary CT angiography. Heart 2009;95(13):1056–60.
[8] Gottlieb I, Miller JM, Arbab-Zadeh A, Dewey M, Clouse ME, Sara L, et al. The absence of coronary calcification does Not exclude obstructive coronary artery disease or the need for revascularization in patients referred for conventional coronary angiography. J Am Coll Cardiol 2010;55(7):627–34.
[9] Rubinshtein R, Gaspar T, Halon DA, Goldstein J, Peled N, Lewis BS. Prevalence and extent of obstructive coronary artery disease in patients with zero or low calcium score undergoing 64-slice cardiac multidetector computed tomography for evaluation of a chest pain syndrome. Am J Cardiol 2007;99(4):472–5.
[10] Redberg RF. What is the prognostic value of a zero calcium score? J Am Coll Cardiol 2010;55(7):635–6.
[11] Youssef G, Budoff MJ. Coronary artery calcium scoring, what is answered and what questions remain. Cardiovasc Diagn Ther 2012;2(2):94–105.
[12] Agatston AS, Janowitz WR, Hildner FJ, Zusmer NR, Viamonte Jr M, Detrano R. Quantification of coronary artery calcium using ultrafast computed tomography. J Am Coll Cardiol 1990;15(4):827–32.
[13] Abunassar JG, Yam Y, Chen L, D'Mello N, Chow BJ. Usefulness of the Agatston score=0 to exclude ischemic cardiomyopathy in patients with heart failure. Am J Cardiol 2011;107(3):428–32.
[14] Greenland P, Bonow RO, Brundage BH, Budoff MJ, Eisenberg MJ, Grundy SM, et al. ACCF/AHA 2007 clinical expert consensus document on coronary artery calcium scoring by computed tomography in global cardiovascular risk assessment and in evaluation of patients with chest pain: a report of the American College of Cardiology Foundation Clinical Expert Consensus Task Force (ACCF/AHA Writing Committee to Update the 2000 Expert Consensus Document on Electron Beam Computed Tomography) developed in collaboration with the Society of Atherosclerosis Imaging and Prevention and the Society of Cardiovascular Computed Tomography. J Am Coll Cardiol 2007;49(3):378–402.
[15] Villines TC, Hulten EA, Shaw LJ, Goyal M, Dunning A, Achenbach S, et al. Prevalence and severity of coronary artery disease and adverse events among symptomatic patients with coronary artery calcification scores of zero undergoing coronary computed tomography angiography: results from the CONFIRM (Coronary CT Angiography Evaluation for Clinical Outcomes: An International Multicenter) registry. J Am Coll Cardiol 2011;58(24):2533–40.
[16] Nieman K, Galema TW, Neefjes LA, Weustink AC, Musters P, Moelker AD, et al. Comparison of the value of coronary calcium detection to computed tomographic

angiography and exercise testing in patients with chest pain. Am J Cardiol 2009;104(11):1499–504.
[17] Mouden M, Timmer JR, Reiffers S, Oostdijk AH, Knollema S, Ottervanger JP, et al. Coronary artery calcium scoring to exclude flow-limiting coronary artery disease in symptomatic stable patients at low or intermediate risk. Radiology 2013;269(1):77–83.
[18] Shaw LJ, Hausleiter J, Achenbach S, Al-Mallah M, Berman DS, Budoff MJ, et al. Coronary computed tomographic angiography as a gatekeeper to invasive diagnostic and surgical procedures: results from the multicenter CONFIRM (coronary CT angiography evaluation for clinical outcomes: an international multicenter) registry. J Am Coll Cardiol 2012;60(20):2103–14.
[19] Gould KL, Kirkeeide RL, Buchi M. Coronary flow reserve as a physiologic measure of stenosis severity. J Am Coll Cardiol 1990;15(2):459–74.
[20] Uren NG, Crake T. Resistive vessel function in coronary artery disease. Heart 1996;76(4):299–304.
[21] Tonino PA, De Bruyne B, Pijls NH, Siebert U, Ikeno F, van' t Veer M, et al. Fractional flow reserve versus angiography for guiding percutaneous coronary intervention. N Engl J Med 2009;360(3):213–24.
[22] Tonino PA, Fearon WF, De Bruyne B, Oldroyd KG, Leesar MA, Ver Lee PN, et al. Angiographic versus functional severity of coronary artery stenoses in the FAME study fractional flow reserve versus angiography in multivessel evaluation. J Am Coll Cardiol 2010;55(25):2816–21.
[23] Emond M, Mock MB, Davis KB, Fisher LD, Holmes Jr DR, Chaitman BR, et al. Long-term survival of medically treated patients in the coronary artery surgery study (CASS) registry. Circulation 1994;90(6):2645–57.
[24] Falk E, Fuster V. Angina pectoris and disease progression. Circulation 1995;92(8):2033–5.
[25] Leschka S, Alkadhi H, Wildermuth S, Marincek B. Multi-detector computed tomography of acute abdomen. Eur Radiol 2005;15(12):2435–47.
[26] Raff GL, Gallagher MJ, O'Neill WW, Goldstein JA. Diagnostic accuracy of noninvasive coronary angiography using 64-slice spiral computed tomography. J Am Coll Cardiol 2005;46(3):552–7.
[27] Herzog C, Zwerner PL, Doll JR, Nielsen CD, Nguyen SA, Savino G, et al. Significant coronary artery stenosis: comparison on per-patient and per-vessel or per-segment basis at 64-section CT angiography. Radiology 2007;244(1):112–20.
[28] Ropers D, Rixe J, Anders K, Kuttner A, Baum U, Bautz W, et al. Usefulness of multidetector row spiral computed tomography with 64- x 0.6-mm collimation and 330-ms rotation for the noninvasive detection of significant coronary artery stenoses. Am J Cardiol 2006;97(3):343–8.
[29] Mowatt G, Cook JA, Hillis GS, Walker S, Fraser C, Jia X, et al. 64-Slice computed tomography angiography in the diagnosis and assessment of coronary artery disease: systematic review and meta-analysis. Heart 2008;94(11):1386–93.
[30] Vanhoenacker PK, Heijenbrok-Kal MH, Van Heste R, Decramer I, Van Hoe LR, Wijns W, et al. Diagnostic performance of multidetector CT angiography for assessment of coronary artery disease: meta-analysis. Radiology 2007;244(2):419–28.
[31] Abdulla J, Abildstrom SZ, Gotzsche O, Christensen E, Kober L, Torp-Pedersen C. 64-multislice detector computed tomography coronary angiography as potential alternative to conventional coronary angiography: a systematic review and meta-analysis. Eur Heart J 2007;28(24):3042–50.
[32] Hachamovitch R, Di Carli MF. Nuclear cardiology will remain the "gatekeeper" over CT angiography. J Nucl Cardiol 2007;14(5):634–44.

[33] Budoff MJ, Dowe D, Jollis JG, Gitter M, Sutherland J, Halamert E, et al. Diagnostic performance of 64-multidetector row coronary computed tomographic angiography for evaluation of coronary artery stenosis in individuals without known coronary artery disease: results from the prospective multicenter ACCURACY (assessment by coronary computed tomographic angiography of individuals undergoing invasive coronary angiography) trial. J Am Coll Cardiol 2008;52(21):1724–32.

[34] Miller JM, Rochitte CE, Dewey M, Arbab-Zadeh A, Niinuma H, Gottlieb I, et al. Diagnostic performance of coronary angiography by 64-Row CT. N Engl J Med 2008;359(22):2324–36.

[35] Meijboom WB, Meijs MFL, Schuijf JD, Cramer MJ, Mollet NR, van Mieghem CAG, et al. Diagnostic accuracy of 64-slice computed tomography coronary angiography: a prospective, multicenter, multivendor study. J Am Coll Cardiol 2008;52(25):2135–44.

[36] Chow BJ, Freeman MR, Bowen JM, Levin L, Hopkins RB, Provost Y, et al. Ontario multidetector computed tomographic coronary angiography study: field evaluation of diagnostic accuracy. Arch Intern Med 2011;171(11):1021–9.

[37] Chow BJ, Abraham A, Wells GA, Chen L, Ruddy TD, Yam Y, et al. Diagnostic accuracy and impact of computed tomographic coronary angiography on utilization of invasive coronary angiography. Circ Cardiovasc Imaging 2009;2(1):16–23.

[38] Fujimoto S, Kondo T, Narula J. Evaluation of plaque morphology by coronary CT angiography. Cardiol Clin 2012;30(1):69–75.

[39] Nicholls SJ, Sipahi I, Schoenhagen P, Wisniewski L, Churchill T, Crowe T, et al. Intravascular ultrasound assessment of novel antiatherosclerotic therapies: rationale and design of the acyl-CoA:cholesterol acyltransferase intravascular atherosclerosis treatment evaluation (ACTIVATE) study. Am Heart J 2006;152(1):67–74.

[40] Leber AW, Knez A, von Ziegler F, Becker A, Nikolaou K, Paul S, et al. Quantification of obstructive and nonobstructive coronary lesions by 64-slice computed tomography: a comparative study with quantitative coronary angiography and intravascular ultrasound. J Am Coll Cardiol 2005;46(1):147–54.

[41] Naghavi M, Libby P, Falk E, Casscells SW, Litovsky S, Rumberger J, et al. From vulnerable plaque to vulnerable patient: a call for new definitions and risk assessment strategies: part II. Circulation 2003;108(15):1772–8.

[42] Naghavi M, Libby P, Falk E, Casscells SW, Litovsky S, Rumberger J, et al. From vulnerable plaque to vulnerable patient: a call for new definitions and risk assessment strategies: part I. Circulation 2003;108(14):1664–72.

[43] Voros S, Rinehart S, Qian Z, Joshi P, Vazquez G, Fischer C, et al. Coronary atherosclerosis imaging by coronary CT angiography: current status, correlation with intravascular interrogation and meta-analysis. JACC Cardiovasc Imaging 2011;4(5):537–48.

[44] Narula J, Finn AV, Demaria AN. Picking plaques that pop. J Am Coll Cardiol 2005;45(12):1970–3.

[45] Braunwald E. Epilogue: what do clinicians expect from imagers? J Am Coll Cardiol 2006;47(8 Suppl):C101–3.

[46] Motoyama S, Kondo T, Anno H, Sugiura A, Ito Y, Mori K, et al. Atherosclerotic plaque characterization by 0.5-mm-slice multislice computed tomographic imaging. Circ J 2007;71(3):363–6.

[47] Motoyama S, Sarai M, Harigaya H, Anno H, Inoue K, Hara T, et al. Computed tomographic angiography characteristics of atherosclerotic plaques subsequently resulting in acute coronary syndrome. J Am Coll Cardiol 2009;54(1):49–57.

[48] Kashiwagi M, Tanaka A, Kitabata H, Tsujioka H, Kataiwa H, Komukai K, et al. Feasibility of noninvasive assessment of thin-cap fibroatheroma by multidetector computed tomography. JACC Cardiovasc Imaging 2009;2(12):1412–9.

[49] Kolodgie FD, Burke AP, Farb A, Gold HK, Yuan J, Narula J, et al. The thin-cap fibroatheroma: a type of vulnerable plaque: the major precursor lesion to acute coronary syndromes. Curr Opin Cardiol 2001;16(5):285–92.
[50] Morita H, Fujimoto S, Kondo T, Arai T, Sekine T, Matsutani H, et al. Prevalence of computed tomographic angiography-verified high-risk plaques and significant luminal stenosis in patients with zero coronary calcium score. Int J Cardiol 2012;158(2):272–8.
[51] Nakazato R, Gransar H, Berman DS, Cheng VY, Lin FY, Achenbach S, et al. Statins use and coronary artery plaque composition: results from the international multicenter CONFIRM registry. Atherosclerosis 2012;225(1):148–53.
[52] Chow BJ, Small G, Yam Y, Chen L, Achenbach S, Al-Mallah M, et al. Incremental prognostic value of cardiac computed tomography in coronary artery disease using CONFIRM: COroNary computed tomography angiography evaluation for clinical outcomes: an InteRnational Multicenter registry. Circ Cardiovasc Imaging 2011;4(5):463–72.
[53] Min JK, Shaw LJ, Devereux RB, Okin PM, Weinsaft JW, Russo DJ, et al. Prognostic value of multidetector coronary computed tomographic angiography for prediction of all-cause mortality. J Am Coll Cardiol 2007;50(12):1161–70.
[54] Ostrom MP, Gopal A, Ahmadi N, Nasir K, Yang E, Kakadiaris I, et al. Mortality incidence and the severity of coronary atherosclerosis assessed by computed tomography angiography. J Am Coll Cardiol 2008;52(16):1335–43.
[55] Chow BJ, Wells GA, Chen L, Yam Y, Galiwango P, Abraham A, et al. Prognostic value of 64-slice cardiac computed tomography severity of coronary artery disease, coronary atherosclerosis, and left ventricular ejection fraction. J Am Coll Cardiol 2010;55(10):1017–28.
[56] Pen A, Yam Y, Chen L, Dennie C, McPherson R, Chow BJ. Discordance between Framingham risk score and atherosclerotic plaque burden. Eur Heart J 2013;34(14):1075–82.
[57] Ozaki Y, Okumura M, Ismail TF, Motoyama S, Naruse H, Hattori K, et al. Coronary CT angiographic characteristics of culprit lesions in acute coronary syndromes not related to plaque rupture as defined by optical coherence tomography and angioscopy. Eur Heart J 2011;32 (November (22)):2814–23.
[58] Maintz D, Seifarth H, Flohr T, Kramer S, Wichter T, Heindel W, et al. Improved coronary artery stent visualization and in-stent stenosis detection using 16-slice computed-tomography and dedicated image reconstruction technique. Invest Radiol 2003;38(12):790–5.
[59] Maintz D, Burg MC, Seifarth H, Bunck AC, Ozgun M, Fischbach R, et al. Update on multidetector coronary CT angiography of coronary stents: in vitro evaluation of 29 different stent types with dual-source CT. Eur Radiol 2009;19(1):42–9.
[60] Hamon M, Biondi-Zoccai GG, Malagutti P, Agostoni P, Morello R, Valgimigli M, et al. Diagnostic performance of multislice spiral computed tomography of coronary arteries as compared with conventional invasive coronary angiography: a meta-analysis. J Am Coll Cardiol 2006;48(9):1896–910.
[61] Carrabba N, Schuijf J, Graaf F, Parodi G, Maffei E, Valenti R, et al. Diagnostic accuracy of 64-slice computed tomography coronary angiography for the detection of in-stent restenosis: a meta-analysis. J Nucl Cardiol 2010;17(3):470–8.
[62] Pugliese F, Weustink AC, Van Mieghem C, Alberghina F, Otsuka M, Meijboom WB, et al. Dual source coronary computed tomography angiography for detecting in-stent restenosis. Heart 2008;94(7):848–54.
[63] de Graaf FR, Schuijf JD, van Velzen JE, Boogers MJ, Kroft LJ, de Roos A, et al. Diagnostic accuracy of 320-row multidetector computed tomography coronary angiography to noninvasively assess in-stent restenosis. Invest Radiol 2010;45(6):331–40.

[64] Pflederer T, Marwan M, Renz A, Bachmann S, Ropers D, Kuettner A, et al. Noninvasive assessment of coronary in-stent restenosis by dual-source computed tomography. Am J Cardiol 2009;103(6):812–7.
[65] Kumbhani DJ, Ingelmo CP, Schoenhagen P, Curtin RJ, Flamm SD, Desai MY. Meta-analysis of diagnostic efficacy of 64-slice computed tomography in the evaluation of coronary in-stent restenosis. Am J Cardiol 2009;103(12):1675–81.
[66] Wolk MJ, Bailey SR, Doherty JU, Douglas PS, Hendel RC, Kramer CM, et al. ACCF/AHA/ASE/ASNC/HFSA/HRS/SCAI/SCCT/SCMR/STS 2013 Multimodality appropriate use criteria for the detection and risk assessment of stable ischemic heart disease: A report of the American College of Cardiology Foundation Appropriate Use Criteria Task Force, American Heart Association, American Society of Echocardiography, American Society of Nuclear Cardiology, Heart Failure Society of America, Heart Rhythm Society, Society for Cardiovascular Angiography and Interventions, Society of Cardiovascular Computed Tomography, Society for Cardiovascular Magnetic Resonance, and Society of Thoracic Surgeons. J Am Coll Cardiol 2014;63(4):380–406.
[67] Meyer TS, Martinoff S, Hadamitzky M, Will A, Kastrati A, Schömig A, et al. Improved noninvasive assessment of coronary artery bypass grafts with 64-slice computed tomographic angiography in an unselected patient population. J Am Coll Cardiol 2007;49(9):946–50.
[68] Malagutti P, Nieman K, Meijboom WB, van Mieghem CAG, Pugliese F, Cademartiri F, et al. Use of 64-slice CT in symptomatic patients after coronary bypass surgery: evaluation of grafts and coronary arteries. Eur Heart J 2007;28(15):1879–85.
[69] Nazeri I, Shahabi P, Tehrai M, Sharif-Kashani B, Nazeri A. Assessment of patients after coronary artery bypass grafting using 64-slice computed tomography. Am J Cardiol 2009;103(5):667–73.
[70] Small GR, Yam Y, Chen L, Ahmed O, Al-Mallah M, Berman DS, et al. Prognostic assessment of coronary artery bypass patients with 64-slice computed tomography angiography: anatomical information is incremental to clinical risk prediction. J Am Coll Cardiol 2011;58(23):2389–95.
[71] Steigner ML, Mitsouras D, Whitmore AG, Otero HJ, Wang C, Buckley O, et al. Iodinated contrast opacification gradients in normal coronary arteries imaged with prospectively ECG-gated single heart beat 320-detector row computed tomography. Circ Cardiovasc Imaging 2010;3(2):179–86.
[72] Choi JH, Koo BK, Yoon YE, Min JK, Song YB, Hahn JY, et al. Diagnostic performance of intracoronary gradient-based methods by coronary computed tomography angiography for the evaluation of physiologically significant coronary artery stenoses: a validation study with fractional flow reserve. Eur Heart J Cardiovasc Imaging 2012;13(12):1001–7.
[73] Chow BJ, Kass M, Gagne O, Chen L, Yam Y, Dick A, et al. Can differences in corrected coronary opacification measured with computed tomography predict resting coronary artery flow? J Am Coll Cardiol 2011;57(11):1280–8.
[74] Stuijfzand W, Danad I, Raijmakers P, Marcu B, Heymans M, Van Kuijk C, et al. Additional value of transluminal attenuation gradient in coronary computed tomography angiography to predict hemodynamic significance of coronary artery stenosis. JACC Cardiovasc Imaging 2014;7(April (4)):374–86.
[75] Wong DTL, Ko BS, Cameron JD, Nerlekar N, Leung MCH, Malaiapan Y, et al. Transluminal attenuation gradient in coronary computed tomography angiography is a novel noninvasive approach to the identification of functionally significant coronary artery stenosis: a comparison with fractional flow reserve. J Am Coll Cardiol 2013;61(12):1271–9.

[76] Berman DS, Stoebner RA, Dey D. Combined anatomy and physiology on coronary computed tomography Angiography: a step or two in the right direction. J Am Coll Cardiol 2014;63(18):1913–5.

[77] De Bruyne B, Pijls NHJ, Kalesan B, Barbato E, Tonino PAL, Piroth Z, et al. Fractional flow reserve–guided PCI versus medical therapy in stable coronary disease. N Engl J Med 2012;367(11):991–1001.

[78] Interventions DwtscotEAfPC, Members ATF, Wijns W, Kolh P, Danchin N, Di Mario C, et al. Guidelines on myocardial revascularization: the task force on myocardial revascularization of the European Society of Cardiology (ESC) and the European Association for Cardio-Thoracic Surgery (EACTS). Eur Heart J 2010;31(20):2501–55.

[79] Pijls NH, De Bruyne B. Coronary pressure measurement and fractional flow reserve. Heart 1998;80(6):539–42.

[80] Hau WK. Fractional flow reserve and complex coronary intervention. J Chin Med Assoc 2004;67(9):433–8.

[81] Rybicki FJ, Otero HJ, Steigner ML, Vorobiof G, Nallamshetty L, Mitsouras D, et al. Initial evaluation of coronary images from 320-detector row computed tomography. Int J Cardiovasc Imaging 2008;24(5):535–46.

[82] Koo BK, Erglis A, Doh JH, Daniels DV, Jegere S, Kim HS, et al. Diagnosis of ischemia-causing coronary stenoses by noninvasive fractional flow reserve computed from coronary computed tomographic angiograms. Results from the prospective multicenter DISCOVER-FLOW (Diagnosis of Ischemia-Causing Stenoses Obtained Via Noninvasive Fractional Flow Reserve) study. J Am Coll Cardiol 2011;58(19):1989–97.

[83] Nørgaard BL, Leipsic J, Gaur S, Seneviratne S, Ko BS, Ito H, et al. Diagnostic performance of noninvasive fractional flow reserve derived from coronary computed tomography angiography in suspected coronary artery DiseaseThe NXT trial (analysis of coronary blood flow using CT angiography: next steps). J Am Coll Cardiol 2014;63(12):1145–55.

[84] Min JK, Berman DS, Budoff MJ, Jaffer FA, Leipsic J, Leon MB, et al. Rationale and design of the DeFACTO (Determination of Fractional Flow Reserve by Anatomic Computed Tomographic AngiOgraphy) study. J Cardiovasc Comput Tomogr 2011;5(5):301–9.

[85] Min JK, Koo BK, Erglis A, Doh JH, Daniels DV, Jegere S, et al. Usefulness of noninvasive fractional flow reserve computed from coronary computed tomographic angiograms for intermediate stenoses confirmed by quantitative coronary angiography. Am J Cardiol 2012;110(7):971–6.

[86] Min JK, Leipsic J, Pencina MJ, Berman DS, Koo BK, van Mieghem C, et al. Diagnostic accuracy of fractional flow reserve from anatomic CT angiography. JAMA 2012;308(12):1237–45.

[87] Koo B-K, Erglis A, Doh J-H, Daniels DV, Jegere S, Kim H-S, et al. Diagnosis of ischemia-causing coronary stenoses by noninvasive fractional flow reserve computed from coronary computed tomographic AngiogramsResults from the prospective multicenter DISCOVER-FLOW (diagnosis of ischemia-causing stenoses obtained Via noninvasive fractional flow reserve) study. J Am Coll Cardiol 2011;58(19):1989–97.

[88] Norgaard BL, Leipsic J, Gaur S, Seneviratne S, Ko BS, Ito H, et al. Diagnostic performance of noninvasive fractional flow reserve derived from coronary computed tomography angiography in suspected coronary artery disease: the NXT trial (Analysis of Coronary Blood Flow Using CT Angiography: Next Steps). J Am Coll Cardiol 2014;63(12):1145–55.

[89] George RT, Mehra VC, Chen MY, Kitagawa K, Arbab-Zadeh A, Miller JM, et al. Myocardial CT perfusion imaging and SPECT for the diagnosis of coronary artery disease: a head-to-head comparison from the CORE320 multicenter diagnostic performance study. Radiology 2014;272(2):407–16.
[90] Techasith T, Cury RC. Stress myocardial CT perfusion: an update and future perspective. JACC Cardiovasc Imaging 2011;4(8):905–16.
[91] Ko BS, Cameron JD, Defrance T, Seneviratne SK. CT stress myocardial perfusion imaging using multidetector CT–a review. J Cardiovasc Comput Tomogr 2011;5(6):345–56.
[92] Dwivedi G, Dowsley TF, Chow BJ. Assessment of cardiac computed tomography-myocardial perfusion imaging - promise and challenges. Circ J 2012;76(3):544–52.
[93] Tandon V, Hall D, Yam Y, Al-Shehri H, Chen L, Tandon K, et al. Rates of downstream invasive coronary angiography and revascularization: computed tomographic coronary angiography vs. Tc-99m single photon emission computed tomography. Eur Heart J 2012;33(6):776–82.
[94] Hachamovitch R, Nutter B, Hlatky MA, Shaw LJ, Ridner ML, Dorbala S, et al. Patient management after noninvasive cardiac ImagingResults from SPARC (study of myocardial perfusion and coronary anatomy imaging roles in coronary artery disease). J Am Coll Cardiol 2012;59(5):462–74.
[95] Min JK, Hachamovitch R, Rozanski A, Shaw LJ, Berman DS, Gibbons R. Clinical benefits of noninvasive testing: coronary computed tomography angiography as a test case. JACC Cardiovasc Imaging 2010;3(3):305–15.
[96] Hlatky MA, Shilane D, Hachamovitch R, Dicarli MF, Investigators S. Economic outcomes in the study of myocardial perfusion and coronary anatomy imaging roles in coronary artery disease registry: the SPARC study. J Am Coll Cardiol 2014;63(10):1002–8.
[97] Shaw LJ, Marwick TH, Zoghbi WA, Hundley WG, Kramer CM, Achenbach S, et al. Why all the focus on cardiac imaging? JACC Cardiovasc Imaging 2010;3(7):789–94.
[98] Chow BJ, Green RE, Coyle D, Laine M, Hanninen H, Leskinen H, et al. Computed tomographic coronary angiography for patients with heart failure (CTA-HF): a randomized controlled trial (IMAGE HF Project 1-C). Trials 2013;14:443.
[99] Goldstein JA, Gallagher MJ, O'Neill WW, Ross MA, O'Neil BJ, Raff GL. A randomized controlled trial of multi-slice coronary computed tomography for evaluation of acute chest pain. J Am Coll Cardiol 2007;49(8):863–71.
[100] Goldstein JA, Chinnaiyan KM, Abidov A, Achenbach S, Berman DS, Hayes SW, et al. The CT-STAT (coronary computed tomographic angiography for systematic triage of acute chest pain patients to treatment) trial. J Am Coll Cardiol 2011;58(14):1414–22.
[101] Hoffmann U, Truong QA, Schoenfeld DA, Chou ET, Woodard PK, Nagurney JT, et al. Coronary CT angiography versus standard evaluation in acute chest pain. N Engl J Med 2012;367(4):299–308.
[102] Litt HI, Gatsonis C, Snyder B, Singh H, Miller CD, Entrikin DW, et al. CT angiography for safe discharge of patients with possible acute coronary syndromes. N Engl J Med 2012;366(15):1393–403.
[103] Hoffmann U, Bamberg F, Chae CU, Nichols JH, Rogers IS, Seneviratne SK, et al. Coronary computed tomography angiography for early triage of patients with acute chest pain: the ROMICAT (Rule Out Myocardial Infarction using Computer Assisted Tomography) trial. J Am Coll Cardiol 2009;53(18):1642–50.
[104] Hulten EA, Carbonaro S, Petrillo SP, Mitchell JD, Villines TC. Prognostic value of cardiac computed tomography angiography: a systematic review and meta-analysis. J Am Coll Cardiol 2011;57(10):1237–47.

[105] Hulten E, Pickett C, Bittencourt MS, Villines TC, Petrillo S, Di Carli MF, et al. Outcomes after coronary computed tomography angiography in the emergency DepartmentA systematic review and meta-analysis of randomized, controlled trials. J Am Coll Cardiol 2013;61(8):880–92.

[106] Taylor AJ, Cerqueira M, Hodgson JM, Mark D, Min J, O'Gara P, et al. ACCF/SCCT/ACR/AHA/ASE/ASNC/NASCI/SCAI/SCMR 2010 Appropriate Use Criteria for Cardiac Computed TomographyA Report of the American College of Cardiology Foundation Appropriate Use Criteria Task Force, the Society of Cardiovascular Computed Tomography, the American College of Radiology, the American Heart Association, the American Society of Echocardiography, the American Society of Nuclear Cardiology, the North American Society for Cardiovascular Imaging, the Society for Cardiovascular Angiography and Interventions, and the Society for Cardiovascular Magnetic Resonance. J Am Coll Cardiol 2010;56(22):1864–94.

[107] Skinner JS, Smeeth L, Kendall JM, Adams PC, Timmis A. Chest pain guideline development G. NICE guidance Chest pain of recent onset: assessment and diagnosis of recent onset chest pain or discomfort of suspected cardiac origin. Heart 2010;96(12):974–8.

[108] American College of Cardiology Foundation Task Force on Expert Consensus Documents, Hundley WG, Bluemke DA, Finn JP, Flamm SD, Fogel MA, et al. ACCF/ACR/AHA/NASCI/SCMR 2010 expert consensus document on cardiovascular magnetic resonance: a report of the American College of Cardiology Foundation Task Force on Expert Consensus Documents. Circulation 2010;121(22):2462–508.

[109] Chiribiri A, Botnar RM, Nagel E. Magnetic resonance coronary angiography: where are we today? Curr Cardiol Rep 2013;15(2):328.

[110] Galjee MA, van Rossum AC, Doesburg T, van Eenige MJ, Visser CA. Value of magnetic resonance imaging in assessing patency and function of coronary artery bypass grafts: an angiographically controlled study. Circulation 1996;93(4):660–6.

[111] Pennell DJ. Cardiovascular magnetic resonance. Circulation 2010;121(5):692–705.

[112] Wintersperger BJ, von Smekal A, Engelmann MG, Knez A, Penzkofer HV, Laub G, et al. Contrast media enhanced magnetic resonance angiography for determining patency of a coronary bypass. A comparison with coronary angiography. Fortschr Geb Rontgenstr Nuklearmed 1997;167(6):572–8.

[113] Bedaux WL, Hofman MB, Vyt SL, Bronzwaer JG, Visser CA, van Rossum AC. Assessment of coronary artery bypass graft disease using cardiovascular magnetic resonance determination of flow reserve. J Am Coll Cardiol 2002;40(10):1848–55.

[114] Maintz D, Aepfelbacher FC, Kissinger KV, Botnar RM, Danias PG, Heindel W, et al. Coronary MR angiography: comparison of quantitative and qualitative data from four techniques. AJR Am J Roentgenol 2004;182(2):515–21.

[115] Nguyen P, Yang P. MR angiography coronaries and great vessels. In: Dilsizian V, Pohost GM, editors. Cardiac CT: PET and MR. Wiley-Blackwell; 2010. p. 154–95, http://au.wiley.com/WileyCDA/WileyTitle/productCd-1405185538.html.

[116] Kim WY, Danias PG, Stuber M, Flamm SD, Plein S, Nagel E, et al. Coronary magnetic resonance angiography for the detection of coronary stenoses. N Engl J Med 2001;345(26):1863–9.

[117] Kato S, Kitagawa K, Ishida N, Ishida M, Nagata M, Ichikawa Y, et al. Assessment of coronary artery disease using magnetic resonance coronary angiography: a national multicenter trial. J Am Coll Cardiol 2010;56(12):983–91.

[118] Schuetz GM, Zacharopoulou NM, Schlattmann P, Dewey M. Meta-analysis: noninvasive coronary angiography using computed tomography versus magnetic resonance imaging. Ann Intern Med 2010;152(3):167–77.

[119] Manning WJ, Chan RH. Coronary magnetic resonance imaging coming of age. J Am Coll Cardiol 2012;60(22):2323–4.
[120] Yoon YE, Kitagawa K, Kato S, Ishida M, Nakajima H, Kurita T, et al. Prognostic value of coronary magnetic resonance angiography for prediction of cardiac events in patients with suspected coronary artery disease. J Am Coll Cardiol 2012;60(22):2316–22.
[121] Greenwood JP, Maredia N, Younger JF, Brown JM, Nixon J, Everett CC, et al. Cardiovascular magnetic resonance and single-photon emission computed tomography for diagnosis of coronary heart disease (CE-MARC): a prospective trial. Lancet 2012;379(9814):453–60.
[122] Plein S, Greenwood JP, Ridgway JP, Cranny G, Ball SG, Sivananthan MU. Assessment of non–ST-segment elevation acute coronary syndromes with cardiac magnetic resonance imaging. J Am Coll Cardiol 2004;44(11):2173–81.
[123] Bettencourt N, Ferreira N, Chiribiri A, Schuster A, Sampaio F, Santos L, et al. Additive Value of magnetic resonance coronary angiography in a comprehensive cardiac magnetic resonance stress-rest protocol for detection of functionally significant coronary artery disease: a pilot study. Circ Cardiovasc Imaging 2013;6:730–38, published online before print July 5 2013. http://dx.doi.org/10.1161/CIRCIMAGING.113.000280.
[124] Sommer T, Hackenbroch M, Hofer U, Schmiedel A, Willinek WA, Flacke S, et al. Coronary MR angiography at 3.0 T versus that at 1.5 T: initial results in patients suspected of having coronary artery disease. Radiology 2005;234(3):718–25.
[125] Hamdan A, Asbach P, Wellnhofer E, Klein C, Gebker R, Kelle S, et al. A prospective study for comparison of MR and CT imaging for detection of coronary artery stenosis. JACC Cardiovasc Imaging 2011;4(1):50–61.
[126] Lockie T, Nagel E, Redwood S, Plein S. Use of cardiovascular magnetic resonance imaging in acute coronary syndromes. Circulation 2009;119(12):1671–81. http://dx.doi.org/10.1161/CIRCULATIONAHA.108.816512 [Review].
[127] Manning WJ, Li W, Edelman RR. A preliminary report comparing magnetic resonance coronary angiography with conventional angiography. N Engl J Med 1993;328:828–32 [25.03.93].

Atherosclerotic plaque

P. Singh*, A. Tawakol†
*Weill Cornell Medical College, New York Presbyterian Hospital, New York, NY, USA;
†Harvard Medical School, Massachusetts General Hospital, Boston, MA, USA

8.1 Introduction

Atherosclerosis is a chronic inflammatory disease [1]. Although great strides have been made in the diagnosis and management of atherosclerotic cardiovascular disease (CVD), overall mortality due to underlying atherosclerosis remains a leading cause of death in industrialized countries [2,3]. For example, more than one-third of all deaths in the United States are attributed to CVD, including atherosclerotic coronary disease and stroke [2]. By 2030, it is projected that more than 148 million of the US population would have heart disease. Given the gravity of this situation, it is of paramount importance to improve cardiac risk assessment in order to identify at-risk individuals. Significant advances have been made over the past decade in noninvasive cardiac imaging, permitting earlier detection of vascular atherosclerotic disease beyond conventional risk calculator assessments. The ability to directly visualize atherosclerotic plaque has spawned further efforts to refine imaging-based detection of plaque with ultrasound (US), computed tomography (CT), magnetic resonance imaging (MRI), single-photon emission computed tomography (SPECT), and positron emission tomography (PET). This chapter will focus on the utility and applications of noninvasive imaging modalities—US, CT, MRI, SPECT, and PET—and their individual, yet complementary roles in the detection and characterization of atherosclerotic plaque.

It is well documented that atherosclerotic plaque rupture is the underlying pathophysiologic mechanism governing the majority of CVD complications, including myocardial infarction (MI), stroke, and sudden cardiac death [4]. Despite contemporary guideline-based management for at-risk and established CAD patients, cardiovascular events persist at an alarming rate. This risk is thought to be due to unabated systemic inflammation [5]. Inflammation is at the crossroads of atherosclerotic plaque initiation, progression, and complications from atherothrombosis [4]. There are many notable steps in the inflammatory cascade that lends to atherogenesis: endothelial cell damage, up-regulation of endothelium adhesion molecules, accumulation of oxidized lipoproteins, monocyte recruitment and subsequent foam cell formation, angiogenesis, microcalcifications, and apoptosis. Unperturbed, these highly coordinated molecular and cellular events result in plaque destabilization. This end event is mediated by activated inflammatory cells, notably macrophages, which release degradative enzymes and confer an increased risk for plaque rupture. In addition to inflammation, other plaque properties such as presence of thin-cap fibroatheroma and lipid-rich necrotic core define an inflamed or high-risk plaque, which are the culprit lesions responsible for vascular atherothrombosis and adverse CV events [6–9].

Accordingly, early detection of both atherosclerotic disease and high-risk plaques is crucial to abating the total burden of CVD and its potential clinical complications [3,10]. In this regard, the use of noninvasive imaging techniques offer substantial advantage over standard CV risk calculators or invasive modalities, by affording the assessment of both anatomical and functional atherosclerosis parameters before the onset of clinical manifestations.

8.2 Non-invasive imaging of atherosclerosis

8.2.1 Carotid artery ultrasound

Carotid ultrasound allows visualization of the carotid arteries with an axial and lateral resolution of 0.044 and 0.25 mm, respectively. Intima-media thickness (IMT) is represented by the measured longitudinal distance between: (1) lumen-to-intima, and (2) media-to-adventitia boundaries [11]. The identification of a carotid atherosclerotic plaque is defined as focal IMT thickness of 50% or >0.5 mm relative to the adjacent arterial wall, or alternatively, an absolute IMT > 1.5 mm [12]. Carotid IMT (CIMT) using ultrasound, with standardized protocols and excellent sonographers and readers, lends to highly reproducible IMT measurements [13].

Another form of carotid ultrasound involves the use of injected contrast, intravascular microbubbles, which permit the visualization of micro- and macro-vasculature, and notably, intraplaque neovascularization [14], as validated by histopathologic exam. Neovascularization occurs early in atherogenesis, whereby the formation of leaky micro-vessels within plaque pose an increased risk for hemorrhage and potentiation of inflammation, leading to plaque instability [15] (Figure 8.1). As such, detection of neovascularization by contrast-enhanced ultrasound (CEUS) is a potential marker of high-risk atheromatous lesions. The diagnostic yield of CEUS has been explored in a few studies. In one such study, CEUS with perflubutane was used in 50 patients prior to carotid endarterectomy. We measured enhanced intensity and assessed the correlation between contrast effect and histopathology, comparing symptomatic and asymptomatic plaques. In both symptomatic and asymptomatic plaques, the correlation between CEUS based intensity in the plaque shoulder was associated with neovessel density ($P < 0.01$; $\rho = 0.43$). Furthermore, CEUS intensity of the plaque shoulder was greater in ruptured plaques than those without ($P < 0.05$), and in symptomatic versus asymptomatic plaques ($P < 0.01$). These compelling results warrant larger longitudinal studies to explore the potential prognostic utility of CEUS.

Another advance in ultrasound plaque imaging involves the use of 3-dimensional (3D) ultrasound imaging, which builds upon many of the core principles of ultrasound imaging. This ultrasound technique enables not only visualization of carotid plaque, but more accurately quantifies plaque size and vessel volume. Plaque volume, as assessed with 3D ultrasound, has been shown to be a more robust metric than CIMT alone; hence, a highly sensitive means to detect plaque progression, by over two orders of magnitude more than IMT [16–18]. Since atherosclerotic plaque increases in size faster longitudinally than it thickens, employing 3D ultrasound allows for smaller sample sizes in the serial assessment of an intervention on plaque progression

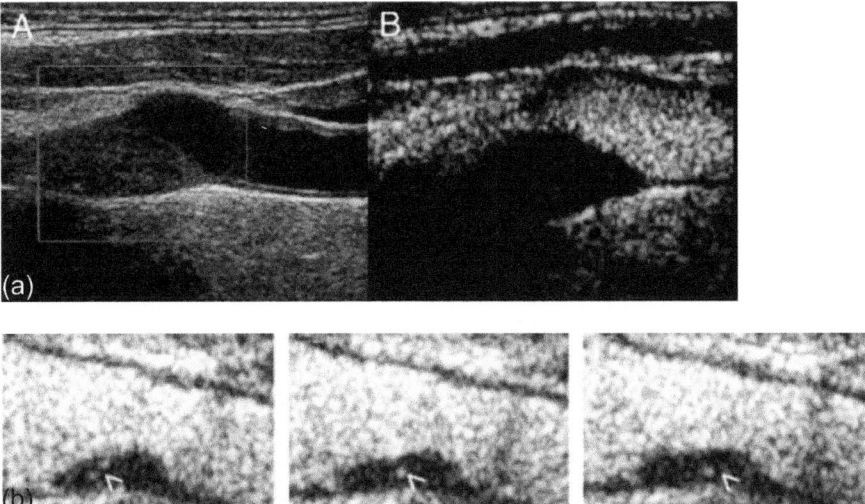

Figure 8.1 (a) Plaque without contrast-agent enhancement. (A) Large, predominantly hypoechoic plaque, at the origin of the internal carotid artery. (B) No plaque enhancement can be detected by contrast-enhanced ultrasound imaging. (b) Contrast enhanced plaque. Three consecutive frames of contrast-enhanced ultrasound imaging of an atherosclerotic lesion in the carotid bulb, showing contrast microbubbles (*arrowhead*) within the plaque. Corresponding micrograph showed a hemorrhagic fibrocalcific plaque with an eccentric large necrotic core occupying approximately 60% of the plaque area. Adapted from Ref. [15].

[18]. Thus, the role of 3D ultrasound plaque imaging in drug trials may prove to be cost-effective and lead to more testing of novel pharmacotherapeutics. Moreover, 3D ultrasound holds predictive and incremental value to coronary artery calcium scoring (CACS) [14], a well-accepted biomarker of CAD that carries prognostic value. The ability of 3D-CIMT to predict subsequent CVD events is actively being studied in the BioImage study (clinicaltrials.gov NCT00738725) and the ability to detect high-risk plaque features in the Canadian Atherosclerosis Imaging Network (NCT01456403).

8.2.1.1 CIMT and cardiovascular risk

The value of CIMT measures is buttressed by a strong association between increased CIMT and major traditional cardiac risk factors [19,20]. Furthermore, epidemiological studies have demonstrated substantial predictive value of CIMT for future CVD events, independent of well-recognized traditional cardiovascular risk factors [21]. The net reclassification index (NRI) is significant with the addition of maximum CIMT of the internal carotid artery ($P < 0.001$). Additional IMT indices have also been investigated. For example, in the Atherosclerosis Risk in Communities (ARIC) study, the presence of plaque in addition to increased CIMT improved the NRI by 9.9% [22]. Notably, the presence of hypoechoic plaques (indicative of lipid-rich content), has been shown to be an independent predictor of CV death [23,24].

8.2.1.2 CIMT and clinical trials

CIMT is used to quantify the degree of early atherosclerosis and to monitor the extent of modulation in response to novel therapies, in particular those that target lipids and blood pressure. In one study, a significant reduction in CIMT progression during statin therapy [25] was demonstrated. Although there was no regression of plaque in a separate study, a greater reduction of IMT progression was observed in response to intensification of statin therapy [26]. The results of these CIMT based trials are concordant with the results of clinical outcomes in clinical studies [27,28]. Despite these promising results with anti-lipid therapy, these results have not been replicated with anti-hypertensives or non-statin agents [29]. Additional studies using plaque-imaging ultrasound techniques are necessary to determine the overall utility and prognostic vale of this technology among the landscape of other imaging modalities, to be discussed in this chapter.

Advantages of ultrasound technology, in comparison to CT, MRI, and nuclear imaging, rest in its broader availability and lower cost profile. Importantly, ultrasound-based plaque imaging affords a reproducible measurement that does not involve any radiation exposure. It has demonstrable value in predicting future CV risk, independent of traditional CV risk factors. For all these reasons, plaque imaging by ultrasound (i.e., CIMT, 3D ultrasound, CEUS) is an attractive modality to employ in the risk assessment of early atherosclerosis in patients.

8.3 Computed tomography

8.3.1 Coronary artery calcium scoring

CACS can be performed by noncontrast-enhanced computed tomography [30]. CACS is a relatively simple technique associated with a low radiation dose in the range of ~1 mSv [31]. The conventional Agatston score is calculated by measuring areas with a CT attenuation value above 130HU (Hounsfield units), multiplying each calcified lesion by a factor related to the maximum attenuation value, and then adding up the per-slice scores to acquire a total calcium score. Alternative measures of coronary calcium, the calcium volume, the calcium mass, or calcium density may be more reproducible or provide incremental prognostic value [32]. Nevertheless, because of its long existence and familiarity, the Agatston score remains the most frequently reported coronary calcium measure, and correlates well with overall atherosclerotic burden. In the general population, the calcium score increases with age, is higher in men than women, and appears to vary by race.

8.3.1.1 CACS and cardiovascular risk

Multiple studies have investigated the prognostic value of the relationship between CACS and atherosclerosis [33,34]. For example, in one of the largest studies, inclusive of 25,253 asymptomatic middle-age men and women, coronary calcium score predicted all-cause mortality and did so more accurately than traditional CAD risk factors [35]. In addition to this large population study, in the Multiethnic Study of Atherosclerosis (MESA), increasing CACS portended a higher risk of future major adverse cardiovascular events (MACE). In MESA, 6724 asymptomatic individuals were compared to individuals with zero CACS. The results demonstrated that CACS of 1–100, 101–300 and >300 are associated with a 3.6-, 7.7- and 9.7-fold increased risk of MACE at 3.8 years, respectively [36]. These findings are independent of age, gender, or ethnicity [37]. In addition, recent data from MESA has shown that although higher CACS scores are associated with increased MACE, a lower density of calcified plaque is associated with lower MACE [38]. Future studies are required to determine the incremental predictive utility of CT densities.

Not only is CACS a robust independent predictor of CV mortality, but the presence of CAC provides incremental value beyond Framingham risk estimates, as well as various biomarkers, for prediction of CV events and mortality [39]. In a study of 4609 asymptomatic individuals, CAC progression provided incremental value in predicting all-cause mortality over baseline score, time between scans, demographics, and CV risk factors [40]. Lastly, the detection of CAC has potential clinical benefits by earlier initiation of therapeutic lifestyle changes and/or medical therapy, or patient compliance, although a direct effect of calcium scanning on outcome has not yet been demonstrated [41–43]. As it stands, current guidelines consider calcium scanning useful to further risk stratify patients at intermediate risk by conventional risk factors. Cohort studies have demonstrated that a calcium score improves risk estimation in these intermediate risk patients, with potentially more effective allocation of preventive measures.

8.3.1.2 CACS and clinical trials

Over the past two decades, a number of published studies used CACS progression as an endpoint. In one of these studies, a randomized controlled outcome trial [41], the utility of CACS to identify patients who may derive benefit from medical treatment was studied. This study, the St. Francis Heart Study, comprised 1005 asymptomatic individuals with CACS >80th percentile that were age- and gender-adjusted. At 4.3 years, treatment with atorvastatin 20 mg/dl reduced low-density lipoprotein cholesterol by 39% ($P<0.0001$), and triglycerides by 11% ($P=0.02$), while reducing clinical endpoints (coronary death, nonfatal MI, coronary revascularization, ischemic stroke, and peripheral arterial surgery) by 30% (6.9% vs. 9.9%, $P=0.08$). These latter clinical event rates were related to baseline CACS and were markedly reduced in a subgroup of subjects with a baseline CACS >400 (8.7% vs. 15.0% (42% reduction), $P=0.04$).

Another study evaluated the progression of subclinical atherosclerosis in 177 asymptomatic postmenopausal women using no hormone replacement therapy (HRT), combined therapy, and estrogen alone in an observational study design. Calcium progression was $14.6\pm21\%$ in women taking any hormone therapy ($n=97$), whereas calcium progression rates in nonusers ($n=80$) was higher at $22.3\pm32\%$. Relative to the nonuser group, HRT treatment inhibited the progression of atherosclerosis by 35% ($P=0.01$). Of the women on HRT ($n=97$) on estrogen replacement only ($n=62$), the annual increase in calcium scores was 63% lower ($9\pm22\%$) compared to those on estrogen plus progestin, rates similar to the nonuser group. These findings were independent of age, CV risk factors, statin use, or baseline CACS. The results of this observational CT study align with the Women Health Initiative, demonstrating that combined estrogen plus progestin imparts a significant increase in CV risk in asymptomatic women.

Based on these results, it is plausible that a baseline calcium scan assessment may hold clinical value in the prediction of future CV risk and guiding initiation of anti-lipid therapy (independent of serum lipid profile). Additional longitudinal studies addressing this issue need to be performed.

8.3.2 Coronary CT angiography

Coronary CT angiography (CCTA) is a noninvasive technique to image the coronary arteries, whereby the identification of not only coronary calcium but also coronary luminal stenosis afford valuable diagnostic and prognostic utility [44]. Over the past decade, technological improvements in spatial resolution (225–750 µm) and temporal resolution (75–125 ms), allow visualization of the epicardial coronary arteries in a 1–5 s breath hold. Indices of diagnostic accuracy for stenosis detection exhibit a sensitivity of 95% and specificity of 83%, on a per-patient level [45].

Despite these technological advances in CCTA, the risk of renal dysfunction (from iodinated contrast) and exposure to ionizing radiation exist. However, these radiation-related risks have been ameliorated with various technical innovations, including ECG-triggered roentgen output modulation, body-size-dependent tube voltage modification, prospective ECG-triggered scan protocols, shorter scan ranges, iterative reconstruction algorithms, and automatic exposure control [46,47]. These measures allow for routine cardiac CT at radiation doses of ~2–4 mSv, but may be reduced below 1 mSv in selected patients.

8.3.2.1 CCTA and cardiovascular risk

CCTA is also a robust noninvasive imaging modality that can directly visualize atherosclerotic plaque. Similar to coronary calcium, the presence of atherosclerosis on CCTA is associated with a worse clinical outcome. Although the number of >50% stenosed vessels has the strongest predictive value, it has been demonstrated that patients with <50% obstructive atherosclerotic plaque also have a worse outcome compared to patients with normal coronary arteries. For example, the CCTA Evaluation for Clinical Outcomes (CONFIRM), a large, prospective, open-label, international multicenter dynamic observational registry of patients who underwent CCTA [48], demonstrated the prognostic value of CCTA findings, with a dose–response relationship of increasing extent of CAD, severity of coronary luminal stenosis, to incident mortality and MACE (Figure 8.2), with prognostic value beyond traditional risk factors (TRFs). In a meta-analysis of 42 studies, the sensitivity and specificity of CCTA to identify any coronary arterial plaque was 93% and 92%, respectively [50]. Despite the robust ability to noninvasively identify coronary atheroma, at this moment, there are no clear recommendations on the risk interpretation and subsequent management of patients with (nonobstructive) coronary plaque.

In addition to quantifying plaque burden, CCTA affords detailed imaging of the coronary arterial wall, and thus, anatomical characterization of atherosclerotic plaque.

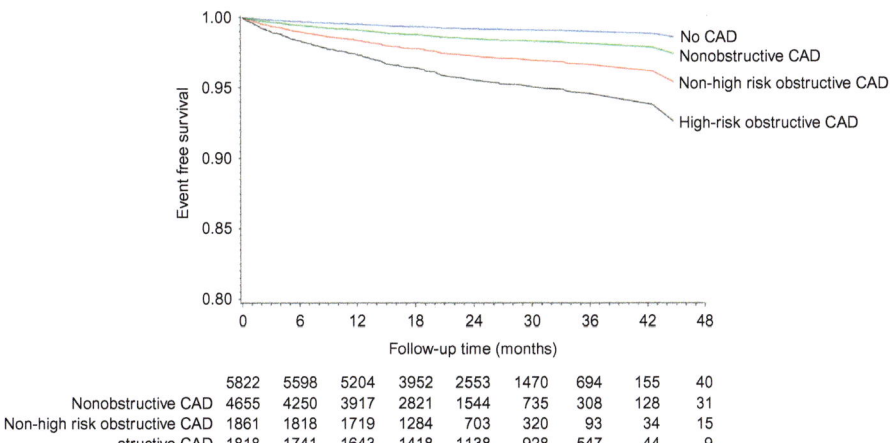

Figure 8.2 Prognostic utility of CCTA assessment of CAD severity. All-cause mortality-free survival by coronary artery disease (CAD) severity for patients without coronary atherosclerosis (blue line), nonobstructive CAD (green line), non-high-risk CAD (red line), and high-risk CAD (black line); $P<0.001$.
Adapted from Ref. [49].

High-risk plaque features such as, low attenuation plaque, i.e., attenuation values below 30HU, positive remodeling, and the napkin-ring sign, i.e., low plaque core attenuation value with a rim of higher attenuation, have been shown to correlate with worsened prognosis [51,52] (Figure 8.3). In one such study, CCTA was performed in human donor hearts to determine the histologic corollaries of advanced coronary atherosclerotic plaques. In a multivariate analysis, necrotic core area (OR=1.9), non-core plaque area (OR=1.6), and total vessel area (OR=0.9) independently predicted the appearance of the napkin-ring sign (a high-risk plaque feature) on CCTA. In another study, plaque composition by CCTA was shown to enhance the predictive capacity for adverse coronary events [53]. In a study of 368 patients, who presented with acute chest pain and had documented stenosis on CCTA, a CT-based score of morphologic coronary lesion characteristics (positive remodeling, spotty calcification, stenosis length, plaque volume) had good discriminatory value for detecting ACS during hospital admission. Additional studies have demonstrated that characterization of atherosclerotic plaque provides incremental predictive value for CV events independent of coronary stenosis and traditional risk factors alone [54]. The ability of CCTA to delineate plaque composition has been shown to strongly correlate with intravascular ultrasound (IVUS), optical coherence tomography (OCT) and histology.

8.3.2.2 Emerging tissue and biological characterization techniques with CT

A major focus of molecular imaging technology has been on identifying high-risk atheroma. Though this approach has been borne out mostly with PET imaging (to be discussed later), there is emerging data that CT molecular imaging holds promise for

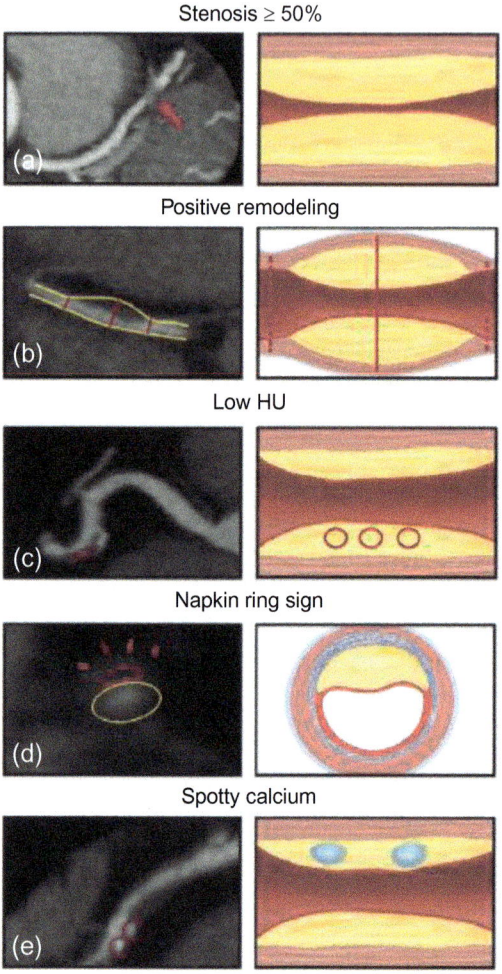

Figure 8.3 High-risk coronary plaque and significant stenosis on CT. (a) Severe stenosis of the mid left anterior descending coronary artery (red arrow). (b) Positive remodeling: noncalcified plaque with positive remodeling in the distal right coronary artery. Two dotted red lines indicate the vessel diameters at the proximal and distal reference areas (both 1.8 mm); and the central red line demonstrates the maximal vessel diameter in the mid portion of the plaque (2.7 mm). The remodeling index is 1.5. (c) Low Hounsfield units (HU) plaque: partially calcified plaque in the mid right coronary artery with low <30 HU plaque. The red circles demonstrate three such regions. (d) Napkin-ring sign: napkin-ring sign plaque in the mid left anterior descending coronary artery. Schematic cross-sectional view of the napkin-ring sign. The red line demonstrates the central low HU area of the plaque adjacent to the lumen (yellow ellipse) surrounded by a peripheral rim of the higher CT attenuation (red arrows). (e) Spotty calcium: partially calcified plaque in the mid right coronary artery with spotty calcification (diameter <3 mm in all directions; red circles). Adapted from Refs. [51,52].

high-risk plaque identification. Based on the fact that macrophages play a key role in atherogenesis and progression, in a preclinical model of atherosclerosis, the CT iodine-based contrast agent N1177, which accumulates in macrophages, was tested to determine its ability to localize to plaque *in vivo* and allow for it detection noninvasively with CT [55]. This study demonstrated that N1177-enhanced CT showed increased aortic wall enhancement in atherosclerotic rabbits compared to control rabbits (10.0 ± 5.2 vs. 2.0 ± 2.1 HU, respectively; $P < 0.05$). In addition, the atherosclerotic rabbits underwent [18] FDG, PET imaging, which demonstrated higher standardized uptake values (SUV) in the aortic wall of versus controls (0.61 ± 0.12 vs. 0.21 ± 0.02; $P < 0.05$). Altogether, the intensity of enhancement in the aortic wall measured with N1177-CT correlated with FDG uptake/ ($r = 0.61$, $P < 0.001$) and macrophage density on immunohistology ($r = 0.63$, $P < 0.001$).

In another study, spectral CT or multicolor CT was used in combination with gold HDL nanoparticle contrast agent (Au-HDL), for characterization of macrophage burden, calcification, and stenosis of atherosclerotic plaques [56]. Apolipoprotein E knockout (apo E-KO) mice were used as the model for atherosclerosis, while wild-type mice served as controls. Macrophage targeting by Au-HDL was confirmed by transmission electron microscopy and confocal microscopy of aortic sections. The results showed that multicolor CT enabled differentiation of Au-HDL accumulation in the aorta. Microscopy of aortic sections revealed that Au-HDL was primarily localized in macrophages. The results of these studies show that CT, when paired with contrast agents, may yield valuable information about atherosclerotic plaque composition. Pilot studies in humans are needed to determine translatability of the findings from the above studies.

8.3.2.3 CCTA and clinical trials

CCTA plaque imaging has so far not been used extensively as a (surrogate) endpoint in large clinical trials. Reproducibility of coronary plaque quantification by CCTA between observers and particularly between examinations has been a challenge as a result of limited (spatial) resolution in relation to the small volumetric changes over time, although improvement has been made with contemporary technology. In a phase-2 multicenter study of patients with recent ACS, CCTA performed at baseline and 24 weeks demonstrated reductions in new coronary plaque formation and noncalcified plaque volumes, in those randomized to anti-inflammatory 5-lipoxygenase inhibitor therapy [57]. In another study, serial CCTA was performed in 32 patients (26 men, ages 64.3 ± 8.5 years) to investigate the effect of statin treatment on coronary plaque morphology. Twenty-four patients received fluvastatin after the baseline CCTA, and eight subjects who refused statin treatment served as controls. After a median interval of 12 months, all vessels were examined, and demonstrated that statins decreased low attenuation plaque volume. Similar findings were seen in the New Age II Pilot Study, whereby treatment with atorvastatin 20 mg significantly reduced noncalcified plaque burden ($23 \pm 14\%$ annual decrease). Other studies using CCTA to evaluate interval plaque modulation in response to statins are ongoing.

8.3.3 Magnetic resonance imaging

Magnetic resonance imaging (MRI) is a noninvasive, nonionizing imaging modality that provides multiparameter and multiplanar 3D data. The physics of MRI are extensively described in Chapter 6. Briefly, MRI is based on the resonance of protons, which have been subjected to a magnetic field upon exposure to radiofrequency pulse. The MR signal intensity from the relaxation time of the protons is governed by the biochemical environment of protons in the respective tissue. Specific weighted spectral sequences, including T1, T2, and proton density, provide high contrast and allows for tissue characterization. These different contrasts allow for separating tissues based on their chemical and biological composition [58]. In regard to atherosclerosis imaging, MR angiography uses time-of-flight or contrast-enhanced sequences to provide a high signal and resolution, which produces a bright lumen signal, allowing for the assessment of luminal arterial stenosis. Current MRI scanners can achieve in-plane spatial resolution of $250 \times 250\,\mu m^2$ for the carotid arteries, $800 \times 800\,\mu m^2$ for the aorta, and $460 \times 460\,\mu m^2$ for the coronary arteries with a slice thickness of 2–5 mm [59].

However, a significant advance of MRI rests in its ability to perform cross-sectional arterial imaging and to characterize plaque components within the vessel wall. For example, black-blood imaging, by suppressing the signal of the blood, provides a high contrast between the interface of the vessel wall and lumen, allowing for arterial wall measurements and plaque assessment. Data from multiple contrast weightings enables characterization of fibrosis, lipid cores, hemorrhage, or calcification within atherosclerotic plaque.

Beyond the anatomical information provided by morphological spectral sequences, the use of dynamic contrast-enhanced sequences allows for the assessment of functional information as it relates to plaque pathobiology. Neovascularization and macrophage accumulation are characteristic biological effects of inflammation within an atherosclerotic plaque [60,61]. MRI contrast agents migrate away from the blood pool and diffuse into plaque, thereby modifying the relaxation time. Gadolinium accumulates in interstitial tissues and enhances the signal, whereas nanoparticulate contrast agents such as ultrasmall superparamagnetic particles of iron oxide (USPIO) accumulate in macrophages and decrease the signal intensity [62]. Blood-suppression techniques, in addition to fast scanning sequences, have promulgated the development of 3D isotropic sequences, resulting in greater signal-to-noise ratio and high spatial resolution to 0.7 mm [63–65], aiding better characterization of plaque constituents.

Furthermore, increase in Tesla field strength (i.e., 1.5-T to 3-T) improves the signal-to-noise ratio [66] for plaque morphology and composition identification, and shorter scan times. Lastly, MRI's major advantage compared to other imaging modalities is the absence of ionizing radiation facilitating its use to serially monitor disease progression and therapeutic efficacy [67].

8.3.3.1 MRI and cardiovascular risk

Plaque characterization by MRI has been histologically validated in humans in the carotid arteries after endarterectomy [68]. MRI's ability to provide quantitative measures on plaque size and composition highlights MRI's potential to yield prognostic information about future clinical events (REFs). Studies have demonstrated that MRI is superior to biomarkers for the identification of subclinical atherosclerosis [69]. In this regard, MRI may potentially lead to refinement of traditional CV risk stratification calculators for future MACE in asymptomatic patients [70].

MRI-based prospective studies [71–75] have shown that atherosclerotic plaque characteristics associated with future clinical events were thin fibrous caps (hazard ratio [HR] 17.0), intraplaque hemorrhage (HR 5.2), lipid/necrotic core area (HR for 10% increase 1.6), and maximum wall thickness (hazard ratio for a 1-mm increase, 1.6). More recent studies have underlined the critical importance of intraplaque hemorrhage in the prediction of downstream clinical events [73–75] (Figure 8.4).

8.3.3.2 MRI and clinical trials

Since MRI is noninvasive and suited for serial imaging, it has been used as the end point in clinical studies. The accuracy of MRI in evaluation of the arterial wall *in vivo* was first explored in 1999 to determine the effect of a drug on plaque progression in rabbits [76]. After this proof-of-principle study, MRI transitioned to monitoring of plaque progression preclinical studies to human pharmaceutical clinical trials. Plaque morphological features such as plaque thickness, volume, and luminal area were inevitably surmounted by more detailed measures of plaque composition. The ability of *in vivo* MRI to monitor changes of plaque components longitudinally was recently used to assess the effects of several drugs [77–79]. Moreover, in drug trials, functional parameters of plaque have been assessed by utilizing molecular imaging MR

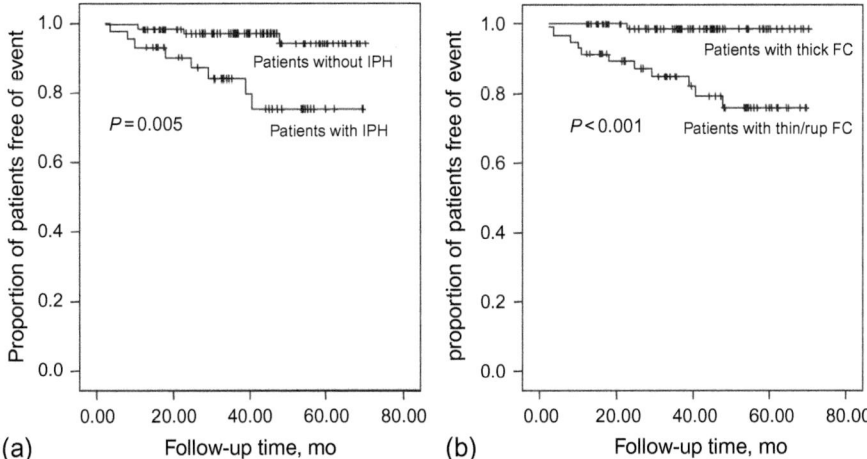

Figure 8.4 Predictive value of intraplaque hemorrhage and thin/ruptured fibrous cap in carotid arteries. Survival of proportion of patients remaining free of ipsilateral cerebrovascular events for subjects with (lower curve) and without (upper curve) intraplaque hemorrhage (a) and thin or ruptured fibrous cap (b) identified by MRI. IPH, intraplaque hemorrhage; FC, fibrous cap.
Reprinted from Ref. [71].

techniques to assess neovascularization by dynamic contrast enhancement or inflammation by novel contrast agents [80].

Multiple MRI contrast agents have been developed to image various steps of atherogenesis, such as endothelial cell activation [81], macrophage accumulation [82,83], apoptosis [84], angiogenesis [85], and thrombosis [81,86,87]. Of these mostly experimental nanoparticulate probes, USPIO have been validated for the inflammation imaging within plaque by histology in humans [88,89]. USPIO are phagocytosed by plaque macrophages, which results in a loss of MR signal intensity [82]. This advancement in the field of MR molecular imaging has resulted in the use of USPIO in a randomized controlled trial to determine the effects of a novel drug on atherosclerotic plaque inflammation [90].

8.3.4 Positron emission tomography

8.3.4.1 Inflammation and cardiovascular risk

Multiple studies have now established an inextricable link between increased inflammation and heightened risk for CV disease. Biomarkers of inflammation, including adhesion proteins, pro-inflammatory cytokines, markers of activated macrophages, and C-reactive protein, have all been shown to increases CV risk. Adding fuel to the fire, it was recently shown that a MI incites pre-existing atherosclerosis, hence resulting in enhanced vascular risk for a subsequent CV event [91]. Both preclinical and clinical studies have shown that plaques causing a CV event exhibit a lipid-rich necrotic core and an eroded thin-fibrous cap as a culmination of inflammatory cell infiltration, where macrophages are notable mediators. Moreover, several epidemiological studies have highlighted a strong connection between CAD and chronic inflammatory diseases, including systemic lupus erythematosus [92], rheumatoid arthritis [93], and psoriasis [94]. Germane to the linkage between inflammation and CV risk, noninvasive imaging of inflammation shows promise to identifying high-risk atherosclerotic plaques.

8.3.4.2 PET imaging of inflammation

The most commonly used PET radiotracer in plaque imaging is ^{18}fluorine-2-deoxy-D-glucose (FDG). The biologic basis for FDG accumulation is rested on its uptake by metabolically active, glucose-requiring cells. Activated inflammatory cells need and metabolize greater quantities of glucose and accordingly up-regulate surface membrane glucose transporter proteins (GLUT) to meet this demand. Upon FDG entry into a cell, it becomes phosphorylated by hexokinase to FDG-6-phosphate. In contrast to glucose-6-phosphate, FDG-6-phosphate is not further metabolized. This results in metabolic trapping of ^{18}FDG-6-PO$_4$ in proportion to its activated metabolic state [95]. Notably, inflammatory cells exhibit a higher rate of glucose uptake than noninflammatory cells within the plaque [96]. Exploitation of this specific property of inflammatory cells allows for imaging-based detection of inflammation. Glucose metabolism (a metric of FDG uptake) has been shown to have a strong relationship with the underlying activation state of inflammatory cells, especially macrophages. The majority of studies suggest that macrophage glycolytic flux (a determinant of FDG uptake) is increased with classical and innate but not alternative activation [97], although some data suggests hypoxia governs FDG uptake rather that glucose consumption [98]. Others have also demonstrated that classically activated M1 (pro-inflammatory) polarized macrophages compared to alternatively activated M2 (anti-inflammatory) macrophages, leads to augmented FDG uptake [99] via increased expression of glycolytic genes in M1 versus M2 macrophages. These data illustrates that cellular FDG accumulation is both a reliable measure of inflammation and proatherogenic M1 (pro-inflammatory) macrophages.

8.3.4.3 PET and clinical trials

Since the first study demonstrating a robust correlation between FDG uptake with macrophage accumulation, activated macrophages, and macrophage infiltration into the arterial wall [100–102], multiple other studies substantiated this finding [101,102]. In the proof-of-concept study, subjects underwent FDG-PET imaging prior to carotid endarterectomy and then FDG uptake was analyzed in relation to corresponding histological sections [100]. After these initial studies, a number of other studies demonstrated a robust correlation with the FDG signal and high-risk plaque characteristics [103]. Also, multiple trials have been performed and show that measurements of arterial wall FDG uptake have excellent interobserver variability [104], and are modifiable by pharmacological interventions targeting plaque inflammation [105–107]. Several other studies have illustrated that FDG uptake is strongly associated with cardiovascular risk factors [108–110], circulating pro-inflammatory serum biomarkers [108,109], recent and future atherothrombotic events [111–115] (Figure 8.5).

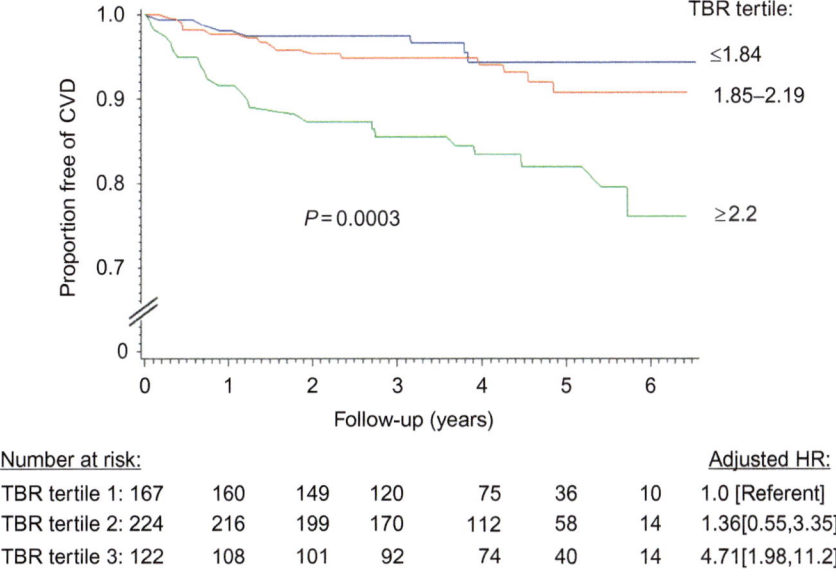

Figure 8.5 FDG uptake predicts risk of cardiovascular disease. Kaplan–Meier survival curve demonstrating that the highest TBR (target-to-background ratio) tertile carries the greatest CV risk compared to the lowest tertile, even after adjustment for major traditional risk factors. Reprint from Ref. [111].

To date, there have been several multicenter randomized controlled trials (RCTs) utilizing serial FDG-PET imaging to monitor signal modulation of novel drug therapies as it relates to atherosclerotic inflammation. For example, these studies have assessed the impact of both novel and FDA approved compounds such as lipoprotein-associated phospholipase A2 inhibitor [116], p38 mitogen-activated protein kinase [117], pioglitazone [118], atorvastatin [119], dalcetrapib [107], and rheumatologic-based therapy [120], on atherosclerotic inflammation (Figure 8.5).

Thus far, the results of FDG-PET based RCTs have been consistent with the results from clinical outcome trials [121–124]. With this in mind, major advantages exist for PET imaging-based studies, whereby these trials require a smaller sample size to detect a potential clinically translatable benefit, and are more economical than mega clinical outcomes studies, which are longer in duration and carry a greater budget. Nevertheless, although the PET signal may be a useful surrogate imaging biomarker of CV risk, large prospective studies need to be carried out to elucidate the role of FDG-PET imaging in predicting clinical CV events.

8.3.5 Novel radiotracers—PET and SPECT

Atherosclerosis is a complex inflammatory disorder involving a myriad of biologic pathways. Recent advances in fluorination chemistry and other radiotracer technology have brought to fruition PET-compatible novel tracers targeted to various pathobiologic processes. For example, tracers targeting vascular cell adhesion molecules [125], matrix metalloproteinases [126], apoptotic caspases [127], mitochondrial translocator proteins (i.e., PK11195 or TSPO) [128], integrin receptors, and apolipoproteins [129], are but a few being investigated.

Many of the above biologic pathways can be probed not only with PET tracers imaging, but also with SPECT radioactive tracers. For example, in murine carotid arteries, a technetium-99m based integrin tracer that binds to monocytes and macrophages has been shown to strongly correlate with vascular inflammation [130]. In another preclinical study, apolipoprotein-deficient mice underwent SPECT imaging with an [101] in-labeled tracer targeting activated MMPs, which significantly correlated with aortic macrophage content. General advantages of SPECT over PET include greater availability, lower cost, and more trained personnel. However, PET offers higher spatial resolution and a broader repertoire of biologic radiotracers, which are paramount for accurate imaging of relatively small anatomical structures, such as the arterial wall and atherosclerotic plaque.

A significant milestone in PET imaging recently came to fruition with coronary imaging of high-risk plaques using sodium fluoride, ^{18}F-NaF. This novel tracer provides a measure of active calcification [131]. In a prospective clinical trial, patients with MI ($n=40$) and stable angina ($n=40$) underwent both ^{18}F-NaF and ^{18}F-FDG PET-CT, and invasive coronary angiography. ^{18}F-NaF uptake correlated with high-risk plaque features on histological carotid endarterectomy specimens in patients with symptomatic carotid disease, and with intravascular ultrasound in patients with stable angina. Notably, ^{18}F-NaF uptake (tissue-to-background ratio) was higher in culprit versus non-culprit coronary plaques in patients with acute MI (Figure 8.6).

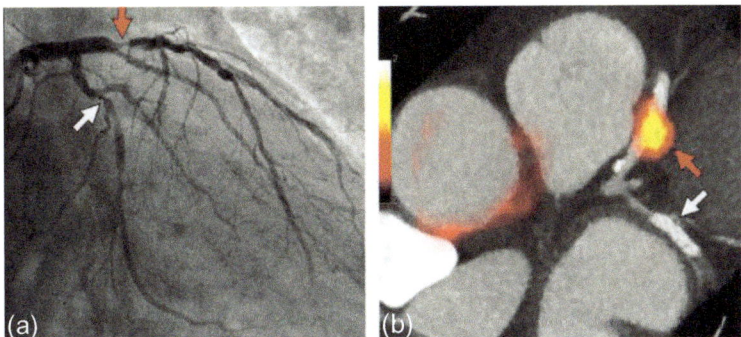

Figure 8.6 ^{18}F-fluoride focal uptake in acute coronary lesion. Patient with anterior non-ST-segment elevation myocardial infarction with (a) culprit (red arrow; left anterior descending artery) and non-culprit (white arrow; circumflex artery) lesions on invasive coronary angiography. Both lesions were stented during the index admission. Only the culprit lesion demonstrated increased ^{18}F-NaF uptake (^{18}F-NaF, tissue-to-background ratios, culprit 2.03 vs. reference segment 1.08 [88% increase]) on PET-CT (b) after percutaneous coronary intervention. Reprinted from Ref. [131].

This is the first noninvasive imaging method to identify and localize ruptured and otherwise high-risk plaques within the coronary vasculature. Prospective studies are needed to clarify the potential and promising clinical utility that ^{18}F-NaF may offer in CV risk algorithms.

8.4 Conclusions

Advances in imaging technologies have enabled enhanced characterization of atherosclerotic plaques. Characterization of atheroma may prove valuable in identifying novel effective therapies as well as refining cardiac risk stratification in a manner that aligns with personalization of care to patients based on their risk profile. The path ahead for clinical implementation of noninvasive imaging of atherosclerosis is challenging; however, with dedicated efforts to improving and standardizing the acquisition protocols and interpretation, a seamless integration into the practice of clinical medicine is on the horizon.

References

[1] Libby P. Inflammation in atherosclerosis. Nature 2002;420:868–74.
[2] Go AS, Mozaffarian D, Roger VL, Benjamin EJ, Berry JD, Borden WB, et al. Executive summary: heart disease and stroke statistics—2013 update: a report from the American Heart Association. Circulation 2013;127:143–52.
[3] Vedanthan R, Fuster V. Disease prevention: the moving target of global cardiovascular health. Nat Rev Cardiol 2009;6:327–8.

[4] Libby P, Ridker PM, Maseri A. Inflammation and atherosclerosis. Circulation 2002;105:1135–43.
[5] Cannon CP, Braunwald E, McCabe CH, Rader DJ, Rouleau JL, Belder R, et al. Intensive versus moderate lipid lowering with statins after acute coronary syndromes. N Engl J Med 2004;350:1495–504.
[6] Muller JE, Abela GS, Nesto RW, Tofler GH. Triggers, acute risk factors and vulnerable plaques: the lexicon of a new frontier. J Am Coll Cardiol 1994;23:809–13.
[7] Libby P, Schoenbeck U, Mach F, Selwyn AP, Ganz P. Current concepts in cardiovascular pathology: the role of LDL cholesterol in plaque rupture and stabilization. Am J Med 1998;104:14S–8S.
[8] Davies MJ, Woolf N, Rowles P, Richardson PD. Lipid and cellular constituents of unstable human aortic plaques. Basic Res Cardiol 1994;89(Suppl. 1):33–9.
[9] Kolodgie FD, Burke AP, Farb A, Gold HK, Yuan J, Narula J, et al. The thin-cap fibroatheroma: a type of vulnerable plaque: the major precursor lesion to acute coronary syndromes. Curr Opin Cardiol 2001;16:285–92.
[10] Schindler TH, Zhang XL, Vincenti G, Mhiri L, Lerch R, Schelbert HR. Role of PET in the evaluation and understanding of coronary physiology. J Nucl Cardiol 2007;14:589–603.
[11] Naik V, Gamad RS, Bansod PP. Carotid artery segmentation in ultrasound images and measurement of intima-media thickness. Biomed Res Int 2013;2013:801962.
[12] Touboul PJ, Hennerici MG, Meairs S, Adams H, Amarenco P, Bornstein N, et al. Mannheim carotid intima-media thickness and plaque consensus (2004–2006–2011). An update on behalf of the advisory board of the 3rd, 4th and 5th watching the risk symposia, at the 13th, 15th and 20th European Stroke Conferences, Mannheim, Germany, 2004, Brussels, Belgium, 2006, and Hamburg, Germany, 2011. Cerebrovasc Dis 2012;34:290–6.
[13] Bots ML, Mulder PG, Hofman A, van Es GA, Grobbee DE. Reproducibility of carotid vessel wall thickness measurements. The Rotterdam study. J Clin Epidemiol 1994;47:921–30.
[14] Coli S, Magnoni M, Sangiorgi G, Marrocco-Trischitta MM, Melisurgo G, Mauriello A, et al. Contrast-enhanced ultrasound imaging of intraplaque neovascularization in carotid arteries: correlation with histology and plaque echogenicity. J Am Coll Cardiol 2008;52:223–30.
[15] Moreno PR, Purushothaman KR, Sirol M, Levy AP, Fuster V. Neovascularization in human atherosclerosis. Circulation 2006;113:2245–52.
[16] Spence JD. Ultrasound measurement of carotid plaque as a surrogate outcome for coronary artery disease. Am J Cardiol 2002;89:10B–5B discussion 15B–16B.
[17] Spence JD, Eliasziw M, DiCicco M, Hackam DG, Galil R, Lohmann T. Carotid plaque area: a tool for targeting and evaluating vascular preventive therapy. Stroke 2002;33:2916–22.
[18] Ainsworth CD, Blake CC, Tamayo A, Beletsky V, Fenster A, Spence JD. 3D ultrasound measurement of change in carotid plaque volume: a tool for rapid evaluation of new therapies. Stroke 2005;36:1904–9.
[19] Sibal L, Agarwal SC, Home PD. Carotid intima-media thickness as a surrogate marker of cardiovascular disease in diabetes. Diabetes Metab Syndr Obes 2011;4:23–34.
[20] Lande MB, Carson NL, Roy J, Meagher CC. Effects of childhood primary hypertension on carotid intima media thickness: a matched controlled study. Hypertension 2006;48:40–4.

[21] Polak JF, Pencina MJ, Pencina KM, O'Donnell CJ, Wolf PA, D'Agostino Sr. RB. Carotid-wall intima-media thickness and cardiovascular events. N Engl J Med 2011;365:213–21.
[22] Nambi V, Chambless L, Folsom AR, He M, Hu Y, Mosley T, et al. Carotid intima-media thickness and presence or absence of plaque improves prediction of coronary heart disease risk: the ARIC (Atherosclerosis Risk In Communities) study. J Am Coll Cardiol 2010;55:1600–7.
[23] Sirico G, Spadera L, De Laurentis M, Brevetti G. Carotid artery disease and stroke in patients with peripheral arterial disease. The role of inflammation. Monaldi archives for chest disease=Archivio Monaldi per le malattie del torace/Fondazione clinica del lavoro, IRCCS [and] Istituto di clinica tisiologica e malattie apparato respiratorio, Universita di Napoli, Secondo ateneo 2009;72:10–7.
[24] Brevetti G, Sirico G, Giugliano G, Lanero S, De Maio JI, Luciano R, et al. Prevalence of hypoechoic carotid plaques in coronary artery disease: relationship with coexistent peripheral arterial disease and leukocyte number. Vasc Med 2009;14:13–9.
[25] Crouse 3rd JR, Raichlen JS, Riley WA, Evans GW, Palmer MK, O'Leary DH, et al. Effect of rosuvastatin on progression of carotid intima-media thickness in low-risk individuals with subclinical atherosclerosis: the METEOR Trial. JAMA 2007;297:1344–53.
[26] Yu CM, Zhang Q, Lam L, Lin H, Kong SL, Chan W, et al. Comparison of intensive and low-dose atorvastatin therapy in the reduction of carotid intimal-medial thickness in patients with coronary heart disease. Heart 2007;93:933–9.
[27] Tsimikas S, Witztum JL, Miller ER, Sasiela WJ, Szarek M, Olsson AG, et al. High-dose atorvastatin reduces total plasma levels of oxidized phospholipids and immune complexes present on apolipoprotein B-100 in patients with acute coronary syndromes in the MIRACL trial. Circulation 2004;110:1406–12.
[28] Schwartz GG, Olsson AG, Ezekowitz MD, Ganz P, Oliver MF, Waters D, et al. Effects of atorvastatin on early recurrent ischemic events in acute coronary syndromes: the MIRACL study: a randomized controlled trial. JAMA 2001;285:1711–8.
[29] Lonn EM, Gerstein HC, Sheridan P, Smith S, Diaz R, Mohan V, et al. Effect of ramipril and of rosiglitazone on carotid intima-media thickness in people with impaired glucose tolerance or impaired fasting glucose: STARR (STudy of Atherosclerosis with Ramipril and Rosiglitazone). J Am Coll Cardiol 2009;53:2028–35.
[30] Ferencik M, Ferullo A, Achenbach S, Abbara S, Chan RC, Booth SL, et al. Coronary calcium quantification using various calibration phantoms and scoring thresholds. Invest Radiol 2003;38:559–66.
[31] Hoffmann U, Massaro JM, Fox CS, Manders E, O'Donnell CJ. Defining normal distributions of coronary artery calcium in women and men (from the Framingham Heart Study). Am J Cardiol 2008;102:1136–41, 1141 e1.
[32] Criqui MH, Denenberg JO, Ix JH, McClelland RL, Wassel CL, Rifkin DE, et al. Calcium density of coronary artery plaque and risk of incident cardiovascular events. JAMA 2014;311:271–8.
[33] Hulten E, Bittencourt MS, Ghoshhajra B, O'Leary D, Christman MP, Blaha MJ, et al. Incremental prognostic value of coronary artery calcium score versus CT angiography among symptomatic patients without known coronary artery disease. Atherosclerosis 2014;233:190–5.
[34] Moselewski F, O'Donnell CJ, Achenbach S, Ferencik M, Massaro J, Nguyen A, et al. Calcium concentration of individual coronary calcified plaques as measured by multidetector row computed tomography. Circulation 2005;111:3236–41.

[35] Budoff MJ, Shaw LJ, Liu ST, Weinstein SR, Mosler TP, Tseng PH, et al. Long-term prognosis associated with coronary calcification: observations from a registry of 25,253 patients. J Am Coll Cardiol 2007;49:1860–70.

[36] Nasir K, McClelland RL, Blumenthal RS, Goff Jr. DC, Hoffmann U, Psaty BM, et al. Coronary artery calcium in relation to initiation and continuation of cardiovascular preventive medications: The Multi-Ethnic Study of Atherosclerosis (MESA). Circ Cardiovasc Qual Outcomes 2010;3:228–35.

[37] Budoff MJ, Nasir K, McClelland RL, Detrano R, Wong N, Blumenthal RS, et al. Coronary calcium predicts events better with absolute calcium scores than age-sex-race/ethnicity percentiles: MESA (Multi-Ethnic Study of Atherosclerosis). J Am Coll Cardiol 2009;53:345–52.

[38] Budoff MJ, Young R, Lopez VA, Kronmal RA, Nasir K, Blumenthal RS, et al. Progression of coronary calcium and incident coronary heart disease events: MESA (Multi-Ethnic Study of Atherosclerosis). J Am Coll Cardiol 2013;61:1231–9.

[39] Otaki Y, Arsanjani R, Gransar H, Cheng VY, Dey D, Labounty T, et al. What have we learned from CONFIRM? Prognostic implications from a prospective multicenter international observational cohort study of consecutive patients undergoing coronary computed tomographic angiography. J Nucl Cardiol 2012;19:787–95.

[40] Budoff MJ, Hokanson JE, Nasir K, Shaw LJ, Kinney GL, Chow D, et al. Progression of coronary artery calcium predicts all-cause mortality. JACC Cardiovasc Imaging 2010;3:1229–36.

[41] Arad Y, Goodman KJ, Roth M, Newstein D, Guerci AD. Coronary calcification, coronary disease risk factors, C-reactive protein, and atherosclerotic cardiovascular disease events: the St Francis Heart Study. J Am Coll Cardiol 2005;46:158–65.

[42] Blankstein R, Dorbala S. Adding calcium scoring to myocardial perfusion imaging: does it alter physicians' therapeutic decision making? J Nucl Cardiol 2010;17:168–71.

[43] Bybee KA, Lee J, Markiewicz R, Longmore R, McGhie AI, O'Keefe JH, et al. Diagnostic and clinical benefit of combined coronary calcium and perfusion assessment in patients undergoing PET/CT myocardial perfusion stress imaging. J Nucl Cardiol 2010;17:188–96.

[44] Cho I, Chang HJ, Sung JM, Pencina MJ, Lin FY, Dunning AM, et al. Coronary computed tomographic angiography and risk of all-cause mortality and nonfatal myocardial infarction in subjects without chest pain syndrome from the CONFIRM Registry (coronary CT angiography evaluation for clinical outcomes: an international multicenter registry). Circulation 2012;126:304–13.

[45] Achenbach S, Goroll T, Seltmann M, Pflederer T, Anders K, Ropers D, et al. Detection of coronary artery stenoses by low-dose, prospectively ECG-triggered, high-pitch spiral coronary CT angiography. JACC Cardiovasc Imaging 2011;4:328–37.

[46] Ghoshhajra BB, Engel LC, Karolyi M, Sidhu MS, Wai B, Barreto M, et al. Cardiac computed tomography angiography with automatic tube potential selection: effects on radiation dose and image quality. J Thorac Imaging 2013;28:40–8.

[47] Ghoshhajra BB, Engel LC, Major GP, Goehler A, Techasith T, Verdini D, et al. Evolution of coronary computed tomography radiation dose reduction at a tertiary referral center. Am J Med 2012;125:764–72.

[48] Min JK, Dunning A, Lin FY, Achenbach S, Al-Mallah MH, Berman DS, et al. Rationale and design of the CONFIRM (COronary CT Angiography EvaluatioN For Clinical Outcomes: An InteRnational Multicenter) Registry. J Cardiovasc Comput Tomogr 2011;5:84–92.

[49] Lee AM, Beaudoin J, Engel LC, Sidhu MS, Abbara S, Brady TJ, et al. Assessment of image quality and radiation dose of prospectively ECG-triggered adaptive dual-source coronary computed tomography angiography (cCTA) with arrhythmia rejection algorithm in systole versus diastole: a retrospective cohort study. Int J Cardiovasc Imaging 2013;29:1361–70.

[50] Fischer C, Hulten E, Belur P, Smith R, Voros S, Villines TC. Coronary CT angiography versus intravascular ultrasound for estimation of coronary stenosis and atherosclerotic plaque burden: a meta-analysis. J Cardiovasc Comput Tomogr 2013;7:256–66.

[51] Maurovich-Horvat P, Schlett CL, Alkadhi H, Nakano M, Otsuka F, Stolzmann P, et al. The napkin-ring sign indicates advanced atherosclerotic lesions in coronary CT angiography. JACC Cardiovasc Imaging 2012;5:1243–52.

[52] Seifarth H, Schlett CL, Nakano M, Otsuka F, Karolyi M, Liew G, et al. Histopathological correlates of the napkin-ring sign plaque in coronary CT angiography. Atherosclerosis 2012;224:90–6.

[53] Ferencik M, Schlett CL, Ghoshhajra BB, Kriegel MF, Joshi SB, Maurovich-Horvat P, et al. A computed tomography-based coronary lesion score to predict acute coronary syndrome among patients with acute chest pain and significant coronary stenosis on coronary computed tomographic angiogram. Am J Cardiol 2012;110:183–9.

[54] Motoyama S, Sarai M, Narula J, Ozaki Y. Coronary CT angiography and high-risk plaque morphology. Cardiovasc Interv Ther 2013;28:1–8.

[55] Hyafil F, Cornily JC, Rudd JH, Machac J, Feldman LJ, Fayad ZA. Quantification of inflammation within rabbit atherosclerotic plaques using the macrophage-specific CT contrast agent N1177: a comparison with 18F-FDG PET/CT and histology. J Nucl Med 2009;50:959–65.

[56] Cormode DP, Roessl E, Thran A, Skajaa T, Gordon RE, Schlomka JP, et al. Atherosclerotic plaque composition: analysis with multicolor CT and targeted gold nanoparticles. Radiology 2010;256:774–82.

[57] Tardif JC, L'Allier PL, Ibrahim R, Gregoire JC, Nozza A, Cossette M, et al. Treatment with 5-lipoxygenase inhibitor VIA-2291 (Atreleuton) in patients with recent acute coronary syndrome. Circ Cardiovasc Imaging 2010;3:298–307.

[58] Choudhury RP, Fuster V, Fayad ZA. Molecular, cellular and functional imaging of atherothrombosis. Nat Rev Drug Discov 2004;3:913–25.

[59] Wilensky RL, Song HK, Ferrari VA. Role of magnetic resonance and intravascular magnetic resonance in the detection of vulnerable plaques. J Am Coll Cardiol 2006;47:C48–56.

[60] McCarthy MJ, Loftus IM, Thompson MM, Jones L, London NJ, Bell PR, et al. Angiogenesis and the atherosclerotic carotid plaque: an association between symptomatology and plaque morphology. J Vasc Surg 1999;30:261–8.

[61] Redgrave JN, Gallagher P, Lovett JK, Rothwell PM. Critical cap thickness and rupture in symptomatic carotid plaques: the oxford plaque study. Stroke 2008;39:1722–9.

[62] Kerwin WS, O'Brien KD, Ferguson MS, Polissar N, Hatsukami TS, Yuan C. Inflammation in carotid atherosclerotic plaque: a dynamic contrast-enhanced MR imaging study. Radiology 2006;241:459–68.

[63] Qiao Y, Steinman DA, Qin Q, Etesami M, Schar M, Astor BC, et al. Intracranial arterial wall imaging using three-dimensional high isotropic resolution black blood MRI at 3.0 Tesla. J Magn Reson Imaging 2011;34:22–30.

[64] Balu N, Yarnykh VL, Chu B, Wang J, Hatsukami T, Yuan C. Carotid plaque assessment using fast 3D isotropic resolution black-blood MRI. Magn Reson Med 2011;65:627–37.

[65] Makhijani MK, Balu N, Yamada K, Yuan C, Nayak KS. Accelerated 3D MERGE carotid imaging using compressed sensing with a hidden Markov tree model. J Magn Reson Imaging 2012;36:1194–202.
[66] Underhill HR, Yarnykh VL, Hatsukami TS, Wang J, Balu N, Hayes CE, et al. Carotid plaque morphology and composition: initial comparison between 1.5- and 3.0-T magnetic field strengths. Radiology 2008;248:550–60.
[67] Li F, Yarnykh VL, Hatsukami TS, Chu B, Balu N, Wang J, et al. Scan-rescan reproducibility of carotid atherosclerotic plaque morphology and tissue composition measurements using multicontrast MRI at 3T. J Magn Reson Imaging 2010;31:168–76.
[68] Saam T, Ferguson MS, Yarnykh VL, Takaya N, Xu D, Polissar NL, et al. Quantitative evaluation of carotid plaque composition by in vivo MRI. Arterioscler Thromb Vasc Biol 2005;25:234–9.
[69] Tardif JC, Lesage F, Harel F, Romeo P, Pressacco J. Imaging biomarkers in atherosclerosis trials. Circ Cardiovasc Imaging 2011;4:319–33.
[70] Heinonen TM, Aamer M, Marshall C, Black DM, Tardif JC. Cardiovascular biomarkers and surrogate end points: key initiatives and clinical trial challenges. Expert Rev Cardiovasc Ther 2012;10:989–94.
[71] Isobe S, Tsimikas S, Zhou J, Fujimoto S, Sarai M, Branks MJ, et al. Noninvasive imaging of atherosclerotic lesions in apolipoprotein E-deficient and low-density-lipoprotein receptor-deficient mice with annexin A5. J Nucl Med 2006;47:1497–505.
[72] Takaya N, Yuan C, Chu B, Saam T, Underhill H, Cai J, et al. Association between carotid plaque characteristics and subsequent ischemic cerebrovascular events: a prospective assessment with MRI – initial results. Stroke 2006;37:818–23.
[73] Altaf N, Beech A, Goode SD, Gladman JR, Moody AR, Auer DP, et al. Carotid intraplaque hemorrhage detected by magnetic resonance imaging predicts embolization during carotid endarterectomy. J Vasc Surg 2007;46:31–6.
[74] Altaf N, Daniels L, Morgan PS, Auer D, MacSweeney ST, Moody AR, et al. Detection of intraplaque hemorrhage by magnetic resonance imaging in symptomatic patients with mild to moderate carotid stenosis predicts recurrent neurological events. J Vasc Surg 2008;47:337–42.
[75] Singh N, Moody AR, Gladstone DJ, Leung G, Ravikumar R, Zhan J, et al. Moderate carotid artery stenosis: MR imaging-depicted intraplaque hemorrhage predicts risk of cerebrovascular ischemic events in asymptomatic men. Radiology 2009;252:502–8.
[76] McConnell MV, Aikawa M, Maier SE, Ganz P, Libby P, Lee RT. MRI of rabbit atherosclerosis in response to dietary cholesterol lowering. Arterioscler Thromb Vasc Biol 1999;19:1956–9.
[77] Dong L, Kerwin WS, Chen H, Chu B, Underhill HR, Neradilek MB, et al. Carotid artery atherosclerosis: effect of intensive lipid therapy on the vasa vasorum–evaluation by using dynamic contrast-enhanced MR imaging. Radiology 2011;260:224–31.
[78] Zhao XQ, Dong L, Hatsukami T, Phan BA, Chu B, Moore A, et al. MR imaging of carotid plaque composition during lipid-lowering therapy a prospective assessment of effect and time course. JACC Cardiovasc Imaging 2011;4:977–86.
[79] Yamaguchi M, Sasaki M, Ohba H, Mori K, Narumi S, Katsura N, et al. Quantitative assessment of changes in carotid plaques during cilostazol administration using three-dimensional ultrasonography and non-gated magnetic resonance plaque imaging. Neuroradiology 2012;54:939–45.
[80] Lobatto ME, Fayad ZA, Silvera S, Vucic E, Calcagno C, Mani V, et al. Multimodal clinical imaging to longitudinally assess a nanomedical anti-inflammatory treatment in experimental atherosclerosis. Mol Pharm 2010;7:2020–9.

[81] Nahrendorf M, Jaffer FA, Kelly KA, Sosnovik DE, Aikawa E, Libby P, et al. Noninvasive vascular cell adhesion molecule-1 imaging identifies inflammatory activation of cells in atherosclerosis. Circulation 2006;114:1504–11.
[82] Ruehm SG, Corot C, Vogt P, Kolb S, Debatin JF. Magnetic resonance imaging of atherosclerotic plaque with ultrasmall superparamagnetic particles of iron oxide in hyperlipidemic rabbits. Circulation 2001;103:415–22.
[83] Amirbekian V, Lipinski MJ, Briley-Saebo KC, Amirbekian S, Aguinaldo JG, Weinreb DB, et al. Detecting and assessing macrophages in vivo to evaluate atherosclerosis noninvasively using molecular MRI. Proc Natl Acad Sci U S A 2007;104:961–6.
[84] van Tilborg GA, Vucic E, Strijkers GJ, Cormode DP, Mani V, Skajaa T, et al. Annexin A5-functionalized bimodal nanoparticles for MRI and fluorescence imaging of atherosclerotic plaques. Bioconjug Chem 2010;21:1794–803.
[85] Winter PM, Morawski AM, Caruthers SD, Fuhrhop RW, Zhang H, Williams TA, et al. Molecular imaging of angiogenesis in early-stage atherosclerosis with alpha(v)beta3-integrin-targeted nanoparticles. Circulation 2003;108:2270–4.
[86] Flacke S, Fischer S, Scott MJ, Fuhrhop RJ, Allen JS, McLean M, et al. Novel MRI contrast agent for molecular imaging of fibrin: implications for detecting vulnerable plaques. Circulation 2001;104:1280–5.
[87] Sirol M, Fuster V, Badimon JJ, Fallon JT, Moreno PR, Toussaint JF, et al. Chronic thrombus detection with in vivo magnetic resonance imaging and a fibrin-targeted contrast agent. Circulation 2005;112:1594–600.
[88] Kooi ME, Cappendijk VC, Cleutjens KB, Kessels AG, Kitslaar PJ, Borgers M, et al. Accumulation of ultrasmall superparamagnetic particles of iron oxide in human atherosclerotic plaques can be detected by in vivo magnetic resonance imaging. Circulation 2003;107:2453–8.
[89] Trivedi RA, U-King-Im JM, Graves MJ, Cross JJ, Horsley J, Goddard MJ, et al. In vivo detection of macrophages in human carotid atheroma: temporal dependence of ultrasmall superparamagnetic particles of iron oxide-enhanced MRI. Stroke 2004;35:1631–5.
[90] Tang TY, Howarth SP, Miller SR, Graves MJ, Patterson AJ, JM UK-I, et al. The ATHEROMA (Atorvastatin Therapy: Effects on Reduction of Macrophage Activity) Study. Evaluation using ultrasmall superparamagnetic iron oxide-enhanced magnetic resonance imaging in carotid disease. J Am Coll Cardiol 2009;53:2039–50.
[91] Dutta P, Courties G, Wei Y, Leuschner F, Gorbatov R, Robbins CS, et al. Myocardial infarction accelerates atherosclerosis. Nature 2012;487:325–9.
[92] Asanuma Y, Oeser A, Shintani AK, Turner E, Olsen N, Fazio S, et al. Premature coronary-artery atherosclerosis in systemic lupus erythematosus. N Engl J Med 2003;349:2407–15.
[93] Maradit-Kremers H, Nicola PJ, Crowson CS, Ballman KV, Gabriel SE. Cardiovascular death in rheumatoid arthritis: a population-based study. Arthritis Rheum 2005;52:722–32.
[94] Gelfand JM, Neimann AL, Shin DB, Wang X, Margolis DJ, Troxel AB. Risk of myocardial infarction in patients with psoriasis. JAMA 2006;296:1735–41.
[95] Camici P, Araujo LI, Spinks T, Lammertsma AA, Kaski JC, Shea MJ, et al. Increased uptake of 18F-fluorodeoxyglucose in postischemic myocardium of patients with exercise-induced angina. Circulation 1986;74:81–8.
[96] Leppanen O, Bjornheden T, Evaldsson M, Boren J, Wiklund O, Levin M. ATP depletion in macrophages in the core of advanced rabbit atherosclerotic plaques in vivo. Atherosclerosis 2006;188:323–30.
[97] Rodriguez-Prados JC, Traves PG, Cuenca J, Rico D, Aragones J, Martin-Sanz P, et al. Substrate fate in activated macrophages: a comparison between innate, classic, and alternative activation. J Immunol 2010;185:605–14.

[98] Folco EJ, Sheikine Y, Rocha VZ, Christen T, Shvartz E, Sukhova GK, et al. Hypoxia but not inflammation augments glucose uptake in human macrophages: implications for imaging atherosclerosis with 18fluorine-labeled 2-deoxy-D-glucose positron emission tomography. J Am Coll Cardiol 2011;58:603–14.

[99] Satomi T, Ogawa M, Mori I, Ishino S, Kubo K, Magata Y, et al. Comparison of contrast agents for atherosclerosis imaging using cultured macrophages: FDG versus ultrasmall superparamagnetic iron oxide. J Nucl Med 2013;54:999–1004.

[100] Tawakol A, Migrino RQ, Bashian GG, Bedri S, Vermylen D, Cury RC, et al. In vivo ^{18}F-fluorodeoxyglucose positron emission tomography imaging provides a noninvasive measure of carotid plaque inflammation in patients. J Am Coll Cardiol 2006;48:1818–24.

[101] Pedersen SF, Graebe M, Fisker Hag AM, Hojgaard L, Sillesen H, Kjaer A. Gene expression and 18FDG uptake in atherosclerotic carotid plaques. Nucl Med Commun 2010;31:423–9.

[102] Graebe M, Pedersen SF, Borgwardt L, Hojgaard L, Sillesen H, Kjaer A. Molecular pathology in vulnerable carotid plaques: correlation with [18]-fluorodeoxyglucose positron emission tomography (FDG-PET). Eur J Vasc Endovasc Surg 2009;37:714–21.

[103] Figueroa AL, Subramanian SS, Cury RC, Truong QA, Gardecki JA, Tearney GJ, et al. Distribution of inflammation within carotid atherosclerotic plaques with high-risk morphological features: a comparison between positron emission tomography activity, plaque morphology, and histopathology. Circ Cardiovasc Imaging 2012;5:69–77.

[104] Rudd JH, Myers KS, Bansilal S, Machac J, Rafique A, Farkouh M, et al. (18) Fluorodeoxyglucose positron emission tomography imaging of atherosclerotic plaque inflammation is highly reproducible: implications for atherosclerosis therapy trials. J Am Coll Cardiol 2007;50:892–6.

[105] Tahara N, Kai H, Ishibashi M, Nakaura H, Kaida H, Baba K, et al. Simvastatin attenuates plaque inflammation: evaluation by fluorodeoxyglucose positron emission tomography. J Am Coll Cardiol 2006;48:1825–31.

[106] Ishii H, Nishio M, Takahashi H, Aoyama T, Tanaka M, Toriyama T, et al. Comparison of atorvastatin 5 and 20 mg/d for reducing F-18 fluorodeoxyglucose uptake in atherosclerotic plaques on positron emission tomography/computed tomography: a randomized, investigator-blinded, open-label, 6-month study in Japanese adults scheduled for percutaneous coronary intervention. Clin Ther 2010;32:2337–47.

[107] Fayad ZA, Mani V, Woodward M, Kallend D, Abt M, Burgess T, et al. Safety and efficacy of dalcetrapib on atherosclerotic disease using novel non-invasive multimodality imaging (dal-PLAQUE): a randomised clinical trial. Lancet 2011;378:1547–59.

[108] Rudd JH, Myers KS, Bansilal S, Machac J, Woodward M, Fuster V, et al. Relationships among regional arterial inflammation, calcification, risk factors, and biomarkers: a prospective fluorodeoxyglucose positron-emission tomography/computed tomography imaging study. Circ Cardiovasc Imaging 2009;2:107–15.

[109] Kim TN, Kim S, Yang SJ, Yoo HJ, Seo JA, Kim SG, et al. Vascular inflammation in patients with impaired glucose tolerance and type 2 diabetes: analysis with 18F-fluorodeoxyglucose positron emission tomography. Circ Cardiovasc Imaging 2010;3:142–8.

[110] Joly L, Djaballah W, Koehl G, Mandry D, Dolivet G, Marie PY, et al. Aortic inflammation, as assessed by hybrid FDG-PET/CT imaging, is associated with enhanced aortic stiffness in addition to concurrent calcification. Eur J Nucl Med Mol Imaging 2009;36:979–85.

[111] Rudd JH, Warburton EA, Fryer TD, Jones HA, Clark JC, Antoun N, et al. Imaging atherosclerotic plaque inflammation with [18F]-fluorodeoxyglucose positron emission tomography. Circulation 2002;105:2708–11.
[112] Rogers IS, Nasir K, Figueroa AL, Cury RC, Hoffmann U, Vermylen DA, et al. Feasibility of FDG imaging of the coronary arteries: comparison between acute coronary syndrome and stable angina. JACC Cardiovasc Imaging 2010;3:388–97.
[113] Rominger A, Saam T, Wolpers S, Cyran CC, Schmidt M, Foerster S, et al. 18F-FDG PET/CT identifies patients at risk for future vascular events in an otherwise asymptomatic cohort with neoplastic disease. J Nucl Med 2009;50:1611–20.
[114] Saam T, Rominger A, Wolpers S, Nikolaou K, Rist C, Greif M, et al. Association of inflammation of the left anterior descending coronary artery with cardiovascular risk factors, plaque burden and pericardial fat volume: a PET/CT study. Eur J Nucl Med Mol Imaging 2010;37:1203–12.
[115] Figueroa AL, Abdelbaky A, Truong QA, Corsini E, MacNabb MH, Lavender ZR, et al. Measurement of arterial activity on routine FDG PET/CT images improves prediction of risk of future CV events. JACC Cardiovasc Imaging 2013;6:1250–9.
[116] Tawakol A, Singh P, Rudd JH, Soffer J, Cai G, Vucic E, et al. Effect of treatment for 12 weeks with rilapladib, a lipoprotein-associated phospholipase A2 inhibitor, on arterial inflammation as assessed with 18F-fluorodeoxyglucose-PET imaging. J Am Coll Cardiol 2014;63:86–8.
[117] Elkhawad M, Rudd JH, Sarov-Blat L, Cai G, Wells R, Davies LC, et al. Effects of p38 mitogen-activated protein kinase inhibition on vascular and systemic inflammation in patients with atherosclerosis. JACC Cardiovasc Imaging 2012;5:911–22.
[118] Mizoguchi M, Tahara N, Tahara A, Nitta Y, Kodama N, Oba T, et al. Pioglitazone attenuates atherosclerotic plaque inflammation in patients with impaired glucose tolerance or diabetes a prospective, randomized, comparator-controlled study using serial FDG PET/CT imaging study of carotid artery and ascending aorta. JACC Cardiovasc Imaging 2011;4:1110–8.
[119] Tawakol A, Fayad ZA, Mogg R, Alon A, Klimas MT, Dansky H, et al. Intensification of Statin Therapy Results in a Rapid Reduction in Atherosclerotic Inflammation: Results of A Multi-Center FDG-PET/CT Feasibility Study. J Am Coll Cardiol 2013;62:909–17.
[120] Maki-Petaja KM, Elkhawad M, Cheriyan J, Joshi FR, Ostor AJ, Hall FC, et al. Anti-tumor necrosis factor-alpha therapy reduces aortic inflammation and stiffness in patients with rheumatoid arthritis. Circulation 2012;126:2473–80.
[121] Erdmann E, Dormandy JA, Charbonnel B, Massi-Benedetti M, Moules IK, Skene AM, et al. The effect of pioglitazone on recurrent myocardial infarction in 2,445 patients with type 2 diabetes and previous myocardial infarction: results from the PROactive (PROactive 05) Study. J Am Coll Cardiol 2007;49:1772–80.
[122] Schwartz GG, Olsson AG, Abt M, Ballantyne CM, Barter PJ, Brumm J, et al. Effects of dalcetrapib in patients with a recent acute coronary syndrome. N Engl J Med 2012;367:2089–99.
[123] LaRosa JC, Grundy SM, Waters DD, Shear C, Barter P, Fruchart JC, et al. Intensive lipid lowering with atorvastatin in patients with stable coronary disease. N Engl J Med 2005;352:1425–35.
[124] Investigators S, White HD, Held C, Stewart R, Tarka E, Brown R, et al. Darapladib for preventing ischemic events in stable coronary heart disease. N Engl J Med 2014;370:1702–11.

[125] Nahrendorf M, Keliher E, Panizzi P, Zhang H, Hembrador S, Figueiredo JL, et al. 18F-4V for PET-CT imaging of VCAM-1 expression in atherosclerosis. JACC Cardiovasc Imaging 2009;2:1213–22.

[126] Matusiak N, van Waarde A, Bischoff R, Oltenfreiter R, van de Wiele C, Dierckx RA, et al. Probes for non-invasive matrix metalloproteinase-targeted imaging with PET and SPECT. Curr Pharm Des 2013;19:4647–72.

[127] Limpachayaporn P, Schafers M, Schober O, Kopka K, Haufe G. Synthesis of new fluorinated, 2-substituted 5-pyrrolidinylsulfonyl isatin derivatives as caspase-3 and caspase-7 inhibitors: nonradioactive counterparts of putative PET-compatible apoptosis imaging agents. Bioorg Med Chem 2013;21:2025–36.

[128] Gaemperli O, Shalhoub J, Owen DR, Lamare F, Johansson S, Fouladi N, et al. Imaging intraplaque inflammation in carotid atherosclerosis with 11C-PK11195 positron emission tomography/computed tomography. Eur Heart J 2012;33:1902–10.

[129] Kawachi E, Uehara Y, Hasegawa K, Yahiro E, Ando S, Wada Y, et al. Novel molecular imaging of atherosclerosis with gallium-68-labeled apolipoprotein A-I mimetic peptide and positron emission tomography. Circ J 2013;77:1482–9.

[130] Razavian M, Marfatia R, Mongue-Din H, Tavakoli S, Sinusas AJ, Zhang J, et al. Integrin-targeted imaging of inflammation in vascular remodeling. Arterioscler Thromb Vasc Biol 2011;31:2820–6.

[131] Joshi NV, Vesey AT, Williams MC, Shah AS, Calvert PA, Craighead FH, et al. 18F-fluoride positron emission tomography for identification of ruptured and high-risk coronary atherosclerotic plaques: a prospective clinical trial. Lancet 2014;383:705–13.

Myocardial ischemia

K. Goetschalckx*, F.E. Rademakers[†]
*University Hospitals Leuven, Leuven, Belgium; [†]KU Leuven, Leuven, Belgium

Abbreviations

BOLD	blood–oxygen-level-dependent
CAD	coronary artery disease
CFR	coronary flow reserve
CTCA	computed tomography coronary angiography
ECHO	echocardiography
FFR	fractional flow reserve
ICA	invasive coronary angiography
IHD	ischemic heart disease
IVUS	intravascular ultrasound
MR	magnetic resonance
MRA	magnetic resonance imaging angiography
MRS	magnetic resonance spectroscopy
OCT	optical coherence tomography
PET	positron emission tomography
PTP	pretest probability
SCAD	stable coronary artery disease
SPECT	single-photon emission computer tomography

9.1 Pathophysiology of ischemia

Ischemia is caused by the imbalance between *oxygen demand* by and *oxygen supply* to the myocardial cells. *Oxygen demand* is determined by contractility, heart rate, and wall tension (preload and afterload), the latter depending mainly on cavity pressure and size. *Oxygen supply* occurs exclusively over the coronary circulation: in contrast to many other tissues in the human body, oxygen extraction (arterio—venous oxygen difference) by the cardiomyocytes is near maximal, so that variation in blood supply is the only variable to adjust oxygen delivery and keep it in balance with oxygen demand. The other variable, i.e., the oxygen carrying capacity of the blood, can be abnormal in some diseases (=hypoxemia f.i. due to lung disease or anemia), but in general it is coronary flow and its distribution over the coronary tree that defines oxygen delivery to the myocardial cells. The primary symptom of ischemia is angina, but patients can have ischemia without angina (silent ischemia) and present with other consequences of ischemia, such as arrhythmia, sudden cardiac death, or left ventricular dysfunction. A local release of vasoactive substances, such as adenosine, is induced by ischemia and is thought to play a role in the formation of collaterals and in ischemic preconditioning (cf. Figure 9.1).

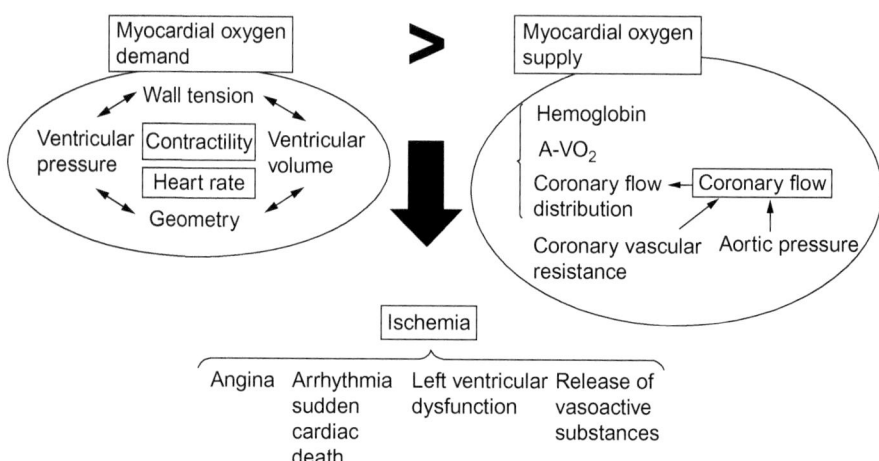

Figure 9.1 Myocardial ischemia. Myocardial ischemia occurs if oxygen demand exceeds oxygen supply to the myocardial cells. Oxygen demand is determined by contractility and heart rate, but also by geometrical factors such as ventricular volume, pressure, and wall tension. Myocardial oxygen supply is mainly determined by coronary flow and its distribution, but also by the oxygen carrying capacity of the blood (hemoglobin) and the ventilatory and pulmonary function. Ischemia can result in angina, but also in arrhythmia, sudden cardiac death, or left ventricular dysfunction.

Coronary blood flow is determined by the aortic pressure on one hand, mainly during diastole when intramyocardial pressure is low, and on the other hand, coronary vascular resistance over the entire coronary vasculature, which consists of the coronary epicardial branches (1), the microvasculature (mainly the arterioles) (2) and the capillary bed (3) (cf. Figure 9.2). The coronary vascular resistance can be pathologically increased structurally or functionally at each of the three levels, thereby potentially causing ischemia.

(1) At the epicardial level, a coronary artery stenosis can be caused by an atheroma, thrombus, and/or vasospasm (Figure 9.3). Atheromatosis is the most prevalent cause of increased coronary vascular resistance impeding oxygen supply. Histologically, a stable atheroma shows less frequent erosion or rupture of the endothelial lining than a vulnerable plaque causing an acute coronary syndrome. The lesions are typically fibrotic, poorly cellular, with small necrotic cores, thick fibrous caps, and little or no overlying thrombus (Figure 9.4) [2].

(2) In normal coronary vasculature under resting conditions, the microvascular resistance is quite high due to a certain degree of vasoconstriction of the arterioles and the sphincters. This allows for autoregulation of the myocardial blood flow by vasodilation of this microvascular bed to compensate for f.i. an epicardial stenosis or low blood pressure (cf. Figure 9.5). Vasodilation can be induced by local release of endothelium-dependent or -independent vasoactive substances, such as respectively nitric oxide or adenosine, resulting in a direct local relaxation of smooth muscle cells in the vessel wall (cf. Figure 9.6). Normal endothelial function contributes to vasodilation by nitric oxide release from the endothelium as a response to increased shear stress, whereas endothelial dysfunction will result in vasospasm. A disturbance of the local adenosine metabolism can also be a dysfunctional factor by impaired vasodilation. Increased vasoconstriction, impaired, or inhomogenous vasodilation (steal-effect) in the microvascular bed occurs in f.i. syndrome X patients or in diabetics with microvascular dysfunction [1].

Myocardial ischemia

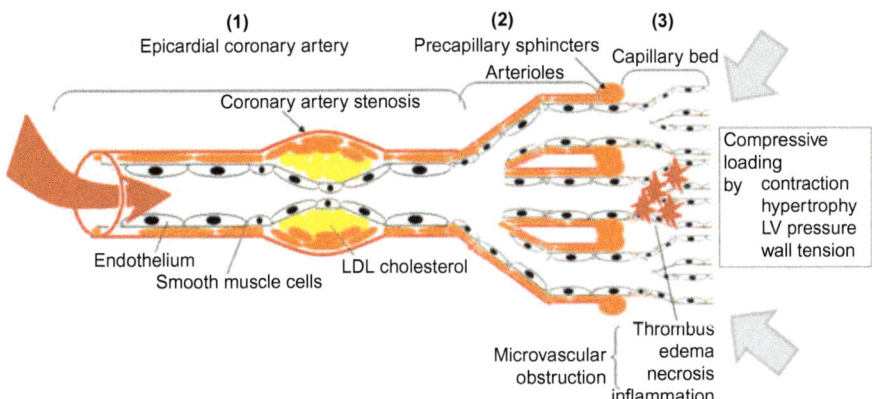

Figure 9.2 Coronary vascular resistance. Coronary vascular resistance is determined by (1) the coronary epicardial branches, (2) the microvasculature, mainly the arterioles and the precapillary sphincters, and (3) the capillary bed. It can be pathologically increased at each of these three levels by a functional or structural disturbancy, thereby potentially causing ischemia.

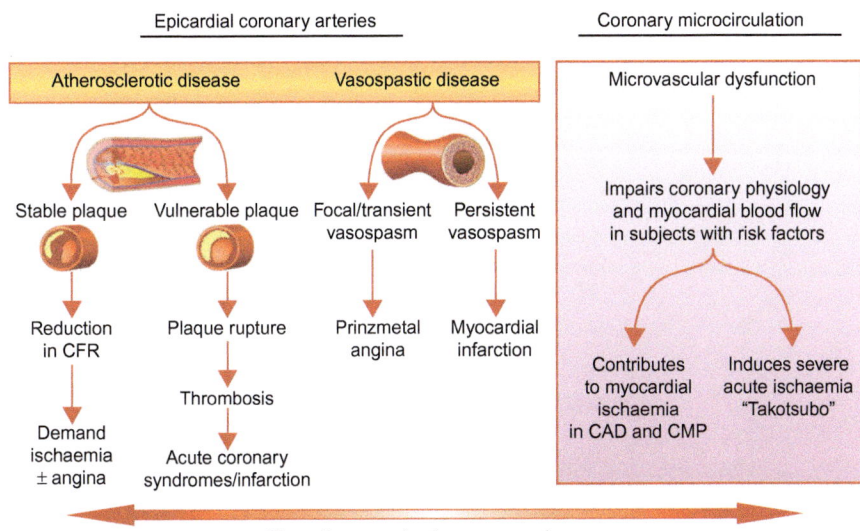

Figure 9.3 Mechanisms of myocardial ischemia. In addition to atherosclerotic and vasospastic disease, coronary microvascular dysfunction has emerged as a "third" mechanism of myocardial ischemia. It can occur alone or in combination with atherosclerotic and/or vasospastic disease and can lead to transient myocardial ischemia as in patients with CAD or cardiomyopathy or to severe acute ischemia as observed in Takotsubo syndrome. From Ref. [1].

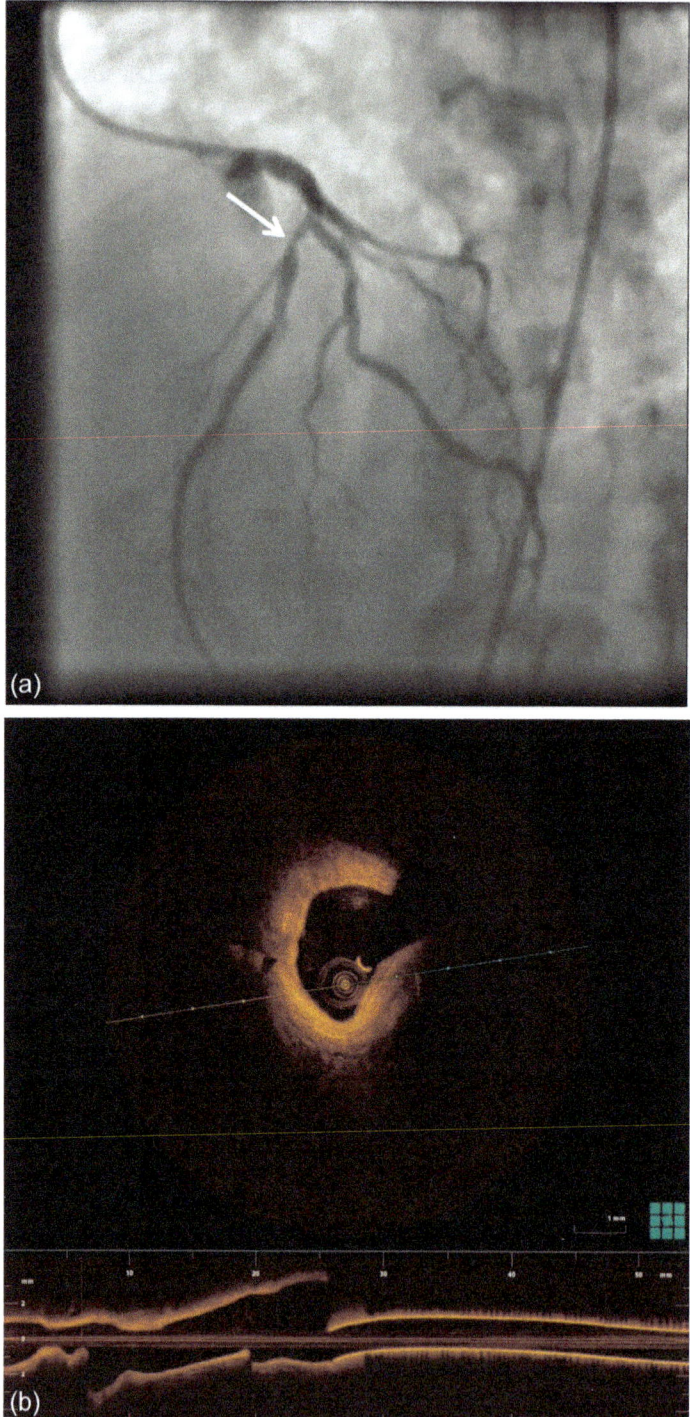

Figure 9.4 Coronary angiography of a 59-year-old man with a stenosis on the mid-LAD (white arrow). OCT shows an intact endothelium over a stable atheroma. FFR was 0.85. The patient was treated conservatively.
With courtesy of Tom Adriaenssens, MD, PhD, University Hospital Leuven, Belgium.

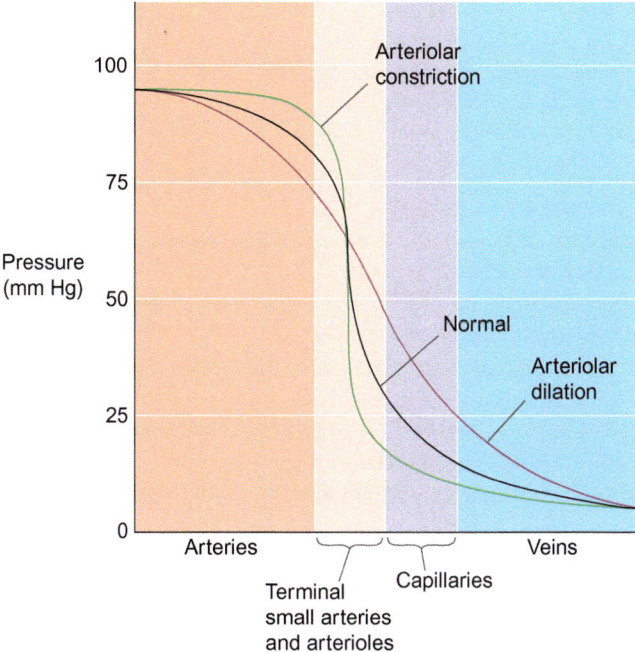

Figure 9.5 Microvascular resistance. In normal coronary vasculature, the microvascular resistance is quite high by maintaining a certain degree of vasoconstriction of the arterioles and the sphincters. This allows for autoregulation of the myocardial blood flow, by vasodilation of this microvascular bed to compensate for f.i. an epicardial stenosis or low blood pressure. From Boron & Boulpaep textbook Physiology.

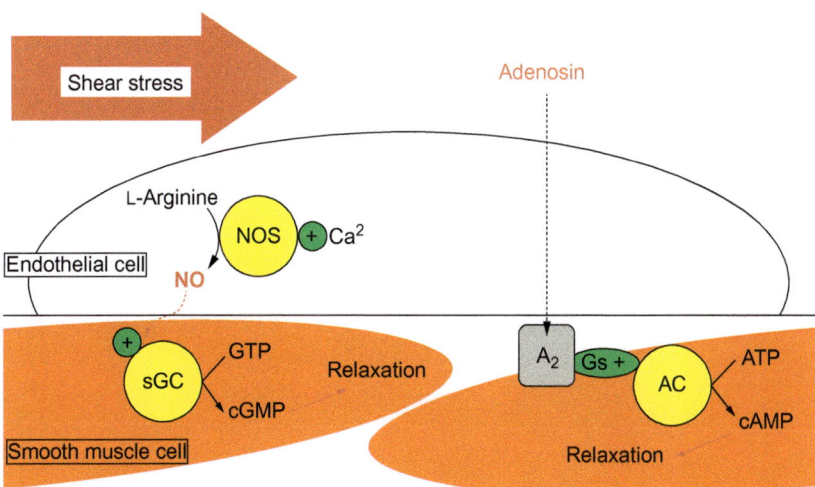

Figure 9.6 Vasorelaxation. Vasodilation can be induced by local release of endothelium-dependent (shear stress) or -independent vasoactive substances, such as respectively nitric oxide or adenosin, resulting in a direct local relaxation of smooth muscle cells in the vessel wall.

(3) A relative deficit of capillaries can occur in left ventricular hypertrophy; microvascular obstruction can result from cellular necrosis, edema, inflammation, and/or thrombus as in acute myocardial infarction. Myocardial blood flow depends on coronary blood flow, but local mechanical factors such as myocardial contraction and left ventricular pressure also influence perfusion pressure, resulting in a transmural myocardial perfusion gradient, with the subendocardium being most vulnerable to ischemia.

Clinical circumstances causing an increase in oxygen demand are f.i. exercise, stress, emotion, and cold exposure. In case diastolic aortic pressure is low, such as in aortic insufficiency or in elderly with isolated systolic hypertension and left ventricular hypertrophy, ischemia can occur in the absence of a severe epicardial coronary artery stenosis. Also shortening of the duration of diastole at higher heart rate, f.i. in case of anemia or in patients with atrial fibrillation with rapid ventricular response, can cause subendocardial ischemia, especially in hypertrophic ventricles. So the actual occurrence of angina can vary in a given patient and can occur even at rest in patients with stable epicardial lesions or microvascular dysfunction, making it difficult to distinguish these from vasospastic angina or even an acute coronary syndrome, only on the basis of symptoms and the circumstances of their occurrence. Epicardial atherosclerosis and microvascular dysfunction are relatively stable structural and functional alterations, that are associated with fairly stable angina or other ischemic alterations such as ECG-changes, starting at a certain level of exercise intensity.

Vasospasm on the other hand, is a transitory phenomenon that often occurs at rest with preserved effort tolerance (Prinzmetal angina). Vasospasm can occur in apparently normal or atherosclerotic coronary arteries, it can be (multi)focal or diffuse, and it is caused most often by vasoconstrictor stimuli acting on hyperreactive smooth muscle cells, although endothelial dysfunction can reinforce the problem. Invasive administration of acetylcholine provoking vasoconstriction by direct stimulation of smooth muscle cells, instead of vasodilation by NO-release from the endothelium, would indicate endothelial dysfunction, whereas ergonovine administration can induce vasospasm by hyperreactive smooth muscle cell contraction [3].

Very often these different coronary abnormalities co-exist in one patient and cause ischemia by a combination of effects. A new concept of ischemic heart disease (IHD) puts myocardial ischemia at the center of our attention and critical coronary stenosis, vasospasm, and microvascular dysfunction in the margin as one of many contributors to myocardial ischemia (cf. Figures 9.3 and 9.7).

9.1.1 The ischemic cascade

The consequences of a transient imbalance between blood/oxygen supply and metabolic demand occur in a predictable temporal sequence, involving (1) insufficient myocardial perfusion resulting in (2) abnormal metabolism with increased H^+ and K^+ concentration in the venous blood that drains the ischemic territory, (3) signs of ventricular diastolic and subsequently systolic dysfunction with regional wall motion abnormalities, (4) development of ST–T changes, and (5) cardiac ischemic pain (angina). This ischemic cascade explains why imaging techniques that identify abnormalities in perfusion, metabolism, or cardiac mechanics are more sensitive than ECG signs or symptoms in detecting ischemia (cf. Figure 9.8).

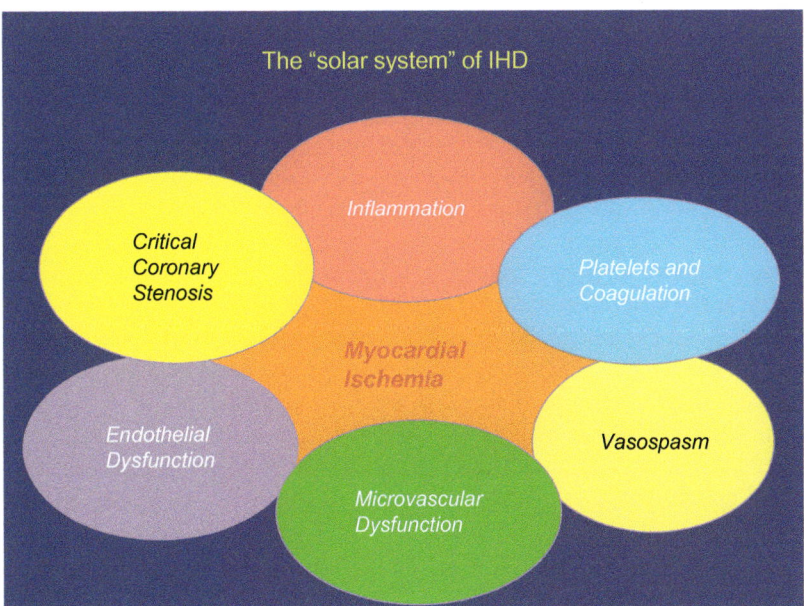

Figure 9.7 Proposed paradigm shift in ischemic heart disease (IHD). This new concept of ischemic heart disease puts myocardial ischemia at the center of our approach and critical coronary stenosis on the side as one of many contributors to myocardial ischemia. From [4].

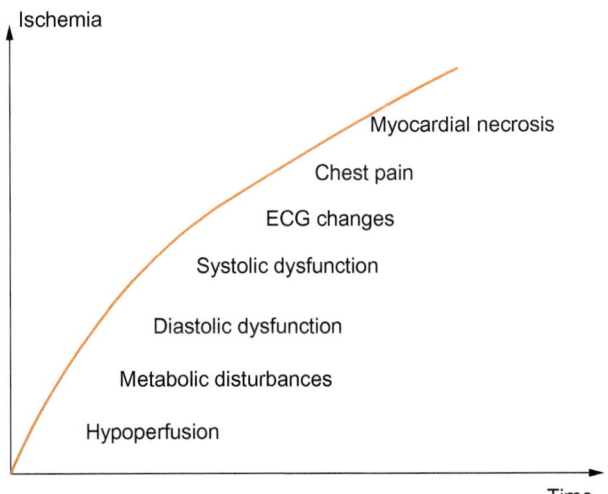

Figure 9.8 The ischemic cascade occurs in a predictable temporal sequence, involving insufficient myocardial perfusion resulting in abnormal metabolism, regional wall motion abnormalities, development of ST–T changes, and angina. This explains why imaging techniques that identify abnormalities in perfusion, metabolism, or cardiac mechanics are more sensitive than ECG signs or symptoms in detecting ischemia.

9.2 Invasive diagnosis of ischemia

9.2.1 Anatomy of coronary artery disease

Invasive coronary angiography (ICA) remains the "gold standard" in depicting epicardial coronary artery disease (CAD). However, the imaging information is only about the lumen, and not the plaque, let alone the consequences of the structural abnormality.

This plaque can be characterized invasively by intravascular ultrasound (IVUS) or optical coherence tomography (OCT). IVUS demonstrates the full thickness of the plaque (except in the presence of extensive subintimal calcification), but its resolution is insufficient to measure cap thickness, whereas OCT penetration is much more limited (1 mm), but its greater resolution allows for reliable identification of subintimal lipidic plaques and precise measurement of the fibrous cap, the two key elements characterizing vulnerable plaques (cf. Figure 9.6). Both techniques have greatly added to our understanding of the natural history of coronary atherosclerosis and offer, to some extent, "virtual histology" (cf. Chapter 8).

Alternatively, coronary anatomy may be visualized noninvasively by coronary computed tomography angiography (CTCA) or magnetic resonance imaging angiography (MRA) (see Chapters 5–8).

All these anatomical techniques provide information about the lumen and/or the plaque surrounding the lumen but do not address function of the epicardial coronary arteries or the condition of the microvasculature.

9.2.2 Ischemia

In stable patients, diagnosing the presence of CAD should be differentiated from diagnosing the presence of ischemia, caused by obstructive CAD and/or microvascular dysfunction [5]. Due to the lack of a linear relationship between epicardial coronary artery stenosis and coronary flow, there is a need for a functional evaluation of the severity of epicardial stenoses and microvascular dysfunction. The more variable causes of ischemia, i.e., vasospasm, warrant a specific diagnostic scheme using provocation tests.

Two methods to invasively determine the functional significance of a lesion are coronary flow reserve (CFR) and fractional flow reserve (FFR). Although these concepts are related, they measure different components of the system of epicardial vessels, microvasculature, and the dependent myocardium. More recently, an instantaneous wave-free ratio (iFR) has shown to be equivalent to FFR, without the need for adenosine administration [6].

The absolute CFR is defined as the ratio of hyperemic to basal coronary blood flow and can be measured invasively by Doppler velocity or thermodilution methods, or noninvasively by measuring Doppler velocities echocardiographically or by measuring myocardial perfusion reserve (ratio of stress over rest perfusion) quantitatively or semiquantitatively with positron emission tomography (PET), magnetic resonance imaging, or transthoracic contrast echocardiography (ECHO).

In a patient with an epicardial coronary artery stenosis, the release of ischemic metabolites, such as adenosine, within the under-perfused myocardium downstream to the stenotic artery, results in dilation of the distal arterioles and precapillary sphincters. This compensatory vasodilation favors local perfusion but at the price of "consuming" part of the normally available flow reserve. At a perfusion pressure of about 50 mmHg, the coronary resting flow is preserved due to maximal downstream vasodilatation but no further flow reserve is available (cf. Figure 9.9).

Due to numerous influencing factors, CFR has a high interindividual variability (cf. Figure 9.10). Healthy subjects have an absolute CFR of 3.5–5, whereas patients with a significant epicardial stenosis have a CFR $\approx$ 2–2.5. Patients with a CFR < 2 have an adverse prognosis, even in the absence of epicardial disease, because in that case CFR indicates severe microvascular disease [7,8]. Flow reserve values between 2.5 and 3.5 are difficult to interpret but may indicate milder forms of coronary microvascular dysfunction, with and without associated epicardial disease. In this respect it is important to take into account the presence of diffuse disease and coronary artery remodeling. Diffuse disease both in the absence or presence of any focal stenosis will have a significant supplementary negative impact on CFR. Adaptive remodeling on the other

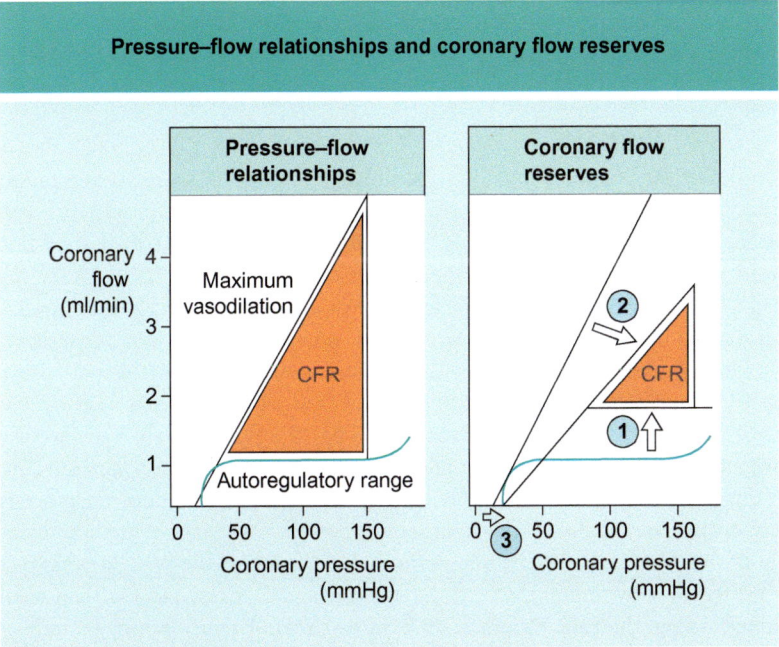

Figure 9.9 (1) CFR diminishes with an increased metabolism of the myocardium, f.o. by increased blood pressure, heart rate, or contractility. (2) CFR decreases with decreased vasodilatory capacity. This is mostly due to an epicardial coronary artery stenosis but it can also be caused by impaired microvascular vasodilation such as in elderly or by microvascular dysfunction in f.i. diabetes. (3) CFR can be reduced by an increased opening/closing pressure at the capillary level, such as in left ventricular hypertrophy, or in dilated cardiomyopathy with increased wall tension.
From Gould et al., Critical coronary stenosis, page 87, © 1994, with permission of ExcerptaMedica Inc.

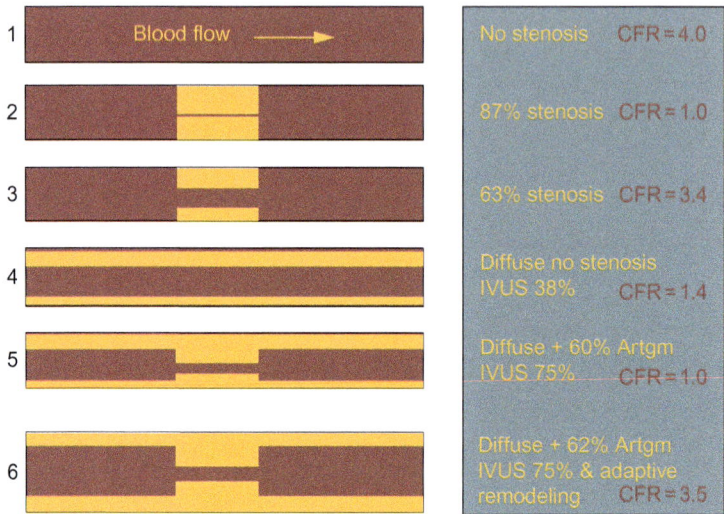

Figure 9.10 Schematic illustrating limitations of anatomic measures of stenosis severity by ICA or IVUS, due to diffuse disease with and without remodeling compared to coronary flow reserve.
From Ref. [5].

hand, will partially "compensate" for the presence of a focal stenosis and reduce the impact on CFR [5].

The complexity of interpreting this "multi-factorial" CFR led to the use of the more simple FFR method in determining the significance of an epicardial stenosis, making to a large extent abstraction from distal microvasculature. The FFR is defined as the ratio of the maximal hyperemic flow in the diseased epicardial coronary artery over the hypothetical maximal hyperemic flow in this artery in case there was no disease. It is based on the assumption that at maximal vasodilation, vascular resistance of the coronary artery is minimal and constant for both the hypothetical and the diseased situation, so that coronary flow is mainly driven by pressure. In a normal coronary artery, this pressure equals aortic pressure, whereas in a diseased coronary artery, the pressure drops over the epicardial stenosis and therefore equals the pressure measured distally of this stenosis. FFR is then defined as the ratio of the post-stenotic over the aortic pressure at hyperemia, which can be measured invasively and can easily be interpreted. When the FFR becomes ≤ 0.8, downstream perfusion may be inadequate. Again, there is no linear relationship between the severity of an angiographic stenosis and the reduction in FFR it causes, stressing the inadequacy of mere anatomical evaluation to identify the impact on perfusion (cf. Figure 9.4).

9.2.3 Relationship between myocardial perfusion and FFR

How, then, is the relationship between CFR (which represents an integrated parameter of myocardial perfusion) and FFR? As can be seen in Figure 9.11a, no clear CFR–FFR relationship is found in this broad scatter. This indicates that, although

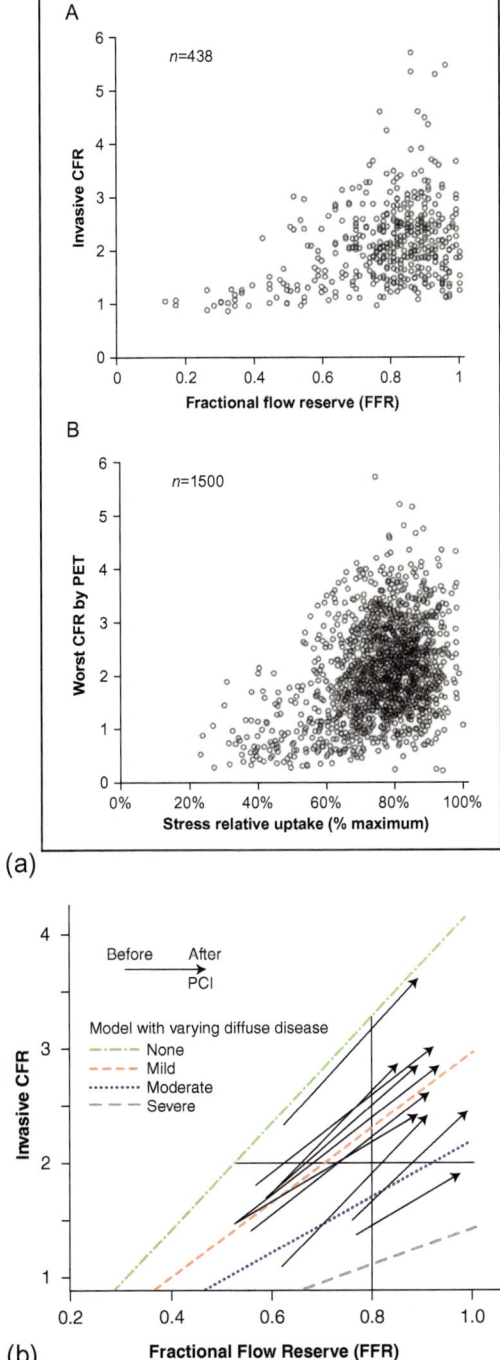

Figure 9.11 (a) No clear CFR–FFR relationship is found in this broad scatter. However, by taking into account the presence of diffuse disease, the CFR–FFR relationship is revealed as illustrated in (b). In the absence of diffuse disease, the relationship between CFR and FFR (before vs. after PCI) is linear and along the upper green diagonal. With an increasing amount of diffuse disease, the slope of the CFR–FFR relationship becomes less and less.
Source: J Am Coll Cardiol Img 2012;5:193–202.

FFR is a functional measurement of ischemia as compared to the anatomical methods, it does not reflect microvasculature and distal coronary flow. Therefore, noninvasive imaging modalities measuring myocardial perfusion can still differ from FFR as a "gold standard" for the detection of ischemia, due to fundamental differences in pathophysiology, rather than shortcomings of methodology [9]. However, by taking into account the presence of diffuse disease, the CFR–FFR relationship is revealed as illustrated in the next graph (Figure 9.11b). From this pathophysiologic framework, it is clear that in case FFR is <0.8 and CFR is <2, both values are concordantly reduced and the patient would benefit from revascularization, whereas a FFR>0.8 and CFR>2 would indicate a nearly normal situation, making revascularization unnecessary. In case there is a FFR>0.8, but CFR<2, angiography mostly confirms diffuse coronary disease rather than a focal stenosis, making this patient not eligible for a revascularization procedure. This leaves us with the situation of a lesion with FFR<0.8 but CFR>2, indicating a significant focal lesion, but adequate CFR, possibly due to positive, adaptive remodeling, where one could question the necessity to intervene on the lesion.

FFR-guided PCI has been shown to be superior to angiographic-guided PCI (based on angiographic judgment of stenosis severity alone) in patients with multivessel disease, for the endpoint of death, nonfatal myocardial infarction, and repeat revascularization at 1 and 2 years (FAME 1) [10,11]. In coronary artery stenoses with FFR<0.8, revascularization by PCI on top of optimal medical therapy (OMT) was shown to be superior to OMT alone at 1 and 2 years of follow-up, by decreasing the need for urgent revascularization (FAME 2) [12,13]. Recently, the use of FFR has been upgraded to a Class IA recommendation in multivessel PCI in the ESC Guidelines on coronary revascularization [14].

The decision whether to revascularize a patient should be based on the presence of a significant obstructive coronary artery stenosis, the amount of related ischemia, and the expected benefit to prognosis and/or symptoms. There are many clinical, anatomical, technical, and environmental factors that contribute to this decision-making. Therefore, the treatment should preferentially be an individualized clinical judgment with consensual decision of a heart team [14].

9.2.4 Heart team discussion

A heart team consists of an interventional cardiologist, a cardiac surgeon, and, according to the European guidelines, preferentially also a noninvasive cardiologist to obtain integrated, active decision making between groups of physicians with diverse expertise and the patient. In certain instances, other providers such as primary care physicians, intensivists, or anesthesiologists can also be involved.

Although no studies have proven superiority of using a heart team instead of making decisions by ourselves, guidelines recommend heart team discussions because people working together in a multidisciplinary manner may reach better decisions by consensus than any individual alone, especially when it involves weighing complicated treatments, such as coronary revascularization, with various risks and benefits. Furthermore, using a heart team can improve timeliness and consistency of decisions when multiple providers are likely to be involved, allow better coordinated treatment plans to be developed (e.g., "hybrid" revascularization procedures), minimize concerns related to physician self-referral, enhance patient enrollment in research protocols, and increase educational opportunities.

9.3 Noninvasive detection and quantification of ischemia

9.3.1 The concept of pretest probability

Recommendations to decide on the appropriateness of the various diagnostic modalities as well as to establish the prognosis of the patient and make the appropriate therapeutic choices rely heavily on estimates of the prevalence of significant CAD in populations characterized by sex, age, and symptoms. On the other hand, the patient with his/her comorbidities and quality of life contributes to the likelihood of potential revascularization.

When there is no indication for a specific ischemia treatment (primary prevention), risk charts such as SCORE or Framingham can be applied to decide on the need for risk modification [14]. When CAD is suspected and a revascularization treatment is considered if appropriate, an estimation of CAD-probability is relevant for further diagnostic and/or treatment strategy planning. The pretest probability (PTP) conforms to a Bayesian approach, allowing for the calculation of an individualized post-test probability. By using a diagnostic test (f.i. stress imaging modality), an intermediate and therefore indecisive PTP is turned into a low or high post-test probability guiding further treatment. Recent estimates based on CTCA registries of the prevalence of obstructive epicardial CAD in patients with typical or atypical angina are substantially lower than the Diamond and Forrester estimates from 1979, though (cf. Figure 9.12) [15]. In contrast, in patients

PTP <15%   PTP 16-65%   PTP 66-85%   PTP > 85%

Age	Typical angina		Atypical angina		Non-angingal pain	
	Men	Women	Men	Women	Men	Women
30–39	59	28	29	10	18	5
40–49	69	37	38	14	25	8
50–59	77	47	49	20	34	12
60–69	84	58	59	28	44	17
70–79	89	68	69	37	54	24
>80	93	76	78	47	65	32

Figure 9.12 Clinical PTP of obstructive CAD in patients with stable chest pain symptoms. From Ref. [15].

with non-anginal chest pain, the prevalence of obstructive CAD as assessed by coronary CTCA may be higher than previously expected. In fact, these coronary CTCA data suggest that there may be little difference in the prevalence of obstructive CAD across the three groups of chest pain. So using PTPs from registries with referred patients may overestimate the true PTP in patients presenting in a primary care environment.

If the *pretest probability (PTP) is less than 15%*, other causes for symptoms should be explored, including functional coronary disease, and the risk profile of the patient should be established, as mentioned before, to decide on primary preventive measures.

If the *PTP is more than 85%* the diagnosis of stable CAD is so likely that one can immediately proceed to risk stratification to decide on therapy (revascularization or not).

The 15% and 85% cut-offs follow from the overall sensitivity and specificity of imaging-based diagnostic methods lying around 85%. This means that 15% of all tests will be false, so that it is better in patients with a PTP below 15% or above 85% NOT to perform a test.

In the *intermediate PTP between 15% and 85%*, noninvasive diagnostic testing is appropriate to convert intermediate PTP into low or high post-test probability (respectively low and high likelihood of CAD), guiding further treatment (cf. Figure 9.13) [14].

Multiple factors contribute to the decision of which diagnostic test will be best in answering the diagnostic question on the one hand, in the particular patient with his/her comorbidities on the other hand. As a general guide in choosing the stressor, exercise is preferred in case a patient is able to exercise, except if there are already significant wall motion abnormalities at rest (dobutamine preferred) or LBBB (a vasodilator such as dipyridamole preferred).

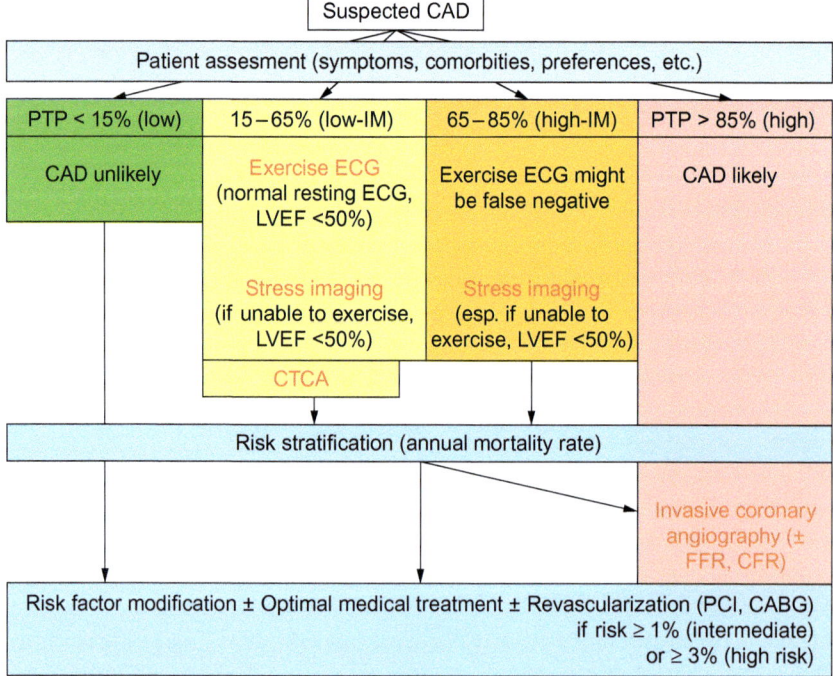

Figure 9.13 Diagnostic strategy according to PTP.

In case the patient has a *low-intermediate PTP between 15% and 50%*, CTCA can be used to rule out significant disease. This can be of particular interest in women, where exercise ECG has less diagnostic accuracy compared with men, which is in part related to impaired exercise capacity, but also to ST-segment abnormalities due to hormonal changes, and lower QRS voltage. With current CT technologies for reducing radiation dose, CTCA can be routinely acquired using 1 mSv or less of radiation.

In patients able to exercise, with a *low-intermediate PTP of 15–65%* and a normal resting ECG and LVEF ≥ 50%, *exercise ECG* is a good option, but even in these patients stress imaging is preferred if available. In case the LVEF is <50%, *exercise stress imaging* is preferred and exercise ECG is only considered when stress imaging is not available. In patients able to exercise, with a *high-intermediate PTP of 65–85%*, *exercise stress imaging* is preferred. In patients who cannot exercise, *pharmacological stress imaging* is preferred if PTP is between 15% and 85% (cf. Figure 9.13).

If the diagnostic test is negative, turning the intermediate PTP into a low post-test probability of CAD, further strategy is as for patients with a *low likelihood of CAD*: other causes for symptoms should be explored, including functional coronary disease, and the risk profile of the patient should be established, as mentioned before, to decide on primary preventive measures. Optimal medical treatment can be considered in case functional coronary disease is likely.

If the diagnostic test is positive, the diagnosis of CAD is established and further strategy is as for patients with a *high likelihood of CAD* from the start: patient factors and risk stratification will determine the opportunity of the patient being revascularized. If the patient does not want any invasive investigation or treatment, risk factor modification and optimal medical treatment will be offered. If the patient's comorbidities allow for invasive strategy and revascularization, and if the patient agrees to this strategy if appropriate, then ICA can be performed provided that risk stratification is not low (annual mortality rate < 1%; cf. Figure 9.14).

If the diagnostic test is unclear, the choice between a second noninvasive test or ICA is to be made. In case a CTCA was indecisive, f.i. because of technical problems or in patients with heavy calcifications (Agatston score > 400), one should proceed to stress imaging, because the information obtained will also serve risk stratification. In case a stress imaging modality was indecisive, depending on the patient and the circumstances, a second stress imaging modality or a CTCA or ICA can be performed.

9.3.2 Stress ECG

As mentioned before, ischemia gradually occurs in a predictable temporal sequence, with the development of ST–T changes rather late in the ischemic cascade. This explains why ECG signs are less sensitive in detecting ischemia (cf. Figures 9.8 and 9.15). *Exercise ECG* is a completely noninvasive, broadly available, low-cost, well-established and time-honored technique, and despite its inferior performance as compared with modern stress imaging techniques, it is still indicated for a low-intermediate PTP of 15–65% in patients with a normal resting ECG; however, the guidelines do underline the superiority of noninvasive stress imaging when local expertise and availability permits their use (cf. Figure 9.13). One must, on the other hand, acknowledge that there are no prospective, randomized data demonstrating that this superior diagnostic performance translates into superior outcomes [14,16].

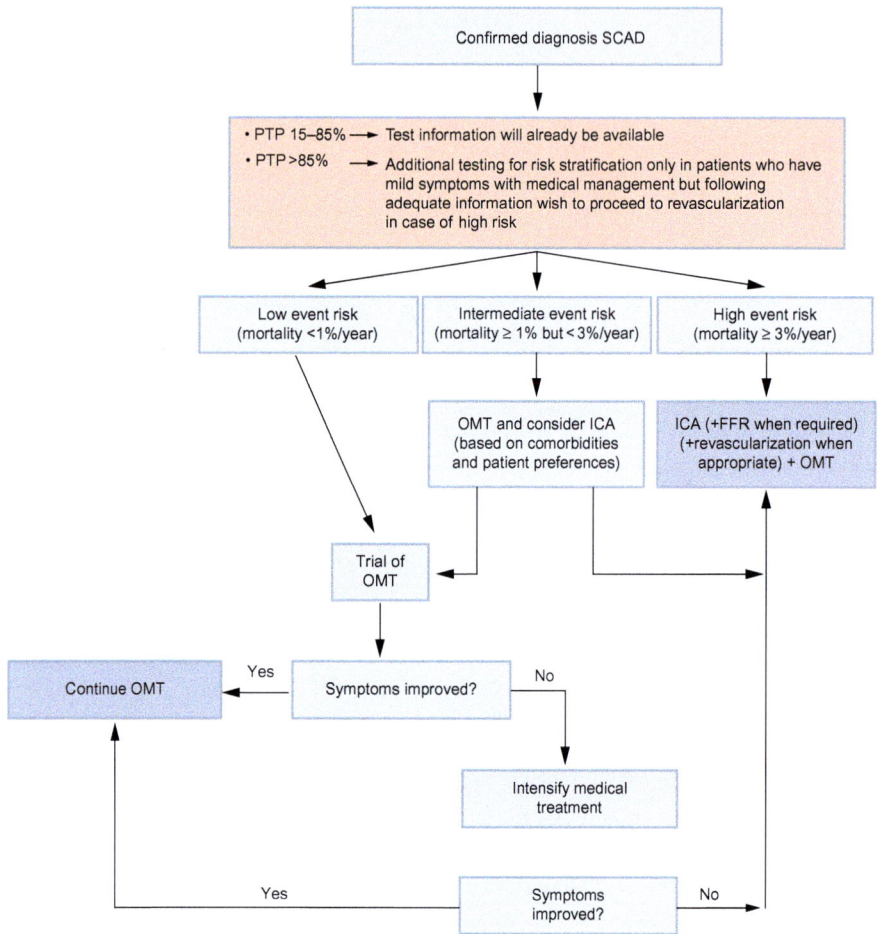

Figure 9.14 Management based on risk determination for prognosis in patients with chest pain and suspected SCAD.
From Ref. [14].

9.3.3 Noninvasive imaging modalities

9.3.3.1 Metabolism

In the ischemic cascade, insufficient myocardial perfusion results in abnormal myocardial metabolism quite early. Therefore, imaging modalities detecting abnormalities in myocardial metabolism are theoretically expected to have high sensitivity for ischemia.

Cardiac magnetic resonance spectroscopy

On average, the heart cycles 10 tons of blood each day using 100,000 heartbeats, resulting in an enormous ATP requirement of about 6 kg a day. Free fatty acids and glucose contribute to ATP synthesis in a ratio of 3:1 in normal situations. The creatine kinase system (PCr) acts as an important energy buffer, providing the heart with energy when

Test modality	Sensitivity (%)	Specificity (%)
Exercise ECG[a]	45–50	85–90
Exercise stress echocardiography	80–85	80–88
Exercise stress SPECT	73–92	63–87
Dobutamine stress echocardiography	79–83	82–86
Dobutamine stress MRI[b]	79–88	81–91
Vasodilator stress echocardiography	72–79	92–95
Vasodilator stress SPECT	90–91	75–84
Vasodilator stress MRI[b]	67–94	61–85
CT coronary angiography	95–99	64–83
Vasodilator stress PET	81–97	74–91

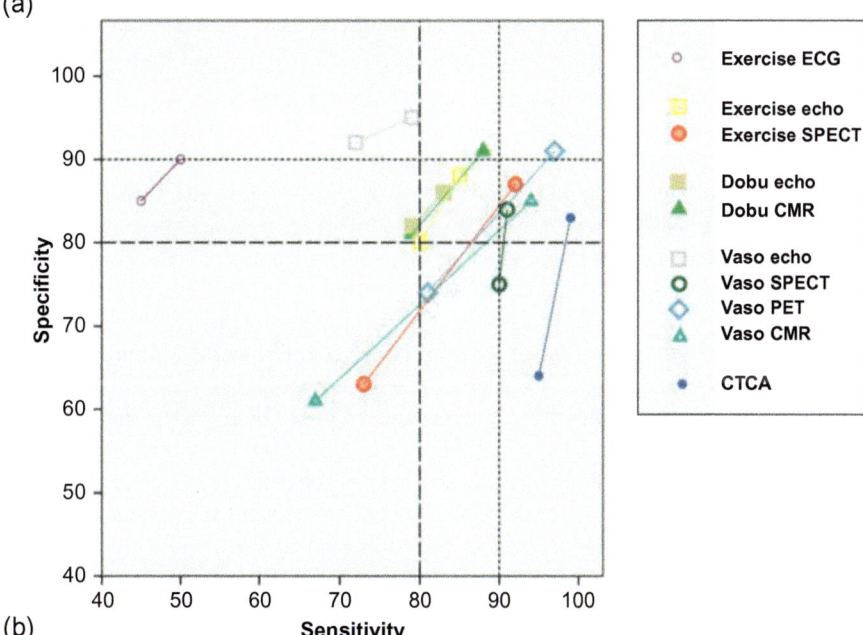

Figure 9.15 (a and b) Sensitivity and specificity of tests commonly used to diagnose the presence of obstructive SCAD. (a) [a]Results without/with minimal referral bias. [b]Results obtained in populations with medium-to-high prevalence of disease without compensation for referral bias. [c]Results obtained in populations with low-to-medium prevalence of disease. The range is mostly determined by local expertise and patient characteristics. (b) Striped and dotted bars indicate sensitivity and specificity of both respectively 80% and 90%. Diagnostic test situated above the dotted line are considered very specific, and diagnostic tests situated at the right side of the dotted line are considered very sensitive. Adapted from Ref. [14].

the demand outweighs the supply. Such a situation results in a decreased PCr concentration and increased ADP concentration, whereas ATP concentrations are held constant.

MRS is able to measure PCr and ATP-peaks. The PCr peak and a combination of the three peaks of ATP are used to calculate the PCr/ATP ratio. This ratio is the most commonly used parameter in 31P-MRS of the heart. In ischemia, ATP synthesis cannot meet the ATP requirement, resulting in a decrease in the PCr/ATP ratio.

MRS of the heart has been performed using 1.5 and 3.0 T magnetic resonance (MR) systems, and recently even using ultra-high 7 T MR systems.

A major drawback of the application of cardiac magnetic resonance spectroscopy (CMRS) in general, although significant in IHD, is the low spatial resolution. Since IHD does not involve the whole myocardium, information on localization of the ischemic or infarcted area is hard to establish with the current techniques. Overcoming these issues with, for example, higher field imaging or hyperpolarization could pave the way for CMRS to be of diagnostic relevance, most notably in patients with suspected IHD without coronary artery stenosis on ICA. Moreover, CMRS could be of use in patients to discriminate between viable and non-viable myocardium [17]. Presently, however, CMRS is a research tool with no established clinical indications.

Positron emission tomography, single-photon emission computed tomography

Ischemia may cause reduction of fatty acid utilization and shift from fatty acid to glucose utilization. Such metabolic shift may persist shortly after recovery of ischemia. Glucose metabolism is most easily imaged using 2-fluorodeoxyglucose (FDG) labeled with fluorine-18 (^{18}F). Free fatty acids (e.g., palmitic acid), but also acetate have been labeled with carbon-11 (^{11}C), limiting their use in clinical practice. Acetate has been proposed as a tracer of oxidative metabolism because its early rapid clearance from the myocardium is related to oxygen consumption. PET imaging combining perfusion with myocardial metabolism using ^{18}F-fluorodeoxyglucose (^{18}F FDG) is an accurate standard for assessment of myocardial hibernation and risk stratification of patients with left ventricular dysfunction of ischemic etiology.

15-(p-Iodophenyl)-3R,S-methyl pentadecanoic acid (BMIPP) is an iodinated branch-chain fatty acid used by single-photon emission computer tomography (SPECT), showing BMIPP uptake in ischemic myocardium. Ischemia shifts the source of myocardial energy from aerobic metabolism driven by fatty acid oxidation to anaerobic metabolism, where glucose utilization through anaerobic glycolysis becomes pivotal for energy production. These metabolic changes are imprinted onto ischemic myocardium for up to 30 h after the ischemic episode and can be visualized by reduced BMIPP uptake, a phenomenon termed "ischemic memory." According to a review of mostly retrospective studies, an abnormal finding on BMIPP imaging is significantly associated with future cardiovascular outcomes across the spectrum of CAD, with BMIPP imaging with the patient at rest being particularly useful for the risk stratification of patients with acute chest pain [18].

Nitrate-enhanced Tc-sestamibi and thallium redistribution imaging are widely used for viability assessment, but metabolic imaging techniques are rarely used to detect myocardial ischemia in clinical practice.

9.3.3.2 Anatomy

Computed tomography coronary angiography-derived ischemic parameters

Computed tomography coronary angiography (CTCA) is by nature an anatomical test with accurate information of the presence and severity of coronary atherosclerotic lesions.

State of the art technology requires at least 64-slice CT [19]. The technique has high sensitivity and negative predictive value for the detection of angiographic CAD (cf. Figure 9.15) [20]. The assessment of coronary artery bypass grafts is highly accurate, but the evaluation of the native coronary vessels in post-bypass patients is difficult and prone to false positive findings [21,22]. The technique is also less reliable in patients with stents [23]. CTCA allows for quantification of atherosclerotic plaque burden and obstructive CAD, particularly in the proximal segments. It therefore carries an incremental prognostic value beyond clinical risk factors [24]. For a more detailed description on the role of CTCA the reader is referred to Chapters 5 and 7 of this textbook.

Functional information on hemodynamic severity of coronary lesions currently escapes standard CTCA, unless adjunctive novel techniques such as $CTCA_{FFR}$ or CT perfusion (CTP) are employed. In CT-FFR software creates a 3D model of the coronary tree from ordinary CTCA examinations with no modification to imaging protocols, no additional image acquisition, and no additional radiation (see Chapter 5) [25]. Maps of coronary blood flow are created computationally, based on principles of myocardial mass and resting coronary flow applied to the measurement of vessel size at CT, in order to demonstrate the flow impact of a stenosis (Figure 9.16). Current CT-FFR applications require transfer of data to an off-site laboratory, several hours of processing on a supercomputer, and a turn-around time of approximately 24 h. CT-FFR was compared against the gold standard invasive FFR in 252 patients in the DeFACTO trial, showing a significant improvement in accuracy, specificity, and positive predictive value, with no sacrifice in sensitivity and negative predictive value compared to

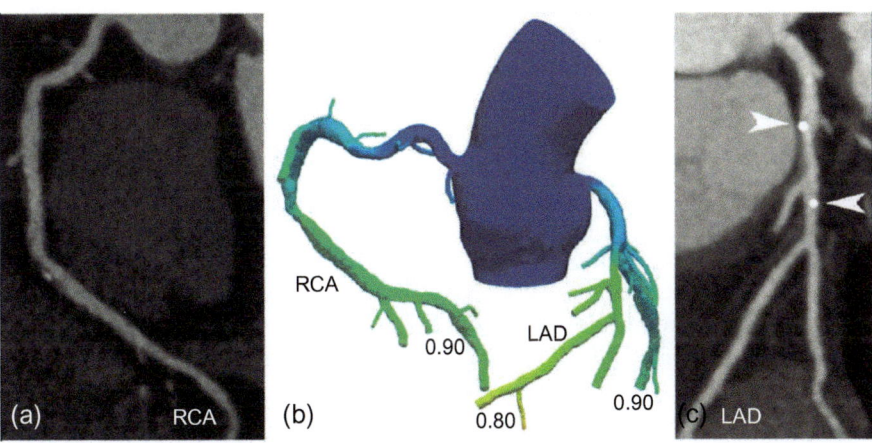

Figure 9.16 CT angiography shows a moderate, partially calcified stenosis in the distal RCA (a). The left coronary artery has been treated previously with a bioresorbable scaffold (c). After 18 months only, the platinum indicators remain visible (arrow heads). CTCA derived fractional flow reserve was performed, and simulated FFR values are displayed by color along the coronary arteries (b). Despite moderate, non-calcified restenosis of the LAD there is no significant pressure drop. Only at the distal LAD the FFR reaches the threshold of 0.80. The lesion in the right coronary does not result in a significant FFR drop.
Figure courtesy of Koen Nieman Erasmus Medical Center, Rotterdam, The Netherlands.

CTCA [25]. The findings suggest that CT-FFR could potentially eliminate the need for risky and costly invasive evaluation and treatment in some patients, especially those at intermediate risk of heart disease, leading to better clinical outcomes and lower costs. Nonetheless, the DeFACTO trial failed to reach the primary efficacy endpoint defined as a diagnostic accuracy significantly above 70% compared to invasive FFR. Recently, a second updated CT-FFR software version with improved image segmentation and refined physiological models has been released and validated in the HeartFlow-NXT trial [26]. Adding CT-FFR to CTCA alone increased particularly the specificity (from 34% to 79%) and positive predictive value (40–65%) for diagnosing flow-limiting coronary lesions.

Transluminal attenuation gradients (TAG) have recently raised some attention as an adjunctive tool to estimate hemodynamic severity of coronary stenoses from standard CTCA images. This approach allows estimating functional significance based on the rate by which intraluminal contrast attenuation decreases along a coronary vessel downstream from a given stenosis (see Chapter 5). First small reports suggest a reasonably good correlation of TAG with invasive FFR measurements and with the presence of ischemia on CTP [27,28]. However, this technique is still at an early phase of clinical validation.

Finally, CT-based dynamic myocardial function, perfusion, and late phase myocardial enhancement imaging is feasible and discussed later in this chapter (see also Chapters 5 and 10) [29–31].

9.3.3.3 Perfusion and function

While metabolism during stress could be obtained by nuclear techniques and CMRS, neither is clinically used during stress to that end, leaving perfusion and function as the main diagnostic parameters to detect ischemia.

Perfusion, being earlier in the ischemic cascade (Figure 9.8), is more sensitive than function, so that smaller areas of ischemia can be picked up by perfusion imaging than by functional imaging. Conversely, *functional imaging*, reflecting a larger area of ischemia, is more specific and carries a worse prognosis.

Perfusion and perfusion defects can be detected preferably using a vasodilating stressor by nuclear techniques, such as SPECT and PET, by contrast ECHO, by stress perfusion magnetic resonance (CMR), or stress CTP. Wall motion abnormalities can preferably be induced by exercise or dobutamine (dipyridamole is less sensitive) and detected by ECHO and CMR. The respective sensitivities and specificities are given in Figure 9.15.

SPECT

SPECT is one of the oldest and best-established techniques for the assessment of myocardial perfusion. Most frequently used tracers for regional perfusion are thallium-201, 99mTc-sestamibi, or 99mTc-tetrofosmin (see Chapter 3). SPECT employs induction of flow heterogeneities by a physical or pharmacological stressor to unmask areas of ischemic myocardium compared to normal remote territories. Perfusion defects may be fixed (identical perfusion defect at rest and stress images) or reversible (perfusion defect on stress images normalizes on rest images) representing myocardial scar or ischemia, respectively (Figure 9.17). An important advantage of SPECT over cross-sectional imaging techniques (CMR, CTP) is that full 3D coverage of the left ventricle is obtained without gaps between slices and including the apex (more recently, full 3D perfusion coverage has also been developed in CMR, cf. infra). Commercially available software packages allow semiquantitative assessment of myocardial perfusion using summed perfusion scores, % extent of perfusion defect, or total perfusion deficit. A large body of evidence has established a high accuracy of myocardial perfusion SPECT to detect CAD with an average sensitivity of 87–89% and an average specificity of 73–75% [14].

However, SPECT is susceptible to artifacts from nonuniform photon attenuation and scattering, which explains the lower specificity. This can be improved by adding attenuation correction methods (X-ray based or transmission scans) and gated SPECT (see Chapter 3). Gated SPECT allows an assessment of regional wall motion abnormalities, left ventricular volumes, and ejection fraction and helps to discriminate between attenuation artifacts and true areas of myocardial scar. In SPECT, evaluation of function is inferior to perfusion analysis, but post-ischemic stunning may be detectable in severely ischemic areas, if ECG-gating is performed for stress images, while fixed perfusion

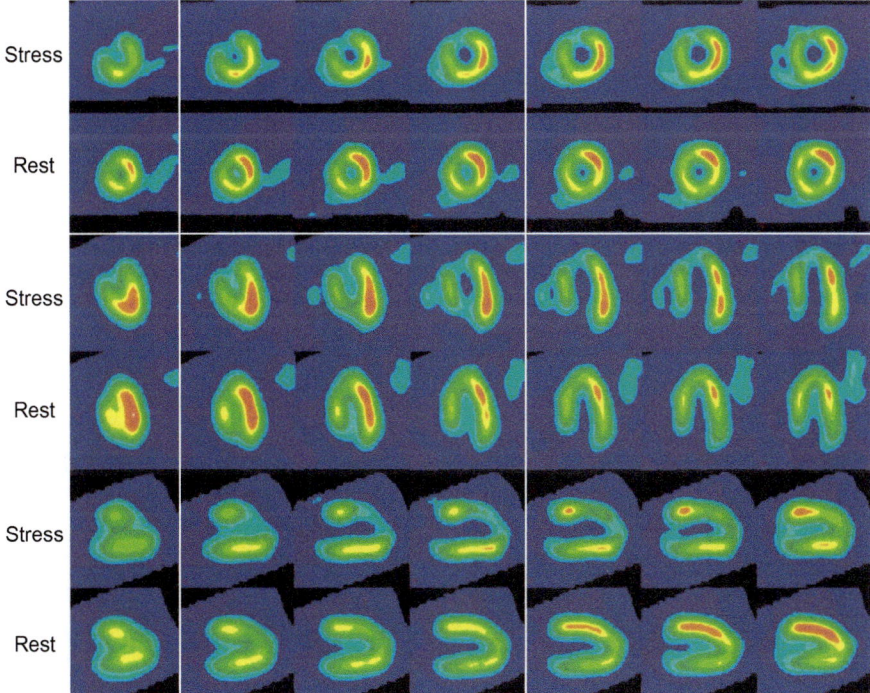

Figure 9.17 SPECT-image of ischemia. Stress-images show reduced perfusion in the anterior wall and the apex.
With courtesy of Olivier Gheysens, MD, PhD, University Hospital Leuven, Belgium.

defects are usually associated with regional wall motion abnormalities on gated rest images. Additional high-risk criteria on SPECT include transient ischemic dilation, increased lung uptake, reduced post-stress ejection fraction, and abnormal right ventricular myocardial uptake. The drawbacks of SPECT include a high-radiation dose (ranging from 10 mSv with 99mTc-labeled tracers to 25 mSv with Thallium), limiting its use for serial follow-up, especially in young women. Additionally, obese subjects are susceptible to more photon attenuation artifacts and noninterpretable scans. Furthermore, myocardial perfusion SPECT does not provide absolute myocardial blood flow, but only relative perfusion defects, i.e., ischemic territories compared to remote myocardium. Due to this intrinsic limitation, SPECT may underestimate the extent of disease in multivessel disease with globally reduced myocardial perfusion. On the other hand, impaired renal function is never, and claustrophobia rarely, a contraindication for SPECT.

Positron emission tomography

PET perfusion imaging has several advantages over SPECT: a higher spatial resolution (4–7 mm with PET compared to 8–10 mm with SPECT), more robust methods of attenuation correction and lower radiation exposure. Although direct head-to-head comparisons between SPECT and PET are scarce, these theoretical advantages of PET seem to translate into an increased diagnostic accuracy particularly with a higher sensitivity [32] (Figure 9.18). Moreover, PET is the gold standard for quantifying myocardial perfusion in absolute terms (ml/min/g) both at rest and stress, allowing for calculation of myocardial perfusion reserve (as a noninvasive alternative for CFR). Quantification may increase the diagnostic accuracy by enhancing substantially the sensitivity without loss of specificity, and in addition improves detection of multivessel disease [33]. The most common tracers of myocardial perfusion are Rubidium-82 (82Rb), Nitrogen-13 ammonia (^{13}N-ammonia), and Oxygen-15 labeled water (^{15}O-water; see Chapter 4). The majority of perfusion tracers (except for ^{82}Rb) have short physical half-lives, which require an onsite cyclotron for immediate production and administration. This limitation may be overcome by the recent introduction of a novel ^{18}F-labeled myocardial perfusion imaging (^{18}F-labeled Flurpiridaz) with promising features for perfusion imaging with PET [34]. The main drawback of PET is related to limited availability and expertise and higher costs of this technique.

Stress echocardiography

Stress echocardiography (SE) is a widely accepted method for the diagnostic and prognostic assessment of IHD. SE is the combination of 2D/3D ECHO with an exercise or pharmacological (or electrical) stress [35]. The diagnostic endpoint for the detection of myocardial ischemia is the induction of a transient worsening in regional function during stress. Extensive ischemia at a low-stress level identifies high-risk patients for which an ICA is reasonable. The accuracy of SE for detection of significant coronary stenosis ranges from 80% to 90%, exceeding that of the exercise ECG (especially in women and patients with LV hypertrophy), and being comparable to that of stress myocardial perfusion scintigraphy. The interpretation of the test can be limited by the quality of 2D images (endocardial definition), the failure to reach the target heart rate, and the difficulties to identify subtle changes in regional function in patients with extensive myocardial dyssynergy.

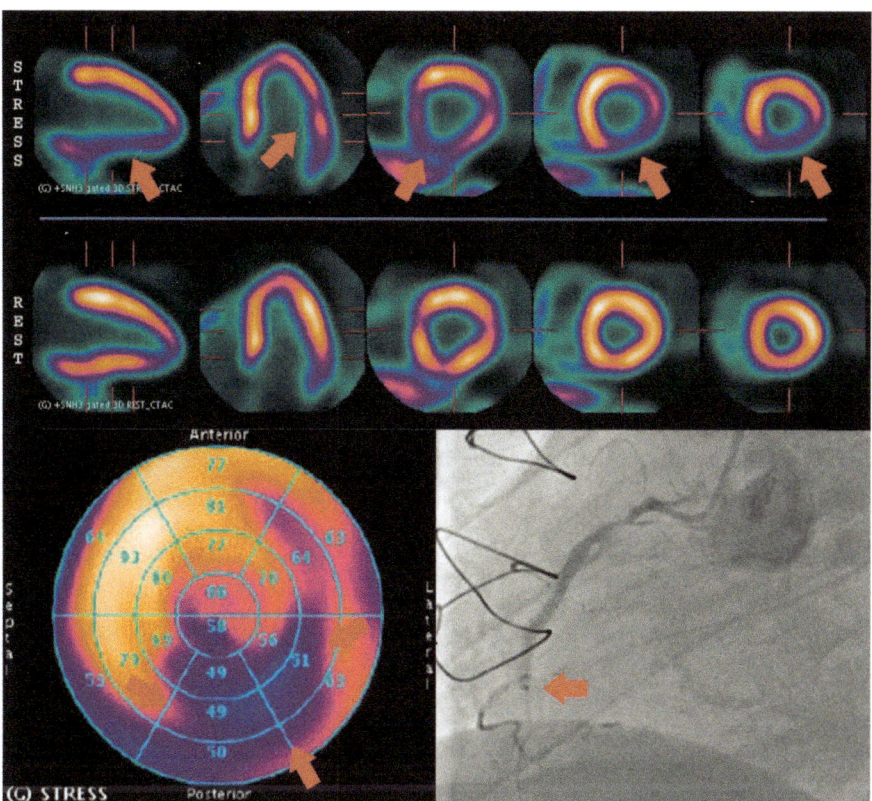

Figure 9.18 PET-image of ischemia. Myocardial perfusion PET study at stress (upper row) and rest (lower row) using $^{13}N-NH_3$ shows a large reversible inferior and inferolateral perfusion defect (ischemia) (red arrows). The stress perfusion polar map (left lower corner) helps to determine location and extent of ischemia (red arrows). On invasive angiography, the culprit lesion was an occluded right coronary artery (RCA). The saphenous vein graft on the RCA was also occluded (not shown).
Courtesy of Olivier Clerc and Philipp A Kaufmann, University Hospital Zurich, Switzerland.

Conventional echocardiographic assessment of regional myocardial function is based on the measurement of wall thickening and does not provide information regarding the transmural distribution of contractile performance. However, Doppler-based tissue velocity measurements, frequently referred to as tissue Doppler or myocardial Doppler, and speckle tracking on the basis of displacement measurements, can overcome this limitation. These techniques show a reduced or missing regional systolic longitudinal and circumferential shortening and radial thickening in ischemic myocardium [36]. Postsystolic shortening (evaluating longitudinal strain) after aortic valve closure is a common finding in acute ischemia [37] (Figure 9.19). 3D Speckle tracking ECHO can measure all three spatial components of the myocardial displacement vector to allow for accurate assessment of regional ventricular dynamics. Nevertheless, it still requires rigorous validation and testing [36].

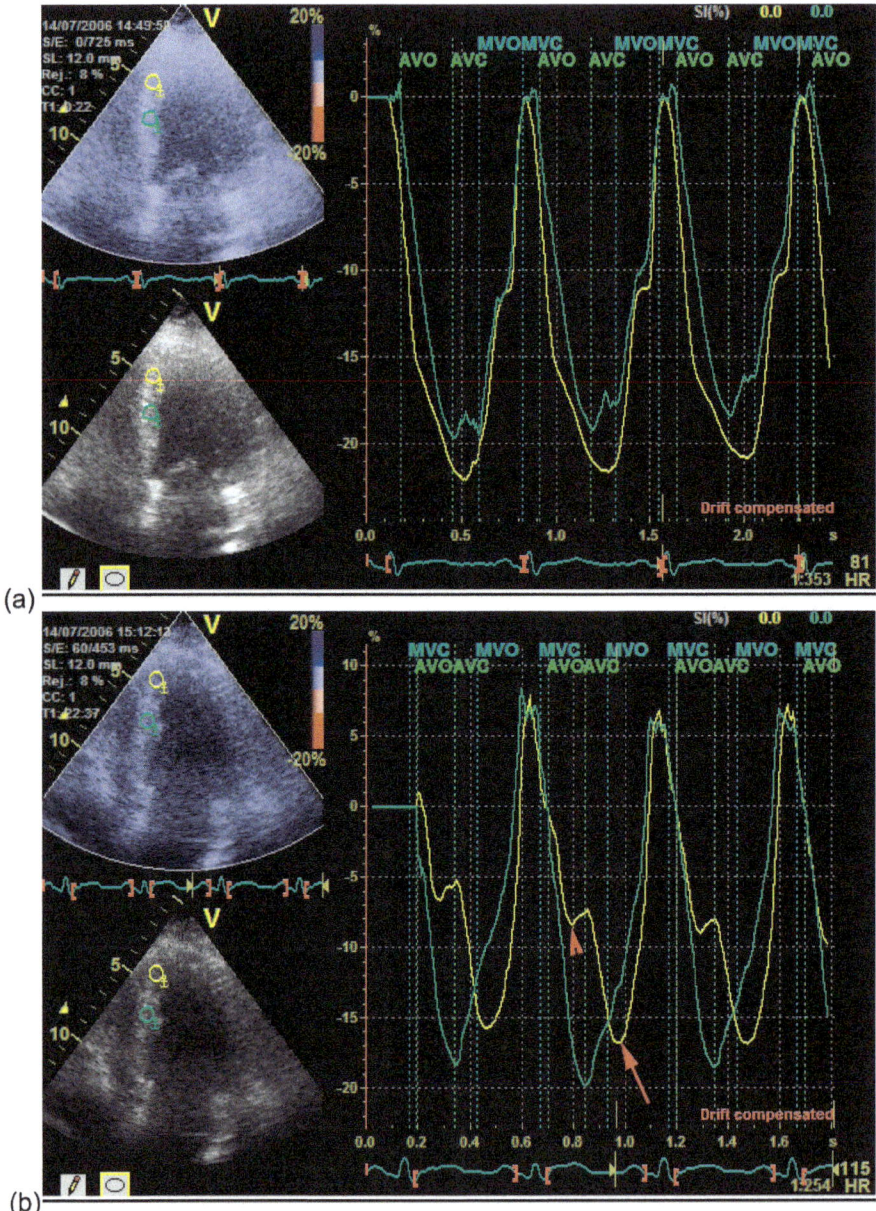

Figure 9.19 SE doppler-based tissue velocity measurements at rest (a) and during stress (b) show a reduced systolic longitudinal shortening in the systolic phase (arrowhead), and postsystolic shortening (arrow) after aortic valve closure in ischemia provoked by dobutamine stress.
With courtesy of Jens-Uwe Voigt, MD, PhD, University Hospital Leuven, Belgium.

In patients with limited echogenicity, the use of LV contrast opacification (microbubbles, i.e., Sonovue®) improves the diagnostic accuracy of the test [38,39] (see Chapter 2). Of note, contrast SE can be performed with 3D-acquisition techniques [40,41]. To some extent, when used with contrast administration, SE also gives the opportunity to assess function and perfusion simultaneously, both during rest and stress [42]. It can determine perfusion for visual analysis, but also semiquantitative and absolute quantification of myocardial perfusion are possible, allowing for calculation of myocardial perfusion reserve (see Chapter 2). However, myocardial contrast perfusion ECHO is not clinically penetrated yet; universal reimbursement for contrast agents for this purpose would be a significant step forward [43]. Measuring CFR with ECHO is possible by measuring Doppler velocity in the proximal LAD at rest and during e.g., dipyridamole or adenosine stress. This technique is limited to the LAD though and performed in only few centers (see Chapter 2) [44].

Stress CMR

CMR can determine both perfusion and function during rest and stress by successive sequences; however, in clinical practice, usually only one stressor is used, favoring one of both techniques, with the choice depending on the clinical question and the patient's cofactors [45]. Stress perfusion images are generally acquired during simultaneous infusion of a vasodilator agent, whereas inotropic (and physical) stress can be used for the imaging of wall motion abnormalities (see also Chapter 6). Stress CMR has high spatial resolution and high accuracy in detecting ischemia (cf. Figures 9.20 and 9.21) [32]. It offers important incremental information over clinical risk factors and resting wall motion abnormalities [46]. Dobutamine stress CMR with assessment of inducible wall motion abnormalities follows the same principles as SE. Diagnostic performance is similar in patients with good image quality and far better with CMR in patients with bad echogenicity [47]. Clinically dobutamine stress CMR is less frequently used than perfusion CMR, but it has the advantage that no gadolinium contrast is needed (f.i. in case of nephrogenic fibrosis). On the other hand, contrast can be administered at peak dobutamine stress for perfusion evaluation as well.

Myocardial perfusion CMR tracks the myocardial contrast passage of an intravenously injected bolus of gadolinium-based contrast agent. Temporal changes in signal intensities are measured and fitted to signal-intensity curves and allow myocardial blood flow (see Chapter 6) to be quantified. Visual, semiquantitative and quantitative perfusion analysis is possible, but in clinical practice only visual evaluation of perfusion defects has penetrated.

Visual CMR perfusion analysis requires high expertise, as can be appreciated by the large differences in perfusion CMR accuracy between single and multicentre studies [48,49]. In a head-to-head comparison of CMR and SPECT, the large single-center CE-MARC study found higher overall diagnostic performance of CMR for the diagnosis of CAD defined by QCA [48]. The sensitivity, negative predictive values and receiver operator characteristics were also significantly higher for CMR stress perfusion compared to SPECT. MR-IMPACT II was the first large multicenter trial comparing CMR and SPECT for the detection of myocardial ischemia [49]. In this study, the sensitivity of myocardial perfusion CMR was superior, but the specificity inferior to SPECT for the detection

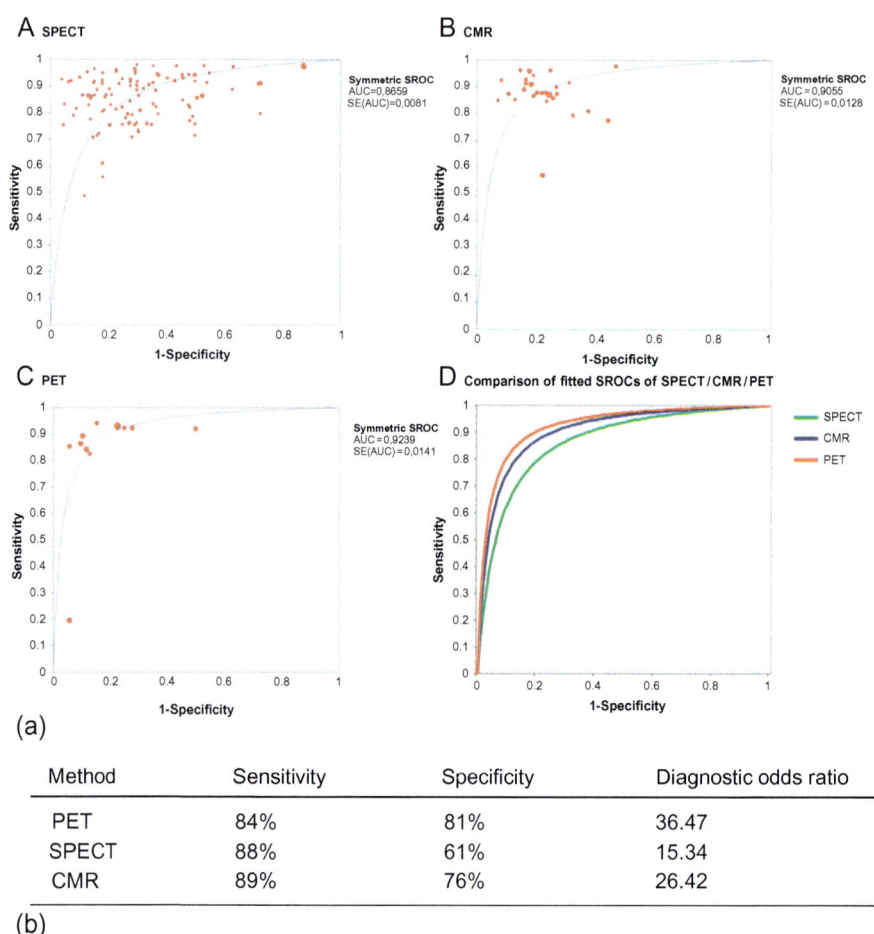

Figure 9.20 (a) SPECT, CMR, and PET for Detecting CAD. Diagnostic performance of (A) SPECT, (B) CMR, and (C) PET for the detection of CAD on a patient-based level: graphic display of diagnostic accuracy with summary receiver-operating characteristics (SROC) curves. Each dot represents a single study, with the size of the dot directly proportional to the sample size of the study. The area under the curve (AUC) reflects the overall diagnostic performance and is expressed as a value between 0 and 1, with higher values indicating better test performance. The AUC was 0.8659, 0.9055, and 0.9239 for SPECT, CMR, and PET, respectively. (D) Fitted SROC curves for direct comparison of the diagnostic performance of SPECT (green line), CMR (blue line), and PET (red line). (b) Mean sensitivity–specificity values and diagnostic odds ratio for PET compared with SPECT and CMR for the diagnosis of myocardial ischemia.
From Ref. [32].

of CAD on QCA. Myocardial perfusion CMR has also been compared with invasive measurements of ischemia with a sensitivity of 89.1% and specificity of 84.9% reported against FFR in a meta-analysis of seven studies [50]. Novel full-volume 3D perfusion sequences (kt sense) for CMR allows full volumetric coverage of the left ventricle during first-pass perfusion imaging to be obtained, with a sensitivity, specificity, and diagnostic accuracy of 90%, 82%, and 87%, respectively, and high inter-study reproducibility [51].

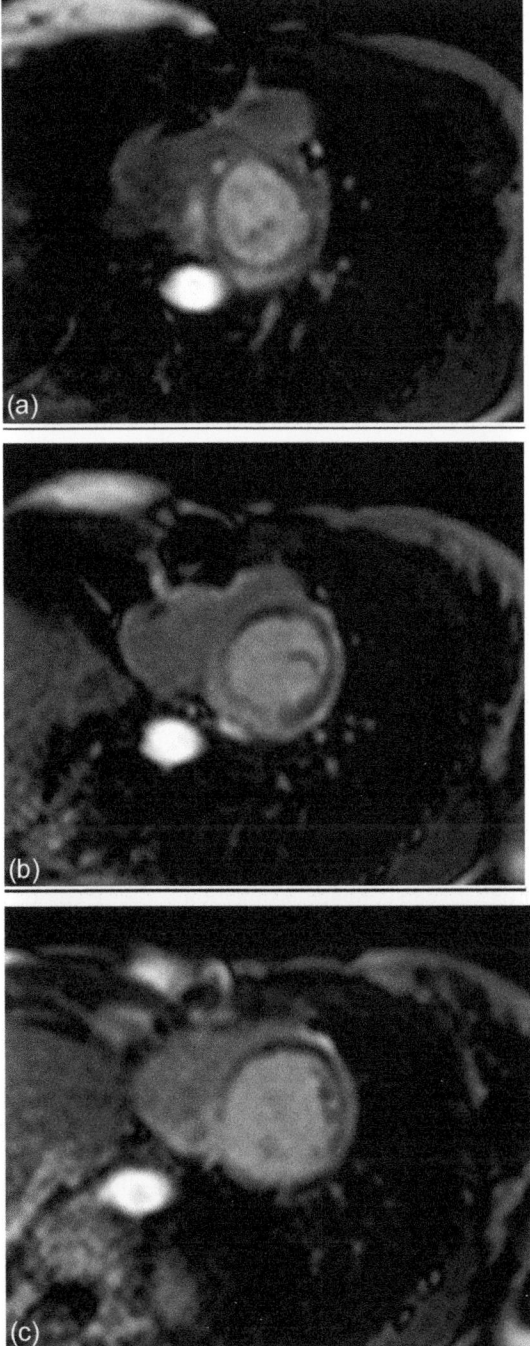

Figure 9.21 Stress CMR with dipyridamole. (a–c) Three slices from left ventricular basis toward the apex. An extensive perfusion defect can be appreciated in the basal slices (a and b) from anteroseptal over anterior to the lateral wall, and in the midventricular slice (c) in the septal and anterior wall.
Goetschalckx K, Bogaert J, University Hospital Leuven, Belgium.

Quantitative analysis of CMR myocardial perfusion reserve has been compared in 1.5 and 3 T CMR in a small study, showing a superior diagnostic accuracy at 3 T, with higher sensitivity (90.5% vs. 61.9%) and specificity (100% vs. 76.9%) [52].

A novel method for semiautomated quantitative analysis of transmural perfusion gradients (TPG) has shown good reproducibility and good correlation with ICA. The TPG diagnostic threshold of 20% was as accurate as visual assessment by experts, but was validated against FFR in one small patient group only [53].

CT perfusion

CT-based dynamic myocardial function and perfusion imaging is feasible, but at this time is still limited by artifacts (partial volume, motion, breathing artifacts) and high-radiation dose. Myocardial ischemia can be assessed with CT based on the first pass of iodinated contrast agents through the myocardium during maximal hyperemia with a vasodilating agent (CTP). Static CTP is performed by obtaining perfusion images at a single time-point during myocardial contrast passage (Figure 9.22). For dynamic CTP, image acquisition is repeated at predefined intervals to cover the entire passage of contrast through the right ventricle, the left ventricle, and the myocardium. Temporal changes in contrast enhancement are measured by time-attenuation curves and allow myocardial blood flow to be quantified [30,31] (see Chapter 5). Only small single-center trials have validated CTP against more established perfusion imaging techniques such as SPECT, PET, and CMR and against invasive angiography with FFR [54]. A recent multicentric head-to-head comparison of CTP and SPECT (with blinded core lab image analysis) showed a superior diagnostic accuracy of CTP (driven by a significantly higher sensitivity) for detecting angiographically significant CAD [55]. However, specificity was higher for SPECT, indicating that CTP may still be subject to artifacts. CTP should always be performed on a CT scanner with single-beat acquisition capabilities. Even so, image acquisition for CTP can be challenging as it requires careful timing to obtain optimal myocardial contrast, and image quality may be further affected by beam-hardening artifacts. Radiation dose may vary from 2 to 12 mSv depending on the protocol used [56].

Hybrid cardiac SPECT/CT, PET/CT, PET/MR, and stress CMR/CTCA imaging

Combining imaging modalities for simultaneous dual scanning is called a "hybrid" technique (see Chapter 3). "Anatomical" CAD-imaging is combined with "functional" ischemia-imaging modalities as in SPECT/CT and PET/CT. In cardiac imaging, the hybrid scanners are not used routinely because of the difficulty in predicting a priori which patients would benefit from the dual scanning. A sequential diagnostic approach is often applied in clinical practice, with additional scans (CTCA or SPECT) performed only if the results of the initial modality are equivocal. However, when CTCA is performed first in a patient population with high-intermediate pretest probability, a lot of patients will need perfusion imaging. The integrated use of SPECT or PET and CTCA by co-registration and fusion of acquired images, either stand-alone or combined, offers incremental diagnostic value beyond that of either device alone and that of side-by-side analysis in patients at intermediate risk for CAD. Integration of dual imaging appears to improve both the identification of the culprit vessel and the diagnostic confidence for categorizing intermediate lesions and equivocal perfusion

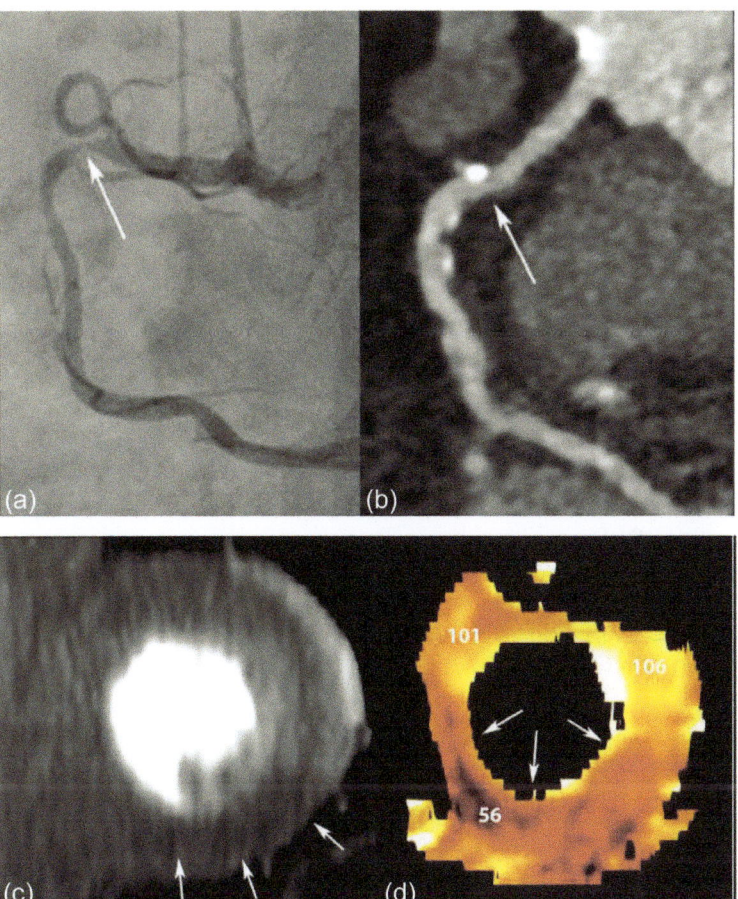

Figure 9.22 Patient with severe stenosis (arrow) of the proximal right coronary artery on invasive angiography (a). CT angiography is affected by motion artifacts but shows diffuse atherosclerotic disease (b). Using adenosine for vasodilation, a dynamic perfusion CT is performed. The raw images (at a single instant) show lower myocardial attenuation (c). From the sequence of images acquired during contrast passage the myocardial blood flow can be calculated and is expressed in ml/100cc/min. Although the anterior wall is inclompletely interpretable, the MBF map shows that myocardial blood flow in the inferior wall is only 56 ml/100 ml/min, compared to more than 100 ml/100 ml/min in the anterior septum and lateral wall (d).
Figure courtesy of Koen Nieman, Erasmus Medical Center, Rotterdam, The Netherlands.

defects, and provides added diagnostic information in almost one-third of patients as compared to side-by-side analysis, thus optimizing management decisions [57].

One of the obvious limitations of hybrid imaging is related to patient radiation dose.

It is anticipated that the ongoing prospective multicenter trials such as SPARC and EVINCI will bring important information about the prognostic value and post-test resource utilization of SPECT, PET, and CTCA in current clinical practice [58,59]. This is of utmost importance, since a recent trial has shown that imaging leads to imaging, but does not necessarily improve outcome [60].

More recently, also PET/MR has been developed. The main differences of PET/MR compared with PET/CT are the reduction of radiation dose, the improvement of soft tissue resolution, but limited means of imaging the coronaries, and extended examination times. Technical obstacles are still to be overcome, but PET/MR appears now to be a very promising modality for improved tissue characterization in the assessment of myocardial viability/hibernation, atherosclerotic plaque imaging, and for assessing novel therapeutic strategies such as cell and gene therapies [61].

Novel full-volume 3D perfusion sequences (kt sense) for CMR allow full volumetric coverage of the left ventricle to be obtained during first-pass perfusion imaging, which can be fused with CTCA information. First case reports of this technique are promising as CMR provides a high spatial resolution (higher in-plane resolution than PET or SPECT) with no added radiation exposure [51].

BOLD-CMR

A non-contrast enhanced CMR technique is blood–oxygen-level-dependent (BOLD) cardiac MR, which images the change in blood flow related to energy use by myocardial cells. BOLD uses the change in magnetization between oxygen-rich and oxygen-poor blood as its basic measure for tissue oxygenation. This measure is frequently corrupted by noise from various sources; hence, statistical procedures are used to extract the underlying signal. This technical drawback has limited the clinical interest for BOLD-CMR, with only few studies in small numbers of patients [62].

9.3.3.4 Stressor

Besides the choice of parameter (perfusion, function) and modality (ECHO, SPECT, PET, CMR), also the type of stress has an impact (cf. Figures 9.23 and 9.24). *Exercise*

Dipyridamole	**Adenosine**	**Dobutamine**

Hypotension
 	
Bradycardia
 	
Major complications 0,07%
  Short asystoly
  Acute myocardial infarction
  Acute pulmonary edema
  Sustained VT
 	
Total: 1,2%
	In 9256 patients:
	
	Minor side effects 81%
	  Flushing, feeling warm
	  Headache
	  Angina
	  Dizziness
	  Dyspnea
	  Abdominal discomfort
	
	Bronchospasm 0.07%
	
	AV-Block I 2.9%
	AV-Block II 2.6%
	AV-Block III 0.8%
	
	Hypotension 7%
	
	Hyperventilation 14%
		In 1000 patients (incl. positive tests):
		
		Sustained VT 1 (0.1%)
		Non-sustained VT 4 (0.4%)
		Parox AF 16 (1.6%)
		Transient AV block II 2:1 2(0.2%)
		Severe increase in BP >240/120
		                                 5 (0.5%)
		
		Decrease in syst BP >40 mmHg
		                                 5 (0.5%)
		
		Nausea 31 (3.1%)
		
		Total 64 (6.4%)

Contra-indications DIP/AD: - Intrinsic asthma, severe CoPD - 2nd/3th degree AV block - Hypotension (BPs < 90 mmHg)	- Carbamazepine - Heart transplant, elderly: DIP safer than AD	**Contra-indications Dobu:** Arrhythmias
Picano et al. [86]	Cerqueira et al. [87]	Wahl et al. [88]

Figure 9.23 Risk and adverse effects of pharmacological stressors used to detect ischemia.

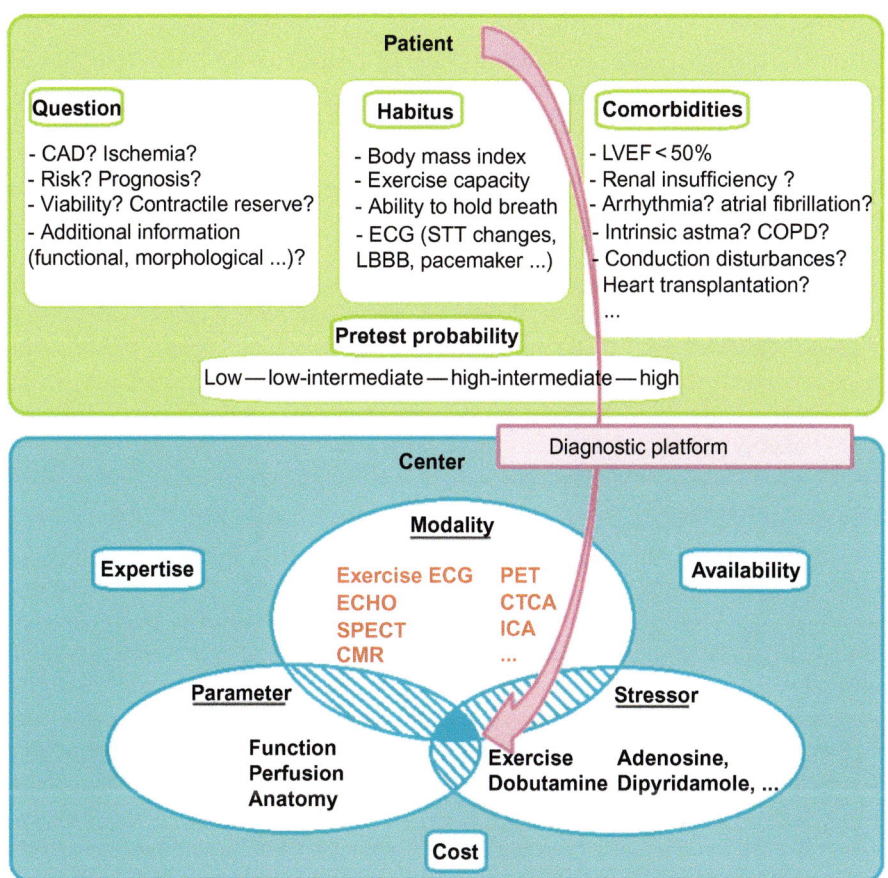

Figure 9.24 Diagnostic platform. This multidisciplinary group of "imagers" of the various modalities decides on the choice and sequence of tests, which will answer the clinical question with the least risk for the patient, the least cost for society, and the best information content to decide on further therapeutic options.

stress is the most physiological stressor and better reflects real live conditions, offering causal information on the patient's symptoms and on the level at which symptoms and/or ischemia sets in. Exercise offers not only further stress of the heart (increase of venous return) but also additional physiological data, such as heart rate and blood pressure, and prognostic information based on overall exercise capacity. This is of particular value in situations where ischemia can hardly be provoked by pharmacological vasodilators, such as in abnormal congenital coronary arteries with interarterial course running between the pulmonary trunc and the aorta or myocardial bridging of a coronary artery.

Pharmacological stress is indicated if the patient is unable to exercise, but it is also more convenient for ECHO, CMR, and PET.

So the value of gaining physiological exercise data should be weighed against improved image quality by reducing movement using pharmacological stress. In case of

LBBB, pacemaker rhythm, or pre-existing resting wall motion abnormalities, pharmacological stress is preferred above exercise. In the case of LBBB and pacemaker rhythm, the likelihood of stress perfusion studies being false positive in the LAD and septal territories is less with vasodilators (adenosine, dipyridamole, regadenoson) than with exercise or dobutamine, which both increase the heart rhythm to a greater extent. Regadenoson is being increasingly used as the preferred pharmacologic stress agent with good clinical results both for visual and for quantitative analysis in nuclear and MR perfusion studies [63,64]. Some concerns are raised about safety (asystole) [65,66], but there is no good evidence that this occurs more often with regadenoson than with other vasodilator agents. Dobutamine is of particular interest in case there are pre-existing wall motion abnormalities, because a biphasic response can be evaluated. At low-dose dobutamine, an improvement in contractility indicates contractile reserve, as in hibernating myocardium, whereas persisting akinesia would indicate lack of viability. At a higher dose, decrease of contractility indicates ischemia.

9.3.3.5 Center

Of course the availability of the different imaging modalities at the local center, as well as the local expertise, cost considerations, and reimbursement will influence decision making. While all modalities and parameters can be shown in small comparative studies, to have some advantage over other combinations, the overall results of sensitivity and specificity in larger studies or in meta-analyses do not allow us at this moment to state with any certainty that one combination of modality and parameter has a significant advantage over another combination. Referral bias is another reason why it seems inappropriate for the moment to prefer one test over another. Local expertise and availability, as well as the specifics of the patients, are more relevant in making the choice, which should preferably be done by a multidisciplinary team (cf. diagnostic platform) (cf. Figure 9.25).

9.3.3.6 Patient

And then there is the patient with his/her preferences, habitus, and comorbidities influencing the choice of the diagnostic modality. Is the patient able to exercise or not; is he/she willing to enter the magnet and to be submitted to contrast or radiation; are there contra-indications to a pharmacological stressor or to the magnet; what is the expected echogenicity of the patient (emphysema, obesity…); what is the size of the patient (will he/she fit in the MR?); does the patient have voluminous breasts (attenuation SPECT), renal insufficiency (risk of nephrogenic systemic fibrosis), or atrial fibrillation (triggering problem MR); can the patient hold his/her breath (CTCA, MR); is the ECG normal (PM, LBBB,…), etc. (cf. Figures 9.24 and 9.25).

In *women*, exercise ECG has less diagnostic accuracy compared with men, which is in part related to impaired exercise capacity but also to ST-segment abnormalities due to hormonal changes and lower QRS voltage. In SPECT, soft tissue attenuation due to voluminous breast tissue or obesity is more often a problem in women than in men. Moreover, women have a smaller heart size and, consequently, potentially smaller myocardial areas with reduced perfusion that may be missed due to the limited spatial

Myocardial ischemia

Diagnostic test	Diagnosis of CAD Sens. (%)	Spec. (%)	Resolution	Function	Perfusion	Viability	Radiation	Availability	Cost	Advantages	Disadvantages
Exercise ECG	45–50	85–90	0	0	0	0	0	+++++	Very low	Wide access	
Exercise ECHO	80–85	80–88	++	+++	+/-*	0	0	+++	Low		
Dobu ECHO	79–83	82–86	+++	++++	+/-*	+++	0	++++	Low	Portability	Operator-dependent
Vasodil. ECHO	72–79	92–95	+++	++	++	0	0	+++	Low	Portability	Operator-dependent
Exercise SPECT	73–92	63–87	+	+	+++	+	High	++++	Moderate	Extensive data	
Vasodil. SPECT	90–91	75–84	+	+	+++	+	High	++++	Moderate	Extensive data	
Dobu MR	79–88	81–91	++++	+++++	+	+++++	0	++	High	No contrast needed, unless scar imaging	Contraindications magnet quality impaired in case of arrhythmia
Vasodil. MR	67–94	61–85	+++++	++	++++	++++	0	++	High	Scar imaging	Limited 3D analysis of ischemia
CTCA	95–99	64–83	+++	+/-*	+/-*	0	Low	+++	Moderate	High NPV in low PTP	Low NPV in high PTP quality impaired in arrhythmia, tachycardia, calcification
Vasodil. PET	81–97	74–91	++	+	+++++	+++++	Moderate	+	High	Perfusion quantification	

* Not in clinical practice yet

Figure 9.25 Summarizing table of diagnostic imaging technique characteristics.

resolution of SPECT. Obesity and voluminous breast tissue may also be a problem for stress ECHO. Pharmacological stress testing using dobutamine or dipyridamole can be preferred in women with reduced exercise capacity. Cardiac MRI has been able to demonstrate subendocardial hypoperfusion in women with chest pain without obstructive CAD. In the only head-to-head comparison to date, perfusion CMR was shown to have better diagnostic performance in women than SPECT, with smaller heart size the main determinant in the lower SPECT performance [67].

Similarly, in *diabetics*, circular subendocardial hypoperfusion as a sign of microvascular dysfunction can be visualized by adenosine or dipyridamole perfusion MRI.

In diabetics, as well as in the *elderly*, a more diffuse and severe disease can be expected, including a higher prevalence of left main stenosis or three-vessel disease. Theoretically, these could be missed by relative perfusion techniques such as SPECT and perfusion MRI, but diagnostic accuracy was shown to be as high in more severe disease states with cardiac MRI [68]. In the elderly, there is a higher number of false negative results, due to limited functional capacity, so pharmacological stress can be preferred. On the other hand, the number of false positive results is higher, due to the higher prevalence of confounders such as prior myocardial infarction, left ventricular hypertrophy, etc.

9.3.3.7 Clinical question

Last but not least, the clinical question is to be thought of carefully beforehand and should guide us through all the cofactors in decision making. Is it anatomy we want to visualize (e.g., for technical aspects of the technique for revascularization), or is it ischemia quantification that is required (e.g., for risk stratification in the decision whether to revascularize)? Is there a need for additional imaging information, such as concomitant diagnosis of valve disease, or viability assessment? Is there a need to visualize or calculate microvascular dysfunction (CFR, myocardial perfusion reserve), etc. (cf. Figure 9.24)?

9.3.3.8 Cost-effectiveness

The clinical use of imaging technologies has caused worldwide significant increases in healthcare expenditures. National healthcare insurers have called upon providers to limit the use of imaging to appropriate indications and to select strategies with proven cost-effectiveness. Unfortunately, robust cost-effectiveness data for cardiac ischemia testing is scarce. Moreover, reimbursement for different imaging techniques varies significantly across countries, which makes it difficult to generalize cost-effectiveness assumptions. The END study used propensity matching to compare a large cohort of patients referred for either gate-keeper myocardial perfusion imaging or upfront angiography—this non-randomized study demonstrated a significant cost-reduction in the nuclear arm [69]. Compared to standard exercise tread mill testing, SPECT appears more cost-effective in patients with intermediate and high pretest probability for CAD, while in low-pretest probability patients (and low-risk women) the tread mill test is more cost-effective [70,71]. In a randomized comparison of SPECT, stress ECHO, and stress perfusion CMR as the initial imaging strategy, the clinical 2-year outcome was similar for the three strategies. However, SPECT appeared marginally superior to the two other strategies with regard to cost-effectiveness [72].

9.3.3.9 Hypothetical examples

In a male patient with intermediate PTP and suspicion of ischemia based on dyspnea during exercise who has only moderate echogenicity because of obesity, with doubt about left ventricular function and the severity of mitral or aortic valve disease: CMR would be preferable to offer this information. As a stressor, exercise would be best, but depending on local expertise, dobutamine might be preferable for better image quality. During stress, not only wall motion abnormalities should be evaluated, but looking at the mitral valve is of great relevance.

In a 50-year-old female with low-intermediate PTP and suspicion of ischemia because of atypical pain while jogging, a CTCA might be the most appropriate way to exclude CAD, added with computational "FFR" in case a coronary artery stenosis is detected with doubt about its functional relevance. Alternatively, an exercise TTE can be chosen.

In a 60-year-old male patient with known CAD, past myocardial infarction, and recurrence of angina, quantification of current ischemia as well as viability information is desirable. This can be offered by ECHO, SPECT, PET, and CMR, depending on local expertise and availability. CMR can be chosen with dobutamine to evaluate contractile reserve at low dose and quantification of ischemia by the number of dysfunctional segments at high dose. In case of extensive pre-existing wall motion abnormalities or a LBBB, a perfusion CMR with a vasodilator would be preferable, with viability evaluation by transmurality of delayed contrast enhancement.

9.4 Diagnostic platform

One might consider, therefore, the concept of a diagnostic platform: the clinician does not order a specific test, but rather asks a specific question (is there ischemia, how much, which territory) and the diagnostic platform, consisting of a multidisciplinary group of "imagers" of the various modalities, decides on the choice and, possibly, sequence of tests that will answer the clinical question with the least risk for the patient, the least cost for society, and the best information content to decide on further therapeutic options. An integrated answer is provided to the clinician, rather than the results of separate tests, which often are not congruent, and sometimes even contradictory, leaving the clinician without a clear answer and escalating further (often invasive) testing, increasing the overall cost and risk (cf. Figure 9.24).

While the diagnostic accuracy of most imaging modalities is largely dependent on local expertise (explaining the large discrepancies in diagnostic accuracy of one modality between single-center and multicenter trials, or between different modalities in one center), the composition of such a diagnostic platform will depend on the local situation and should mainly follow from expertise rather than specialty training. As emphasized above, local expertise and availability, as well as the specifics of the patients, are more relevant to make the choice of diagnostic modality, independent of other considerations but the highest quality for the patient, i.e., best result for least cost and risk (cf. Figures 9.24 and 9.25).

9.5 Risk stratification and prognosis

While determination of diagnosis and prognosis were considered together in previous versions of the guidelines, the newest international guidelines both in the United States and in Europe first establish the presence of ischemia and subsequently judge the extent and prognosis to come to a decision on therapeutic management (cf. Figure 9.14) [14,73].

When there is no indication for specific ischemia treatment (primary prevention), risk charts such as SCORE or Framingham can be applied to decide on the need for risk modification. Besides this global risk estimation, calcium scoring and CTCA can individualize risk by providing information on coronary calcification or coronary anatomy and plaque distribution. CTCA has a very strong negative predictive value, useful in excluding significant epicardial coronary disease in patients where this is the most relevant part of the clinical question.

In patients with stable obstructive CAD and ischemia, a decision about the need for revascularization is to be made. Whereas in the acute setting there is absolutely no debate about the benefit of revascularization, in stable ischemia there is less evidence for this approach, except for left main disease and proximal LAD stenosis [74]. In patients with non-left main stable CAD and stenosis arteriographically suitable for revascularization, those undergoing revascularization procedures had no benefit on mortality, coronary events, or angina over OMT-treated patients [75,76]. In these trials, however, there was a big selection bias, plus a significant crossover from the OMT to the invasively treated arm. In a SPECT-substudy of patients who underwent serial myocardial perfusion imaging, adding PCI to OMT resulted in greater ischemia reduction compared with OMT alone, with ischemia reduction being related to lower risk for death or myocardial infarction, particularly if baseline ischemia was moderate to severe [77]. However, from a later COURAGE post-hoc substudy dividing the patients into those with mild and those with moderate to severe ischemia on baseline SPECT, the extent of site-defined ischemia did not predict adverse events and did not alter treatment effectiveness [78]. But randomized trials are scarce, and the vast majority of evidence supporting the use of imaging prior to revascularization procedures comes from large retrospective trials: Hachamovitch and colleagues demonstrated in 10,627 propensity-matched patients, that those with moderate to large myocardial ischemia (defined as $\geq 10\%$ ischemic LV) had better outcome with revascularization compared to medical therapy (cardiac death rate 2.0% vs. 6.7% for patients with $\geq 20\%$ ischemia) [79] (Figure 9.26). However, the opposite was the case in patients with normal MPI (or only mild ischemia) (6.3% vs. 0.7%). The superiority of revascularization over medical therapy in patients with $\geq 10\%$ ischemia (and likewise the potential harm of revascularization over medical therapy in the absence of significant ischemia) was maintained over a follow-up period of 8.7 ± 3.3 years [80]. An ongoing trial called ISCHEMIA will hopefully shed more light on the issue whether stable ischemia needs to be revascularized or not [81].

Awaiting these results, at this moment, the need for revascularization is based on risk estimation. High risk is defined as an all-cause annual mortality of >3%,

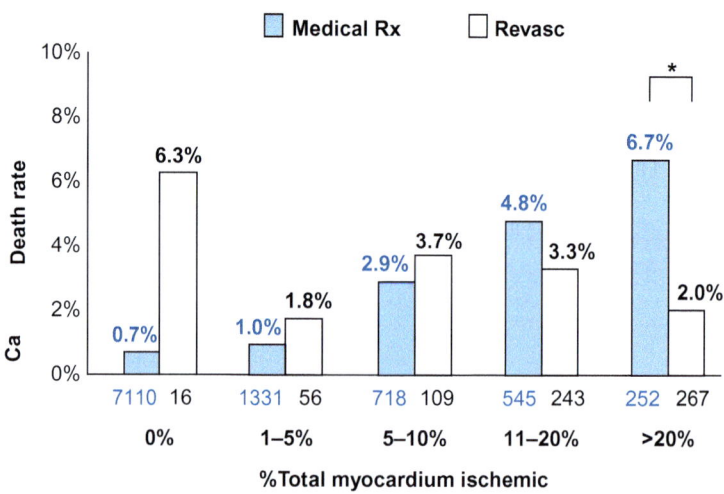

Figure 9.26 Observed cardiac death rates over the follow-up period in patients undergoing revascularization (Revasc) vs. medical therapy (Medical Rx) as a function of the amount of inducible ischemia. Increase in cardiac death frequency as a function of inducible ischemia, $P<0.0001$.
From Ref. [79].

intermediate risk ≥1% but ≤3%, while low risk is linked to an annual mortality <1% [14]. One can base this risk assessment on different parameters: clinical evaluation, ventricular function, extent of ischemia during stress testing, and coronary anatomy. For patients who already underwent a diagnostic imaging modality, the information to establish prognosis will already be available. For patients with a PTP > 85% additional testing can be performed unless severity of symptoms or other information already suggests high-risk coronary anatomy, in which case medical therapy should be initiated and invasive testing offered immediately. Risk categories for ischemia imaging with different modalities are given in Table 9.1.

In the setting without epicardial coronary artery stenosis, the assessment of CFR or MPR has also been used to assess prognosis. Invasive measures of CFR in patients with chest pain and normal coronary angiograms predict increased mortality [8]. PET-measured MPR was an independent predictor of deterioration and death in patients with hypertrophic cardiomyopathy [82], dilated cardiomyopathy, and patients with suspected or known CAD [83], whereas a preserved value could exclude high-risk CAD [84]. Echocardiographically LAD-dopplered CFR was an independent predictor of death in patients with non-ischemic dilated cardiomyopathy [85]. So patients with a reduced CFR do have ischemia and will be at increased risk for arrhythmias and sudden death, despite normal coronary angiograms. Whether treatment will have an impact on this outcome, however, is less clear form randomized trials.

Table 9.1 Risk stratification based on imaging

SPECT, PET	High risk	Area of ischemia > 10% of the LV myocardium or ≥2/17 segments
	Intermediate risk	Area of ischemia between 1 and 10% of the LV myocardium or 1/17 segments
	Low risk	No ischemia
Stress ECHO	High risk	≥3/17 dysfunctional segments during dobutamine stimulation
	Intermediate risk	Between 1/17 and 2/17 dysfunctional segments during dobutamine stimulation
	Low risk	No dysfunctional segments
CMR	High risk	≥2/16 segments[a] with new perfusion defects or ≥3/17 dysfunctional segments during dobutamine stimulation
	Intermediate risk	1/16 segments with new perfusion defects or between 1/17 and 2/17 dysfunctional segments during dobutamine stimulation
	Low risk	No ischemia

SPECT, single-photon emission computed tomography; PET, positron emission computed tomography; ECHO, echocardiography; CMR, cardiac magnetic resonance; LV, left ventricular.
[a]Note that for first-pass perfusion CMR the established myocardial segmentation model is a 16-segment instead of a 17-segment model, since the apex is not included in standard perfusion protocols.
Adapted from 2013 ESC guidelines on the management of stable CAD [11].

9.6 Noninvasive follow-up of the patient with known coronary artery disease

While no firm data exist to warrant follow-up stress imaging testing, re-testing may be considered after the "warranty" period of the test has expired, which is considered 3 years for most tests, although it probably is closer to 5 years for SPECT. When symptoms appear or change, additional testing is required to reestablish prognosis and guide therapy. Whether patients have had revascularization does not change this overall scheme, but imaging testing is preferred over exercise testing in patients with previous revascularisation. Class IIb level C evidence is available to suggest 6 month stress imaging after PCI or CABG to detect restenosis or graft occlusion [14].

References

[1] Crea F, Camici PG, Bairey Merz CN. Coronary microvascular dysfunction: an update. Eur Heart J 2014;35(17):1101–11.
[2] Sakakura K, Nakano M, Otsuka F, Ladich E, Kolodgie FD, Virmani R. Pathophysiology of atherosclerosis plaque progression. Heart Lung Circ 2013;22:399–411.
[3] Takagi Y, Takahashi J, Yasuda S, et al. Prognostic stratification of patients with vasospastic angina. A comprehensive clinical risk score developed by the Japanese Coronary Spasm Association. J Am Coll Cardiol 2013;62:1144–53.
[4] Marzilli M, Merz CN, Boden WE, Bonow RO, Capozza PG, Chilian WM, et al. Obstructive coronary atherosclerosis and ischemic heart disease: an elusive link. J Am Coll Cardiol 2012;60:951–6.
[5] Gould KL. Does coronary flow trump coronary anatomy? J Am Coll Cardiol Cardiovasc Imaging 2009;2(8):1009–23.
[6] Jeremias A, Maehara A, Généreux P, et al. Multicenter core laboratory comparison of the instantaneous wave-free ratio and resting Pd/Pa with fractional flow reserve. The RESOLVE Study. J Am Coll Cardiol 2014;63(13):1253–61.
[7] Schächinger V, Britten MB, Zeiher AM. Prognostic impact of coronary vasodilator dysfunction on adverse long-term outcome of coronary heart disease. Circulation 2000;101:1899–906.
[8] Pepine CJ, Anderson RD, Sharaf BL, et al. Coronary microvascular reactivity to adenosine predicts adverse outcome in women evaluated for suspected ischemia: results from the National Heart, Lung and Blood Institute WISE (Women's Ischemia Syndrome Evaluation) study. J Am Coll Cardiol 2010;55:2825–32.
[9] Melikian N, De Bondt P, Tonino P, De Winter O, Wyffels E, Bartunek J, et al. Fractional flow reserve and myocardial perfusion imaging in patients with angiographic multivessel coronary artery disease. JACC Cardiovasc Interv 2010;3(3):307–14.
[10] Tonino PAL, De Bruyne B, Pijls NHJ, Siebert U, Ikeno F, van't Veer M, et al. Fractional flow reserve versus angiography for guiding percutaneous coronary intervention. N Engl J Med 2009;360(3):2013–224.
[11] Sels JWEM, Tonino PAL, Siebert U, et al. Fractional flow reserve in unstable angina and non-ST-segment elevation myocardial infarction: experience from the FAME (Fractional flow reserve versus Angiography for Multivessel Evaluation) study. JACC Cardiovasc Interv 2011;4(11):1183–9.

[12] De Bruyne B, Fearon WF, Pijls NH, Barbato E, Tonino P, Piroth Z, et al. Fractional flow reserve-guided PCI for stable coronary artery disease. N Engl J Med 2014;371(13):1208–17.
[13] De Bruyne B, Pijls NH, Kalesan B, Barbato E, Tonino PA, Piroth Z, et al. Fractional flow reserve-guided PCI versus medical therapy in stable coronary artery disease. N Engl J Med 2012;367(11):991–1001.
[14] Task Force Members: Montalescot G, Sechtem U, Achenbach S, Andreotti F, Arden C, Budaj A, et al. ESC guidelines on the management of stable coronary artery disease: the Task Force on the management of stable coronary artery disease of the European Society of Cardiology. Eur Heart J 2013;34(38):2949–3003.
[15] Genders TS, Steyerberg EW, Alkadhi H, Leschka S, Desbiolles L, Nieman K, et al. A clinical prediction rule for the diagnosis of coronary artery disease: validation, updating, and extension. Eur Heart J 2011;32:1316–30.
[16] Shaw LJ, Tandon S, Rosen S, et al. Evaluation of suspected ischemic heart disease in symptomatic women. Can J Cardiol 2014;30(7):729–37.
[17] Bizino MB, Hammer S, Lamb HJ. Metabolic imaging of the human heart: clinical application of magnetic resonance spectroscopy. Heart 2014;100(11):881–90. http://dx.doi.org/10.1136/heartjnl-2012-302546.
[18] Inaba Y, Bergmann SR. Prognostic value of myocardial metabolic imaging with BMIPP in the spectrum of coronary artery disease: a systematic review. J Nucl Cardiol 2010;17:61–70.
[19] Min L, Xiang-min D, Zhao-hui P, Juan D, Li L. The diagnostic performance of coronary artery angiography with 64-MSCT and post 64-MSCT: systematic review and meta-analysis. PLoS One 2014;9(1):e84937. http://dx.doi.org/10.1371/journal.pone.0084937.
[20] Budoff MJ, Dowe D, Jollis JG, et al. Diagnostic performance of 64-multidetector row coronary competud tomographic angiography for evaluation of conoary computed tomographic angiography for evalutation of coronary artery stenosis in individuals without known coronary artery disease: results from the prospective multicenter ACCURACY (Assessment by Coronary Computed Tomographic Angiography of Individuals Undergoing Invasive Coronary Angiography) trial. J Am Coll Cardiol 2008;52:1724–32.
[21] Ropers D, Pohle FK, Kuettner A, et al. Diagnostic accuracy of noninvasive coronary angiography in patients after bypass surgery using 64-slice spiral computed tomography with 330-ms gantry rotation. Circulation 2006;114:2334–41.
[22] Wuestink AC, Nieman K, Pugliese F, et al. Diagnostic accuracy of computed tomography angiography in patients after bypass grafting: comparison with invasive angiography. JACC Cardiovasc Imaging 2009;2:816–24.
[23] Kumbhani DJ, Ingelmo CP, Schoenhagen P, et al. Meta-analysis of diagnostic efficacy of 64-slice computed tomography in the evaluation of coronary in-stent restenosis. Am J Cardiol 2009;103:1675–81.
[24] Hadamitzky M, Achenbach S, Al-Mallah M, et al. Optimized prognostic score for coronary computed tomographic angiography: results from the CONFIRM registry (Coronary CT Angiography EvaluatioN For Clinical Outcomes: An InteRnational Multicenter Registry). J Am Coll Cardiol 2013;62(5):468–76.
[25] Min JK, Leipsic J, Pencina MJ, et al. Diagnostic accuracy of fractional flow reserve from anatomic CT angiography. JAMA 2012;308:1989–97.
[26] Nørgaard BL, Leipsic J, Gaur S, et al. Diagnostic performance of noninvasive fractional flow reserve derived from coronary computed tomography angiography in suspected coronary artery disease. The NXT Trial (analysis of coronary blood flow using CT angiography: next steps). J Am Coll Cardiol 2014;63(12):1145–55.

[27] Wong DT, Ko BS, Cameron JD, Nerlekar N, Leung MC, Malaiapan Y, et al. Transluminal attenuation gradient in coronary computed tomography angiography is a novel noninvasive approach to the identification of functionally significant coronary artery stenosis: a comparison with fractional flow reserve. J Am Coll Cardiol 2013;61(12):1271–9.
[28] Wong DTL, Ko BS, Cameron JD, et al. Comparison of diagnostic accuracy of combined assessment using adenosine stress computed tomography perfusion + computed tomography angiography with transluminal attenuation gradient + computed tomography angiography against invasive fractional flow reserve. J Am Coll Cardiol 2014;63(18):1904–12.
[29] Srichai MB, Chandarana H, Donnino R, et al. Diagnostic accuracy of cardiac computed tomography angiography for myocardial infarction. World J Radiol 2013;5(8):295–303.
[30] Bamberg F, Becker A, Schwarz F, et al. Detection of hemodynamiccaly significant coronary artery stenosis: incremental diagnostic value of dynamic CT-based myocardial perfusion imaging. Radiology 2011;260:689–98.
[31] Bamberg F, Marcus RP, Becker A, et al. Dynamic myocardial CT perfusion imaging for evaluation of myocardial ischemia as determined by MR imaging. JACC Cardiovasc Imaging 2014;7:257–77. http://dx.doi.org/10.1016/j.jcmg.2013.06.008, pii: S1936-878X(13)00731-6.
[32] Jaarsma C, Leiner T, Bekkers SC, et al. Diagnostic performance of noninvasive myocardial perfusion imaging using single-photon emission computed tomography, cardiac magnetic resonance, and positron emission tomography imaging for the detection of obstructive coronary artery disease. A meta-analysis. J Am Coll Cardiol 2012;59(19):1719–28.
[33] Hajjiri MM, Leavitt MB, Zheng H, Spooner AE, Fischman AJ, Gewirtz H. Comparison of positron emission tomography measurement of adenosine stimulated absolute myocardial blood flow versus relative myocardial tracer content for physiological assessment of coronary artery stenosis severity and location. JACC Cardiovasc Imaging 2009;2(6):751–8.
[34] Berman DS, Maddahi J, Tamarappoo BK, et al. Phase II safety and clinical comparison with single-photon emission computed tomography myocardial perfusion imaging for detection of coronary artery Disease. Flurpiridaz F 18 Positron Emission Tomography. J Am Coll Cardiol 2013;61:469.
[35] Sicari R, Nihoyannopoulos P, Evangelista A. Stress echocardiography expert consensus statement—executive summary. European Association of Echocardiography (EAE). Eur Heart J 2009;30:278–89.
[36] Mor-Avi V, Lang RM, Badano LP, et al. Current and evolving echocardiographic techniques for the quantitative evaluation of cardiac mechanics: ASE/EAE consensus statement on methodology and indications endorsed by the Japanese Society of Echocardiography. J Am Soc Echocardiogr 2011;24:277–313.
[37] Voigt JU, Exner B, Schmiedehausen K, et al. Strain-rate imaging during dobutamine stress echocardiography provides objective evidence of inducible ischemia. Circulation 2003;107:2120–6.
[38] Senior R, Moreo A, Gaibazzi N, et al. Comparison of sulfur hexafluoride microbubble (SonoVue)-enhanced myocardial contrast echocardiography with gated single-photon emission computed tomography for detection of significant coronary artery disease: a large European multicenter study. J Am Coll Cardiol 2013;62(15):1353–61.
[39] Plana JC, MIkati IA, Kokainish H, et al. A randomized cross-over study for evaluation of the effect of image optimization with contrast on the diagnostic accuracy of dobutamine echocardiography in coronary artery disease: The OPTIMIZE Trial. JACC Cardiovasc Imaging 2008;2:145–52.

[40] Aggeli C, Giannopoulos G, Misovoulos P, et al. Real-time three-dimensional dobutamine stress echocardiography for coronary artery disease diagnosis: validation with coronary angiography. Heart 2009;93:672–5.
[41] Lang RM, Badano LP, Tsang W, et al. EAE/ASE recommendations for image acquisition and display using three-dimensional echocardiography. J Am Soc Echocardiogr 2012;13:1–46.
[42] Senior R, Shah BN. Myocardial contrast echocardiography for simultaneous assessment of function and perfusion in real time: a technique comes of age. Circulation 2012;126:1182–4.
[43] Bhattacharyya S, Chehab O, Khattar R, et al. Stress echocardiography in clinical practice: a United Kingdom National Health Service Survey on behalf of the British Society of Echocardiography. Eur Heart J Cardiovasc Imaging 2014;15:158–63.
[44] Kasprzak JD, Weiner-Mik P, Nouri A, et al. Transthoracic measurement of left coronary artery flow reserve improves the diagnostic value of routine dipyridamole-atropine stress echocardiogram. Arch Med Sci 2013;9(5):802–7.
[45] Paetsch I, Jahnke C, Wahl A, et al. Comparison of dobutamine stress magnetic resonance, adenosine stress magnetic resonance, and adenosine stress magnetic resonance perfusion. Circulation 2004;110:835–42.
[46] Jahnke C, Nagel E, Gebker R, et al. Prognostic value of cardiac magnetic resonance stress tests. Adenosine stress perfusion and dobutamine stress wall motion imaging. Circulation 2007;115:1769–76.
[47] Nagel E, Lehmkuhl HB, Klein C, et al. Influence of image quality on the diagnostic accuracy of dobutamine stress magnetic resonance imaging in comparison with dobutamine stress echocardiography for the noninvasive detection of myocardial ischemia. Z Kardiol 1999;88(9):622–30 [German].
[48] Greenwood JP, Maredia N, Younger JF, et al. Cardiovascular magnetic resonance and single-photon emission computed tomography for diagnosis of coronary heart disease (CE-MARC): a prospective trial. Lancet 2012;379(9814):453–60.
[49] Schwitter J, Wacker CM, Wilke N, et al. MR-IMPACT II: Magnetic resonance imaging for myocardial perfusion assessment in coronary artery disease trial: perfusion-cardiac magnetic resonance vs. single-photon emission computed tomography for the detection of coronary artery disease: a comparative multicentre, multivendor trial. Eur Heart J 2013;34(10):775–81.
[50] Desai RR, Jha S. Diagnostic performance of cardiac stress perfusion MRI in the detection of coronary artery disease using fractional flow reserve as the reference standard: a meta-analysis. AJR Am J Roentgenol 2013;201(2):W245–52.
[51] Manka R, Paetsch I, Kozerke S, et al. Whole-heart dynamic three-dimensional magnetic resonance perfusion imaging for the detection of coronary artery disease defined by fractional flow reserve: determination of volumetric myocardial ischaemic burden and coronary lesion location. Eur Heart J 2012;33(16):2016–24.
[52] Bernhardt P, Walcher T, Rottbauer W, et al. Quantification of myocardial perfusion reserve at 1.5 and 3.0 Tesla: a comparison to fractional flow reserve. Int J Cardiovasc Imaging 2012;28:2049–56.
[53] Chiribiri A, Hautvast GLTF, Lockie T, et al. Assessment of coronary artery stenosis severity and location. Quantitative analysis of transmural perfusion gradients by high-resolution MRI versus FFR. J Am Coll Cardiol Img 2013;6:600–9.
[54] Rossi A, Merkus D, Klotz E, et al. Stress myocardial perfusion: imaging with multidetector CT. Radiology 2014;270(1):25–46.

[55] George RT, Mehra VC, Chen MY, et al. Myocardial CT perfusion imaging and SPECT for the diagnosis of coronary artery disease: a head-to-head comparison from the CORE320 multicenter diagnostic performance study. Radiology 2014;272(2):407–16.
[56] Blankstein R, Shturman LD, Rogers IS. Adenosine-induced stress myocardial perfusion imaging using dual-source cardiac computed tomography. J Am Coll Cardiol 2009;54:1072–84.
[57] Flotats A, Knuuti J, Gutberlet M, et al. Hybrid cardiac imaging: SPECT/CT and PET/CT. A joint position statement by the European Association of Nuclear Medicine (EANM), the European Society of Cardiac Radiology (ESCR) and the European Council of Nuclear Cardiology (ECNC). Eur J Nucl Med Mol Imaging 2011;38:201–12.
[58] Hachamovitch R, Johnson JR, Hlatky MA, et al. The study of myocardial perfusion and coronary anatomy imaging roles in CAD (SPARC): design, rationale, and baseline patient characteristics of a prospective, multicenter observational registry comparing PET, SPECT, and CTA for resource utilization and clinical outcomes. J Nucl Cardiol 2009;16:935–48.
[59] Evaluation of Integrated Cardiac Imaging in Ischemic Heart Disease (EVINCI). NCT00979199; ESC Press Office Public release date: 26-Jun-2012.
[60] Safavi KC, Dharmarajan K, Venkatesh AK, et al. Hospital variation in the use of non-invasive cardiac imaging and its association with downstream testing, interventions, and outcomes. JAMA Intern Med 2014;174(4):546–53. http://dx.doi.org/10.1001/jamainternmed.2013.14407.
[61] Anagnostopoulos C, Georgakopoulos A, Pianou N, et al. Assessment of myocardial perfusion and viability by positron emission tomography. Int J Cardiol 2013;167:1737–49.
[62] Luu J, Harker J, Guensch D, et al. FUnctinal significance of Blood Oxygen Level Dependent (BOLD) imaging in patients with coronary artery disease – a validation study using fractional flow reserve. J Cardiovasc Magn Reson 2011;13(Suppl. 1):92–3.
[63] Mahmarian JJ, Peterson LE, Xu J, Cerqueira MD, et al. Regadenoson provides perfusion results comparable to adenosine in heterogeneous patient populations: A quantitative analysis from the ADVANCE MPI trials. J Nucl Cardiol 2015;22(2):248–61, PubMed PMID:25287737.
[64] Abbasi SA, Heydari B, Shah RV, et al. Risk stratification by regadenoson stress magnetic resonance imaging in patients with known or suspected coronary artery disease. Am J Cardiol 2014;114(8):1198–203. http://dx.doi.org/10.1016/j.amjcard.2014.07.041, Epub 2014 Jul 30. PubMed PMID: 25173444.
[65] Hage FG. Regadenoson for myocardial perfusion imaging: is it safe? J Nucl Cardiol 2014;21(5):871–6. http://dx.doi.org/10.1007/s12350-014-9922-4, Epub 2014 Jun 19. PubMed PMID: 24939324.
[66] Rosenblatt J, Mooney D, Dunn T, Cohen M. Asystole following regadenoson infusion in stable outpatients. J Nucl Cardiol 2014;21(5):862–8. http://dx.doi.org/10.1007/s12350-014-9898-0, Epub 2014 May 31. PubMed PMID: 24879452.
[67] Greenwood JP, Motwani M, Maredia N, et al. Comparison of cardiovascular magnetic resonance and single-photon emission computed tomography in women with suspected coronary artery disease from the clinical evaluation of magnetic resonance imaging in coronary heart disease (CE-MARC) trial. Circulation 2014;129(10):1129–38.
[68] Patel AR, Antkowiak PF, Nandalur KR, et al. Assessment of advanced coronary artery disease. Advantages of quantitative cardiac magnetic resonance perfusion analysis. J Am Coll Cardiol 2010;56:561–9.

[69] Shaw LJ, Hachamovitch R, Berman DS, et al. The economic consequences of available diagnostic and prognostic strategies for the evaluation of stable angina patients: an observational assessment of the value of precatheterization ischemia. J Am Coll Cardiol 1999;33:661–9.
[70] Sabharwal NK, Stoykova B, Taneja AK, et al. A randomized trial of exercise treadmill ECG versus stress SPECT myocardial perfusion imaging as an initial diagnostic strategy in stable patients with chest pain and suspected CAD: cost analysis. J Nucl Cardiol 2007;14:174–86.
[71] Shaw LJ, Mieres JH, Hendel RH, et al. Comparative effectiveness of exercise electrocardiography with or without myocardial perfusion single photon emission computed tomography in women with suspected coronary artery disease. Results from the What Is the Optimal Method for Ischemia Evaluation in Women (WOMEN) trial. Circulation 2011;124:1239–49.
[72] Thom H, West NEJ, Hughes V, et al. Cost-effectiveness of initial stress cardiovascularMR, stress SPECT or stress echocardiography as a gate-keeper test, compared with upfront invasive coronary angiography in the investigation and management of patients with stable chest pain: mid-term outcomes from the CECaT randomised controlled trial. BMJ Open 2014;4(2), e003419.
[73] Fihn SD, Gardin JM, et al. 2012 ACCF/AHA/ACP/AATS/PCNA/SCAI/STS Guideline for the diagnosis and management of patients with stable ischemic heart disease: executive summary. J Am Coll Cardiol 2012;60(24):2564–603.
[74] Caracciolo EA, Davis KB, Sopko G, et al. Comparison of surgical and medical group survival in patients with left main coronary artery disease. Long-term CASS experience. Circulation 1995;91:2325–34.
[75] Boden WE, O'Rourke RA, Teo KK, et al. Optimal medical therapy with or without PCI for stable coronary disease. N Engl J Med 2007;356:1503–16.
[76] The Bari 2D Study Group. A randomized trial of therapies for type 2 diabetes and coronary artery disease. N Engl J Med 2009;360:2503–15.
[77] Shaw LJ, Berman DS, Maron DJ, et al. Optimal medical therapy with or without percutaneous coronary intervention to reduce ischemic burden. Results from the Clinical Outcomes Utilizing Revacularization and AGgressive drug Evaluation (COURAGE) trial nuclear substudy. Circulation 2008;117:1283–91.
[78] Shaw LJ, Weintraub WS, Maron DJ, et al. Baseline stress myocardial perfusion imaging results and outcomes in patients with stable ischemic heart disease randomized to optimal medical therapy with or without percutaneous coronary intervention. Am Heart J 2012;164:243–50.
[79] Hachamovitch R, Hayes SW, Friedman JD, et al. Comparison of the short-term survival benefit associated with revascularization compared with medical therapy in patients with no prior coronary artery disease undergoing stress myocardial perfusion single photon emission computed tomography. Circulation 2003;107:2900–7.
[80] Hachamovitch R, Rozanski A, Shaw LJ, et al. Impact of ischaemia and scar on the therapeutic benefit derived from myocardial revascularization vs. medical therapy among patients undergoing stress-rest myocardial perfusion scintigraphy. Eur Heart J 2011;32:1012–24.
[81] International Study if Comparative Health Effectiveness with Medical and Invasive Approaches (ISCHEMIA). ClinicalTrials.gov NCT01471522.
[82] Camici PG, Olivotto I, Rimoldi OE. The coronary circulation and blood flow in left ventricular hypertrophy. J Mol Cell Cardiol 2012;52(4):857–64.

[83] Gaemperli O, Kaufmann PA. Why quantify myocardial perfusion. Curr Cardiovasc Imaging Rep 2012;5(3):133.

[84] Naya M, Murthy VL, Taqueti VR, Foster CR, Klein J, Garber M, et al. Preserved coronary flow reserve effectively excludes high-risk coronary artery disease on angiography. J Nuc Med 2014;55:248–55.

[85] Rigo F, Ciampi Q, Ossena G, et al. Prognostic value of left and right coronary flow reserve assessment in nonischemic dilated cardiomyopathy by transthoracic Doppler echocardiography. J Card Fail 2011;17:39–46.

[86] Picano E, Landi P, Bolognese L, Chiarandà G, Chiarella F, Seveso G, et al. Prognostic value of dipyridamole echocardiography early after uncomplicated myocardial infarction: a large-scale, multicenter trial. The EPIC Study Group. Am J Med 1993;95(December (6)):608–18.

[87] Cerqueira MD, Verani MS, Schwaiger M, Heo J, Iskandrian AS. Safety profile of adenosine stress perfusion imaging: results from the Adenoscan Multicenter Trial Registry. J Am Coll Cardiol 1994;23(February (2)):384–9.

[88] Wahl A, Paetsch I, Gollesch A, Roethemeyer S, Foell D, Gebker R, et al. Safety and feasibility of high-dose dobutamine-atropine stress cardiovascular magnetic resonance for diagnosis of myocardial ischaemia: experience in 1000 consecutive cases. Eur Heart J 2004;25(July (14)):1230–6.

Myocardial infarction

10

A. Flotats*, B.L. Gerber†, S. Gurunathan‡, A. Mahnken§,
T.A. Magalhães¶, C.E. Rochitte¶, R. Senior‡
*Hospital de la Santa Creu i Sant Pau, Universitat Autònoma de Barcelona, Barcelona, Spain; †Cliniques Universitaires St. Luc Université Catholique de Louvain, Brussels, Belgium; ‡Royal Brompton Hospital, Imperial College, London, UK; §Philipps University, Marburg, Germany; ¶Hospital do Coração, HCOR, University of São Paulo Medical School, São Paulo, Brazil

10.1 Introduction

Acute myocardial infarction (MI) is defined as death of the myocytes (myocardial necrosis) in a clinical setting consistent with acute myocardial ischemia [1]. Echocardiography, nuclear imaging techniques, CMR, and CT play an important role in detecting and following patients with acute MI (AMI).

10.1.1 Pathophysiology of AMI

AMI is most often caused by acute coronary artery plaque rupture and thrombosis, but it may also occur due to vasospasm, myocardial supply-demand imbalance with or without associated stable coronary artery disease (CAD), or after revascularization procedures. AMI develops generally when myocardial ischemia lasts for more than 20 min. Because myocardial workload is higher and perfusion is less in sub-endocardial areas, infarcts spread in a wavefront phenomenon from sub-endocardial to epicardial layers with increasing duration of ischemia [2] (Figure 10.1). Complete transmural necrosis of the ischemic area of risk usually occurs when ischemia lasts longer than 4–6 h, depending on the severity of the coronary artery occlusion, the presence of collateral circulation, preconditioning, and the individual oxygen demand/supply balance. Intermittent durations of ischemia less than 4–6 h result therefore in incomplete mostly subendocardial necrosis, in which part of the area at risk remains viable. This concept is fundamental to current revascularization therapy of AMI. Indeed, modern treatment strategies of AMI aim at opening the infarct-related artery as quickly as possible, in order to reduce the duration of ischemia and to save viable myocardium in the risk area. The importance of saving such viable myocardium was underscored by the recent OAT trial [3], which demonstrated no benefit of opening the infarct-related artery by PCI in patients having suffered an STEMI more than 3 days ago, likely because in such subacute STEMI the window of action for saving residual viable myocardium had expired. Experimental studies showed that additional myocardial injury may occur at the time of reperfusion or shortly thereafter [4]. This suggests

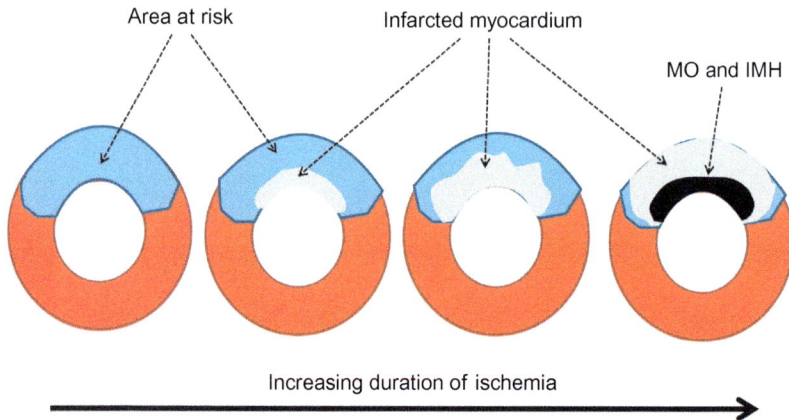

Figure 10.1 Pathophysiology of MI: ischemia wave-front phenomenon of myocardial infarction. MO = microvascular obstruction. IMH = intramyocardial hemorrhage

that the relation between risk area and final MI size for a given duration of occlusion could be still modified at the time of reperfusion by administration of "cardioprotective" drugs; however, clinically, none of such drugs are currently available.

By histology, AMI is characterized by coagulation and contraction band necrosis of myocytes. In addition, AMI leads to the destruction of the extracellular matrix, and in the center of large infarcts, to destruction and occlusion of the microvasculature (the so-called no-reflow phenomenon) [5], may be complicated by intramyocardial hemorrhage (Figure 10.2). Non-infarcted post-ischemic areas may present with myocyte and interstitial edema. Subsequent to the acute injury is a complex healing process occurring in several different phases both in the infarcted area, the MI border zone, and in remote non-infarcted areas [7,8]. In the infarcted area, after an initial inflammatory phase leading to detersion of dead myocytes and other cellular debris, follows a proliferative phase characterized by neoangiogenesis and myofibroblast proliferation aiming to reconstitute a new extracellular matrix. Finally, MI healing is concluded when mature fibroblasts deposit a solid collagen-based extracellular scar (replacement fibrosis), approximately 4 weeks after the acute injury. During the phase of MI healing, the left ventricle (LV) can undergo significant remodeling (Figures 10.3 and 10.4) caused by different underlying mechanisms: In the first days after infarction, the infarcted area may present significant expansion through sliding of myocytes during the inflammatory phase before collagen deposition has stabilized the extracellular matrix. This occurs particularly in areas where the extracellular matrix and microvasculature have been heavily damaged, such as in areas of microvascular obstruction. At later times, border zone and remote myocardium present left ventricular remodeling also occurring through adaptive hypertrophy of non-infarcted cardiomyocytes and extracellular matrix. These processes can continue for several months after AMI. Unfavorable MI healing and excessive remodeling may result in infarct thinning, ventricular dilatation, functional mitral regurgitation, and ultimately heart failure (HF).

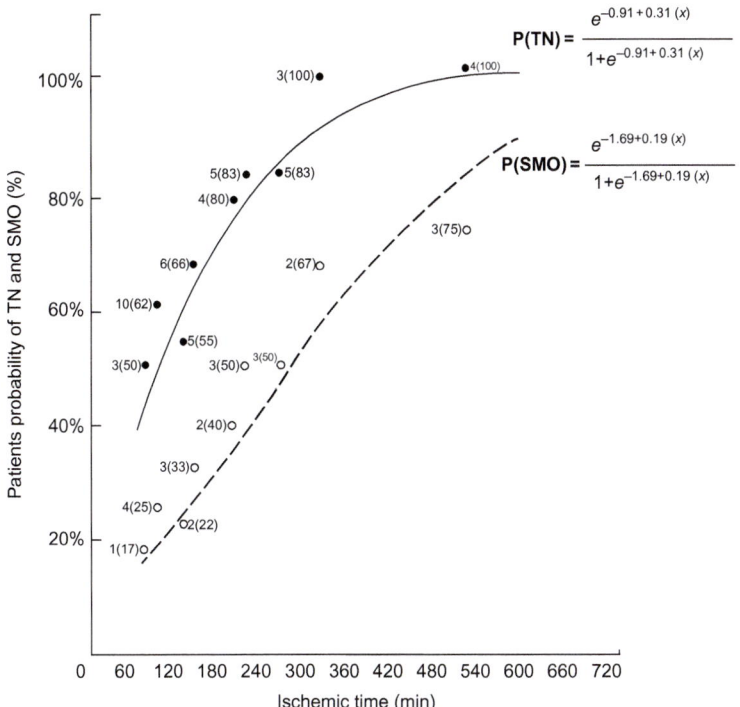

Figure 10.2 Relationship between ischemic time and probability of transmural necrosis (TN) or severe microvascular dysfunction (SMO) assessed with logistic regression model. Filled circles observed TN rate expressed in number (%); open circles observed SMO rate expressed in number (%) post-MI remodeling.
Reproduced with permissions from Ref. [6].

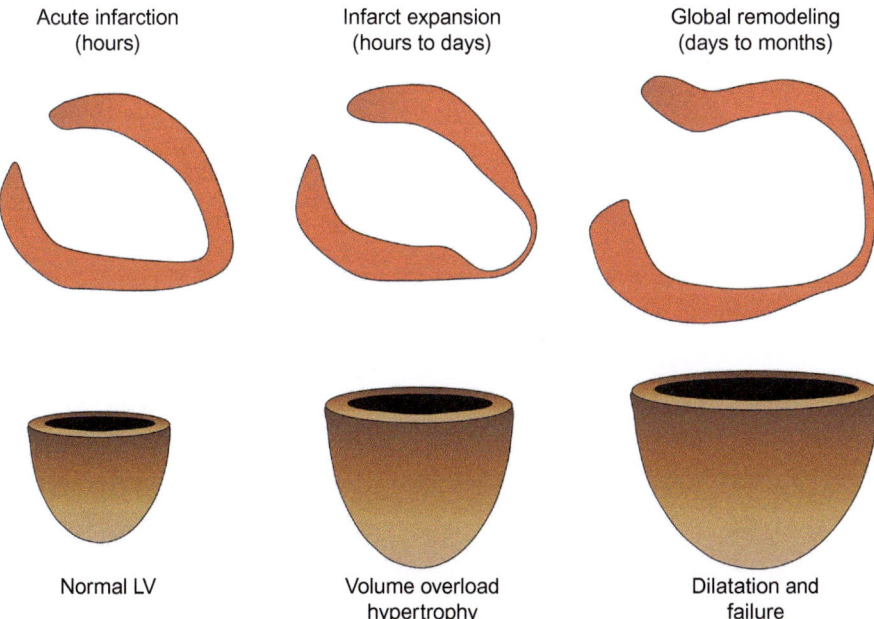

Figure 10.3 Post-MI LV remodeling.

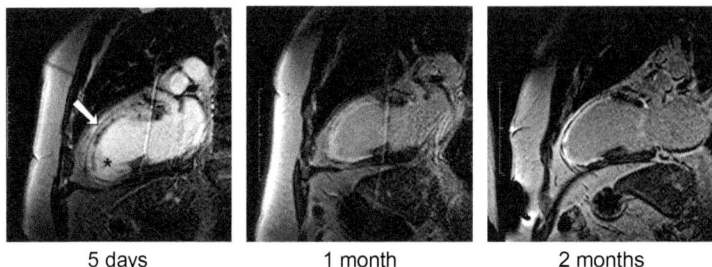

| 5 days | 1 month | 2 months |

Figure 10.4 Contrast-enhanced MR demonstrating progressive changes occurring during infarct healing of a large anterior MI over a 2-month period (arrow indicates no-reflow, * infarcted area). Area of no-reflow disappears after 1 month, over time, the infarcted area thins and the ventricle slightly enlarges due to remodeling.

10.1.2 Principles of detection of MI and associated phenomena by imaging techniques

Imaging techniques can detect AMI by various principles (Table 10.1) based on the different phenomena occurring during the ischemic cascade (Figure 10.5). Most often, AMI is revealed indirectly by demonstrating the presence of new regional wall motion abnormalities (WMA) or of new fixed perfusion defects. These features are, however non-specific, since they may occur also in acute other diseases mimicking acute coronary syndromes (ACSs), such as aborted MI with myocardial stunning, Takutsubo cardiomyopathy, myocarditis, etc. Definite detection of myocardial necrosis is allowed by late gadolinium-enhanced (LGE) CMR (and late contrast enhancement on MDCT) in typical subendocardial or transmural location corresponding to the distribution of coronary arteries. Myocardial necrosis can also be detected by ^{99m}Tc-pyrophosphate or ^{111}In-antimyosin antibody imaging, which are, however, rarely used today because of their inability to early identify the occurrence of the acute event. Fibrosis in chronic scars may also be identified by echocardiography as regions with higher ultrasound reflection [15].

The quantification of MI size (Figure 10.6) is traditionally performed in research studies by measuring Tc-99m sestamibi defect size [16]. This approach is, however, only valid for a first AMI. Measurements of ejection fraction or regional wall motion score at 6 weeks or later after AMI provide indirect measurements of MI size with good correlation to sestamibi defect. LGE CMR is currently the most accurate technique for measuring MI size; however, the actual size may depend on the cutoff value of signal intensity on LGE images that is used, and recent data suggests that LGE CMR performed very early after AMI may overestimate MI size [17] as opposed to measurement performed later than 10 days. By combining LGE and T2-weighted imaging, CMR may also separate acute from chronic MI.

Microvascular obstruction (Figure 10.7) is a phenomenon frequently associated with large infarcts and can be detected as perfusion defects in patients after reperfusion of epicardial coronary arteries. It may be revealed by various imaging techniques, in particular contrast-echocardiography, CMR, and CT. It is fairly specific,

Table 10.1 Aspects of myocardial infarcts revealed by different imaging techniques

	WMA	Global LV function	Ischemia	Coronary artery occlusion	Infarcted myocardium	Measurement of infarct size	MVO	Infarct hemorrhage	Area at risk
Echocardiography	++	+++	Possible with stress	–	–	Indirectly by WMS. EF	++ with CE	–	Possible with intracoronary CE
SPECT	+	++	+++	–	Possible with infarct avid tracers (rarely used)	Indirectly by perfusion defect	–	–	Possible before reperfusion
PET	+	+	+++	–		Indirectly by perfusion defect/FDG defect	–	–	Theoretically possible before reperfusion
MR	+++	+++	Possible with stress	+	Late enhancement	Area of LGE	++	Possible with T2/T2* T1 map	Possible by T2 imaging
CT	+–	+	Possible with stress	++	Late enhancement	Area of late-enhancement	+++		–

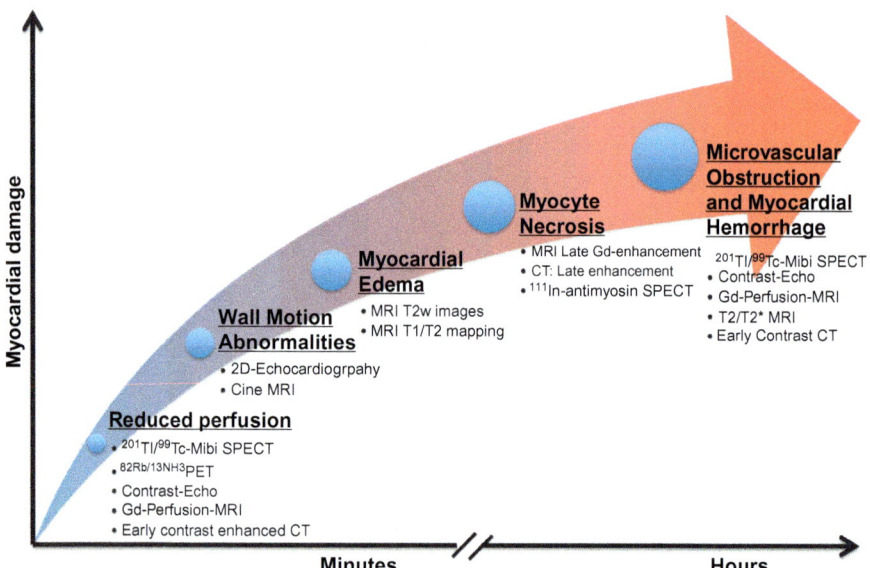

Figure 10.5 Pathophysiology of the ischemic cascade and what imaging techniques detect in acute myocardial infarction. The first process to occur is acute reduction of myocardial perfusion; this can be depicted by nuclear imaging, MR, CT, or contrast echo. Reduction of wall motion follows rapidly and can be detected by echo or cine CMR. Myocardial edema is the last reversible stage in ischemic cascade and can be identified by T2 or T1 CMR. With the progressive increase of duration, myocyte death occurs. This can be detected by late Gd and contrast-enhanced CT, and by indium antimyosine imaging. Destruction of the microvasculature and intramyocardial hemorrhage marks the most severe stage of necrosis and can be detected by nuclear perfusion imaging, contrast echo, MR, or CT.

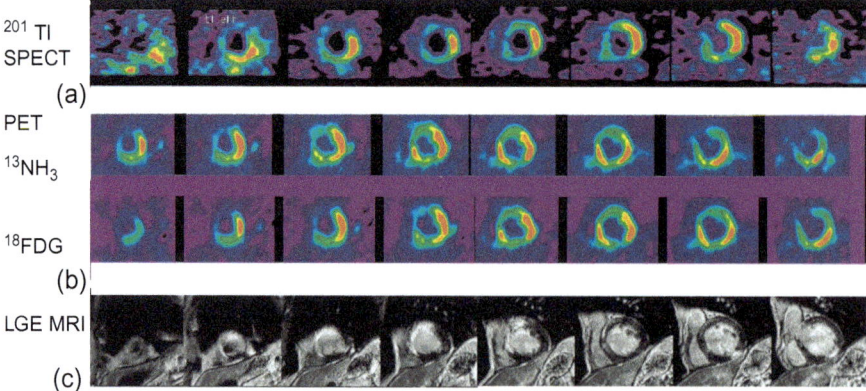

Figure 10.6 Evaluation of infarct size in a patient with a large anterior and small posterior MI by different modalities. Representative short-axis images by (a) rest 201-Tl SPECT, (b) NH_3-FDG PET, (c) late gadolinium enhanced CMR.

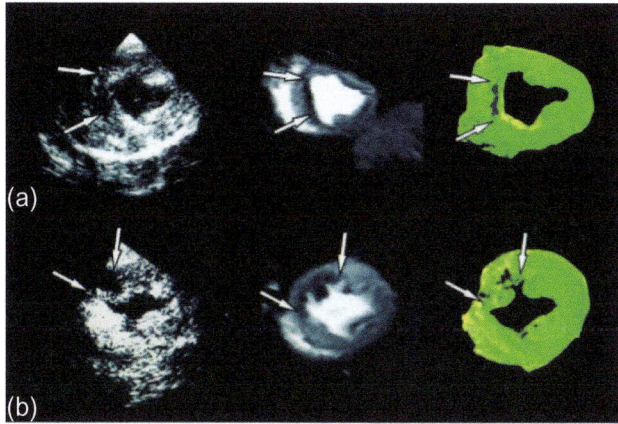

Figure 10.7 Evaluation of microvascular obstruction by contrast echo (left panels), contrast-enhanced CMR (middle panel).
Reproduced with permission from Ref. [18].

but not sensitive of AMI. It persists only for approximately 4–6 weeks after MI, and disappears thereafter, so it can provide additional information on the age of MI. Also, microvascular obstruction was shown to be an important predictor of events and left ventricular remodeling [6,19].

The area at risk of infarcts (Figure 10.8) can be measured by intracoronary contrast echocardiography in the catheter laboratory. It can also be quantified by nuclear imaging if the tracer is injected prior to opening the occluded artery and images are

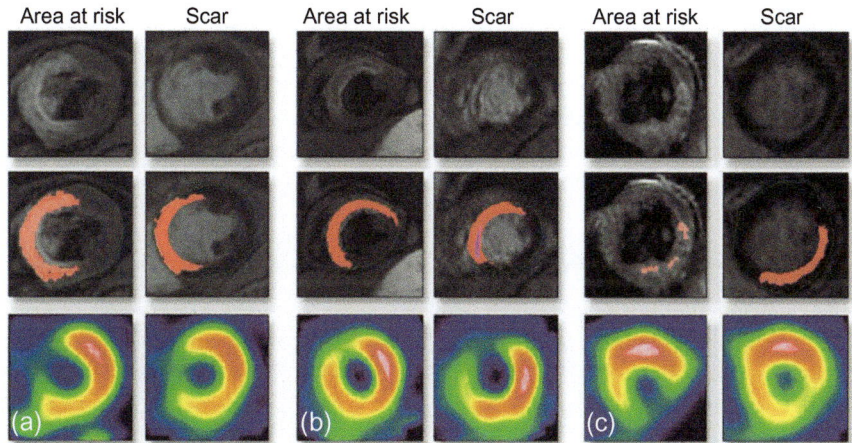

Figure 10.8 Evaluation of risk area with T2 weighted CMR and scar using late gadolinium enhancement by CMR and nuclear imaging. The top row shows CMR images, the middle panel shows the same images with the area at risk and scar delineated in red and the bottom row shows stress and rest nuclear perfusion images.
Reproduced with permission from Ref. [20].

acquired thereafter. These approaches are, however, rarely feasible in clinical practice and remain confined to research studies. A posteriori, that is, after revascularization, the area of edema by T2 weighted MR or non-enhanced T1 mapping provides an estimate of the initial area at risk. This seems to be possible up to several days after the acute event; however, controversy remains on the exact underlying mechanisms. Comparison of MI area and area at risk (AAR) allows an estimate of *myocardial salvage* [21] of revascularization therapy.

10.1.3 Role of imaging techniques in AMI in clinical practice

Imaging techniques play a major role in diagnosis, follow-up, and prognosis of patients with AMI. Clinically, *diagnosis of AMI* is usually performed by a combination of clinical symptoms (i.e., chest pain or ischemic equivalents such as dyspnea or fatigue), electrocardiographic (ECG) findings such as new significant ST–T wave changes (either ST elevation or depression), development of pathological Q waves, or new left bundle-branch block and detection of rise and/or fall of biomarkers of myocardial necrosis, and in particular of troponin I or T. For the detection of STEMI, the ECG by itself is most often diagnostic, and the decision to reperfuse should not be delayed by imaging studies. Yet in some patients, and in particular in those with non-interpretable ECG such as left bundle block, or paced rhythm, the diagnosis of MI may be uncertain and may benefit from non-invasive imaging techniques to support the diagnosis of AMI. Because of its availability and ease, echocardiography is usually the technique of choice for this purpose. Also in the setting of suspected NSTEMI with normal or borderline ECG, patients may benefit from imaging studies to confirm the diagnosis and estimate the severity of ischemic injury prior to treatment initiation.

Imaging techniques play an even more important role in detecting *complications of AMI*. Indeed, the acute phase of MI may be complicated by HF and shock, due to severe left ventricular dysfunction, or mechanical complications such as papillary muscle rupture and acute mitral regurgitation, or left ventricular septal or free wall rupture and tamponade. Echocardiography is the technique of choice for detection of these complications. Patients with AMI can also develop intraventricular thrombi complicated by systemic embolization or stroke. This may be detected by echocardiography, but more sensitively by CMR or MDCT.

The long-term *prognosis of patients with AMI* is mainly determined by the magnitude size of the initial injury (MI size), by the severity of left ventricular remodeling, and by the extent of myocardial ischemia in the remote areas subtended by the stenosed artery, in particular in patients who have undergone thrombolysis and who have not been fully revascularized (Figure 10.9). In clinical practice, LV ejection fraction (LVEF) and end-systolic volume are some of the most important predictors of prognosis in patients after acute ST- and NSTEMI [23,24]. Indeed, numerous studies have demonstrated that reduced LVEF predicts mortality, both due to HF and to arrhythmia [26]. Yet because a substantial amount of myocardium after AMI may present reversible injury due to acute stunning, the initial severity of left ventricular dysfunction can overestimate true MI size and the final degree of left ventricular dysfunction. Therefore, the true MI size is more closely estimated by LVEF late (3–6 months) post AMI than by early LVEF.

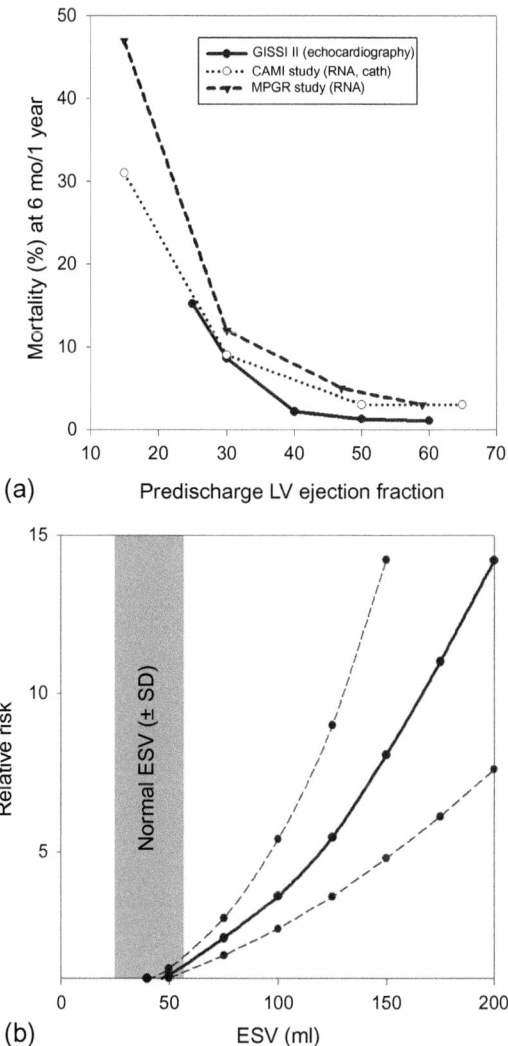

Figure 10.9 Risk of mortality according to global ejection fraction and end systolic volume. (a) Redrawn with data from Refs. [22–24]. (b) Reproduced with permission from White et al. [25].

Also, in the acute phase of MI, viability imaging by nuclear imaging, stress echo, or direct MI size measurement by CMR/MDCT can better predict prognosis than severity of contractile dysfunction. The identification of microvascular obstruction and hemorrhage appears to have additional prognostic value.

Finally, imaging may *also direct treatment*. Patients with initial large infarcts and depressed ejection fraction require more clinical attention and benefit from more aggressive treatment with ACE inhibitors and beta blockers. Those who develop large ventricles due to adverse post MI remodeling and who present persistent low LVEF have substantial risk of subsequent development of HF and high risk of sudden cardiac death from ventricular arrhythmia. The MADIT-II trial demonstrated benefit of automated implantable cardioverter defibrillator (AICD) implantation in those patients. Therefore, it is necessary to evaluate the magnitude of remodeling and measurement of LVEF by cardiac imaging, 2–3 months after MI, allowing identification of high-risk patients who may benefit from AICD implantation for primary prevention. Also, nuclear myocardial innervation imaging appears to be a promising approach to identify such patients at high risk of sudden cardiac death after MI; however, this approach has not been validated for treatment selection. Finally, stress imaging techniques play an important role in detecting ischemia due to progression of coronary artery stenosis or due to in-stent restenosis post MI and to direct revascularization therapy in these patients.

10.2 Echocardiography

10.2.1 Introduction

Because of its wide availability, and its portability to the emergency room and intensive care unit, echocardiography remains the most commonly used imaging technique in patients with AMI. It allows comprehensive evaluation not only of regional wall motion and global systolic and diastolic function, but also of valve function in patients with AMI. It also allows detection of complications such as pericardial effusion, myocardial and pericardial rupture, and intraventricular thrombus. It is therefore useful not only for the initial diagnosis, but also for the follow-up of patients with AMI, and provides important prognostic information in these patients.

10.2.2 Echocardiographic techniques in use in patients with AMI

To date, echocardiography offers a multitude of techniques for assessment of patients with AMI. *Standard 2D echocardiography* still remains the most commonly used imaging technique and allows for the comprehensive evaluation of the dimensions of the left and right ventricles, and of their systolic global and regional function, as well as imaging of the pericardium. *Doppler and tissue Doppler imaging* of mitral flow patterns allows the evaluation of diastolic function and left ventricular filling pressures. *Color, pulse, and continuous wave* Doppler imaging allows the evaluation of valve function. *Contrast echocardiography* enhances discrimination between myocardial tissue and the blood pool by opacifying the LV cavity with contrast agents, which consist of gas-filled microbubbles surrounded by a shell (see Chapter 2). Commercially available contrast agents for use are Optison, Definity, and Sonovue. These are referred to as the second-generation contrast agents and allow accurate assessment of regional and global LV function (Figure 10.10). Contrast enhancement is also recommended in patients requiring confirmation or exclusion of LV structural abnormalities and intracardiac masses and for the

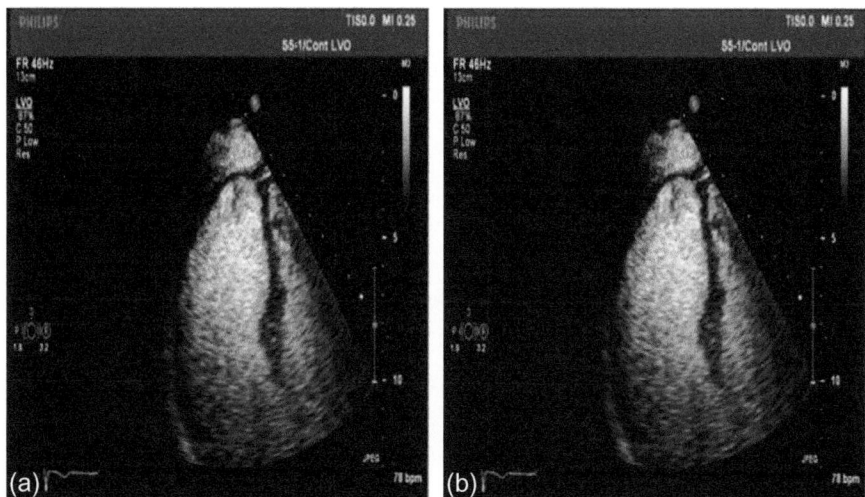

Figure 10.10 Apical three-chamber view from a subject with suboptimal endocardial visualization (a) improving dramatically after 0.3 mg of sonovue contrast injection (b).

assessment of myocardial perfusion (discussed in detail in Chapter 2) and detection of microvascular obstruction in AMI. *Myocardial deformation imaging* (MDI) using either tissue Doppler-based or 2-dimensional speckle tracking-based methods (Figure 10.11) (see Chapter 2) allows computation of regional and global myocardial strain and strain rate, parameters of regional and global of contractile function, which are believed to have higher reproducibility than 2D-LVEF. *3D echocardiography* offers advantages in the assessment of LV volumes and LVEF (Figure 10.12). Unlike 2DE, it eliminates the need for geometric modeling, which is inaccurate in the presence of aneurysms, asymmetrical LVs, and WMA, which commonly occur in patients with AMI. Several studies comparing real-time 3-dimensional echocardiography with widely accepted reference techniques such as radionuclide ventriculography and CMR have demonstrated higher levels of agreement and reproducibility in comparison to 2DE [28]. Recently, RT3DE with contrast enhancement was found to be comparable to CMR for accuracy and reproducibility of LV volumes and LVEF and superior to unenhanced images [29].

10.2.3 Role of echocardiography in AMI

10.2.3.1 Detection of AMI and ACSs in the emergency department

In patients presenting to the emergency department (ED) with possible MI, both the assessment of global [30] and regional WMA [31] enhance risk stratification and may facilitate rapid decision making. Diagnostic uncertainty remains even if resting LV function is normal when patients present several hours after chest pain with

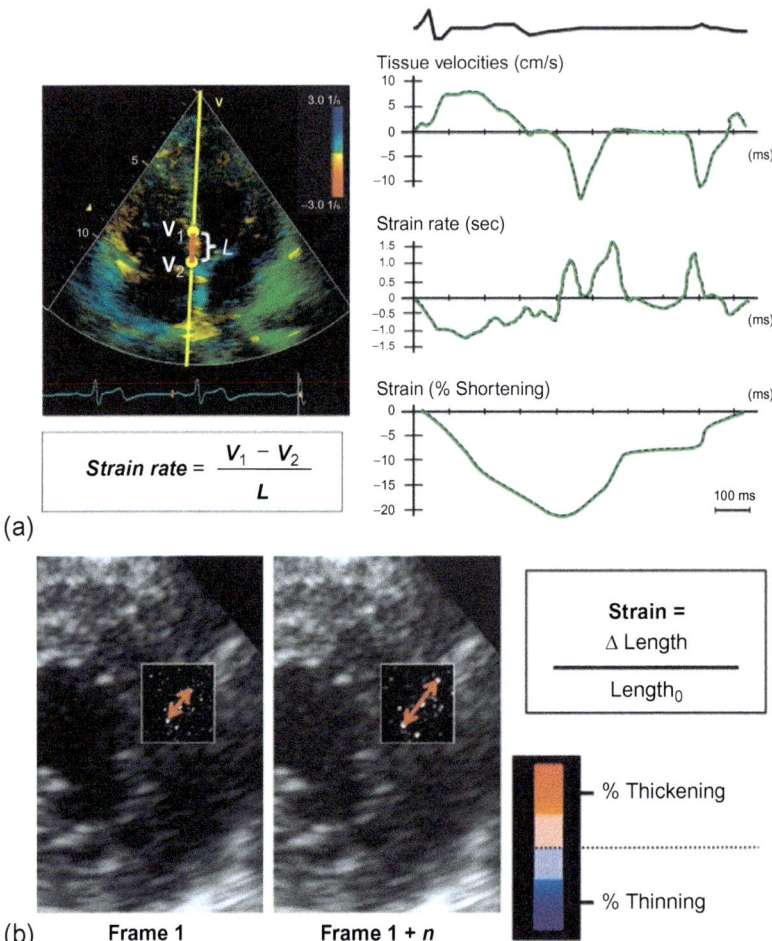

Figure 10.11 (a) Strain imaging in a normal subject. Examples of tissue Doppler imaging velocity, strain rate, and strain curves for a cardiac cycle from a subject with normal cardiac function. L, length; V, velocity. Reproduced with permission from Ref. [27]. (b) Speckle tracking strain by echocardiography diagram of speckle tracking strain from 2-dimensional short-axis echocardiographic images.
Reproduced with permission from Ref. [27].

non-diagnostic ECG, negative troponins, and an intermediate clinical risk score (TIMI score). In this population, stress echocardiography may be potentially useful in risk stratification and rapid discharge of patients with a normal stress echocardiogram. In 839 such patients, stress echocardiography performed within 24 h of admission was able to risk stratify patients during follow-up. In the first year, the event rate was 0.5% and 6.6% in the normal and abnormal stress echocardiography groups, respectively. Over 70% of patients could be discharged within 24 h with a normal stress echocardiogram [32].

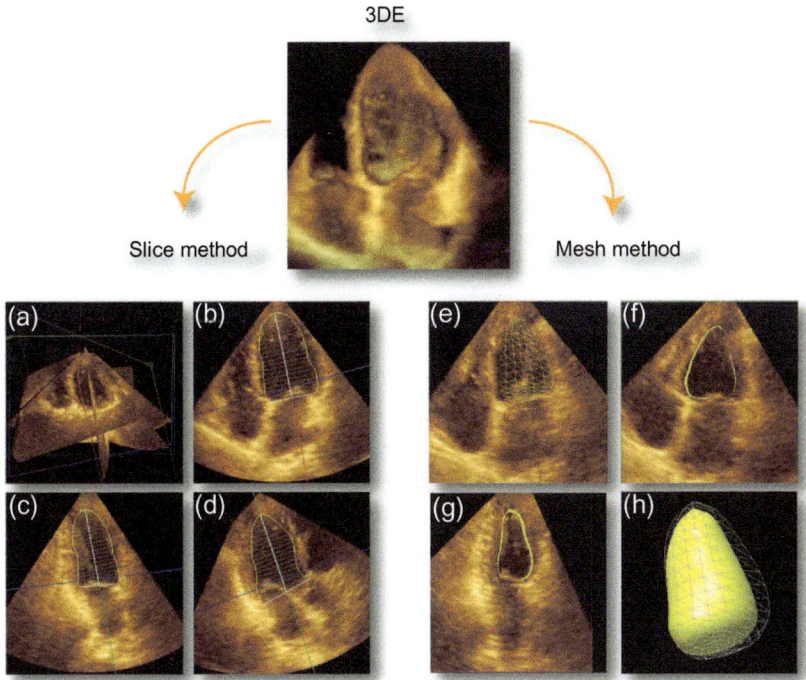

Figure 10.12 Examples of three-dimensional echocardiographic analysis using mesh and slices. Volumes can be obtained from three-dimensional echocardiographic (3DE) datasets by one of two methods. With the first, equally spaced slices are traced in end-systole and end-diastole and combined to obtain volumes (three traced slices are shown in a–d). The second method uses automated software to generate a 3D mesh from points identified on the four- and two-chamber views (e–h).
Reproduced with permission from Ref. [28].

Contrast defects by MCE allow the identification of AAR during arterial occlusion [33]. Recent work demonstrated the prognostic value of MCE in patients presenting to the ED with chest pain syndromes and non-diagnostic ECGs.

In a large single-center study in over 1000 patients in with chest pain and non-diagnostic ECG [34], adding regional function assessment by MCE increased the prognostic information of the clinical and ECG variables significantly for predicting early events occurring within 48 h. When myocardial perfusion assessment was added, additional information was obtained. Also, when patients without early events were followed up for a median of 7.7 months, those with normal perfusion and function had excellent prognosis, whereas those in whom both were abnormal had the worst outcome. Intermediate outcome was noted in those with normal perfusion despite abnormal function (Figure 10.13). In another study in 532 patients presenting to the ED, regional function on MCE provided incremental information over modified TIMI scores for predicting intermediate (<30 days) and late (>30 days) events. In patients with abnormal regional function, myocardial

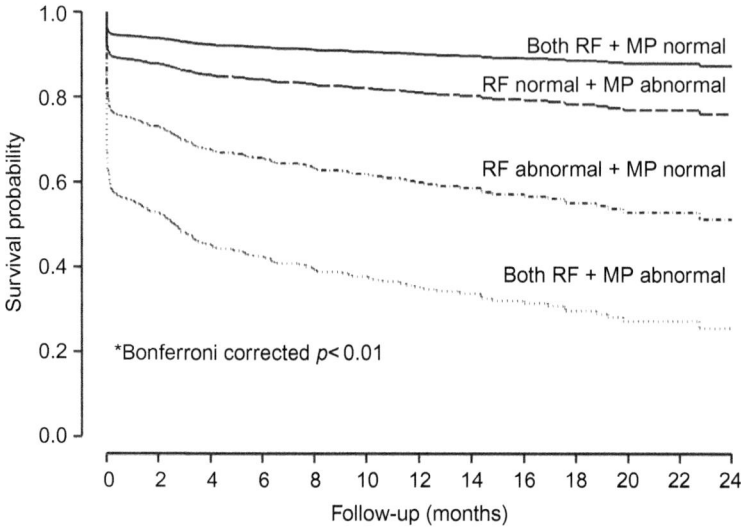

Figure 10.13 Adjusted survival probabilities for patients with different combinations of RF and MP values. *Bonferroni corrected $p < 0.01$ indicated there were significant differences in survival probabilities between any two groups.
Reproduced with permission from Ref. [34].

perfusion further classified those into intermediate- and high-risk groups. The full TIMI score (after troponin levels became available) could not improve on these results at any follow-up time point [35].

10.2.3.2 Assessment of microvascular obstruction and reperfusion in patients with established AMI

No reflow as assessed by MCE has been found to be an important predictor of LV remodeling, LV dysfunction, and adverse cardiac events in patients with established STMI. Initially, this was demonstrated using intracoronary MCE, where such imaging is performed within the first hour following PPCI. In a study of 199 patients, MCE was performed on average 15 min following PPCI. No reflow occurred in 40% of patients, and this population had higher CK levels than those without MCE no-reflow [36]. Also in patients with anterior MI, where no-reflow phenomenon identified by this technique was associated with higher incidence of pericardial effusion, early and late HF and increase in LV end diastolic volume during the convalescent period [37]. Subsequently, these results were also reproduced for intravenous MCE with second- or third-generation contrast agents. In a small number of patients, MCE performed within 24 h of AMI treated by primary PCI (PPCI) was the best predictor of LV remodeling at 1 month over clinical and angiographic parameters, with a sensitivity and specificity of 88% and 74%, respectively [38]. More recently, a larger multicenter study has produced similar results [39]. The optimal timing to assess no-reflow by intravenous MCE is at 48 h.

Here, the coronary hyperemia has settled and the dynamic character of the microcirculation has abated. One study examined patients at 24 h and 3–5 days after PCI following AMI. Intravenous MCE performed at 3–5 days correlated more strongly with contractile reserve than MCE at 24 h [40].

10.2.3.3 Risk stratification after MI

Prognosis after AMI depends on residual LV dysfunction, extent and degree of residual myocardial viability, and ischemia (at the site of MI or remote territory).

LV function

As for other techniques, LV function assessed by echocardiography strongly predicts outcome following AMI [41]. Several studies have shown that contrast-enhanced determination of LV volumes and function are more accurate and reproducible than nonenhanced echocardiography using CMR as the gold standard [42,43]. In a post-AMI study by Lim, LVEF determined by contrast-enhanced echocardiography with low-power real-time imaging was found to be more accurate compared with unenhanced echocardiography [44]. The importance of accurate assessment of LVEF is not only for risk stratification, but also accurate delivery of life-saving, invasive treatments.

Assessment of viability and ischaemia

In patients with AMI, DSE allows for detection of myocardial ischemia and viability in regions with abnormal resting function (see Chapter 11) by four different responses. (1) biphasic response—an increase in contractile function and wall thickening at low dose, with deterioration of systolic function with higher dose (Figure 10.14), indicating both viability and ischemia; (2) uniphasic—an improvement in function at low dose that persists or further improves into high dose, indicating myocardial viability; (3) worsening of resting wall function, indicating ischemia; or (4) no change in function, indicating scar. The biphasic response has the higher predictive value (72%) for improvement of regional recovery [46] than uniphasic response, since this latter pattern can be present not only in jeopardized myocardium, but also in subendocardial scar or remodeled myocardium with no flow-limiting stenosis. Although the interpretation of wall motion is subjective, and there is significant intra- and interobserver variability with DSE, in the clinical setting, the diagnostic accuracy of DSE is good with 85% sensitivity and 79% specificity for the identification of regional functional recovery [47] after AMI.

Adding tissue Doppler deformation measurements with DSE was shown to provide additional benefit over wall motion in predicting functional recovery [48–50]. Hanekom showed that the addition of strain rate imaging enhanced the sensitivity of dobutamine echocardiography (82% vs. 73%) for assessing myocardial viability, without affecting the specificity [50]. Few studies have examined the role of speckle tracking during stress testing.

Deformation imaging has also been shown to predict myocardial viability at rest. Zhang performed tissue Doppler strain rate measurements and contrast-enhanced CMR to assess the extent and transmurality of scar in the immediate post MI period.

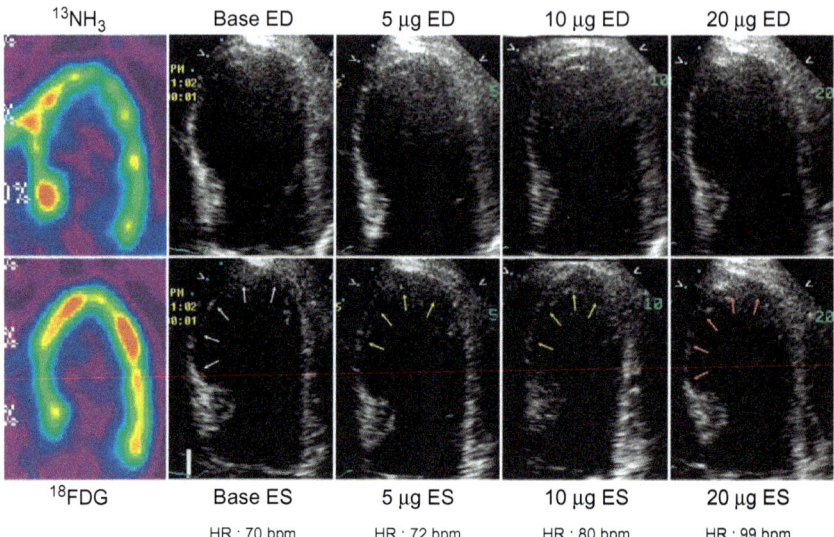

Figure 10.14 Inotropic response to dobutamine in dysfunctional segments (white arrows) with normal rest flow ($^{13}NH_3$) and F-18-fluorodeoxyglucose (^{18}FDG) uptake. The upper row shows images obtained from the apical four-chamber view in end-diastole at baseline and during the infusion of 5, 10, and 20 µg kg^{-1} min^{-1} of dobutamine. The lower row shows the corresponding end-systolic images. The yellow arrows indicate segments improving function, whereas red arrows indicate deteriorating segments. The sequence illustrates a typical biphasic response in the distal septum and the apex. Since blood flow and FDG uptake are normal in these segments, this is an example of chronically stunned myocardium.
Reproduced with permission from Ref. [45].

Peak myocardial deformation by SRI was able differentiate transmural from non-transmural MI, and thereby the extent of non-viable myocardium [51]. In 147 AMI patients, global longitudinal strain was able to predict viability and LV recovery with sensitivity 86% and specificity 74% [52].

The assessment of viability assumes that viable myocardium requires a preserved micro-vasculature. This can be accurately assessed by MCE, with its excellent spatial resolution (Figure 10.15). The absence of myocardial contrast enhancement on MCE should indicate areas that lack viability, and tissue necrosis. This was verified in 20 patients with ischemic cardiomyopathy undergoing CABG, in which MCE was performed within 24 h of surgery. Myocardial signal intensity (an index of myocardial blood volume) closely correlated with microvascular density and capillary area on pre-procedural MCE. An inverse correlation was demonstrated between the degree of myocardial fibrosis, and myocardial intensity [54]. The role of MCE in predicting regional and global wall motion recovery after AMI is well documented. In 96 AMI patients with a patent infarct related artery, failure of myocardial replenishment within 10 cardiac cycles during high-power imaging resulted in lack of recovery of function in 84% of the time [55]. Similarly in patients with recent AMI and occluded infarct-related artery (IRA), MCE accurately evaluates

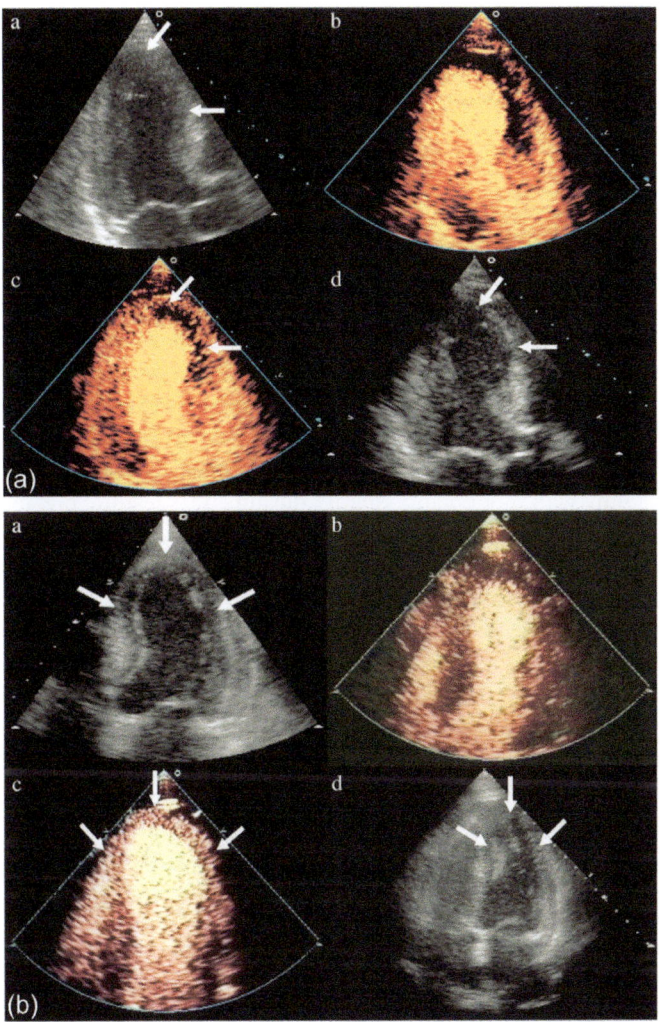

Figure 10.15 (a) End-systolic frames of the apical three-chamber view showing: (Aa) akinetic mid-anterior septum and apex (arrows); (Ab) complete destruction of myocardial contrast immediately after a high mechanical index pulse on MCE; (Ac) lack of contrast opacification of the dysynergic segments, even at 15 cardiac cycles (arrows); (Ad) lack of functional recovery at 12 weeks despite revascularization (arrows). (b) End-systolic frames of the apical four-chamber view showing: (Ba) akinetic mid-septum, apex, and mid-lateral segments (arrows); (Bb) complete destruction of myocardial contrast immediately after a high mechanical index pulse on MCE; (Bc) homogenous contrast opacification of the dysynergic segments by 15 cardiac cycles (arrows); (Bd) functional recovery at 12 weeks after revascularization (arrows).
Reproduced with permission from Ref. [53].

collateral blood flow and contractile reserve [56]. In a study by Janardhanan, 50 patients underwent low power continuous MCE 7–10 days after AMI. Myocardial segments that did not replenish within 10–15 cardiac cycles following microbubble destruction showed significantly less contractile reserve after revascularization compared with those segments that replenished. Contrast intensity measured in this way had a predictive value of 90% for the presence of contractile reserve. The absence of contrast enhancement predicted the absence of contractile reserve in 90% of cases (Figure 10.6) [57].

There is excellent agreement between MCE and DSE in predicting LV functional recovery [58]. Senior et al. assessed the incremental value of MCE in addition to low-dose dobutamine for the assessment of viability post MI [59]. The presence of contrast enhancement in segments with no contractile response resulted in improvement in function compared with segments with no contrast enhancement. MCE thus predicted viability in this group of patients with no contractile response to dobutamine. Perfusion abnormalities appear earlier in the ischemic cascade, followed by wall motion abnormality during stress testing, making perfusion more sensitive.

Although LVEF is a powerful predictor of outcome, the extent and intensity of the perfusion defect is a superior predictor of recovery of LV function. This underscores the fact that perfusion, not wall motion abnormality, accurately differentiates stunned from necrotic myocardium. MCE performed 7–10 days post MI predicts the transmural extent of AMI as assessed by CMR [60], and predicts cardiovascular outcomes immediately following AMI [26]. 99 patients post thrombolysis underwent MCE at 7 ± 2 days and were followed up for 46 ± 16 months. The extent of residual myocardial viability was an independent predictor of cardiac death and cardiac death or AMI. A Contrast Defect Index of <1.86 and <1.67 predicted survival and survival or absence of re- current AMI in 99% and 95% of the patients, respectively [26].

The accuracy of vasodilator MCE for detecting flow-limiting coronary artery stenosis in suspected coronary artery has been confirmed in several studies. A 73-patient study demonstrated the ability of Dipyridamole MCE to detect residual IRA stenosis and presence of remote flow-limiting CAD in patients with recent STEMI and thrombolysis (Figure 10.16). Sensitivities for the detection of >50% IRA stenosis and MVD were 88% and 72%, respectively [61].

10.3 Nuclear imaging

10.3.1 Introduction

Nuclear imaging allows the assessment of the major predictors of subsequent patient outcome after AMI, including MI size, LVEF, LV volumes, and the presence and extent of residual myocardial ischemia [62] and therefore also plays an important role in the initial evaluation and risk stratification of patients surviving AMI, as well as in guiding and monitoring subsequent patient management.

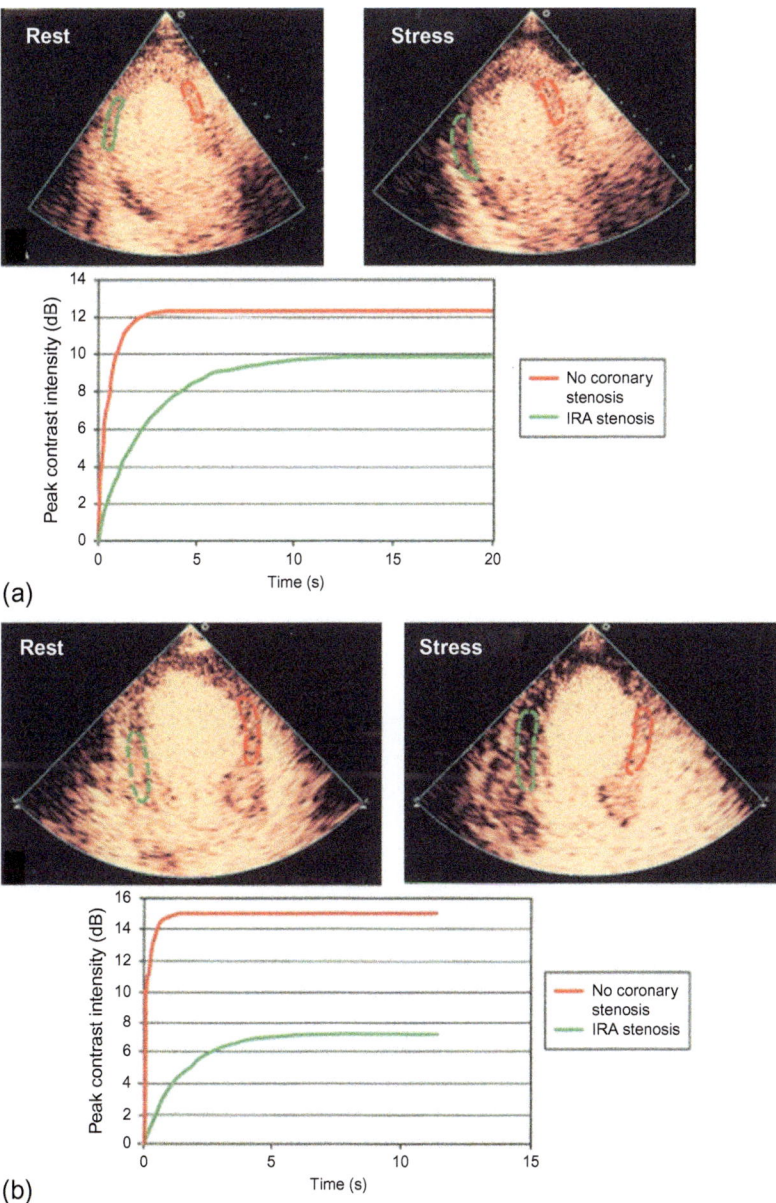

Figure 10.16 (a) Apical three-chamber view shows reversible perfusion defect (posterior wall) at the infarct site. (b) Apical three-chamber view shows reversible perfusion defect in the remote, normally contracting mid-posterior segment in a patient with an anterior acute myocardial infarction. (Graphs) Replenishment curves demonstrate reduced peak contrast intensity (MBV—α) and rate of replenishment (myocardial blood velocity—β) during stress, suggesting residual infarct-related artery (IRA) stenosis (A) and multivessel disease (B). Red indicates no coronary stenosis; green indicates significant coronary stenosis.
Reproduced with permission from Ref. [53].

10.3.2 Principles of AMI imaging by nuclear imaging

Nuclear cardiac imaging can detect MI by demonstrating fixed perfusion defects present both at stress and rest myocardial perfusion imaging (MPI) (Figure 10.17). It also allows measurement of myocardial ejection fraction on gated MPI (Figure 10.17) or radionuclide angiography. Myocardial damage can also be directly detected with infarct

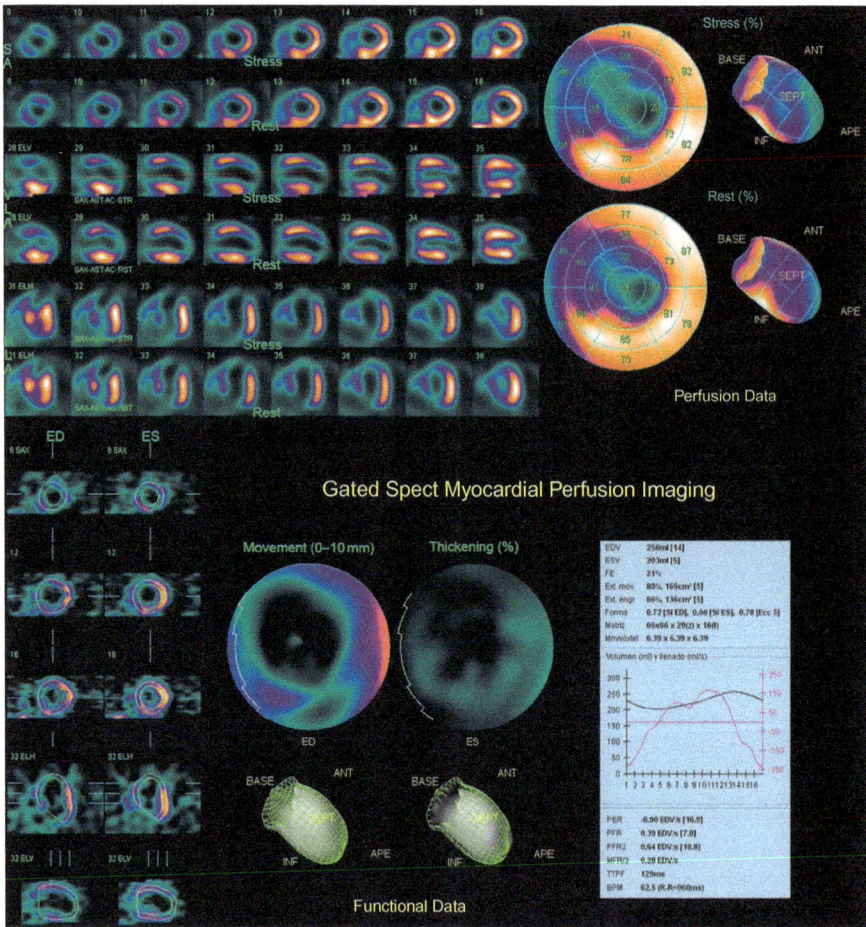

Figure 10.17 Stress/rest gated SPECT myocardial perfusion imaging of a patient with an extensive myocardial infarction. The upper part of the figure shows the left ventricle (LV) perfusion data (slices, polar maps, and 3D displays). The bottom part of the figure shows the functional data. There is LV dilatation with a fixed defect (infarction) compressing 27% of the LV (mid and apical anteroseptal segments as well as the apical lateral and apical inferior segments and the apex); with mild reversibility (ischemia) in the mid anteroseptal segment. There is generalized hypokinesis (LV ejection fraction 21%) as well as akinesis and decreased systolic thickening of the area, showing reduced tracer uptake. SA, short-axis slices (extending from the apex to the base); VLA, vertical long-axis slices (extending from the septum to the lateral wall); HLA, horizontal long-axis slices (extending from the inferior wall to the anterior wall); ED, end-diastole at mid LV; ES, end-systole at LV.

avid tracers. Finally abnormalities of cardiac sympathetic innervation in infarcted areas can be detected by ^{123}I-metaiodobenzylguanidine (^{123}I-mIBG) scintigraphy.

10.3.2.1 Myocardial perfusion imaging

As discussed in Chapter 3, MPI with gated single-photon emission tomography (SPECT) evaluates relative myocardial blood volume at rest and stress. Resting MPI defect size has shown to accurately assess MI size. Animal studies with ^{99m}Tc-sestamibi and ^{99m}Tc-tetrofosmin demonstrate close correlation between their respective initial myocardial uptake and occluded flows by microspheres, and the gradient in count activity between normally perfused and infarcted zones remains relatively constant over time [63–65]. Therefore, quantitative assessment of the total LV perfusion defect size, the extent of inducible ischemia, and the degree of LV dysfunction is possible with a single imaging technique.

MI size has been quantitated on MPI using a standardized approach [66] based on cardiac phantom studies [67]. The feasibility of performing multicentre trials using MPI in patients with AMI was demonstrated in a cardiac phantom experiment, which showed that the measured MI size closely correlated with the actual phantom defect size with an average absolute error of <3% of the LV [68]. The quantitation was not subject to differences in camera, collimator, or imaging routine [68]. In one large trial, 98% of 1184 studies provided analyzable end point data [69].

In addition, a close association between MI size measured by MPI and various parameters related with MI size used clinically has been published, including LVEF, LV end-systolic volume, LV regional wall motion, and enzyme release [16].

A close association between fibrosis in human hearts and MI size assessed by MPI has been described. The defect of tracer uptake measured by *ex vivo* MPI of myocardial slices from explanted human hearts showed a close association with the quantitation of fibrosis by pathology in a cardiac transplantation study [70]. Likewise, a good correlation between *in vivo* MPI defect size and the amount of fibrosis has been found on myocardial biopsies [71].

Although measurements of global and regional LV function are often used clinically in the estimation of MI size, these measurements are less direct and are influenced by the presence of arrhythmias, cardiomyopathies, valvular heart disease, and ventricular loading.

10.3.2.2 Infarct avid tracers

MI avid imaging evolved from ^{99m}Tc-pyrophosphate to ^{111}In-labeled monoclonal antimyosin antibodies and, more recently, ^{99m}Tc-glucarate [72].

^{99m}Tc-pyrophosphate is a polyphosphate derivative, first introduced for bone scanning, which bounds to the necrotic myocardium in relation to the presence of residual MBF or the redevelopment of MBF to the infarcted region, predominantly targeting the sequestered calcium phosphate deposited in the mitochondria of the infarcted or severely injured myocardium [73]. The process thus occurs within a few hours of the acute event if the infarct-related artery is patent, or later (≥ 12 h) if the vessel remains occluded. Maximum infarct uptake occurs 24–72 h later, and usually lasts for 6–10 days [73].

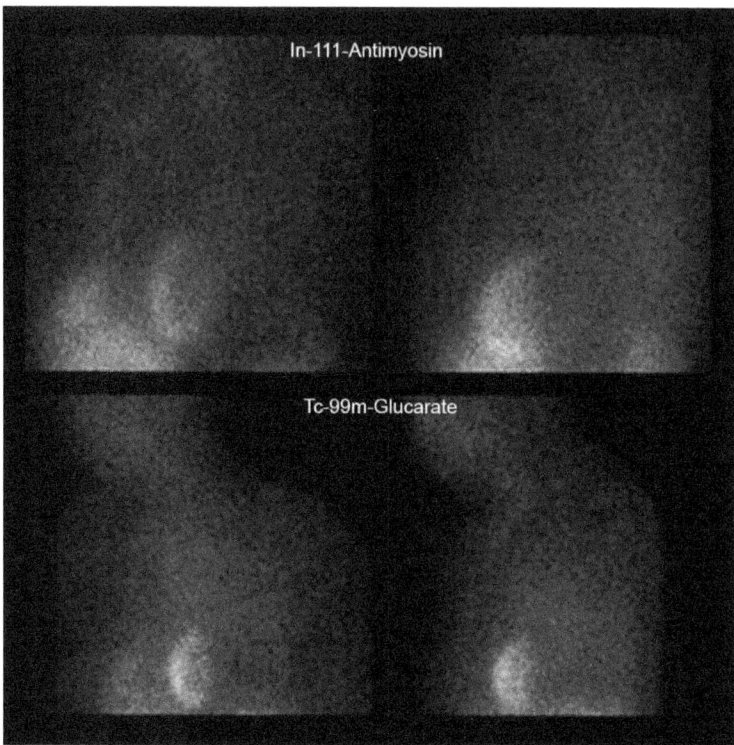

Figure 10.18 45° and 70° LAO images of a patient with an extensive anteroseptal and apical myocardial infarction showing matched uptake of ^{111}In-antimyosin and ^{99m}Tc-glucarate.

^{111}In-labeled murine monoclonal antimyosin Fab antibody fragments (R11D10-Fab) target specifically and with high affinity the intracellular heavy chain of cardiac myosin exposed to extracellular fluid by loss of cell membrane integrity [72] (Figure 10.18).

The sensitivity and specificity of both tracers for AMI detection vary depending on MI size and the timing of imaging, but in the appropriate setting have generally provided similar sensitivity results (87–98% for Q wave MI, and 78–84% for non-Q wave MI) [72], with ^{111}In-antimyosin being more specific (85–96%) [72,74]. In contrast to ^{99m}Tc-pyrophosphate, ^{111}In-antimyosin uptake is maximum in areas with severe flow impairment [73]. This difference may be explained considering that antimyosin antibodies remain in the plasma much longer time than pyrophosphate does, which is rapidly cleared from the blood due to bone uptake and renal clearance, thus antimyosin would have a greater opportunity to interact with necrotic tissue. However ^{111}In-antimyosin uptake is more intense in MI with reperfusion than in those MI with persistent coronary occlusion. The time interval between ^{111}In-antimyosin administration and effective visualization of the target necrotic myocardial region has been a major clinical concern because of the delayed blood-pool clearance of ^{111}In-antimyosin. In reperfused canine models, the experimental MI could be visualized relatively soon after the administration of ^{111}In-antimyosin, although visualization of nonreperfused infarcts took longer time.

The uptake of ^{111}In-antimyosin by infarcted myocardium may persist for as long as 9 months after the acute event [75], although the intensity of uptake tends to decrease with time. Slow clearance of such a large and insoluble molecule as myosin by granulocytes may account for this persistent uptake. Thus, the use of ^{111}In-antimyosin scintigraphy to differentiate acute from old myocardial injury occurring within 1 year should be interpreted using all available clinical information.

Although these two infarct avid tracers are effective in localizing MI, they have limited clinical value due to their inability to early identify the occurrence of the acute event for an early use of interventions aimed at myocardial salvage. ^{99m}Tc-glucarate has been reported to be useful in this setting. Glucaric acid is a six-carbon dicarboxylic acid sugar, natural endogenous end-catabolite of UDP-glucose that can be labeled with ^{99m}Tc [76]. ^{99m}Tc-glucarate does not accumulate in ischemic or old necrotic tissues. The proposed mechanism of ^{99m}Tc-glucarate localization in MI is through collateral circulation and/or diffusion across sarcolemmal breaches owing to its avidity for the positively charged histones within disintegrated nuclei and reduced subcellular organelles proteins in necrotic myocytes [72].

^{99m}Tc-glucarate distribution in the central necrotic zone closely parallels the distribution of ^{111}In-antimyosin (Figure 10.18), contrarily to ^{99m}Tc-pyrophosphate, which principally accumulates peripherally to the necrosis, where residual MBF is highest. ^{99m}Tc-glucarate by comparison appears to have less dependence on residual MBF for tracer delivery, and a rapid uptake into either reperfused or nonreperfused necrotic myocardium, with a relative rapid blood-flow clearance, which allows imaging within 1–2 h of injection [72]. However, since ^{99m}Tc-glucarate predominantly targets the positively charged histones, which disintegrate fairly rapidly, the clinical window for ^{99m}Tc-glucarate uptake appears to be limited to 9 h after the onset of an AMI. This time window may allow differentiation of acute from recent MI [72]. If early ^{99m}Tc-glucarate uptake in AMI with persistently occluded infarct related coronary artery is confirmed in clinical studies, it may help to direct the use of thrombolytic therapy in patients presenting with equivocal diagnosis, as well as to differentiate acute from old MI. Neither ^{99m}Tc-glucarate nor ^{111}In-antimyosin are commercially available currently.

10.3.2.3 Innervation imaging (^{123}I-mIBG)

Imaging cardiac autonomic nervous system has shown to be of value in the assessment of patients with different cardiac disorders, especially in those with HF, where it has an independent prognostic value and provides a potential tool for improving patient management [77].

^{123}I-mIBG is the most used tracer for cardiac innervation imaging. Cardiac ^{123}I-mIBG uptake and retention is reflected, with good reliability [78,79], by the heart to mediastinum ratio (HMR) at early (15 min) and late (4 h) planar images and the washout rate (WR) between them. The late HMR reflects the relative distribution of sympathetic nerve terminals, offering the global information about neuronal function resulting from uptake, storage and release. The WR is an index of the sympathetic tone [77].

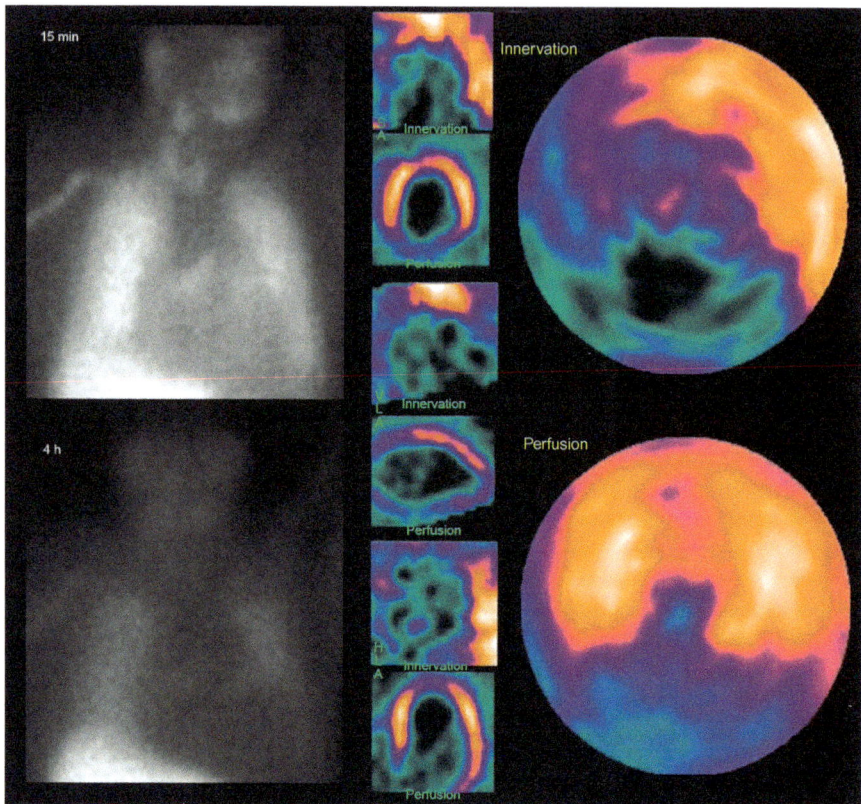

Figure 10.19 Anterior planar images at 15 min and 4 h after ^{123}I-MIBG injection, showing extremely reduced cardiac sympathetic innervation of a patient with an old inferior myocardial infarction and heart failure (NYHA class III, left ventricular ejection fraction 15%), candidate to ICD placement. Innervation (4 h) and perfusion SPECT slices at mid left ventricle and polar maps show an extensive innervation defect compressing the inferior, septal, and inferolateral walls as well as the apex. The defect is less pronounced in the perfusion study. SA, short-axis slices; VLA, vertical long-axis slices; HLA, horizontal long-axis slices.

The sympathetic nervous tissue is more sensitive to ischemia than the myocardial tissue. ^{123}I-mIBG uptake is significantly reduced in areas of MI and adjacent noninfarcted regions (Figure 10.19), as well as in areas with acute and chronic ischemia. Reinnervation late after MI in periinfarct regions has been demonstrated by reappearance of ^{123}I-mIBG uptake, which may be in part responsible for the improvement of function. It is likely that ischemia induces damage to sympathetic neurons which may take a long time to regenerate resulting in decreased ^{123}I-mIBG uptake [77]. This characteristic may be important in the pathophysiology of HF and arrhythmias [80] and offers potential for ^{123}I-mIBG imaging at rest for the detection of sporadic transient ischemic attacks such as those of vasospastic angina, and for the evaluation of the AAR in the subacute phase of ACSs by revealing more extensive defects than MPI at rest, as well as a marker of reversible ischemia in patients with contraindications for stress MPI.

10.3.3 Prognostic value of nuclear imaging in AMI

Scintigraphic size of MI has shown to predict subsequent survival following the acute event. MI size as determined by resting MPI is frequently used as a surrogate marker for mortality in clinical trials assessing therapies during acute MI [62].

In addition, LVEF and LV volumes can be accurately measured with gated SPECT MPI [81], which is important since LVEF is still the single best long-term predictor of mortality in survivors of AMI, irrespective of initial therapy during ST elevation MI (STEMI). It should be taken into account that if the LVEF is measured within the first 2 weeks after MI, cardiac risk could be overestimated because of the presence of myocardial stunning that may subsequently resolve over the ensuing 1–2 months. LV enlargement is also related with increased mortality in patients with AMI, particularly when coexisting with myocardial dysfunction (LVEF < 50%) [25].

The amount of tracer uptake predicts the response of myocardium with abnormal function to subsequent revascularization in chronic CAD, and the recovery of myocardium after reperfusion therapy for AMI. The mismatch between MI size and LV function after reperfusion therapy in AMI identified myocardial stunning in both retrospective [82] and prospective [83] studies. MPI infarct size measured at discharge predicts short-term patient mortality in both single-center [84] and multicenter [85] studies. In the largest study among 1181 patients, MI size assessment by MPI at 1–2 weeks after MI was significantly associated with 6-month mortality [86]. Furthermore, two different randomized trials have shown a corresponding improvement in clinical outcome in association with treatment that reduces MI size as determined by means of serial MPI with ^{99m}Tc-sestamibi [87,88].

The presence and extent of residual myocardial ischemia are strong predictors of cardiac events and improve risk stratification beyond that provided by clinical variables or the extent of CAD. The assessment of total and ischaemic perfusion defects and LVEF by means of MPI allows risk stratification of individual patients and early hospital discharge [89,90]. Patients with AMI and preserved LV function and no residual ischemia are at very low risk, which is no further reduced with coronary revascularization [91]. Likewise, PCI of an occluded infarct-related artery does not improve outcome over medical therapy in patients who have depressed LV function and minimal or no residual ischemia [3].

Pharmacologic vasodilators such as adenosine, regadenoson, and dipyridamole can be administered safely within 1–2 days of AMI, allowing very early risk stratification based on MPI results and thereby expediting appropriate patient care [89].

In patients with STEMI treated with primary PCI in the current era of interventional cardiology, MPI could be used to identify viable myocardium within the MI zone, to assess for ischemia outside the MI zone in those patients with multivessel CAD, and to predict recovery in LV function in those with myocardial stunning. In addition, patients not treated with primary PCI are also good candidates for noninvasive risk stratification using MPI. Regarding viability assessment, ^{18}F-fluorodeoxyglucose (FDG) metabolic imaging with positron emission tomography (PET) in conjunction with MBF imaging with ^{13}N ammonia (NH_3) or ^{82}Rb has become a recognized clinical standard [92].

10.3.3.1 Positron emission tomography

PET offers the unique opportunity to quantitatively measure physiological parameters such as absolute MBF (using NH_3, ^{15}O, water or ^{82}Rb), oxidative (using ^{11}C acetate) and glucose metabolism (using FDG) in post-infarcted myocardium, allowing better understanding of the underlying pathophysiology of infarcted, stunned, and hibernating myocardium [93]. In clinical practice, the typical assessment of myocardial viability using PET relies rather on a semiquantitative comparison of regional myocardial perfusion by either ^{13}N ammonia or ^{82}Rb and glucose utilization using FDG in the dysfunctional myocardium relative to remote normally functioning myocardium (see Chapter 11 for a more detailed discussion of myocardial viability assessment). Different perfusion/metabolism patterns have been described in dysfunctional myocardium and related to recovery of myocardial function: Infarcted non-viable myocardium typically presents with reduced perfusion and concomitant reduced or absence of FDG uptake (the so called perfusion-metabolism match) pattern. Under fasted conditions and after glucose load, dysfunctional myocardium with preserved viability has been shown to present either both normal perfusion and FDG uptake, or a pattern of moderate reduced perfusion with increased FDG uptake (perfusion-metabolism mismatch pattern), since dysfunctional hibernated or postischemic stunned myocardium displays preferential use of glucose rather than free fatty acids as metabolic substrate. Alternative protocols to standardize myocardial glucose uptake other than oral glucose loading include the more time-consuming hyperinsulinemic euglycemic clamp or administration of nicotinic acid, which blocks lipid utilization by the heart. Several studies have examined the value of detection of viability by NH_3-FDG PET for predicting recovery of LV function after AMI and demonstrated high accuracy of the technique [94].

As discussed above, myocardial sympathetic innervation is an important determinant of prognosis (LV remodeling, HF, and arrhythmic events) after MI. ^{11}C-metahydroxyephedrine (^{11}C-HED) is a structural radiolabeled analog of norepinephrine and allows interrogating presynaptic catecholamine reuptake (which is reduced either with increased sympathetic drive, or with rarification of sympathetic nerve endings). The recent PAREPET study [95] demonstrated in 204 survivors of AMI that reduced myocardial ^{11}C-HED uptake (meaning sympathetic denervation) was a strong and independent predictor of sudden cardiac death over a follow-up of 4.1 years. Such information may allow an improvement in risk stratification in AMI survivors and in the selection of those at higher risk for AICD implantation.

10.3.4 Future directions in nuclear imaging of AMI

The role of nuclear cardiac imaging in AMI continues to evolve. New imaging devices with higher spatial and contrast resolution are being developed [96], with capability to detect subendocardial MI, as well as to quantify the MI size with increased confidence, which will enhance the assessment of dysfunctional myocardial states associated with depressed myocardial flow, i.e., differentiation between hibernating myocardium and nontransmural MI. Furthermore, new tracers for PET MPI are also being developed, with higher myocardial extraction than that of SPECT tracers and closer linearity with MBF [97]. Additionally, potential advantages of PET over SPECT include higher resolution and sensitivity, as well as robust attenuation correction and absolute quantification of MBF, with higher accuracy than SPECT in the diagnosis of CAD [98]. Furthermore, all these developments allow a shortening of the acquisition protocols and/or lowering of patient radiation exposure. The advent of hybrid SPECT/CT and PET/CT equipment offers the additional clinical advantages of evaluating coronary calcium and myocardial anatomy (including non-invasive CT angiography) together with myocardial function and myocardial perfusion in a single imaging procedure. Finally, the development of new tracers for vascular imaging of the coronary bed may also allow the identification of vulnerable plaques and better predict which patients with cardiovascular risks factors are likely to have a subsequent cardiac event.

Recently hybrid PET/CMR imaging systems are being developed. This novel assembly combines the high soft tissue contrast of CMR with the high molecular sensitivity of PET. While their advantages over conventional PET/CT scanners have not been proven systematically yet, for cardiac imaging PET/CMR may offer some interesting avenues: The high soft tissue contrast of CMR allows for differentiation of myocardial integrity and cine imaging allows for accurate assessment of myocardial wall motion. Late gadolinium enhancement is useful in distinguishing infarcted from viable myocardium. In combination with FDG and NH_3 PET, integrated PET/CMR may offer interesting possibilities to distinguish infarcted or necrotic from viable underperfused myocardium [99].

10.4 CMR imaging

10.4.1 Introduction

The role of CMR in the diagnosis of AMI has been increasing over the last decade. New techniques including edema quantification and detection of myocardium at risk as well as refinements in identification of fibrosis enabled not only diagnosis of small infarcts, but also the differentiation of MI from other acute chest pain syndromes with altered biomarkers, such as myocarditis and Takotsubo cardiomyopathy. The most recent consensus document defining MI [1] highlighted the importance of CMR in the detection of both acute and chronic MI due to its accuracy in identifying WMA and the high accuracy of LGE CMR in detecting myocardial necrosis.

10.4.2 Principles of MI imaging by CMR

CMR is a versatile modality that allows different approaches for detection of myocardial damage at different time points. Considering that myocardial damage is a sequence of events ranging from WMA to myocardial necrosis, different CMR methods are used to identify these alterations, according to the onset of symptoms. Figure 10.4 exemplifies that CMR can be used to track the evolution of myocardial damage over time.

10.4.2.1 First-pass perfusion images

The assessment of myocardial perfusion in CMR for detection of significant coronary stenosis has been validated in unicenter and multicenter trials. T1-weighted fast gradient-echo sequences (with echo-planar images when available for faster acquisition times) produce high contrast/high resolution images to analyze first pass dynamic myocardial perfusion. In the setting of an ACS, rest perfusion images can highlight hypoperfused areas related to the culprit vessel, even in the absence of fibrosis detected by LGE images. Although rest/stress myocardial perfusion CMR protocols were developed for patients in the investigation of stable CAD, this technique can identify the impaired rest myocardial blood flow in patients with ACS. In chronic infarcts, both rest and stress images may show hypointense areas that match with fibrotic areas identified by LGE images, although due to residual contrast and variability in the blood supply to infarcted tissue, perfusion CMR is not reliable on its own in identifying MI.

10.4.2.2 Wall motion abnormalities

New regional WMA are an early alteration in the myocardial ischemic cascade. Cine CMR imaging offers excellent resolution images and is widely accepted as the gold standard for global and regional myocardial function assessment. However, small infarcts are not usually associated with contractile dysfunction, and other pathologies such as myocarditis can be related to WMA, which denotes that these findings should not be a cornerstone in the definition of an AMI. On the other hand, analysis of regional myocardial function is crucial to define other diagnosis, such as stress (Takotsubo) cardiomyopathy. Additionally, there are data showing the role of WMA for detecting patients with ACSs, even in absence of biomarkers of necrosis, with an accuracy of 82%, when using the analysis of myocardial thickening [100]. More recently, other pulse sequences that can be used to analyze myocardial function (SENC, DENSE, phase velocity) have been proposed; however, more studies validating these new techniques are needed.

10.4.2.3 Quantification of myocardial area at risk and myocardial salvage

Two CMR approaches have been proposed for estimation of "area at risk": endocardial surface area (ESA) of LGE images and T2W detection of edema. The ESA of LGE is an indirect measure of AAR, based on the assumption of the "wavefront phenomenon" [2] that myocardial injury extends from the subendocardial to subepicardial layers with no or minimum lateral extension. Using this principle, the AAR is estimated as the ratio of endocardial extent of necrosis (identified by LGE images) and the total endocardial circumference. This method has shown excellent correlation ($r=0.90$) to at risk myocardium estimated angiographically using the Myocardial Jeopardy Index [101], but other studies did not find favorable results using this approach [102,103], probably because ESA would underestimate the myocardial salvage in aborted infarctions [102].

T2-weighted images (T2W) using double inversion-recovery fast spin echo can detect myocardial edema, a marker of acute injury [104], and thus determine myocardial

AAR. Previous studies supported the use of T2W images in the identification of ACSs in the emergency department. Cury et al. [105] implemented a comprehensive protocol including T2W images, first-pass perfusion, cine function, late gadolinium-enhancement images, and assessment of left ventricular wall thickness for evaluation of acute chest pain. They found that the addition of T2W and left ventricular wall thickness increased the overall accuracy from 84% to 93% ($p<0.01$). Fuernau et al. [102] showed a good correlation between AAR estimated by T2W images and angiography ($r=0.87$), but only modest correlation between ESA and angiographically estimated AAR ($r=0.44$). Figure 10.20 shows a representative case of myocardial edema related to AMI.

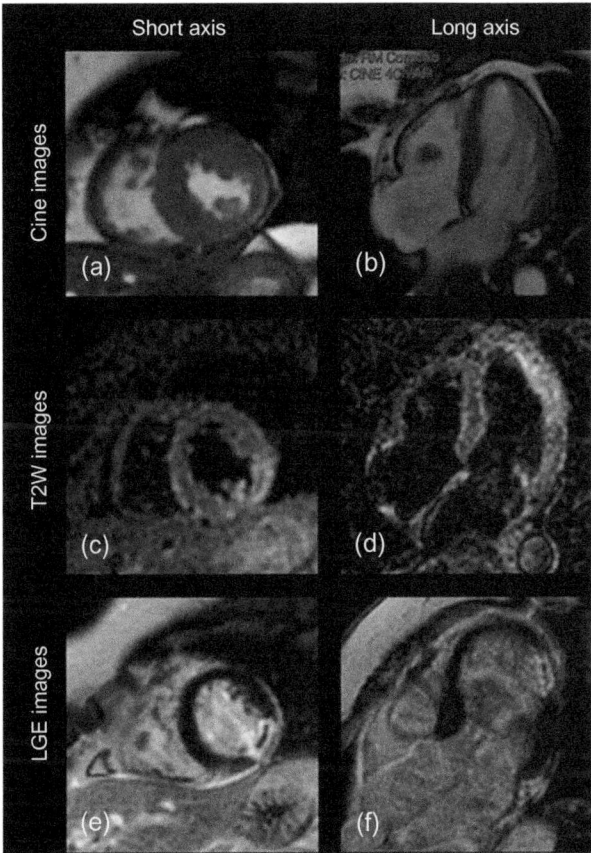

Figure 10.20 Representative case of a patient with acute MI in CMR. (a) Short axis cine image (systole) showing a regional contractile deficit in inferolateral wall (white arrow). (b) Long axis four-chamber view showing a mass in right ventricle, a potential source of emboli in this case, which may have caused the infarct (arrowhead). (c–d) In T2W images, there is an area of hyperintense signal in inferolateral wall, suggesting edema related to the myocardial infarct (arrows). (e–f) Area of myocardial necrosis with microvascular obstruction is seen in LGE images in inferolateral wall. LGE, late gadolinium enhanced images; MI, myocardial infarction; T2W, T2-weighted images.

By comparing methods of estimation of AAR (T2W images, ESA) and the final MI size with LGE images, CMR can detect myocardial salvage index (MSI). This is calculated as the proportion of salvaged AAR (AAR—final MI size)/AAR and is a marker of treatment efficacy (successful reperfusion) [21].

Other approaches to determine acute myocardial damage, AAR, and salvageable myocardium are currently under investigation. *In vivo quantification of T2 times by T2 maps* demonstrated that infarcted areas have significantly higher T2 times compared to the remote myocardium [106]. Pre-contrast T1 mapping techniques have also shown promising results in dogs, with excellent correlation with myocardial blood flow assessed by microspheres [107].

10.4.2.4 Myocardial necrosis—LGE images

LGE CMR acquired 5–15 after intravenous administration of gadolinium has become the reference method for *in vivo* imaging of MI. The late enhancement phenomenon is dependent on the kinetics and distribution volume of the gadolinium chelates in the infarcted area and in healthy myocardium. These contrast agents have extravascular distribution volume (see Chapter 11). While in remote myocardium gadolinium diffuses throughout the extracellular space and cannot cross the intact sarcolemmal membranes, in the infarcted area there is an increase in gadolinium concentration (due to the expansion of extracellular space) and longer washout times. The excellent spatial resolution (near 1 mm) and high contrast-to-noise ratios between the myocardium and the scar (about 300–500%) provided by current pulse sequences allow a precise estimation of infarcted area and inform also the transmurality of a given MI (Figure 10.6).

LGE has been extensively validated against histopathological studies in animal models [108–110]. Amado et al. [108] showed an excellent correlation ($R^2 = 0.94$, $p < 0.001$) of MI size by LGE with triphenyltetrazolium chloride pathology, using a semi-automated tool (full-width at half-maximum). In humans, MI detection by LGE had its validation by PET studies [111,112], and has shown its superiority over SPECT, due to its ability to detect very small areas of MI [109].

10.4.2.5 Microvascular obstruction—the "no-reflow" phenomenon

CMR can also detect microvascular obstruction in the setting of an AMI, as perfusion defects after injection of contrast (Figure 10.7). Considering that gadolinium cannot reach the necrotic core and areas of microvascular obstruction, the result is a dark area within a hyperenhanced infarcted area on first-pass perfusion early or late post gadolinium or LGE images [113]. Although the size of no-reflow phenomenon decreases when imaging is performed later after contrast injection, the higher in-plane resolution of early and late gadolinium images favors these techniques over first-pass perfusion imaging to identify and quantify microvascular obstruction.

10.4.3 Clinical implication and prognostic results of CMR in AMI

Preliminary clinical studies using CMR for myocardial salvage quantification showed consistent results to predict clinical outcome [114,115]. Eitel et al. [114] followed up a cohort of 208 patients who suffered AMI for a median of 18.5 months.

They found that overall mortality and major cardiovascular events were significantly lower among those patients with a MSI above the median group (2 vs. 12 deaths, $p = 0.001$, and 7 vs. 26 events, $p < 0.001$, respectively). Although the metrics of myocardial salvage by CMR is promised, there is no consensus about the best protocol to define the AAR. Additionally, more studies are required to define the role of CMR in the assessment of myocardial AAR, salvageable area and clinical implications.

One of the most powerful predictors of prognosis and myocardial viability related to AMI is the identification of fibrosis and its characteristics in LGE images (see Chapter 11). In early 2000, Kim et al. presented the concept of transmurality in the prediction of contractile recovery after revascularization [116]. They performed contrast enhanced CMR with LGE images in 50 patients with ventricular dysfunction referred to coronary revascularization. In 804 dysfunctional myocardial segments (severe hypokinesia, akinesia, or dyskinesia), the likelihood of functional recovery decreased significantly with the increase of transmural extension of fibrosis—in the group of segments with no LGE, 78% of them had contractile recovery; on the other hand, only one in 58 segments with more than 75% of infarcted tissue had contractile recovery ($p < 0.001$). Other studies identified the effect of scar size detected by LGE on left ventricular remodeling and ejection fraction, with a positive linear correlation between scar size and ventricular volumes [117,118], and a negative linear correlation with ejection fraction [119].

Quantification of scar and its characteristics plays an important role in prediction of induced arrhythmias after an AMI [119]. Schmidt et al. [120] did not find an association of scar mass after MI with inducible arrhythmias during electrophysiological study or device testing, but they showed that quantification of tissue heterogeneity (grey zone) in the MI boundaries was strongly associated to inducible monomorphic ventricular tachycardia.

The presence of myocardial fibrosis on LGE images, even if related to unrecognized MIs, is a marker of major cardiovascular events and mortality on follow-up [121,122]. Roes et al. [123] prospectively analyzed a cohort of 231 patients with previous MI referred for a clinical CMR study. Although LVEF and LV volumes were associated with mortality in follow-up, scar size was the strongest predictor of events. LGE is not a simple measure of presence or absence of viability; it can also identify microvascular obstruction, a robust marker of poor prognosis [37,124]. Wu et al. performed a CMR in 44 patients within 16 days after an AMI. The presence of microvascular obstruction (even after MI size was controlled for) was a robust marker of complications, scar formation, and left ventricular remodeling [125].

In the clinical scenario, another important role of CMR in the evaluation of AMI is the identification of complications, including ventricular septal rupture, free wall rupture, right ventricular involvement, acute pericarditis, aneurysm, and/or pseudoaneurysm and thrombus (Figures 10.21 and 10.22) (although echocardiography remains the first-choice technique to identify early post-ischemic complications). The particular advantages of CMR are its higher sensitivity for identification of thrombi and the better differentiation of true from pseudoaneurysm, Most importantly, it may distinguish MI from other conditions mimicking ACSs, such as myocarditis and Takutsubo cardiomyopathy (Figure 10.23).

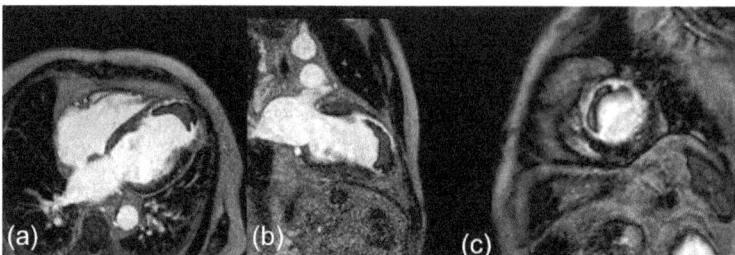

Figure 10.21 Example of left ventricular thrombus on late gadolinium enhanced images (a) four-chamber view, (b) two-chamber view, (c) short-axis view. The infarct is shown as bright hyperenhanced region. The thrombus does not take up contrast and therefore presents as an additional black structure in the cavity.

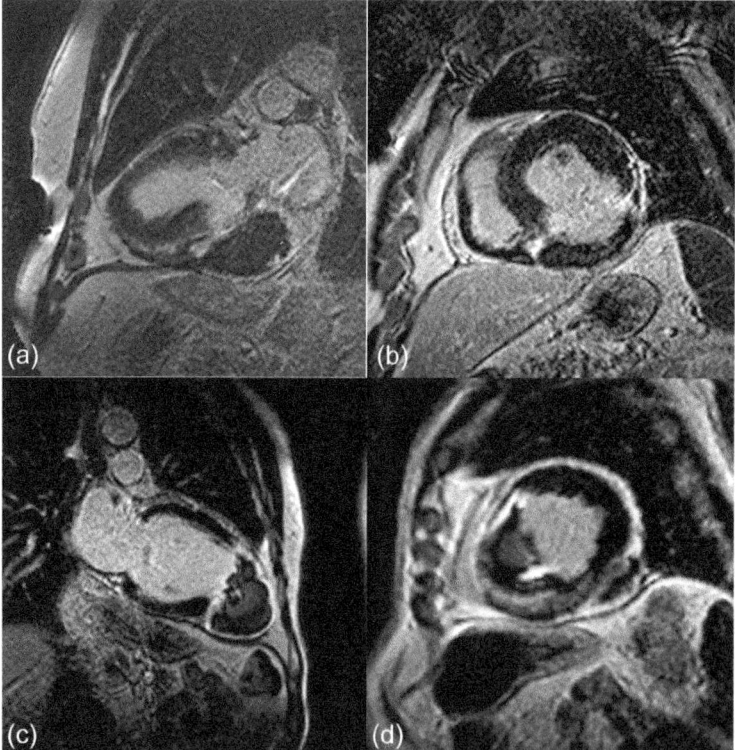

Figure 10.22 Example of two cases of LV pseudoanevrysms with massive thrombus post MI by late-gadolinium-enhanced CMR. (a and b) Two-chamber long-axis and short-axis slices in a case of inferior infarct complicated by LV-pseudoaneurysm. (c and d) Two-chamber long-axis and short-axis slices anterior-apical infarct complicated by LV-pseudoaneurysm. The infarcted area is hyperenhanced and severely thinned with rupture of continuity into the pericardium. A huge thrombus appearing as black mass fills out the ruptured area.

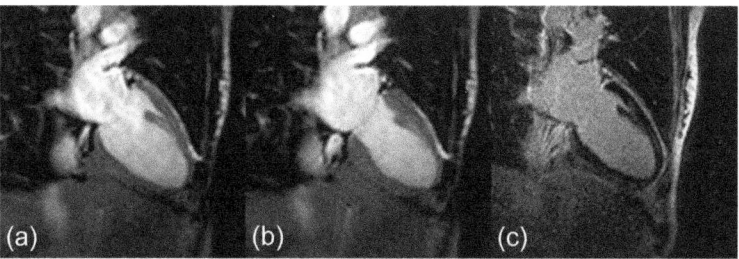

Figure 10.23 Example of Takutsubo cardiomyopathy. Cine images in diastole and systole (a and b) show apical akinesia. Late gadolinium enhanced CMR images (c) shows absence of necrosis.

10.4.4 CMR in evaluation of AMI—future directions

The unique ability of edema detection by CMR can be useful in evaluation of AMI. Refinements in the current protocols, including emerging pulse sequences, shortening scan times, and improving image resolution and contrast-to-noise ratios may provide a alternative modality to confirm acute myocardial injury in the earlier phases of MI, particularly in those cases with no ST elevation and unidentifiable troponins.

Myocardial mapping methods (T1, T2, and T2*) are set to play an ever-increasing clinical role in more precise delineation of AAR, no-reflow area, and infarction. Also it is under investigation whether these techniques allow assessment of MI without injection of contrast. As the methodology matures and is standardized, mapping methods are expected to provide quantitative and objective measures of infarct size, AAR, and infarct characteristics such as hemorrhage.

Coronary imaging is available for anatomic evaluation using 3D whole-heart T2-weighted SSFP sequence with ECG gating and respiratory gating. However, current technology cannot provide in-plane resolution to quantify stenosis severity in distal epicardial arteries [126]. Most importantly, there are preliminary data showing promising results of CMR in the identification of markers of vulnerable coronary plaques [127,128].

MR spectroscopy is an imaging technique that uses the resonance of other atoms besides hydrogen (e.g., ^{33}P, ^{23}Na, ^{13}C) to generate *in vivo* metabolic information. Under severe ischemic injury, the phosphocreatine/ATP ratio and phosphocreatine levels decrease in myocardium, and MR spectroscopy can detect these alterations [129,130]. Future improvements in spatial resolution and implementation of higher magnetic fields would allow the application of this technique in the identification of viable myocardium. Novel methods such as hyperpolarized MRI are in preclinical and clinical testing and may offer new opportunities for *in vivo* metabolic imaging, with many applications anticipated in the imaging of MI.

10.5 Multidetector CT

10.5.1 Introduction

Over the past decade, computed tomography (CT) imaging of AMI became a readily available, though rarely used, tool in clinical routine. The nowadays robust technique of coronary CT angiography was the driver of cardiac CT's rapid development. Starting from anecdotal case reports, several authors systematically investigated the use of cardiac CT for the visualization of AMI. The idea of viability imaging, however, dates back for more than 4 decades, when early clinical observations indicated that ventricular function may recover after CABG surgery. Direct visualization of MI was the most appealing concept, as it permits treatment planning and prediction of an individual patient's prognosis.

Starting in the late 1970s, different CT approaches to the assessment of MI and myocardial viability were developed. While conventional CT imaging techniques were technically insufficient for reliably imaging the heart, electron beam CT (EBCT), with its high temporal resolution, proved a valid tool for the assessment of the myocardium in MI. At that time the basic concepts of unenhanced, arterial, and late-phase CT imaging of MI were tested. For various reasons, none of these CT techniques made it to clinical routine practice.

The most recent addition in imaging of AMI is multi-detector row CT (MDCT). While MDCT is now widely used for the visualization of the coronary arteries, it also allows for the assessment of left ventricular function, myocardial perfusion, and myocardial viability. Although it is currently not considered appropriate for imaging of myocardial viability [131], MDCT holds a unique potential as a comprehensive and cost-effective imaging strategy for simultaneously assessing coronary arteries and myocardial viability. Moreover, it offers an alternative imaging approach to magnetic resonance (MR) imaging for the ever-increasing patient population with metallic implants, particularly cardiac pacemakers or deep brain stimulators.

10.5.2 CT techniques for imaging of AMI

CT angiography has been shown to be an effective tool for ruling out AMI in patients with low-to-intermediate risk for CAD presenting with chest pain to the emergency room [132–134]. This approach makes use of the high negative predictive value of CT to rule CAD by direct visualization of coronary artery lumen in such patient with chest pain. Moreover a variety of CT approaches have been developed for direct visualization of AMI. All of these approaches aim toward the direct visualization of the infarcted myocardium, while in chronic MI additional indirect approaches such as unenhanced CT for assessing fatty infiltrations or calcifications or measurement of end-diastolic wall thickness from arterial phase CT images are commonly used as surrogate parameters of myocardial viability. Basically, there are three different approaches for direct visualization of the infarcted myocardium in AMI:

- Unenhanced CT for imaging myocardial edema
- Arterial phase CT for visualizing perfusion defects
- Late-phase CT for depicting non-viable myocardium

10.5.2.1 Unenhanced CT for imaging myocardial edema

AMI is associated with myocardial edema. This fact is long exploited by CMR imaging for differentiating acute from chronic MI. Edema in the infarction zone was first visualized by CT in 1977, when a marked reduction in CT-values was confirmed as a

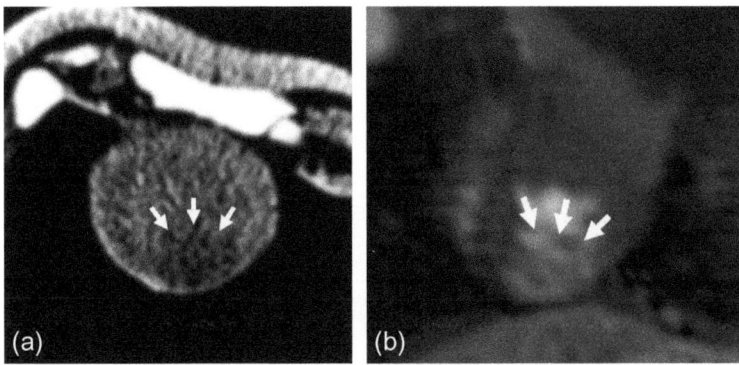

Figure 10.24 Unenhanced CT in interventionally induced acute MI in pig shows a markedly hypodense area of the inferior left ventricular myocardium (a, arrows). This hypodensity corresponds to edema as seen on T2-weighted MR imaging (b, arrows). The presence of acute MI was confirmed by TTC staining and histology.

CT correlate of edema [135]. At that time, however, it could only be visualized in an ex-vivo setting, and this knowledge was soon forgotten. It was only recently that *in-vivo* visualization of myocardial edema by means of CT was proven feasible in an animal model of AMI [136] (Figure 10.24). The area presenting with edema usually exceeds the area of delayed myocardial contrast enhancement on CT as well as on CMR scans. The edematous myocardium without delayed contrast enhancement has been suggested to correspond to the peri-infarction zone, which may benefit from revascularization therapy.

This approach suffers from several relevant limitations. Most importantly, the contrast resolution of CT is poor and on unenhanced scans, CT values differ only by about 12–25 Hounsfield units (HU) between healthy and infarcted myocardium. Moreover, the areas of edema are not to be confused with strongly hypodense areas on unenhanced CT scans, as they are known to occur in chronic or healed MI (the latter representing subendocardial lipomatous metaplasia late after AMI) [137]. Consequently, this technique has not been adopted into clinical routine practice, but it is potentially helpful to interpret findings on unenhanced CT scans in patients suffering from acute chest pain (Figure 10.25).

10.5.2.2 Arterial phase CT for visualizing perfusion defects

Visualization of hypoenhancing myocardium from arterial phase CT is the oldest and the most straightforward approach for the detection of MI [138]. Arterial phase CT data are acquired during the contrast materials' first pass and therefore contain information on myocardial perfusion. Reduced contrast enhancement, in other words, hypoenhancement, is due to impaired blood flow and is therefore a potential surrogate of MI. This is a quite robust finding, and even with ungated sequential CT, it provided an acceptably reliable surrogate for the assessment of myocardial injury. Various reports on the successful application of arterial phase CT for imaging MI were published as early as the late 1970s. Limitations in spatial and temporal resolution with the constant

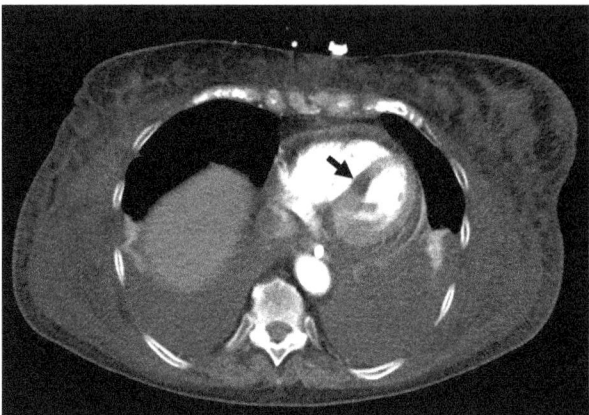

Figure 10.25 71-year-old female with a history of pulmonary embolism (PE). The patient underwent ungated contrast enhanced CT for exclusion of another episode of PE. Arterial phase CT shows a septal perfusion deficit (arrow) corresponding to acute MI.

motion artifacts and the inability to compute multiplanar reformats depiction of the myocardium, particularly of the inferior wall of the LV, meant that the method was previously insufficient for clinical routine practice.

The excellent spatial and temporal resolution of modern MDCT in combination with advanced techniques for ECG synchronization has overcome these limitations. As coronary CT angiography can also be described as arterial phase imaging; these developments fostered the revival of arterial phase CT for assessing the myocardium.

The direct relation between MI, missing perfusion, and hypoenhancement on arterial phase CT has been described in several animal models of AMI. Hoffmann et al. reported that arterial phase MDCT detected all areas of experimentally induced MI by a significant reduction of myocardial CT attenuation when compared to healthy myocardium [139].

Several researchers transferred these experimental findings to clinical imaging (Tables 10.2 and 10.3). Taken from clinical routine imaging, Nikolaou et al. retrospectively investigated coronary CT angiographies of 106 patients of whom 13 patients suffered AMI. In this setting, MDCT provided a sensitivity of 77% for the detection of AMI. A similar sensitivity of 75% was reported from another retrospective trial comparing arterial phase MDCT with SPECT [14]. In a more comprehensive approach, including hypoperfused myocardium and WMA as detected from ECG-gated MDCT, Cury et al. reported a sensitivity of 94% and a specificity of 97% for the detection of any MI [12]. The excellent temporal resolution of modern CT scanners even permits the use of ungated MDCT for detecting myocardial perfusion deficits (Figure 10.25). Consequently, several groups were able to identify MI from CT pulmonary angiograms in patients with acute chest pain with sensitivities and specificities of 67% and up to 91%, respectively [140,141]. Several studies reported an underestimation in infarct size as determined by MDCT [10,142]. As a potential explanation, part of the

Table 10.2 Selection of patient studies on the detection of acute MI from arterial phase CT

References	Patients acute MI/total	Reference	Sensitivity (%)	Specificity (%)	Attenuation MI (HU)	Attenuation healthy (HU)
[9]	18/69[a]	Clinical	83	95	8–87	66–147
[10]	110/448[b]	CMR	83	91	59 ± 17	101 ± 14
[11]	16 acute 13 chronic	Clinical	– –	– –	26 ± 26 −13 ± 37	73 ± 14
[12]	34/102	SPECT	–	–	50 ± 12	99 ± 14
[13]	24/35	Clinical	96	–	–	–
[14]	15/122	SPECT	75	98	–	–

[a] Ungated CT.
[b] Segment based analysis.

Table 10.3 Selection of clinical studies on late-phase CT for assessing acute MI

Reference	Patient/segment	Reference	MI Age	Delay (min)	Agreement (κ)	Attenuation MI (HU)	Attenuation healthy (HU)
[10]	28/448	CMR	Acute	15	0.878	108±16	75±11
[147]	16/256	CMR	Acute	10		97±11	131±16
	21/336	CMR	Chronic	10			
[148]	19/323	CMR	Acute	5	0.8	134±6	96±3
				10		118±5	81±3
[149]	15	CMR	Acute	7	0.99	93±15	72±10
[124]	107/1819	SPECT	Acute	10	0.702	–	–
[150]	11/187	CMR	Acute	7	0.85	100±10	73±7

There is a good agreement between late-phase CT and MR imaging and SPECT as standards of reference.

reperfused necrotic myocardium enhances normally during the first-pass but presents with hyperenhancement on late-phase imaging. Consequently, hypoattenuated areas on arterial phase CT represent only a fraction of AMI [10].

Moreover, the extent of a perfusion deficit detected on arterial phase CT also has prognostic value. Shapiro et al. found that the transmural extent of hypoperfused areas as determined from arterial phase CT is to some degree related with functional recovery [143]. In this study, segments with 25% transmural extent of perfusion deficit at baseline had no worsening of wall motion, while 89% of patients with 75% perfusion deficit showed worsening of wall motion over time (Figure 10.27a). Thus, assessing myocardium for perfusion deficits from coronary CT angiography is a promising tool for the evaluation of AMI, without applying additional radiation dose. However, this approach is limited as perfusion deficits on arterial phase CT are not only found in AMI, but also in other conditions with hypoattenuation either due to coronary stenosis or occlusion, MI, microvascular obstruction, lipomatous metaplasia, or any combination of these entities. Therefore, it is not yet possible to differentiate AMI from viable hypoperfused myocardium by use of a single arterial phase CT scan. So far clinical correlation is needed to establish the aetiology of hypoattenuating myocardium on arterial phase MDCT images.

10.5.2.3 Late-phase CT for depicting non-viable myocardium

While arterial phase imaging is the most obvious approach for the CT assessment of the myocardium, its value is limited, as it does not provide direct information on myocyte injury. Delayed myocardial contrast enhancement is seen in areas where myocytes have lost cellular membrane integrity and therefore are irreversibly damaged. In the late 1970s, CT imaging of AMI by means of delayed contrast enhancement has been proven feasible. Initial observations from animal experiments were followed by several reports on the use of late-phase CT for the assessment of AMI. However, CT imaging of AMI was superseded by CMR and became forgotten.

With the introduction of MDCT, late-phase CT of the heart for assessing AMI has been rediscovered (Figure 10.26). Several animal studies proved the feasibility and reliability of late-phase CT in AMI in comparison with accepted standards of reference [144,145]. These studies demonstrated a good correlation between the size of AMI on late-phase CT and CMR or TTC staining. This experimental experience was followed by several human studies confirming the concept of late-phase CT imaging for assessing myocardial viability [10,146]. All of these clinical studies reported excellent agreement between late-phase CT and CMR or SPECT as standard of reference (Table 10.3). In late-phase CT for AMI, some technical issues need to be considered, as contrast-to-noise ratio (CNR) of delayed myocardial contrast enhancement is markedly lower when compared to CMR. In order to achieve sufficient image quality, the use of low kV scans and administration of 0.5–0.75 g of iodine/kg bodyweight is recommended.

Delayed myocardial contrast enhancement is typically assessed from a second (late-phase) CT scan obtained 5–15 min after routine coronary CT angiography [145,147], with late-phase imaging providing additional information on viability

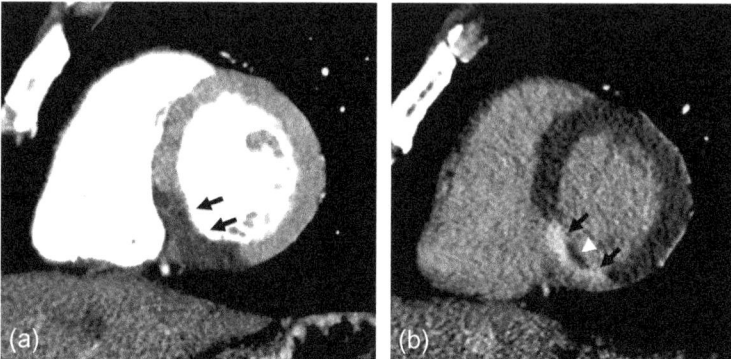

Figure 10.26 64-year-old male patient with acute MI. Arterial phase CT obtained from coronary CT angiography depicts a transmural hypoattenuation of the infero-septal myocardium without wall thinning (a, arrows). This finding is indicative of acute MI. Late-phase CT shows a corresponding area with delayed myocardial contrast enhancement (b, black arrows). Inside the region of delayed myocardial contrast enhancement there is a hypodense area corresponding to microvascular obstruction or "no-reflow" (white arrowhead). This combination is associated with a poor prognosis for functional recovery.

(see Chapter 5). However, delayed myocardial contrast enhancement as seen on CT is not specific for MI and is also seen in other cardiac pathologies, such as dilated cardiomyopathy, myocarditis, and sarcoidosis. Therefore, arterial and late-phase images need to be interpreted together. Moreover, different combinations of early hypoattenuation and delayed hyperenhancement have different prognostic meaning [151,152].

The presence of transmural perfusion defects on arterial phase CT was shown to be a better predictor of persistent myocardial dysfunction than transmural delayed myocardial contrast enhancement [153]. This might be due to the so-called "no-reflow" phenomenon. On late-phase CT imaging, "no-reflow" areas remain hypoattenuating surrounded by a hyperenhancing rim of infarcted myocardium (Figure 10.27b). These residual perfusion defects were shown to be the strongest predictor of persistent myocardial dysfunction in reperfused AMI [153]. Accordingly, Koyama et al. reported that global left ventricular function and wall thickness on follow-up examinations in patients with AMI was best in a group with delayed myocardial contrast enhancement, but without early or residual perfusion defects [151]. In another study assessing the impact of different contrast patterns on functional recovery, Lessick et al. reported that persistent myocardial dysfunction is clearly related to the presence of both early perfusion defects and delayed myocardial contrast enhancement (Figure 10.26) [152].

Delayed myocardial contrast enhancement may not only be assessed after coronary CT angiography. It also presents after invasive coronary angiography and percutaneous coronary intervention (PCI) using the intra-arterially applied contrast material from coronary angiography for late-phase contrast enhanced CT. Unfortunately, this approach is rarely used because it poses a logistical challenge: CT imaging needs to be performed about 30 min after the PCI in patients with reperfused AMI.

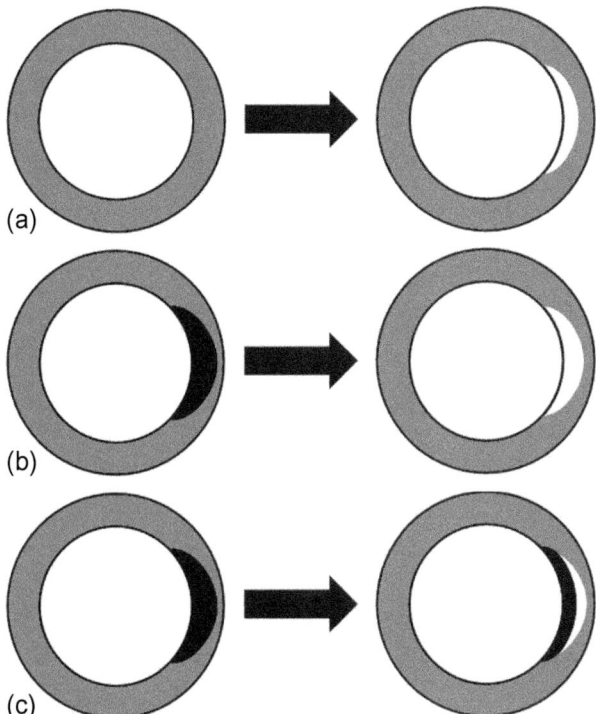

Figure 10.27 Arterial (left) and late-phase CT images (right) should be read side-by-side, as ischemic injury presents with different contrast enhancement patterns. These patterns provide information on the individual patients prognosis after acute MI. Left ventricular function are likely to improve in patients without perfusion deficit on arterial phase images but delayed myocardial contrast enhancement (a, white regions). Prognosis worsens if there are areas of hypoattenuation (black regions) on arterial phase CT with corresponding areas of delayed myocardial contrast enhancement on late-phase CT (b). Poorest long-term results are seen in patients with perfusion deficit on arterial phase images and hypoattenuating areas on late-phase CT images, corresponding to so-called no-reflow areas (c).

10.5.3 Future directions in CT imaging: dual energy CT

Dual-energy CT (DECT) is one of most recent developments in CT technology. It uses two datasets with different kV settings obtained at almost the same time either by rapid kV switching [154] by using data from two different tube-detector systems in dual-source CT [155] or by using energy specific multi-layer detectors. The use of different energies with different X-ray spectra gave way for tissue differentiation. It is particularly well suited to separate iodine and thereby the iodine-based end of the angiographic procedure. Otherwise, wash-out of the contrast material may limit image quality and subsequently the diagnostic value.

This approach was first reported for ungated CT in an attempt to establish a correlation between delayed myocardial contrast enhancement and myocardial blood flow in the ischemically injured region. Habis et al. showed 97% accuracy with 99% positive and 79% negative predictive values of CT imaging after PCI for detecting segments with viable myocardium [156]. Subsequent studies confirmed the validity of this approach in comparison with ^{201}Thallium SPECT and LGE CMR [157,158]. This technique can reliably distinguish transmural from subendocardial MI, and this approach provides an attractive option for assessing the individual patient's prognosis immediately after PCI for AMI [159]. There is only very limited data on this approach; however, it may permit very early risk stratification contrast media by its unique X-ray absorption characteristics at different kV levels.

For the evaluation of AMI, DECT may be used as an advanced tool for either arterial or late-phase CT. Most experience with DECT has been gathered in the assessment of myocardial perfusion deficits in CAD. In comparison with SPECT, an overall sensitivity of 92%, specificity of 93%, with 93% accuracy was reported for detecting any type of myocardial perfusion deficits [155]. Data on DECT in AMI are scarce. An animal study in six dogs by Zhang et al. found arterial phase DECT to be moderately superior to single-energy detection of AMI from arterial phase scans. A recent study in a canine model from the same group confirmed these findings in comparison with SPECT. Most recently, the capability of arterial phase DECT for assessing angiogenesis in different stages of MI was investigated. Pang et al. showed a good correlation between microvessel density and myocardial iodine concentration as measured by DECT [160]. However, so far there is only a single case report using DECT for the direct imaging assessment of AMI [161], indicating the almost non-existing role of this technique in clinical routine.

10.6 Guidelines for use of imaging in AMI

Current guidelines [162–165] suggest that emergency echocardiography can sometimes be useful to assist in making the diagnosis of AMI in uncertain cases (ESC Class II level C). It should, however, never delay transfer for angiography for STEMI, nor should angiography be delayed in suspected STEMI when imaging is unavailable or when doubt persists after imaging (ESC Class I level B). In contrast, in patients with NSTEMI, ESC guidelines suggest that echocardiography should be performed in all patients to evaluate regional and global LV function and to rule in or rule out differential diagnoses (Class I level C). Urgent echocardiography is considered the technique of choice in any patients with AMI/ACS presenting with cardiogenic shock, to detect mechanical complications and assess systolic function and loading conditions (Class I level B). ESC guidelines advocate coronary CT angiography as an alternative to invasive angiography to exclude ACS when there is a low to intermediate likelihood of CAD and when troponin and ECG are inconclusive (Class I level B). In patients without recurrence of pain, normal ECG findings, negative troponins tests, and a low risk score, a noninvasive stress test for inducible ischemia may be recommended before deciding on an invasive strategy.

For risk stratification in patients after reperfused STEMI current AHA/ACC and ESC guidelines indicate measurement of LVEF to be performed in all patients prior to discharge (ESC Class I—level of evidence B, AHA/ACC Class I—level C). The AHA/

ACC guidelines do not express preferences for any imaging technique, however ESC guidelines advocate echocardiography as the preferred modality (Class I level B), and CMR as an alternative (Class IIb level C). Also, guidelines recommend that patients with an initially reduced LVEF who are possible candidates for ICD therapy should undergo reevaluation of LVEF 40 or more days after discharge to evaluate whether EF remains lower than 35% (ESC Class I Level A and AHA/ACC Class I level B).

In patients with STEMI who did not undergo coronary angiography, i.e., patients who underwent thrombolysis for reperfusion, current guidelines recommend noninvasive testing for ischemia to be performed before discharge to assess the presence and extent of inducible ischemia (AHA/ACC Class I level B AHA/ACC). Also, they suggest that noninvasive testing for ischemia might be considered before discharge to evaluate the functional significance of a noninfarct artery stenosis previously identified at angiography (AHA/ACC Class IIb Level of Evidence: C) and to guide the postdischarge exercise prescription (Class IIb Level of Evidence: C). No preference for imaging technique is expressed, and nuclear imaging, stress echocardiography, or stress CMR could be equally useful for this purpose.

Finally, viability testing using stress myocardial perfusion scintigraphy, stress echocardiography, PET, or CMR is recommended for patients with multivessel disease or in whom revascularization of other vessels is considered (ESC Guidelines Class I Level A).

10.7 Conclusion

Imaging techniques are central in the management of patients with AMI. They allow key diagnostic and outcome measures during and after AMI. Echocardiography is the most available, versatile, and comprehensive technique and is therefore employed in the majority of patients with AMI, both in the acute phase to estimate left ventricular function and during follow-up to evaluate remodeling and final infarct size. It is also the technique of choice to screen for complications of AMI. Nuclear imaging plays an important role in the evaluation of patients for residual or recurring ischemia after revascularization. CMR and CT are rapidly evolving imaging techniques, offering comprehensive examination strategies for evaluation of patients with known or suspected AMI. CMR is particularly useful for infarct imaging and distinction from other pathologies in ACS with angiographically normal coronary arteries. Both CT and CMR allow for complementary information not offered by other modalities, and their use may be required in the context of more complex diagnostic situations.

References

[1] Thygesen K, Alpert JS, Jaffe AS, Simoons ML, Chaitman BR, White HD, et al. Third universal definition of myocardial infarction. J Am Coll Cardiol 2012;60:1581–98.
[2] Reimer KA, Jennings RB. The "wavefront phenomenon" of myocardial ischemic cell death. II. Transmural progression of necrosis within the framework of ischemic bed size (myocardium at risk) and collateral flow. Lab Invest 1979;40:633–44.

[3] Hochman JS, Lamas GA, Buller CE, Dzavik V, Reynolds HR, Abramsky SJ, et al. Coronary intervention for persistent occlusion after myocardial infarction. N Engl J Med 2006;355:2395–407.
[4] Ambrosio G, Tritto I. Reperfusion injury: experimental evidence and clinical implications. Am Heart J 1999;138:S69–75.
[5] Kloner RA, Ganote CE, Jennings RB. The "no-reflow" phenomenon after temporary coronary occlusion in the dog. J Clin Invest 1974;54:1496–508.
[6] Tarantini G, Razzolini R, Cacciavillani L, Bilato C, Sarais C, Corbetti F, et al. Influence of transmurality, infarct size, and severe microvascular obstruction on left ventricular remodeling and function after primary coronary angioplasty. Am J Cardiol 2006;98:1033–40.
[7] Gonzalez A, Ravassa S, Beaumont J, Lopez B, Diez J. New targets to treat the structural remodeling of the myocardium. J Am Coll Cardiol 2011;58:1833–43.
[8] Gajarsa JJ, Kloner RA. Left ventricular remodeling in the post-infarction heart: a review of cellular, molecular mechanisms, and therapeutic modalities. Heart Fail Rev 2011;16:13–21.
[9] Gosalia A, Haramati LB, Sheth MP, Spindola-Franco H. CT detection of acute myocardial infarction. AJR Am J Roentgenol 2004;182:1563–6.
[10] Mahnken AH, Koos R, Katoh M, Wildberger JE, Spuentrup E, Buecker A, et al. Assessment of myocardial viability in reperfused acute myocardial infarction using 16-slice computed tomography in comparison to magnetic resonance imaging. J Am Coll Cardiol 2005;45:2042–7.
[11] Nieman K, Cury RC, Ferencik M, Nomura CH, Abbara S, Hoffmann U, et al. Differentiation of recent and chronic myocardial infarction by cardiac computed tomography. Am J Cardiol 2006;98:303–8.
[12] Cury RC, Nieman K, Shapiro MD, Butler J, Nomura CH, Ferencik M, et al. Comprehensive assessment of myocardial perfusion defects, regional wall motion, and left ventricular function by using 64-section multidetector CT. Radiology 2008;248:466–75.
[13] Nagao M, Matsuoka H, Kawakami H, Higashino H, Mochizuki T, Uemura M, et al. Myocardial ischemia in acute coronary syndrome: assessment using 64-MDCT. AJR Am J Roentgenol 2009;193:1097–106.
[14] Rubinshtein R, Miller TD, Williamson EE, Kirsch J, Gibbons RJ, Primak AN, et al. Detection of myocardial infarction by dual-source coronary computed tomography angiography using quantitated myocardial scintigraphy as the reference standard. Heart 2009;95:1419–22.
[15] Montant P, Chenot F, Goffinet C, Poncelet A, Vancraeynest D, Pasquet A, et al. Detection and quantification of myocardial scars by contrast-enhanced 3D echocardiography. Circ Cardiovasc Imaging 2010;3:415–23.
[16] Gibbons RJ, Valeti US, Araoz PA, Jaffe AS. The quantification of infarct size. J Am Coll Cardiol 2004;44:1533–42.
[17] Engblom H, Hedstrom E, Heiberg E, Wagner GS, Pahlm O, Arheden H. Rapid initial reduction of hyperenhanced myocardium after reperfused first myocardial infarction suggests recovery of the peri-infarction zone: one-year follow-up by MRI. Circ Cardiovasc Imaging 2009;2:47–55.
[18] Wu KC, Kim RJ, Bluemke DA, Rochitte CE, Zerhouni EA, Becker LC, Lima JA. Quantification and time course of microvascular obstruction by contrast-enhanced echocardiography and magnetic resonance imaging following acute myocardial infarction and reperfusion. J Am Coll Cardiol 1998;32:1756–64.

[19] Gerber BL, Rochitte CE, Melin JA, McVeigh ER, Bluemke DA, Wu KC, et al. Microvascular obstruction and left ventricular remodeling early after acute myocardial infarction. Circulation 2000;101:2734–41.
[20] Hadamitzky M, Langhans B, Hausleiter J, Sonne C, Kastrati A, Martinoff S, Schömig A, Ibrahim T. The assessment of area at risk and myocardial salvage after coronary revascularization in acute myocardial infarction: comparison between CMR and SPECT. JACC Cardiovasc Imaging 2013;6:358–69.
[21] Botker HE, Kaltoft AK, Pedersen SF, Kim WY. Measuring myocardial salvage. Cardiovasc Res 2012;94:266–75.
[22] Volpi A, de VC, Franzosi MG, et al. Determinants of 6-month mortality in survivors of myocardial infarction after thrombolysis. Results of the GISSI-2 data base. The Ad hoc Working Group of the Gruppo Italiano per lo Studio della Sopravvivenza nell'Infarto Miocardico (GISSI)-2 Data Base. Circulation 1993;88:416–29.
[23] Rouleau JL, Talajic M, Sussex B, Potvin L, Warnica W, Davies RF, et al. Myocardial infarction patients in the 1990s – their risk factors, stratification and survival in Canada: the Canadian Assessment of Myocardial Infarction (CAMI) Study. J Am Coll Cardiol 1996;27:1119–27.
[24] Risk stratification and survival after myocardial infarction. N Engl J Med 1983;309:331–6.
[25] White HD, Norris RM, Brown MA, Brandt PW, Whitlock RM, Wild CJ. Left ventricular end-systolic volume as the major determinant of survival after recovery from myocardial infarction. Circulation 1987;76:44–51.
[26] Dwivedi G, Janardhanan R, Hayat SA, Swinburn JM, Senior R. Prognostic value of myocardial viability detected by myocardial contrast echocardiography early after acute myocardial infarction. J Am Coll Cardiol 2007;50:327–34.
[27] Gorcsan III J, Tanaka H. Echocardiographic assessment of myocardial strain. J Am Coll Cardiol 2011;58:1401–13.
[28] Dorosz JL, Lezotte DC, Weitzenkamp DA, Allen LA, Salcedo EE. Performance of 3-dimensional echocardiography in measuring left ventricular volumes and ejection fraction: a systematic review and meta-analysis. J Am Coll Cardiol 2012;59:1799–808.
[29] Hoffmann R, Barletta G, von BS, Vanoverschelde JL, Kasprzak J, Greis C, et al. Analysis of left ventricular volumes and function: a multicenter comparison of cardiac magnetic resonance imaging, cine ventriculography, and unenhanced and contrast-enhanced two-dimensional and three-dimensional echocardiography. J Am Soc Echocardiogr 2014;27:292–301.
[30] Sabia P, Abbott RD, Afrookteh A, Keller MW, Touchstone DA, Kaul S. Importance of two-dimensional echocardiographic assessment of left ventricular systolic function in patients presenting to the emergency room with cardiac-related symptoms. Circulation 1991;84:1615–24.
[31] Sabia P, Afrookteh A, Touchstone DA, Keller MW, Esquivel L, Kaul S. Value of regional wall motion abnormality in the emergency room diagnosis of acute myocardial infarction. A prospective study using two-dimensional echocardiography. Circulation 1991;84:I85–92.
[32] Shah BN, Balaji G, Alhajiri A, Ramzy IS, Ahmadvazir S, Senior R. Incremental diagnostic and prognostic value of contemporary stress echocardiography in a chest pain unit: mortality and morbidity outcomes from a real-world setting. Circ Cardiovasc Imaging 2013;6:202–9.

[33] Kaul S, Pandian NG, Okada RD, Pohost GM, Weyman AE. Contrast echocardiography in acute myocardial ischemia: I. In vivo determination of total left ventricular "area at risk". J Am Coll Cardiol 1984;4:1272–82.
[34] Rinkevich D, Kaul S, Wang XQ, Tong KL, Belcik T, Kalvaitis S, et al. Regional left ventricular perfusion and function in patients presenting to the emergency department with chest pain and no ST-segment elevation. Eur Heart J 2005;26:1606–11.
[35] Tong KL, Kaul S, Wang XQ, Rinkevich D, Kalvaitis S, Belcik T, et al. Myocardial contrast echocardiography versus Thrombolysis In Myocardial Infarction score in patients presenting to the emergency department with chest pain and a nondiagnostic electrocardiogram. J Am Coll Cardiol 2005;46:920–7.
[36] Iwakura K, Ito H, Kawano S, Shintani Y, Yamamoto K, Kato A, et al. Predictive factors for development of the no-reflow phenomenon in patients with reperfused anterior wall acute myocardial infarction. J Am Coll Cardiol 2001;38:472–7.
[37] Ito H, Maruyama A, Iwakura K, Takiuchi S, Masuyama T, Hori M, et al. Clinical implications of the 'no reflow' phenomenon. A predictor of complications and left ventricular remodeling in reperfused anterior wall myocardial infarction. Circulation 1996;93:223–8.
[38] Greaves K, Dixon SR, Fejka M, O'Neill WW, Redwood SR, Marber MS, et al. Myocardial contrast echocardiography is superior to other known modalities for assessing myocardial reperfusion after acute myocardial infarction. Heart 2003;89:139–44.
[39] Galiuto L, Garramone B, Scara A, Rebuzzi AG, Crea F, La TG, et al. The extent of microvascular damage during myocardial contrast echocardiography is superior to other known indexes of post-infarct reperfusion in predicting left ventricular remodeling: results of the multicenter AMICI study. J Am Coll Cardiol 2008;51:552–9.
[40] Balcells E, Powers ER, Lepper W, Belcik T, Wei K, Ragosta M, et al. Detection of myocardial viability by contrast echocardiography in acute infarction predicts recovery of resting function and contractile reserve. J Am Coll Cardiol 2003;41:827–33.
[41] Nicolosi GL, Latini R, Marino P, Maggioni AP, Barlera S, Franzosi MG, et al. The prognostic value of predischarge quantitative two-dimensional echocardiographic measurements and the effects of early lisinopril treatment on left ventricular structure and function after acute myocardial infarction in the GISSI-3 Trial. Gruppo Italiano per lo Studio della Sopravvivenza nell'Infarto Miocardico. Eur Heart J 1996;17:1646–56.
[42] Malm S, Frigstad S, Sagberg E, Larsson H, Skjaerpe T. Accurate and reproducible measurement of left ventricular volume and ejection fraction by contrast echocardiography: a comparison with magnetic resonance imaging. J Am Coll Cardiol 2004;44:1030–5.
[43] Hundley WG, Kizilbash AM, Afridi I, Franco F, Peshock RM, Grayburn PA. Administration of an intravenous perfluorocarbon contrast agent improves echocardiographic determination of left ventricular volumes and ejection fraction: comparison with cine magnetic resonance imaging. J Am Coll Cardiol 1998;32:1426–32.
[44] Lim TK, Burden L, Janardhanan R, Ping C, Moon J, Pennell D, et al. Improved accuracy of low-power contrast echocardiography for the assessment of left ventricular remodeling compared with unenhanced harmonic echocardiography after acute myocardial infarction: comparison with cardiovascular magnetic resonance imaging. J Am Soc Echocardiogr 2005;18:1203–7.
[45] Nihoyannopoulos P, Vanoverschelde JL. Myocardial ischaemia and viability: the pivotal role of echocardiography. Eur Heart J 2011;32:810–9.
[46] Sicari R, Nihoyannopoulos P, Evangelista A, Kasprzak J, Lancellotti P, Poldermans D, et al. Stress echocardiography expert consensus statement: European Association of Echocardiography (EAE) (a registered branch of the ESC). Eur J Echocardiogr 2008;9:415–37.

[47] Rizzello V, Poldermans D, Bax JJ. Assessment of myocardial viability in chronic ischemic heart disease: current status. Q J Nucl Med Mol Imaging 2005;49:81–96.
[48] Cianfrocca C, Pelliccia F, Pasceri V, Auriti A, Guido V, Mercuro G, et al. Strain rate analysis and levosimendan improve detection of myocardial viability by dobutamine echocardiography in patients with post-infarction left ventricular dysfunction: a pilot study. J Am Soc Echocardiogr 2008;21:1068–74.
[49] Hanekom L, Cho GY, Leano R, Jeffriess L, Marwick TH. Comparison of two-dimensional speckle and tissue Doppler strain measurement during dobutamine stress echocardiography: an angiographic correlation. Eur Heart J 2007;28:1765–72.
[50] Hanekom L, Jenkins C, Jeffries L, Case C, Mundy J, Hawley C, et al. Incremental value of strain rate analysis as an adjunct to wall-motion scoring for assessment of myocardial viability by dobutamine echocardiography: a follow-up study after revascularization. Circulation 2005;112:3892–900.
[51] Zhang Y, Chan AK, Yu CM, Yip GW, Fung JW, Lam WW, et al. Strain rate imaging differentiates transmural from non-transmural myocardial infarction: a validation study using delayed-enhancement magnetic resonance imaging. J Am Coll Cardiol 2005;46:864–71.
[52] Mollema SA, Delgado V, Bertini M, Antoni ML, Boersma E, Holman ER, et al. Viability assessment with global left ventricular longitudinal strain predicts recovery of left ventricular function after acute myocardial infarction. Circ Cardiovasc Imaging 2010;3:15–23.
[53] Hayat SA, Senior R. Myocardial contrast echocardiography in ST elevation myocardial infarction: ready for prime time? Eur Heart J 2008;29:299–314.
[54] Shimoni S, Frangogiannis NG, Aggeli CJ, Shan K, Quinones MA, Espada R, et al. Microvascular structural correlates of myocardial contrast echocardiography in patients with coronary artery disease and left ventricular dysfunction: implications for the assessment of myocardial hibernation. Circulation 2002;106:950–6.
[55] Swinburn JM, Lahiri A, Senior R. Intravenous myocardial contrast echocardiography predicts recovery of dysynergic myocardium early after acute myocardial infarction. J Am Coll Cardiol 2001;38:19–25.
[56] Janardhanan R, Burden L, Senior R. Usefulness of myocardial contrast echocardiography in predicting collateral blood flow in the presence of a persistently occluded acute myocardial infarction-related coronary artery. Am J Cardiol 2004;93:1207–11.
[57] Janardhanan R, Swinburn JM, Greaves K, Senior R. Usefulness of myocardial contrast echocardiography using low-power continuous imaging early after acute myocardial infarction to predict late functional left ventricular recovery. Am J Cardiol 2003;92:493–7.
[58] Huang WC, Chiou KR, Liu CP, Lin SL, Lee D, Mar GY, et al. Comparison of real-time contrast echocardiography and low-dose dobutamine stress echocardiography in predicting the left ventricular functional recovery in patients after acute myocardial infarction under different therapeutic intervention. Int J Cardiol 2005;104:81–91.
[59] Senior R, Swinburn JM. Incremental value of myocardial contrast echocardiography for the prediction of recovery of function in dobutamine nonresponsive myocardium early after acute myocardial infarction. Am J Cardiol 2003;91:397–402.
[60] Janardhanan R, Moon JC, Pennell DJ, Senior R. Myocardial contrast echocardiography accurately reflects transmurality of myocardial necrosis and predicts contractile reserve after acute myocardial infarction. Am Heart J 2005;149:355–62.
[61] Janardhanan R, Senior R. Accuracy of dipyridamole myocardial contrast echocardiography for the detection of residual stenosis of the infarct-related artery and multivessel disease early after acute myocardial infarction. J Am Coll Cardiol 2004;43:2247–52.
[62] Mahmarian JJ, Dwivedi G, Lahiri T. Role of nuclear cardiac imaging in myocardial infarction: postinfarction risk stratification. J Nucl Cardiol 2004;11:186–209.

[63] Verani MS, Jeroudi MO, Mahmarian JJ, Boyce TM, Borges-Neto S, Patel B, et al. Quantification of myocardial infarction during coronary occlusion and myocardial salvage after reperfusion using cardiac imaging with technetium-99 m hexakis 2-methoxyisobutyl isonitrile. J Am Coll Cardiol 1988;12:1573–81.
[64] Glover DK, Ruiz M, Koplan BA, Watson DD, Beller GA. 99mTc-tetrofosmin assessment of myocardial perfusion and viability in canine models of coronary occlusion and reperfusion. J Nucl Med 1999;40:142–9.
[65] Vesely MR, Dilsizian V. Nuclear cardiac stress testing in the era of molecular medicine. J Nucl Med 2008;49:399–413.
[66] Gibbons RJ, Verani MS, Behrenbeck T, Pellikka PA, O'Connor MK, Mahmarian JJ, et al. Feasibility of tomographic 99mTc-hexakis-2-methoxy-2-methylpropyl-isonitrile imaging for the assessment of myocardial area at risk and the effect of treatment in acute myocardial infarction. Circulation 1989;80:1277–86.
[67] O'Connor MK, Hammell T, Gibbons RJ. In vitro validation of a simple tomographic technique for estimation of percentage myocardium at risk using methoxyisobutyl isonitrile technetium 99 m (sestamibi). Eur J Nucl Med 1990;17:69–76.
[68] O'Connor MK, Gibbons RJ, Juni JE, O'Keefe Jr. J, Ali A. Quantitative myocardial SPECT for infarct sizing: feasibility of a multicenter trial evaluated using a cardiac phantom. J Nucl Med 1995;36:1130–6.
[69] Effects of RheothRx on mortality, morbidity, left ventricular function, and infarct size in patients with acute myocardial infarction. Collaborative Organization for RheothRx Evaluation (CORE). Circulation 1997;96:192–201.
[70] Medrano R, Lowry RW, Young JB, Weilbaecher DG, Michael LH, Afridi I, et al. Assessment of myocardial viability with 99mTc sestamibi in patients undergoing cardiac transplantation. A scintigraphic/pathological study. Circulation 1996;94:1010–7.
[71] Maes AF, Borgers M, Flameng W, Nuyts JL, van de Werf F, Ausma JJ, et al. Assessment of myocardial viability in chronic coronary artery disease using technetium-99 m sestamibi SPECT. Correlation with histologic and positron emission tomographic studies and functional follow-up. J Am Coll Cardiol 1997;29:62–8.
[72] Flotats A, Carrio I. Non-invasive in vivo imaging of myocardial apoptosis and necrosis. Eur J Nucl Med Mol Imaging 2003;30:615–30.
[73] Khaw BA. The current role of infarct avid imaging. Semin Nucl Med 1999;29:259–70.
[74] Johnson LL, Seldin DW, Becker LC, LaFrance ND, Liberman HA, James C, et al. Antimyosin imaging in acute transmural myocardial infarctions: results of a multicenter clinical trial. J Am Coll Cardiol 1989;13:27–35.
[75] Tamaki N, Yamada T, Matsumori A, Yoshida A, Fujita T, Ohtani H, et al. Indium-111-antimyosin antibody imaging for detecting different stages of myocardial infarction: comparison with technetium-99 m-pyrophosphate imaging. J Nucl Med 1990;31:136–42.
[76] Orlandi C, Crane PD, Edwards DS, Platts SH, Bernard L, Lazewatsky J, et al. Early scintigraphic detection of experimental myocardial infarction in dogs with technetium-99 m-glucaric acid. J Nucl Med 1991;32:263–8.
[77] Flotats A, Carrio I. Cardiac neurotransmission SPECT imaging. J Nucl Cardiol 2004;11:587–602.
[78] Veltman CE, Boogers MJ, Meinardi JE, Al Younis I, Dibbets-Schneider P, Van der Wall EE, et al. Reproducibility of planar (123)I-meta-iodobenzylguanidine (MIBG) myocardial scintigraphy in patients with heart failure. Eur J Nucl Med Mol Imaging 2012;39:1599–608.
[79] Jacobson AF, Matsuoka DT. Influence of myocardial region of interest definition on quantitative analysis of planar 123I-mIBG images. Eur J Nucl Med Mol Imaging 2013;40:558–64.

[80] Fallavollita JA, Canty Jr. JM. Dysinnervated but viable myocardium in ischemic heart disease. J Nucl Cardiol 2010;17:1107–15.
[81] Abidov A, Germano G, Hachamovitch R, Berman DS. Gated SPECT in assessment of regional and global left ventricular function: major tool of modern nuclear imaging. J Nucl Cardiol 2006;13:261–79.
[82] Christian TF, Behrenbeck T, Pellikka PA, Huber KC, Chesebro JH, Gibbons RJ. Mismatch of left ventricular function and infarct size demonstrated by technetium-99 m isonitrile imaging after reperfusion therapy for acute myocardial infarction: identification of myocardial stunning and hyperkinesia. J Am Coll Cardiol 1990;16:1632–8.
[83] Christian TF, Gitter MJ, Miller TD, Gibbons RJ. Prospective identification of myocardial stunning using technetium-99 m sestamibi-based measurements of infarct size. J Am Coll Cardiol 1997;30:1633–40.
[84] Miller TD, Christian TF, Hopfenspirger MR, Hodge DO, Gersh BJ, Gibbons RJ. Infarct size after acute myocardial infarction measured by quantitative tomographic 99mTc sestamibi imaging predicts subsequent mortality. Circulation 1995;92:334–41.
[85] Miller TD, Hodge DO, Sutton JM, Grines CL, O'Keefe JH, DeWood MA, et al. Usefulness of technetium-99 m sestamibi infarct size in predicting posthospital mortality following acute myocardial infarction. Am J Cardiol 1998;81:1491–3.
[86] Burns RJ, Gibbons RJ, Yi Q, Roberts RS, Miller TD, Schaer GL, et al. The relationships of left ventricular ejection fraction, end-systolic volume index and infarct size to six-month mortality after hospital discharge following myocardial infarction treated by thrombolysis. J Am Coll Cardiol 2002;39:30–6.
[87] Schomig A, Kastrati A, Dirschinger J, Mehilli J, Schricke U, Pache J, et al. Coronary stenting plus platelet glycoprotein IIb/IIIa blockade compared with tissue plasminogen activator in acute myocardial infarction. Stent versus Thrombolysis for Occluded Coronary Arteries in Patients with Acute Myocardial Infarction Study Investigators. N Engl J Med 2000;343:385–91.
[88] Kastrati A, Mehilli J, Dirschinger J, Schricke U, Neverve J, Pache J, et al. Myocardial salvage after coronary stenting plus abciximab versus fibrinolysis plus abciximab in patients with acute myocardial infarction: a randomised trial. Lancet 2002;359:920–5.
[89] Mahmarian JJ, Shaw LJ, Filipchuk NG, Dakik HA, Iskander SS, Ruddy TD, et al. A multinational study to establish the value of early adenosine technetium-99 m sestamibi myocardial perfusion imaging in identifying a low-risk group for early hospital discharge after acute myocardial infarction. J Am Coll Cardiol 2006;48:2448–57.
[90] Mahmarian JJ, Dakik HA, Filipchuk NG, Shaw LJ, Iskander SS, Ruddy TD, et al. An initial strategy of intensive medical therapy is comparable to that of coronary revascularization for suppression of scintigraphic ischemia in high-risk but stable survivors of acute myocardial infarction. J Am Coll Cardiol 2006;48:2458–67.
[91] Ellis SG, Mooney MR, George BS, da Silva EE, Talley JD, Flanagan WH, et al. Randomized trial of late elective angioplasty versus conservative management for patients with residual stenoses after thrombolytic treatment of myocardial infarction. Treatment of Post-Thrombolytic Stenoses (TOPS) Study Group. Circulation 1992;86:1400–6.
[92] Allman KC. Noninvasive assessment myocardial viability: current status and future directions. J Nucl Cardiol 2013;20:618–37.
[93] Vanoverschelde JL, Wijns W, Borgers M, Heyndrickx G, Depre C, Flameng W, et al. Chronic myocardial hibernation in humans. From bedside to bench. Circulation 1997;95:1961–71.

[94] Bax JJ, Poldermans D, Elhendy A, Boersma E, Rahimtoola SH. Sensitivity, specificity, and predictive accuracies of various noninvasive techniques for detecting hibernating myocardium. Curr Probl Cardiol 2001;26:141–86.

[95] Fallavollita JA, Heavey BM, Luisi Jr. AJ, Michalek SM, Baldwa S, Mashtare Jr. TL, et al. Regional myocardial sympathetic denervation predicts the risk of sudden cardiac arrest in ischemic cardiomyopathy. J Am Coll Cardiol 2014;63:141–9.

[96] Garcia EV. Physical attributes, limitations, and future potential for PET and SPECT. J Nucl Cardiol 2012;19(Suppl. 1):S19–29.

[97] Berman DS, Maddahi J, Tamarappoo BK, Czernin J, Taillefer R, Udelson JE, et al. Phase II safety and clinical comparison with single-photon emission computed tomography myocardial perfusion imaging for detection of coronary artery disease: flurpiridaz F 18 positron emission tomography. J Am Coll Cardiol 2013;61:469–77.

[98] Flotats A, Bravo PE, Fukushima K, Chaudhry MA, Merrill J, Bengel FM. (8)(2)Rb PET myocardial perfusion imaging is superior to (9)(9)mTc-labelled agent SPECT in patients with known or suspected coronary artery disease. Eur J Nucl Med Mol Imaging 2012;39:1233–9.

[99] Rischpler C, Nekolla SG, Beer AJ. PET/MR imaging of atherosclerosis: initial experience and outlook. Am J Nucl Med Mol Imaging 2013;3:393–6.

[100] Kwong RY, Schussheim AE, Rekhraj S, Aletras AH, Geller N, Davis J, et al. Detecting acute coronary syndrome in the emergency department with cardiac magnetic resonance imaging. Circulation 2003;107:531–7.

[101] Ortiz-Perez JT, Meyers SN, Lee DC, Kansal P, Klocke FJ, Holly TA, et al. Angiographic estimates of myocardium at risk during acute myocardial infarction: validation study using cardiac magnetic resonance imaging. Eur Heart J 2007;28:1750–8.

[102] Fuernau G, Eitel I, Franke V, Hildebrandt L, Meissner J, de WS, et al. Myocardium at risk in ST-segment elevation myocardial infarction comparison of T2-weighted edema imaging with the MR-assessed endocardial surface area and validation against angiographic scoring. JACC Cardiovasc Imaging 2011;4:967–76.

[103] Wright J, Adriaenssens T, Dymarkowski S, Desmet W, Bogaert J. Quantification of myocardial area at risk with T2-weighted CMR: comparison with contrast-enhanced CMR and coronary angiography. JACC Cardiovasc Imaging 2009;2:825–31.

[104] Abdel-Aty H, Zagrosek A, Schulz-Menger J, Taylor AJ, Messroghli D, Kumar A, et al. Delayed enhancement and T2-weighted cardiovascular magnetic resonance imaging differentiate acute from chronic myocardial infarction. Circulation 2004;109:2411–6.

[105] Cury RC, Shash K, Nagurney JT, Rosito G, Shapiro MD, Nomura CH, et al. Cardiac magnetic resonance with T2-weighted imaging improves detection of patients with acute coronary syndrome in the emergency department. Circulation 2008;118:837–44.

[106] Giri S, Chung YC, Merchant A, Mihai G, Rajagopalan S, Raman SV, et al. T2 quantification for improved detection of myocardial edema. J Cardiovasc Magn Reson 2009;11:56.

[107] Ugander M, Bagi PS, Oki AJ, Chen B, Hsu LY, Aletras AH, et al. Myocardial edema as detected by pre-contrast T1 and T2 CMR delineates area at risk associated with acute myocardial infarction. JACC Cardiovasc Imaging 2012;5:596–603.

[108] Amado LC, Gerber BL, Gupta SN, Rettmann DW, Szarf G, Schock R, et al. Accurate and objective infarct sizing by contrast-enhanced magnetic resonance imaging in a canine myocardial infarction model. J Am Coll Cardiol 2004;44:2383–9.

[109] Wagner A, Mahrholdt H, Holly TA, Elliott MD, Regenfus M, Parker M, et al. Contrast-enhanced MRI and routine single photon emission computed tomography (SPECT) perfusion imaging for detection of subendocardial myocardial infarcts: an imaging study. Lancet 2003;361:374–9.

[110] Kim RJ, Fieno DS, Parrish TB, Harris K, Chen EL, Simonetti O, et al. Relationship of MRI delayed contrast enhancement to irreversible injury, infarct age, and contractile function. Circulation 1999;100:1992–2002.
[111] Klein C, Nekolla SG, Bengel FM, Momose M, Sammer A, Haas F, et al. Assessment of myocardial viability with contrast-enhanced magnetic resonance imaging: comparison with positron emission tomography. Circulation 2002;105:162–7.
[112] Kuhl HP, Beek AM, van der Weerdt AP, Hofman MB, Visser CA, Lammertsma AA, et al. Myocardial viability in chronic ischemic heart disease: comparison of contrast-enhanced magnetic resonance imaging with (18)F-fluorodeoxyglucose positron emission tomography. J Am Coll Cardiol 2003;41:1341–8.
[113] Rochitte CE, Lima JA, Bluemke DA, Reeder SB, McVeigh ER, Furuta T, et al. Magnitude and time course of microvascular obstruction and tissue injury after acute myocardial infarction. Circulation 1998;98:1006–14.
[114] Eitel I, Desch S, de WS, Fuernau G, Gutberlet M, Schuler G, et al. Long-term prognostic value of myocardial salvage assessed by cardiovascular magnetic resonance in acute reperfused myocardial infarction. Heart 2011;97:2038–45.
[115] Eitel I, Desch S, Fuernau G, Hildebrand L, Gutberlet M, Schuler G, et al. Prognostic significance and determinants of myocardial salvage assessed by cardiovascular magnetic resonance in acute reperfused myocardial infarction. J Am Coll Cardiol 2010;55:2470–9.
[116] Kim RJ, Wu E, Rafael A, Chen EL, Parker MA, Simonetti O, et al. The use of contrast-enhanced magnetic resonance imaging to identify reversible myocardial dysfunction. N Engl J Med 2000;343:1445–53.
[117] Kaandorp TA, Lamb HJ, Viergever EP, Poldermans D, Boersma E, Van der Wall EE, et al. Scar tissue on contrast-enhanced MRI predicts left ventricular remodelling after acute infarction. Heart 2007;93:375–6.
[118] Orn S, Manhenke C, Anand IS, Squire I, Nagel E, Edvardsen T, et al. Effect of left ventricular scar size, location, and transmurality on left ventricular remodeling with healed myocardial infarction. Am J Cardiol 2007;99:1109–14.
[119] Bello D, Fieno DS, Kim RJ, Pereles FS, Passman R, Song G, et al. Infarct morphology identifies patients with substrate for sustained ventricular tachycardia. J Am Coll Cardiol 2005;45:1104–8.
[120] Schmidt A, Azevedo CF, Cheng A, Gupta SN, Bluemke DA, Foo TK, et al. Infarct tissue heterogeneity by magnetic resonance imaging identifies enhanced cardiac arrhythmia susceptibility in patients with left ventricular dysfunction. Circulation 2007;115:2006–14.
[121] Kim HW, Klem I, Shah DJ, Wu E, Meyers SN, Parker MA, et al. Unrecognized non-Q-wave myocardial infarction: prevalence and prognostic significance in patients with suspected coronary disease. PLoS Med 2009;6, e1000057.
[122] Kwong RY, Chan AK, Brown KA, Chan CW, Reynolds HG, Tsang S, et al. Impact of unrecognized myocardial scar detected by cardiac magnetic resonance imaging on event-free survival in patients presenting with signs or symptoms of coronary artery disease. Circulation 2006;113:2733–43.
[123] Roes SD, Kelle S, Kaandorp TA, Kokocinski T, Poldermans D, Lamb HJ, et al. Comparison of myocardial infarct size assessed with contrast-enhanced magnetic resonance imaging and left ventricular function and volumes to predict mortality in patients with healed myocardial infarction. Am J Cardiol 2007;100:930–6.
[124] Chiou KR, Huang WC, Peng NJ, Huang YL, Hsiao SH, Chen KH, et al. Dual-phase multi-detector computed tomography assesses jeopardised and infarcted myocardium subtending infarct-related artery early after acute myocardial infarction. Heart 2009;95:1495–501.

[125] Wu KC, Zerhouni EA, Judd RM, Lugo-Olivieri CH, Barouch LA, Schulman SP, et al. Prognostic significance of microvascular obstruction by magnetic resonance imaging in patients with acute myocardial infarction. Circulation 1998;97:765–72.
[126] Sakuma H, Ichikawa Y, Chino S, Hirano T, Makino K, Takeda K. Detection of coronary artery stenosis with whole-heart coronary magnetic resonance angiography. J Am Coll Cardiol 2006;48:1946–50.
[127] Kawasaki T, Koga S, Koga N, Noguchi T, Tanaka H, Koga H, et al. Characterization of hyperintense plaque with noncontrast T(1)-weighted cardiac magnetic resonance coronary plaque imaging: comparison with multislice computed tomography and intravascular ultrasound. JACC Cardiovasc Imaging 2009;2:720–8.
[128] Korosoglou G, Weiss RG, Kedziorek DA, Walczak P, Gilson WD, Schar M, et al. Noninvasive detection of macrophage-rich atherosclerotic plaque in hyperlipidemic rabbits using "positive contrast" magnetic resonance imaging. J Am Coll Cardiol 2008;52:483–91.
[129] Neubauer S, Krahe T, Schindler R, Horn M, Hillenbrand H, Entzeroth C, et al. 31P magnetic resonance spectroscopy in dilated cardiomyopathy and coronary artery disease. Altered cardiac high-energy phosphate metabolism in heart failure. Circulation 1992;86:1810–8.
[130] Kalil-Filho R, de Albuquerque CP, Weiss RG, Mocelim A, Bellotti G, Cerri G, et al. Normal high energy phosphate ratios in "stunned" human myocardium. J Am Coll Cardiol 1997;30:1228–32.
[131] Taylor AJ, Cerqueira M, Hodgson JM, Mark D, Min J, O'Gara P, et al. ACCF/SCCT/ACR/AHA/ASE/ASNC/NASCI/SCAI/SCMR 2010 Appropriate Use Criteria for Cardiac Computed Tomography. A Report of the American College of Cardiology Foundation Appropriate Use Criteria Task Force, the Society of Cardiovascular Computed Tomography, the American College of Radiology, the American Heart Association, the American Society of Echocardiography, the American Society of Nuclear Cardiology, the North American Society for Cardiovascular Imaging, the Society for Cardiovascular Angiography and Interventions, and the Society for Cardiovascular Magnetic Resonance. Circulation 2010;122:e525–55.
[132] Goldstein JA, Chinnaiyan KM, Abidov A, Achenbach S, Berman DS, Hayes SW, et al. The CT-STAT (Coronary Computed Tomographic Angiography for Systematic Triage of Acute Chest Pain Patients to Treatment) trial. J Am Coll Cardiol 2011;58:1414–22.
[133] Litt HI, Gatsonis C, Snyder B, Singh H, Miller CD, Entrikin DW, et al. CT angiography for safe discharge of patients with possible acute coronary syndromes. N Engl J Med 2012;366:1393–403.
[134] Hoffmann U, Truong QA, Schoenfeld DA, Chou ET, Woodard PK, Nagurney JT, et al. Coronary CT angiography versus standard evaluation in acute chest pain. N Engl J Med 2012;367:299–308.
[135] Wittenberg J, Powell Jr. WM, Dinsmore RE, Miller SW, Maturi RA. Computerized tomography of ischemic myocardium: quantitation of extent and severity of edema in an in vitro canine model. Invest Radiol 1977;12:215–23.
[136] Mahnken AH, Bruners P, Bornikoel CM, Kramer N, Guenther RW. Assessment of myocardial edema by computed tomography in myocardial infarction. JACC Cardiovasc Imaging 2009;2:1167–74.
[137] Winer-Muram HT, Tann M, Aisen AM, Ford L, Jennings SG, Bretz R. Computed tomography demonstration of lipomatous metaplasia of the left ventricle following myocardial infarction. J Comput Assist Tomogr 2004;28:455–8.

[138] Adams DF, Hessel SJ, Judy PF, Stein JA, Abrams HL. Computed tomography of the normal and infarcted myocardium. AJR Am J Roentgenol 1976;126:786–91.
[139] Hoffmann U, Millea R, Enzweiler C, Ferencik M, Gulick S, Titus J, et al. Acute myocardial infarction: contrast-enhanced multi-detector row CT in a porcine model. Radiology 2004;231:697–701.
[140] Lessick J, Ghersin E, Dragu R, Litmanovich D, Mutlak D, Rispler S, et al. Diagnostic accuracy of myocardial hypoenhancement on multidetector computed tomography in identifying myocardial infarction in patients admitted with acute chest pain syndrome. J Comput Assist Tomogr 2007;31:780–8.
[141] Moore W, Fields J, Mieczkowski B. Multidetector computed tomography pulmonary angiogram in the assessment of myocardial infarction. J Comput Assist Tomogr 2006;30:800–3.
[142] Sanz J, Weeks D, Nikolaou K, Sirol M, Rius T, Rajagopalan S, et al. Detection of healed myocardial infarction with multidetector-row computed tomography and comparison with cardiac magnetic resonance delayed hyperenhancement. Am J Cardiol 2006;98:149–55.
[143] Shapiro MD, Sarwar A, Nieman K, Nasir K, Brady TJ, Cury RC. Cardiac computed tomography for prediction of myocardial viability after reperfused acute myocardial infarction. J Cardiovasc Comput Tomogr 2010;4:267–73.
[144] Buecker A, Katoh M, Krombach GA, Spuentrup E, Bruners P, Gunther RW, et al. A feasibility study of contrast enhancement of acute myocardial infarction in multislice computed tomography: comparison with magnetic resonance imaging and gross morphology in pigs. Invest Radiol 2005;40:700–4.
[145] Baks T, Cademartiri F, Moelker AD, Weustink AC, van Geuns RJ, Mollet NR, et al. Multislice computed tomography and magnetic resonance imaging for the assessment of reperfused acute myocardial infarction. J Am Coll Cardiol 2006;48:144–52.
[146] Paul JF, Wartski M, Caussin C, Sigal-Cinqualbre A, Lancelin B, Angel C, et al. Late defect on delayed contrast-enhanced multi-detector row CT scans in the prediction of SPECT infarct size after reperfused acute myocardial infarction: initial experience. Radiology 2005;236:485–9.
[147] Gerber BL, Belge B, Legros GJ, Lim P, Poncelet A, Pasquet A, et al. Characterization of acute and chronic myocardial infarcts by multidetector computed tomography: comparison with contrast-enhanced magnetic resonance. Circulation 2006;113:823–33.
[148] Jacquier A, Boussel L, Amabile N, Bartoli JM, Douek P, Moulin G, et al. Multidetector computed tomography in reperfused acute myocardial infarction. Assessment of infarct size and no-reflow in comparison with cardiac magnetic resonance imaging. Invest Radiol 2008;43:773–81.
[149] Nieman K, Shapiro MD, Ferencik M, Nomura CH, Abbara S, Hoffmann U, et al. Reperfused myocardial infarction: contrast-enhanced 64-Section CT in comparison to MR imaging. Radiology 2008;247:49–56.
[150] Wang, et al. Low dose prospective ECG-gated delayed enhanced dual-source computed tomography in reperfused acute myocardial infarction comparison with cardiac magnetic resonance. Eur J Radiol 2011;80:326–30.
[151] Koyama Y, Matsuoka H, Mochizuki T, Higashino H, Kawakami H, Nakata S, et al. Assessment of reperfused acute myocardial infarction with two-phase contrast-enhanced helical CT: prediction of left ventricular function and wall thickness. Radiology 2005;235:804–11.

[152] Lessick J, Dragu R, Mutlak D, Rispler S, Beyar R, Litmanovich D, et al. Is functional improvement after myocardial infarction predicted with myocardial enhancement patterns at multidetector CT? Radiology 2007;244:736–44.

[153] Kim T, Choi BJ, Kang DK, Sun JS. Assessment of myocardial viability using multidetector computed tomography in patients with reperfused acute myocardial infarction. Clin Radiol 2012;67:754–65.

[154] So A, Hsieh J, Imai Y, Narayanan S, Kramer J, Procknow K, et al. Prospectively ECG-triggered rapid kV-switching dual-energy CT for quantitative imaging of myocardial perfusion. JACC Cardiovasc Imaging 2012;5:829–36.

[155] Ruzsics B, Lee H, Zwerner PL, Gebregziabher M, Costello P, Schoepf UJ. Dual-energy CT of the heart for diagnosing coronary artery stenosis and myocardial ischemia-initial experience. Eur Radiol 2008;18:2414–24.

[156] Habis M, Capderou A, Ghostine S, Daoud B, Caussin C, Riou JY, et al. Acute myocardial infarction early viability assessment by 64-slice computed tomography immediately after coronary angiography: comparison with low-dose dobutamine echocardiography. J Am Coll Cardiol 2007;49:1178–85.

[157] Sato A, Hiroe M, Nozato T, Hikita H, Ito Y, Ohigashi H, et al. Early validation study of 64-slice multidetector computed tomography for the assessment of myocardial viability and the prediction of left ventricular remodelling after acute myocardial infarction. Eur Heart J 2008;29:490–8.

[158] Habis M, Capderou A, Sigal-Cinqualbre A, Ghostine S, Rahal S, Riou JY, et al. Comparison of delayed enhancement patterns on multislice computed tomography immediately after coronary angiography and cardiac magnetic resonance imaging in acute myocardial infarction. Heart 2009;95:624–9.

[159] Sato A, Nozato T, Hikita H, Akiyama D, Nishina H, Hoshi T, et al. Prognostic value of myocardial contrast delayed enhancement with 64-slice multidetector computed tomography after acute myocardial infarction. J Am Coll Cardiol 2012;59:730–8.

[160] Pang LF, Zhang H, Lu W, Yang WJ, Xiao H, Xu WQ, et al. Spectral CT imaging of myocardial infarction: preliminary animal experience. Eur Radiol 2013;23:133–8.

[161] Hamilton-Craig C, Seltmann M, Ropers D, Achenbach S. Myocardial viability by dual-energy delayed enhancement computed tomography. JACC Cardiovasc Imaging 2011;4:207–8.

[162] O'Gara PT, Kushner FG, Ascheim DD, Casey Jr. DE, Chung MK, de Lemos JA, et al. 2013 ACCF/AHA guideline for the management of ST-elevation myocardial infarction: a report of the American College of Cardiology Foundation/American Heart Association Task Force on Practice Guidelines. Circulation 2013;127:e362–425.

[163] Anderson JL, Adams CD, Antman EM, Bridges CR, Califf RM, Casey Jr. DE, et al. ACC/AHA 2007 guidelines for the management of patients with unstable angina/non ST-elevation myocardial infarction: a report of the American College of Cardiology/American Heart Association Task Force on Practice Guidelines (Writing Committee to Revise the 2002 Guidelines for the Management of Patients With Unstable Angina/Non ST-Elevation Myocardial Infarction): developed in collaboration with the American College of Emergency Physicians, the Society for Cardiovascular Angiography and Interventions, and the Society of Thoracic Surgeons: endorsed by the American Association of Cardiovascular and Pulmonary Rehabilitation and the Society for Academic Emergency Medicine. Circulation 2007;116:e148–304.

[164] Steg PG, James SK, Atar D, Badano LP, Blomstrom-Lundqvist C, Borger MA, et al. ESC Guidelines for the management of acute myocardial infarction in patients presenting with ST-segment elevation. Eur Heart J 2012;33:2569–619.
[165] Hamm CW, Bassand JP, Agewall S, Bax J, Boersma E, Bueno H, et al. ESC Guidelines for the management of acute coronary syndromes in patients presenting without persistent ST-segment elevation: The Task Force for the management of acute coronary syndromes (ACS) in patients presenting without persistent ST-segment elevation of the European Society of Cardiology (ESC). Eur Heart J 2011;32:2999–3054.

Myocardial viability

A.J. Ludman*, C.D. Anagnostopoulos†, P. Leeson‡, F. Pugliese§, S.E. Petersen§
*Royal Devon & Exeter NHS Foundation Trust, Exeter, UK; †Biomedical Research Foundation Academy of Athens, Athens, Greece; ‡University of Oxford, Oxford, UK; §The London Chest Hospital, London, UK

11.1 Background, terms, and definitions

11.1.1 Introduction

With advancing technology, non-invasive imaging has gone through exponential growth and myocardial viability assessment is now possible using several different imaging modalities with numerous different techniques. Echocardiography, computed tomography (CT), single-photon emission computed tomography (SPECT), cardiovascular magnetic resonance (CMR), and even positron emission tomography (PET) imaging have become much more widely accessible, meaning patients may now undergo a number of different imaging studies prior to decisions on invasive treatments and particularly revascularisation therapy. The differentiation between infarcted, non-viable myocardium and regions that are still viable has been an area of extensive research and debate over several decades; however, the clinical role of viability information is still controversial. This chapter will define viability in its different forms, compare and contrast the non-invasive imaging modalities most commonly used, and discuss the clinical context where knowledge of viability may inform clinical decisions at a patient level. Areas of ongoing research and emerging new imaging methods will be highlighted and discussed. We are able to gather huge quantities of information from non-invasive imaging studies of viability, and by doing this we hope to limit the risks of invasive procedures and treatments to those who are likely to gain benefit and reduce the number of unnecessary or unsuccessful interventions. Increasingly, cardiac surgeons and physicians are required to be able to assimilate information from several different forms of viability studies and it is important to understand the strengths and weaknesses of the different modalities (Table 11.1), as well as the usefulness of this data at a patient level.

11.1.2 Ischaemic heart disease and heart failure

Deaths from coronary artery disease (CAD) have been falling in the Western world over the past few decades due to progressive advances in primary and secondary prevention as well as improvements in acute treatments of myocardial infarction (MI). However, CAD remains the cause of death in 1 in 6 Americans [1] and 1 in 5 Europeans [2], and although survival is improving, approximately 20% of over 65-year-olds will

Table 11.1 Comparison of the different imaging modalities used for myocardial viability assessment

Imaging technique	Main physical property imaged	Advantages	Disadvantages	LV segmental recovery Sensitivity	LV segmental recovery Specificity	Global LV functional improvement Sensitivity	Global LV functional improvement Specificity
LDDSE	Contractile reserve	Relative low cost, availability, few contraindications	Image quality variable, operator dependent	79%	78%	57%	73%
SPECT							
Thallium-201 Technetium-99 sestamibi or Tetrofosmin	Myocyte membrane integrity	Availability, many years experience	Limited resolution, radiation dose	87% 83%	54% 65%	84% 84%	53% 68%
PET							
FDG	Glucose metabolism	High accuracy	Radiation dose, cost, limited availability, patient preparation	92%	63%	83%	64%
CMR							
LGE	Scar/interstitial space	High accuracy, reproducible, lack of radiation	Limited availability, gadolinium relatively contraindicated in severe renal dysfunction, contraindicated with metallic implants	84%	63%	–	–
LDD	Contractile reserve	Good image quality, no contraindication in renal dysfunction	Relatively long procedure, claustrophobia	81%	91%	–	–

LDDSE: low dose dobutamine stress echo, LGE: late gadolinium enhancement, CMR: cardiac magnetic resonance, LDD: low dose dobutamine, SPECT: single photon emission computed tomography, PET: positron emission tomography.

subsequently develop heart failure within 5 years of a first MI [1]. Approximately two-thirds of cases of systolic heart failure are caused by CAD [3], and the overall mortality for people diagnosed with heart failure remains 50% at 5 years [1]. Therefore, it is clear that there is still significant room for improvement in the treatment of this group of patients. The ability to predict who will benefit from revascularisation therapies is an attractive prospect that may help target interventions appropriately. An assessment of myocardial viability has become integral to this process, although the ideal method of assessment remains controversial.

11.1.3 Viable myocardium

Viable myocardium is commonly used as an umbrella term that may describe many different myocardial entities, including normal, myopathic, ischaemic, or partially infarcted. However, the term "viable myocardium" is particularly important when that area is dysfunctional, and implies capacity for improvement if the insult (usually ischaemia) is corrected and differentiates from areas that are non-viable and will not recover function. The identification of viable and non-viable myocardium *should* allow the direction of therapies to provide most benefit for the risk of the intervention. Of course, how to decide whether myocardium is viable, and what intervention may be of benefit, are not always straightforward questions to answer and will be discussed in this chapter.

11.1.4 Myocardial cell death

Ischaemia is the most common cause of myocyte death. Myocyte dysfunction occurs very early following the onset of ischaemia and irreversible cell death occurs in a matter of minutes. During an MI the progression of injury is described as a "wave front" proceeding from endocardium to epicardium [4] (see Chapter 10). In theory, in the absence of reperfusion, all myocardium subtended by the occluded artery will become infarcted – a transmural MI. However, in chronic coronary arterial disease, the development of extensive collateral vessels may allow a large vessel to occlude with minimal resultant infarction. Increasingly, reperfusion therapy is administered, aborting the MI, leaving an infarct which has progressed only partway between endo- and epicardium. It is most commonly in these cases that an assessment of viability is required but is also most challenging. Whether or not to offer revascularisation to a dysfunctional and partially infarcted myocardial territory is the key question that non-invasive imaging attempts to answer.

11.1.5 Myocardial stunning

As discussed above, myocardial ischaemia does not always result in cell death. "Stunning" of the myocardium represents myocardial dysfunction which persists following a period of non-lethal myocardial ischaemia, despite restoration of coronary blood flow. Therefore there is a "mismatch" between the normal perfusion and abnormal contraction. Stunning may also occur following exercise-induced ischaemia in the setting of critical coronary stenosis or following cardiac surgery and cardioplegic cardiac arrest [5,6]. Importantly, this form of myocardial dysfunction will resolve over time. The exact mechanism remains to be elucidated but it is thought that oxygen-derived free-radical formation, transient intracellular calcium overload, and excitation–contraction uncoupling result in contractile dysfunction which recovers gradually [7,8].

11.1.6 Myocardial hibernation

This situation arises in the face of chronic ischaemia or repeated episodes of stunning where the myocardium adapts to enter a low energy usage state as a protective mechanism from infarction [9–12] but which results in contractile dysfunction (see Figure 11.1 for some of the postulated pathophysiological mechanisms of myocardial stunning and hibernation). In contrast to early definitions, resting flow in hibernating myocardial segments may not be decreased to the extent that would account for the degree of contractile dysfunction. In most cases, there is impairment of myocardial per-

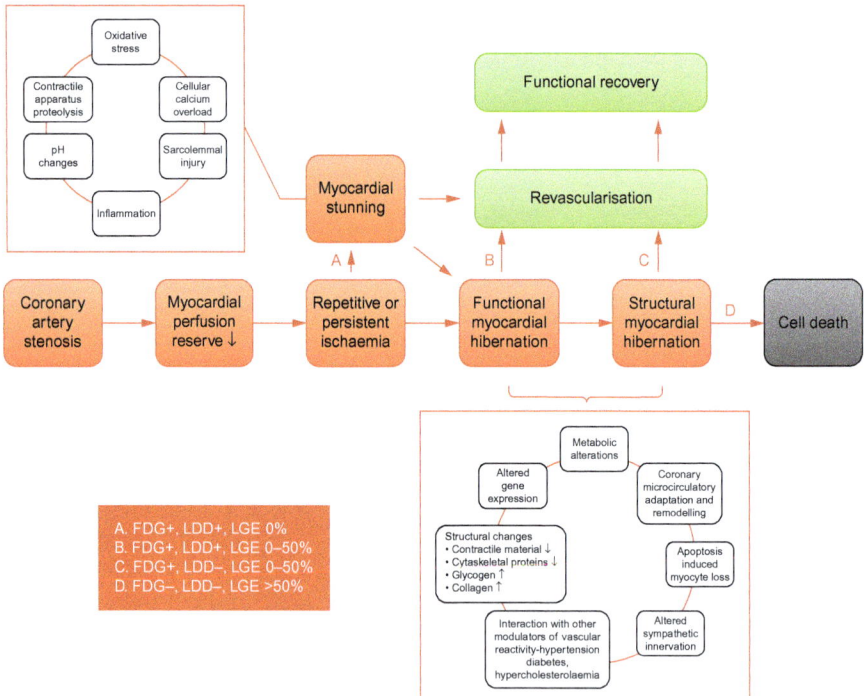

Figure 11.1 Some of the postulated pathophysiological mechanisms associated with myocardial stunning and progressive myocardial hibernation. Representative patterns of findings from ^{18}F FDG PET, low-dose dobutamine stress (LDD), and late gadolinium enhancement (LGE) CMR at different stages are shown at points A–D. Note that as the duration of myocardial hibernation prolongs, pathological changes become increasingly structural rather than functional and the myocardium may cease to respond to low-dose dobutamine and eventually will no longer take up FDG. Eventually, in the absence of reperfusion, myocyte cell death may occur; however, the timing and extent will be variable in each individual. See text for further details and references.

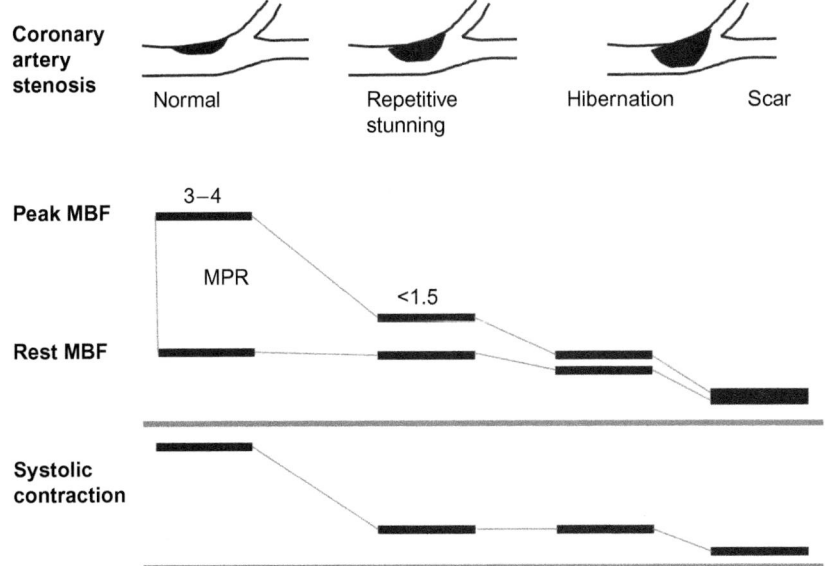

Figure 11.2 Relative myocardial blood flow (MBF) and myocardial perfusion reserve (MPR) associated with increasing coronary artery stenosis and the impact on myocardial systolic contraction.

fusion reserve (MPR), with reduction of resting perfusion seen in only the most severe cases (Figure 11.2). Hibernation describes a spectrum with chronic repetitive stunning showing normal or near normal resting perfusion and impaired MPR at one end and reduced resting perfusion at the other. In order to recover function in hibernating myocardium, coronary revascularisation is required which restores an adequate MPR.

11.1.7 Clinical setting

In the clinical arena, away from the controlled conditions of the laboratory, stunning and hibernation may be encountered together or separately in a number of conditions. For instance, even if an acute MI is treated rapidly with primary percutaneous coronary intervention or thrombolysis, significant LV dysfunction may result. This will be composed of an established infarct which will not be salvageable and probably a component of myocardial stunning in surrounding tissue which will recover over hours to days. In the more chronic presentation of heart failure due to ischaemic heart disease, there is likely to be a contribution from established infarction and, due to ongoing persistent ischaemia, other areas will have entered a hibernating state. Other conditions may include congenital defects leading to ischaemic myocardium, such as anomalous left coronary artery from the pulmonary artery or occasionally severe valvular disease. On a case-by-case basis, it is the diagnosis of the underlying pathology and then the clarification of the relative contributions of viable (stunned or hibernating) and non-viable myocardium by multimodality imaging which may guide future therapy and evaluate associated risks and benefits.

11.2 Multimodality imaging for myocardial viability assessment

Since the discovery that a MI did not have to result in complete tissue death [13], the concept of viable and non-viable areas of myocardium has become increasingly important. The search for reliable markers of viability predates this, however, as the clinical question of viability is relevant not only in the acute phase of a MI but also with chronic ischaemia. Early studies in cardiac surgery demonstrated improvement in LV function following revascularisation even in some akinetic territories thought to be completely infarcted [14]. Early assessments of viability were largely based on ECG criteria – estimating infarct size with measurement of ST segment elevation height [15] or chronically with the presence of Q waves. The use of invasive left ventriculography was also common but it was recognised that dysfunction did not always mean non-viable and detailed conclusions from this technique were limited. However, the presence of contractile reserve had been identified with an epinephrine challenge, the so-called epinephrine ventriculogram [16]. Cardiac enzyme quantification (mainly creatine kinase release) was also used [17]. Whilst this correlates to infarct size, and may be a useful surrogate end-point in clinical trials, it does not allow an assessment of residual viable tissue in an individual. Thereafter, the ideal non-invasive imaging technique to measure infarct size and to establish whether residual myocardium is viable or not has been pursued with vigour [18].

11.2.1 Morphology

All imaging techniques allow some descriptive assessment of the left ventricle and some morphological features may give early clues to viability. It has been recognised for some time that myocardial cell death leads to thinning of the ventricle wall [19,20] and reduced residual viable myocardium. On this basis, severe regional thinning with contractile dysfunction maybe detected by several different imaging modalities and represents an indicator of viability. Echocardiography is often the first line investigation used (it is widely available, portable and does not require radiation) and will give the first information regarding viability. Nuclear techniques tend not to be used for morphology alone due to limited spatial resolution, whereas CMR excels in this area with excellent spatial resolution and unlimited image planes, allowing straightforward and accurate wall thickness measurement (Figure 11.3). In patients where poor acoustic windows make echocardiography impossible or where an implantable cardiac device renders CMR unfeasible, cardiac CT is an alternative option. Using retrospective gating to image throughout the cardiac cycle, or prospective gating with padded acquisition windows to include end-systole and end-diastole, it is possible to acquire whole-heart data very rapidly with CT. In post-processing, regions of interest can be drawn in a similar fashion to CMR around the LV/RV endo- and epicardium at end-systole and end-diastole in order to calculate end-diastolic volume, end-systolic volume, and myocardial volume which can be converted to mass. CT measures compare favourably to that of CMR, with $r=0.95–0.97$ for LV measures and $r=0.94–0.97$ for RV volumes, using a 16 slice CT scanner [21], and $r=0.89–0.96$ for LV volumes

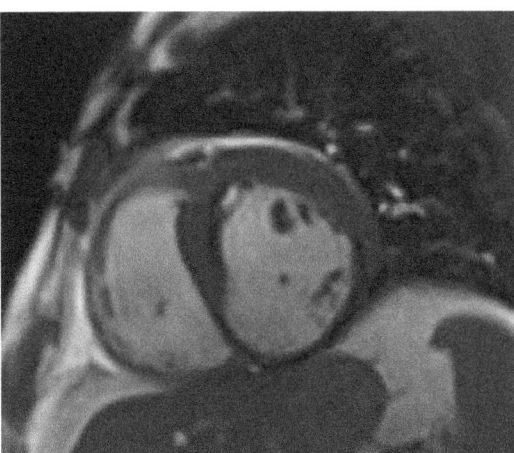

Figure 11.3 Still image from a LV short-axis CMR cine sequence demonstrating a thinned inferior wall due to myocardial infarction.

and mass measures and $r=0.7–0.88$ for RV volumes and mass using a dual-source CT scanner with low radiation (20%) during the majority of the acquisition time [22]. Technically, in order to achieve good definition of the interventricular septum and RV cavity, it is important not to wash out the contrast from the RV and so a mixed saline/contrast "chaser" can be used, following the initial contrast bolus in order to avoid this.

With echocardiography, chronic MI will eventually produce a thinned and "echo bright" appearance of the myocardium. In a group of 45 patients, a LV segmental wall thickness of <6mm gave a sensitivity of 94%, specificity of 48%, and negative predictive value of 93% for non-recovery of function following revascularisation, although the reverse was not true, as a value >6mm was not predictive of viability [23]. A recent CMR study has cast some doubt on this relatively straightforward parameter. Of 201 patients studied, 18% with a thinned myocardial wall (end-diastolic wall thickness <5.5mm) were found to have limited scar burden in this area using late gadolinium imaging. There was poor correlation between wall thickness and scar extent ($r=-0.22$) and the likelihood of recovery following revascularisation was reliably predicted only by the scar extent and not by regional thinning [24]. In addition, the presence of Q waves or collateral flow on angiography did not reliably predict the extent of scar tissue. Therefore, myocardial thickness may be an early indicator of viability in some patients but additional information is required in order to make clinical decisions.

11.2.2 Contractile reserve

Whilst a regional wall motion abnormality may provide the first indicator of previous myocardial injury, it is not always possible to reliably distinguish between stunned, hibernating, or completely infarcted myocardium under rest conditions. However, the response of severely hypokinetic or akinetic segments to stress may allow an assessment of viability by demonstrating whether the area has contractile reserve. Although low-level exercise stress can be used, dobutamine pharmacological stress is the most commonly used method and may be used alongside echocardiography or CMR. To avoid increasing myocardial oxygen demand and provoking more profound hypokinesis, a low dose (typically 5–10 mcg/kg/min) is used, aiming to provide inotropic effects without significant chronotropic response. If additional information regarding ischaemia is required, then doses up to 40 mcg/kg/min with additional atropine may be used, in order to reach a target heart rate of 85% of the predicted maximum for age. Echo is the more traditional modality and is particularly reliant on good acoustic windows, even more so than resting echo, as subtle changes in wall motion may be crucial. If two contiguous LV segments are incompletely visualised then the use of blood pool contrast agents is recommended [25], which can significantly improve the endocardial border visualisation and may allow a combined perfusion assessment (see Chapter 2). The "classic" response of dysfunctional but viable myocardium to dobutamine stress is biphasic, with an initial increase in contractility at low dose but with a worsening of contractility at higher doses due to developing ischaemia (Figure 11.4). This biphasic response is most associated with segmental functional recovery following revascularisation [26]; however, other responses may be seen (Figure 11.5).

Continued functional improvement through low and high doses of dobutamine suggests a limited infarct which has produced a resting regional wall motion abnormality

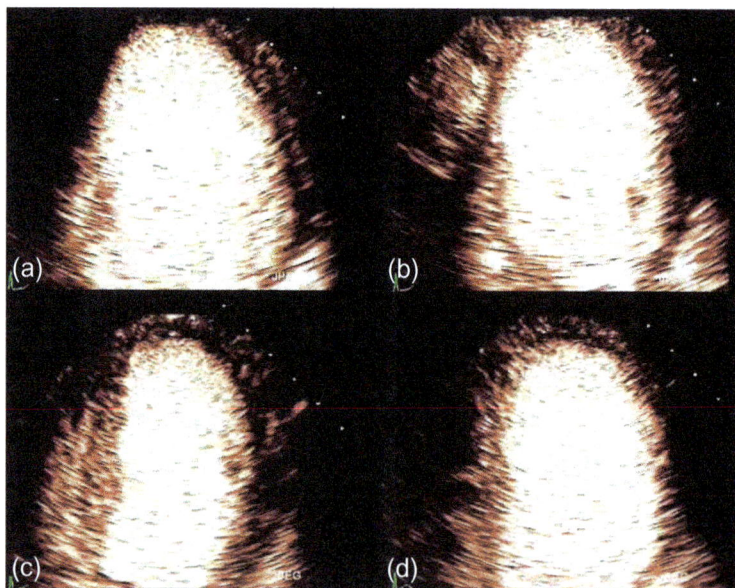

Figure 11.4 Apical two-chamber views at end-systole from a contrast-enhanced dobutamine stress echo study demonstrating a biphasic response. At rest (a) the ventricle is dilated with poor systolic contraction which progressively improves in all territories with 5 mcg/kg/min (b) and 10 mcg/kg/min (c) of dobutamine but which deteriorates again with 20 mcg/kg/min dobutamine (d). This suggests hibernation of the inferior and anterior walls and the presence of significant stenoses in the coronary arteries supplying these territories. With thanks to Dr Navtej Chahal.

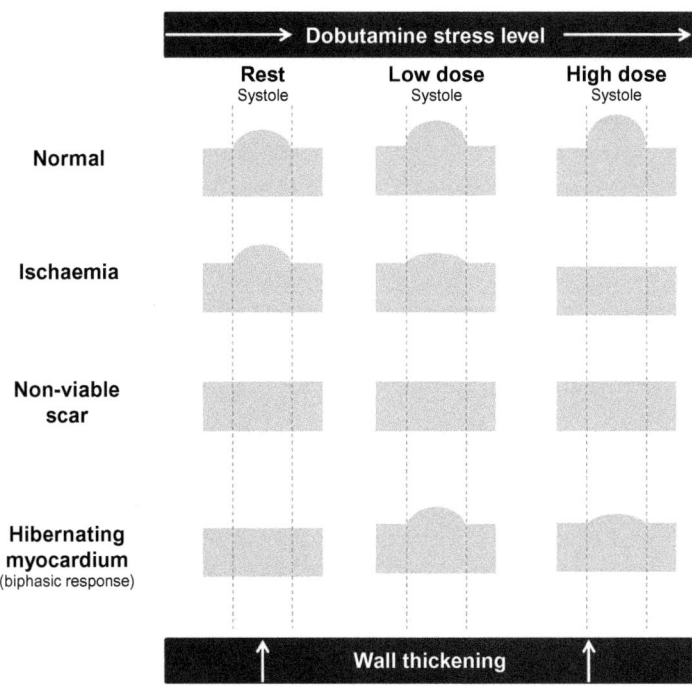

Figure 11.5 Different myocardial responses to dobutamine stress testing. The reduction in wall thickening with ischaemia may be variable in degree and timing.

but is not ischaemic. No response to dobutamine may mean that the segment is non-viable and will not recover function once revascularised; however, caution should be exercised in cases of critical ischaemia, where even low doses of dobutamine may cause a further reduction in myocardial blood flow, preventing any apparent initial improvement of contraction in viable tissue. These segments often have mild reduction in resting perfusion with avid uptake of FDG or SPECT tracers and almost completely exhausted MPR which prevents the segments from increasing their oxygen consumption upon inotropic stimulation and hence from increasing their contractile function. Apart from the exhaustion of MPR, other factors, such as the presence and severity of cardiomyocytic alterations or down-regulation of beta-adrenoceptors, may also contribute to the lack of contractile reserve in apparently viable segments.

Dobutamine stress techniques evaluating contractile reserve in general have slightly lower sensitivities than perfusion modalities but with higher specificity. Pooled analysis of 1121 patients using low-dose dobutamine stress echo (LDDSE) to predict regional improvement in function following revascularisation gave a weighted mean sensitivity of 79% and specificity of 78% which improves to 83% and 79% respectively when high-dose dobutamine is used [27]. Tissue Doppler (see Chapter 2) has been used with some success to try and give objective measures to viability assessment [28]. Although increasing the sensitivity in this study, angle dependency and an increased examination time have prevented this being adopted routinely.

Low-dose dobutamine used as part of a CMR study to evaluate viability allows the attractive prospect of being able to evaluate infarct extent (see infarct imaging below), visualise un-infarcted areas and test for contractile reserve in one sitting. Technically this is performed in a similar fashion to DSE with an incremental increase in dobutamine dose from typically 5–10 mcg/kg/min. At rest, and with each dose increment, three short axis and three long axis cine images are acquired and assessed for regional wall motion. For ischaemia assessment, it is possible to administer gadolinium-based contrast agents at peak stress (40 mcg/kg/min) to assess for inducible perfusion defects with first pass perfusion. This may help improve the specificity [29] for diagnosis of coronary disease, but whether this adds additional weight to a viability decision is unknown.

A meta-analysis of nine small studies using LDD CMR calculated the mean weighted sensitivity and specificity as 81% (95% CI: 73–86%) and 91% (95% CI: 84–95%), whereas the PPV and NPV were 93% (95% CI: 87–97%) and 75% (95% CI: 65–83%), respectively. The weighted overall accuracy for this technique in isolation was 84% (95% CI: 82–86%) [30].

Finally, low-dose dobutamine has been combined with nitrate enhanced, sestamibi, and ECG-gated SPECT in order to assess LV regional wall motion, and has good agreement with LDDSE [31]. Inability to assess segments with low tracer uptake limits use in some patients, but in general, wall motion and LVEF can also be accurately assessed during a viability/perfusion study by SPECT or PET [32].

11.2.3 Membrane integrity

Myocardial perfusion scintigraphy (MPS) relies on the fact that the tracer is taken up by intact cardiac myocytes but not myocardial scar. SPECT MPS is a well-established and widely available technique. 201-Thallium is not only a perfusion agent but also a tracer of myocardial viability due to the reliance of tracer uptake on both myocardial blood flow and sarcolemmal integrity (see Chapter 3). It has therefore been used widely for identifying myocardial viability and hibernation. Various imaging criteria have been proposed for the identification of viable myocardium. The most commonly used is the ratio of radiotracer uptake in the relevant region to the uptake seen in the best-perfused area of the myocardium. There is a direct relationship between tracer uptake and amount of viable myocardium and an inverse relationship with the amount of connective tissue. Myocardial viability is considered clinically significant when the detected tracer uptake exceeds 50% of the maximum in the myocardium. This criterion is highly specific, if there is coexisting ischemia at rest. As thallium redistribution may be slow or incomplete in regions of reduced perfusion, the usual stress/redistribution protocol can underestimate myocardial viability and additional steps may be required. These include late redistribution imaging at 8–72 h after stress injection, reinjection of tracer at rest after redistribution imaging, and a resting injection on a separate day with both early (20 min) and delayed imaging (4 h) (Figure 11.6).

MIBI and tetrofosmin have also been used for the detection of viable and hibernating myocardium. In theory, these tracers may underestimate viability in areas with reduced resting perfusion because they do not redistribute and cannot thus allow independent distinction of perfusion and viability. Some studies have therefore found ^{201}Tl SPECT MPS to be a more sensitive test for the assessment of viability (Figure 11.7).

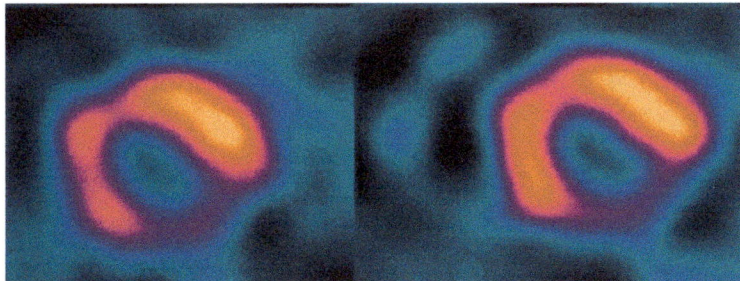

Figure 11.6 Rest and redistribution Thallium-201 scintigraphy. Early (20 min – left panel) and late (4 h – right panel) resting short-axis images demonstrating a mildly reversible defect in the anteroseptal region as well as a fixed abnormality at the inferolateral wall. The appearances are compatible with myocardial hibernation in the anteroseptal region and partial thickness myocardial infarction in the inferolateral region.
Reproduced with the permission of Elsevier from Ref. [33].

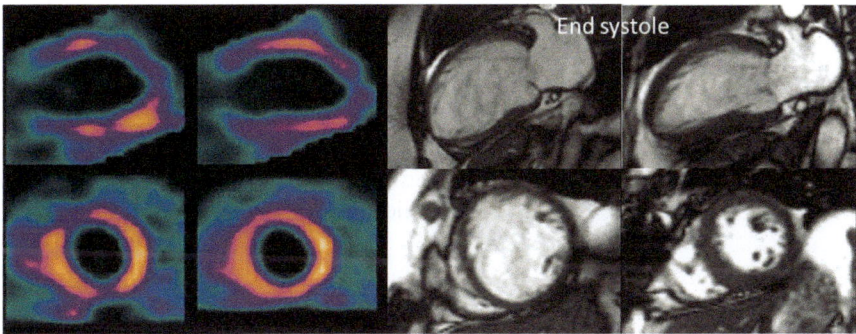

Figure 11.7 An example of a large area of anteroapical myocardial stunning which is reversed following revascularisation. Tc-99m tetrofosmin myocardial perfusion images demonstrating inducible ischaemia in the anteroapical wall. Viability is well maintained in this area exhibiting tracer uptake greater than 50% of the maximum in the LV myocardium. The cine CMR images are at end-systole before and after CABG and show regional thinning and contractile dysfunction of the anterior wall. Following CABG, there is a significant reduction in end-systolic cavity size and improvement in wall thickening, and therefore improvement in LVEF.

However, the use of sublingual nitrates improves resting perfusion and thus the detection of myocardial viability using technetium tracers. An important advantage of using MIBI or tetrofosmin SPECT is the ability to perform ECG gating and thus assess ventricular function. Whichever tracer is used, SPECT assessments have generally higher sensitivity but poorer specificity when compared with DSE for the detection of myocardial viability. Pooled analysis of 40 studies (1119 patients) using thallium-201 to predict the segmental recovery of function calculated the weighted mean sensitivity and specificity to be 87% and 54% respectively, with positive and negative predictive values (PPV or NPV) of 67% and 79% respectively [27]. Similar analysis of 25 studies (721 patients) using technetium-99 sestamibi or tetrofosmin found a sensitivity and specificity of 83% and 65% respectively, with PPV and NPV of 74% and 76%, respectively [27]. The generally lower specificity for regional recovery of function may not be such a critical disadvantage because other factors, such as the improvement of symptoms and prognosis after revascularisation, are more important than the exact prediction of improvement of regional wall systolic function. The higher sensitivity of SPECT is likely to be due to the reliance of tracer uptake on myocyte membrane integrity, which may be preserved even after loss of myocyte contractile reserve. The use of a 50% threshold of maximal myocardial uptake to identify viability may contribute to the poorer specificity and SPECT cannot assess transmurality of an infarct. It may also encounter difficulties when there is severe global myocardial ischaemia, as the assessment of relative perfusion relies on at least one segment with normal blood flow. This situation is uncommon but obviously important not to miss, and so other signs, such as transient LV dilatation during stress, must be considered.

11.2.4 Infarct imaging

Once again, the visualisation and quantification of MI in humans has been the domain of the radionuclide techniques (and largely SPECT) for several decades; however, the choice of technique has grown substantially with the development of PET–CT, CMR and increasingly cardiac CT (see Chapter 10). This section will discuss the ability of these techniques to detect and image MI.

SPECT derived measures of infarct size have good correlation against pathological specimens in animals [34,35], cardiac enzymes, and prognosis in chronic [36] and acute [37] MI. SPECT MPS has been used in patients with acute MI to estimate the area at risk and subsequently myocardial salvage. For this purpose, the most appropriate radiotracers are MIBI or tetrofosmin, administered before reperfusion. Due to their non-significant redistribution, imaging can be performed after the acute event when the patient is stable, but the information obtained represents the perfusion conditions that existed in the myocardium before reperfusion. Repeat injection of radiotracer and imaging a few days later allows the difference between the two images to be calculated, giving the amount of myocardium salvaged. Areas with reduced uptake, in comparison to presumed normal areas of myocardium, are considered infarcted. The amount of reduction in uptake indicates viability (with $\geq 50\%$ reduction commonly indicating lack of viability), but it is not possible to assess transmurality or visualise any residual rim of un-infarcted myocardium. Resolution of small or subendocardial infarcts is limited, and whilst it is possible to estimate the percentage of myocardium infarcted, the difficulty in visualising the epicardial border necessitates extrapolation in these areas. SPECT is useful in new onset heart failure in differentiating ischaemic from non-ischaemic cardiomyopathy, but when defects are found in patients with unobstructed epicardial coronary arteries, beyond distribution of the defects, SPECT may not add considerably to the differential diagnosis [38].

PET–CT imaging has significantly better resolution than SPECT (4–7 vs. 8–10 mm respectively) and therefore can detect smaller infarcts; however, its use in the acute setting has been limited. PET is an excellent option for viability assessment in patients with LV dysfunction of ischaemic aetiology, as discussed later in this chapter.

CMR is now widely regarded as the gold standard imaging technique with which to image MI. The technique relies upon the increased extracellular volume which is present in the infarcted area due to myocyte death and progressive fibrosis. A gadolinium chelate administered intravenously will perfuse the myocardium and over a few minutes fill the myocardial extracellular space. Gadolinium-based contrast does not cross intact cell membranes and so remains extracellular and will "wash out" more slowly from the infarct than from normal myocardium. Using an inversion recovery fast gradient echo sequence, the maximum signal contrast between infarct and normal myocardium is sought, which produces a hyperenhanced infarcted area with "nulled" normal myocardium appearing black when imaged in the "late" phase (between 10 and 20 min following contrast administration) [39] (Figure 11.8). CMR offers spatial resolution of 1–2 mm and measured infarct size correlates perfectly ($R=0.99$) with pathological specimens [40].

The infarct size detected by late gadolinium enhancement (LGE) correlates with clinical measures of infarction [41] as well as clinical outcomes in acute [42] and chronic MI [43]. In comparison to the radionuclide techniques, the rate of detection

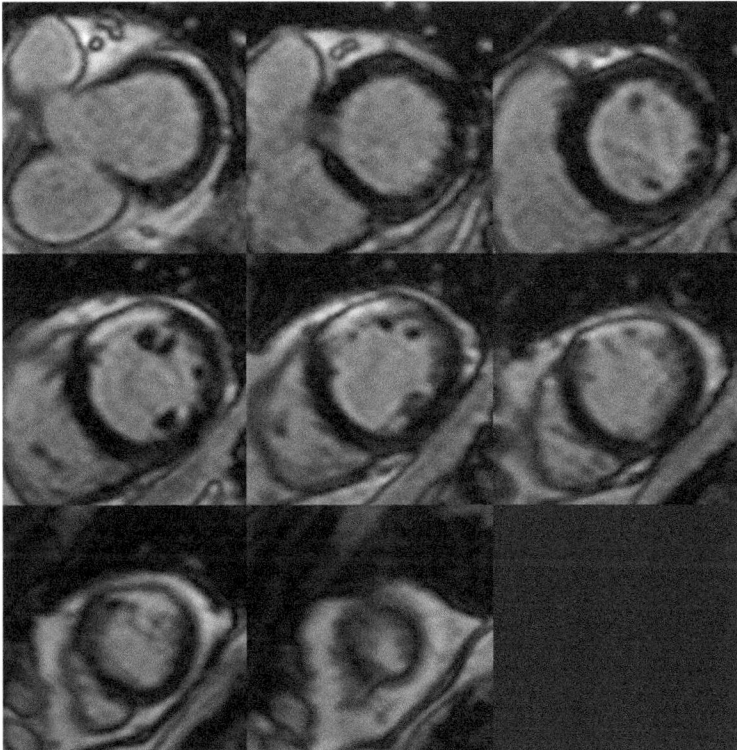

Figure 11.8 A "stack" of short-axis CMR images demonstrating late gadolinium enhancement of the mid to apical anterior LV wall. This is approximately 75% transmurality, suggesting a very low likelihood of functional recovery following revascularisation. With thanks to Dr Filip Zemrak.

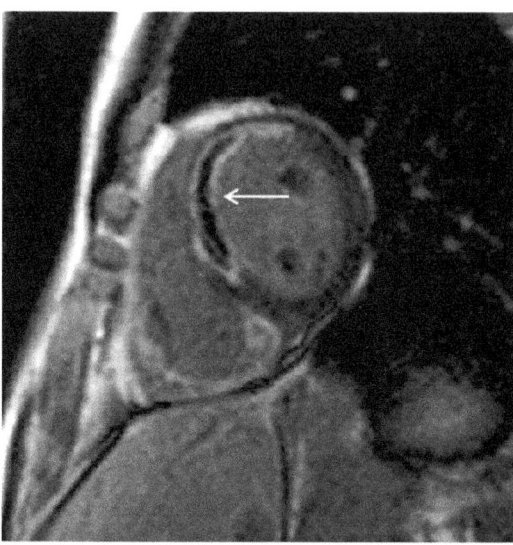

Figure 11.9 An acute transmural anteroseptal myocardial infarction imaged with late gadolinium enhanced CMR. Note the hypointense core of microvascular obstruction ringed by brightly enhanced infarcted myocardium.

of infarction between SPECT [44,45], PET and CMR is similar but CMR has significantly better sensitivity to detect smaller, subendocardial infarcts [46,47].

The resolution and tissue characterisation capability of CMR is also allowing new insights into infarct pathology with descriptions of the border zone between normal and infarcted myocardium [48] and characteristics within the infarct such as microvascular obstruction [49] (Figure 11.9). Contrast-enhanced CMR is not specific to MI; the high spatial resolution allows precise delineation of the areas of enhancement; the pattern of which can be a signal of alternative non-ischaemic pathology and therefore very useful in the evaluation of patients with de novo heart failure [50]. The lack of ionising radiation makes CMR a very attractive tool with which to follow the evolution of myocardial infarcts either clinically or as part of a trial of new treatment.

The ability to assess the transmurality of an MI by CMR has important implications for viability (Figure 11.10). The seminal paper by Kim et al. established the inverse link between transmural extent of an infarct detected by LGE and subsequent improvement in function. Using a scale of 0, $\leq 25\%$, 26–50%, 51–75%, and >75% transmurality in 50 patients prior to revascularisation by CABG or PCI, dysfunctional segments of myocardium that had >75% transmural infarction had almost no chance (1/58) of recovery of function at a mean follow-up of 79 ± 36 days. Segments with >50% transmural infarction also had a very small (13/124) chance of recovery; however, those with <50% had a good chance of recovering (256/329 for 0%, 109/183 for 1–25%, and 46/110 for 26–50%) [51]. These findings were subsequently replicated in acute MI [52] and in chronic MI and CABG [53], and have been widely adopted into CMR reporting (Figure 11.11). However, it is important to note that the segmental models used in these studies were more extensive (e.g., eight short axis slices with

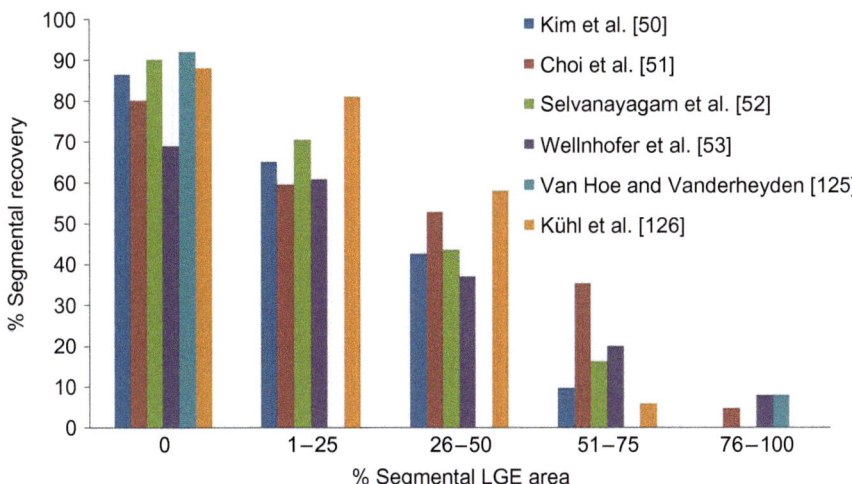

Figure 11.10 Percentage of segments with severe hypokinesia, akinesia, or dyskinesia that improved in function following revascularisation versus extent of segmental late gadolinium enhancement [51–54,125,126]; Van Hoe and Vanderheyden [125] did not report data divided for quartiles 1–75% but overall saw a 43% segmental recovery in this group. Kim et al. [51], Selvanayagam et al. [53] and Kühl et al. [126] reported 0% segmental recovery for 76–100% segmental LGE area.

8 or 12 segments each) than the standard 17 segment model of the LV commonly used (Figure 11.12), and so caution must be used in clinical practice to avoid the wrong conclusion. Also, a lack of contrast enhancement does not guarantee recovery. The reasons for this are not always clear, but may include incomplete revascularisation, peri-procedural injury, or an additional underlying cardiomyopathy. Pooled analysis of 5 studies using delayed contrast-enhanced CMR to predict segmental recovery of function found a weighted mean sensitivity and specificity of 84% and 63%, respectively [27]. The number of patients studied so far is relatively small, but it is evident that precise demarcations of viable/non-viable tissue linked to CMR-derived infarct transmurality are somewhat artificial, and rather there is probably a continuum of viability that will also be governed by other factors. A rim of unenhanced sub-epicardial myocardium greater than 3–4 mm seems also to suggest recovery of function following revascularisation, but additional predictive power can be gained by evaluating contractile reserve as well in these patients [55,56]. Therefore, in cases where the transmural extent of infarction is between 26% and 75% it may be important to consider information from a number of imaging modalities [54].

Pushed by advancing CMR techniques and by widening availability of cardiac CT, there has been renewed interest in the use of CT to visualise areas of MI with a technique similar to that of delayed enhancement CMR (Figure 11.13). Altered "wash-in", "wash-out" kinetics of the iodine based contrast in areas of infarction or replacement fibrosis will produce an area of hyperenhancement when imaged approximately 5–20 min following administration. The contrast is thought to accumulate in

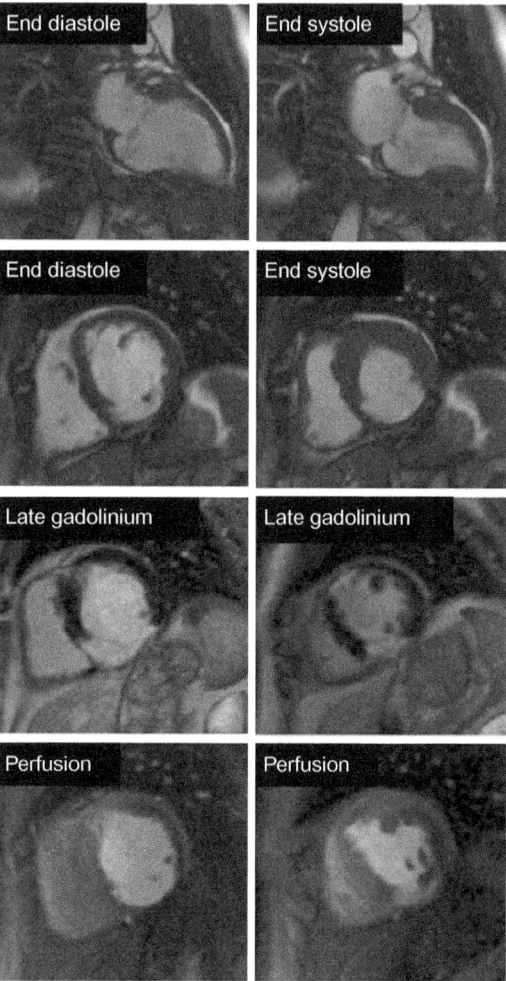

Figure 11.11 A 52-year-old male with moderately impaired LV systolic function and symptoms of dyspnoea and exertional angina. Invasive coronary angiography (not shown) demonstrates a patent LAD, occluded RCA and severe proximal stenosis in the left circumflex. CMR images in the top two rows show preserved wall motion in the anterior and lateral walls but a thinned and akinetic inferior wall. The third row shows two short-axis LV views with late gadolinium enhancement, demonstrating a near transmural inferior infarct (considered non-viable), a limited anterior infarct (<50% transmurality, considered viable), and no infarct in the lateral wall. The bottom row demonstrates perfusion defects following adenosine stress in the inferior and anterior walls which match the areas of infarction as well as an extensive defect in the lateral wall. Given the lack of viability in the inferior wall, with no significant ischaemia beyond the infarcted area, the patient went on to have targeted intervention to the LCx artery along with optimisation of his medical therapy.

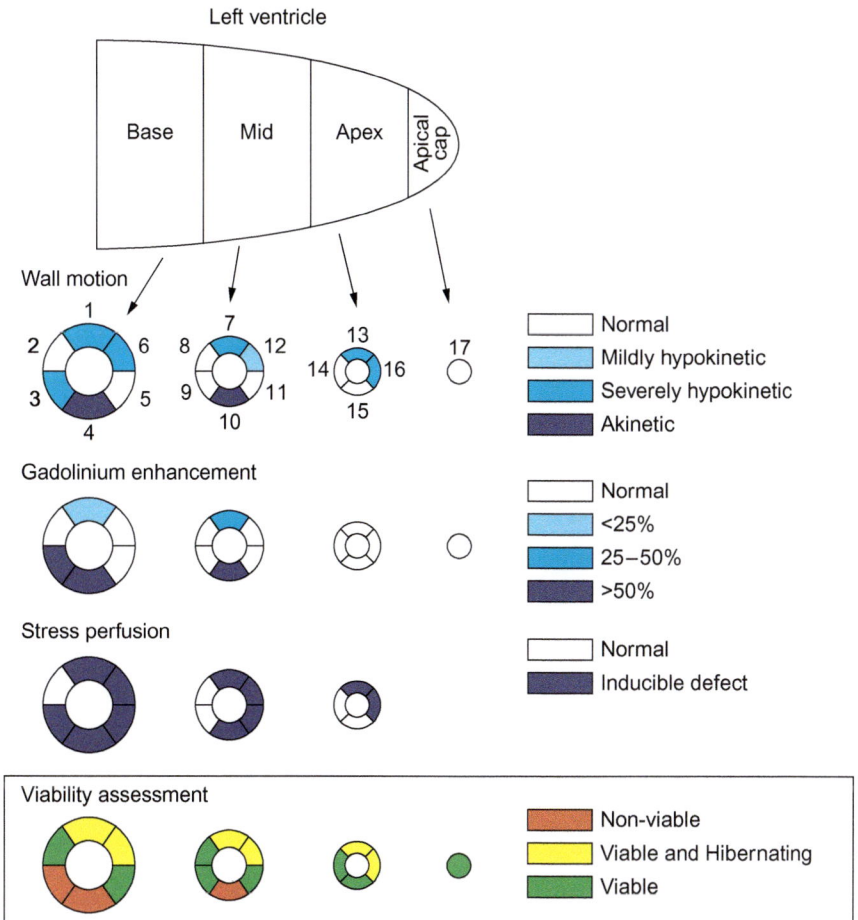

Figure 11.12 An example of a viability and perfusion chart that can be used in clinical practice. Note in this example there is a near transmural myocardial infarction of the basal inferoseptal and inferior segments and mid inferior segment with severe hypokinesia or akinesia. There is an inducible perfusion defect in these segments but this is matched by near transmural infarction and so these segments are non-viable. There is a limited anterior myocardial infarction with an extensive perfusion defect in the anterior and lateral walls from base to apex with hypokinesia of the basal to mid anterior and anterolateral segments and of the apical anterior and lateral segments. This suggests significant remaining viability and ischaemic myocardium in the anterior and lateral walls and there is a good chance that function will recover following revascularisation.

the expanded extracellular space in areas of infarction or replacement fibrosis [57]. Overall, experience in clinical settings remains relatively small, but CT correlates highly with pathological specimens [58] and CMR [59] in animal models of acute and chronic infarction. Initial experience in humans was also very positive with early studies in patients following acute MI demonstrating excellent correlation of CT infarct

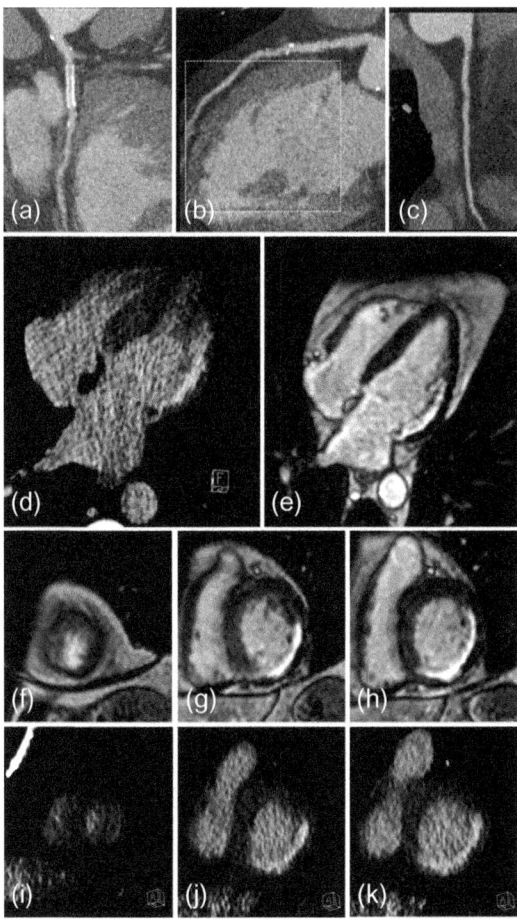

Figure 11.13 CT coronary angiography multi-planar reformatted images with CT delayed contrast enhancement of a myocardial infarction compared to CMR gadolinium late enhancement. (a) Patent stent in the proximal left circumflex artery. (b) Patent left anterior descending artery with minor calcified plaque. (c) Right coronary artery with minor plaque disease. (d) Delayed contrast imaging by CT in a four-chamber view demonstrating hyperenhancement of the basal to mid lateral wall. (e) Late gadolinium enhancement by CMR in the same patient. (f–h) Late gadolinium enhancement by CMR and by delayed contrast-enhanced CT (i–k) in short axis confirming a 50–75% transmural myocardial infarction involving the basal to mid inferior and lateral walls.

quantification with CMR [60,61] and SPECT [62]. Enterprisingly, some investigators have made use of the iodine contrast load that patients receive during PCI for acute MI and performed delayed-phase CT in the period directly after the last contrast injection [63, 64]. CT assessment of infarct size derived viability (using <50% transmurality as viable and >50% as non-viable) correlated well to DSE with 98% sensitivity and 94% specificity [63] and transmural infarcts were associated with increased adverse remodeling and hospitalisations for heart failure [64]. However, away from the acute setting in a population of 105 symptomatic patients with intermediate to high pre-test probability of CAD, CT had only moderate ability to detect MI by delayed enhancement (sensitivity 53%, specificity 98%) versus CMR and did not add incremental value to the CT angiogram and perfusion study [65]. Promisingly, the additional radiation dose was small for the delayed imaging and in some patients image quality was very good (e.g., patients weighing <80 kg), so, with refinement, CT is still likely to have a role in imaging infarction, but further work will need to be done in order to clarify where and when.

11.2.5 Metabolic assessment

The myocardium has a high energy demand and under physiological conditions the majority of energy comes from the oxydation of fatty acids. In ischaemia, oxydation of fatty acids is suppressed and there is increased glycolysis and glycogen breakdown. Clinical myocardial metabolic imaging for viability therefore centres on glucose and fatty acid metabolism. There are two main techniques which study viability in the clinical setting using these metabolic pathways and will be discussed below.

The most established technique uses 2-fluorodeoxyglucose labelled with fluorine-18 (^{18}F FDG) to image glucose metabolism with PET and has been regarded as the "gold standard" for detection of myocardial hibernation since at least 1986 [66] (for detailed procedural technique, see [67]). Dysfunctional myocardial segments with higher FDG uptake compared to that of ^{13}N-ammonia or ^{82}Rb (mismatch between perfusion and metabolism) represent hibernating myocardium while reduction of both perfusion and metabolism suggests the presence of scarring (Figure 11.14). In cases of myocardial stunning, perfusion is normal or almost normal while the ^{18}F FDG uptake is variable. Indeed, this may even be reduced compared to perfusion (reverse mismatch). This pattern has been observed in situations of repetitive stunning, following revascularisation early post-MI when the myocardium is stunned, in patients with LBBB and in some patients with diabetes.

Pooled analysis of 24 studies (756 patients) demonstrated a weighted mean sensitivity and specificity of 92% and 63% respectively for prediction of recovery of segmental contractile function [27] (Table 11.1). In addition, ^{18}F FDG imaging may also allow identification of viability in some patients, despite lack of contractile reserve on DSE [69] and in one study had a particularly impressive negative predictive value (100%) for lack of segmental functional recovery [70]. From a practical perspective, the established post-processing software, with largely automatic and objective calculation of ischaemic burden and viability extent makes PET very attractive for viability assessment. Although definitely increasing in availability, widespread use has been limited by cost, centre expertise, logistic arrangements for tracers, and concern around additional radiation dose (~10.8 mSv for a stress/rest ^{82}Rb/^{18}F FDG examination), although this may be of limited concern in older people with chronic heart failure.

11.2.5.1 BMIPP fatty acid metabolism

^{123}I-(p-iodophenyl)-3-(R,S)-methylpentadecanoic acid, (^{123}I-BMIPP) is a radio-iodinated fatty acid analogue which is taken up into the myocyte and incorporated into the

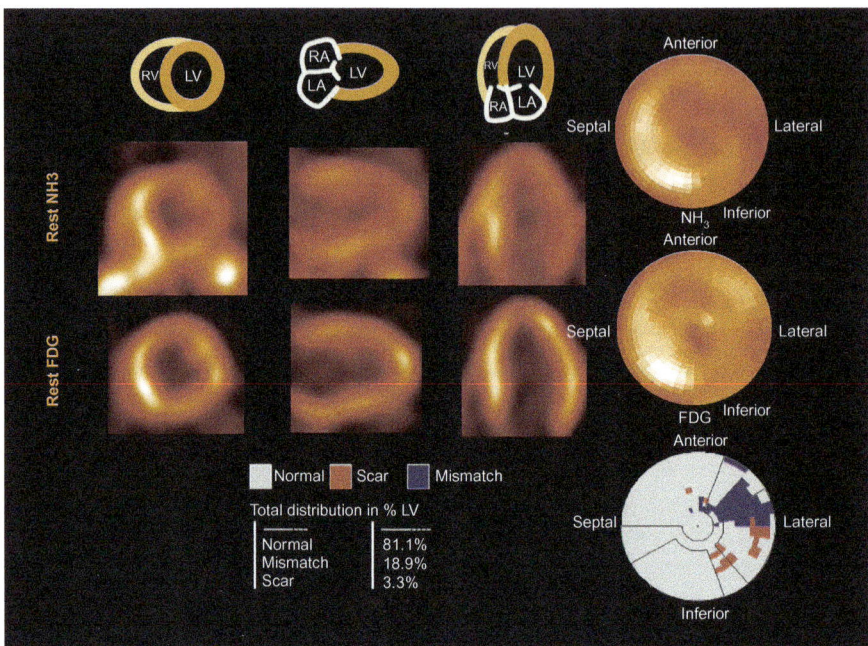

Figure 11.14 A 68-year-old male with known CAD, previous myocardial infarctions, impaired LV function, and multiple previous PCIs underwent a PET study for assessment of myocardial viability. Analysis of the resting ^{13}N-ammonia and ^{18}F FDG tomographic images and polar maps shows a large mismatch between perfusion and metabolism (19% of the total myocardial mass) in the anterolateral region compatible with hibernating myocardium. There is an area with minor match inferolaterally (indicative of very limited myocardial damage involving only 3.1% of the total myocardial mass) but otherwise well preserved perfusion and viability in the LV myocardium. ^{18}F FDG, ^{18}F-fluorodeoxyglucose; CAD, coronary artery disease; LV, left ventricle; PCI, percutaneous coronary intervention; PET, positron emission tomography, RV, right ventricle; RA, right atrium; LA, left atrium).
Modified with the permission of Elsevier from Ref. [68].

triglyceride pool. Its molecular structure prevents rapid catabolism and so has good characteristics for clinical imaging. In the acute phase following a revascularised MI, BMIPP SPECT imaging has been successfully used to demonstrate the amount of myocardial salvage that has occurred and in acute coronary syndromes to represent jeopardised ("at risk") myocardium with links to future adverse events [71,72]. In patients with chronic ischaemic LV dysfunction the presence of a mismatch (reduced BMIPP activity in comparison to perfusion level) correlates well with LDDSE to suggest viable territory [73]. In a small number of patients the combined use of ^{201}Tl and BMIPP to predict regional functional recovery following revascularisation gave a sensitivity of 80% and specificity of 62% [74]. Combining ^{18}F FDG and BMIPP allows a differential to be evaluated between glucose and fatty acid metabolism (preserved or increased glucose metabolism with reduced fatty acid metabolism) and predicts viability in the most severely dysfunctional segments which show the most improvement in function once revascularised [75]. However, this study only evaluated segments supplied by the left coronary artery which were only revascularised if viability had been demonstrated and BMIPP did not add greatly over ^{18}F FDG results, hence the generalisability to clinical practice is limited.

In conclusion, BMIPP gives an interesting insight to the myocardial metabolism in viability but as yet has mainly been studied in Japan and has not demonstrated reproducible incremental value in the clinical setting over other established techniques.

11.3 The role of myocardial viability assessment in clinical decision-making

11.3.1 Heart failure and ischaemic heart disease – to revascularise or not to revascularise?

Whether patients with significant systolic dysfunction due to ischaemic heart disease should undergo revascularisation of stenosed or occluded coronary arteries has remained one of the most contentious issues in cardiology for several decades. Patients with severe LV systolic dysfunction are at relatively high risk of peri-procedural morbidity and mortality and so it is important to understand who to subject to this risk in order to maximise the reward. Early studies of CABG versus medical therapy in patients with reduced LVEF (>34% but <50%) demonstrated a large survival benefit over 7 years of follow-up [76], but it was hoped that viability assessment may identify those likely to benefit the most. Subsequently, there were a number of largely retrospective, cohort-based studies evaluating this issue. The presence of viability by any imaging modality (although mainly DSE and nuclear techniques) appeared to confer a significantly improved outcome in those undergoing revascularisation. A meta-analysis of 24 studies including 3088 patients, with viability tested by thallium perfusion imaging, ^{18}F FDG metabolic imaging, or DSE concluded that in patients with viable myocardium revascularisation resulted in a 79.6% relative reduction in annual mortality compared to medical treatment (absolute risk, 16% vs. 3.2%, $p<0.0001$) (Table 11.2). The beneficial effect of revascularisation on survival in patients with viability appeared to correlate to the severity of LV dysfunction. However, patients with no imaging evidence of viability gained no benefit from revascularisation [77]. Despite the retrospective nature of the original studies, the weight of this apparent benefit was difficult to argue with and viability assessment became established in international guidelines. An updated meta-analysis published in 2007 confirmed the previously made conclusions as well as added data for CMR [27]. Whilst there were small variations between the different modalities (discussed previously), in general, patients with viability undergoing revascularisation had significantly improved mortality versus medical therapy and patients without viability gained limited if any benefit. Notably, the worst prognosis was found in patients with demonstrable viability receiving only medical therapy. In addition, patients with viability gained the most improvement in symptoms and exercise tolerance. A separate meta-analysis, of similar studies, identified an optimal threshold for percentage of viable myocardium

Table 11.2 Summary of the main studies evaluating the effect of viability imaging on mortality

Reference	Imaging modality	Study design	Number of participants	Effect on mortality
Allman et al. [77]	DSE, 201 Tl-MPS, FDG-PET	Meta-analysis of retrospective studies	3088	79.6% relative reduction in annual mortality with revascularisation versus medical treatment in those with evidence of myocardial viability (absolute risk, 16% vs. 3.2%, $p < 0.0001$)
Schinkel et al. [27]	DSE, MPS (201 Tl and 99 Tc), FDG-PET	Meta-analysis of retrospective studies	3640	Pooled analysis of annual mortality (revascularisation/medical treatment): With viability 3.5%/11.25%; without viability 9%/9%
Beanlands et al. [78]	FDG-PET	Prospective, randomised, controlled	430	Primary intention-to-treat analysis: No benefit of FDG-PET on mortality (HR for cardiac death 0.72; 95% CI 0.40–1.3; $p = 0.25$)
Bonow et al. [79]	DSE, SPECT	Sub-group analysis of patients who had undergone viability testing having previously been randomised to CABG or medical therapy	601	The presence of viability had no significant effect on mortality following adjustment for baseline confounders (HR 0.64; 95% CI 0.48–0.86; $p = 0.21$)

CABG: coronary artery bypass graft surgery, DSE: dobutamine stress echo, MPS: myocardial perfusion scintigraphy, SPECT: single photon emission computed tomography, PET: positron emission tomography.

which led to an increase in survival with revascularisation of ~25% for PET, ~35% for stress echo, and ~38% for SPECT [80]. These values were considerably higher than the mismatch threshold of 7% for PET identified in the substudy of PET and Recovery following Revascularisation (PARR-2) study [81] (discussed below) and of >5% in another retrospective analysis [82], highlighting the uncertainty in this area and the limitations of retrospective data. The extent of hibernating myocardium required to render revascularisation successful in substantially increasing LVEF also varies between studies. A consistent theme is that LVEF is likely to increase with successful revascularisation of increasing numbers of hibernating segments [83] and that significant residual viability is required (at least 20%). By SPECT and CMR, thresholds of 8 and 10 segments of viable/normal myocardium have been suggested, below which no significant increase in LVEF is seen post revascularisation by CABG [84,85]. However, others [86] have reported that mortality is improved even if no increase in LVEF occurs, with benefit conferred by reduced ischaemic events or fatal arrhythmia; thus emphasising the importance of adequately powered studies with hard end-points rather than surrogate markers. As in many of these studies, the revascularisation decision making process was not randomised, confounders not always adequately adjusted for, and the quality of the medical therapy was unverified. Accordingly, doubts about the optimal treatment strategy persisted and it was evident that a prospective randomised trial with up-to-date medical therapy was required. Unfortunately, recruiting to studies of this nature was difficult [87], possibly in some quarters it was felt that the benefit of revascularisation had already been proven. Similarly, it is difficult to conduct studies of viability when the decision to revascularise includes the viability information, as physician bias may intervene without strict adherence to protocols. This was found in the PARR-2 study [78] where there was significant clinician deviation (25% of patients) from the recommendations of the PET studies performed. In this study, patients with severe LV dysfunction being investigated for heart failure, transplantation, or revascularisation were recruited and underwent ^{18}F FDG PET ischaemia/viability assessment (with ^{82}Rb or NH_3 as the perfusion tracer) (Table 11.2), if it may have been useful to the clinician. Patients had already been stratified to those having recent angiography against those who had not, but the results of the PET meant that a significant number of patients then underwent angiography, having not done so before. In the standard treatment arm, physicians did not have access to the PET data but other viability studies could be considered. Overall, the study did not report a statistically significant difference in the primary outcome of time to first major cardiac event, but in a post-hoc analysis, when revascularisation was performed based on the viability findings, there was a significant benefit to PET guided therapy with a hazard ratio of 0.62 (95% CI 0.42–0.93, $p=0.019$) of a major adverse cardiac event at 1 year.

The Surgical Treatment of IsChaemic Heart failure (STICH) study [88] was expected to resolve the ongoing equipoise (Table 11.2). Although a complex study with a number of aims, the main hypothesis was to test the outcome of patients with severe LV dysfunction and coronary disease randomised to CABG and optimal medical therapy or optimal medical therapy alone. It was originally intended that all patients would have an imaging assessment of viability, but in the end, only about half the patients enrolled were assessed by either DSE or SPECT (601) with varying protocols and outcomes reported separately [79]. From the main study, there was no significant difference in the primary outcome of all-cause mortality over the 6 years follow-up, although there was a significant reduction in the secondary end-point of cardiovascular mortality and hospitalisations over this time period (hazard ratio with CABG, 0.74; 95% CI, 0.64–0.85; $p < 0.001$). Unfortunately, in the viability sub-study, patients were not randomised to their viability study, there was significant variation in SPECT protocol across the centres, and the definition of significant viability varied (defined as at least 11 remaining viable segments by SPECT but as 5 dysfunctional segments with contractile reserve by DSE). Therefore, importantly, in the SPECT group, patients were included with viable myocardium that was not dysfunctional and so this study did not necessarily investigate the benefit of revascularising hibernating myocardium. Overall, after adjustment for baseline variables there was no difference in outcome between those undergoing revascularisation versus optimal medical therapy whether they had evidence of viability or not. Extensive discussion and debate of these findings ensued, but as of yet, there is no clear answer. The STICH study has emphasised the benefit of modern medical therapy and so this should always be optimised. Going forward, in this group of patients who often have significant co-morbidity it is difficult to prescribe a single revascularisation strategy to test in a prospective trial, and trying to prove a potentially small incremental benefit over modern medical therapy is challenging. Whether the added sensitivity and specificity of CMR or PET would have changed the result is also commonly debated [89]. It is hoped, once again, that ongoing trials such as the IMAGE-HF study will resolve this daily clinical dilemma [90].

Until we have further randomised trial evidence regarding revascularisation in patients with severe systolic dysfunction, any data from viability testing should be incorporated to an individualised patient decision. Ideally this should be in the context of a multi-disciplinary "heart team" including experts in surgery, coronary intervention, imaging techniques, and heart failure. The relative risks of an intervention must be weighed against the comorbidities, extent of coronary disease, the extent of ischaemic and hibernating myocardium, the need for valve surgery, and, of course, the preference of the patient. Both the ESC and AHA/ACC heart failure guidelines utilise the findings from the STICH studies to allow revascularisation in this group to potentially reduce cardiovascular mortality and morbidity (AHA/ACC IIa B) [3,91]. The precise place of viability testing remains to be determined.

11.3.2 Heart failure and ischaemic heart disease – should the presence of viability alter medical management?

The Christmas study [92] investigated whether patients with heart failure due to ischaemic heart disease and evidence of hibernating myocardium (defined as 2 or more segments with a contraction–perfusion mismatch by echo and MPS) would benefit more from carvedilol use than patients without evidence of hibernation. 305 patients were randomised to incrementally titrated carvedilol or placebo in a double-blinded manner. Interestingly, the incidence of significant hibernation in this cohort based on their definition was 59%. Although carvedilol significantly improved the ejection fraction versus placebo at the 6-month follow-up, there was no significant difference in EF when divided by presence or absence of hibernating myocardium (+3.6% vs. +2.9% in hibernators and non-hibernators respectively). Whilst well conducted, the study was criticised for its definition of viability [93], it did not attempt to detect myocardial stunning, and it is notable that 43% of non-hibernators also had a myocardial segment which matched study criteria for hibernation. Therefore, given the substantial benefit of beta-blockers in heart failure, and in the absence of absolute contraindications, these should be used regardless and in-spite of any viability assessment or revascularisation therapy. Similarly, there is currently no evidence that other medical therapies should be altered depending on the presence or absence of viable myocardium, and all patients should be titrated to maximal tolerated doses of guideline recommended therapy [3,91].

11.3.3 Heart failure and ischaemic heart disease – should the presence of viability alter implantable device therapy?

11.3.3.1 Implantable cardiac defibrillator

A number of studies have explored this issue but given the direct relation between the amount of myocardial scar and the amount of myocardial viability it may often be difficult to differentiate independent effects. Extent of viability was inversely related to incidence of ventricular tachycardia (VT) in 57 patients with cardiomyopathy (24 due to IHD) evaluated by SPECT imaging prior to cardiac resynchronisation therapy with defibrillator implantation [94]. Each viable segment gave an odds ratio (OR) for VT of 0.66 (95% CI 0.53–0.85, $p=0.001$) and viability of the segment adjacent to the LV lead placement gave an OR of 0.9 (95% CI 0.85–0.97, $p=0.003$). Studies with CMR have clearly demonstrated a relation between total amount of myocardial scar and arrhythmia irrespective of aetiology [95]. It is not clear, however, whether the extent of remaining viability modifies this risk or whether other factors may contribute. Other factors may include the amount of residual viable but denervated myocardium. Although areas of MI are generally denervated, surrounding viable myocardium may be as well. Using a tracer of sympathetic activity (^{11}C-meta-hydroxyephedrine, ^{11}C-HED) it is possible to image these areas with PET. In a prospective, observational cohort study, 204 patients eligible for ICD implantation underwent PET imaging for sympathetic activity, perfusion, and viability. A strong correlation was found between areas of denervated and denervated but viable myocardium. There was an increasing risk of sudden cardiac death by 6.7% for every 1% increase in viable but denervated myocardium [96]. Prospective studies to investigate whether this technique can aid risk stratification for sudden cardiac death in ischaemic heart disease will be required, however, before this becomes useful in planning ICD therapy.

11.3.3.2 Cardiac resynchronisation therapy

Approximately 30% of patients judged suitable for CRT will not respond. Viability assessment may help in identifying non-responders or assist in improving implantation to improve the likelihood of response. Extent of viability appears to be directly linked to improved CRT response as well as the presence of myocardial viability at the LV lead site, no matter whether measured by SPECT [97,98], echo [99,100], or CMR [101,102]. Imaging studies are now looking at the integration of dyssynchrony data with venous anatomy and myocardial scar in order to improve outcomes. A small study using CMR to guide the position of the LV lead to the latest activated LV segment, relative to the venous anatomy, and away from areas of scar produced a 92% response rate from 20 patients (reduction in LV end-systolic volume by >15% on echo) [103]. A larger study is underway in order to establish whether similar approaches can be successful on a wider scale [104].

11.3.4 Heart failure and valvular disease – does viability assessment help?

The timing of valvular intervention in patients with impaired LV systolic function is a common and difficult clinical problem. Predicting which patients will recover LV function with non-invasive imaging techniques may help in the decision making process. There are extensive international guidelines [105,106] on the timing of valve surgery; however, whether imaging of myocardial viability is useful remains controversial. In aortic stenosis (AS) and severe LV dysfunction, dobutamine stress echo may assist in diagnosing true severe AS, and the presence of contractile reserve appears to correlate with improved operative mortality but does not accurately predict post-operative improvement in LV function [107]. The extent of ischaemic myocardial scar detected by LGE CMR in patients undergoing valve intervention for severe AS predicts adverse remodelling (as expected) [108], but in the majority of patients the mechanism of LV dysfunction attributable to AS is through chronically raised afterload. One element of the adaptive response to this is the development of diffuse myocardial fibrosis, which is now detectable by CMR and does not significantly regress following surgery [109]. Therefore, intuitively, intervention prior to the development of significant fibrosis may improve post-operative response and beneficial remodelling; however, this remains to be studied and the optimal technique is not yet clear [110].

In mitral regurgitation, the presence or absence of contractile reserve by exercise echocardiography is linked to post-operative LV ejection fraction; however, in general, LV ejection fraction improved even in those patients without contractile reserve, meaning that this parameter is unable to predict outcomes at a patient level [111]. LDDSE and exercise echo have been used to try and predict the likelihood of recovery of LV function following valve replacement in severe aortic regurgitation. Failure to reduce end-systolic volume or increase EF on exercise correlates to LV dysfunction post-operatively [112] and the presence or absence of contractile reserve cannot be inferred from resting LV dimensions [113]. Therefore, it has been suggested that exercise stress echo may allow better stratification of patients who would benefit from earlier valve surgery [114]; however, this approach remains to be tested.

11.4 Current research, emerging techniques, and hybrid imaging

Despite the current uncertainty regarding the exact role of viability testing, there continues to be confidence that in the correct patient it will assist in clinical decision making. This section will briefly discuss some areas that have particular potential.

Echo-based techniques are attractive for a number of reasons but particularly due to wide availability, portability, relatively low cost, and lack of ionising radiation. As such, there is considerable ongoing research in this area for a method which will identify viable/non-viable myocardium.

One such technique uses myocardial integrated backscatter, which is the broadband scattering of frequencies from the myocardium when ultrasound echocardiography is applied. The mean integrated backscatter from an operator-defined region of interest can be plotted in decibels against time to give the temporal cyclic variation of backscatter. As the backscatter varies during the cardiac cycle and with different tissue characteristics, investigators have attempted to apply this technique to viability assessment. In order to compare parameters between studies and populations, a number of summary measures of integrated backscatter are used. These most commonly include the magnitude of cyclic variation of integrated backscatter (MVIB), which is the maximum range of backscatter measured throughout the cardiac cycle; and the normalised time delay, which is expressed as the time between the beginning of the QRS complex to the nadir of backscatter measures, divided by the QT interval. The MVIB is reduced in ischaemic or infarcted myocardium as compared to normal myocardium and may return to normal following reperfusion [115]. In patients with dysfunctional myocardial segments, it appears to correlate well with viability determined by FDG-PET but less well with contractile reserve determined by dobutamine stress echo [116]. Angle dependency has limited the myocardial segments that this technique can be reliably applied to and as yet there are no normal values defined. Therefore, as a non-invasive technique it has significant potential but cannot yet be reliably used in clinical practice.

Multimodality techniques of deformation imaging are also hoped to provide additional information.

Speckle tracking (see Chapter 2) derived values on 2D echo for longitudinal strain have been correlated to transmural extent of infarct on DE-CMR. In heart failure due to chronic ischaemic heart disease, a regional longitudinal strain value of −4.5% differentiated between no infarct and transmural infarct with a sensitivity and specificity of 81% [117]. In acute MI however, a value of −11.5% has been reported [118] with similar accuracy. Tissue tagging applied to dobutamine CMR is able to demonstrate reduced circumferential strain in non-viable territories at rest and with dobutamine [119]. Further work in larger cohorts will be required to refine the accuracy of these techniques in intermediate infarct extents, reduce inter-operator variability, and apply results on an individual patient basis.

An exciting prospect is the increasing use of a combination of imaging modalities or "hybrid imaging" (see Chapter 3 and 4). Hybrid SPECT, PET/CT, or even MRI/CT may allow simultaneous assessment of areas of viability or scar along with the coronary artery anatomy, thereby facilitating a targeted revascularisation strategy. The combination of PET with CMR has excellent soft tissue resolution to define precise myocardial scar and the high-molecular signal sensitivity of PET, allowing detailed characterisation of the myocardium (Figure 11.15). Technical challenges remain in combining different imaging modalities, and relative costs remain high; however, the combination of imaging techniques to bring together different strengths may well provide the best route forwards [120].

Advances in metabolic imaging may allow us further insights at a cellular level. Using MR spectroscopy, it is possible to measure the molecules responsible for myocyte energy. Clinically the largest experience is with the ^{31}P nucleus; this allows detection of large reductions in phosphocreatine-to-adenosine triphosphate ratio in infarcted and non-viable tissue compared to healthy controls [121]. The technique is limited by availability, the expertise required, and technical aspects, including acquisition time and spatial resolution, but has the potential to give information on cellular energetics without ionising radiation.

An alternative approach is to investigate electrolyte differences in viable versus infarcted myocardium with myocardial sodium MRI. In the acute phase of an infarct, loss of cell membrane integrity and failure of cellular homeostasis results in intracellular sodium accumulation as well as myocardial oedema and increased total sodium content. In chronic MI, the expansion in extracellular space results in ^{23}Na accumulation whereas normal values remain in stunned, hibernating, or normal myocardium. Small studies have demonstrated the ability to identify infarction and viable myocardium in animal and human models [122,123], and variations in technique allow the separation of intracellular from extracellular signals which may help in differentiating oedema from infarction in the acute phase [124]. However, this technique is far from ready for widespread clinical use as high field strength scanners are recommended and reagents safe for routine human use need to be developed.

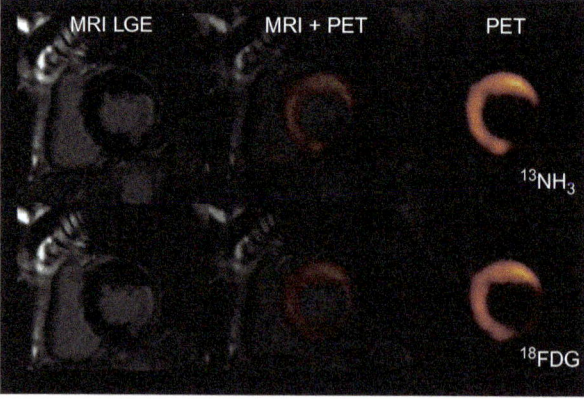

Figure 11.15 A hybrid PET/MR examination using late gadolinium enhancement MRI as a marker of fibrotic tissue with high spatial resolution, ^{13}N-ammonia PET to measure myocardial perfusion and ^{18}F FDG to delineate myocardial viability in a patient 1 week after infarction and successful intervention. Note the non-transmural LGE pattern and the higher ^{18}F FDG compared to ^{13}N-ammonia uptake. MRI, magnetic resonance imaging; ^{18}F FDG, ^{18}F-fluorodeoxyglucose, PET, positron emission tomography.
Modified with the permission of Elsevier from Ref. [68].

11.4.1 Looking to the future

The future is likely to see persistent development in all imaging modalities, aiming to refine all areas of viability assessment. The use of DSE is likely to remain strong due to its relatively low cost and widespread availability. However, as newer technologies become more available, it is likely that combinations of techniques will reveal the most sensitive results with both imaging of the scar extent as well as assessment of the metabolic and functional reserve of the residual un-infarcted myocardium. Prospective, truly randomised studies are required in defined patient groups in order to end the ongoing uncertainty of the role that viability assessment has in clinical decisions on an individual patient basis.

11.5 Conclusion

Multimodality non-invasive imaging of myocardial viability is coming of age, and it is now commonplace for patients to undergo several different imaging studies in the course of their investigation. Medical practitioners need to be able to assimilate the information received from the different imaging modalities in order to offer the best advice to the patient. Likewise, the imaging practitioner must be aware of rapid developments in all aspects of cardiac imaging and be able to recommend the right test, at the right time, for the right patient. As we continue to gain smaller and smaller incremental benefits with advancing therapies, precise imaging techniques are likely to become more and more valuable to choose the correct patients, guide the intervention, and then follow the results. The extent of myocardial viability and of myocardial scar give strong prognostic information, but the exact role that viability assessment should have in determining revascularisation strategy in LV dysfunction remains to be clarified. The results of ongoing prospective studies are eagerly awaited, which, it is hoped, will resolve this daily clinical dilemma.

Acknowledgements

The authors would like to thank The Royal Brompton Hospital CMR Unit, Dr Stephan Nekolla, Dr Filip Zemrak, and Dr Navtej Chahal for assistance with images.

References

[1] Roger VL, Go AS, Lloyd-Jones DM, Benjamin EJ, Berry JD, Borden WB, et al. Heart disease and stroke statistics—2012 update a report from the American Heart Association. Circulation 2012;125:e2–e220. http://dx.doi.org/10.1161/CIR.0b013e31823ac046.

[2] Nichols M, Townsend N, Scarborough P, Rayner M. Cardiovascular disease in Europe 2014: epidemiological update. Eur Heart J 2014;35(42):2950–9. http://dx.doi.org/10.1093/eurheartj/ehu299.

[3] McMurray JJV, Adamopoulos S, Anker SD, Auricchio A, Böhm M, Dickstein K, et al. ESC guidelines for the diagnosis and treatment of acute and chronic heart failure 2012: the task force for the diagnosis and treatment of acute and chronic heart failure 2012 of the European Society of Cardiology. Developed in collaboration with the Heart Failure Association (HFA) of the ESC. Eur J Heart Fail 2012;14:803–69. http://dx.doi.org/10.1093/eurjhf/hfs105.

[4] Reimer KA, Lowe JE, Rasmussen MM, Jennings RB. The wavefront phenomenon of ischemic cell death. 1. Myocardial infarct size vs duration of coronary occlusion in dogs. Circulation 1977;56:786–94.

[5] Braunwald E, Kloner RA. The stunned myocardium: prolonged, postischemic ventricular dysfunction. Circulation 1982;66:1146–9.

[6] Ambrosio G, Betocchi S, Pace L, Losi MA, Perrone-Filardi P, Soricelli A, et al. Prolonged impairment of regional contractile function after resolution of exercise-induced angina. Evidence of myocardial stunning in patients with coronary artery disease. Circulation 1996;94:2455–64.

[7] Bolli R, Marbán E. Molecular and cellular mechanisms of myocardial stunning. Physiol Rev 1999;79:609–34.

[8] Camici PG, Dutka DP. Repetitive stunning, hibernation, and heart failure: contribution of PET to establishing a link. Am J Physiol Heart Circ Physiol 2001;280:H929–36.

[9] Diamond GA, Forrester JS, deLuz PL, Wyatt HL, Swan HJ. Post-extrasystolic potentiation of ischemic myocardium by atrial stimulation. Am Heart J 1978;95:204–9.

[10] Rahimtoola SH. The hibernating myocardium. Am Heart J 1989;117:211–21.

[11] Elsässer A, Schlepper M, Klövekorn WP, Cai WJ, Zimmermann R, Müller KD, et al. Hibernating myocardium: an incomplete adaptation to ischemia. Circulation 1997;96:2920–31.

[12] Canty JM, Suzuki G. Myocardial perfusion and contraction in acute ischemia and chronic ischemic heart disease. J Mol Cell Cardiol 2012;52:822–31. http://dx.doi.org/10.1016/j.yjmcc.2011.08.019.

[13] Maroko PR, Kjekshus JK, Sobel BE, Watanabe T, Covell JW, Ross J, et al. Factors influencing infarct size following experimental coronary artery occlusions. Circulation 1971;43:67–82.

[14] Rees G, Bristow JD, Kremkau EL, Green GS, Herr RH, Griswold HE, et al. Influence of aortocoronary bypass surgery on left ventricular performance. N Engl J Med 1971;284:1116–20. http://dx.doi.org/10.1056/NEJM197105202842002.

[15] Reid PR, Taylor DR, Kelly DT, Weisfeldt ML, Humphries JO, Ross RS, et al. Myocardial-infarct extension detected by precordial ST-segment mapping. N Engl J Med 1974;290:123–8. http://dx.doi.org/10.1056/NEJM197401172900302.

[16] Horn HR, Teichholz LE, Cohn PF, Herman MV, Gorlin R. Augmentation of left ventricular contraction pattern in coronary artery disease by an inotropic catecholamine. The epinephrine ventriculogram. Circulation 1974;49:1063–71.

[17] Sobel BE, Shell WE. Serum enzyme determinations in the diagnosis and assessment of myocardial infarction. Circulation 1972;45:471–82. http://dx.doi.org/10.1161/01.CIR.45.2.471.

[18] Goldstein RA. Wanted: dead or alive—the search for markers of myocardial viability. J Am Coll Cardiol 1990;16:486–8. http://dx.doi.org/10.1016/0735-1097(90)90607-Q.

[19] Dubnow MH, Burchell HB, Titus JL. Postinfarction ventricular aneurysm: a clinicomorphologic and electrocardiographic study of 80 cases. Am Heart J 1965;70:753–60. http://dx.doi.org/10.1016/0002-8703(65)90331-5.

[20] Roberts CS, Maclean D, Maroko P, Kloner RA, Roberts CS, Maclean D, Maroko P, Kloner RA. Early and late remodeling of the left ventricle after acute myocardial infarction. Am J Cardiol 1984;54:407–10. http://dx.doi.org/10.1016/0002-9149(84)90206-6.

[21] Raman SV, Shah M, McCarthy B, Garcia A, Ferketich AK. Multi-detector row cardiac computed tomography accurately quantifies right and left ventricular size and function compared with cardiac magnetic resonance. Am Heart J 2006;151:736–44. http://dx.doi.org/10.1016/j.ahj.2005.04.029.

[22] Takx RAP, Moscariello A, Schoepf UJ, Barraza Jr JM, Nance Jr JW, Bastarrika G, et al. Quantification of left and right ventricular function and myocardial mass: comparison of low-radiation dose 2nd generation dual-source CT and cardiac MRI. Eur J Radiol 2012;81:e598–604. http://dx.doi.org/10.1016/j.ejrad.2011.07.001.

[23] Cwajg JM, Cwajg E, Nagueh SF, He ZX, Qureshi U, Olmos LI, et al. End-diastolic wall thickness as a predictor of recovery of function in myocardial hibernation: relation to rest-redistribution T1-201 tomography and dobutamine stress echocardiography. J Am Coll Cardiol 2000;35:1152–61.

[24] Shah DJ, Kim HW, James O, Parker M, Wu E, Bonow RO, et al. Prevalence of regional myocardial thinning and relationship with myocardial scarring in patients with coronary artery disease. J Am Med Assoc 2013;309:909–18. http://dx.doi.org/10.1001/jama.2013.1381.

[25] Senior R, Becher H, Monaghan M, Agati L, Zamorano J, Vanoverschelde JL, et al. Contrast echocardiography: evidence-based recommendations by European Association of Echocardiography. Eur J Echocardiogr 2009;10:194–212. http://dx.doi.org/10.1093/ejechocard/jep005.

[26] Afridi I, Qureshi U, Kopelen HA, Winters WL, Zoghbi WA. Serial changes in response of hibernating myocardium to inotropic stimulation after revascularization: a dobutamine echocardiographic study. J Am Coll Cardiol 1997;30:1233–40.

[27] Schinkel AFL, Bax JJ, Poldermans D, Elhendy A, Ferrari R, Rahimtoola SH. Hibernating myocardium: diagnosis and patient outcomes. Curr Probl Cardiol 2007;32:375–410. http://dx.doi.org/10.1016/j.cpcardiol.2007.04.001.

[28] Rambaldi R, Poldermans D, Bax JJ, Boersma E, Elhendy A, Vletter W, et al. Doppler tissue velocity sampling improves diagnostic accuracy during dobutamine stress echocardiography for the assessment of viable myocardium in patients with severe left ventricular dysfunction. Eur Heart J 2000;21:1091–8. http://dx.doi.org/10.1053/euhj.1999.1857.

[29] Lubbers DD, Janssen CHC, Kuijpers D, van Dijkman PRM, Overbosch J, Willems TP, et al. The additional value of first pass myocardial perfusion imaging during peak dose of dobutamine stress cardiac MRI for the detection of myocardial ischemia. Int J Cardiovasc Imaging 2008;24:69–76. http://dx.doi.org/10.1007/s10554-006-9205-5.

[30] Romero J, Xue X, Gonzalez W, Garcia MJ. CMR imaging assessing viability in patients with chronic ventricular dysfunction due to coronary artery disease: a meta-analysis of prospective trials. JACC Cardiovasc Imaging 2012;5:494–508. http://dx.doi.org/10.1016/j.jcmg.2012.02.009.

[31] Leoncini M, Marcucci G, Sciagrà R, Frascarelli F, Traini AM, Mondanelli D, et al. Nitrate-enhanced gated technetium 99m sestamibi SPECT for evaluating regional wall motion at baseline and during low-dose dobutamine infusion in patients with chronic coronary artery disease and left ventricular dysfunction: comparison with two-dimensional echocardiography. J Nucl Cardiol Off Publ Am Soc Nucl Cardiol 2000;7:426–31. http://dx.doi.org/10.1067/mnc.2000.108029.

[32] Rajappan K, Livieratos L, Camici PG, Pennell DJ. Measurement of ventricular volumes and function: a comparison of gated PET and cardiovascular magnetic resonance. J Nucl Med Off Publ Soc Nucl Med 2002;43:806–10.
[33] Underwood SR, Anagnostopoulos C. Nuclear cardiology. In: Grainger RG, Allison DJ, Adam A, Dixon AK, editors. Diagnostic radiology. 4th ed. London: Churchill Livingstone; 2001. p. 21–40.
[34] Caldwell JH, Williams DL, Harp GD, Stratton JR, Ritchie JL. Quantitation of size of relative myocardial perfusion defect by single-photon emission computed tomography. Circulation 1984;70:1048–56.
[35] Wolfe CL, Lewis SE, Corbett JR, Parkey RW, Buja LM, Willerson JT. Measurement of myocardial infarction fraction using single photon emission computed tomography. J Am Coll Cardiol 1985;6:145–51.
[36] Hurrell DG, Milavetz J, Hodge DO, Gibbons RJ. Infarct size determination by technetium 99m sestamibi single-photon emission computed tomography predicts survival in patients with chronic coronary artery disease. Am Heart J 2000;140:61–6. http://dx.doi.org/10.1067/mhj.2000.105104.
[37] Byrne RA, Ndrepepa G, Braun S, Tiroch K, Mehilli J, Schulz S, et al. Peak cardiac troponin-T level, scintigraphic myocardial infarct size and one-year prognosis in patients undergoing primary percutaneous coronary intervention for acute myocardial infarction. Am J Cardiol 2010;106:1212–7. http://dx.doi.org/10.1016/j.amjcard.2010.06.050.
[38] Soman P, Lahiri A, Mieres JH, Calnon DA, Wolinsky D, Beller GA, et al. Etiology and pathophysiology of new-onset heart failure: evaluation by myocardial perfusion imaging. J Nucl Cardiol Off Publ Am Soc Nucl Cardiol 2009;16:82–91. http://dx.doi.org/10.1007/s12350-008-9010-8.
[39] Klein C, Schmal TR, Nekolla SG, Schnackenburg B, Fleck E, Nagel E. Mechanism of late gadolinium enhancement in patients with acute myocardial infarction. J Cardiovasc Magn Reson 2007;9:653–8.
[40] Kim RJ, Fieno DS, Parrish TB, Harris K, Chen EL, Simonetti O, et al. Relationship of MRI delayed contrast enhancement to irreversible injury, infarct age, and contractile function. Circulation 1999;100:1992–2002.
[41] Ingkanisorn WP, Rhoads KL, Aletras AH, Kellman P, Arai AE. Gadolinium delayed enhancement cardiovascular magnetic resonance correlates with clinical measures of myocardial infarction. J Am Coll Cardiol 2004;43:2253–9.
[42] Larose E, Rodés-Cabau J, Pibarot P, Rinfret S, Proulx G, Nguyen CM, et al. Predicting late myocardial recovery and outcomes in the early hours of ST-segment elevation myocardial infarction traditional measures compared with microvascular obstruction, salvaged myocardium, and necrosis characteristics by cardiovascular magnetic resonance. J Am Coll Cardiol 2010;55:2459–69. http://dx.doi.org/10.1016/j.jacc.2010.02.033.
[43] Kelle S, Roes SD, Klein C, Kokocinski T, de Roos A, Fleck E, et al. Prognostic value of myocardial infarct size and contractile reserve using magnetic resonance imaging. J Am Coll Cardiol 2009;54:1770–7. http://dx.doi.org/10.1016/j.jacc.2009.07.027.
[44] Ibrahim T, Nekolla SG, Hornke M, Bulow HP, Dirschinger J, Schomig A, et al. Quantitative measurement of infarct size by contrast-enhanced magnetic resonance imaging early after acute myocardial infarction – comparison with single-photon emission tomography using Tc-99m-sestamibi. J Am Coll Cardiol 2005;45:544–52.
[45] Lund GK, Stork A, Saeed M, Bansmann MP, Gerken JH, Müller V, et al. Acute myocardial infarction: evaluation with first-pass enhancement and delayed enhancement MR imaging compared with ^{201}Tl SPECT imaging. Radiology 2004;232:49–57. http://dx.doi.org/10.1148/radiol.2321031127.

[46] Wagner A, Mahrholdt H, Holly TA, Elliott MD, Regenfus M, Parker M, et al. Contrast-enhanced MRI and routine single photon emission computed tomography (SPECT) perfusion imaging for detection of subendocardial myocardial infarcts: an imaging study. Lancet 2003;361:374–9.
[47] Klein C, Nekolla SG, Bengel FM, Momose M, Sammer A, Haas F, et al. Assessment of myocardial viability with contrast-enhanced magnetic resonance imaging: comparison with positron emission tomography. Circulation 2002;105:162–7.
[48] Yan AT, Shayne AJ, Brown KA, Gupta SN, Chan CW, Luu TM, et al. Characterization of the peri-infarct zone by contrast-enhanced cardiac magnetic resonance imaging is a powerful predictor of post-myocardial infarction mortality. Circulation 2006;114:32–9.
[49] Wu KC, Zerhouni EA, Judd RM, Lugo-Olivieri CH, Barouch LA, Schulman SP, et al. Prognostic significance of microvascular obstruction by magnetic resonance imaging in patients with acute myocardial infarction. Circulation 1998;97:765–72.
[50] Assomull RG, Shakespeare C, Kalra PR, Lloyd G, Gulati A, Strange J, et al. Role of cardiovascular magnetic resonance as a gatekeeper to invasive coronary angiography in patients presenting with heart failure of unknown etiology. Circulation 2011;124:1351–60. http://dx.doi.org/10.1161/CIRCULATIONAHA.110.011346.
[51] Kim RJ, Wu E, Rafael A, Chen EL, Parker MA, Simonetti O, et al. The use of contrast-enhanced magnetic resonance imaging to identify reversible myocardial dysfunction. N Engl J Med 2000;343:1445–53. http://dx.doi.org/10.1056/NEJM200011163432003.
[52] Choi KA, Kim RJ, Gubernikoff G, Vargas JD, Parker M, Judd RA. Transmural extent of acute myocardial infarction predicts long-term improvement in contractile function. Circulation 2001;104:1101–7.
[53] Selvanayagam JB, Kardos A, Francis JM, Wiesmann F, Petersen SE, Taggart DP, et al. Value of delayed-enhancement cardiovascular magnetic resonance imaging in predicting myocardial viability after surgical revascularization. Circulation 2004;110:1535–41. http://dx.doi.org/10.1161/01.CIR.0000142045.22628.74.
[54] Wellnhofer E, Olariu A, Klein C, Gräfe M, Wahl A, Fleck E, et al. Magnetic resonance low-dose dobutamine test is superior to SCAR quantification for the prediction of functional recovery. Circulation 2004;109:2172–4. http://dx.doi.org/10.1161/01.CIR.0000128862.34201.74.
[55] Kirschbaum SW, Rossi A, van Domburg RT, Gruszczynska K, Krestin GP, Serruys PW, et al. Contractile reserve in segments with nontransmural infarction in chronic dysfunctional myocardium using low-dose dobutamine CMR. JACC Cardiovasc Imaging 2010;3:614–22. http://dx.doi.org/10.1016/j.jcmg.2010.03.007.
[56] Glaveckaite S, Valeviciene N, Palionis D, Skorniakov V, Celutkiene J, Tamosiunas A, et al. Value of scar imaging and inotropic reserve combination for the prediction of segmental and global left ventricular functional recovery after revascularisation. J Cardiovasc Magn Reson Off J Soc Cardiovasc Magn Reson 2011;13:35. http://dx.doi.org/10.1186/1532-429X-13-35.
[57] Schuleri KH, George RT, Lardo AC. Applications of cardiac multidetector CT beyond coronary angiography. Nat Rev Cardiol 2009;6:699–710. http://dx.doi.org/10.1038/nrcardio.2009.172.
[58] Lardo AC, Cordeiro MAS, Silva C, Amado LC, George RT, Saliaris AP, et al. Contrast-enhanced multidetector computed tomography viability imaging after myocardial infarction: characterization of myocyte death, microvascular obstruction, and chronic scar. Circulation 2006;113:394–404. http://dx.doi.org/10.1161/CIRCULATIONAHA.105.521450.

[59] Baks T, Cademartiri F, Moelker AD, Weustink AC, van Geuns R-J, Mollet NR, et al. Multislice computed tomography and magnetic resonance imaging for the assessment of reperfused acute myocardial infarction. J Am Coll Cardiol 2006;48:144–52. http://dx.doi.org/10.1016/j.jacc.2006.02.059.

[60] Mahnken AH, Koos R, Katoh M, Wildberger JE, Spuentrup E, Buecker A, et al. Assessment of myocardial viability in reperfused acute myocardial infarction using 16-slice computed tomography in comparison to magnetic resonance imaging. J Am Coll Cardiol 2005;45:2042–7. http://dx.doi.org/10.1016/j.jacc.2005.03.035.

[61] Gerber BL, Belge B, Legros GJ, Lim P, Poncelet A, Pasquet A, et al. Characterization of acute and chronic myocardial infarcts by multidetector computed tomography: comparison with contrast-enhanced magnetic resonance. Circulation 2006;113:823–33. http://dx.doi.org/10.1161/CIRCULATIONAHA.104.529511.

[62] Paul J-F, Wartski M, Caussin C, Sigal-Cinqualbre A, Lancelin B, Angel C, et al. Late defect on delayed contrast-enhanced multi-detector row CT scans in the prediction of SPECT infarct size after reperfused acute myocardial infarction: initial experience. Radiology 2005;236:485–9. http://dx.doi.org/10.1148/radiol.2362040912.

[63] Habis M, Capderou A, Ghostine S, Daoud B, Caussin C, Riou J-Y, et al. Acute myocardial infarction early viability assessment by 64-slice computed tomography immediately after coronary angiography: comparison with low-dose dobutamine echocardiography. J Am Coll Cardiol 2007;49:1178–85. http://dx.doi.org/10.1016/j.jacc.2006.12.032.

[64] Sato A, Hiroe M, Nozato T, Hikita H, Ito Y, Ohigashi H, et al. Early validation study of 64-slice multidetector computed tomography for the assessment of myocardial viability and the prediction of left ventricular remodelling after acute myocardial infarction. Eur Heart J 2008;29:490–8. http://dx.doi.org/10.1093/eurheartj/ehm630.

[65] Bettencourt N, Ferreira ND, Leite D, Carvalho M, Ferreira Wda S, Schuster A, et al. CAD detection in patients with intermediate-high pre-test probability: low-dose CT delayed enhancement detects ischemic myocardial scar with moderate accuracy but does not improve performance of a stress-rest CT perfusion protocol. JACC Cardiovasc Imaging 2013;6:1062–71. http://dx.doi.org/10.1016/j.jcmg.2013.04.013.

[66] Tillisch J, Brunken R, Marshall R, Schwaiger M, Mandelkern M, Phelps M, et al. Reversibility of cardiac wall-motion abnormalities predicted by positron tomography. N Engl J Med 1986;314:884–8. http://dx.doi.org/10.1056/NEJM198604033141405.

[67] Dilsizian V, Bacharach SL, Beanlands RS, Bergmann SR, Delbeke D, Gropler RJ, et al. PET myocardial perfusion and metabolism clinical imaging. J Nucl Cardiol 2009;16:651. http://dx.doi.org/10.1007/s12350-009-9094-9.

[68] Anagnostopoulos C, Georgakopoulos A, Pianou N, Nekolla SG. Assessment of myocardial perfusion and viability by positron emission tomography. Int J Cardiol 2013;167(5):1737–49.

[69] Cornel JH, Bax JJ, Elhendy A, Visser FC, Boersma E, Poldermans D, et al. Agreement and disagreement between "metabolic viability" and "contractile reserve" in akinetic myocardium. J Nucl Cardiol Off Publ Am Soc Nucl Cardiol 1999;6:383–8.

[70] Schmidt M, Voth E, Schneider CA, Theissen P, Wagner R, Baer FM, et al. F-18-FDG uptake is a reliable predictory of functional recovery of akinetic but viable infarct regions as defined by magnetic resonance imaging before and after revascularization. Magn Reson Imaging 2004;22:229–36. http://dx.doi.org/10.1016/j.mri.2003.07.006.

[71] Mochizuki T, Murase K, Higashino H, Miyagawa M, Sugawara Y, Kikuchi T, et al. Ischemic "memory image" in acute myocardial infarction of ^{123}I-BMIPP after reperfusion therapy: a comparison with ^{99m}Tc-pyrophosphate and ^{201}Tl dual-isotope SPECT. Ann Nucl Med 2002;16:563–8.

[72] Inaba Y, Bergmann SR. Prognostic value of myocardial metabolic imaging with BMIPP in the spectrum of coronary artery disease: a systematic review. J Nucl Cardiol Off Publ Am Soc Nucl Cardiol 2010;17:61–70. http://dx.doi.org/10.1007/s12350-009-9157-y.

[73] Hambÿe AS, Vaerenberg MM, Dobbeleir AA, Van den Heuvel PA, Franken PR. Abnormal BMIPP uptake in chronically dysfunctional myocardial segments: correlation with contractile response to low-dose dobutamine. J Nucl Med Off Publ Soc Nucl Med 1998;39:1845–50.

[74] Yasugi N, Koyanagi S, Ohzono K, Sakai K, Matsumoto T, Sako S, et al. Comparative study of dobutamine stress echocardiography and dual single-photon emission computed tomography (thallium-201 and I-123 BMIPP) for assessing myocardial viability after acute myocardial infarction. Circ J Off J Jpn Circ Soc 2002;66:1132–8.

[75] Sato H, Iwasaki T, Toyama T, Kaneko Y, Inoue T, Endo K, et al. Prediction of functional recovery after revascularization in coronary artery disease using (18)F-FDG and (123) I-BMIPP SPECT. Chest 2000;117:65–72.

[76] Passamani E, Davis KB, Gillespie MJ, The CASS Principal Investigators and Their Associates. A randomized trial of coronary artery bypass surgery: survival of patients with a low ejection fraction. N Engl J Med 1985;312:1665–71. http://dx.doi.org/10.1056/NEJM198506273122603.

[77] Allman KC, Shaw LJ, Hachamovitch R, Udelson JE. Myocardial viability testing and impact of revascularization on prognosis in patients with coronary artery disease and left ventricular dysfunction: a meta-analysis. J Am Coll Cardiol 2002;39:1151–8.

[78] Beanlands RSB, Nichol G, Huszti E, Humen D, Racine N, Freeman M, et al. F-18-fluorodeoxyglucose positron emission tomography imaging-assisted management of patients with severe left ventricular dysfunction and suspected coronary disease: a randomized, controlled trial (PARR-2). J Am Coll Cardiol 2007;50:2002–12. http://dx.doi.org/10.1016/j.jacc.2007.09.006.

[79] Bonow RO, Maurer G, Lee KL, Holly TA, Binkley PF, Desvigne-Nickens P, et al. Myocardial viability and survival in ischemic left ventricular dysfunction. N Engl J Med 2011;364:1617–25. http://dx.doi.org/10.1056/NEJMoa1100358.

[80] Inaba Y, Chen JA, Bergmann SR. Quantity of viable myocardium required to improve survival with revascularization in patients with ischemic cardiomyopathy: a meta-analysis. J Nucl Cardiol Off Publ Am Soc Nucl Cardiol 2010;17:646–54. http://dx.doi.org/10.1007/s12350-010-9226-2.

[81] D'Egidio G, Nichol G, Williams KA, Guo A, Garrard L, deKemp R, et al. Increasing benefit from revascularization is associated with increasing amounts of myocardial hibernation: a substudy of the PARR-2 trial. JACC Cardiovasc Imaging 2009;2:1060–8. http://dx.doi.org/10.1016/j.jcmg.2009.02.017.

[82] Uebleis C, Hellweger S, Laubender RP, Becker A, Sohn H-Y, Lehner S, et al. The amount of dysfunctional but viable myocardium predicts long-term survival in patients with ischemic cardiomyopathy and left ventricular dysfunction. Int J Cardiovasc Imaging 2013;29:1645–53. http://dx.doi.org/10.1007/s10554-013-0254-2.

[83] Bax JJ, Maddahi J, Poldermans D, Elhendy A, Schinkel A, Boersma E, et al. Preoperative comparison of different noninvasive strategies for predicting improvement in left ventricular function after coronary artery bypass grafting. Am J Cardiol 2003;92:1–4. http://dx.doi.org/10.1016/S0002-9149(03)00454-5.

[84] Pagano D, Townend JN, Littler WA, Horton R, Camici PG, Bonser RS. Coronary artery bypass surgery as treatment for ischemic heart failure: the predictive value of viability assessment with quantitative positron emission tomography for symptomatic and functional outcome. J Thorac Cardiovasc Surg 1998;115:791–9.

[85] Pegg TJ, Selvanayagam JB, Jennifer J, Francis JM, Karamitsos TD, Dall'Armellina E, et al. Prediction of global left ventricular functional recovery in patients with heart failure undergoing surgical revascularisation, based on late gadolinium enhancement cardiovascular magnetic resonance. J Cardiovasc Magn Reson Off J Soc Cardiovasc Magn Reson 2010;12:56. http://dx.doi.org/10.1186/1532-429X-12-56.
[86] Samady H, Elefteriades JA, Abbott BG, Mattera JA, McPherson CA, Wackers FJ. Failure to improve left ventricular function after coronary revascularization for ischemic cardiomyopathy is not associated with worse outcome. Circulation 1999;100:1298–304.
[87] Cleland JGF, Calvert M, Freemantle N, Arrow Y, Ball SG, Bonser RS, et al. The heart failure revascularisation trial (HEART). Eur J Heart Fail 2011;13:227–33. http://dx.doi.org/10.1093/eurjhf/hfq230.
[88] Velazquez EJ, Lee KL, Deja MA, Jain A, Sopko G, Marchenko A, et al. Coronary-artery bypass surgery in patients with left ventricular dysfunction. N Engl J Med 2011;364:1607–16. http://dx.doi.org/10.1056/NEJMoa1100356.
[89] Srichai MB, Jaber WA. Viability by MRI or PET would have changed the results of the STICH trial. Prog Cardiovasc Dis 2013;55:487–93. http://dx.doi.org/10.1016/j.pcad.2013.01.005.
[90] O'Meara E, Mielniczuk LM, Wells GA, deKemp RA, Klein R, Coyle D, et al. Alternative imaging modalities in ischemic heart failure (AIMI-HF) IMAGE HF Project I-A: study protocol for a randomized controlled trial. Trials 2013;14:218. http://dx.doi.org/10.1186/1745-6215-14-218.
[91] Yancy CW, Jessup M, Bozkurt B, Butler J, Casey DE, Drazner MH, et al. 2013 ACCF/AHA guideline for the management of heart failure a report of the American College of Cardiology Foundation/American Heart Association Task Force on Practice Guidelines. Circulation 2013; 128:e240–327. http://dx.doi.org/10.1161/CIR.0b013e31829e8776.
[92] Cleland JGF, Pennell DJ, Ray SG, Coats AJ, Macfarlane PW, Murray GD, et al. Myocardial viability as a determinant of the ejection fraction response to carvedilol in patients with heart failure (CHRISTMAS trial): randomised controlled trial. Lancet 2003;362:14–21.
[93] Köszegi Z, Balogh E. Myocardial dysfunction: hibernation and remodelling. Lancet 2003;362:1416–7. http://dx.doi.org/10.1016/S0140-6736(03)14649-1.
[94] Zižek D, Cvijić M, Ležaić L, Salobir BG, Zupan I. Impact of myocardial viability assessed by myocardial perfusion imaging on ventricular tachyarrhythmias in cardiac resynchronization therapy. J Nucl Cardiol Off Publ Am Soc Nucl Cardiol 2013;20:1049–59. http://dx.doi.org/10.1007/s12350-013-9795-y.
[95] Gao P, Yee R, Gula L, Krahn AD, Skanes A, Leong-Sit P, et al. Prediction of arrhythmic events in ischemic and dilated cardiomyopathy patients referred for implantable cardiac defibrillator: evaluation of multiple scar quantification measures for late gadolinium enhancement magnetic resonance imaging. Circ Cardiovasc Imaging 2012;5:448–56. http://dx.doi.org/10.1161/CIRCIMAGING.111.971549.
[96] Fallavollita JA, Heavey BM, Luisi Jr. AJ, Michalek SM, Baldwa S, Mashtare Jr TL, et al. Regional myocardial sympathetic denervation predicts the risk of sudden cardiac arrest in ischemic cardiomyopathy. J Am Coll Cardiol 2013; http://dx.doi.org/10.1016/j.jacc.2013.07.096, Epub ahead of print.
[97] Ypenburg C, Schalij MJ, Bleeker GB, Steendijk P, Boersma E, Dibbets-Schneider P, et al. Extent of viability to predict response to cardiac resynchronization therapy in ischemic heart failure patients. J Nucl Med Off Publ Soc Nucl Med 2006;47:1565–70.
[98] Ypenburg C, Schalij MJ, Bleeker GB, Steendijk P, Boersma E, Dibbets-Schneider P, et al. Impact of viability and scar tissue on response to cardiac resynchronization

therapy in ischaemic heart failure patients. Eur Heart J 2007;28:33–41. http://dx.doi.org/10.1093/eurheartj/ehl379.
[99] Lim P, Bars C, Mitchell-Heggs L, Roiron C, Elbaz N, Hamdaoui B, et al. Importance of contractile reserve for CRT. Eur Eur Pacing Arrhythm Card Electrophysiol J Work Groups Card Pacing Arrhythm Card Cell Electrophysiol Eur Soc Cardiol 2007;9:739–43. http://dx.doi.org/10.1093/europace/eum117.
[100] Becker M, Zwicker C, Kaminski M, Napp A, Altiok E, Ocklenburg C, et al. Dependency of cardiac resynchronization therapy on myocardial viability at the LV lead position. JACC Cardiovasc Imaging 2011;4:366–74. http://dx.doi.org/10.1016/j.jcmg.2011.01.010.
[101] Chalil S, Foley PWX, Muyhaldeen SA, Patel KCR, Yousef ZR, Smith REA, et al. Late gadolinium enhancement-cardiovascular magnetic resonance as a predictor of response to cardiac resynchronization therapy in patients with ischaemic cardiomyopathy. Europace 2007;9:1031–7. http://dx.doi.org/10.1093/europace/eum133.
[102] Leyva F, Foley PWX, Chalil S, Ratib K, Smith REA, Prinzen F, et al. Cardiac resynchronization therapy guided by late gadolinium-enhancement cardiovascular magnetic resonance. J Cardiovasc Magn Reson Off J Soc Cardiovasc Magn Reson 2011;13:29. http://dx.doi.org/10.1186/1532-429X-13-29.
[103] Shetty AK, Duckett SG, Ginks MR, Ma Y, Sohal M, Bostock J, et al. Cardiac magnetic resonance-derived anatomy, scar, and dyssynchrony fused with fluoroscopy to guide LV lead placement in cardiac resynchronization therapy: a comparison with acute haemodynamic measures and echocardiographic reverse remodelling. Eur Heart J Cardiovasc Imaging 2012; 14(7):692–97. http://dx.doi.org/10.1093/ehjci/jes270.
[104] Sommer A, Kronborg MB, Poulsen SH, Böttcher M, Nørgaard BL, Bouchelouche K, et al. Empiric versus imaging guided left ventricular lead placement in cardiac resynchronization therapy (imaging CRT): study protocol for a randomized controlled trial. Trials 2013;14:113. http://dx.doi.org/10.1186/1745-6215-14-113.
[105] Joint Task Force on the Management of Valvular Heart Disease of the European Society of Cardiology (ESC), European Association for Cardio-Thoracic Surgery (EACTS), Vahanian A, Alfieri O, Andreotti F, Antunes MJ, et al. Guidelines on the management of valvular heart disease (version 2012). Eur Heart J 2012;33:2451–96. http://dx.doi.org/10.1093/eurheartj/ehs109.
[106] Bonow RO, Carabello BA, Chatterjee K, de Leon AC, Faxon DP, Freed MD, et al. ACC/AHA 2006 guidelines for the management of patients with valvular heart disease a report of the American College of Cardiology/American Heart Association Task Force on Practice Guidelines (writing committee to revise the 1998 guidelines for the management of patients with valvular heart disease): developed in collaboration with the Society of Cardiovascular Anesthesiologists: endorsed by the Society for Cardiovascular Angiography and Interventions and the Society of Thoracic Surgeons. Circulation 2006;114:e84–231. http://dx.doi.org/10.1161/CIRCULATIONAHA.106.176857.
[107] Quere J-P, Monin J-L, Levy F, Petit H, Baleynaud S, Chauvel C, et al. Influence of preoperative left ventricular contractile reserve on postoperative ejection fraction in low-gradient aortic stenosis. Circulation 2006;113:1738–44. http://dx.doi.org/10.1161/CIRCULATIONAHA.105.568824.
[108] Fairbairn TA, Steadman CD, Mather AN, Motwani M, Blackman DJ, Plein S, et al. Assessment of valve haemodynamics, reverse ventricular remodelling and myocardial fibrosis following transcatheter aortic valve implantation compared to surgical aortic valve replacement: a cardiovascular magnetic resonance study. Heart 2013;99:1185–91. http://dx.doi.org/10.1136/heartjnl-2013-303927.

[109] Flett AS, Sado DM, Quarta G, Mirabel M, Pellerin D, Herrey AS, et al. Diffuse myocardial fibrosis in severe aortic stenosis: an equilibrium contrast cardiovascular magnetic resonance study. Eur Heart J Cardiovasc Imaging 2012; http://dx.doi.org/10.1093/ehjci/jes102.
[110] Moon JC, Messroghli DR, Kellman P, Piechnik SK, Robson MD, Ugander M, et al. Myocardial T1 mapping and extracellular volume quantification: a Society for Cardiovascular Magnetic Resonance (SCMR) and CMR Working Group of the European Society of Cardiology consensus statement. J Cardiovasc Magn Reson Off J Soc Cardiovasc Magn Reson 2013;15:92. http://dx.doi.org/10.1186/1532-429X-15-92.
[111] Lee R, Haluska B, Leung DY, Case C, Mundy J, Marwick TH. Functional and prognostic implications of left ventricular contractile reserve in patients with asymptomatic severe mitral regurgitation. Heart 2005;91:1407–12. http://dx.doi.org/10.1136/hrt.2004.047613.
[112] Tam JW, Antecol D, Kim HH, Yvorchuk KJ, Chan KL. Low dose dobutamine echocardiography in the assessment of contractile reserve to predict the outcome of valve replacement for chronic aortic regurgitation. Can J Cardiol 1999;15:73–9.
[113] Park S-J, Enriquez-Sarano M, Song J-E, Lee Y-J, Ha M-R, Chang S-A, et al. Contractile reserve determined on exercise echocardiography in patients with severe aortic regurgitation. Circ J Off J Jpn Circ Soc 2013;77:2390–8.
[114] Lancellotti P, Magne J. Stress echocardiography in regurgitant valve disease. Circ Cardiovasc Imaging 2013;6:840–9. http://dx.doi.org/10.1161/CIRCIMAGING.113.000474.
[115] Wickline SA, Thomas 3rd. LJ, Miller JG, Sobel BE, Perez JE. Sensitive detection of the effects of reperfusion on myocardium by ultrasonic tissue characterization with integrated backscatter. Circulation 1986;74:389–400.
[116] Komuro K, Yamada S, Mikami T, Yoshinaga K, Noriyasu K, Goto K, et al. Sensitive detection of myocardial viability in chronic coronary artery disease by ultrasonic integrated backscatter analysis. J Am Soc Echocardiogr 2005;18:26–31. http://dx.doi.org/10.1016/j.echo.2004.08.019.
[117] Roes SD, Mollema SA, Lamb HJ, van der Wall EE, de Roos A, Bax JJ. Validation of echocardiographic two-dimensional speckle tracking longitudinal strain imaging for viability assessment in patients with chronic ischemic left ventricular dysfunction and comparison with contrast-enhanced magnetic resonance imaging. Am J Cardiol 2009;104:312–7. http://dx.doi.org/10.1016/j.amjcard.2009.03.040.
[118] Cimino S, Canali E, Petronilli V, Cicogna F, Luca LD, Francone M, et al. Global and regional longitudinal strain assessed by two-dimensional speckle tracking echocardiography identifies early myocardial dysfunction and transmural extent of myocardial scar in patients with acute ST elevation myocardial infarction and relatively preserved LV function. Eur Heart J Cardiovasc Imaging 2013;14:805–11. http://dx.doi.org/10.1093/ehjci/jes295.
[119] Bree D, Wollmuth JR, Cupps BP, Krock MD, Howells A, Rogers J, et al. Low-dose dobutamine tissue-tagged magnetic resonance imaging with 3-dimensional strain analysis allows assessment of myocardial viability in patients with ischemic cardiomyopathy. Circulation 2006;114:I33–6. http://dx.doi.org/10.1161/CIRCULATIONAHA.105.000885.
[120] Rischpler C, Nekolla SG, Dregely I, Schwaiger M. Hybrid PET/MR imaging of the heart: potential, initial experiences, and future prospects. J Nucl Med Off Publ Soc Nucl Med 2013;54:402–15. http://dx.doi.org/10.2967/jnumed.112.105353.
[121] Beer M, Machann W, Sandstede J, Buchner S, Lipke C, Köstler H, et al. Energetic differences between viable and non-viable myocardium in patients with recent myocardial

infarction are not an effect of differences in wall thinning—a multivoxel (31)P-MR-spectroscopy and MRI study. Eur Radiol 2007;17:1275–83. http://dx.doi.org/10.1007/s00330-006-0492-y.

[122] Horn M, Weidensteiner C, Scheffer H, Przyklenk K, von Kienlin M, Neubauer S. Use of ^{23}Na MRS to discriminate viable from non viable tissue: experimental studies. Magma 2000;11:42–3.

[123] Beer M, Sandstede J, Pabst T, Landschütz W, Harre K, von Kienlin M, et al. Assessment of myocardial viability by ^{31}P-MR-spectroscopy and ^{23}Na-MR imaging. Magma 2000;11:44–6.

[124] Aguor ENE, van de Kolk CWA, Arslan F, Nederhoff MGJ, Doevendans PAFM, Pasterkamp G, et al. ^{23}Na chemical shift imaging and Gd enhancement of myocardial edema. Int J Cardiovasc Imaging 2013;29:343–54. http://dx.doi.org/10.1007/s10554-012-0093-6.

[125] Van Hoe L, Vanderheyden M. Ischemic cardiomyopathy: value of different MRI techniques for prediction of functional recovery after revascularisation. AJR Am J Roentgenol 2004;182 (January (1)):95–100.

[126] Kuhl HP, Lipke CS, Krombach GA, Katoh M, Battenberg TF, Nowak B, et al. Assessment of reversible myocardial dysfunction in chronic ischaemic heart disease: comparison of contrast-enhanced cardiovascular magnetic resonance and a combined positron emission tomography-single photon emission computed tomography imaging protocol. Eur Heart J 2006;27 (April (7)):846–53.

Contractile function and heart failure

E. Donal[*,†], E. Galli[*,†], M. Lederlin[*], A. Manrique[‡,§]
[*]CHU Rennes, Rennes, France; [†]LTSI, INSERM 1099, Université Rennes-1, Rennes, France;
[‡]CHU de Caen, Caen, France; [§]Université de Caen Basse-Normandie, Caen, France

12.1 Introduction

Heart failure (HF) is a growing problem worldwide. Almost 6 million Americans and 15 million Europeans have HF [1,2]. Normal ventricular function requires coordinated electrical activation and contraction but also appropriate pre- and after-loads. Given the 3D pattern of ventricular activation and contraction, the assessment of mechanical activation using conventional imaging methods is complex [1,3]. Several imaging techniques might be necessary in HF patients. For instance, the most prevalent etiology of HF is coronary artery disease. In that context, one must assess myocardial viability (and sometimes ischemia) using stress echocardiography, stress nuclear medical imaging, or cardiac magnetic resonance (CMR) [2,4,5]. CMR provides imaging of the scar (subendocardial or transmural or patchy, according to the etiology). With regards to the objective of this chapter of contractility in HF, one might also be aware of the potential usefulness of innervation imaging for best adapting the treatment strategy in HF patients [6,7]. This nuclear technique might help to best select patients requiring an intra-cardiac defibrillator (ICD).

HF is complex. There are several etiologies and clinical expressions reported in guidelines for HF with depressed ejection fraction (EF) and HF with preserved EF when the left ventricular (LV) EF ≥50%. For dealing with this complexity and multiplicity of the HF syndrome, imaging is no longer thought of as a single and mono parametric approach. One has to use a combination of techniques for a precise diagnosis and, hopefully, a greater individualization of patients' treatment strategies [8].

That is not clearly demonstrated yet; it is efforts remain necessary to affirm the key role of imaging techniques for best treating patients with HF even if the role of imaging is to increase guideline after guideline for HF [2]. For instance, the impact of cardiac resynchronization therapy (CRT) on global systolic and diastolic performance in dyssynchronous hearts provides an interest in understanding the physiological background for optimal LV performance. Unfortunately, contradictory results have been published, and even if the subject is still in debate, imaging techniques are not key in the indication of CRT [9–12]. The complexity of LV function assessment in HF patients is related to the complexity of heart anatomy and of electromechanical interaction and to the load dependency of all the parameters that are obtained in clinical practice [3,13,14].

One must thus keep testing imaging techniques in trials in order to demonstrate their key role. Also, imaging techniques have to be available, cost-effective, robust, and feasible; also, they are performed by only a very few experts.

The starting point for this chapter about HF and contractility is based on the work of Torrent-Guasp et al. [15]. This author showed that both ventricles consist of a single myofiber band extending from the right ventricular (RV) muscle just below the pulmonary artery to the LV muscle where it attaches to the aorta; it is twisted and wrapped into a double helical coil during evolutionary and embryological development. In this construct, sequential activation and contraction beginning in fibers near the pulmonary artery and spreading toward the aortic end of the band might explain the pattern of ejection and suction needed for ventricular output and filling. Disease resulting from ischemic or non-ischemic mechanisms may produce architectural distortion and create a more spherical ventricular shape.

The counter-directional arrangement of muscle fibers helps maintain stability and minimizes energy expenditure. For quantification of fiber orientation, the helix and transverse angles were introduced by Streeter and Hanna [16]. The helix angle represents the angle between the circumferential axis and the projection of the myofiber onto the circumferential-longitudinal plane. The myofiber helix angle changes continuously from the subendocardium to the subepicardium, from a right- to a left-handed helix, typically ranging from $-60°$ at the subendocardium to $60°$ at the subepicardium [17,18]. All the descriptions proposed, especially by Torrent-Guasp et al., have been confirmed using advanced imaging techniques and CMR, in particular. Diffusion-tensor magnetic resonance imaging has confirmed that myocardial fibers within the ventricular mass are arranged in layers of counter-wound helices, encircling the ventricular cavities [19,20]. Evidence suggests that the configuration of these fibers serves to equalize stresses and strains across the thick-walled ventricle, allowing an optimal mechanical functioning of the heart throughout the cardiac cycle [21]. Nevertheless, if the anatomy seems clearly described, and if one knows approximately how the heart is activated, there is still a lot of mystery, and ongoing work is attempting to deal with the key problem of the coupling between the electrical activation (first) and the mechanical consequence (electromechanical coupling).

In this chapter, we first summarize the echocardiographic capabilities for assessing cardiac function or contractility (global and regional). We will distinguish the assessment of the left and the right ventricles. Then, we will discuss CMR and nuclear imaging approaches that are usually complementary for the best management of any single patient with HF (chronic). Clearly, all imaging modalities should not be used in every individual patient. One will probably use echocardiography for the initial assessment and the follow-up. CMR and nuclear imaging will be used afterward and less frequently for the etiologic diagnosis and to assist in the treatment strategy and/or the prognosis assessment. Also, cardiac CT can provide accurate indices of global LV function. While the technique is not the first-choice modality for this, it can provide a third alternative when echocardiography and CMR are inconclusive or contra-indicated [22].

12.2 Echocardiographic approach to the LV contractility

During a cardiac cycle, the LV wall shortens, thickens, and twists along the long axis. Shortening and thickening can be quantified by measuring regional strains. Strain or myocardial deformation from developing forces is expressed as either the fractional or the percent change from the original dimension [17,18]. Positive radial strains represent wall thickening (radial deformation), whereas negative strains represent segment shortening (e.g., circumferential shortening, longitudinal shortening, and fiber shortening) [14].

Three perpendicular axes orienting the global geometry of the LV define the local cardiac coordinate system: radial, circumferential, and longitudinal.

Echocardiographic techniques like tissue Doppler imaging have excellent temporal resolution (± 4 ms) and could be used for the assessment of myocardial deformations [14] (see Chapter 2).

The base and apex of the LV rotate in opposite directions. Twist defines the base to apex gradient in the rotation angle along the longitudinal axis of the LV and is expressed in degrees per centimeter [9,23]. Torsion and twist are equivalent terms. Torsion can also be expressed as the axial gradient in the rotation angle multiplied by the average of the outer radii in apical and basal cross-sectional planes, thereby representing the shear deformation angle on the epicardial surface (unit degrees or radians) [23]. This normalization can be used as a method for comparing torsion for different sizes of LV. When the apex-to-base difference in LV rotation is not normalized, the absolute difference (also in degrees or radians) is stated as the net LV twist angle [24].

Speckle-tracking echocardiography (STE) has emerged as an alternative technique [25] (see Chapter 2). The robustness and the clinical applicability of that technique are nowadays only validated for the assessment of global longitudinal strain [26,27]. When considering regional longitudinal strains, there are inaccuracies according to the software used. Longitudinal LV mechanics, which are predominantly governed by the subendocardial region, are the most vulnerable component of LV mechanics and therefore most sensitive to the presence of myocardial disease. The first of them is the ischemic etiology that will affect first the subendocardium. The mid-myocardial and epicardial function may remain relatively unaffected or weakly affect in patients with HF and preserved LV EF. Circumferential strain and twist may remain normal or show exaggerated compensation for preserving LV systolic performance. Increase in cardiac muscle stiffness, however, may cause progressive delay in LV untwisting. Loss of early diastolic longitudinal relaxation and delayed untwisting attenuate LV diastolic performance, producing elevation in LV filling pressures and a phase of predominant diastolic dysfunction, although the LV EF may remain normal. The diagnostic of these HF with preserved ejection that most affect the subendocardium could be very difficult and might require submaximal exercise stress echocardiographies [28]. It has not been proposed in past recommendation, but that could change [29].

On the other hand, an acute transmural insult (like a myocardial infarction) or progression of disease results in concomitant mid-myocardial and subepicardial dysfunction, leading to a reduction in LV circumferential and twist mechanics and a reduction in LV EF. Assessment of myocardial function, therefore, can be tailored per the clinical goals. The detection of altered longitudinal function alone may suffice if the overall goal of analysis is to detect the presence of early myocardial disease. Further characterization of radial strains, circumferential strains, and torsional function provides assessment of the transmural disease burden and provides pathophysiologic insight into the mechanism of LV dysfunction [30]. For instance, the pathophysiologic process such as radiation that affects both the pericardium and the subendocardial region may produce attenuation of both longitudinal (first) and circumferential (afterwards) LV function [31]. Several studies have reported the strain values in patients with systolic HF (Table 12.1), HF with preserved LV EF, and hypertrophied cardiomyopathies. The data proposed in Table 12.1 are rather convergent; however, these measurements of LV systolic longitudinal strains are not used or proposed in guidelines such as in those for HF with preserved LV EF.

As a rule of thumb, a global longitudinal strain less than -17% is an independent parameter of severity of the cardiomyopathy [33]. In HF with preserved LV EF, the prognostic cut-off that is most frequently reported is -16% [38].

In more complex cardiomyopathies like those induced by anthracyclins, it seems that as soon as the global longitudinal strain is less than -19%, physicians have to carefully monitor the patients. Studies are ongoing to know whether dedicated treatments like ACE-inhibitor and B-blockers should be introduced [26].

Although strain data are valuable in patients with systolic HF, the indication for an ICD or a biventricular pace maker remains dependent upon the degree of LV dysfunction as determined by the LV EF (Figures 12.1 and 12.2). The LV EF should be measured, according to recommendations using the apical four- and two-chamber views using the Simpson method. The M mode should not be used especially in hearts having a spherical remodeling.

In the present and even more in the very near future, real-time 3D echocardiography (RT3DE) should improve the robustness and reproducibility of the echo data [39–41]. It is not yet available everywhere (see Chapter 2). Still, improvements in transducer are required for the actual transfer of the 3D approach in clinical practice. Feasibility remains lower than for the 2D approach [42,43]. It has been demonstrated that in patients in whom serial examinations are obtained, the 3D echocardiographic approach is the most reliable [39,44].

Other approaches are available (Figures 12.1–12.4) [25,45]. Pulse tissue Doppler is the most relevant and is a way for assessing LV longitudinal systolic function as well as MAPSE.

In addition to these measurements (LV EF required, global longitudinal strain, or pulse tissue Doppler), one must measure the LV stroke volume (Doppler and volumetric approaches) for estimating the cardiac output and finally the efficacy of this LV contractility to eject enough blood in the arterial tree (Figure 12.5).

Also, as already mentioned, stress tests might be required to look for contractile reserve, in particular. Without going into much detail in regard to the technique, dobu-

Table 12.1 Principal studies published in the field of heart failure with depressed LV ejection fraction

Study	n	Population	End-point	Follow-up duration	GLS prognostic value	LV EF in the population (month)
Bertini et al. [32]	1060	Ischemic cardiomyopathies	Death, cardiovascular hospitalization	31 months	−11.5%	Median = 34(25–58)
Mignot et al. [33]	147	Heart failure	idem	>12-months	−7%	Mean = 29.9 ± 8.9
Donal et al. [34]	140	Heart failure	idem	38 months	−8%	Mean = 30 ± 9%
Nahum et al. [35]	125	Heart failure	idem	8.8 ± 6	−9%	Mean = 31 ± 10%
Lacoviello et al. [36]	308	Heart failure	et idem + maligant arrhythmias	26 ± 13		
Cho et al. [37]	201	Heart failure	Cardiac death + cardiovascular hospitalization	39 ± 17	Not available −10.7% for mean circumferential strain	Mean = 34 ± 13%

GLS, global longitudinal strain.

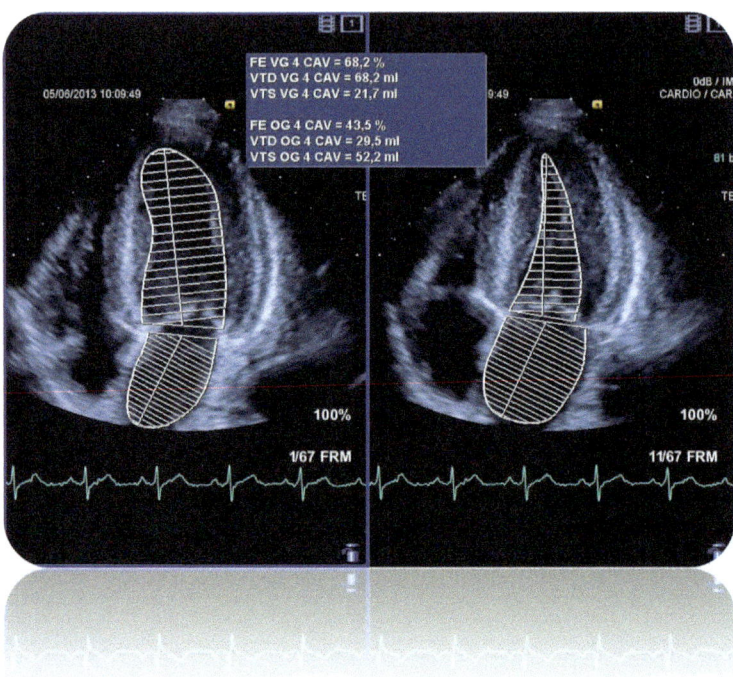

Figure 12.1 Automatic measurement of left ventricular volumes in systole and diastole for an automatic calculation of the ejection fraction (Simpson method).

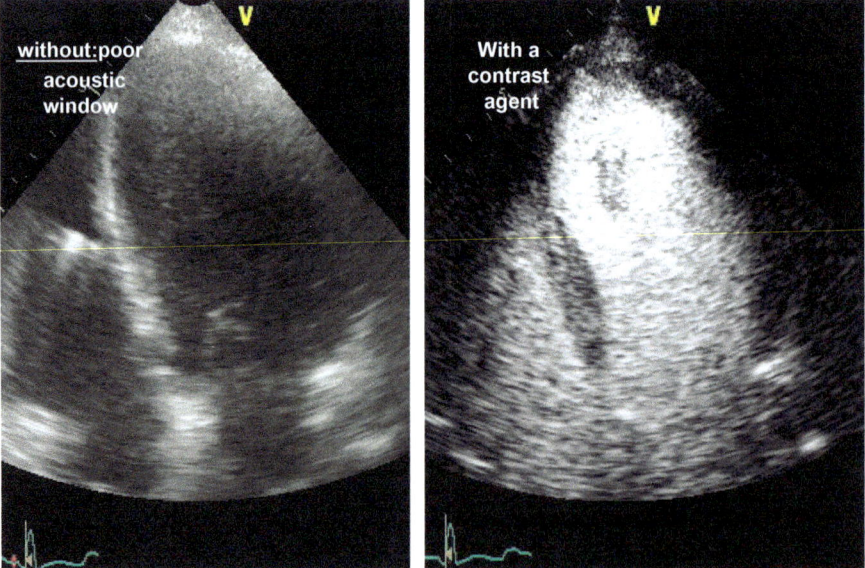

Figure 12.2 Use of an ultrasonic contrast agent to improve the echocardiographic detection of left ventricular endocardial borders. It will help to best quantify the left ventricular geometry and systolic function.

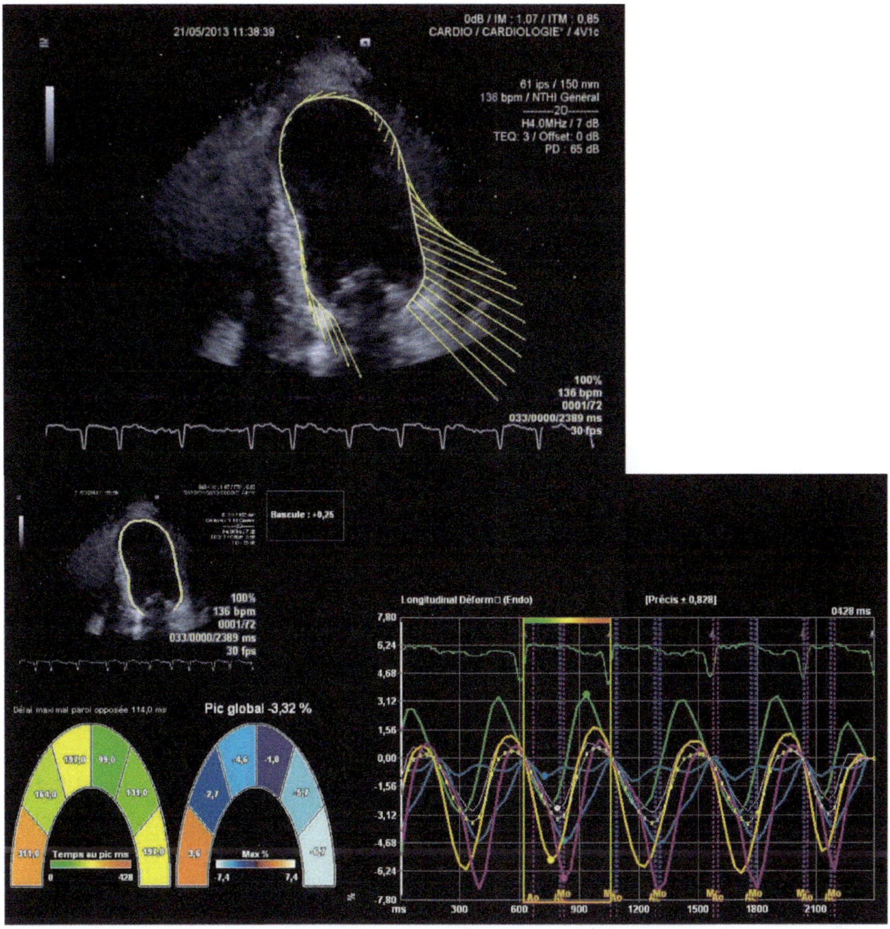

Figure 12.3 Assessment of regional and global left ventricular longitudinal strain.

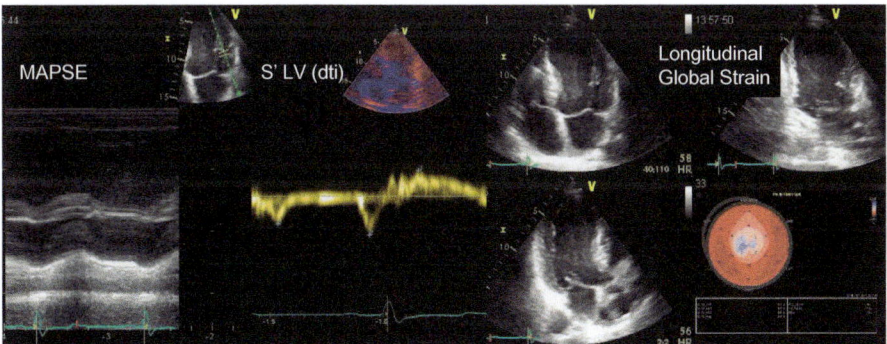

Figure 12.4 Assessment of the longitudinal component of the left ventricular systolic function. MAPSE: mitral annular plan systolic excursion measured by M-mode; S': pulse tissue Doppler recording systolic and diastolic velocities and s' is corresponding to the systolic peak velocity of the displacement of the mitral annulus; longitudinal global strain: assessment of the longitudinal deformation of the whole left ventricle using the speckle tracking technique.

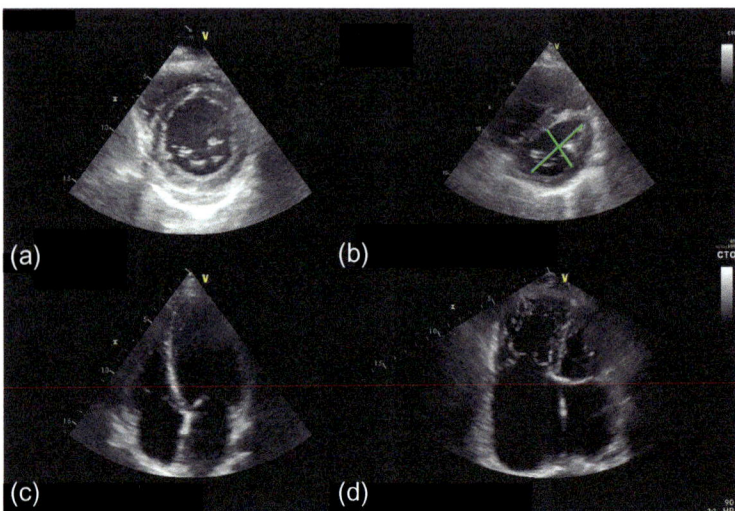

Figure 12.5 Right ventricular shape in normal and pathological condition. Under normal loading conditions, the right ventricle (RV) appears crescent-shaped in cross section (a) and triangular-shaped in the sagittal plane (c), and the interventricular septum is concave toward the LV in both systole and diastole. In condition of RV pressure and volume overload, left deviation of the interventricular septum may occur, which causes a reduction of the LV cavity and LV function impairment (b and d). In this patient, an end-dyastolic LV sphericity index (LV major axis/LV minor axis) = 2 (b), identifies a severe alteration of LV morphology due to severe pulmonary hypertension.

tamine could be used, but submaximal exercise stress echocardiography is probably the ideal approach to test the systolic response and the diastolic response of the failing heart. In HF with preserved ejection, the absence of systolic and diastolic reserve has already been mentioned. In ischemic heart disease, it has to be tested; sometimes, one is "surprised" to observe that without any acute ischemia, the exercise unmasks a dynamic functional mitral regurgitation that might be very useful for understanding the symptoms and is perhaps the best treatment of a patient with systolic HF [46].

In addition to the assessment of viability or contractile reserve, it might be necessary to look for myocardial ischemia. The techniques are the same as in a non-failing heart, being nevertheless aware of the risk of maximal dobutamine stress test in patients with a failing heart (risk of ventricular arrhythmia, in particular).

12.3 Assessment of RV function

Until recently, the function of the RV in HF has been mostly ignored. A 2006 report of the National Heart, Lung, and Blood Institute identified a gap between RV research efforts that is far from being filled [47]. Historically, the concept of a secondary role of the RV in circulation has been supported by the experimental evidence that ablation of the RV was not associated with significant alteration in systemic circulation or venous pressure [48]. This evidence seemed cemented by the introduction of the Fontan procedure for complex congenital heart disease in 1968, a technique that directly connects the right atrium to the pulmonary artery, thus "bypassing" the RV [49]. In spite of this fact, RV dysfunction is associated with increased morbidity and mortality in HF [50] and in various heart diseases, such as myocardial infarction [51], pulmonary arterial hypertension (PAH) [52], and cardiac surgery [53] after heart transplantation [54] or LV-assisted device implantation [55]. It is important to underline that the evaluation of RV function has often been limited to the estimation of pulmonary artery pressure (PAP). Actually, even if PAH and RV dysfunction are often joined, a normal RV function may coexist with increased PAP, even if the occurrence of RV is associated with a poor prognosis.

12.3.1 Anatomical and myofibers architecture

In the normal heart, the RV is the most anteriorly situated cardiac chamber and lies immediately behind the sternum. With respect to the LV, where the mitral and aortic valve are in continuity, one with the other, in the RV, a ventriculo-infundibular fold separates the tricuspid and the pulmonary valve, distinguishing the RV inlet from the RV outflow tract and determining the complex anatomy of the RV. Actually, the RV appears triangular in the sagittal plane and crescent shaped in cross section (Figure 12.5). RV shape, as far as RV function, is also influenced by the position of the interventricular septum. Under normal loading and electrical conditions, the septum is concave toward the LV in both systole and diastole, but left deviation of the septum may occur in condition of RV pressure and volume overload, leading to alteration of both RV and LV functions. As far as the architecture of myofibril is concerned, the RV wall is composed of two muscle layers. The superficial fibers are arranged more or less circumferentially in a direction that is parallel to the atrioventricular (AV), while the deep layer is characterized by longitudinally oriented fibers [56] and is responsible for the essentially longitudinal contraction of the RV.

12.3.2 RV function physiology

The alteration in RV function in pathological condition can be explained by looking at the particular physiology of this cardiac chamber. During fetal life, the RV provides blood to the lower body and placenta, supplying only a modest amount of blood to the lungs and thus working as a "systemic ventricle." After birth, the primary function of the RV is to receive systemic venous return and to pump it into the pulmonary arteries. The reduction in pulmonary vascular resistance transforms RV physiology and morphology, and the RV becomes a low-pressure chamber [57,58] connected in series with the LV and pumping on average the same effective stroke volume.

Several differences exist between LV and RV contraction. Because of its myocardial structure and its bullet shape, LV contraction is due to a concentric contraction of the walls associated to a twisting motion of the heart. RV contracts by three separate mechanisms: inward movement of the free wall, which produces a bellows effect; contraction of the longitudinal fibers, which shortens the long axis; and traction on the free wall at the points of attachment, secondary to LV contraction. Interestingly, because of the greater surface to volume ratio of the RV, a greater EF is produced by a small change in surface area. This means that shortening of the RV is greater in longitude than in radius, and that a smaller inward motion of the lateral wall is required to equal LV stroke volume [59]. The low impedance pulmonary circulation explains the very brief isovolumic contraction time of the RV and allows the RV to eject the blood into the pulmonary artery even after the onset of RV relaxation. This late ejection, or "hangout period," explains the triangular-shaped RV pressure-volume loop [60] and makes the identification of RV end-systole difficult.

The reduced mass and wall stress of the RV cause the RV to have a lower oxygen demand with respect to the LV. Moreover, in the LV, myocardial perfusion occurs predominantly in diastole when intramyocardial tissue pressure falls below aortic root pressure. Because of an intramyocardial tissue pressure that is below aortic root pressure throughout the cardiac cycle, coronary blood supply to the RV is continuous in the condition of normal afterload. Because of its particular physiology, changes in afterload and preload strongly affect RV morphology and function, leading to RV dilatation, reduced performance, and failure.

12.3.2.1 Response of the right ventricle to chronically increased volume

RV volume overload due to interatrial shunts or tricuspid or pulmonic regurgitation is normally well tolerated, and evident in patients with volume overload due to congenital heart disease [61]. Initially, chronic volume overload causes RV dilatation and does not appear to impair contractile function that is preserved according to the Frank–Starling law. At a later stage, volume overload induces significant regional overexpression of growth factors like angiotensin II, insulin-like growth factor-I, and endothelin-1, with a corresponding increase of myocyte diameter and length and collagen deposition [62]. The development of RV fibrosis is detrimental because it has been associated with an adverse clinical outcome in patients with congenital heart disease. This vicious cycle of collagen deposition and RV dilatation is associated with a rise in RV pressure [63] and with an impairment in further increase in volume, either due to pericardial constraint or because of the shared architecture of the RV and LV. In this phase, additional increments in RV volume recruit minimal increments in RV free wall surface area and causes flattening and then bulging of the interventricular septum toward the LV, with development of biventricular failure.

12.3.2.2 Response of the right ventricle to acutely increased afterload

Being a "low-pressure" chamber, even small changes in afterload can reduce RV contractile performance and lower cardiac output, as evident in the setting of acute pulmonary embolism or acute lung failure. The RV cannot tolerate an acute increase in pulmonary pressure above 40–60 mmHg. As firstly described by Guyton et al. in 1954, a rapid increase in afterload induces a rise in RV contractility mediated by an homeomeric auto-regulation of the Anrep effect and by the release of endogenous catecholamines [64]. With further increase in afterload, the RV begins to dilate and recruit function via the Frank–Starling mechanism. In this condition, the thin RV free wall experiences a rise in wall tension with increments in RV pressure. Moreover, the

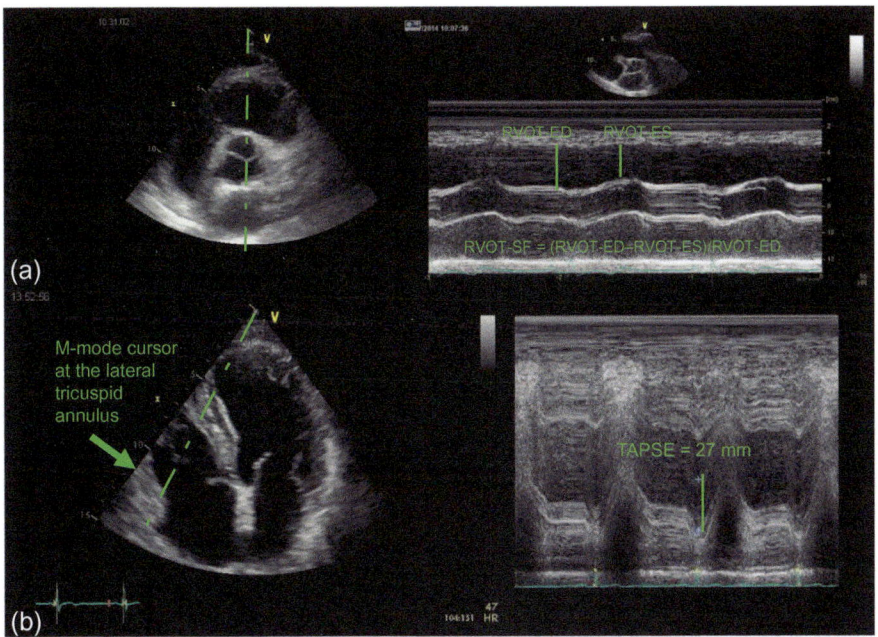

Figure 12.6 Right ventricular outflow tract shortening fraction and tricuspid annular plane systolic excursion measurement. ED, end-diastole ES; end-systole; right ventricular outflow tract (RVOT); TAPSE, tricuspid annular plane systolic excursion.

prevalent longitudinal contraction of the RV causes an increase in RV radius during systole (Figure 12.6) that causes a shape-dependent increase in wall stress according to the Laplace law [65], contributing to RV ischaemia and RV failure. Once all the mechanisms of contractile reserve are exhausted, systemic pressure begins to fall, causing a sudden catastrophic hemodynamic collapse.

12.3.2.3 Response of the right ventricle to chronically increased afterload

In the case of chronic increase in LV afterload, RV can maintain adequate output over prolonged periods but develops detrimental remodeling and injury that ultimately affect its long-term function [66]. The RV adaptation to chronic overload is characterized by the development of RV hypertrophy and by the re-expression of the fetal phenotype, with a shift from α- to β-myosin heavy chains and an increase in adrenergic receptors and phosphodiesterase type 5-expression [67]. These structural changes are associated with concomitant alterations in myocardial contraction patterns, with increased circumferential contractions with respect to longitudinal shortening, thereby preserving cardiac output [68]. However, with disease progression, RV dilatation, fibrosis, and increase in wall stress and end-diastolic pressure develop, leading to a reduction in cardiac output and finally to RV failure.

12.3.2.4 Mechanical and functional interdependence between RV and LV

LV and RV function are intimately linked. The ventricles share common injury mechanisms and myocardial fibers. From an anatomical point of view, the RV and the LV are attached through a common septum and share the pericardial space. As showed in experimental evidences, >50% of the normal RV mechanical work is generated by LV contraction, and changes in RV volume lead to substantial reduction of LV performance. This interdependence is evident also in the clinical setting. For example, in PAH, RV failure induces leftward displacement of the interventricular septum, impeding LV filling [69]. In this condition, the prolonged RV contraction and shortened filling times alter both RV output an LV preload, leading to adverse ventricular–ventricular interaction [66]. Also, the pericardium contributes substantially to this interventricular cross talk. As demonstrated by Brookes et al., with an intact, incompliant pericardium, acute RV dilatation leads to a reduction in LV size and contractility, which is only partially restored after pericardial release [70]. Moreover, maladaptative responses to a pathogenic mechanism like fibrosis and apoptosis or pathogenic mechanisms are often activated in both ventricles as showed in patients with dilated cardiomyopathy [71], PAH [72], ventricular non-compaction [73], or arrhythmogenic RV dysplasia.

12.3.2.5 RV function in HF

RV dysfunction in common in patients with HF, being detected in about one-third of patients with both preserved and reduced LV EF [74]. In the case of ischemic aetiology, the prevalence of RV dysfunction is lower in (about 16%), probably because the primary pathologic process affecting the LV contributes also to RV dysfunction [71]. Whatever is the cause of LV failure, concomitant RV dysfunction always portends a poor prognosis [52,75]. In HF developing after myocardial infarction, RV dysfunction is a major risk factor for death, HF, and stroke and is a strong predictor of re-infarction and hospitalization. In HFpEF, RV remodeling, indicated by RV free-wall hypertrophy and RV dysfunction, is associated with a poor prognosis and is a strong predictor of survival. In patients with dilated cardiomyopathy, RV dysfunction is associated with elevated BNP levels, increased congestion, reduced renal function, and poor exercise tolerance [76] and is a powerful independent predictor of transplant-free survival and adverse HF outcomes [74]. All these data confirm the fundamental role of the RV in the whole-heart physiology and highlight the need for a systematic assessment of RV function in daily clinical practice.

12.3.3 Echocardiographic assessment

Echocardiographic assessment of the RV is complicated by the complex geometry of this chamber, the pronounced trabeculation that compromises accurate endocardial delineation, and the anterior position that often limits echo image quality. More than one projection is needed for a comprehensive evaluation of RV structure. Moreover, even if the congenital heart disease is beyond the scope of this chapter, some morphological characteristics allow the identification of the RV in case of uncertainty: the visualization of the typical trabeculation, the position of septal the tricuspid leaflet valve that is more apical with respect to the anterior mitral leaflet, and the presence of the moderator band and of a septal papillary muscle.

12.3.3.1 Evaluation of RV dimension

The measure of RV dimensions is fundamental for further evaluation of RV function and PAP. According to 2D echocardiography, left parasternal long axis (PLAX), parasternal short-axis (PSAX), left parasternal RV inflow, apical four-chamber, modified apical four-chamber, and subcostal views provide images for the comprehensive assessment of RV systolic and diastolic function and RV systolic pressure (RVSP) (Figure 12.7). Table 12.1 summarizes the main acoustic windows and referral limits for the right heart evaluation.

12.3.3.2 Evaluation of RV function

Because of its complex shape, biplane method is not useful for the estimation of RV function [77]. Several methods of evaluation of RV have therefore been developed using 2D echocardiography [78].

2D echocardiographic parameters

RVOT shortening fraction (RVOT-SF) expresses the percentage changes in RVOT diameter during diastole and systole according to the following formula (%): [(end-diastole RVOT − end-systole RVOT-ES)/end-diastole RVOT]. These measures are obtained in PLAX view, at the base of the heart, using M-mode echocardiography [78]. A RVOT-FS value of $61 \pm 13\%$ is considered normal. RVOT-FS correlates well with RV longitudinal function, pulmonary pressure gradient, and RV-right atrial (RA)

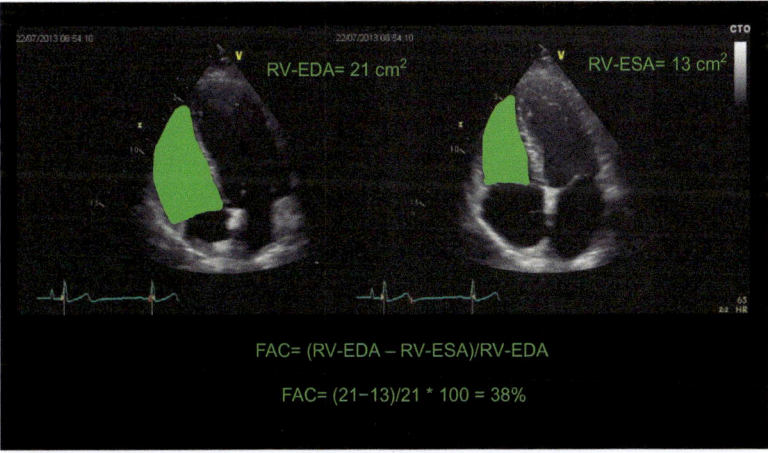

Figure 12.7 Fractional area change measurement. EDA, end-diastolic area; ESA, end-systolic area; FAC, fractional area change; RV, right ventricle.

pressure gradient. Care should be taken during measurements because some inaccuracies may results from oblique plane acquisition.

RV fractional area change (RVFAC) evaluates the percentage changes in RV area between diastole and systole. RV end-diastolic area (RV-EDA) and RV end-systolic area (RV-ESA) are obtained in apical four-chamber view, and RVFAC is calculated view according to the following formula (%): [(RV-EDA − RV-ESA)/RV-EDA]. A value of RVFAC of 35% is considered normal. This measure is limited by the difficult delineation of RV endocardial border, particularly in the case of highly trabeculated RV. In spite of these facts, several studies have shown the correlation of RV-FAC with RV function estimated by cardiac magnetic resonance imaging (MRI), and its prognostic the value in patients with HF chronic obstructive pulmonary disease, myocardial infarction, and pulmonary embolism [78].

Tricuspid annular plane systolic excursion (TAPSE) is the most used parameter of RV function evaluation. This is because it is easily measured from an apical four-chamber view, using an M-mode cursor passing through the lateral side of the RV annulus and evaluates the extent of systolic motion of the lateral portion of the tricuspid ring towards the apex (Figure 12.8). A value of TAPSE ≥ 17 is considered normal. As with other regional methods, it assumes that the displacement of the basal and adjacent segments in the apical four-chamber view is representative of the function of the entire right ventricle, an assumption that is not valid if there are regional RV wall motion abnormalities or in the case of conditions that affect the overall cardiac motion, as in the case of surgery. Other limitations of TAPSE are its angle

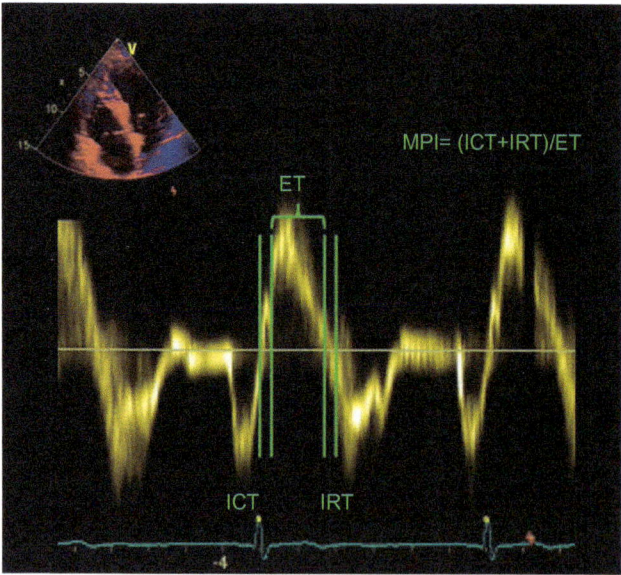

Figure 12.8 Right ventricular myocardial performance index measured using tissue Doppler imaging. ET, ejection time; ICT, isovolumic contraction time; IRT, isovolumic relaxation time; MPI, myocardial performance index.

Contractile function and heart failure

and load dependency. TASPE is well correlated with RV function estimated by radio-isotopic methods, but not with MRI-derived EF [78]. In spite of this fact, TAPSE mm has been identified as a stronger prognostic predictor in patients with HF and reduced or preserved LV EF [79].

Myocardial Performance Index (MPI or Tei index) is an index of RV function than combines diastolic and systolic parameters. As for the LV, it is the ratio between the sum of isovolumic contraction and relaxation time and ejection time [80]. The right-sided MPI can be obtained by two methods: the pulsed Doppler method and the tissue Doppler method. In the pulsed Doppler method, the ET is measured with pulsed Doppler positioned at the RV outflow (Figure 12.9). Normal values for MPI are 0.28 ± 0.04 with increased values associated with RV dysfunction. Even if useful in the follow-up of patients with previous pulmonary embolism and PAH [81].

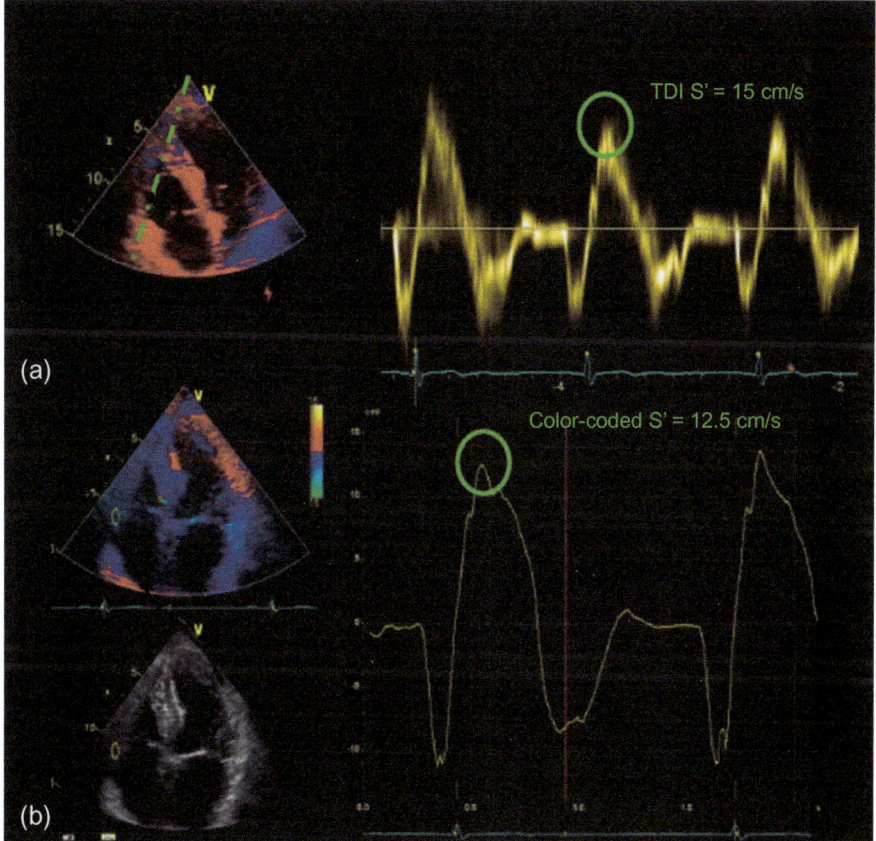

Figure 12.9 Lateral tricuspid annulus velocity measured using tissue Doppler (a) and colour-coded tissue Doppler (b). In the case of tissue Doppler imaging, the cursor is posed at the lateral tricuspid annulus level in real time (a). If color-coded tissue Doppler velocity is measured (b), the color-coded data are acquired and then the measure of the lateral tricuspid annulus velocity is obtained offline.

TEI index is difficult to measure in patients with normal RV function because of the extremely brief isovolumic period [80], and in patients with increased RA pressure because the reduced isovolumic relaxation time causes a pseudonormalization of the index. [82,83].

Tissue Doppler-derived parameters

Doppler tissue imaging (DTI) and color Doppler imaging (CDI) are often used to assess the longitudinal displacement of the lateral tricuspid annulus in the four-chamber view. The obtained parameter is termed RV S' or RV excursion velocity [82,83].

DTI S' represents the peak systolic velocity of lateral tricuspid annulus. DTI S' is normal if ≥11.5 cm/s and is index of RV dysfunction if <10 cm/s, particularly in young subjects. A reduced S' is a predictor of poor prognosis in patients with HF and reduced or preserved LV EF and myocardial infarction.

Color-coded tissue Doppler yields 20% ~ lower velocities with respect to DTI S', because the encoded data represent mean velocities. Mean annular velocities average is between 9.3 and 11 cm/s at the lateral tricuspid annulus. Doppler velocities are easy to obtain and widely used for the estimation of RV function, even if limited data are available regarding normative values in wide cohorts of patients [78]. DTI has also several limitations: as for all Doppler techniques, DTI is load dependent and a good alignment of the ultrasound beam; the region of interest is mandatory to avoid underestimation of velocities. DTI velocities may be affected by overall cardiac motion and by tethering of the adjacent myocardial segment. Moreover, S' velocity assumes that the function of a single segment represents the function of the entire RV, which is not likely in conditions that include regionality [78].

Myocardial isovolumic acceleration time (IVA) is a DTI-derived index that is supposed to be less dependent on loading conditions in a physiological range. It is calculated as the ratio between maximum systolic velocity and time to maximum systolic velocity (Figure 12.10). Studies have shown that an IVA measured in the basal segment of the RV free wall of >1.1 m/s^2 correlates well with MRI RVEF >45% [82,83]. In spite of these facts, current guidelines for the evaluation of the right heart do not recommend IVA as a screening parameter for RV systolic function in the general echocardiography laboratory population and no reference value has been recommended.

Other techniques to evaluate RV function

STE is a relatively newer technique that provides non-Doppler, relatively angle-independent measurement of myocardial deformation and LV systolic and diastolic dynamics [45]. By estimating spatial gradients in myocardial velocities between features (i.e., the "speckles") oriented in the same plane and at a known distance apart, STE allows for the semi-automated quantification of myocardial deformation (strain and strain rate) in the three spatial directions (longitudinal, radial, and circumferential) [45,82,83].

With respect to Doppler techniques, STE is not angle dependent, is less influenced by preload and afterload, and can provide an estimate of "whole" RV function. Nevertheless, STE is affected by a low temporal resolution and its reliability depends on optimal image quality [45]. Strain and SR correlate well with radionuclide RV EF [83]. Cut-off points of systolic strain and SR at the basal RV free wall are of less

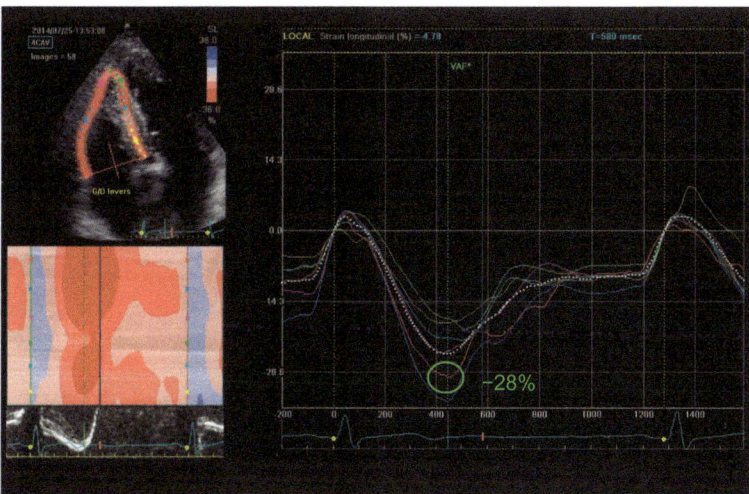

Figure 12.10 Right ventricular function evaluation through STE. Evaluation of right ventricular (RV) function through the calculation of basal RV free wall strain. In this patient, a normal RV function was detected with basal RV free wall strain value of −28%.

than −25% and $4\,s^{-1}$, respectively. STE abnormalities of the RV have been detected in COPD (pulmonary hypertension), amyloidosis, and congenital heart diseases and associated with a poor prognosis. Moreover, RV systolic function assessed by 2D strain and strain-rate has proved to be sensitive enough to detect early alterations of RV function in patients with systemic sclerosis and normal pulmonary pressures. Even if extremely promising, STE application is not recommended for routine evaluation of RV function; rather, it is addressed only at experienced laboratories and for research purposes [82] (Figure 12.10).

RT3DE [84] allows a comprehensive analysis of heart volumes and function avoiding geometric assumption and foreshortening, thus representing an ideal method for the evaluation of the complex RV structure and function. Good correlation between RT3DE and CMR for the calculation of RV volumes and EF has been reported. Pitfalls and limitations of this method include the patient's inability to cooperate for breath-hold, arrhythmias, the larger footprint and size of matrix-array transducer, dependence on optimal acoustic quality, and the need for specific training. In addition, even if increasing data are available regarding normal reference values for RV volumes and EF using RT3DE, further studies exploring RV function and geometry by RT3DE in different pathological conditions are still necessary for the application of this method in routine clinical practice.

12.4 Assessment of contractile function by CMR

CMR imaging has long been proven to be accurate and reproducible for measuring ventricular volumes and derived quantitative parameters of cardiac function [85–87].

Contrary to planar echocardiography or projection imaging techniques, ventricular volume assessment using CMR does not rely on geometric assumptions, thus leading to more accuracy and reproducibility [88,89]. In addition, CMR is very safe and increasingly available and the assessment of contractile function is well standardized. For these reasons, CMR is currently considered the standard of reference for evaluation of cardiac volumes and systolic function [90].

12.4.1 CMR sequence

Routine CMR assessment of contractile function is based on breath-hold ECG-triggered balanced steady-state free precession (b-SSFP) sequence, offering an excellent compromise between contrast, temporal, and spatial resolution. No gadolinium is necessary to obtain a consistent, good contrast between dark ventricular walls and bright blood pool. Moreover, b-SSFP sequences are less susceptible to spin-dephasing effects (i.e., signal loss due to high velocity or complex blood flow) than conventional gradient echo sequences [91]. The temporal resolution of b-SSFP sequence is typically 40 ms, which permits the acquisition of 20–25 images per slice throughout the cardiac cycle. With the use of parallel imaging, scanning time for a sequence can be reduced to less than 10 s, thereby allowing acquisition during one breath-hold for most patients. Additionally, non-Cartesian techniques, such as k-space radial filling, are now widely implemented to further speed up acquisition. Slice thickness is generally in the range of 7 mm with 3-mm interslice gap and a typical in-plane spatial resolution of 1.5 mm.

Most commonly, cine MRI is performed using retrospective ECG gating so that data is acquired during the whole R–R interval. A multiphase cine loop is then reconstructed, permitting assessment of cardiac motion throughout the entire cardiac cycle. Cine loops are acquired in different planes, including, at the least, four-chamber, two-chamber, left or RV outflow tract views, and three short-axis slices at base, mid-ventricle, and apex levels. Alternatively, prospective ECG gating may allow shorter scan duration but does not cover the entire cardiac cycle, leading to a loss of information at the end of the R–R interval. For patients who cannot hold their breath, real-time free-breathing acquisition without ECG triggering may be employed, at the cost of lower spatial and temporal resolution [92]. It has been recently demonstrated that a significant gain in spatiotemporal resolution could be achieved by the use of radial real-time k–t SENSE imaging [93].

12.4.2 Global contractile function

Quantitative assessment of contractile function requires a stack of contiguous short-axis slices covering the whole ventricle from level of AV valves to apex. Commercially available software allows either manual or semi-automated delineation of both epicardial and endocardial borders at each slice and at each phase of the cardiac cycle (Figure 12.1). End-diastolic and end-systolic volumes are then automatically calculated as the summation of endocardial planimetry. Stroke volume and EF are easily derived from the values of end-diastolic and end-systolic volumes. For the purpose of measuring contractile function, including papillary muscles and endocardial muscular trabeculations in the cavity volume (i.e., blood pool) is generally recommended for a faster and more reproducible approach [94–96]. However, when measuring ventricular mass, especially in patients with LV hypertrophy, papillary muscles and trabeculations should be included in myocardial volume [97]. Another issue in assessing ventricular volumes is the movement of the base of the heart toward the apex during the cardiac cycle, due to longitudinal systolic shortening. This so-called through-plane motion needs to be taken into account when contouring ventricles in order not to overestimate end-systolic ventricular volumes [98]. Because of its thinner wall with complex trabecular structure, RV mass calculation is harder than that of LV (Figure 12.11). However, CMR remains the most accurate technique for RV volumetric analysis [58,99]. It should also be mentioned that the end-systolic and end-diastolic frames may not be the same for right and left ventricles and thus need to be selected independently.

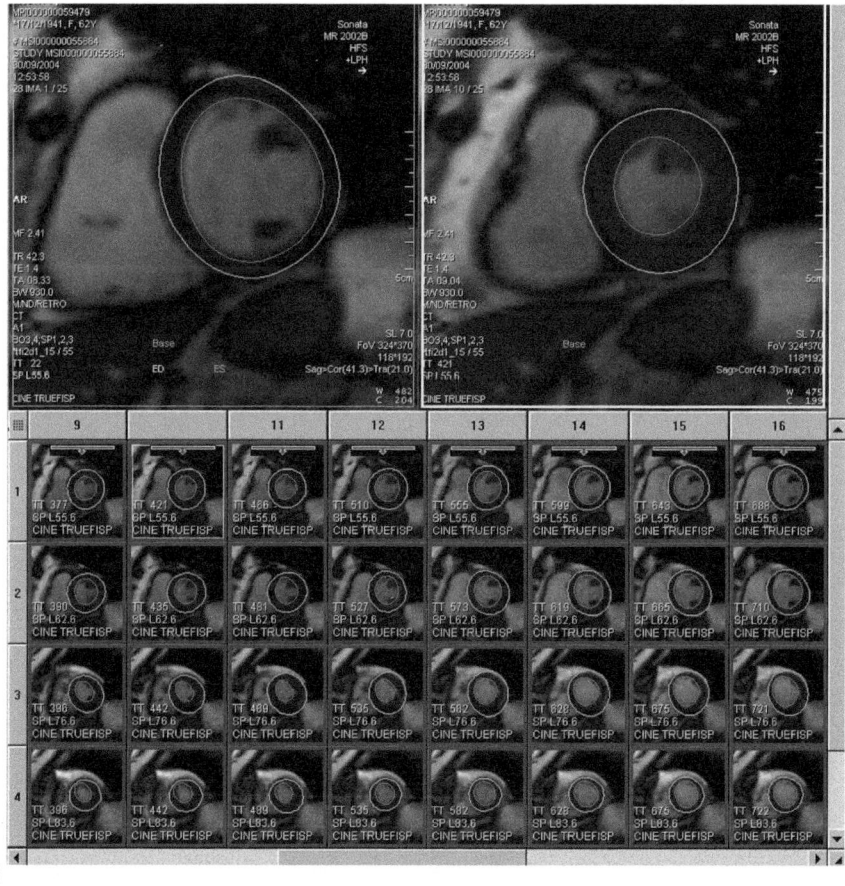

Figure 12.11 (a) LV segmentation;

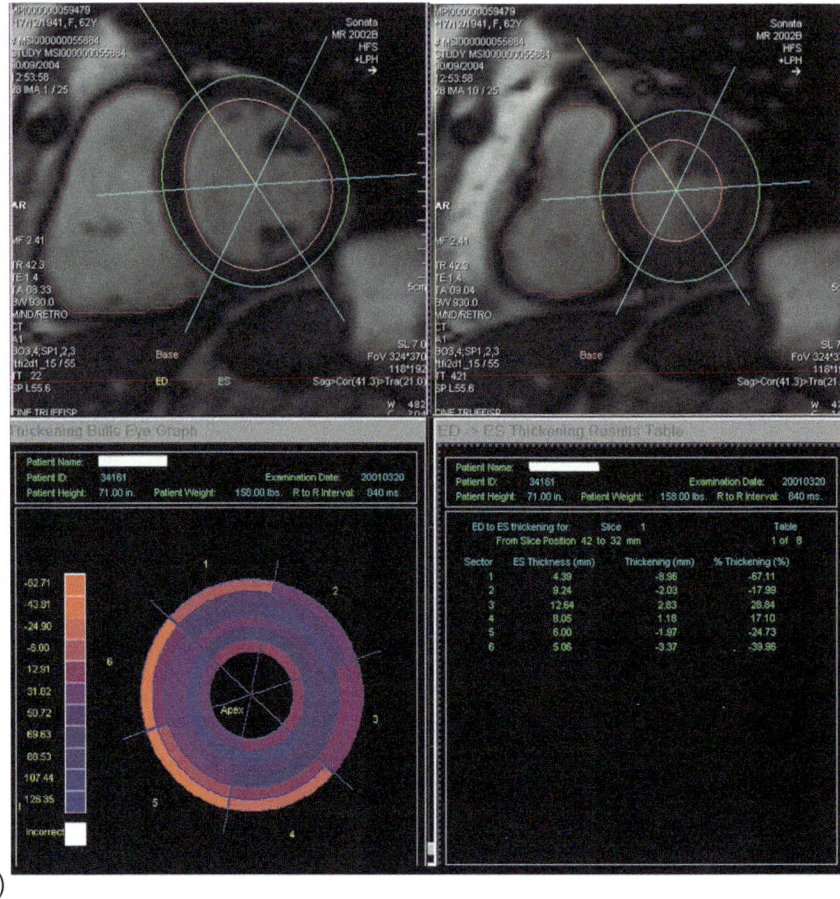

Figure 12.11, Cont'd (b) Results for the LV segmentation.

Besides volume measurements with cine b-SSFP imaging, a direct assessment of ventricular stroke volume can be obtained using phase-contrast MRI [100,101]. Phase-contrast velocity imaging is based on the properties of phase images in which pixel intensity is proportional to velocity. It allows the blood flow passing through the aortic root or the pulmonary artery to be quantified, and thus the stroke volume to be calculated, provided that mitral or tricuspid valves are competent, respectively. Because it does not provide information on ventricular volumes and regional contractility, phase-contrast imaging is rarely used in daily practice for evaluation of contractile function, but is mostly employed for quantifying shunts and valvular diseases.

12.4.3 Regional contractile function

Assessment of regional contractile function consists in analyzing wall motion and wall thickening. Wall motion analysis is routinely performed visually, using a grading system (normokinesia, hypokinesia, akinesia, dyskinesia). Wall thickening can be easily quantified [102] through delineation of endocardial and epicardial borders on short-axis images, as described above. A centerline technique allows the values of absolute or relative wall thickening to be obtained for each myocardial segment (Figure 12.2).

Further quantitative analysis of myocardial motion and thickening can be achieved by CMR myocardial tagging and phase-contrast imaging. Tagging consists of applying various spatial modulation of magnetization (SPAMM) perpendicularly to the imaging plane, thus creating a grid of dark lines superimposed on the b-SSFP image [103]. These tags displace and deform with ventricular motion and therefore may serve as internal landmarks that can be processed using dedicated software to calculate regional myocardial strain [104,105] or rotational deformation [106]. Strain-encoded MRI is a variant of conventional CMR tagging that uses planar SPAMM not perpendicular but parallel to the imaging plane in order to provide longitudinal strain from short-axis images [107–109]. CMR tagging may also be used to estimate regional EF of the different segments of the left ventricle [110]. More recently, a method called feature tracking has been introduced that allows calculation of strain parameters from standard SSFP cine images using similar principles to speckle tracking echocardiography [115]. Feature tracking CMR avoids the need for additional acquisition of tagging data or tissue phase mapping and shows good agreement with these methods.

Another approach for measuring segmental contractility is phase-contrast myocardial velocity imaging. Besides measuring flow velocity in blood vessels, phase-contrast imaging can be used to measure myocardial velocity. It allows myocardial tissue tracking with high spatiotemporal resolution in all spatial directions, which is an advantage over Doppler tissue imaging [111,112]. CMR is therefore an attractive method for the assessment of regional myocardial motion using either tagging, feature tracking or tissue phase mapping.

12.5 Assessment of ventricular function using radionuclide techniques

12.5.1 Introduction

The quantitative assessment of LV systolic function has been the first achievement of radionuclide imaging using planar equilibrium angiography. Since the late 1990s, the development of gated single-photon emission tomography (SPECT) imaging as an adjunct for myocardial perfusion imaging has enabled the assessment of perfusion along with the determination of regional and global LV function in the same examination. Although this later technique has now replaced planar radionuclide angiography (RNA) in many situations, the combination of tomographic acquisition with red blood cell (RBC) labeling yields the opportunity to assess both left and RV function using gated blood pool SPECT.

12.5.2 Planar equilibrium RNA

RNA techniques, known as gated blood pool scans, multigated acquisition (MUGA), or equilibrium RNA, are recognized for monitoring cardiac function, especially in the context of drug-induced cardiotoxicity.

The advantages of RNA include a high reliability (nuclear imaging has a long and well-established track record of reliable results in monitoring the cardiac effects of chemotherapy, accuracy, and precision of measurements of LV systolic function and reproducibility in the determination of LVEF), well-established standard for monitoring LV function, and a relative operator independence. However, RNA is not as readily available as echocardiography and lacks the ability to collect information on anatomical details of the heart, valves, diastolic function, and pulmonary pressure.

12.5.2.1 Principle and acquisition

Although first-pass imaging has been widely used in the past, RNA is now performed by equilibrium techniques. The radiopharmaceuticals for equilibrium measurements should have an unchanging concentration in the blood pool during the acquisition period. Only 99mTc-labeled red cells and albumin meet this criteria. The ease of use is better with albumin, which is available as a multi-dose kit, but the target to background activity ratio is better with RBC, providing a better image contrast. RBC are labeled in vivo with the consecutive intravenous injections of stannous pyrophosphate and then of 99mTc-pertechnetate (555–1110 MBq) 30 min later, preferably in the opposite arm. This procedure results in a mean RBC labeling of greater than 95% during the first hour after pertechnetate injection. ECG gated data are recorded 5–10 min after the injection of 99mTc-pertechnetate, during 800–1000 cardiac cycles, to produce an averaged cardiac cycle with a high resolution. For EF measurement, images are acquired in the left anterior oblique ("best septal") view to allow the separation between left and right ventricle, for a preset count of 300–400 kcts/frame. A 5–15° cranio-caudal tilt may be used to avoid the interposition of the atria. The division of the RR interval into at least 16 frames per cycle provides adequate temporal resolution for the assessment of resting systolic function. Premature beats lead to changes in heart rate during the acquisition and may underestimate EF. In this situation, arrhythmia filtering can be used to reject beats outside of a specified RR interval (usually 20% around the mean RR interval), with both extrasystolic and post extrasystolic beats excluded.

12.5.2.2 Image analysis

The EF is calculated by dividing the stroke counts by the background corrected end-diastolic counts, and is highly reproducible [48,49]. The EF is best calculated using a count-based technique. It is derived from the ventricular time–activity curves, which parallel the angiographic time–volume curve. This method is independent of geometric models and allows the use of automatic edge detection programs to compute the EF from the left anterior oblique images on equilibrium angiography with high accuracy and reproducibility.

After correction for background counts, EF is computed as $EF = (EDC - ESC)/EDC$, where EDC is end-diastolic counts, and ESC is end-systolic counts.

Fourier analysis is used to provide functional images (amplitude and phase) of the heart by approximating the time–activity curve with the first Fourier harmonic, a sine function with a period identical to the period of the cardiac cycle. The phase image reflects the timing of regional ejection and is not determined solely by any particular cardiac event, but depends on function in general.

The principle of phase analysis programs is to assign a phase angle to each pixel of the phase image, derived from the first Fourier harmonic of time. The phase angle corresponds to the relative sequence and pattern of ventricular contraction during the cardiac cycle. Color-encoded phase images with corresponding histograms are generated and scintigrams are also intensity-coded for amplitude, the other parameter of Fourier first harmonic study. To help interpretation, phase images are generated for cardiac regions using a continuous color scale, corresponding to phase angles from 0° to 360°. Mean phase angles may be computed for LV and RV blood pools as the arithmetic mean phase angle for all pixels in both ventricular regions of interest. Interventricular contractile synchrony is then measured as the absolute difference between LV and RV mean phase angles. Intraventricular contractile synchrony in each ventricle is assessed as the standard deviation of the mean phase angle for the LV and RV blood pools. Multiharmonic Fourier filtering (using 2 or 3 harmonics) has been reported to increase the sensitivity for diagnosing limited focal contraction abnormalities [50].

12.5.2.3 Results and normal values

The lower limit of normal EF using RNA is 50% for the left ventricle and lower (40%) for the right ventricle [51,52], with a high reproducibility of the results [48]. In patients with HF, phase analysis has been used to demonstrate that LV asynchrony is a powerful predictor of long-term outcome [113]. A decreased RNA RV EF is associated with a poor clinical outcome in patients with HF [54].

RNA remains widely used for monitoring LV function in patients receiving potentially cardiotoxic chemotherapy. Because of the well-established reproducible results, RNA has compared favorably with 2D echocardiography for monitoring LV systolic function [55] in this task. Based on RNA, serial LV EF monitoring during doxorubicin therapy for preventing HF was proposed over 30 years ago and reduced the incidence of doxorubicin-induced HF [51]. The efficacy of RNA in this setting has never been denied [56,57].

12.5.3 Gated blood pool SPECT

In the last decade, software packages dedicated to the segmentation of gated blood pool SPECT acquisitions have been developed and validated, making possible the clinical use of this technique [58,60]. After RBC labeling according to an in vivo protocol, image acquisition requires a dual-head gamma-camera equipped with a low-energy high-resolution collimator to collect images at 32 views over a 180 noncircular orbit, using a 8- to 16-interval gating, 25–40 s per view, and a 64×64 matrix.

The tomographic approach of blood pool imaging allows the assessment of ventricular volumes, with a high accuracy compared to MRI [61,62,114] for both left and right ventricles. Moreover, gated blood pool SPECT has an excellent inter-exam precision and reliability for the measurement of LV function [64].

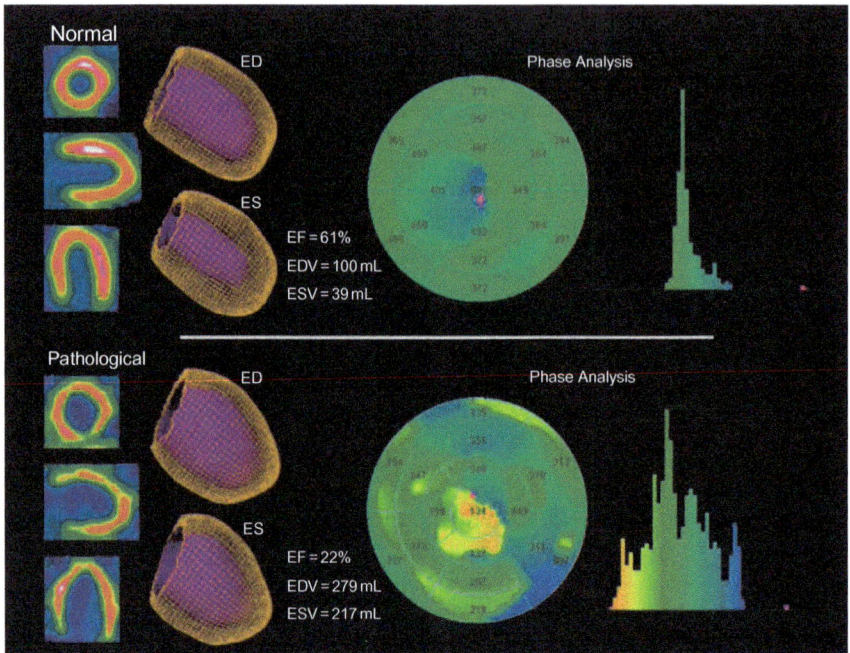

Figure 12.12 Gated blood pool SPECT(Normal Phase Analysis and Pathological Phase Analysis)

Phase analysis is feasible and allows the diagnosis of diffuse and localized arrhythmogenic RV dysplasia [65], creating a new method for a comprehensive biventricular assessment. However, the prognostic value of gated blood pool SPECT, especially for RV function, remains to be established (Figure 12.12).

12.5.4 Perfusion gated SPECT

ECG-gated myocardial perfusion SPECT was developed in the late 1980s and has rapidly evolved into a standard for myocardial perfusion imaging. 99mTc-labeled perfusion radiopharmaceuticals provide higher count rates and stable myocardial distribution with time compared to thallium, and permit the evaluation of regional myocardial wall motion and wall thickening throughout the cardiac cycle. Furthermore, validated automated software is available to quantify LV volumes and EF, providing additional information to perfusion studies.

12.5.4.1 Principle and acquisition

A gated myocardial perfusion SPECT is usually performed using 8 to 16 frames per RR interval per projection. However, 16-frame gating is preferred to avoid an overestimation of end-systolic volumes resulting in the underestimation of EF that is documented when using an 8-interval gating [66]. As for blood pool imaging, it is recommended to reject extrasystolic and post extrasystolic beats using a 20–50% acceptance window.

The acquired data are reconstructed and displayed in a cinematic format to allow the reader to assess wall motion and thickening, which is related to the apparent systolic count increase.

12.5.4.2 Post-processing

For global LV function assessment, validated computer software uses gated reconstructed short-axis images in order to estimate endocardial and epicardial volumes for all intervals of the cardiac cycle. EF is then automatically derived from the end-diastolic and end-systolic volumes. The three most widely distributed software packages for LV function analysis are third-party software proposed by gamma-camera and/or postprocessing workstations vendors: QGS (Cedars-Sinai), 4D-MSPECT (University of Michigan), and the Emory Cardiac Toolbox (Emory University). Most software allows for the manual correction of left ventricle reconstruction limits in case of operator discrepancy, especially in regions with severe perfusion defects or when the mitral valve plane is involved in the defect.

In addition, most of these software programs propose validated options for the assessment of intraventricular mechanical asynchrony using Fourier analysis of perfusion ECG-gated data. 3D sampling is performed on each temporal frame of the gated short-axis image to detect regional maximum counts. The first harmonic Fourier function is used to approximate the wall thickening data to calculate a phase angle for each region. Once the phase angles of all regions are obtained, a phase distribution is generated and displayed in a polar map or histogram. Using this technique, phase standard deviation (the standard deviation of the onset of mechanical contraction phase distribution) and phase histogram bandwidth (the width of the histogram band, including 95% of the 3D samples) are two quantitative indices to assess LV global mechanical dyssynchrony [67]. Figure 12.1 shows an example of phase analysis in a normal patient and in a patient with dilated cardiomyopathy and intraventricular mechanical asynchrony.

12.5.4.3 Results and normal values

Perfusion gated has been widely validated against several reference techniques (echocardiography, contrast angiography, CMR) for the assessment of LV volumes and EF [68] and the performance of the main software packages has been validated as well. If it is documented that they provide LV function values that are slightly different, it is also documented that these methods showed close correlation with each other [69–71].

Most importantly, EDV, ESV, and LVEF determined by gated SPECT (with several software programs) agree with a wide range of CMR [72]. In clinical practice, algorithm-inherent over- or underestimation of volumes and EF should be accounted for, and an interchangeable use of different software packages should be avoided. Moreover, these results encourage nuclear cardiology laboratories to establish their own normal values for their currently used method and gamma-cameras, using data acquired in patients with low prescan likelihood of coronary artery disease. Compared to echocardiography, it is important to note that gated SPECT, which is based on the acquisition of the 3D myocardial distribution of a perfusion tracer, is better correlated to 3D than to conventional 2D echocardiography [73].

The prognostic impact of LV function with regard to long-term survival is well documented using a variety of techniques for functional assessment, and gated SPECT imaging has also found an important role in the risk assessment of patients with known or suspected coronary artery disease. In their early study, the group from Cedars Sinai [74] demonstrated among a large series of 1690 consecutive patients that an EF <45% (i.e., below the normal limit calculated in patients with a low prescan likelihood of coronary artery disease) was associated with a reduced survival, independently of the perfusion defect size. In addition, patients with normal end-systolic volumes (i.e., <70 mL in this publication) or a normal EF ($\geq$45%) had a very low cardiac mortality rate. The same group demonstrated that EF was most predictive of death, while the amount of ischemia was the best predictor of nonfatal myocardial infarction [75].

Phase analysis of gated perfusion SPECT is an evolving technique for measuring LV mechanical dyssynchrony. Phase analysis is automatic, and has been shown to have high reproducibility and repeatability. The LV dyssynchrony parameters measured by phase analysis have been shown to be independent from the type of camera used, the type of image reconstruction, or the clinically relevant tracer doses [67]. Preliminary results have also shown good correlation with echocardiography for assessment of LV mechanical dyssynchrony [76–78]. This technique has been validated for the assessment of ventricular asynchrony, and preliminary results suggest that it would be a useful tool for assessing candidates for CRT. The technique is now ready to be assessed in multi-center, randomized, prospective clinical trials as a clinical approach to consistently predicting CRT response in HF patients.

References

[1] Buckberg GD, Weisfeldt ML, Ballester M, et al. Left ventricular form and function: scientific priorities and strategic planning for development of new views of disease. Circulation 2004;110:e333–6.

[2] McMurray JJ, Adamopoulos S, Anker SD, et al. ESC Guidelines for the diagnosis and treatment of acute and chronic heart failure 2012: The Task Force for the Diagnosis and Treatment of Acute and Chronic Heart Failure 2012 of the European Society of Cardiology. Developed in collaboration with the Heart Failure Association (HFA) of the ESC. Eur Heart J 2012;33:1787–847.

[3] Sengupta PP, Krishnamoorthy VK, Korinek J, et al. Left ventricular form and function revisited: applied translational science to cardiovascular ultrasound imaging. J Am Soc Echocardiogr 2007;20:539–51.

[4] Gurunathan S, Ahmed A, Senior R. The benefits of revascularization in chronic heart failure. Current heart failure reports; 2014.

[5] Shah BN, Senior R. Role of viability imaging in the post-STICH era. Curr Opin Cardiol 2014;29:145–51.

[6] Bax JJ, Kraft O, Buxton AE, et al. 123 I-mIBG scintigraphy to predict inducibility of ventricular arrhythmias on cardiac electrophysiology testing: a prospective multicenter pilot study. Circ Cardiovasc Imaging 2008;1:131–40.

[7] Flotats A, Carrio I, Agostini D, et al. Proposal for standardization of ^{123}I-metaiodobenzylguanidine (MIBG) cardiac sympathetic imaging by the EANM

Cardiovascular Committee and the European Council of Nuclear Cardiology. Eur J Nucl Med Mol Imaging 2010;37:1802–12.
[8] Kirchhof P, Sipido KR, Cowie MR, et al. The continuum of personalized cardiovascular medicine: a position paper of the European Society of Cardiology. Eur Heart J 2014;35:3250–7.
[9] Sengupta PP, Khandheria BK, Korinek J, et al. Apex-to-base dispersion in regional timing of left ventricular shortening and lengthening. J Am Coll Cardiol 2006;47:163–72.
[10] Beshai JF, Grimm RA, Nagueh SF, et al. Cardiac-resynchronization therapy in heart failure with narrow QRS complexes. N Engl J Med 2007;357:2461–71.
[11] European Heart Rhythm Association, European Society of Cardiology, Heart Rhythm Society, et al. EHRA/HRS expert consensus statement on cardiac resynchronization therapy in heart failure: implant and follow-up recommendations and management. Heart Rhythm 2012;9:1524–76.
[12] Chung ES, Leon AR, Tavazzi L, et al. Results of the predictors of response to CRT (PROSPECT) trial. Circulation 2008;117:2608–16.
[13] Bijnens B, Claus P, Weidemann F, Strotmann J, Sutherland GR. Investigating cardiac function using motion and deformation analysis in the setting of coronary artery disease. Circulation 2007;116:2453–64.
[14] Bijnens BH, Cikes M, Claus P, Sutherland GR. Velocity and deformation imaging for the assessment of myocardial dysfunction. Eur J Echocardiogr 2009;10:216–26.
[15] Torrent-Guasp F, Kocica MJ, Corno AF, et al. Towards new understanding of the heart structure and function. Eur J Cardiothorac Surg 2005;27:191–201.
[16] Streeter Jr DD, Hanna WT. Engineering mechanics for successive states in canine left ventricular myocardium. II. Fiber angle and sarcomere length. Circ Res 1973; 33:656–64.
[17] Sengupta PP, Tajik AJ, Chandrasekaran K, Khandheria BK. Twist mechanics of the left ventricle: principles and application. JACC Cardiovasc Imaging 2008;1:366–76.
[18] Sengupta PP, Korinek J, Belohlavek M, et al. Left ventricular structure and function: basic science for cardiac imaging. J Am Coll Cardiol 2006;48:1988–2001.
[19] Scollan DF, Holmes A, Winslow R, Forder J. Histological validation of myocardial microstructure obtained from diffusion tensor magnetic resonance imaging. Am J Physiol 1998;275:H2308–18.
[20] Arts T, Costa KD, Covell JW, McCulloch AD. Relating myocardial laminar architecture to shear strain and muscle fiber orientation. Am J Physiol Heart Circ Physiol 2001;280:H2222–9.
[21] Walker CA, Spinale FG. The structure and function of the cardiac myocyte: a review of fundamental concepts. J Thorac Cardiovasc Surg 1999;118:375–82.
[22] Arsanjani R, Berman DS, Gransar H, et al. Left ventricular function and volume with coronary CT angiography improves risk stratification and identification of patients at risk for incident mortality: results from 7758 patients in the prospective multinational CONFIRM observational cohort study. Radiology 2014;273:70–7.
[23] Sengupta PP, Khandheria BK, Narula J. Twist and untwist mechanics of the left ventricle. Heart Fail Clin 2008;4:315–24.
[24] Bertini M, Sengupta PP, Nucifora G, et al. Role of left ventricular twist mechanics in the assessment of cardiac dyssynchrony in heart failure. JACC Cardiovasc Imaging 2009;2:1425–35.
[25] Geyer H, Caracciolo G, Abe H, et al. Assessment of myocardial mechanics using speckle tracking echocardiography: fundamentals and clinical applications. J Am Soc Echocardiogr 2010;23:351–69, quiz 453–5.

[26] Thavendiranathan P, Poulin F, Lim KD, Plana JC, Woo A, Marwick TH. Use of myocardial strain imaging by echocardiography for the early detection of cardiotoxicity in patients during and after cancer chemotherapy: a systematic review. J Am Coll Cardiol 2014;63:2751–68.
[27] Abraham T, Kass D, Tonti G, et al. Imaging cardiac resynchronization therapy. JACC Cardiovasc Imaging 2009;2:486–97.
[28] Donal E, Thebault C, Lund LH, et al. Heart failure with a preserved ejection fraction additive value of an exercise stress echocardiography. Eur Heart J Cardiovasc Imaging 2012;13:656–65.
[29] Erdei T, Smiseth OA, Marino P, Fraser AG. A systematic review of diastolic stress tests in heart failure with preserved ejection fraction, with proposals from the EU-FP7 MEDIA study group. Eur J Heart Fail 2014;16:1345–61.
[30] Yu CM, Sanderson JE, Marwick TH, Oh JK. Tissue Doppler imaging a new prognosticator for cardiovascular diseases. J Am Coll Cardiol 2007;49:1903–14.
[31] Wang J, Nagueh SF. Current perspectives on cardiac function in patients with diastolic heart failure. Circulation 2009;119:1146–57.
[32] Bertini M, Ng AC, Antoni ML, et al. Global longitudinal strain predicts long-term survival in patients with chronic ischemic cardiomyopathy. Circ Cardiovasc Imaging 2012;5:383–91.
[33] Mignot A, Donal E, Zaroui A, et al. Global longitudinal strain as a major predictor of cardiac events in patients with depressed left ventricular function: a multicenter study. J Am Soc Echocardiogr 2010;23:1019–24.
[34] Donal E, Coquerel N, Bodi S, et al. Importance of ventricular longitudinal function in chronic heart failure. Eur J Echocardiogr 2011;12:619–27.
[35] Nahum J, Bensaid A, Dussault C, et al. Impact of longitudinal myocardial deformation on the prognosis of chronic heart failure patients. Circ Cardiovasc Imaging 2010;3:249–56.
[36] Iacoviello M, Puzzovivo A, Guida P, et al. Independent role of left ventricular global longitudinal strain in predicting prognosis of chronic heart failure patients. Echocardiography 2013;30:803–11.
[37] Cho GY, Marwick TH, Kim HS, Kim MK, Hong KS, Oh DJ. Global 2-dimensional strain as a new prognosticator in patients with heart failure. J Am Coll Cardiol 2009;54:618–24.
[38] Wang J, Khoury DS, Yue Y, Torre-Amione G, Nagueh SF. Preserved left ventricular twist and circumferential deformation, but depressed longitudinal and radial deformation in patients with diastolic heart failure. Eur Heart J 2008;29:1283–9.
[39] Thavendiranathan P, Grant AD, Negishi T, Plana JC, Popovic ZB, Marwick TH. Reproducibility of echocardiographic techniques for sequential assessment of left ventricular ejection fraction and volumes: application to patients undergoing cancer chemotherapy. J Am Coll Cardiol 2013;61:77–84.
[40] Jenkins C, Moir S, Chan J, Rakhit D, Haluska B, Marwick TH. Left ventricular volume measurement with echocardiography: a comparison of left ventricular opacification, three-dimensional echocardiography, or both with magnetic resonance imaging. Eur Heart J 2009;30:98–106.
[41] Hare JL, Jenkins C, Nakatani S, Ogawa A, Yu CM, Marwick TH. Feasibility and clinical decision-making with 3D echocardiography in routine practice. Heart 2008;94:440–5.
[42] Muraru D, Badano LP, Peluso D, et al. Comprehensive analysis of left ventricular geometry and function by three-dimensional echocardiography in healthy adults. J Am Soc Echocardiogr 2013;26:618–28.
[43] Muraru D, Cucchini U, Mihaila S, et al. Left ventricular myocardial strain by three-dimensional speckle-tracking echocardiography in healthy subjects: reference values and analysis of their physiologic and technical determinants. J Am Soc Echocardiogr 2014;27:858–71.

[44] Marwick TH. Application of 3D echocardiography to everyday practice: development of normal ranges is step 1. JACC Cardiovasc Imaging 2012;5:1198–200.
[45] Mor-Avi V, Lang RM, Badano LP, et al. Current and evolving echocardiographic techniques for the quantitative evaluation of cardiac mechanics: ASE/EAE consensus statement on methodology and indications endorsed by the Japanese Society of Echocardiography. Eur J Echocardiogr 2011;12:167–205.
[46] Lancellotti P, Pierard LA. Chronic ischaemic mitral regurgitation: exercise testing reveals its dynamic component. Eur Heart J 2005;26:1816–7.
[47] Voelkel NF, Quaife RA, Leinwand LA, et al. Right ventricular function and failure: report of a National Heart, Lung, and Blood Institute working group on cellular and molecular mechanisms of right heart failure. Circulation 2006;114:1883–91.
[48] Starr I. Clinical studies on incoordination of the circulation, as determined by the response to arising. J Clin Invest 1943;22:813–26.
[49] Fontan F, Baudet E. Surgical repair of tricuspid atresia. Thorax 1971;26:240–8.
[50] Meluzin J, Spinarova L, Hude P, et al. Combined right ventricular systolic and diastolic dysfunction represents a strong determinant of poor prognosis in patients with symptomatic heart failure. Int J Cardiol 2005;105:164–73.
[51] Antoni ML, Scherptong RW, Atary JZ, et al. Prognostic value of right ventricular function in patients after acute myocardial infarction treated with primary percutaneous coronary intervention. Circ Cardiovasc Imaging 2010;3:264–71.
[52] Ghio S, Gavazzi A, Campana C, et al. Independent and additive prognostic value of right ventricular systolic function and pulmonary artery pressure in patients with chronic heart failure. J Am Coll Cardiol 2001;37:183–8.
[53] Ye Y, Desai R, Vargas Abello LM, et al. Effects of right ventricular morphology and function on outcomes of patients with degenerative mitral valve disease. J Thorac Cardiovasc Surg 2014;148:2012–20.
[54] Kendall SW, Bittner HB, Peterseim DS, Campbell KA, Van Trigt P. Right ventricular function in the donor heart. Eur J Cardiothorac Surg 1997;11:609–15.
[55] Patel ND, Weiss ES, Schaffer J, et al. Right heart dysfunction after left ventricular assist device implantation: a comparison of the pulsatile HeartMate I and axial-flow HeartMate II devices. Ann Thorac Surg 2008;86:832–40, discussion 832-40.
[56] Ho SY, Nihoyannopoulos P. Anatomy, echocardiography, and normal right ventricular dimensions. Heart 2006;92(Suppl. 1):i2–13.
[57] Dragulescu A, Friedberg MK, Grosse-Wortmann L, Redington A, Mertens L. Effect of chronic right ventricular volume overload on ventricular interaction in patients after tetralogy of fallot repair. J Am Soc Echocardiogr 2014;27:896–902.
[58] Mertens LL, Friedberg MK. Imaging the right ventricle—current state of the art. Nat Rev Cardiol 2010;7:551–63.
[59] Petitjean C, Rougon N, Cluzel P. Assessment of myocardial function: a review of quantification methods and results using tagged MRI. J Cardiovasc Magn Reson 2005;7:501–16.
[60] Dell'Italia LJ, Walsh RA. Acute determinants of the hangout interval in the pulmonary circulation. Am Heart J 1988;116:1289–97.
[61] Davlouros PA, Niwa K, Webb G, Gatzoulis MA. The right ventricle in congenital heart disease. Heart 2006;92(Suppl. 1):i27–38.
[62] Modesti PA, Polidori G, Bertolozzi I, Vanni S, Cecioni I. Impairment of cardiopulmonary receptor sensitivity in the early phase of heart failure. Heart 2004;90:30–6.
[63] Linardi D, Rungatscher A, Morjan M, et al. Ventricular and pulmonary vascular remodeling induced by pulmonary overflow in a chronic model of pretricuspid shunt. J Thorac Cardiovasc Surg 2014;148:2609–17.

[64] Vitarelli A, Barilla F, Capotosto L, et al. Right ventricular function in acute pulmonary embolism: a combined assessment by three-dimensional and speckle-tracking echocardiography. J Am Soc Echocardiogr 2014;27:329–38.
[65] Greyson CR. Pathophysiology of right ventricular failure. Crit Care Med 2008;36:S57–65.
[66] Friedberg MK, Redington AN. Right versus left ventricular failure: differences, similarities, and interactions. Circulation 2014;129:1033–44.
[67] Nagendran J, Archer SL, Soliman D, et al. Phosphodiesterase type 5 is highly expressed in the hypertrophied human right ventricle, and acute inhibition of phosphodiesterase type 5 improves contractility. Circulation 2007;116:238–48.
[68] Pettersen E, Helle-Valle T, Edvardsen T, et al. Contraction pattern of the systemic right ventricle shift from longitudinal to circumferential shortening and absent global ventricular torsion. J Am Coll Cardiol 2007;49:2450–6.
[69] Gan C, Lankhaar JW, Marcus JT, et al. Impaired left ventricular filling due to right-to-left ventricular interaction in patients with pulmonary arterial hypertension. Am J Physiol Heart Circ Physiol 2006;290:H1528–33.
[70] Brookes C, Ravn H, White P, Moeldrup U, Oldershaw P, Redington A. Acute right ventricular dilatation in response to ischemia significantly impairs left ventricular systolic performance. Circulation 1999;100:761–7.
[71] La Vecchia L, Zanolla L, Varotto L, et al. Reduced right ventricular ejection fraction as a marker for idiopathic dilated cardiomyopathy compared with ischemic left ventricular dysfunction. Am Heart J 2001;142:181–9.
[72] Kitahori K, Murakami A, Takaoka T, Takamoto S, Ono M. Precise evaluation of bilateral pulmonary artery banding for initial palliation in high-risk hypoplastic left heart syndrome. J Thorac Cardiovasc Surg 2010;140:1084–91.
[73] Agmon Y, Connolly HM, Olson LJ, Khandheria BK, Seward JB. Noncompaction of the ventricular myocardium. J Am Soc Echocardiogr 1999;12:859–63.
[74] Gulati A, Ismail TF, Jabbour A, et al. The prevalence and prognostic significance of right ventricular systolic dysfunction in nonischemic dilated cardiomyopathy. Circulation 2013;128:1623–33.
[75] Lam CS, Roger VL, Rodeheffer RJ, Borlaug BA, Enders FT, Redfield MM. Pulmonary hypertension in heart failure with preserved ejection fraction: a community-based study. J Am Coll Cardiol 2009;53:1119–26.
[76] Murninkas D, Alba AC, Delgado D, et al. Right ventricular function and prognosis in stable heart failure patients. J Card Fail 2014;20:343–9.
[77] Lindqvist P, Calcutteea A, Henein M. Echocardiography in the assessment of right heart function. Eur J Echocardiogr 2008;9:225–34.
[78] Rudski LG, Lai WW, Afilalo J, et al. Guidelines for the echocardiographic assessment of the right heart in adults: a report from the American Society of Echocardiography endorsed by the European Association of Echocardiography, a registered branch of the European Society of Cardiology, and the Canadian Society of Echocardiography. J Am Soc Echocardiogr 2010;23:685–713, quiz 86–8.
[79] Guazzi M, Bandera F, Pelissero G, et al. Tricuspid annular plane systolic excursion and pulmonary arterial systolic pressure relationship in heart failure: an index of right ventricular contractile function and prognosis. Am J Physiol Heart Circ Physiol 2013;305:H1373–81.
[80] Tei C, Dujardin KS, Hodge DO, et al. Doppler echocardiographic index for assessment of global right ventricular function. J Am Soc Echocardiogr 1996;9:838–47.
[81] Ogihara Y, Yamada N, Dohi K, et al. Utility of right ventricular Tei-index for assessing disease severity and determining response to treatment in patients with pulmonary arterial hypertension. J Cardiol 2014;63:149–53.

[82] Jurcut R, Giusca S, Ticulescu R, et al. Different patterns of adaptation of the right ventricle to pressure overload: a comparison between pulmonary hypertension and pulmonary stenosis. J Am Soc Echocardiogr 2011;24:1109–17.

[83] Jurcut R, Giusca S, La Gerche A, Vasile S, Ginghina C, Voigt JU. The echocardiographic assessment of the right ventricle: what to do in 2010? Eur J Echocardiogr 2010;11:81–96.

[84] Maffessanti F, Muraru D, Esposito R, et al. Age-, body size-, and sex-specific reference values for right ventricular volumes and ejection fraction by three-dimensional echocardiography: a multicenter echocardiographic study in 507 healthy volunteers. Circ Cardiovasc Imaging 2013;6:700–10.

[85] Longmore DB, Klipstein RH, Underwood SR, et al. Dimensional accuracy of magnetic resonance in studies of the heart. Lancet 1985;1:1360–2.

[86] Sakuma H, Fujita N, Foo TK, et al. Evaluation of left ventricular volume and mass with breath-hold cine MR imaging. Radiology 1993;188:377–80.

[87] Sechtem U, Pflugfelder PW, Gould RG, Cassidy MM, Higgins CB. Measurement of right and left ventricular volumes in healthy individuals with cine MR imaging. Radiology 1987;163:697–702.

[88] Bottini PB, Carr AA, Prisant LM, Flickinger FW, Allison JD, Gottdiener JS. Magnetic resonance imaging compared to echocardiography to assess left ventricular mass in the hypertensive patient. Am J Hypertens 1995;8:221–8.

[89] Grothues F, Moon JC, Bellenger NG, Smith GS, Klein HU, Pennell DJ. Interstudy reproducibility of right ventricular volumes, function, and mass with cardiovascular magnetic resonance. Am Heart J 2004;147:218–23.

[90] Bellenger NG, Burgess MI, Ray SG, et al. Comparison of left ventricular ejection fraction and volumes in heart failure by echocardiography, radionuclide ventriculography and cardiovascular magnetic resonance; are they interchangeable? Eur Heart J 2000;21:1387–96.

[91] Hildebrand LB, Buonocore MH. Fully refocused gradient recalled echo (FRGRE): factors affecting flow and motion sensitivity in cardiac MRI. J Cardiovasc Magn Reson 2002;4:211–22.

[92] Nagel E, Schneider U, Schalla S, et al. Magnetic resonance real-time imaging for the evaluation of left ventricular function. J Cardiovasc Magn Reson 2000;2:7–14.

[93] Muthurangu V, Lurz P, Critchely JD, Deanfield JE, Taylor AM, Hansen MS. Real-time assessment of right and left ventricular volumes and function in patients with congenital heart disease by using high spatiotemporal resolution radial k-t SENSE. Radiology 2008;248:782–91.

[94] Papavassiliu T, Kuhl HP, Schroder M, et al. Effect of endocardial trabeculae on left ventricular measurements and measurement reproducibility at cardiovascular MR imaging. Radiology 2005;236:57–64.

[95] Sievers B, Kirchberg S, Bakan A, Franken U, Trappe HJ. Impact of papillary muscles in ventricular volume and ejection fraction assessment by cardiovascular magnetic resonance. J Cardiovasc Magn Reson 2004;6:9–16.

[96] Winter MM, Bernink FJ, Groenink M, et al. Evaluating the systemic right ventricle by CMR: the importance of consistent and reproducible delineation of the cavity. J Cardiovasc Magn Reson 2008;10:40.

[97] Janik M, Cham MD, Ross MI, et al. Effects of papillary muscles and trabeculae on left ventricular quantification: increased impact of methodological variability in patients with left ventricular hypertrophy. J Hypertens 2008;26:1677–85.

[98] Marcus JT, Gotte MJ, DeWaal LK, et al. The influence of through-plane motion on left ventricular volumes measured by magnetic resonance imaging: implications for image acquisition and analysis. J Cardiovasc Magn Reson 1999;1:1–6.

[99] Sugeng L, Mor-Avi V, Weinert L, et al. Multimodality comparison of quantitative volumetric analysis of the right ventricle. JACC Cardiovasc Imaging 2010;3:10–8.
[100] Devos DG, Kilner PJ. Calculations of cardiovascular shunts and regurgitation using magnetic resonance ventricular volume and aortic and pulmonary flow measurements. Eur Radiol 2010;20:410–21.
[101] Kondo C, Caputo GR, Semelka R, Foster E, Shimakawa A, Higgins CB. Right and left ventricular stroke volume measurements with velocity-encoded cine MR imaging: in vitro and in vivo validation. AJR Am J Roentgenol 1991;157:9–16.
[102] Peshock RM, Rokey R, Malloy GM, et al. Assessment of myocardial systolic wall thickening using nuclear magnetic resonance imaging. J Am Coll Cardiol 1989;14:653–9.
[103] Zerhouni EA, Parish DM, Rogers WJ, Yang A, Shapiro EP. Human heart: tagging with MR imaging—a method for noninvasive assessment of myocardial motion. Radiology 1988;169:59–63.
[104] Garot J, Bluemke DA, Osman NF, et al. Fast determination of regional myocardial strain fields from tagged cardiac images using harmonic phase MRI. Circulation 2000;101:981–8.
[105] Osman NF, Kerwin WS, McVeigh ER, Prince JL. Cardiac motion tracking using CINE harmonic phase (HARP) magnetic resonance imaging. Magn Reson Med 1999;42:1048–60.
[106] Buchalter MB, Weiss JL, Rogers WJ, et al. Noninvasive quantification of left ventricular rotational deformation in normal humans using magnetic resonance imaging myocardial tagging. Circulation 1990;81:1236–44.
[107] Garot J, Lima JA, Gerber BL, et al. Spatially resolved imaging of myocardial function with strain-encoded MR: comparison with delayed contrast-enhanced MR imaging after myocardial infarction. Radiology 2004;233:596–602.
[108] Neizel M, Lossnitzer D, Korosoglou G, et al. Strain-encoded MRI for evaluation of left ventricular function and transmurality in acute myocardial infarction. Circ Cardiovasc Imaging 2009;2:116–22.
[109] Osman NF, Sampath S, Atalar E, Prince JL. Imaging longitudinal cardiac strain on short-axis images using strain-encoded MRI. Magn Reson Med 2001;46:324–34.
[110] Bogaert J, Bosmans H, Maes A, Suetens P, Marchal G, Rademakers FE. Remote myocardial dysfunction after acute anterior myocardial infarction: impact of left ventricular shape on regional function: a magnetic resonance myocardial tagging study. J Am Coll Cardiol 2000;35:1525–34.
[111] Foll D, Jung B, Staehle F, et al. Visualization of multidirectional regional left ventricular dynamics by high-temporal-resolution tissue phase mapping. J Magn Reson Imaging 2009;29:1043–52.
[112] Jung B, Foll D, Bottler P, Petersen S, Hennig J, Markl M. Detailed analysis of myocardial motion in volunteers and patients using high-temporal-resolution MR tissue phase mapping. J Magn Reson Imaging 2006;24:1033–9.
[113] Ye Y, Desai R, Vargas Abello LM, et al. Effects of right ventricular morphology and function on outcomes of patients with degenerative mitral valve disease. J Thorac Cardiovasc Surg 2014;148:2012–20.
[114] Linardi D, Rungatscher A, Morjan M, et al. Ventricular and pulmonary vascular remodeling induced by pulmonary overflow in a chronic model of pretricuspid shunt. J Thorac Cardiovasc Surg 2014;148:2609–17.
[115] Andre F, Steen H, Matheis P, Westkott M, Breuninger K, Sander Y, et al. Age- and gender-related normal left ventricular deformation assessed by cardiovascular magnetic resonance feature tracking. J Cardiovasc Magn Reson 2015;17:25.

Cardiomyopathy

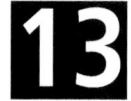

A.J. Baksi, D.J. Pennell
Royal Brompton Hospital, London, UK

13.1 Introduction

13.1.1 Definition and spectrum of disease

The term cardiomyopathy refers to a diverse range of diseases of the heart muscle associated with mechanical and/or electrical dysfunction [1]. These conditions are of particular importance due to their propensity to cause significant morbidity and mortality, frequently through heart failure and arrhythmia. The myocardial disease may be primary or a secondary consequence of a systemic condition. The classification of cardiomyopathies has evolved since the World Health Organisation's description of idiopathic cardiomyopathies [2], largely with the evolution of understanding of these conditions, but this remains somewhat contentious. There is increasing recognition and identification of the genetic basis or contribution to many of the cardiomyopathies, but many questions remain. The most recent classification of the European Society of Cardiology (ESC) is grounded in ventricular morphology and function [3], in contrast to the American Heart Association (AHA) and American College of Cardiology (ACC), whose classification groups the cardiomyopathies into primary cardiomyopathies, which are subdivided depending on whether they are genetic, acquired or mixed, and secondary cardiomyopathies [1]. All classifications have some limitations resulting from the diverse and heterogeneous yet overlapping nature of the cardiomyopathies.

13.1.2 Role and challenges of imaging

Much of the classification of the cardiomyopathies relies on the phenotypic description of the structural and functional changes identified by imaging. There is growing recognition of the phenotypic and genetic overlap amongst cardiomyopathies [4]. As a result, there are a number of challenges in making an accurate diagnosis. Cardiac imaging has become central to the investigation of heart failure aetiology, discrimination between the differential causes of LV hypertrophy, and in informing risk stratification.

The strengths, limitations, and utility of specific techniques are briefly reviewed and then discussed in greater depth with respect to specific conditions. All the imaging techniques have seen considerable advances in their capability due to development of both hardware and software. The technological developments in the cardiac imaging techniques are covered in detail in Part One of this book. Table 13.1 provides a summary comparison of the non-invasive imaging modalities available for the assessment of non-ischaemic cardiomyopathy.

Table 13.1 Comparison of imaging modalities

	Echo	CT	CMR	PET	SPECT
Scan duration	20–30 min	10 min	30–45 min	2 h	1½–2 h
Contraindications	None	Renal failure Pregnancy	MRI-incompatible implants and devices (relative) Pregnancy during first trimester (precautionary)	Pregnancy	Pregnancy
Limitations	Operator dependent. Acoustic window Imaging of apical segments and RV	Radiation Currently not suited for detection of fibrosis, perfusion and wall motion Blood flow cannot be assessed	Availability Lower temporal resolution than echo	Availability Low spatial resolution	Availability Low spatial resolution
Risks	None	Radiation Renal failure Allergy	NSF (with some types of gadolinium-based contrast if severe renal failure)	Radiation Allergy (rare)	Radiation Allergy (rare)
Radiation	None	1–10 mSv (depending on scanner and protocol) 1–2 mSv calcium score only	None	14 mSv (F-18 FDG)	41 mSv (Thallium stress/rest) 9 mSv (Sestamibi)
LV/RV function and volumes	++ 3D echo	+	+++	−	++
Mass quantification	+ (localised hypertrophy can be missed)	+	+++	−	−
Oedema	− (non-specific findings such as wall thickening)	−	+++ (STIR sequences)	+++ FDG (uptake)	+ (non-specific; areas of reduced perfusion)
Fibrosis	−	+	+++	+	−

Adapted from Parsai et al. [90].

While CT has flourished of recent for the assessment of coronary artery disease, perhaps the greatest developments with respect to the imaging of cardiomyopathies have been in cardiovascular magnetic resonance (CMR). With advances in scanner technology and sequences, this technique now offers a "one-stop" shop in the assessment of both ischaemic and non-ischaemic cardiomyopathies.

Specific consideration is given to the imaging of ischaemic heart disease, myocarditis, and contractile function in other chapters in this book.

13.1.3 Echocardiography

Echocardiography remains the initial modality to investigate suspected cardiomyopathy due to its accessibility and availability at relatively low cost. Furthermore, its unrivalled temporal resolution, well-established ability to assess diastolic function, and robust assessment of valvular function, as well as quantitative analysis of features such as strain, have further strengthened its application in the assessment of cardiomyopathy. However, limited ability to clearly discriminate between overlapping phenotypes in cardiomyopathy as well as issues of reproducibility can reduce the power of this technique when applied to myocardial disease. Notably, visualisation of the LV apex and of the right ventricle can be limited on echocardiography and, consequently, some pathologies, such as apical hypertrophic cardiomyopathy, may not be identified. If apical HCM is a possibility, the use of a contrast agent can aid identification of this sometimes subtle pathology (see Chapter 2).

In most patients, optimal endocardial definition allows the echocardiographic assessment of LV function. In the minority of subjects where image quality is suboptimal, it is recommended to use contrast echocardiography for LV opacification [101]. The adjunctive use of contrast echocardiography for enhanced endocardial border definition and more accurate measurement of LV ejection fraction is well described [5,102]. The accuracy of contrast echocardiography remains inferior, even if close, to 3D echocardiography in patients with adequate imaging windows.

With the use of advanced echo techniques such as tissue Doppler imaging (TDI) and speckle-tracking echocardiography (STE), particularly in combination with sophisticated analysis software, regional myocardial function can be accurately assessed by echocardiography [6]. Although parameters such as velocity, strain, and strain rate (the temporal derivative of strain) obtained by these techniques can offer insight into local myocardial deformation, such deformation imaging is unable to discriminate between active and passive myocardial deformation. TDI measures the velocity of myocardial motion, and measurements at the mitral annulus are validated and widely employed to assess both systolic and diastolic left ventricular function [7]. This technique has been applied to the assessment of cardiomyopathy with good effect, notably in HCM, as described later in the chapter [8–10]. Unlike TDI, STE is largely angle-independent and exploits the speckles that are apparent in grayscale B-mode 2D images. It is an offline technique, and again unlike TDI, can measure motion in any direction relative to the probe. Consequently, both the circumferential and radial components of myocardial deformation can be interrogated. 3D speckle tracking is an even more superior technique, often able to incorporate the entire left ventricle in a single scan volume, allowing true interrogation in any direction and also reduced acquisition time. As with 2D speckle tracking imaging, robust data requires good image quality. For both TDI and STE, measurement of longitudinal deformation is more robust than that of radial deformation.

13.1.4 Cardiovascular magnetic resonance

CMR provides a comprehensive assessment of both ischaemic and non-ischaemic cardiomyopathies. In a single scan, typically lasting around 45 min, detailed information can be obtained with regard to cardiovascular anatomy and cardiac function, blood flow, inducible ischaemia due to epicardial coronary disease or microvascular dysfunction, and tissue characterisation. In the assessment of cardiomyopathy, tissue characterisation by CMR, both using native and extrinsic contrast, is particularly powerful. CMR is also not limited by patient echogenicity, and allows imaging in any plane with excellent delineation of the blood–myocardium interface. Despite these advantages, the quality of CMR images can be markedly reduced by the presence of arrhythmia which can interfere with ECG gating and also by patient difficulty performing breath-holds. A small number of patients are unable to tolerate CMR due to severe claustrophobia, but with experienced staff, adaptations to patient positioning, aids such as prism glasses and reassurance, this is rare. An even smaller number of patients are physically too large to comfortably fit in the bore of a standard clinical scanner. Severe renal impairment carries a potential risk of nephrogenic systemic fibrosis following administration of gadolinium-based agents [11], but with appropriate consent, this need not be a bar to contrast use providing the indication is robust such that the benefit of the scan outweighs the potential risk. There are also a number of patients who are unable to undergo CMR due to the presence of metallic implants or devices which are not CMR-safe. Given that increasing numbers of patients with cardiomyopathy who require serial imaging are having device implantation, it is of benefit that CMR conditional pacemaker and ICD devices are increasingly available and employed. In addition, there are guidelines and evidence to support safe MR imaging in patients with conventional devices who meet the criteria and where appropriate experience and precautions exist [12,13].

Diagnosis of cardiomyopathy may require the integration of numerous pieces of information and investigations, but CMR can often be definitive in a single test. For example, increased LV wall thickness may be the consequence of hypertension, aortic stenosis, hypertrophic cardiomyopathy, cardiac amyloidosis, sarcoidosis, Anderson–Fabry disease, aortic coarctation, and athletic conditioning, in addition to numerous other substrates. CMR assessment of LV hypertrophy can allow accurate discrimination between these various causes of a hypertrophic phenotype (Table 13.2). It is established that the assessment of LV mass is best done by CMR [14]. The following briefly summarises the techniques and sequences commonly employed in CMR in the assessment of cardiomyopathy. Greater detail on technological developments in this technique can be found in Chapter 6.

CMR is the gold standard for assessment of ventricular volumes given its accuracy and reproducibility [15–18]. Of all the techniques, it is currently the most able to

Table 13.2 Causes of LV hypertrophy/increased wall thickness

Abnormal loading
- Hypertension
- Aortic stenosis
- Aortic coarctation
Hypertrophic cardiomyopathy (predominantly due to sarcomeric protein gene mutation)
Amyloidosis (Familial ATTR, Wild type TTR (senile), AL amyloidosis)
Sarcoidosis
Lyosomal storage disease (e.g. Anderson–Fabry)
Glycogen storage diseases (Danon, Pompe)
Friedrich's ataxia
Drug-induced (Tacrolimus, hydroxychloroquine, steroids)
Intense athletic conditioning
Noonan syndrome/LEOPARD syndrome/Costello syndrome
Mitochondrial disease

deal with the variable anatomy of the right ventricle and generate robust quantitative assessment of volume and function. The routine practice of quantification of RV volumes and function enhances the accuracy of this.

Differences in LV volumes acquired by different modalities are widely reported such that it is important to be aware that measures obtained by different modalities are not interchangeable. This will consequently impact on eligibility where EF is used as a criteria and the majority of existing literature is based on echocardiographic measurement of EF. Previous studies have highlighted this point, although few have quantified the impact of this in specific relevant populations, either in terms of cost or outcome. The incorporation of CMR assessment in major HF trials is important.

The protocol for CMR assessment of cardiomyopathy is a relatively standard protocol, although this may be modified based on the clinical question. Typically dark-blood anatomical images are acquired using a multi-slice single shot spin-echo sequence (Half-Fourier Acquisition of Single-Shot Turbo Spin Echo, HASTE) in trans-axial, coronal, and sagittal planes. Bright-blood images may be acquired instead or as well using steady-state free precession (SSFP) imaging. Cine-CMR images are then acquired using cine-SSFP imaging to provide functional information.

Tissue characterisation exploits either intrinsic tissue properties (non-contrast tissue characterisation) or the interaction of extrinsic contrast agents (specifically gadolinium-based contrast) with tissues. Specific sequences have been developed to enable the identification of pathological tissue.

Short-tau inversion recovery (STIR) sequences are T2-weighted sequences with increased sensitivity to myocardial fluid content. Signal from flowing blood and fat is suppressed and the physical properties of the sequence are designed to yield high signal in regions of oedematous tissue. Consequently, regions of acute myocyte swelling and interstitial oedema can be identified, although as such are relatively non-specific. The technique can be limited by interference from high signal in regions of low velocity blood flow, notably at the LV apex and in regions of prominent trabeculation, by variation in proximity to the surface coil, low signal-to-noise ratio and the standard sources of artefact. Additionally, interpretation is usually subjective, often informed by comparison with late gadolinium enhancement. The subjectivity and limitation in detecting more global oedema can be improved by comparing myocardial signal intensity with skeletal muscle as a reference or better still by using T2 mapping techniques. Any of the mapping techniques simply creates a spatial representation of a particular signal, be it flow velocity, T2 value, or T1 values.

Recent CMR literature has been dominated by the numerous sequences and techniques which aim to identify diffuse fibrosis through T1 mapping and extracellular volume quantification. T1 parameters can be interrogated either with or without utilisation of a gadolinium-based contrast. The current gold standard technique for non-invasive determination of the ECV is the equilibrium contrast method [19,20]. There is now much data using these techniques, yet they are not universally employed clinically for a variety of reasons. There is currently a wide heterogeneity of protocols and sequences with limited data across vendors [21]. White et al. [22] show that there is a systematic overestimation of ECV in high ECV diseases with bolus only protocols for ECV quantification compared to measurement obtained by the equilibrium contrast method and histology.

T2* sequences exploit the more rapid destruction of signal by iron after radiofrequency excitation to identify myocardial iron loading and are uniquely powerful in this respect.

Gadolinium-based contrast agents are extracellular and can be utilised in CMR in a number of ways to generate additional information. As well as being administered for MR angiography, they can be used in combination with vasodilator stress to assess first pass myocardial perfusion, identifying inducible myocardial ischemia. In the minutes after administration, the presence of gadolinium in the blood pool can identify filling defects due to thrombus, and there may also be discernible changes in myocardial signal intensity in the presence of myocardial pathology. Gadolinium accumulates where there is expansion of the interstitial space and after at least 5 min is allowed for this to occur, LGE imaging can identify areas of myocardial infarction, fibrosis, oedema, or infiltration. The pattern of enhancement can inform both diagnosis and prognosis. This may be one of the most useful tools in informing the aetiology of heart failure in increased LV wall thickness. In the conditions studied so far, the presence of LGE confers an adverse prognosis compared to its absence [23,24].

Tagging sequences superimpose a grid or similar pattern with radiofrequency excitation and allow visualisation of tag deformation. This not only provides readily interpretable subjective information, but can be analysed in a number of software packages to provide quantitative analysis of deformation parameters.

13.1.5 Computed tomography

Multi-detector CT (MDCT) is emerging as a valuable adjunct in the assessment of cardiomyopathy to rule out coronary artery disease in place of invasive angiography, customarily undertaken as part of the assessment of newly diagnosed heart failure. Probably the greatest advance in CT with consequent increase in the utilisation of this technique is in relation to radiation dose reduction (see Chapter 5). Acquisition can take under one minute and is not generally limited by the presence of devices or implants. The strength of CT coronary angiography is in its negative predictive value and consequently should be utilised in those with no more than a low-intermediate probability of significant epicardial coronary artery disease. CT perfusion has recently been introduced as a first-pass contrast technique to assess myocardial ischemia. Although first results with this novel technique are promising, some practical issues still limit the widespread acceptance of this technique, including low myocardial contrast, beam-hardening artefacts, and considerable radiation exposure. Delayed contrast enhancement protocols for demarcating fibrotic scar have also been tested in some experimental settings but are not routine yet, and may be more difficult in diffuse patterns of myocardial fibrosis. The risk of nephropathy associated with the iodine-based contrast agents used for CT can also be limiting. Nonetheless, with its very high isotropic spatial resolution which for the newest devices is lower than 0.3 mm, CT may be a valuable alternative to CMR for certain cardiomyopathies, whenever CMR is contraindicated. Evidence of ventricular dilatation, increased wall thickness, or subclinical myocardial infarction may be noted incidentally at cardiac CT. Cardiac CT with extended exposure throughout the heart cycle allows for assessment of regional and global LV function, myocardial motion and thickening, and measurements of RV parameters, albeit at a higher radiation exposure than conventional CT coronary angiography.

13.1.6 Nuclear imaging

Radionuclide imaging is generally not the first-line modality for the assessment of cardiomyopathies, unless when imaging is considered for excluding ischemic cardiomyopathy. The spatial resolution of current positron emission tomography (PET) or single-photon emission computed tomography (SPECT) is in the range of 4–5 and 8–10 mm, respectively, and therefore these techniques are not suitable for detecting structurally abnormal myocardium (see Chapters 3 and 4). However, radionuclide techniques are notable for their high molecular sensitivity which allows for the detection of radiotracer in nanomolar concentrations. Therefore, these techniques are employed to address specific pathobiological and functional changes in the myocardium that escape anatomical imaging modalities.

^{18}F-fluorodeoxyglucose and ^{67}Gallium are avidly taken up by activated macrophages and therefore allow detection of inflammatory infiltrates, notably in cardiac sarcoidosis. Myocardial perfusion PET with ^{82}rubidium, ^{13}N-NH$_3$ or ^{15}O-H$_2$O allows quantification of myocardial blood flow in mL/min/g, and thereby is considered the gold standard technique to detect microvascular dysfunction. Several cardiomyopathies have been shown to coexist with variable severities of impaired microvascular vasoreactivity, and the most severe forms are generally associated with a worse cardiovascular prognosis. Finally, myocardial sympathetic innervation can be interrogated with radiolabeled structural analogues of norepinephrine (e.g. ^{131}I-meta-iodo-benzylguanidine (MIBG) or ^{11}C-meta-hydroxyephedrine (MHED)). A number of cardiomyopathies (in particular hypertrophic, dilated, and arrhythmogenic right ventricular cardiomyopathy (ARVC)) may be associated with increased sympathetic activity, which in turn has been linked with a higher likelihood of unfavourable ventricular remodelling, progression to heart failure, and a higher risk of arrhythmic events and cardiovascular mortality. However, although radionuclide imaging has enhanced our pathophysiologic understanding of many cardiomyopathies, its use is currently limited to experimental investigations rather than clinical routine. Additional issues are limited availability of radiolabelled compounds, radiation exposure, and costs.

Finally, radionuclide ventriculography (RNV) using either first-pass or blood-pool imaging can be used to quantify left- and/or right ventricular ejection fraction and regional contraction patterns and mechanical synchronicity. With the widespread use of echocardiography and CMR, RNV has lost importance. However, in patients with poor acoustic windows and contraindications to CMR, RNV represents a useful alternative imaging test to measure and quantify ejection fraction.

13.2 Dilated cardiomyopathy

13.2.1 Diagnosis

Dilated cardiomyopathy is defined by left ventricular dilatation and systolic dysfunction in the absence of abnormal loading conditions (namely hypertension or valvular heart disease) or ischaemic heart disease of sufficient severity to explain the observed ventricular derangement. Dilatation and impairment of the right ventricle may also be present, but are not required for the diagnosis. The atria are also commonly dilated.

A dilated cardiomyopathy phenotype (Figure 13.1a and b) may result from a wide variety of causes (including familial, infectious, toxin mediated, metabolic, inflammatory, infiltrative, connective tissue and neuromuscular causes, as well as pregnancy and arrhythmia related). In up to 50% of cases, no aetiology is identified and the disease is termed idiopathic. With increasing identification of genetic substrates [25], now thought to contribute to at least 25% of dilated cardiomyopathies, this label is becoming less prevalent. However, the interplay between genetic and acquired factors requires much further elucidation [99].

Demonstration of LV dilatation (end diastolic diameter >117% predicted value normalised for age, gender, and body surface area) and systolic dysfunction (LVEF <45% and/or fractional shortening <25%) by echocardiography continues to be the mainstay of diagnosis [26]. Typically, there is global hypokinesia. However, regional variation in wall stress or coexisting myocardial infarction may give rise to regional wall motion abnormalities.

An important role of non-invasive imaging in dilated cardiomyopathy relates to exclusion of an ischemic origin. Several techniques have the ability to detect or exclude with high accuracy underlying coronary artery disease, although in many centres, such patients will be submitted to invasive angiography with the ability to perform simultaneously right heart catheterization and measuring pulmonary pressures. CT coronary angiography, however, represents a valuable alternative to invasive angiography in patients with low-to-intermediate likelihood of coronary artery disease [27,28]. However, these patients pose technical challenges to conventional CT coronary angiography: They tend to have higher heart rates, and betablockade may be problematic,

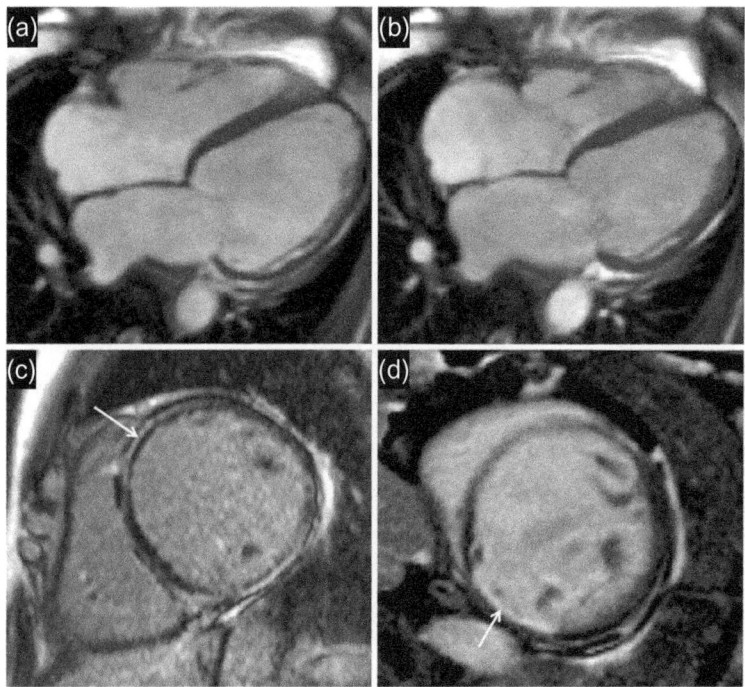

Figure 13.1 Cardiovascular magnetic resonance images of dilated cardiomyopathy. The upper images are bright blood images showing typical dilatation of all 4 cardiac chambers at end diastole (panel a) and end systole (panel b). The lower images are late gadolinium enhancement images. Panel c shows linear midwall replacement fibrosis (arrowed) in the same patient as the upper images. Panel d shows enhancement arising from the subendocardium (arrowed) which corresponds to a region of myocardial infarction.

leading to lower image quality and more motion artefacts. Furthermore, circulation times may be longer, thereby increasing the time for the contrast bolus to arrive in the coronary arteries. This may result in lower signal-to-noise ratios and more difficult scan timing. Furthermore, larger contrast amounts may be required to obtain high image quality with potentially higher nephrotoxicity. A calcium scan may be an alternative, contrast-medium free approach to exclude ischemic CMP. Although non-calcified coronary stenoses are frequently encountered, the probability of extensive CAD (as would be expected in dilated CMP caused by diffuse myocardial ischemia) is extremely rare [29]. Because the specificty of the calcium scan is low, the calcium scan is most effective in patients with a relatively low pre-test probability.

Radionulide myocardial perfusion imaging has demonstrated a high sensitivity and negative predictive value to exclude an ischemic origin in patients with dilated cardiomyopathy [30]. However, specificity is somewhat limited by false positives occurring in the presence of attenuation artefacts or microvascular dysfunction.

Over recent years, the application of CMR to the assessment of DCM has expanded notably due to the accurate and reproducible assessment of cardiac morphology and function and the capability for non-invasive identification of myocardial fibrosis and inflammation, as well as myocardial infarction. The majority of patients with DCM have no LGE. However, midwall myocardial fibrosis (Figure 13.1c) has been found to be present in approximately one-third of DCM patients as identified by LGE and this has been well validated against histological specimens. This midwall LGE is in contrast to the subendocardial or transmural pattern of LGE corresponding to myocardial infarction (Figure 13.1d).

13.2.2 Prognostic imaging markers

Prognostic markers in DCM include clinical factors, biochemical markers, electrophysiological parameters, and haemodynamic parameters. There is now considerable data supporting imaging parameters as powerful prognostic indicators. It has been apparent for some time that echocardiographic assessment of LV remodelling can provide prognostic information in DCM [31]. LV ejection fraction consistently appears as an independent predictor of outcome in the literature [23]. Several other parameters obtained by echocardiography have also been found to confer prognostic information in DCM. These include evidence of RV involvement as assessed by TAPSE [32], the presence of a restrictive filling pattern [33,34] and the severity of mitral regurgitation [103]. Venturi et al. [35] found the effective orifice area of functional mitral regurgitation to be a better predictor of NHYA class and mortality than LV EF.

Both strain and strain rate are reported to be reduced in DCM, again associated with poorer outcome [36].

Assomull et al. [23] have shown late gadolinium enhancement to be an important predictor of adverse outcome. In a cohort of 101 consecutive DCM patients followed up prospectively for 658 ± 355 days for events; 35% had midwall fibrosis as evident on CMR by LGE. This was associated with a higher rate of the predefined primary combined end point of all-cause death and hospitalization for a cardiovascular event (hazard ratio 3.4, $p=0.01$). Midwall fibrosis remained predictive of SCD/VT after correction for baseline differences in left ventricular ejection fraction between the group with and the group without LGE. Wu et al. [37] and Lehrke et al. [38] similarly found the presence of LGE in non-ischaemic cardiomyopathy to be associated with marked increase in cardiac events.

Left atrial size has long been considered a barometer of the cardiovascular system, with both maximum and minimum size carrying prognostic information [39]. Left atrial volume has now been established as a prognostic marker across a number of cardiovascular diseases including DCM [40] and HCM [41]. In a cohort of 483 consecutive DCM patients, Gulati et al. [40] found that an indexed left atrial volume of more than $72\,\text{mL/m}^2$ carried a threefold elevated risk of death or transplantation (HR 3.00; 95% CI 1.92–4.70; $p<0.001$).

While these data highlight the potential value of these parameters in risk stratification, the way these inform patient management requires further consideration and elucidation.

Microvascular dysfunction occurs in dilated cardiomyopathy in the absence of epicardial coronary artery disease and is an important risk factor. Neglia and colleagues reported reduced hyperemic blood flow in patients with dilated cardiomyopathy and an ejection fraction of 34% on average [42]. A low hyperemic blood flow emerged as a strong and independent predictor for cardiac mortality or progression/development of heart failure. A hyperemic blood flow <1.36 mL/min/g increased the risk of death or heart failure by a factor of 3.5.

Abnormal cardiac sympathetic activity is common in dilated cardiomyopathy and plays an important role in the LV remodelling and progression of heart failure, including its complications of arrhythmia and sudden death. Cardiac sympathetic activity can be evaluated by its uptake of radiolabeled catecholamine analogues like MIBG with SPECT. In dilated cardiomyopathy, low MIBG uptake (indicating increased sympathetic innervation) is one of the strongest predictors of outcome (even stronger than EF), and provided independent prognostic information [43,44]. These results have recently been replicated in large multicentric registries [45,46] consisting of a mixed population of nonischemic and ischemic cardiomyoapthies confirming the independent prognostic value of MIBG SPECT of ejection fraction, NYHA functional status, and biomarkers (e.g. pro-BNP).

13.2.3 Non-invasive imaging as a gatekeeper for coronary angiography

Current US guidelines prioritise the identification of coronary anatomy either by invasive angiography or CTCA in the assessment of heart failure and the exclusion of coronary artery disease as a substrate for LV dysfunction is ubiquitous. Given significant reduction in radiation dose, increased availability and advances in image quality, recent years have seen a marked increase in the utilisation of CTCA for this, notably where the likelihood of coronary artery disease is thought to be low given the excellent negative predictive power of this investigation. The identification or exclusion of ischaemic heart disease and flow limiting coronary artery disease is also an area where CMR has much to offer. The ability of CMR to identify myocardial infarction and inducible ischemia in a single test (by LGE and stress perfusion respectively) raises the possibility of using this as a gatekeeper to coronary angiography as proposed by Assomull et al. [47].

It will take either strong evidence or other pressures, perhaps financial to produce a shift from the traditional assessment of invasive coronary imaging in patients with newly diagnosed heart failure. A persistent challenge in functional assessment by DSE, nuclear or perfusion CMR is with false negative and false positive studies. In selecting the appropriate test, it is important to evaluate the pre-test likelihood of the patient having coronary artery disease. The role of CT is for ruling out coronary artery disease given its high negative predictive value, although the development of CT assessment of FFR may see this evolve.

13.2.4 Chemotherapy-related cardiomyopathy

A number of chemotherapeutic regimes are well recognised to carry cardiotoxic side effects. Amongst these, the anthracyclines (doxorubicin, daunorubicin, and epirubicin) and the HER2 receptor modulator Trastuzumab carry significant risk meriting cardiac assessment prior to, during and following therapy. Cardiotoxicity is typically dose dependent and is also influenced by a number of other factors. The prudent application of imaging before, during and after chemotherapy can enable safer use of potentially cardiotoxic agents by identifying LV dysfunction early when chances of reversibility are greater. A recent international consensus statement details recommended multi-modality imaging strategies for surveillance and detection of cardiotoxicity [48]. In this document, cancer therapeutics-related cardiac dysfunction (CTRCD) is defined as a decrease in LVEF of more than 10% points to a value of below 53% (the lower limit of the normal reference range by 2-D echocardiography). Confirmation of this change on repeat study 2–3 weeks after the initial detection of decreased LVEF is recommended. LVEF is the parameter typically used for assessment of LV systolic function and as with other cardiomyopathies, echocardiography with LV volume quantification and LVEF calculation by the modified biplane Simpson's technique is at the core of imaging evaluation. The volumetric method for calculating ejection fraction increases detection of CTRCD that due to some agents may be regional rather than global. CMR and MUGA are also robust options for quantification of LV volumes and ejection, although utilisation of the former may be constrained by limited availability and the latter by the incumbent ionising radiation burden. Bountioukos et al. [49] found that incorporating a wall motion score index obtained by 2-D echocardiography using a 16-segment model increased sensitivity for anthracycline cardiotoxicity, a practice encouraged in the consensus statement. In the same study, Bountioukos et al. found that repetitive assessment of contractile reserve using low-dose dobutamine stress echocardiography did not have incremental value for the early detection of anthracycline cardiotoxicity. Although an asymptomatic reduction in LVEF is the most frequently observed clinical manifestation of cardiotoxicity, LVEF is relatively insensitive to the detection of subclinical myocardial injury. Small changes in LV contractility may not be detected by the 2D echocardiographic assessment of LVEF. Thavendiranathan et al. [50] assess the temporal variability in LVEF by echocardiography in 56 patients undergoing cancer chemotherapy in whom stable LV systolic function was inferred by stability of global longitudinal strain (GLS) at up to 5 time points. They reported the limit of the 95% confidence interval for longitudinal variability of 2-D LVEF management in the asymptomatic patients to be 9.8% (range 9.0–10.8%). Nonetheless, echocardiography remains the method of choice for serial evaluation of patients requiring potentially cardiotoxic agents. If available, 3D echocardiography is preferable for calculation of LVEF. The newer techniques for interrogating systolic function, such as myocardial strain and strain, have much greater sensitivity for changes in myocardial tissue deformation and in CRTCD, as in other conditions, can enable detection of subclinical disease [51,104]. GLS measured by 2-D speckle tracking echocardiography is considered the optimal parameter of myocardial deformation for the early detection of subclinical LV dysfunction as it is not angle dependent, unlike diffusion tensor imaging (DTI). It is recommended that measurements be compared with baseline and that a greater than 15% reduction from baseline indicates clinically significant abnormality [52]. If assessment of GLS is not available, using pulse wave DTI to assess peak systolic velocity (s') of the mitral annulus or M-mode echocardiography to assess mitral annular displacement is recommended.

Loss of torsional motion is an even earlier feature of cardiomyopathy in this setting, and may be evident before loss of longitudinal or radial function or significant reduction in ejection fraction [53]. This can be visualised by echocardiography or CMR and quantified with the use of 2D speckle tracking or myocardial tagging sequences in the respective techniques. Unlike assessment of LV systolic function, assessment of LV diastolic function has not yet been shown to provide prognostic data in this setting but should still be included in the routine echocardiographic assessment of such patients. Additional consideration of CMR or CT is highlighted for the evaluation of primary cardiac tumours or when echocardiographic assessment has been inconclusive in the evaluation of possible constrictive pericarditis.

Some chemotherapeutic agents, for example fluorouracil, bevacizumab, sorafenib, and sunitinib, are recognised to potentially precipitate myocardial ischaemia. Evaluating patients due to receive such agents and who have an intermediate or high pre-test probability for coronary artery disease with stress echocardiography may be of value. Beyond this, the role of dobutamine stress echocardiography in the assessment of patients with CTRCD remains somewhat inconclusive, although using this to assess contractile reserve may be of benefit. Reduction in contractile reserve demonstrated in this manner may allow earlier detection of cardiotoxicity as well as predicting outcome.

13.3 Non-compaction cardiomyopathy

Left ventricular non-compaction (LVNC) is recognised as a distinct cardiomyopathic entity characterised by hypertrabeculation (Figure 13.2) of the left ventricular myocardium resulting from failure or arrested compaction of the myocardium in utero. Consequently the myocardium has a spongy appearance with characteristically excessive trabeculation and deep intra-trabecular recesses [54]. This structure predisposes to thrombus formation as well as to ventricular arrhythmia. In progressive disease, this may cause significant systolic impairment. Although hypertrabeculation may also be evident in the right ventricle, it is typically the LV apex and lateral wall where the features of LVNC are most commonly seen. The relatively thin noncompacted layers often display hypokinesia. Diagnosis is heavily reliant on advanced imaging with echocardiography or CMR. The superior ability of CMR to clearly visualise the apical myocardium is of potential advantage in assessing this condition, although diagnosis is frequently made by echocardiography. There is discrepancy between echo and CMR criteria for non-compaction cardiomyopathy as published by Jenni et al. [55] and Petersen et al. [56], respectively. It is likely that these will be revised in the near future. Diagnosis by echocardiography requires a ratio of non-compacted to compacted myocardium of greater than 2.0 in systole compared to a ratio of >2.3 at end-diastole by CMR. It is also problematic that features of non-compaction are often seen when there is marked LV dilatation, which can make distinguishing primary non-compaction cardiomyopathy from the appearance of non-compaction due to LV

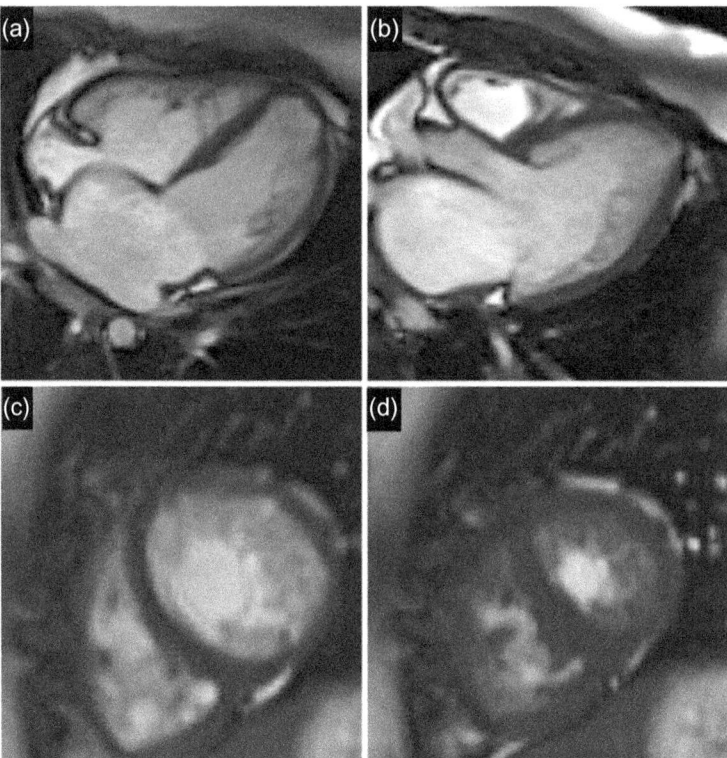

Figure 13.2 Left ventricular non-compaction. The upper images are zoomed 2-dimensional echocardiographic images showing hypertrabeculation of the left ventricle in the four chamber (left) and two-chamber views (right) in left ventricular non-compaction (LVNC). The lower images are cardiovascular magnetic resonance images of LVNC. Panels a to c are end-diastolic bright blood images. In panel a, hypertrabeculation of the left ventricle is evident in the 4-chamber view along with left ventricular and left atrial impairment. Panel b is from the same patient in the LVOT view. Panel c is a short axis view at end-diastole and panel d at end systole.

dilatation difficult. Whilst LVNC may represent a previously under-recognised cause of heart failure, it may be that diagnostic features lack sufficient specificity. Kohli et al. [57] suggest that diagnostic echocardiographic criteria for LVNC may be too sensitive, most notably in Black patients. The use of an appropriate contrast agent is helpful in the identification of ventricular thrombi regardless of technique. Observed to have a largely autosomal dominant inheritance, a genetic basis underlying this condition has been well defined, with mutations defined in three sarcomeric genes [58].

Reduced microvascular vasoreactivity by quantitative ^{13}N-NH_3 PET was reported in LVNC patients, interestingly to similar extent in noncompacted as well as compacted myocardium, and was associated with wall motion abnormalities on echocardiography [59] However, to what degree microvascular dysfunction plays a role in the pathogenesis of LVNC or whether it is merely an epiphenomenon remains unclear.

13.4 Stress (Takotsubo) cardiomyopathy

Stress cardiomyopathy is increasingly identified as a cause of presentation with acute chest pain, typically accompanied by mild elevation of cardiac biomarkers, or acute heart failure. Presentation frequently mimics acute myocardial infarction and hence often results in urgent coronary angiography, given that associated ECG changes can raise suspicion of an acute coronary syndrome. The absence of a culprit lesion in the coronary arteries and an awareness of the differential diagnosis may lead to a left ventriculogram being performed, which is then diagnostic. Some caution should be exercised here as the condition may give rise to apical thrombus. As ever, a careful history may point to the underlying diagnosis and both echocardiography and CMR can be valuable in identifying the characteristic imaging features. It is thought to be most common in post-menopausal women, and classically follows a stressful trigger, which can be emotional, physical, or pharmacological. The typical imaging findings are of "apical ballooning" with akinesia or dyskinesia of the LV apical region together with hypercontractility of the basal segments, giving rise to the term Takotsubo cardiomyopathy because of the similarity in shape of the LV cavity on left ventriculogram or other imaging to the Japanese trap used to catch octopuses. Variant patterns of abnormal contractile function, such as an inverted phenotype with basal hypokinesia have also been observed. The exact underlying pathogenetic mechanism underlying Takotsubo cardiomyopathy is unclear and several theories are debated including microvascular spasm, transient thrombotic occlusion, or left ventricular outflow obstruction. The classic finding of a stressful trigger also suggest an involvement of the cardiac sympathetic system. Indeed several studies with radionuclide imaging using MIBG or MHED have demonstrated abnormal myocardial sympathetic innervation in apical and midventricular areas of patients with Takotsubo cardiomyopathy [60–62]. Appearances on late gadolinium CMR imaging will readily distinguish possible myocardial infarction with coronary recanalisation from stress-induced cardiomyopathy, where there will be intense myocardial enhancement in the setting of myocardial infarction and typically none in the setting of stress-induced cardiomyopathy. A gadolinium study will also identify the presence of apical thrombus in either the LV or RV. It is recognised that there may be significant myocardial oedema in the affected apical region and this can be readily identified by CMR (Figure 13.3). Oedema is also seen in acute myocardial infarction and myocarditis, but the distribution of oedema and the pattern of wall motion abnormality and late gadolinium enhancement will usually allow discrimination between the two conditions. Furthermore, it is emerging that CMR may be particularly advantageous if imaging is performed in the sub-acute phase as the significant myocardial oedema that can occur in the apical region with consequent increase in wall thickness may mimic an apical hypertrophic cardiomyopathy phenotype.

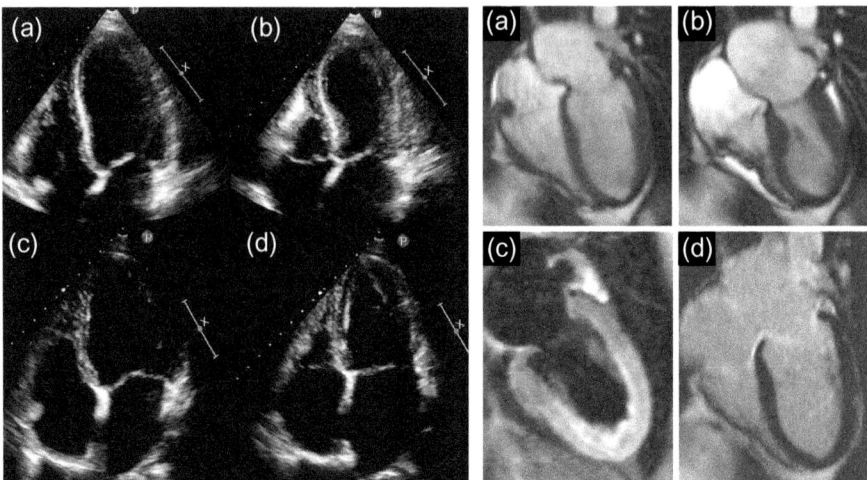

Figure 13.3 Takostusbo (stress) cardiomyopathy. The left images are echocardiographic images of takotsubo cardiomyopathy in the acute phase (upper panels) and following resolution (lower panels). The left hand panels are at end-diastole and the right hand panels at end-systole. In panel b, the characteristic 'apical ballooning' is evident, whereas in pane d, all myocardial segments are thickened normally in systole. The right images are cardiovascular magnetic resonance images during the acute phase of takotsubo cardiomyopathy with bright blood images at end-diastole (panel a) and end-systole (panel b). In the STIR-T2 (oedema) imaging in panel C, higher myocardial signal is evident in the apical half of the ventricle identifying myocardial oedema. In panel d, no late gadolinium enhancement is evident, notably no myocardial infarction.

13.5 Arrhythmogenic (right) ventricular cardiomyopathy

ARVC is an inherited cardiomyopathy that can be diagnostically extremely challenging, but which is important to identify given the potential for sudden cardiac death due to ventricular arrhythmia. Suspicion is frequently aroused by family history, frequent ventricular ectopy, ventricular arrhythmia, and/or unexplained right ventricular dilatation. The typical pathological characteristic of this condition is fibrofatty replacement of the right ventricular myocardium, and it remains a diagnosis which may be undetected until post-mortem examination. ARVC is thought to account for up to 10% of sudden cardiac deaths of those aged under 65 years where a pre-existing diagnosis was not apparent [63].

A detailed discussion of echocardiographic findings in patients meeting the initial Task Force Criteria for ARVD is provided by Yoerger et al. However, diagnosis is currently reliant upon the Modified ARVC Task Force Criteria [64]. The identification of structural and functional alterations by echocardiographic and/or CMR imaging forms an important part of assessment (Figure 13.4). Additional criteria focus on ECG, arrhythmic, and histological parameters as well as family history. Given that CMR offers the current gold standard for assessment of the RV, it is a central component of evaluation for this condition. In the Revised 2010 Task Force Criteria [64],

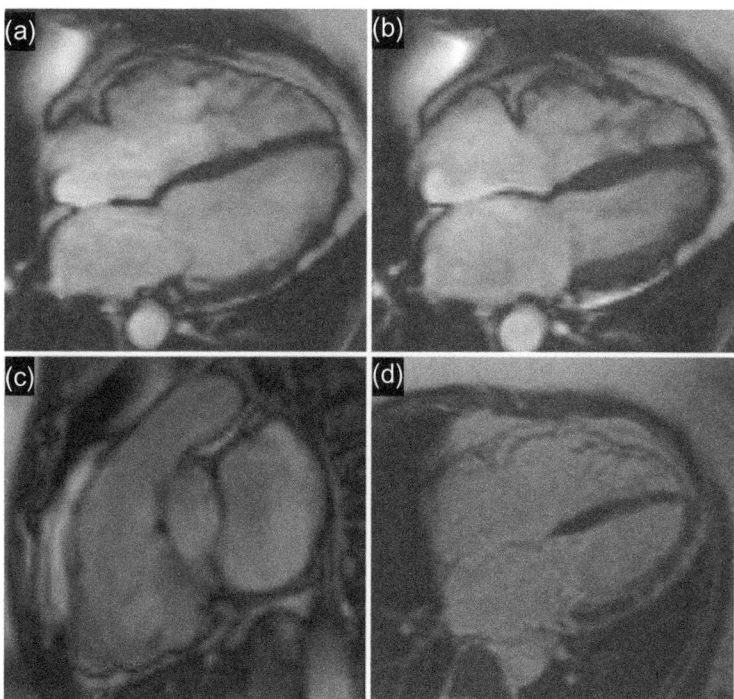

Figure 13.4 Arrhythmogenic right ventricular cardiomyopathy. Cardiovascular magnetic resonance images of ARVC. The upper images show bright blood images at end-diastole (panel a) and end-systole (panel b). The right ventricle is dilated and aneurysms of the free wall are evident at end-systole (panel b). Panel c shows the RVOT view at end-diastole. In panel d, some fatty infiltration of the lateral wall is evident on late gadolinium imaging.

major imaging criteria require the detection of regional RV akinesia or dyskinesia by either 2D echocardiography, CMR, or RV angiography. Alternatively, criteria allow for the identification of aneurysm by echocardiography or angiography or the appearance of dyssynchronous RV contraction by CMR. In addition to one of the aforementioned abnormalities, major echocardiographic criteria require an RVOT diameter measured at end-diastole of 32 mm (19 mm/m^2) or more in the parasternal long-axis view or 36 mm (21 mm/m^2) or more in the parasternal short axis view. Similarly, major CMR criteria require the additional finding of either a BSA indexed RV end-diastolic volume of 110 mL/m^2 or more (in males), 100 mL/m^2 in females, or an RV ejection fraction of 40% or less. Wall thinning and microaneurysm formation, with a "concertina" appearance may be evident. High temporal resolution transaxial cine sequences have been found to be most sensitive for the detection of these wall motion abnormalities [65]. The use of T1-weighted spin echo images is now considered to be less diagnostically helpful as some fatty infiltration of the RV can be observed in normal healthy individuals. The finding of LGE has high diagnostic sensitivity and specificity [65]. Although the distribution of LGE can be variable, it is classically observed in the midwall of the LV inferolateral and inferior walls. This may cause confusion with DCM, although in reality, these conditions likely lie on an overlapping spectrum [4]. Bluemke [66] discusses the difficulties with the CMR diagnosis of ARVC and the strengths and weaknesses of the diagnostic criteria. From a practical point of view, if the right ventricle is normal in size and function, other criteria are reduced in relevance.

Given that changes may be first or most apparent in the left ventricle, there is a growing tendency to refer to this condition as arrhythmogenic cardiomyopathy [105,106]. Lindstrom et al. [107] report a prevalence of left ventricular involvement of 76%.

One of the greatest challenges of ARVC remains identifying those individuals who have active disease and high risk of potentially fatal arrhythmia, but whose imaging is not diagnostic for the condition or potentially entirely normal. This "concealed" phase can also be the most arrhythmogenic. Like a number of the cardiomyopathies, the broad phenotypic spectrum further complicates diagnosis.

State-of-the-art CT scanners deliver sufficient temporal resolution to assess the RV morphology and even regional function, and offer an alternative option in patients whom cannot be imaged sufficiently by echocardiography or MRI. Nakajima et al. [67] evaluated the utility of a system for scoring characteristic CT findings to diagnose ARVC. The system graded fatty tissue, bulging appearance, and dilatation of the right ventricle and then validated the diagnosis against the modified 2010 Task Force criteria. Of the 77 patients studied, the CT criteria diagnosed 23 with definite ARVC and another 4 with borderline ARVC. For the cases determined as definite ARVC, sensitivity was 87%, specificity 94.4%, positive predictive value 87%, and negative predictive value 94.4%.

13.6 Hypertrophic cardiomyopathy

13.6.1 Diagnosis

Hypertrophic cardiomyopathy is the most common inherited cardiomyopathy and the leading cause of sudden death in the young [68]. It is characterised by left ventricular hypertrophy, myocyte disarray, and myocardial fibrosis. Establishing the diagnosis of HCM can be challenging, particularly as hypertension may also be present and the definition of HCM requires that the increased wall thickness should not be attributable to hypertension. Imaging has a central role in distinguishing LVH due to HCM from other causes. Table 13.2 lists the differential causes of increased LV wall thickness.

The mainstay of the diagnosis of HCM is a precise assessment of LV wall thickness. This can be achieved with echocardiography, CMR, or CT. A wall thickness of 15 mm or more in one or more LV myocardial segments without other explanation defines HCM [68]. Lesser degrees of wall thickening may be considered highly suggestive of or suspicious for HCM if accompanied by other clinical indicators, particularly a positive family history. Where a first-degree relative has a definite diagnosis, unexplained wall thickness of 13 mm or more may be considered diagnostic. In children, a z-score for LV wall thickness of greater than 2 (placing them more than 2 standard deviations from the predicted mean) is used for the diagnosis of HCM. In HCM, the hypertrophy typically involves the interventricular septum, but the pattern of hypertrophy and distribution can be highly heterogeneous. Basal septal hypertrophy is commonly seen in the elderly and can contribute to diagnostic difficulty. The emergence of population-based atlases [69] may make discerning pathologically increased wall thickness easier. Challenges can also be created by the RV septomarginal band, which may be erroneously incorporated into measurement, as it may not readily distinguishable from the septal myocardium on lower-quality echocardiography studies. Such erroneous measurement has implications for risk stratification [97]. When assessing wall thickness by echocardiography, it is important that imaging planes are correct to avoid overestimation and multiple views assessed. Wall thickness should be measured in short axis views at end diastole, regardless of which imaging modality is utilised. All LV segments should be assessed, at basal, mid-ventricular, and apical levels. Use of M-mode in the parasternal long axis on echocardiography is discouraged to avoid overestimation of wall thickness if the image plane is oblique. Inability to adequately visualise any segment is an indication to consider adjunctive use of a contrast agent or CMR.

Overall LV mass may not be increased in HCM, particularly in the approximately one-third of HCM patients whose wall thickening is focal and localized to a limited region of the LV [70,71]. Olivotto et al. [108] found that LV mass index was normal in around 20% of subjects with an overt HCM phenotype, promoting the recognition that wall thickness is a more sensitive marker of HCM than mass index, and that elevated mass index should not be required for such a diagnosis to be made. There is evidence to suggest that applying echo TDI to the assessment of diastolic function is able to detect preclinical or early disease in HCM, before increased wall thickness may be apparent. Nagueh et al. [109] reported that myocardial contraction and relaxation as measured by TDI were reduced in the mutant β-myosin heavy chain-glutamic acid transgenic rabbit model of human HCM regardless of whether LVH was present compared to nontransgenic rabbits. They also reported that TDI showed greater sensitivity for the detection of HCM than conventional echocardiographic screening. Data in humans with HCM support the utility of TDI to detect altered diastolic function as an earlier manifestation of HCM prior to the development of LVH [110]. Although mean diastolic myocardial velocities (Ea) were significantly lower in genotype positive individuals with and without HCM compared to normal control subjects, there was considerable overlap between the groups, and this parameter lacked sufficient diagnostic sensitivity in isolation. Ea velocity <15cm combined with LVEF ≥68% was found to be highly predictive of affected genotype without overt manifestations of HCM (specificity 100%, sensitivity 44%). Cardim et al. [8] highlight the potential utility of TDI in the discrimination of athlete's heart from the hypertrophy in HCM with Ea velocities being rapid in the highly compliant ventricle of athlete's with physiological hypertrophy in contrast to the reduced Ea velocities in HCM.

Apical aneurysms are now recognised as a highly relevant finding in HCM, associated with increased adverse events. Maron et al. [72] found apical aneurysms identified by CMR to be present in 2% of HCM patients, although only 57% of these were detected by echocardiography.

HCM can cause left ventricular outflow tract (LVOT) obstruction and echo remains the gold standard for its assessment. Ideally, this should be assessed at rest, during

Valsalva maneuver and during stress (when more patients have symptoms). The optimal stress should be physiological. It is well recognised that pharmacological stressors, notably dobutamine, can themselves induce marked LVOT gradients in the absence of pathology. Not all patients with obstruction have hypertrophy. An LVOT gradient of ≥30 mmHg is defined as obstructive, although generally not considered to be of haemodynamic concern below 50 mmHg. Determining the site and level of the obstruction systematically is of importance, not only to ensure that it is attributed to the correct aetiology, but also such that the most appropriate treatment is considered. Systolic anterior motion of the mitral apparatus or other mitral valve abnormalities may generate LVOTO in the absence of hypertrophy. Echocardiography, ideally with 3D technology, remains the gold standard for assessment of mitral valve and can provide an understanding of the interplay between mitral apparatus and myocardium. Where the mechanism of LVOTO is unclear, TOE and CMR have potential additive value. TOE in particular can also provide valuable perioperative information in patients undergoing septal reduction therapies. Mitral SAM typically produces mid-to-late-systolic mitral regurgitation that has an infero-lateral direction. Left atrial size is a prognostic marker in HCM, and anteroposterior LA diameter is included in the recent risk prediction model for sudden cardiac death [41].

Myocardial fibrosis is very common in hypertrophic cardiomyopathy, and tissue characterisation with CMR gives valuable additional information beyond echocardiography (Figure 13.5). LGE closely correlates with regions of replacement fibrosis,

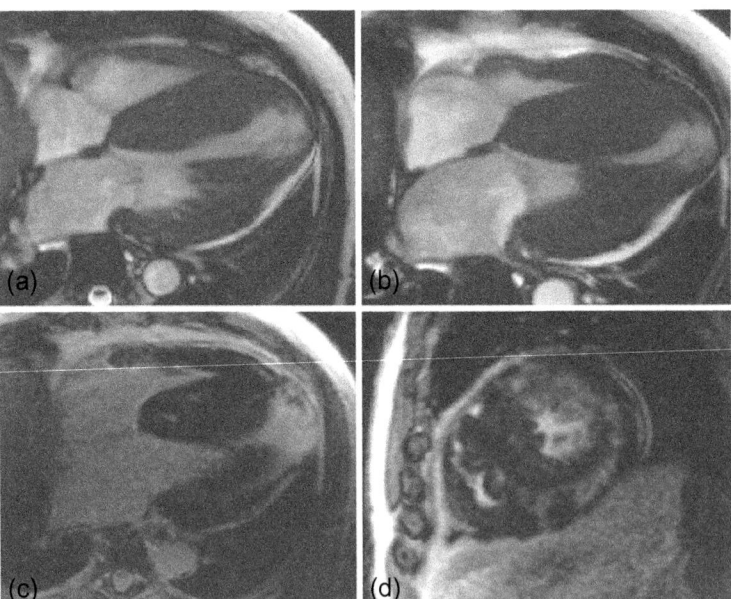

Figure 13.5 Hypertrophic cardiomyopathy with apical aneurysm. Bright blood images at end-diastole (a) and end-systole (b) demonstrating hypertrophy of both ventricles and near mid-cavity obliteration in systole. Late Gadolinium imaging (panels c and d) demonstrated extensive patchy, predominantly midwall fibrosis with transmural infarction of the apex.

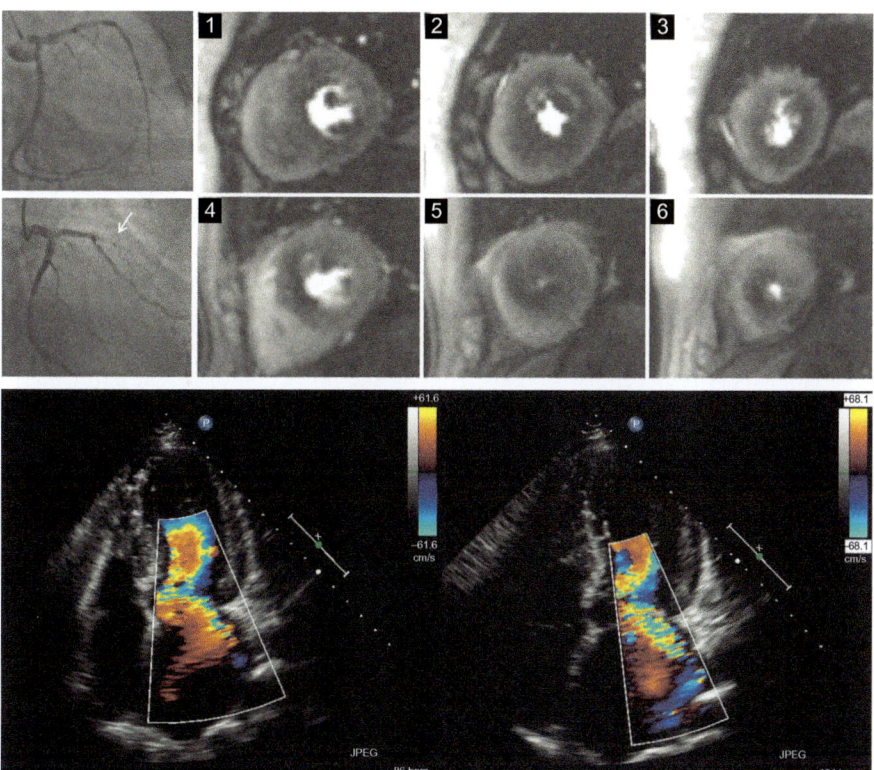

Figure 13.5, Cont'd CMR stress perfusion imaging in hypertrophic cardiomyopathy. The top panels demonstrate microvascular ischaemia in hypertrophic cardiomyopathy in a patient with angiographically normal epicardial left coronary arteries. There is a widespread, near circumferential, subendocardial perfusion defect with peak adenosine stress. The bottom panel shows a patient with HCM and a chronic total occlusion of the left anterior descending artery (arrowed). There is marked ischaemia in the LAD territory with a further subendocardial perfusion defect, most marked at mid ventricular level.
Physiological exercise echocardiography in hypertrophic cardiomyopathy. 4 chamber views in hypertrophic cardiomyopathy with colour Doppler examination at rest (left image) and during physiological exercise stress (right hand image). During the exercise image, the severity of the mitral regurgitation (due to systolic anterior motion of the mitral valve) into the dilated left atrium is visibly greater compared to the resting image.

while interstitial fibrosis may be detected using more novel techniques of T1 mapping. Replacement fibrosis in HCM is typically patchy and predominantly midwall [73]. In minor disease, the RV insertion points are most commonly affected, with fibrosis extending both to the hypertrophied and non-hypertrophied segments. In advanced disease, microinfarctions may manifest as areas of microvascular obstruction, and LGE patterns may become transmural. In these cases of late, burned-out disease, where the ventricle typically dilates, distinction from other cardiomyopathies may be challenging.

The degree of LGE in HCM is likely to also have an increasing role in informing prognosis and risk stratification, but thus far data has not been deemed sufficient to support inclusion of LGE in current risk prediction models. O'Hanlon et al. [24] showed that the presence as well as the extent of LGE predicted a composite endpoint of sudden cardiac death, sustained ventricular tachycardia, and hospitalisation for heart failure. A recent multicentre trial assessing the relation between LGE and cardiovascular outcomes in 1293 HCM patients has also shown percentage LGE to independently predict sudden cardiac death in this population [74]. This has led to the suggestion that the extent of fibrosis should become a further prognostic marker used in risk stratification for ICD therapy. It is increasingly apparent that the absence of LGE does not mean the absence of fibrosis, but only that there is no focal replacement fibrosis. Among the profusion of recent publications validating T1 mapping techniques for the determination of the presence of diffuse fibrosis and quantification of ECV, a number of these have investigated the ability of T1 mapping techniques to identify interstitial fibrosis in HCM. Brouwer et al. [75] compared mean ECV values in 16 HCM patients with 14 healthy controls using a modified Look-Locker Inversion Recovery (MOLLI) pulse sequence. Not only was there no significant difference between the two groups, but there was also no significant difference between mean ECV in the LGE positive HCM patients and LGE negative HCM patients, raising doubts as to the clinical utility of this technique in HCM. Puntmann et al. [76] reported that native T1 values and post-contrast T1 values were able to discriminate between the presumably normal myocardium of 30 normotensive subjects and the presumed diffusely disease myocardium of a cohort of 25 HCM patients as well as a cohort of 27 non-ischaemic cardiomyopathy patients. In HCM, native T1 values appeared to correspond to indexed LV mass. By echocardiography, decreased LV longitudinal strain using tissue Doppler derived strain or 2D speckle tracking imaging in the hypertrophied segments can represent an indirect marker of myocardial fibrosis. Saito et al. [77] studied 2D GLS in 48 HCM patients and found this to be significantly lower in those subjects with LGE by CMR than those without. Recently, Almaas et al. [78] studied 32 HCM patients preoperatively by speckle-tracking strain echocardiography and LGE-CMR ($n=21$) and correlated longitudinal septal strain and percentage LGE with interstitial and replacement fibrosis on histological samples obtained at myectomy. Reduced strain correlated with total ($r=0.50$, $p=0.01$) and interstitial fibrosis ($r=0.40$, $p=0.03$), but not replacement fibrosis ($r=0.28$, $p=0.14$).

Myocardial ischemia is a common and often underappreciated finding in HCM [71]. While epicardial coronary artery disease may occasionally coexist with HCM, the majority of patients with HCM suffer from variable degrees of microvascular dysfunction. Morphological abnormalities of the intramural coronary arterioles (thickening of the intima and/or medial layers of the vessel wall associated with decreased luminal cross-sectional area) represent the primary morphologic substrate for microvascular dysfunction and its consequence of blunted hyperemic myocardial blood flow. Myocardial perfusion PET studies have consistently shown reduced hyperemic myocardial blood flow in hypertrophied as well as non-hypertrophied myocardial areas of HCM patients [79]. Hyperemic blood flow is lowest in areas of increased fibrosis by LGE, suggesting an important association between ischemia, myocardial fibrosis, and LV remodelling [100]. Finally, blunted hyperemic blood flow is associated with higher cardiovascular mortality, unfavourable long-term LV remodelling, and progression to heart failure [80].

Cardiac sympathetic innervation may also play a role in the pathophysiology of HCM: Studies with PET have shown downregulation of postsynaptic beta-adrenoreceptors by ^{11}C-CGP 12177 PET with increased sympathetic activity by reduced presynaptic MHED uptake [81]. However, it is currently unclear how cardiac sympathetic dysfunction is related to clinical risk by LV remodelling, heart failure, and sudden cardiac death, and therefore the technique has not entered the clinical field yet.

Because exclusion of coronary artery disease is not straightforward in patients with HCM, invasive angiography is frequently performed in symptomatic patients. In these patients, who generally have a low pre-test probability, CAD can generally be excluded by coronary CT angiography. Cardiac CT also allows visualisation of the septal perforators, and knowledge of which branch supplies the tissue responsible for LVOT obstruction could become useful in preparation of percutaneous therapy.

13.6.2 Risk stratification

Risk stratification has historically been based on echocardiographic, clinical, and exercise test data. Contemporary risk prediction models are moving from the conventional fixed cut-offs in parameters predictive of risk to incorporate these as continuous variables [41].

13.7 Hypertrophic phenocopies

Part of the challenge of diagnosis in hypertrophic cardiomyopathy is the presence of many phenocopies. The most common of these is hypertensive heart disease with left ventricular hypertrophy. In Anderson–Fabry disease, hypertrophy is typically concentric and may be associated with fibrosis which is readily identified by LGE and is typically seen as midwall fibrosis in the infero-lateral wall (Figure 13.6). However, once fibrosis is established, response to replacement therapy is reduced and can be extremely limited. Although uncommon given the inheritance pattern, Anderson–Fabry disease can occur in females; there is some data that the phenotype in females varies, notably that fibrosis can occur in the absence of hypertrophy [82]. Non-contrast T1 mapping has been applied to successfully identify Anderson–Fabry disease by shorter septal T1 values without overlap with control subjects [83].

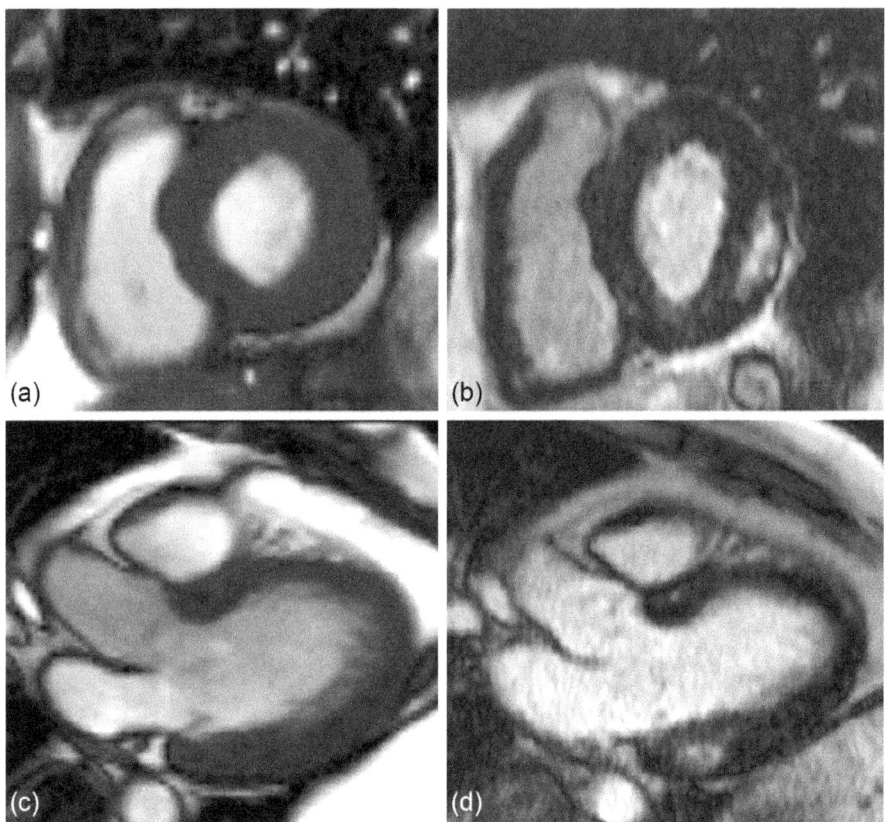

Figure 13.6 Anderson–Fabry's disease. There is largely concentric left ventricular hypertrophy (a and c) with midwall fibrosis, typically localised to the basal lateral wall (panels b and d).

13.8 Infiltrative disease/restrictive cardiomyopathy

Restrictive filling and reduced end-diastolic volume of one or both ventricles in the absence of significant impairment of systolic function characterise restrictive cardiomyopathy. This is a consequence of myocardial disease which may be classified as primary or secondary. Causes of primary restrictive cardiomyopathy include endomyocardial fibrosis, Löeffler's endocarditis, and idiopathic restrictive cardiomyopathy. Infiltrative conditions such as amyloidosos and sarcoidosis are causes of secondary restrictive cardiomyopathy, as are storage diseases such as haemochromatosis and Anderson–Fabry disease. Given that Anderson–Fabry disease is a fully treatable cause of premature mortality, early recognition of this condition is critical. Unsurprisingly, given the characteristic cardiac features which predominantly relate to diastolic function, echocardiography is the mainstay of initial diagnosis in restrictive cardiomyopathy. The characteristic features of increased wall thickness, reduced long axis function, atrial dilatation, and pleural and pericardial effusions may be combined with changes in septal motion and a speckled appearance of the septum that point to a restrictive process such as amyloidosis. However, it can often be difficult to determine the underlying diagnosis with certainty from echocardiography alone. CMR and nuclear imaging offer a significant contribution in diagnosing and characterising the underlying disease, notably in the assessment of cardiac sarcoidosis by PET imaging [111] and amyloidosis by CMR. FDG-PET can identify disease activity, which potentially may not be identified by conventional subjective evaluation of CMR STIR imaging.

13.8.1 Amyloidosis

The deposition of amyloid protein in the myocardium typically results in a restrictive cardiomyopathy, heart failure symptoms, and conduction abnormalities. Echo is usually the first line test in suspected amyloidosis, while endomyocardial biopsy remains the gold standard to confirm the diagnosis. Typical echocardiographic findings are increased ventricular wall thickness, small ventricular cavities, atrial enlargement, and thickening of the interatrial septum. The interventricular septum is often found to have a "speckled" appearance. Pericardial and pleural effusions may also be present. A low-voltage ECG in combination with the above may also strengthen suspicion of this condition. Although CMR may be able to identify cardiac amyloidosis (Figure 13.7), additional assessment by biopsy may be required to importantly confirm the subtype of amyloid disease, as this influences therapy and prognosis. Dungu et al. [84] reported that transmural patterns of LGE on CMR were readily able to distinguish transthyretin-related amyloidosis (ATTR) from light chain (AL) cardiac amyloidosis which typically has circumferential subendocardial LGE. In this study of 97 patients, left ventricular mass was significantly increased in ATTR amyloidosis compared with AL type. LGE was more extensive in ATTR compared with AL amyloidosis and was identified in all but one patient. A transmural pattern of LGE was evident in 90% of ATTR patients compared with 37% of AL patients. In CMR, in addition to the typical features of restrictive cardiomyopathy (biatrial dilatation, reduced long axis function, pleural and pericardial effusions), the abnormal kinetics following gadolinium administration can be diagnostic for cardiac amyloid. Although routinely used by many centres to ensure the optimal inversion time for LGE is selected, the Look-Locker sequence should be seen as a diagnostic sequence in the diagnosis of cardiac amyloidosis. A Look-Locker sequence, also known as a TI scout, is a single breathhold sequence with successive images of the same myocardial slice at incremental inversion times. This is because uniquely in cardiac amyloid, the myocardium nulls before the blood pool, in contrast to the usual nulling of the blood pool at earlier inversion times to the myocardium. T1 mapping with ECV calculation can quantify this phenomenon and has been shown to enable detection of cardiac amyloidosis. Karamitsos et al. [85] found noncontrast myocardial T1 to be significantly elevated in cardiac AL amyloidosis compared to normal subjects, and that this correlated with markers of systolic and diastolic dysfunction. They proposed that this technique may have greater sensitivity than LGE for detection of early disease. Banypersad et al. [86] have found elevated myocardial ECV and native pre-contrast T1 values to be predictive of mortality in AL amyloid. The assessment of the diagnostic utility of T1 values in amyloid is not new [87], but with the recent expansion of interest in T1 mapping, this has been revisited.

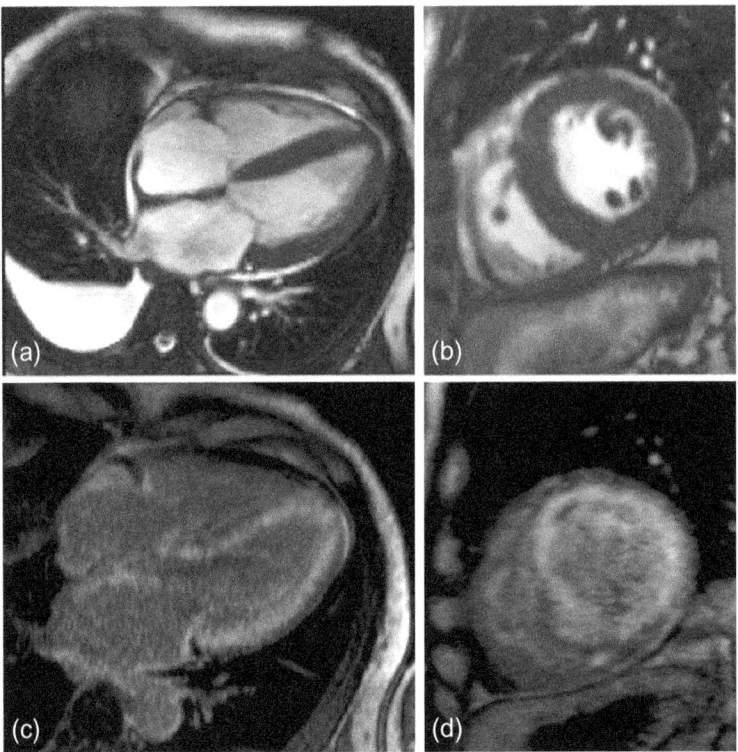

Figure 13.7 Amyloid: Typical CMR appearances of cardiac amyloid demonstrating pleural and pericardial effusions and left ventricular hypertrophy (a and b) and altered gadolinium kinetics, typically circumferential subendocardial late gadolinium enhancement (c and d).

Bisphosphonate compounds (which are routinely used as bone scintigraphy agents) have been shown to accumulate in areas of amyloid deposits. The ^{99m}Tc-labelled bisphononate 3,3-diphosphono-1,2-propanodicarboxylic acid (DPD) is highly sensitive for detecting cardiac involvement in transthyretin (TTR) amyloidosis with reported sensitivities up to 100% on late-phase planar scintigraphy [88,89]. Typical uptake patterns besides cardiac uptake in TTR amyloidosis include increased soft tissue uptake (mainly muscular uptake in the gluteal, shoulder, chest, and abdominal wall regions) with obscuring of bone uptake. Conversely, cardiac uptake is found in less than half of patients with light chain amyloidosis (AL) and uptake is generally less intense. Additionally, AL patients have generally no muscular DPD uptake, while visceral uptake (liver, spleen) may be more common. Hence, planar DPD scintigraphy may have great value to distinguish TTR from other types (mainly AL) of amyloidosis, an issue with important clinical consequences that is often difficult to solve just by clinical assessment or other imaging modalities. Figure 13.8 shows increased uptake of DPD in the heart due to cardiac amyloid on a DPD scan with (left panel) and a fused CT/SPECT image (right panel).

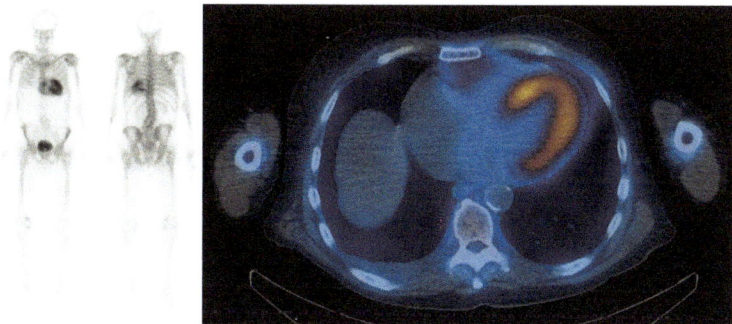

Figure 13.8 Images showing increased uptake of DPD in the heart (arrowed) due to Wild type ATTR cardiac amyloidosis. The image on the left is of a planar DPD scan (anterior and posterior views). The image on the right is of a fused CT/SPECT image. Images courtesy of Dr Ashutosh Wechalekar and Mr David Hutt, National Amyloidosis Centre, University College London.

13.8.2 Sarcoidosis (see also Chapter 15)

The more routine use of cardiac imaging has led to the recognition that myocardial involvement in sarcoidosis is common, being observed in at least 20% of patients, although only about a quarter of these patients have any clinical manifestation of this [90]. Older post-mortem data have suggested that cardiac involvement may be as high as 50% [91]. The aetiology of this multisystem granulomatous condition which typically affects the lungs remains unknown. Nevertheless, early identification of myocardial involvement can facilitate therapeutic intervention to avert the development of cardiac failure and arrhythmia. Reliance on endomyocardial biopsy for diagnosis is not only suboptimal due to its invasive nature; however, the technique also lacks sensitivity outside of advanced disease.

Sarcoid is described as one of the "great mimickers" and should be considered when appearances are unusual or unexplained. Echocardiography can reveal increased wall thickness related to oedema or infiltration and wall thinning due to fibrosis, and identify features suggestive of a restrictive cardiomyopathy in addition to assessing myocardial function, but findings are frequently non-specific and subtle changes may be missed. CMR is able to identify active inflammation, infiltration, and fibrosis, as well as providing other structural and functional information (Figure 13.9). Furthermore, the wide field of view acquired by CMR usually allows visualisation of any mediastinal lymphadenopathy which may be diagnostically helpful.

The appearances of cardiac sarcoidosis can be similar to myocardial infarction. FDG-PET imaging in cardiac sarcoid characteristically shows patchy inflammation. In order to detect this, glucose metabolism must be fully suppressed. Figure 13.10 shows extensive active myocardial inflammation identified by FDG-PET in a patient who could not have CMR due to the presence of an ICD. "Hot areas" on PET may be seen adjacent to the areas of late gadolinium enhancement on CMR in the absence of overtly increased signal on STIR-T2 imaging, suggesting persistent inflammation. It is worth noting also that the absence of late gadolinium enhancement does not guarantee

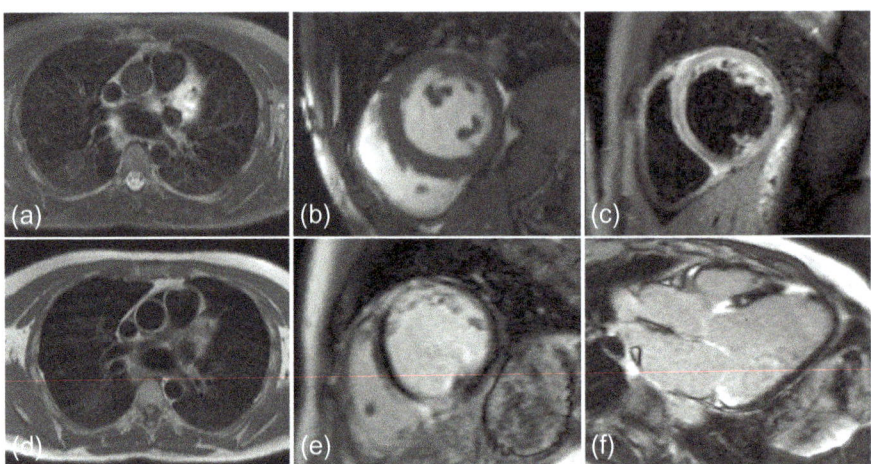

Figure 13.9 Sarcoid: CMR appearances of cardiac sarcoid disease. Panels a and b demonstrate bilateral hilar lymphadenopathy. Negative STIR T2 (oedema) imaging indicates inactive disease (e). Late gadolinium enhancement is typically subepicardial and patchy (d and f).

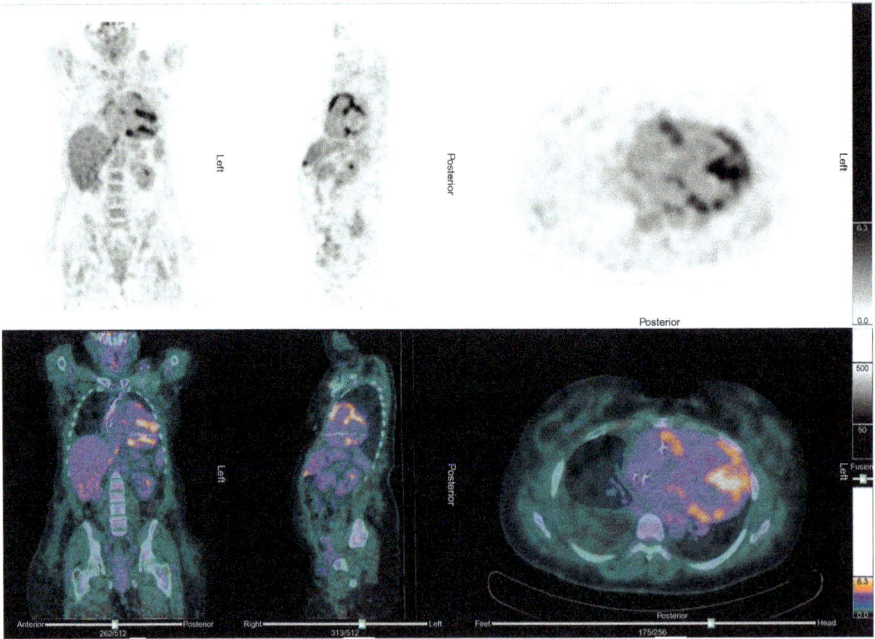

Figure 13.10 FDG-PET in active cardiac sarcoidosis. FDG PET-CT images in patient with known pulmonary sarcoidosis and previously biopsy confirmed cardiac involvement. ICD implanted for VT. The half body FDG PET-CT following metabolic preparation to suppress normal glucose uptake by myocardium shows abnormal patchy FDG uptake in LV and other chambers of heart suggestive of active inflammation in keeping with sarcoidosis. Images courtesy of Dr Kshama Wechalekar, Department of Nuclear Medicine, Royal Brompton and Harefield NHS Foundation Trust.

Cardiomyopathy

the absence of an inflammatory infiltrate, as cellular infiltrate may not show as LGE. Figure 13.9 shows CMR images of cardiac sarcoidosis.

13.9 Cardiac iron overload

Iron loading in the heart has, until recently, been the dominant cause of considerable mortality in β-thalassaemia major (TM). In this condition, recurrent transfusions are necessary within the first years of life to avert life-threatening anaemia. As a consequence, organs including the heart may become overloaded with iron with the potential sequelae of heart failure, which, once manifest, is difficult to treat effectively eliminating associated mortality. Iron loading in the heart may also occur due to haemachromatosis, a hereditary disorder of iron metabolism. The difficulty in identifying cardiac iron loading previously resided in the dissociation between blood or liver markers of iron loading and levels of iron in the heart (Figure 13.11). However, CMR T2* imaging has become established as the technique of choice for the detection of myocardial iron loading (He [92]. The accurate measurement of iron in the heat and

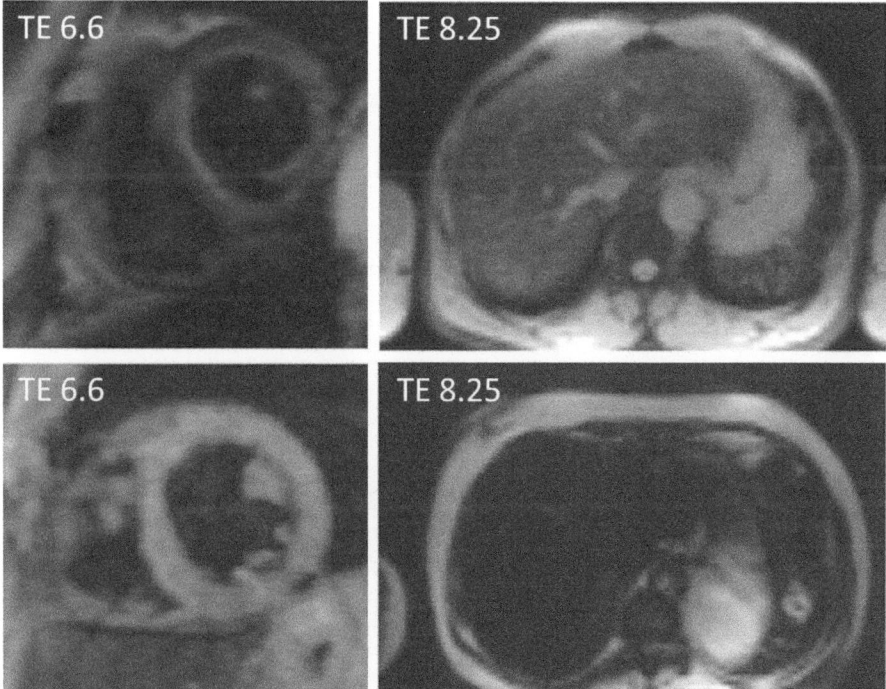

Figure 13.11 T2* assessment of cardiac and hepatic iron loading. T2* imaging in two patients with thalassaemia major. The top panels demonstrate a patient with severe cardiac iron loading and moderate liver iron loading. The bottom panels are show a patient with no cardiac iron loading but severe liver iron loading.

liver can then guide both the requirement for and response to chelation therapy, aiming to prevent organ dysfunction consequent upon iron loading. A cardiac T2* value below 10 ms is currently regarded as the most important predictor of the development of heart failure in this setting [93]. The application of CMR T2* to the detection of myocardial iron loading exemplifies the potential for imaging to powerfully inform clinical management with dramatic impact on disease outcome [94].

CT also has the potential capability to identify high electron density iron loading in the organs. However, in addition to the ionising radiation, unlike CMR, CT has low sensitivity for early iron loading.

13.10　Pericardial constriction

The assessment of pericardial constriction is discussed in detail in Chapter 18 on pericardial disease. Echo is the modality of choice for assessing the physiological impact of pericardial disease, but both CMR and CT have a valuable and potentially important complementary role in imaging and characterising the pericardium in greater detail.

13.11　Limitations of imaging

Despite considerable and remarkable developments in imaging, there remain a number of challenges and limitations. Some of these are unique to particular modalities but others are not currently resolved by any existing technique. Some of the cardiomyopathies have a primarily electrical basis, not identifiable by imaging. Imaging is unable to detect the potentially important concealed phase of disease which may be associated with disease activity culminating in life-threatening arrhythmia. At present, there is no non-invasive surrogate for myocyte disarray.

13.12　Likely future trends

Recent years have seen much interest and research looking beyond LGE on CMR with the performance of T1 mapping and ECV quantification to identify diffuse fibrosis. While this has shown much promise, a number of issues remain with regard to the clinical application of these techniques [21]. The exact role for this technique remains to be determined [95].

Although currently limited by radiation burden, expense and available facilities, the development of hybrid dual-modality imaging wherein CT and nuclear capability is combined within a single piece of equipment may facilitate powerful combined assessment of coronary anatomy, perfusion, function, and metabolism.

Beyond existing reference ranges for two-dimensional parameters, the emergence of three-dimensional atlases such as that described by De Marvao et al. [69] will allow more accurate discrimination of pathological phenotypes from the normal spectrum which can be extremely difficult and also have the potential to reduce the sample sizes required in studies where wall thickness is an important parameter. There is likely to be increased use of three-dimensional imaging and image integration whereby datasets are combined into a single multiparametric model or mapping system.

DTI to study the details of myocardial architecture is an evolving area [98].

It is unlikely that any single parameter will ever be sufficient to adequately stratify risk of sudden cardiac death in cardiomyopathy, and even the best current multivariate models lack predictive power. More complex risk stratification models, with the likely inclusion of clinical genetics, will hopefully further refine our ability to predict risk in cardiomyopathy. The potential of studying the left atrium to inform with regard to ventricular pathology and more global cardiovascular status has been recognised for many years, but the power of this information is continually becoming more apparent.

With the improved survival in a variety of cancers, unfortunately will come increased sequelae of the chemotherapeutic agents used to achieve this. There will be an expanding role for imaging in cardiac oncology for the diagnosis, monitoring, and hopefully prevention of this. A greater understanding of the molecular, pharmacological, and genetic factors resulting in the deleterious effects of chemotherapy and identifying both optimal and hazardous regimes will be important in avoiding the adverse mortality of cancer with the adverse mortality of heart failure. This population will require significant imaging resources, and the propagation of specialist services and clinics is likely to further enhance care.

The growing utilisation of CMR in the cardiomyopathy population, the need for serial study, and also the need to facilitate MRI later in life is coupled to the greater utilisation of CMR compatible devices. We are just beginning to see increased CMR in the presence of conventional devices with appropriate indications and oversight, and this is likely to increase.

Prognosis in heart failure and cardiomyopathy has been dramatically altered by the implantation of automated implantable cardiac defibrillators in those felt at highest risk of life-threatening arrhythmia. However, at present, once such a device is implanted, that patient has historically been subsequently denied CMR as devices are not approved for use in the magnet environment. With the more generalised use of CMR-compatible or conditional pacemakers for use at 1.5 T we are now also seeing the development of ICD devices which will also be approved for use at 1.5 T.

13.13 Conclusions and reflection

Imaging is central to the diagnosis and management of cardiomyopathy. Echocardiography remains the cornerstone of cardiac imaging. However, other modalities, notably CMR, have developed considerable diagnostic power with respect to cardiomyopathy. Despite the numerous available modalities, the diagnosis of cardiomyopathy can still be challenging, particularly given the potential overlap of phenotypes. This chapter describes applications of the modalities to imaging cardiomyopathy and highlights some of the strengths and weaknesses of each technique; however, the precise choice of imaging should still be tailored to the individual patient.

Regardless of the imaging modality employed, interpretation of the findings with respect to appropriate reference ranges is important and normalising to appropriate parameters such as age, gender, ethnic origin, and body surface area which increases sensitivity and specificity. Furthermore, caution should be exercised with the transfer of values across modalities. While it may be reasonable to compare some parameters, others should not be directly compared (e.g. EF derived by echocardiography versus CMR). It is accepted that the normal range for LV volumes differs between genders. It is important to bear in mind that LV volumes and EF derived by echo and CMR are not interchangeable. Hence, it is not necessarily valid to extrapolate the findings of major trials across modalities. This has a potential impact on the choice of device therapy. The optimum CMR-derived value for LVEF in determining benefit from device therapy remains to be established, but is difficult in the face of a wealth of echo-based outcome data. There is the need for large, multicentre, multi-vendor RCTs of parameters that modify outcome. This is especially true for CMR.

While employing multiple imaging modalities has benefits, this brings with it financial costs. There will almost inevitably be a pressure for a single test. The key will be identifying the most appropriate test or combination of tests on an individual patient basis, and that this process is executed intelligently and appropriately. Ultimately, investigation must be tied to outcome. There is a need for contemporary cost-effective analysis of imaging strategies in this setting and evidence that such imaging improves outcome to support its utilisation. With ever-worsening financial pressures, fixed tariffs may force providers to rationalize investigation and utilise fewer modalities per patient.

Cardiomyopathy encompasses a heterogeneous collection of conditions, often on a continuous phenotypic spectrum with frequent phenotypic overlap. The combination of imaging data with the genetic information now readily available through next-generation sequencing is likely to transform understanding and management of cardiomyopathies over the next decades. However, the capability of NGS to identify mutations will likely raise more questions than answers, and accurate phenotyping will remain central to diagnosis and interpretation of genetic information, in combination with detailed and robust interrogation of family history.

Despite advances in genotyping, the accurate description of phenotype is central to the diagnosis and management of cardiomyopathy. Similarly, once a feature potentially representing an inherited cardiomyopathy is identified, close examination of family history is required.

Resources

The website of the European Association of Cardiovascular imaging (www.eacvi.org) contains a wide range of educational material for all non-invasive cardiac imaging modalities.

Multimodality imaging evaluation documents:

HCM [68,96]
Cancer therapy [48]

Modality specific resources:

Echocardiography – www.echopedia.org
CMR – The website of The Society for Cardiovascular Magnetic Resonance (scmr.org) contains a wide variety of educational material
Parsai et al. [90] provides an excellent review of the diagnostic and prognostic value of CMR in non-ischaemic cardiomyopathies
CT – www.scct.org

References

[1] Maron BJ, Towbin JA, Thiene G, et al. Contemporary definitions and classification of the cardiomyopathies: an American Heart Association Scientific Statement from the Council on Clinical Cardiology, Heart Failure and Transplantation Committee; Quality of Care and Outcomes Research and Functional Genomics and Translational Biology Interdisciplinary Working Groups; and Council on Epidemiology and Prevention. Circulation 2006;113:1807.

[2] Anon. Report of the WHO/ISFC task force on the definition and classification of cardiomyopathies. Br Heart J 1980;44(6):672–3. http://dx.doi.org/10.1136/hrt.44.6.672.

[3] Elliott P, Andersson B, Arbustini E, Bilinska Z, Cecchi F, Charron P, et al. Classification of the cardiomyopathies: a position statement from the European Society of Cardiology Working Group on Myocardial and Pericardial Diseases. Eur Heart J 2008;29:270.

[4] Taylor M, Graw S, Sinagra G, Barnes C, Slavov D, Brun F, et al. Genetic variation in titin in ARVC-overlap syndromes. Circulation 2011;124(8):876–85. http://dx.doi.org/10.1161/CIRCULATIONAHA.110.005405.

[5] Galiuto L, Senior R, Becher H. Contrast echocardiography. In: Galiuto L, Badano L, Fox K, Sicari R, Zamorano JL, editors. The EAE textbook of echocardiography. Oxford: Oxford University Press; 2011. p. 99–115.

[6] Mor-Avi V, Lang RM, Badano LP, Belohlavek M, Cardim NM, Derumeaux G, et al. Current and evolving echocardiographic techniques for the quantitative evaluation of cardiac mechanics: ASE/EAE consensus statement on methodology and indications endorsed by the Japanese Society of Echocardiography. Eur J Echocardiogr 2011;12:167–205. http://dx.doi.org/10.1093/ejechocard/jer021.

[7] Ho CY, Solomon SD. A clinician's guide to tissue Doppler imaging. Circulation 2006;113:e396–8.

[8] Cardim N, Oliveira AG, Longo S, Ferreira T, Pereira A, Reis RP, et al. Doppler tissue imaging: regional myocardial function in hypertrophic cardiomyopathy and in athlete's heart. J Am Soc Echocardiogr 2003;16:223–32.

[9] Ho CY, Sweitzer NK, McDonough B, Maron BJ, Casey SA, Seidman JG, et al. Assessment of diastolic function with Doppler tissue imaging to predict genotype in preclinical hypertrophic cardiomyopathy. Circulation 2002;105:2992–7.

[10] Nagueh SF, Bachinski LL, Meyer D, Hill R, Zoghbi WA, Tam JW, et al. Tissue Doppler imaging consistently detects myocardial abnormalities in patients with hypertrophic cardiomyopathy and provides a novel means for an early diagnosis before and independently of hypertrophy. Circulation 2001;104:128–30.

[11] Reiter T, Ritter O, Prince MR, Nordbeck P, Wanner C, Nagel E, et al. Minimizing risk of nephrogenic systemic fibrosis in cardiovascular magnetic resonance. J Cardiovasc Magn Reson 2012;14:31. http://dx.doi.org/10.1186/1532-429X-14-31.

[12] Brignole M, Auricchio A, Baron-Esquivias G, Bordachar P, Boriani G, Breithardt O-A, et al. 2013 ESC Guidelines on cardiac pacing and cardiac resynchronization therapy. Eur Heart J 2013;34:2281–329. http://dx.doi.org/10.1093/eurheartj/eht150.

[13] Nazarian S, Hansford R, Roguin A, Goldsher D, Zviman MM, Lardo AC, et al. A prospective evaluation of a protocol for magnetic resonance imaging of patients with implanted cardiac devices. Ann Intern Med 2011;155:415–24. http://dx.doi.org/10.7326/0003-4819-155-7-201110040-00004.

[14] Myerson SG, Bellenger NG, Pennell DJ. Assessment of left ventricular mass by cardiovascular magnetic resonance. Hypertension 2002;39:750–5.

[15] Bellenger NG, Burgess MI, Ray SG, Lahiri A, Coats ASJ, Cleland JGF, et al. Comparison of left ventricular ejection fraction and volumes in heart failure by echocardiography, radionuclide ventriculography and cardiovascular magnetic resonance. Are they interchangeable? Eur Heart J 2000;21:1387–96.

[16] Bellenger NG, Grothues F, Smith G, Pennell DJ. Quantification of right and left ventricular function by MRI. Herz 2000;25:392–9.

[17] Longmore DB, Klipstein RH, Underwood SR, Firmin DN, Hounsfield GN, Watanabe M, et al. Dimensional accuracy of magnetic resonance in studies of the heart. Lancet 1985;1:1360–2.

[18] Sechtem U, Pflugfelder PW, Gould RG, Cassidy MM, Higgins CB. Measurement of right and left ventricular volumes in healthy individuals with cine MR imaging. Radiology 1987;163:697–702.

[19] Flett AS, Hayward MP, Ashworth MT, Hansen MS, Taylor AM, Elliott PM, et al. Equilibrium contrast cardiovascular magnetic resonance for the measurement of diffuse myocardial fibrosis: preliminary validation in humans. Circulation 2010;122:138–44.

[20] Fontana M, White SK, Banypersad SM, Sado DM, Maestrini V, Flett AS, et al. Comparison of T1 mapping techniques for ECV quantification. Histological validation and reproducibility of ShMOLLI versus multibreath-hold T1 quantification equilibrium contrast CMR. J Cardiovasc Magn Reson 2012;14:88. http://dx.doi.org/10.1186/1532-429X-14-88.

[21] Moon JC, Messroghli DR, Kellman P, Piechnik SK, Robson MD, Ugander M, et al. Myocardial T1 mapping and extracellular volume quantification: a Society for Cardiovascular Magnetic Resonance (SCMR) and CMR Working Group of the European Society of Cardiology consensus statement. J Cardiovasc Magn Reson 2013;15:92. http://dx.doi.org/10.1186/1532-429X-15-92.

[22] White SK, Sado DM, Fontana M, Banypersad SM, Maestrini V, Flett AS, et al. T1 mapping for myocardial extracellular volume measurement by CMR bolus only versus primed infusion technique. J Am Coll Cardiol Img 2013;6(9):955–62. http://dx.doi.org/10.1016/j.jcmg.2013.01.011.

[23] Assomull RG, Prasad SK, Lyne J, Smith G, Burman ED, Khan M, et al. Cardiovascular magnetic resonance, fibrosis, and prognosis in dilated cardiomyopathy. J Am Coll Cardiol 2006;48:1977–85.

[24] O'Hanlon R, Grasso A, Roughton M, Smith G, Alpendurada FD, Wong J, et al. Prognostic significance of myocardial fibrosis in hypertrophic cardiomyopathy. J Am Coll Cardiol 2010;56:867–74.

[25] Hershberger RE, Hedges DJ, Morales A. Dilated cardiomyopathy: the complexity of a diverse genetic architecture. Nat Rev Cardiol 2013;10(9):531–47. http://dx.doi.org/10.1038/nrcardio.2013.105.

[26] Manolio TA, Baughman KL, Rodeheffer R, Pearson TA, Bristow D, Michels VV, et al. Prevalence and etiology of idiopathic dilated cardiomyopathy (summary of a National Heart, Lung, and Blood Institute Workshop). Am J Cardiol 1992;69:1458–66.

[27] Andreini D, Pontone G, Pepi M, et al. Diagnostic accuracy of multidetector computed tomography coronary angiography in patients with dilated cardiomyopathy. J Am Coll Cardiol 2007;49:2044–450.
[28] Patel MR, White RD, Abbara S, Bluemke DA, Herfkens RJ, Picard M, et al. 2013 ACCF/ACR/ASE/ASNC/SCCT/SCMR appropriate utilization of cardiovascular imaging in heart failure: a joint report of the American College of Radiology Appropriateness Criteria Committee and the American College of Cardiology Foundation Appropriate Use Criteria Task Force. J Am Coll Cardiol 2013;61(21):2207–31. http://dx.doi.org/10.1016/j.jacc.2013.02.005.
[29] Abunassar JG, Yam Y, Chen L, D'Mello N, Chow BJ. Usefulness of the Agatston score=0 to exclude ischemic cardiomyopathy in patients with heart failure. Am J Cardiol 2011;107(3):428–32. http://dx.doi.org/10.1016/j.amjcard.2010.09.040.
[30] Klocke FJ, Baird MG, Lorell BH, Bateman TM, Messer JV, Berman DS, et al. ACC/AHA/ASNC guidelines for the clinical use of cardiac radionuclide imaging—executive summary. A report of the American College of Cardiology/American Heart Association Task Force on Practice Guidelines (ACC/AHA/ASNC Committee to Revise the 1995 Guidelines for the Clinical Use of Cardiac Radionuclide Imaging). Circulation 2003;108:1404–18. http://dx.doi.org/10.1161/01.CIR.0000080946.42225.4D.
[31] Douglas PS, Morrow R, Ioli A, Reichek N. Left ventricular shape, afterload and survival in idiopathic dilated cardiomyopathy. J Am Coll Cardiol 1989;13(2):311–5. http://dx.doi.org/10.1016/0735-1097(89)90504-4.
[32] Ghio S, Recusani F, Klersy C, et al. Prognostic usefulness of the tricuspid annular planar systolic excursion in patients with congestive heart failure secondary to idiopathic or ischemic dilated cardiomyopathy. Am J Cardiol 2000;85:837–42.
[33] Faris R, Coats AJ, Henein MY. Echocardiography-derived variables predict outcome in patients with nonischemic dilated cardiomyopathy with or without a restrictive filling pattern. Am Heart J 2002;144:343–50.
[34] Pinamonti B, Zecchin M, Di Lenarda A, Gregori D, Sinagra G, Camerini F. Persistence of restrictive left ventricular filling pattern in dilated cardiomyopathy: an ominous prognostic sign. J Am Coll Cardiol 1997;29:604–12.
[35] Venturi F, Gianfaldoni ML, Melina G, Cecchi A, Petix NR, Monopoli A, et al. Mitral effective regurgitant orifice area versus left ventricular ejection fraction as prognostic indicators in patients with dilated cardiomyopathy and heart failure. Ital Heart J 2004;5(10):755–61.
[36] Jasaityte R, Dandel M, Lehmkuhl H, Hetzer R. Prediction of short-term out-comes in patients with idiopathic dilated cardiomyopathy referred for transplantation using standard echocardiography and strain imaging. Transplant Proc 2009;41:277–80.
[37] Wu KC, Weiss RG, Thiemann DR, Kitagawa K, Schmidt A, Dalal D, et al. Late gadolinium enhancement by cardiovascular magnetic resonance heralds an adverse prognosis in nonischemic cardiomyopathy. J Am Coll Cardiol 2008;51:2414–21.
[38] Lehrke S, Lossnitzer D, Schob M, Steen H, Merten C, Kemmling H, et al. Use of cardiovascular magnetic resonance for risk stratification in chronic heart failure: prognostic value of late gadolinium enhancement in patients with non-ischaemic dilated cardiomyopathy. Heart 2011;97:727–32.
[39] Abhayaratna WP, Seward JB, Appleton CP, Douglas PS, Oh JK, Tajik AJ, et al. Left atrial size physiologic determinants and clinical applications. J Am Coll Cardiol 2006;47:2357–63.
[40] Gulati A, Ismail TF, Jabbour A, Ismail NA, Morarji K, Ali A, et al. Clinical utility and prognostic value of left atrial volume assessment by cardiovascular magnetic resonance

in non-ischaemic dilated cardiomyopathy. Eur J Heart Fail 2013;15(6):660–70. http://dx.doi.org/10.1093/eurjhf/hft019.
[41] O'Mahony C, Jichi F, Pavlou M, Monserrat L, Anastasakis A, Rapezzi C, et al. A novel clinical risk prediction model for sudden cardiac death in hypertrophic cardiomyopathy (HCM risk-SCD). Eur Heart J 2014;35:2010–20.
[42] Neglia D, Michelassi C, Trivieri MG, Sambuceti G, Giorgetti A, Pratali L, et al. Prognostic role of myocardial blood flow impairment in idiopathic left ventricular dysfunction. Circulation 2002;105(2):186–93.
[43] Merlet P, Benvenuti C, Moyse D, Pouillart F, Dubois-Rande JL, Duval AM, et al. Prognostic value of MIBG imaging in idiopathic dilated cardiomyopathy. J Nucl Med 1999;40:917–23.
[44] Momose M, Kobayashi H, Iguchi N, et al. Comparison of parameters of ^{123}I-MIBG scintigraphy for predicting prognosis in patients with dilated cardiomyopathy. Nucl Med Commun 1999;20(6):529–35.
[45] Jacobson AF, Senior R, Cerqueira MD, Wong ND, Thomas GS, Lopez VA, et al. Myocardial iodine-123 meta-iodobenzylguanidine imaging and cardiac events in heart failure results of the prospective ADMIRE-HF (AdreView Myocardial Imaging for Risk Evaluation in Heart Failure) study. J Am Coll Cardiol 2010;55:2212–21.
[46] Nakata T, Nakajima K, Yamashina S, Yamada T, Momose M, Kasama S, et al. A pooled analysis of multicenter cohort studies of ^{123}I-MIBG-imaging of sympathetic innervation for assessment of long-term prognosis in heart failure. JACC Cardiovasc Imaging 2013;6:772–84.
[47] Assomull RG, Shakespeare C, Kalra PR, Lloyd G, Gulati A, Strange J, et al. Role of cardiovascular magnetic resonance as a gatekeeper to invasive coronary angiography in patients presenting with heart failure of unknown etiology. Circulation 2011;124:1351–60. http://dx.doi.org/10.1161/CIRCULATIONAHA.110.011346.
[48] Plana JC, Galderisi M, Barac A, Ewer MS, Ky B, Scherrer-Crosbie M, et al. Expert consensus for multimodality imaging evaluation of adult patients during and after cancer therapy: a report from the American Society of Echocardiography and the European Association of Cardiovascular Imaging. J Am Soc Echocardiogr 2014;27:911–39.
[49] Bountioukos M, Doorduijn JK, Roelandt JRTC, Vourvouri EC, Bax JJ, Schinkel AFL, et al. Repetitive dobutamine stress echocardiography for the prediction of anthracycline cardiotoxicity. Eur J Echocardiogr 2003;4(4):300–5.
[50] Thavendiranathan P, Grant AD, Negishi T, Plana JC, Popovic ZB, Marwick TH. Reproducibility of echocardiographic techniques for sequential assessment of left ventricular ejection fraction and volumes: application to patients undergoing cancer chemotherapy. J Am Coll Cardiol 2013;61:77–84.
[51] Thavendiranathan P, Poulin F, Lim K-D, Plana JC, Woo A, Marwick TH. Use of myocardial strain imaging by echocardiography for the early detection of cardiotoxicity in patients during and after cancer chemotherapy: a systematic review. J Am Coll Cardiol 2014;63:2751–68.
[52] Negishi K, Negishi T, Hare JL, Haluska BA, Plana JC, Marwick TH. Independent and incremental value of deformation indices for prediction of trastuzumab-induced cardiotoxicity. J Am Soc Echocardiogr 2013;26:493–8.
[53] Motoki H, Koyama J, Nakazawa H, Aizawa K, Kasai H, Izawa A, et al. Torsion analysis in the early detection of anthracycline-mediated cardiomyopathy. Eur Heart J Cardiovasc Imaging 2012;13(1):95–103. http://dx.doi.org/10.1093/ejechocard/jer172.

[54] Sarma RJ, Chana A, Elkayam U. Left ventricular noncompaction. Prog Cardiovasc Dis 2010;52:264–73.
[55] Jenni R, Oechslin E, Schneider J, Attenhofer JC, Kaufmann PA. Echocardiographic and pathoanatomical characteristics of isolated left ventricular non-compaction: a step towards classification as a distinct cardiomyopathy. Heart 2001;86(6):666–71.
[56] Petersen SE, Selvanayagam JB, Wiesmann F, Robson MD, Francis JM, Anderson RH, et al. Left ventricular non-compaction: insights from cardiovascular magnetic resonance imaging. J Am Coll Cardiol 2005;46(1):101–5.
[57] Kohli SK, Pantazis AA, Shah JS, Adeyemi B, Jackson G, McKenna WJ, et al. Diagnosis of left-ventricular non-compaction in patients with left-ventricular systolic dysfunction: time for a reappraisal of diagnostic criteria? Eur Heart J 2008;29(1):89–95.
[58] Klaassen S, Probst S, Oechslin E, Gerull B, Krings G, Schuler P, et al. Mutations in sarcomere protein genes in left ventricular noncompaction. Circulation 2008;117(22):2893–901.
[59] Jenni R, Wyss CA, Oechslin EN, Kaufmann PA. Isolated ventricular noncompaction is associated with coronary microcirculatory dysfunction. J Am Coll Cardiol 2002;39:450–4.
[60] Banki NM, Kopelnik A, Dae MW, Miss J, Tung P, Lawton MT, et al. Acute neurocardiogenic injury after subarachnoid hemorrhage. Circulation 2005;112:3314–9. http://dx.doi.org/10.1161/CIRCULATIONAHA.105.558239.
[61] Burgdorf C, von Hof K, Schunkert H, Kurowski V. Regional alterations in myocardial sympathetic innervation in patients with transient left-ventricular apical ballooning (Tako-Tsubo cardiomyopathy). J Nucl Cardiol 2008;15(1):65–72.
[62] Prasad A, Madhavan M, Chareonthaitawee P. Cardiac sympathetic activity in stress induced (Takotsubo)cardiomyopathy. Nat Rev Cardiol 2009;6(6):430–4.
[63] Sen-Chowdhry S, Morgan RD, Chambers JC, McKenna WJ. Arrhythmogenic cardiomyopathy: etiology, diagnosis and treatment. Annu Rev Med 2010;61:233–53.
[64] Marcus FI, McKenna WJ, Sherrill D, Basso C, Bauce B, Bluemke DA, et al. Diagnosis of arrhythmogenic right ventricular cardiomyopathy/dysplasia. Proposed modification of the Task Force Criteria. Circulation 2010;121:1533–41.
[65] Sen-Chowdhry S, Prasad SK, Syrris P, Wage R, Ward D, Merrifield R, et al. Cardiovascular magnetic resonance in arrhythmogenic right ventricular cardiomyopathy revisited: comparison with task force criteria and genotype. J Am Coll Cardiol 2006;48:2132–40.
[66] Bluemke DA. ARVC: imaging diagnosis is still in the eye of the beholder. J Am Coll Cardiol Img 2011;4(3):288–91. http://dx.doi.org/10.1016/j.jcmg.2011.01.007.
[67] Nakajima T, Kimura F, Kajimoto K, Kasanuki H, Hagiwara N. Utility of ECG-gated MDCT to differentiate patients with ARVC/D from patients with ventricular tachyarrhythmias. J Cardiovasc Comput Tomogr 2013;7(4):223–33.
[68] Elliott PM, Anastasakis A, Borger MA, Borggrefe M, Cecchi F, Charron P, et al. 2014 ESC Guidelines on diagnosis and management of hypertrophic cardiomyopathy. The Task Force for the Diagnosis and Management of Hypertrophic Cardiomyopathy of the European Society of Cardiology (ESC). Eur Heart J 2014;35(39):2733–79. http://dx.doi.org/10.1093/eurheartj/ehu284.
[69] De Marvao A, Dawes TJW, Shi W, Minas C, Keenan NG, Diamond T, et al. Population-based studies of myocardial hypertrophy: high resolution cardiovascular magnetic resonance atlases improve statistical power. J Cardiovasc Magn Reson 2014;16:16.
[70] Maron MS, Maron BJ, Harrigan C, et al. Hypertrophic cardiomyopathy phenotype revisited after 50 years with cardiovascular magnetic resonance. J Am Coll Cardiol 2009;54:220–8.

[71] Maron MS, Olivotto I, Maron BJ, Prasad SK, Cecchi F, Udelson JE, et al. The case for myocardial ischemia in hypertrophic cardiomyopathy. J Am Coll Cardiol 2009;54:866–75.

[72] Maron MS, Finley JJ, Bos JM, Hauser TH, Manning WJ, Haas TS, et al. Prevalence, clinical significance, and natural history of left ventricular apical aneurysms in hypertrophic cardiomyopathy. Circulation 2008;118:1541–9.

[73] Rudolph A, Abdel-Aty H, Bohl S, Boye P, Zagrosek A, Dietz R, et al. Noninvasive detection of fibrosis applying contrast-enhanced cardiac magnetic resonance in different forms of left ventricular hypertrophy relation to remodeling. J Am Coll Cardiol 2009;53:284–91.

[74] Chan RH, Maron BJ, Olivotto I, Pencina MJ, Assenza GE, Haas T, et al. Prognostic value of quantitative contrast-enhanced cardiovascular magnetic resonance for the evaluation of sudden death risk in patients with hypertrophic cardiomyopathy. Circulation 2014;130:484–95.

[75] Brouwer WP, Baars EN, Germans T, de Boer K, Beek AM, van der Velden J, et al. In-vivo T1 cardiovascular magnetic resonance study of diffuse myocardial fibrosis in hypertrophic cardiomyopathy. J Cardiovasc Magn Reson 2014;16:28.

[76] Puntmann VO, Voigt T, Chen Z, Mayr M, Karim R, Rhode K, et al. Native T1 mapping in differentiation of normal myocardium from diffuse disease in hypertrophic and dilated cardiomyopathy. J Am Coll Cardiol Img 2013;6(4):475–84.

[77] Saito M, Okayama H, Yoshii T, Higashi H, Morioka H, Hiasa G, et al. Clinical significance of global two-dimensional strain as a surrogate parameter of myocardial fibrosis and cardiac events in patients with hypertrophic cardiomyopathy. Eur Heart J Cardiovasc Imaging 2012;13:617–23.

[78] Almaas VM, Haugaa KH, Strøm EH, Scott H, Smith HJ, Dahl CP, et al. Noninvasive assessment of myocardial fibrosis in patients with obstructive hypertrophic cardiomyopathy. Heart 2014;100(8):631–8. http://dx.doi.org/10.1136/heartjnl-2013-304923.

[79] Camici P, Chiriatti G, Lorenzoni R, Bellina RC, Gistri R, Italiani G, et al. Coronary vasodilation is impaired in both hypertrophied and nonhypertrophied myocardium of patients with hypertrophic cardiomyopathy: a study with nitrogen-13 ammonia and positron emission tomography. J Am Coll Cardiol 1991;17:879–86.

[80] Cecchi F, Olivotto I, Gistri R, Lorenzoni R, Chiriatti G, Camici PG. Coronary microvascular dysfunction and prognosis in hypertophic cardiomyopathy. N Engl J Med 2003;349:1027–35.

[81] Schäfers M, Dutka D, Rhodes CG, Lammertsma AA, Hermansen F, Schober O, et al. Myocardial presynaptic and postsynaptic autonomic dysfunction in hypertrophic cardiomyopathy. Circ Res 1998;82:57–62.

[82] Niemann M, Herrmann S, Hu K, Breunig F, Strotmann J, Beer M, et al. Differences in Fabry cardiomyopathy between female and male patients: consequences for diagnostic assessment. JACC Cardiovasc Imaging 2011;4(6):592–601. http://dx.doi.org/10.1016/j.jcmg.2011.01.020.

[83] Sado DM, White SK, Piechnik SK, Banypersad SM, Treibel T, Captur G, et al. Identification and assessment of Anderson–Fabry disease by cardiovascular magnetic resonance noncontrast myocardial T1 mapping. Circ Cardiovasc Imaging 2013;6:392–8.

[84] Dungu JN, Valencia O, Pinney JH, Gibbs SDJ, Rowczenio D, Gilbertson JA, et al. CMR-based differentiation of AL and ATTR cardiac amyloidosis. J Am Coll Cardiol 2014;7:133–42. http://dx.doi.org/10.1016/j.jcmg.2013.08.015.

[85] Karamitsos TD, Piechnik SK, Banypersad SM, Fontana M, Ntusi NB, Ferreira VM, et al. Noncontrast T1 mapping for the diagnosis of cardiac amyloidosis. J Am Coll Cardiol Img 2013;6:488–97.

[86] Banypersad SM, Fontana M, Maestrini V, Sado DM, Captur G, Petrie A, et al. T1 mapping and survival in systemic light-chain amyloidosis. Eur Heart J 2015;36:244–51. http://dx.doi.org/10.1093/eurheartj/ehu444.

[87] Maceira AM, Joshi J, Prasad SK, Moon JC, Perugini E, Harding I, et al. Cardiovascular magnetic resonance in cardiac amyloidosis. Circulation 2005;111:186–93.

[88] Hutt DF, Quigley AM, Page J, Hall ML, Burniston M, Gopaul D, et al. Utility and limitations of 3,3-diphosphono-1,2-propanodicarboxylic acid (^{99m}Tc-DPD) scintigraphy in systemic amyloidosis. Eur Heart J Cardiovasc Imaging 2014; 15:1289–98. http://dx.doi.org/10.1093/ehjci/jeu107.

[89] Perugini E, Guidalotti PL, Salvi F, Cooke RM, Pettinato C, Riva L, et al. Noninvasive etiologic diagnosis of cardiac amyloidosis using ^{99m}Tc-3,3-diphosphono-1,2-propanodicarboxylic acid scintigraphy. J Am Coll Cardiol 2005;46:1076–84.

[90] Parsai C, O'Hanlon R, Prasad SK, Mohiaddin RH. Diagnostic and prognostic value of cardiovascular magnetic resonance in non-ischaemic cardiomyopathies. J Cardiovasc Magn Reson 2012;14:54.

[91] Silverman K, Hutchins G, Bulkley B. Cardiac sarcoidosis: a clinico-pathological study of 84 in selected patients with systemic sarcoidosis. Circulation 1978;58:1204–11.

[92] He T. Cardiovascular magnetic resonance T2* for tissue iron assessment in the heart. Quant Imaging Med Surg 2014;4(5):407–12. http://dx.doi.org/10.3978/j.issn.2223-4292.2014.10.05.

[93] Pennell DJ, Udelson JE, Arai AE, Bozkurt B, Cohen AR, Galanello R, et al. Cardiovascular function and treatment in β-thalassemia major: a consensus statement from the American Heart Association. Circulation 2013;128:281–308.

[94] Baksi AJ, Pennell DJ. T2* imaging of the heart: methods, applications, and outcomes. Top Magn Reson Imaging 2014;23:13–20.

[95] Kramer CM, Chandrashekhar Y, Narula J. T1 mapping by CMR in cardiomyopathy: a noninvasive myocardial biopsy? J Am Coll Cardiol Img 2013;6(4):532–4. http://dx.doi.org/10.1016/j.jcmg.2013.02.002.

[96] Nagueh SF, Bierig SM, Budoff MJ, Desai M, Dilsizian V, Eidem B, et al. American society of echocardiography clinical recommendations for multimodality cardiovascular imaging of patients with hypertrophic cardiomyopathy. J Am Soc Echocardiogr 2011;24:473–98.

[97] Maron BJ, Spirito P. Implantable defibrillators and prevention of sudden death in hypertrophic cardiomyopathy. J Cardiovasc Electrophysiol 2008;19:1118–26.

[98] Ferreira PF, Kilner PJ, McGill LA, Nielles-Vallespin S, Scott AD, Ho SY, et al. In vivo cardiovascular magnetic resonance diffusion tensor imaging shows evidence of abnormal myocardial laminar orientations and mobility in hypertrophic cardiomyopathy. J Cardiovasc Magn Reson 2014;16:87. http://dx.doi.org/10.1186/s12968-014-0087-8.

[99] Mestroni L, Rocco C, Gregori D, Sinagra G, Lenarda AD, Miocic S, et al. Familial dilated cardiomyopathy: evidence for genetic and phenotypic heterogeneity. J Am Coll Cardiol 1999;34:181–90.

[100] Peterson SE, Jerosch-Herold M, Hudsmith LE, Robson MD, Francis JM, Doll HA, et al. Evidence for microvascular dysfunction in hypertrophic cardiomyopathy: new insights from multiparametric magnetic resonance imaging. Circulation 2007;115(18):2418–25.

[101] Senior R, Becher H, Monaghan M, Agati L, Zamorano J, Vanoverschelde JL, et al. Contrast echocardiography: evidence-based recommendations by European Association of Echocardiography. Eur J Echocardiogr 2009;10:194–212.

[102] Thomson HL, Basmadjian A-J, Rainbird AJ, Razavi M, Avierinos J-F, Pellikka PA, et al. Contrast echocardiography improves the accuracy and reproducibility of left ventricular remodeling measurements. J Am Coll Cardiol 2001;38:867–75.

[103] Junker A, Thayssen P, Nielsen B, Andersen PE. The hemodynamic and prognostic significance of echo-Doppler-proven mitral regurgitation in patients with dilated cardiomyopathy. Cardiology 1993;83(1–2):14–20.

[104] Florescu M, Magda LS, Enescu OA, Jinga D, Vinereanu D. Early detection of epirubicin-induced cardiotoxicity in patients with breast cancer. J Am Soc Echocardiogr 2014;27(1):83–92. http://dx.doi.org/10.1016/j.echo.2013.10.008.

[105] Corrado D, Basso C, Thiene G, McKenna WJ, Davies MJ, Fontaliran F, et al. Spectrum of clinicopathologic manifestations of arrhythmogenic right ventricular cardiomyopathy/dysplasia: a multicenter study. J Am Coll Cardiol 1997;30(6):1512–20.

[106] Sen-Chowdhry S, Syrris P, Prasad SK, Hughes SE, Merrifield R, Ward D, et al. Left-dominant arrhythmogenic cardiomyopathy: an under-recognized clinical entity. J Am Coll Cardiol 2008;52(25):2175–87. http://dx.doi.org/10.1016/j.jacc.2008.09.019.

[107] Lindström L, Nylander E, Larsson H, Wranne B. Left ventricular involvement in arrhythmogenic right ventricular cardiomyopathy - a scintigraphic and echocardiographic study. Clin Physiol Funct Imaging 2005;25(3):171–7.

[108] Olivotto I, Maron MS, Autore C, Lesser JR, Rega L, Casolo G, et al. Assessment and significance of left ventricular mass by cardiovascular magnetic resonance in hypertrophic cardiomyopathy. J Am Coll Cardiol 2008;52(7):559–66. http://dx.doi.org/10.1016/j.jacc.2008.04.047.

[109] Nagueh SF, Kopelen HA, Lim DS, Zoghbi WA, Quinones MA, Roberts R, et al. Tissue Doppler imaging consistently detects myocardial contraction and relaxation abnormalities, irrespective of cardiac hypertrophy, in a transgenic rabbit model of human hypertrophic cardiomyopathy. Circulation 2000;102:1346–50.

[110] Ho CY, Sweitzer NK, McDonough B, Maron BJ, Casey SA, Seidman JG, et al. Assessment of diastolic function with Doppler tissue imaging to predict genotype in preclinical hypertrophic cardiomyopathy. Circulation 2002;105(25):2992–7.

[111] Osborne M, Kolli S, Padera RF, Naya M, Lewis E, Dorbala S, et al. Use of multimodality imaging to diagnose cardiac sarcoidosis as well as identify recurrence following heart transplantation. J Nucl Cardiol 2013;20(2):310–2. http://dx.doi.org/10.1007/s12350-013-9677-3.

Myocarditis

R. Wassmuth*,†, J. Schulz-Menger†,‡
*Oberhavel-Kliniken Hennigsdorf, Hennigsdorf, Germany; †Universitätsmedizin Berlin, A Joint Institution of Charite and Max-Delbruck-Center, Berlin, Germany; ‡HELIOS Klinikum Berlin-Buch, Berlin, Germany

14.1 Clinical background

14.1.1 Etiology and presentation

Acute myocardial inflammation can induce a broad clinical spectrum, from subclinical disease to fulminant acute heart failure [1]. Myocarditis more often affects young male than female or elderly patients [2]. The clinical presentation differs depending on age and gender [3]. Young men often present with acute chest pain similar to myocardial infarction after a few days of airway or intestinal infection (Figure 14.1a and b) [4]. In female patients, the clinical presentation is frequently less obvious and imaging findings are less impressive than in young males. On the other hand, some patients can present with fulminant myocarditis, requiring circulatory support in intensive care [5]. In most cases, acute viral infection is the underlying mechanism, but drug-induced toxicity [6] and autoimmune diseases have also a role and their prevalence as a cause of myocarditis is probably underestimated.

Myocarditis is an important differential diagnosis in acute coronary syndrome or acute heart failure. Non-invasive imaging plays an increasing role in ACS for the differentiation of the underlying injury. Once significant coronary artery disease (CAD) has been excluded, cardiac imaging is often requested to elucidate the reason for elevated troponin [7–10]. The main objective of further testing is the safe and accurate identification of the cause of raised cardiac biomarkers, especially if invasive procedures are to be avoided. The order of the procedures (invasive vs. non-invasive) depends on several conditions, including clinical features and pre-test probability of disease. An intelligent and innovative setting is helpful for speeding up the diagnostic procedure and avoiding unneeded invasive procedures, especially in young patients.

14.1.2 Course of disease

The time course of myocarditis depends on the initiating cause and the patient constitution. The so-called "natural course" of disease typically lasts 5 weeks [11]. In the majority of cases, patients do recover after 3–6 weeks. Prognosis also depends on the type of initial clinical presentation and LV function at baseline [12]. In particular, young male patients with a presentation similar to a myocardial infarction most often

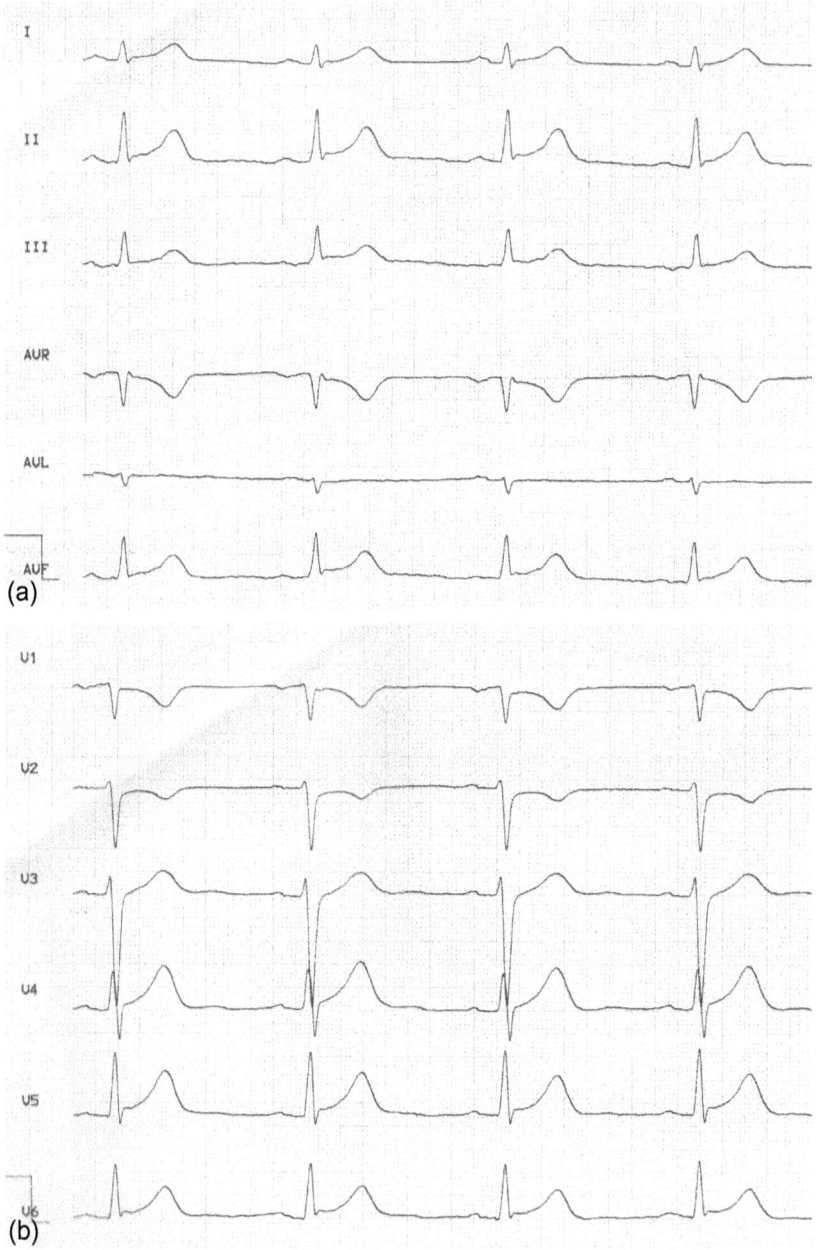

Figure 14.1 A 28 year-old male was admitted with sudden chest pain after 3 days of severe diarrhoea. His EKG showed ST elevation in the inferior (a) and lateral leads (b). Troponin was elevated and further increased up to 9, 4 ng/ml (normal < 0.15 ng/ml).

recover despite troponin elevations [4]. However, some patients may develop dilated cardiomyopathy. In some patients with fulminant myocarditis (mainly young females), ventricular dilatation and hypocontractility persist for several weeks or months but it often eventually recover to a normal or almost normal state [5].

14.2 Biopsy as "the invasive standard"

Endomyocardial biopsy (EMB) is the only method that can identify the underlying cause of myocarditis and differentiate the causative organism [13]. In experienced hands, this invasive procedure has a low risk [14,15]. The indication for EMB in clinical routine is limited due to sample error and the lack of therapeutic consequences. The currently accepted indications are published in a consensus statement of AHA, ACC, and ESC based on the description of 14 clinical scenarios (Table 14.1) [16]. According to guidelines, EMB is

Table 14.1 **Indications for endomyocardial biopsy**

	Clinical scenario	Class of recommendation	Level of evidence
1	New-onset heart failure of 2 weeks' duration associated with a normal-sized or dilated left ventricle and hemodynamic compromise	I	B
2	New-onset heart failure of 2 weeks' to 3 months' duration associated with a dilated left ventricle and new ventricular arrhythmias, second- or third-degree heart block, or failure to respond to usual care within 1 to 2 weeks	I	B
3	Heart failure of 3 months' duration associated with a dilated left ventricle and new ventricular arrhythmias, second- or third-degree heart block, or failure to respond to usual care within 1 to 2 weeks	IIa	C
4	Heart failure associated with a DCM of any duration associated with suspected allergic reaction and/or eosinophilia	IIa	C
5	Heart failure associated with suspected anthracycline cardiomyopathy	IIa	C
6	Heart failure associated with unexplained restrictive cardiomyopathy	IIa	C
7	Suspected cardiac tumors	IIa	C
8	Unexplained cardiomyopathy in children	IIa	C

(*Continued*)

Table 14.1 **Continued**

	Clinical scenario	Class of recommendation	Level of evidence
9	New-onset heart failure of 2 weeks' to 3 months' duration associated with a dilated left ventricle, without new ventricular arrhythmias or second- or third-degree heart block, that responds to usual care within 1 to 2 weeks	IIb	B
10	Heart failure of 3 months' duration associated with a dilated left ventricle, without new ventricular arrhythmias or second- or third-degree heart block, that responds to usual care within 1 to 2 weeks	IIb	C
11	Heart failure associated with unexplained HCM	IIb	C
12	Suspected ARVD/C	IIb	C
13	Unexplained ventricular arrhythmias	IIb	C
14	Unexplained atrial fibrillation	III	C

Reproduced from Ref 16.

indicated especially if it may change management in unexplained heart failure, e.g., in suspected giant cell myocarditis. More data are required to develop new therapeutic strategies based on EMB and non-invasive imaging [17]. It had been suggested that cardiovascular magnetic resonance (CMR) might guide the location of biopsies to increase sensitivity. However, inflammatory lesions often have an intramural or epicardial location less accessible to biopsy. In addition, the biopsy forceps are a rigid tool that cannot be directed to any location indicated by CMR. CMR might indicate whether left ventricular (LV) or right ventricular (RV) myocardial biopsy appears more promising in an individual case, but Yilmaz et al. demonstrated that biopsies did not yield higher sensitivity when taken from regions (septal or lateral wall) with positive late gadolinium enhancement (LGE) by CMR [14]. In addition, they found that combined RV and LV biopsies were more sensitive than samples from one ventricle alone. In acute coronary syndrome without obvious etiology, biopsy and CMR may offer synergistic diagnostic power superior to either approach alone [17]. Myocardial involvement in systemic disorders is more difficult to assess, especially in focal pronounced disease, such as sarcoidosis (see Chapter 15). Therefore, current recommendations are restrictive. EMB in a clinical setting is only indicated if a specific therapeutic consequence is expected mostly depending on patient hemodynamic stability, as indicated in Table 14.1. Research settings will have other degrees of freedom. EMB allows the specific evaluation of the kind of virus and could stratify a specific therapy. But inflammation may be caused by viral and non-viral agents and the diagnostic performance is also related to the scatter of evaluated causes. There is no doubt that EMB as well as all imaging techniques also depends on the experience of the centre.

14.3 Therapeutic options

The therapy depends on the clinical situation of an individual patient. The clinical picture ranges from cardiogenic shock over mild symptoms to asymptomatic disease. A fulminant myocarditis needs full intensive care support, potentially including assist devices. According to EMB guidelines, a specific diagnosis is warranted in these patients. For example, giant cell myocarditis is a rare, but life-threatening condition requiring application of steroids. In nearly all patients, including those with mild symptoms, heart failure medication is administered. The duration and extent of therapy depends on individual circumstances [1]. It is common sense that physical activities should be avoided in the acute stage. Defining the appropriate time of restarting exercise is often difficult [18]. Data regarding this problem are scarce. The only trial is based on mice experiments which indicate that physical activity in myocarditis increased mortality [19].

In patients with myocardial involvement in systemic disorders, an intensification of the applied disease specific medication is usually recommended. A detailed discussion based on clinical stages and/or on the likelihood of the disease was published by Sagar et al. (Table 14.2) [1].

14.4 Imaging

14.4.1 Echocardiography

Echocardiography is an important first-line tool readily available at the bedside, including intensive care units, and is generally the first non-invasive imaging test in suspected myocarditis.

14.4.1.1 Wall motion

Echocardiography can readily assess global and regional wall motion abnormalities. Generally, echocardiographic findings in myocarditis are rather unspecific as described in small patient series and single case reports [5,20–22]. Echocardiography may also be less accurate than, for example, CMR in detecting subtle contractile impairment as are typical for myocarditis (Figure 14.2).

14.4.1.2 Oedema

Acute inflammatory or ischemic myocardial injury results in myocardial oedema detectable as transient regional wall thickening. Even if wall thickening might be a subtle phenomenon, it can be detected by echocardiography [5,20–25]. Grossly affected myocardial segments may occasionally appear brighter than remote myocardium. So far, however, there is no reliable link between echo signal and myocardial texture. If the pericardium is involved in the inflammatory process, a small pericardial effusion may be present and detected by echocardiography.

Table 14.2 **Classification of myocarditis**

	Criteria	Histological confirmation	Biomarker, ECG or Imaging abnormalities needed	Treatment
Possible subclinical acute myocarditis	In the clinical context of possible myocardial injury without cardiovascular symptoms but with at least one of the following 1 Biomarkers of myocardial injury raised 2 ECG findings suggestive of cardiac injury 3 Abnormal cardiac function on echocardiogram or cardiac MRI	Absent	Needed	Not known
Possible acute myocarditis	In the clinical context of possible myocardial injury with cardiovascular symptoms and at least one of the following 1 Biomarkers of myocardial injury raised 2 ECG findings suggestive of cardiac injury 3 Abnormal cardiac function on echocardiogram or cardiac MRI	Absent	Needed	Per clinical syndrome
Definite myocarditis	Histological or immunohistological evidence of myocarditis	Needed	Not needed	Tailored to specific cause

A three-tiered clinical classification for the diagnosis of myocarditis on the basis of level of diagnostic certainty
From Ref 1

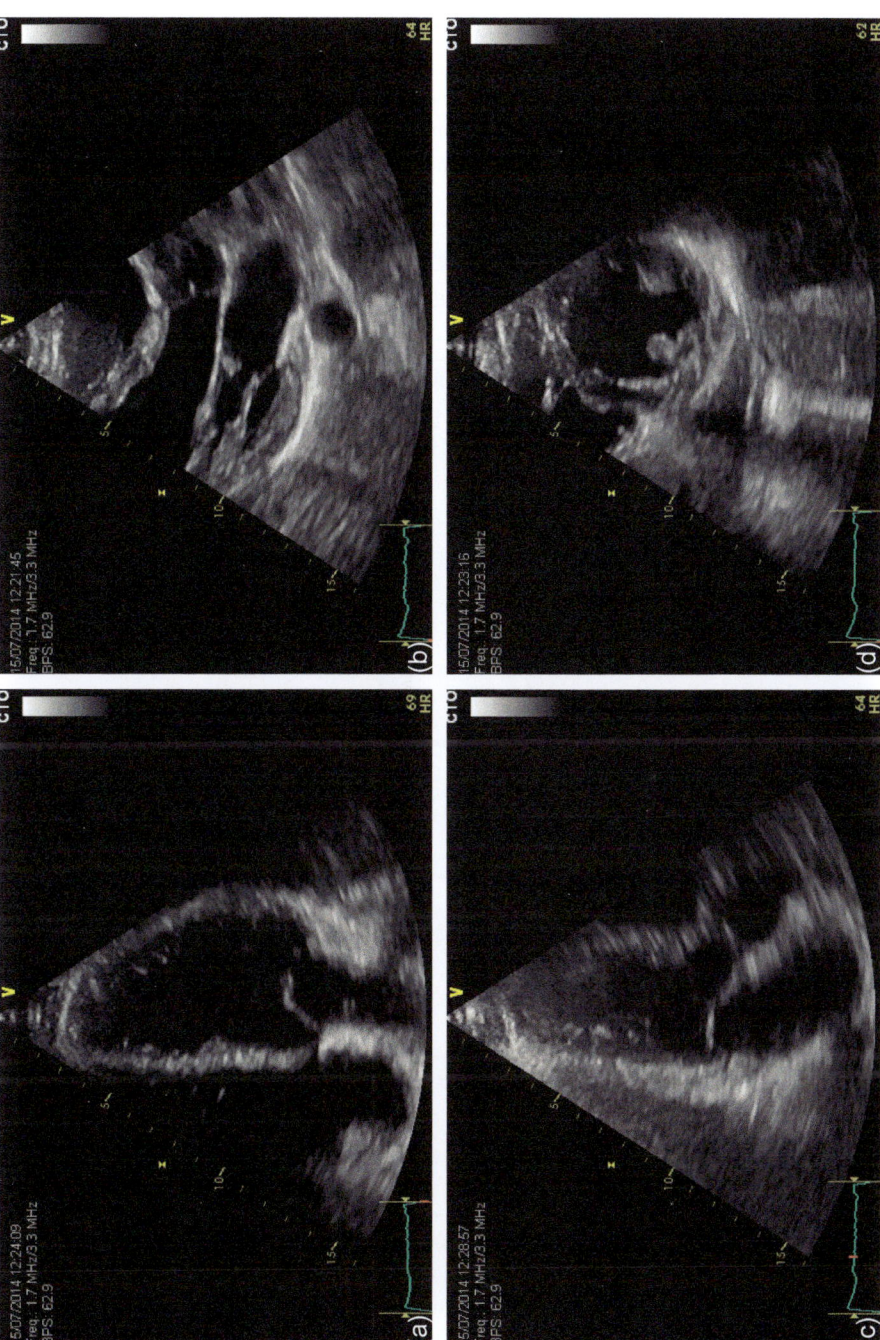

Figure 14.2 Echocardiography showed overall normal LV function in the absence of pericardial effusion. Apical contraction appeared somewhat sluggish.

14.4.1.3 Advanced techniques: strain imaging and tissue Doppler imaging

Ejection fraction, as the most frequently reported parameter for systolic function, overemphasizes radial contraction while early impairment of longitudinal contraction is neglected. Global longitudinal strain has proven to be a stable parameter that detects early impairment in contractility when EF is still normal, e.g., in patients after chemotherapy or with aortic stenosis. In acute myocarditis, initial experience suggests that longitudinal strain can detect myocardial impairment even if ejection fraction is close to normal (Figure 14.3) [26–28]. In addition, markers for diastolic dysfunction like low mitral annular plane systolic excursion (MAPSE), mitral e' or elevated mitral E/e' were found

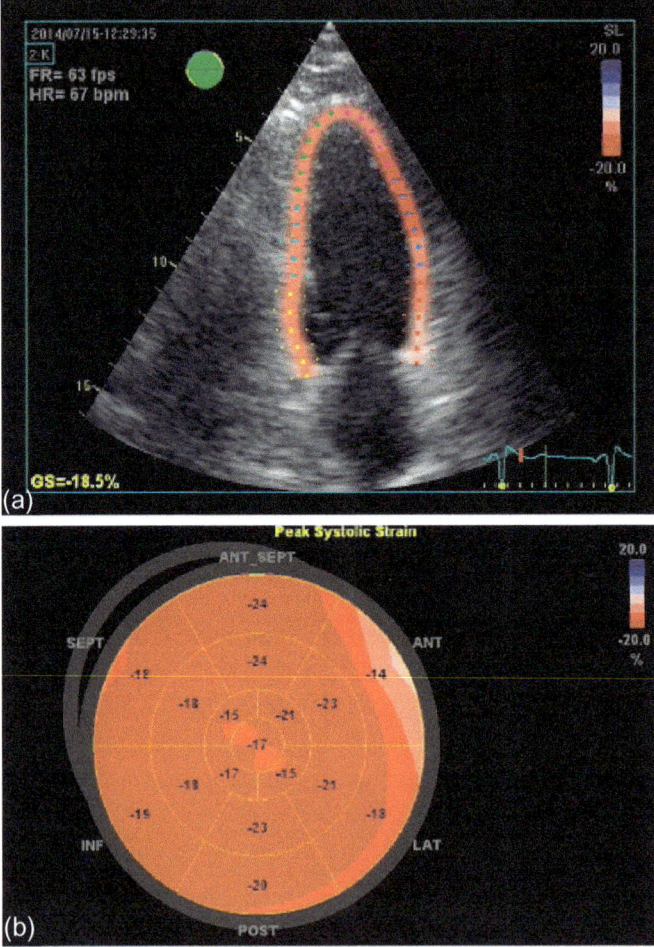

Figure 14.3 Semiautomatic contouring results in strain quantification, based on 2D speckle tracking (A). Global longitudinal strain was normal with −18.5%, but apical segments did show slightly lower values reflecting the visual impression of sluggish apical contraction (B).

in patients with acute myocarditis in the presence of normal left ventricular ejection fraction (LVEF) [29]. Even if a single abnormal parameter may have limited sensitivity for myocardial damage in acute myocarditis, the combination of various advanced echocardiographic markers may be sufficient to reveal subtle myocardial impairment [30].

14.4.2 Nuclear imaging

Different nuclear tracers have been applied to diagnose myocarditis, especially gallium-67 and indium-111-labelled antimyosin antibodies, which have been under evaluation for detecting myocarditis in conjunction with single-photon emission computed tomography (SPECT) [31]. The latter binds specifically to exposed myosin molecules when cellular integrity is lost due to the inflammatory process (see Chapter 10). Sensitivity of antimyosin antibody scanning is reported to be very high, however, with lower specificity, as other cell injury (e.g., myocardial infarction) results in uptake of the tracer. Perfusion SPECT using standard tracers (e.g., 99mTc-tetrofosmin, 99mTc-sestamibi, or 201-Thallium) may reveal defects in the more severe cases of myocarditis (e.g., Chagas disease). Whereas most of the approaches no longer have a place in the clinical routine, PET technology is opening new insights and has the potential to add information. For example, PET can particularly contribute to the diagnosis of myocardial sarcoidosis after applying commercially available tracers [32].

14.4.3 Coronary angiography

The clinical picture of acute ST elevation infarction (STEMI) and acute myocarditis can be similar, and where STEMI is suspected, instant coronary angiography is warranted. Where the clinical picture is strongly suggestive of myocarditis, especially in young males with a history of infection and ECG changes in more than a single coronary territory, non-invasive imaging may be considered as a first line test. If a well-trained CMR unit is in the same hospital and the investigation can be applied immediately, a CMR can be considered. CMR is safe in acute coronary syndrome in experienced hands [10,33] and may provide the diagnosis without requiring invasive angiography [7,9,34]. A typical pattern of epicardial and or patchy late enhancement in the absence of infarction scar may be the basis to defer coronary angiography in a young patient without risk factors for CAD. Alternatively, CAD may be excluded by coronary computed tomography (CT) angiography.

14.4.4 Cardiovascular magnetic resonance

CMR plays an increasing role in the diagnosis and management of myocarditis, mainly due to its unique ability for tissue characterisation and differentiation between ischaemic and non-ischaemic myocardial injury. In addition to the highly accurate assessment of contractile function and morphology, CMR allows assessment of three tissue markers that are relevant in myocarditis: myocardial oedema imaging, hyperaemia and capillary leakage, and myocardial necrosis and fibrosis. Two CMR methods (T2- and early T1-weighted imaging) allow for the detection of oedema. The interpretation is based on a semi-quantitative analysis, and a "cut-off" is given. The use of this cut-off is only reasonable if the detailed technical parameters (sequence-details, coils, field-strengths, contrast-media-characteristics) are respected. Hyperaemia and capillary leakage are assessed with early enhancement (EE) images and irreversible injury can be identified on LGE-images.

14.4.4.1 Diagnostic criteria for myocarditis

Of the available CMR methods, LGE has been the most popular due to high availability, advanced experience due to application in infarction imaging, best comparability between platforms, and highest specificity in myocarditis. The disadvantages of LGE in myocarditis are limited sensitivity and its inability to differentiate between acute and chronic lesions. In 2009, an international expert panel suggested a clinical "routine" protocol for acute myocarditis, the so-called "Lake Louise criteria" [35]. The Lake Louise criteria recommended the use of a multi-parametric CMR protocol to increase sensitivity and specificity compared to the analysis of a single CMR parameter. The authors propose that the CMR study is called positive if 2 or more of the 3 tissue-based criteria are positive (Table 14.3). Furthermore, the combination of T2-weighted imaging, EE, and LGE may help to assess how acute the myocardial damage is [36]. Importantly, CMR findings vary depending on the patients studied. The typical young male patient most often presents with focal oedema and LGE in corresponding locations. Fewer patients may present without LGE and still do have true myocarditis. A subgroup of patients presents with global oedema and increased EE.

Table 14.3 **Diagnostic criteria for myocarditis**

Proposed diagnostic CMR criteria (i.e., Lake Louise Consensus Criteria) for myocarditis
In the setting of clinically suspected myocarditis,* CMR findings are consistent with myocardial inflammation, if at least two of the following criteria are present: (1) Regional or global myocardial SI increase in T2-weighted images (2) Increased global myocardial early gadolinium enhancement ratio between myocardium and skeletal muscle in gadolinium-enhanced T1-weighted images (3) There is at least one focal lesion with nonischemic regional distribution in inversion recovery-prepared gadolinium-enhanced T1-weighted images ("late gadolinium enhancement")
A CMR study is consistent with myocyte injury and/or scar caused by myocardial inflammation if criterion 3 is present.

A repeat CMR study between 1 and 2 weeks after the initial CMR study is recommended if
    None of the criteria are present, but the onset of symptoms has been very recent and there is strong clinical evidence for myocardial inflammation
    One of the criteria is present

The presence of LV dysfunction or pericardial effusion provides additional, supportive evidence for myocarditis.

Reproduced from Friedrich et al. [34].

It is worth noting that the 2009 Lake Louise recommendations did not incorporate mapping techniques nor differentiate in detail between various ways of T2-weighted imaging. Ongoing research is investigating the incremental value of these evolving methods. The different CMR methods used in myocarditis are described in more detail in the following paragraphs.

14.4.4.2 Cine imaging

As described in detail in Table 14.3, the Lake Louise protocol includes cine imaging for the assessment of LV and RV geometry and function, as well as for the detection of pericardial or pleural fluid. Cine-CMR imaging also allows the detection of subtle wall-motion abnormalities, as is typical for acute myocarditis. Less often, severely reduced LV function with global wall motion abnormalities can be seen. It is important to ensure coverage of the basal myocardium, as the myocarditic damage is often found in a basal posterolateral location (Figure 14.4).

14.4.4.3 Oedema imaging

Acute inflammation induces oedema which means more local water accumulation [37]. CMR can visualize water accumulation within the tissue, e.g., by T2-weighted fast spin echo imaging (Figure 14.5a and b) [38]. However, arrhythmias and slow flowing blood may induce a hyperintense signal that must not be mistaken with true oedema. Alternative spin echo [39] or gradient echo techniques [40] are more stable and yield in higher signal-to-noise, however, the contrast-to-noise of STIR is unsurpassed. In acute myocarditis, oedema can be regional or global. Young male patients with a clinical presentation similar to acute infarction often have regional oedema in a lateral or inferior region, whereas women tend to have global oedema. Abnormal findings suggesting regional oedema should be confirmed in a second perpendicular plane or by changing the readout direction to exclude artefacts. Beside directly detecting water accumulation within the tissue, cine CMR can also visualize the subtle

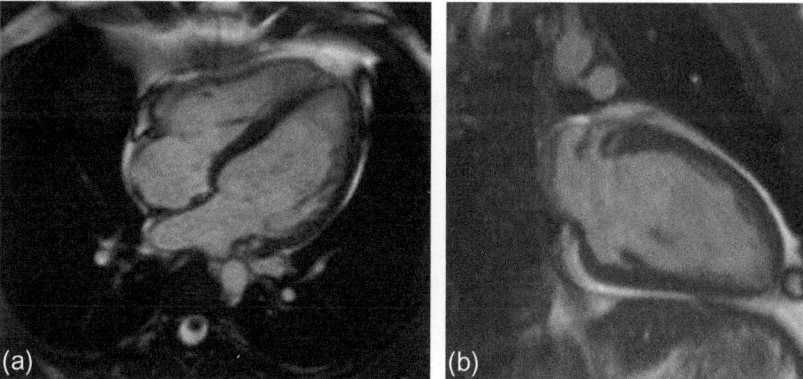

Figure 14.4 The patient underwent CMR 3 days after echocardiography. Steady state free precession cine confirmed good LV function with subtle hypokinesia apical and basal inferior.

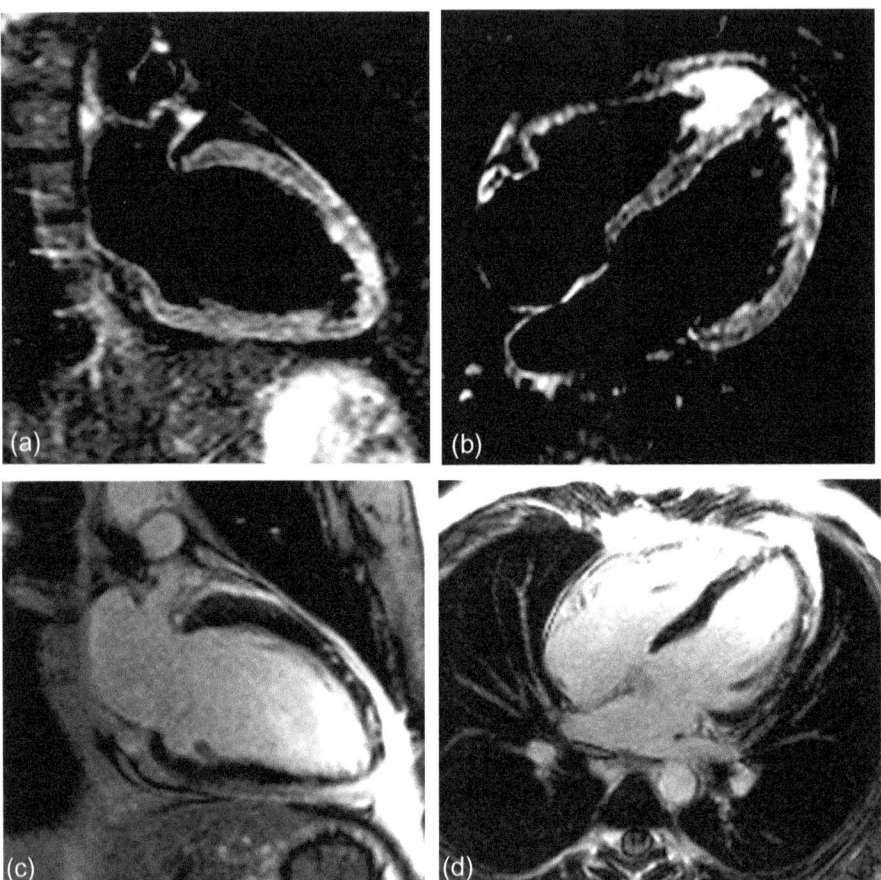

Figure 14.5 Triple inversion short tau inversion recovery T2-weighted fast spin echo (A and B) reveals focal spots of hyperintense signal within the myocardium, most likely reflecting edema. Note the bright signal within the right ventricular apex as well as the bright rim within the LV cavity along the apicolateral wall. These bright areas do not reflect edema but slow flow artefacts. Late Gadolinium enhancement images (C and D) depict small areas of irreversible myocardial damage in the same segments. The lesions are located in the middle of the myocardial wall or in the epicardial portion, thereby differing from myocardial infarction. Due to the typical clinical presentation, the young age of the patient, preserved LV function and the lack of severe wall motion abnormality coronary angiography was not done.

and transient wall thickening that comes with oedema [22,41]. That supports the idea that CMR can also detect global oedema. Care should be applied not to confuse myocardial oedema with hypertrophy. Global oedema can be assessed semi-quantitatively by comparing myocardium to skeletal muscle as a reference structure, as described previously [42]. The published cut-off values are based on dedicated technical parameters (e.g., slice thickness) and should only be used in this setting. The technique is sensitive and reliable enough to detect myocardial changes after alcohol intake under controlled study conditions [43]. Oedema can typically be detected several weeks after onset of the disease. The earlier patients are scanned, the higher the diagnostic yield [44]. Thereby, oedema imaging allows an assessment of how acute the inflammation process is.

14.4.4.4 Early gadolinium enhancement

In acute myocarditis, CMR can detect increased myocardial contrast uptake within the first 5 min after contrast administration, also known as EE, relative enhancement, or early gadolinium enhancement [45]. Typically, a fast spin echo sequence is used to obtain images before and after contrast administration [35]. Slice thickness should be at least 7 mm to allow for sufficient signal-to-noise. The contrast uptake occurs after first-pass perfusion but long before late gadolinium images are acquired. The increased contrast uptake does not occur in normal volunteers and usually normalizes again in patients after about 4 weeks. Visual assessment of EE is difficult. Therefore, semi-quantitative comparison of pre- and post-contrast images is recommended. Myocardial signal increase is compared to signal increase in skeletal muscle. A myocardial signal increase that is five times higher than in skeletal muscle is considered pathologic, whereas in normal subjects, a ratio of about three can be expected. Potential explanations for this phenomenon are hyperemia and capillary leakage within an inflammatory state. So far, there are no experimental data to support this concept. Caution is indicated in inflammatory diseases, including skeletal muscles. If the disease increases skeletal muscle contrast uptake as well, the ratio may become false negative. In clinical routine, EE appears most helpful in female patients without LGE lesions, whereas in typical young male patients, the additional diagnostic value of EE beyond oedema and LGE lesions appears limited [46]. Interestingly, the EE appears helpful in detecting transplant rejection [47].

14.4.4.5 Late gadolinium enhancement

Some, but not all myocarditis patients present with lesions on LGE images (Figure 14.5c and d) [42,48]. The technique is the same as for imaging infarction scars, only the distribution pattern of the lesions differ. In myocarditis, lesions can be found in the central intramural or the outer epicardial part of the myocardial wall. Most often, multiple small lesions strung like a chain of pearls can be found, but confluent epicardial lesions are also common. The posterolateral segment is the one most frequently affected; the anteroseptal wall can be affected as well. The reason for the predominance of the posterolateral distribution is unclear. One group has postulated that the type of virus is associated with a certain spatial distribution pattern [49]; so far this has not been confirmed elsewhere. The lesions are visible early on at initial presentation. They do not allow a differentiation between acute and chronic damage. The typical young male patient with an infarction-like presentation most often recovers without sequelae despite impressive troponin elevations and extensive LGE lesions. The lesions shrink over time and may thereby slowly disappear over the years in some patients. Nevertheless, in a single study including a broader spectrum of patients with a mean age of 52 years, the authors found a relation between LGE lesions and a worse prognosis [50]. One important difference to scar imaging in CAD is the small lesion size. Therefore, LGE imaging in myocarditis requires a high spatial resolution, complete coverage of the left ventricle, and a careful suppression of remote non-affected myocardium.

14.4.4.6 Technical innovations

T1 and T2 mapping techniques allow for direct quantification of tissue properties independent of any reference structures [51]. The diagnosis of diseased myocardium as inflammation has to be based on normal values at different field strengths [52–54]. There are first applications in myocarditis showing that T1 mapping was able to detect myocarditis [22,55,56]. A recent study by Luetkens et al. found that native T1 mapping at 3T was superior compared to the Lake Louise criteria in detecting myocarditis [57]. Early single-centre experience suggests diagnostic value of increased extracellular volume in myocarditis [58], which needs to be confirmed in additional studies. Interestingly, in a recent mapping study at 3T, extracellular volume (ECV) was indeed elevated in acute myocarditis. However, in a receiver operating characteristic (ROC) analysis, elevated ECV did not appear to be diagnostically superior compared to previous CMR markers [57].

14.4.5 Computed tomography

The role of CT in the evaluation of myocarditis is generally limited to the assessment of coronary arteries as an alternative to invasive X-ray angiography. CT can however also provide additional relevant information.

14.4.5.1 LV size and function

LV size and function can in principle be accurately quantified by CT, but this is not a primary indication for cardiac CT unless echo and CMR do not yield diagnostic image quality [59].

14.4.5.2 CT coronary angiography

In selected young myocarditis patients with unusual acute chest pain, coronary CT angiography might be an alternative for coronary catheterization to exclude CAD as the underlying cause.

14.4.5.3 CT late enhancement

The late enhancement technique used in CMR, i.e., acquiring images late after contrast administration to visualize non-viable myocardium, is technically also feasible with CT. Several case reports of acute myocarditis demonstrate that if CMR is not available or feasible, similar images can be acquired with CT and thereby confirm the diagnosis [60–63]. However, with current methods, contrast-to-noise is lower than for LGE CMR. Furthermore, additional radiation exposure and higher doses of contrast medium are required; therefore CT, is currently not the first-choice modality for imaging of late contrast enhancement [64].

Table 14.4 Multimodality imaging in myocarditis

	Echo	CMR	Nuclear imaging	Coronary angiography	CT
LV size and function	Excellent if acoustic window is ok	Excellent	Poor temporal resolution	Rough estimate	No indication
Edema	Subtle wall thickening	Excellent	–	–	–
Permanent lesions	–	Excellent	Poor spatial resolution	–	Low contrast Additional radiation
Exclusion of CAD	–	–	–	Gold standard	Excellent
Particular strenghts	Bedside technique	Combination of functional and tissue information		Acute PCI in CAD	Noninvasive exclusion of CAD
Disadvantages	No tissue characterization			Radiation Invasive	Radiation No functional information

PCI denotes percutaneous coronary intervention. CAD denotes coronary artery disease.

14.4.6 Imaging for follow-up and evolution

Those patients with dilated ventricles or impaired contraction need follow-up to confirm whether and to what extent cardiac function improves after the acute stage of the disease. Whether echocardiography or CMR is preferred for the follow-up depends partly on the acoustic window of an individual patient, local experience, availability of the techniques, and the extent of cardiac abnormality. Due to lower variability, CMR may detect smaller changes in systolic function than echocardiography.

Clinically, it is often challenging to determine when the patient should resume his usual daily activities and in particular sports. There are no specific data whether imaging can contribute to this decision. Common sense suggests that the markers of acute damage like oedema should have normalized before the patient can be sent back to work. On the other hand, patients frequently experience a prolonged phase of impaired exercise capacity despite normalization of all available tests (Figures 14.1–14.5).

14.5 Summary

Myocarditis presents with a high clinical variability, often posing a diagnostic challenge. Imaging can assess the degree of myocardial injury and exclude differential diagnoses, such as acute infarction. The specific strengths and weaknesses of various imaging methods are summarized in Table 14.4. Depending on local availability and expertise, clinicians have to select those tools that best fit the demands of their individual patients. Often a combination of imaging methods will yield in the most useful information, e.g., echocardiography in the very acute and unstable phase of the disease followed by CMR once the patient is stabilized.

References

[1] Sagar S, Liu PP, Cooper Jr LT. Myocarditis. Lancet 2012;379(9817):738–47.
[2] Kyto V, Sipila J, Rautava P. The effects of gender and age on occurrence of clinically suspected myocarditis in adulthood. Heart 2013;99(22):1681–4.
[3] Cocker MS, Abdel-Aty H, Strohm O, Friedrich MG. Age and gender effects on the extent of myocardial involvement in acute myocarditis: a cardiovascular magnetic resonance study. Heart 2009;95(23):1925–30.
[4] Costantini M, Oreto G, Albanese A, Ranieri A, De Fabrizio G, Sticchi I, et al. Presumptive myocarditis with ST-Elevation myocardial infarction presentation in young males as a new syndrome. Clinical significance and long term follow up. Cardiovasc Ultrasound 2011;9:1.
[5] Levenson JE, Kaul DR, Saint S, Nallamothu BK, Gurm HS. Clinical problem-solving. A shocking development. N Engl J Med 2013;369(23):2253–8.
[6] Ronaldson KJ, Taylor AJ, Fitzgerald PB, Topliss DJ, Elsik M, McNeil JJ. Diagnostic characteristics of clozapine-induced myocarditis identified by an analysis of 38 cases and 47 controls. J Clin Psychiatry 2010;71(8):976–81.

[7] Assomull RG, Lyne JC, Keenan N, Gulati A, Bunce NH, Davies SW, et al. The role of cardiovascular magnetic resonance in patients presenting with chest pain, raised troponin, and unobstructed coronary arteries. Eur Heart J 2007;28(10):1242–9.
[8] Gerbaud E, Harcaut E, Coste P, Erickson M, Lederlin M, Labeque JN, et al. Cardiac magnetic resonance imaging for the diagnosis of patients presenting with chest pain, raised troponin, and unobstructed coronary arteries. Int J Cardiovasc Imaging 2012;28(4):783–94.
[9] Wassmuth R. Heart failure in patients with normal coronary anatomy: diagnostic algorithm and disease pattern of various etiologies as defined by cardiac MRI. Cardiovasc Diagn Ther 2012;2(2):128–37.
[10] Plein S, Greenwood JP, Ridgway JP, Cranny G, Ball SG, Sivananthan MU. Assessment of non-ST-segment elevation acute coronary syndromes with cardiac magnetic resonance imaging. J Am Coll Cardiol 2004;44(11):2173–81.
[11] Feldman AM, McNamara D. Myocarditis. N Engl J Med 2000;343(19):1388–98.
[12] D'Ambrosio A, Patti G, Manzoli A, Sinagra G, Di Lenarda A, Silvestri F, et al. The fate of acute myocarditis between spontaneous improvement and evolution to dilated cardiomyopathy: a review. Heart 2001;85(5):499–504.
[13] Cooper Jr LT. Myocarditis. N Engl J Med 2009;360(15):1526–38.
[14] Yilmaz A, Kindermann I, Kindermann M, Mahfoud F, Ukena C, Athanasiadis A, et al. Comparative evaluation of left and right ventricular endomyocardial biopsy: differences in complication rate and diagnostic performance. Circulation 2010;122(9):900–9.
[15] Holzmann M, Nicko A, Kuhl U, Noutsias M, Poller W, Hoffmann W, et al. Complication rate of right ventricular endomyocardial biopsy via the femoral approach: a retrospective and prospective study analyzing 3048 diagnostic procedures over an 11-year period. Circulation 2008;118(17):1722–8.
[16] Cooper LT, Baughman KL, Feldman AM, Frustaci A, Jessup M, Kuhl U, et al. The role of endomyocardial biopsy in the management of cardiovascular disease: a scientific statement from the American Heart Association, the American College of Cardiology, and the European Society of Cardiology. Circulation 2007;116(19):2216–33.
[17] Baccouche H, Mahrholdt H, Meinhardt G, Merher R, Voehringer M, Hill S, et al. Diagnostic synergy of non-invasive cardiovascular magnetic resonance and invasive endomyocardial biopsy in troponin-positive patients without coronary artery disease. Eur Heart J 2009;30(23):2869–79.
[18] Scharhag J, Meyer T. Return to play after acute infectious disease in football players. J Sports Sci 2014;32(13):1237–42.
[19] Kiel RJ, Smith FE, Chason J, Khatib R, Reyes MP. Coxsackievirus B3 myocarditis in C3H/HeJ mice: description of an inbred model and the effect of exercise on virulence. Eur J Epidemiol 1989;5(3):348–50.
[20] Armstrong GT, Plana JC, Zhang N, Srivastava D, Green DM, Ness KK, et al. Screening adult survivors of childhood cancer for cardiomyopathy: comparison of echocardiography and cardiac magnetic resonance imaging. J Clin Oncol 2012;30(23):2876–84.
[21] Felker GM, Boehmer JP, Hruban RH, Hutchins GM, Kasper EK, Baughman KL, et al. Echocardiographic findings in fulminant and acute myocarditis. J Am Coll Cardiol 2000;36(1):227–32.
[22] Ferreira VM, Piechnik SK, Firoozan S, Karamitsos TD, Neubauer S. Acute chest pain and massive LV hypertrophy in a 38-year-old man. Heart 2014;100(4):347.
[23] Tsiamis E, Panagopoulou V, Aggeli C, Toutouzas K, Oikonomou E, Stefanadis C, et al. Segmental myocardial hypokinesis and hypertrophy as initial echocardiographic presentation of myocarditis. Int J Cardiol 2014;176(3):1460–1.

[24] Hiramitsu S, Morimoto S, Kato S, Uemura A, Kubo N, Kimura K, et al. Transient ventricular wall thickening in acute myocarditis: a serial echocardiographic and histopathologic study. Jpn Circ J 2001;65(10):863–6.
[25] Maeder M, Wolber T, Rickli H, Ammann P. Transient left ventricular "hypertrophy" in a woman with meningoencephalitis. Echocardiography 2006;23(7):582–4.
[26] Hsiao JF, Koshino Y, Bonnichsen CR, Yu Y, Miller Jr FA, Pellikka PA, et al. Speckle tracking echocardiography in acute myocarditis. Int J Cardiovasc Imaging 2013;29(2):275–84
[27] Di Bella G, Gaeta M, Pingitore A, Oreto G, Zito C, Minutoli F, et al. Myocardial deformation in acute myocarditis with normal left ventricular wall motion – a cardiac magnetic resonance and 2-dimensional strain echocardiographic study. Circ J 2010;74(6):1205–13.
[28] Escher F, Kasner M, Kuhl U, Heymer J, Wilkenshoff U, Tschope C, et al. New echocardiographic findings correlate with intramyocardial inflammation in endomyocardial biopsies of patients with acute myocarditis and inflammatory cardiomyopathy. Mediators Inflamm 2013;2013:875420.
[29] Lynch M, O'Donnell R, Weintraub NL, Lopez-Candales A. Assessment of mitral annular and velocity vector imaging in acute myopericarditis. Echocardiography 2013;30(8):E227–30.
[30] Khoo NS, Smallhorn JF, Atallah J, Kaneko S, Mackie AS, Paterson I. Altered left ventricular tissue velocities, deformation and twist in children and young adults with acute myocarditis and normal ejection fraction. J Am Soc Echocardiogr 2012;25(3):294–303.
[31] Lopez-Majano V. 67Gallium scintigraphy in myocarditis. Eur J Nucl Med 1982;7(3):141–2.
[32] Soussan M, Brillet PY, Nunes H, Pop G, Ouvrier MJ, Naggara N, et al. Clinical value of a high-fat and low-carbohydrate diet before FDG-PET/CT for evaluation of patients with suspected cardiac sarcoidosis. J Nucl Cardiol 2013;20(1):120–7.
[33] Kwong RL, Schussheim AE, Rekhraj S, Aletras AH, Geller N, Davis J, et al. Detecting acute coronary syndrome in the emergency department with cardiac magnetic resonance imaging. Circulation 2003;107:531–7.
[34] White JA, Fine NM, Gula L, Yee R, Skanes A, Klein G, et al. Utility of cardiovascular magnetic resonance in identifying substrate for malignant ventricular arrhythmias. Circ Cardiovasc Imaging 2012;5(1):12–20.
[35] Friedrich MG, Sechtem U, Schulz-Menger J, Holmvang G, Alakija P, Cooper LT, et al. Cardiovascular magnetic resonance in myocarditis: a JACC white paper. J Am Coll Cardiol 2009;53(17):1475–87.
[36] Zagrosek A, Abdel-Aty H, Boye P, Wassmuth R, Messroghli D, Utz W, ct al. Cardiac magnetic resonance monitors reversible and irreversible myocardial injury in myocarditis. JACC Cardiovasc Imaging 2009;2(2):131–8.
[37] Friedrich MG. Myocardial edema – a new clinical entity? Nat Rev Cardiol 2010;7(5):292–6.
[38] Abdel-Aty H, Zagrosek A, Schulz-Menger J, Taylor AJ, Messroghli D, Kumar A, et al. Delayed enhancement and T2-weighted cardiovascular magnetic resonance imaging differentiate acute from chronic myocardial infarction. Circulation 2004;109(20):2411–6.
[39] Aletras AH, Kellman P, Derbyshire JA, Arai AE. ACUT2E TSE-SSFP: a hybrid method for T2-weighted imaging of edema in the heart. Magn Reson Med 2008;59(2):229–35.
[40] Kellman P, Aletras AH, Mancini C, McVeigh ER, Arai AE. T2-prepared SSFP improves diagnostic confidence in edema imaging in acute myocardial infarction compared to turbo spin echo. Magn Reson Med 2007;57(5):891–7.

[41] Zagrosek A, Wassmuth R, Abdel-Aty H, Rudolph A, Dietz R, Schulz-Menger J. Relation between myocardial edema and myocardial mass during the acute and convalescent phase of myocarditis – a CMR study. J Cardiovasc Magn Reson 2008;10(1):19.
[42] Abdel-Aty H, Boye P, Zagrosek A, Wassmuth R, Kumar A, Messroghli D, et al. Diagnostic performance of cardiovascular magnetic resonance in patients with suspected acute myocarditis: comparison of different approaches. J Am Coll Cardiol 2005;45(11):1815–22.
[43] Zagrosek A, Messroghli D, Schulz O, Dietz R, Schulz-Menger J. Effect of binge drinking on the heart as assessed by cardiac magnetic resonance imaging. JAMA 2010;304(12):1328–30.
[44] Monney PA, Sekhri N, Burchell T, Knight C, Davies C, Deaner A, et al. Acute myocarditis presenting as acute coronary syndrome: role of early cardiac magnetic resonance in its diagnosis. Heart 2011;97(16):1312–8.
[45] Friedrich MG, Strohm O, Schulz-Menger J, Marciniak H, Luft FC, Dietz R. Contrast media-enhanced magnetic resonance imaging visualizes myocardial changes in the course of viral myocarditis. Circulation 1998;97(18):1802–9.
[46] Chu GC, Flewitt JA, Mikami Y, Vermes E, Friedrich MG. Assessment of acute myocarditis by cardiovascular MR: diagnostic performance of shortened protocols. Int J Cardiovasc Imaging 2013;29(5):1077–83.
[47] Taylor AJ, Vaddadi G, Pfluger H, Butler M, Bergin P, Leet A, et al. Diagnostic performance of multisequential cardiac magnetic resonance imaging in acute cardiac allograft rejection. Eur J Heart Fail 2010;12(1):45–51.
[48] Mahrholdt H, Goedecke C, Wagner A, Meinhardt G, Athanasiadis A, Vogelsberg H, et al. Cardiovascular magnetic resonance assessment of human myocarditis: a comparison to histology and molecular pathology. Circulation 2004;109(10):1250–8.
[49] Mahrholdt H, Wagner A, Deluigi CC, Kispert E, Hager S, Meinhardt G, et al. Presentation, patterns of myocardial damage, and clinical course of viral myocarditis. Circulation 2006;114(15):1581–90.
[50] Grun S, Schumm J, Greulich S, Wagner A, Schneider S, Bruder O, et al. Long-term follow-up of biopsy-proven viral myocarditis: predictors of mortality and incomplete recovery. J Am Coll Cardiol 2012;59(18):1604–15.
[51] Giri S, Chung YC, Merchant A, Mihai G, Rajagopalan S, Raman SV, et al. T2 quantification for improved detection of myocardial edema. J Cardiovasc Magn Reson 2009;11(1):56.
[52] von Knobelsdorff-Brenkenhoff F, Prothmann M, Dieringer MA, Wassmuth R, Greiser A, Schwenke C, et al. Myocardial T1 and T2 mapping at 3T: reference values, influencing factors and implications. J Cardiovasc Magn Reson 2013;15(1):53.
[53] Thavendiranathan P, Walls M, Giri S, Verhaert D, Rajagopalan S, Moore S, et al. Improved detection of myocardial involvement in acute inflammatory cardiomyopathies using T2 mapping. Circ Cardiovasc Imaging 2012;5(1):102–10.
[54] Wassmuth R, Prothmann M, Utz W, Dieringer M, von Knobelsdorff-Brenkenhoff F, Greiser A, et al. Variability and homogeneity of cardiovascular magnetic resonance myocardial T2-mapping in volunteers compared to patients with edema. J Cardiovasc Magn Reson 2013;15(1):27.
[55] Ferreira VM, Piechnik SK, Dall'Armellina E, Karamitsos TD, Francis JM, Ntusi N, et al. T(1) mapping for the diagnosis of acute myocarditis using CMR: comparison to T2-weighted and late gadolinium enhanced imaging. JACC Cardiovasc Imaging 2013;6(10):1048–58.
[56] Ferreira VM, Piechnik SK, Dall'Armellina E, Karamitsos TD, Francis JM, Ntusi N, et al. Native T1-mapping detects the location, extent and patterns of acute myocarditis without the need for gadolinium contrast agents. J Cardiovasc Magn Reson 2014;16:36.

[57] Luetkens JA, Doerner J, Thomas DK, Dabir D, Gieseke J, Sprinkart AM, et al. Acute myocarditis: multiparametric cardiac MR imaging. Radiology 2014;273(2):383–92.
[58] Radunski UK, Lund GK, Stehning C, Schnackenburg B, Bohnen S, Adam G, et al. CMR in patients with severe myocarditis: diagnostic value of quantitative tissue markers including extracellular volume imaging. JACC Cardiovasc Imaging 2014;7(7):667–75.
[59] Taylor AJ, Cerqueira M, Hodgson JM, Mark D, Min J, O'Gara P, et al. ACCF/SCCT/ACR/AHA/ASE/ASNC/NASCI/SCAI/SCMR 2010 Appropriate Use Criteria for Cardiac Computed Tomography. A Report of the American College of Cardiology Foundation Appropriate Use Criteria Task Force, the Society of Cardiovascular Computed Tomography, the American College of Radiology, the American Heart Association, the American Society of Echocardiography, the American Society of Nuclear Cardiology, the North American Society for Cardiovascular Imaging, the Society for Cardiovascular Angiography and Interventions, and the Society for Cardiovascular Magnetic Resonance. Circulation 2010;122(21):e525–55.
[60] Schoenhagen P, Dewey M. CT assessment of coronary artery disease: trends and clinical implications. JACC Cardiovasc Imaging 2013;6(10):1072–4.
[61] Brett NJ, Strugnell WE, Slaughter RE. Acute myocarditis demonstrated on CT coronary angiography with MRI correlation. Circ Cardiovasc Imaging 2011;4(3):e5–6.
[62] Axsom K, Lin F, Weinsaft JW, Min JK. Evaluation of myocarditis with delayed-enhancement computed tomography. J Cardiovasc Comput Tomogr 2009;3(6):409–11.
[63] Ferreira ND, Bettencourt N, Rocha J, Leite D, Carvalho M, Teixeira M, et al. Diagnosis of acute myopericarditis by delayed-enhancement multidetector computed tomography. J Am Coll Cardiol 2012;60(9):868.
[64] Bories MC, Nicollet E, Amrar-Vennier F, Gonin S, Goube P, Toussaint M. Contribution of 64-slice cardiac tomodensitometry for non-invasive diagnosis of acute myocarditis. Ann Cardiol Angeiol (Paris) 2012;61(5):317–22.

Systemic diseases

M. Lombardi*, A. Gimelli†, M. Galderisi‡

*IRCCS, Policlinico San Donato, Milan, Italy; †UOC Nuclear Medicine at Fondazione CNR/Regione Toscana 'G. Monasterio', Pisa, Italy; ‡Federico II University Hospital, Naples, Italy

15.1 Arterial systemic hypertension

Arterial systemic hypertension is a well established, leading cardiovascular (CV) risk factor for morbidity and mortality in the general population. Myocardial infarction, heart failure, and sudden death are the main fatal and non-fatal complications in hypertensive patients [1]. The clinical consequences of hypertension on the heart derive from chronic pressure overload, such as to induce left ventricular (LV) structural and functional alterations, which define hypertensive heart disease. The development of LV hypertrophy (LVH) is of hinge importance since it increases the risk for CV outcomes by a factor of 3–5-fold [2]. Hypertensive heart disease is clinically asymptomatic but manifests at a more advanced stage as angina pectoris, dyspnoea, and palpitation. These symptoms can be attributed to a reduced coronary flow reserve (CFR), impaired diastolic function, and arrhythmias [3,4].

Echocardiographic examination is the first-step imaging technique for diagnosing hypertensive heart disease because of its relatively low cost, prompt availability, and suitability for serial examinations and patient follow-up. Echo-Doppler examination is currently used to detect LV remodelling and LVH [5] as well as LV diastolic dysfunction (DD) [6] and also to unmask regional wall motion abnormalities [7] and the onset of coronary artery disease (CAD).

The estimation of LV geometry and LV mass (LVM) has been one of the most studied issues by echocardiography in the epidemiologic studies and treatment trials in the last three decades [8,9]. LV geometric patterns of hypertensive heart are identified according to a classification which combines the values of relative wall thickness (RWT) and LVM index (Figure 15.1) [10]. LVM (indexed for body surface area [BSA] or, better, for height) identifies LVH according to standardized cut-off point values (Table 15.1) [5]. LV concentric remodelling and LVH are independent predictors of morbidity and mortality in the general population [2,11,12]. Reduction of LVM can be obtained by different kinds of anti-hypertensive treatments [13,14] and improves prognosis in hypertensive patients [15–17]. Further information could be added by the calculation of midwall fractional shortening, obtainable by mathematical model from linear measures of LV cavity size and wall thickness at end-diastole and end-systole [18]. Midwall shortening should be preferred to ejection fraction (EF) in the presence of LV concentric geometry, in which the prognostic power of this parameter has been reported [19,20]. The assessment of LV systolic function in hypertensive heart disease,

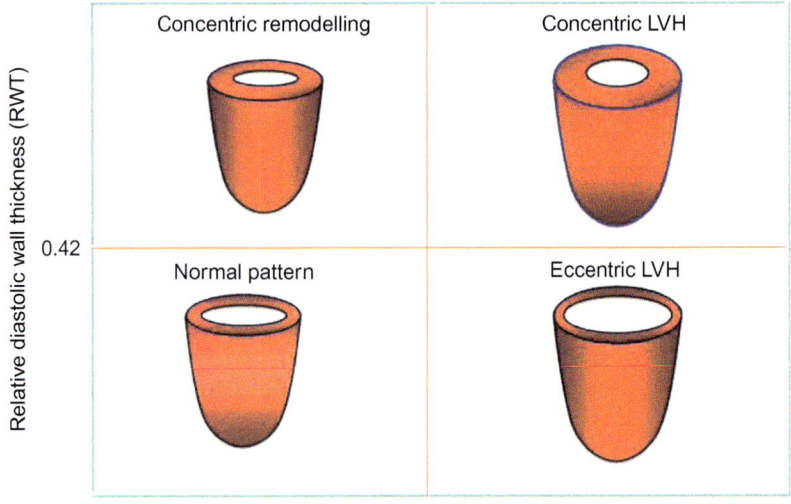

Figure 15.1 Left ventricular geometric patterns in arterial systemnic hypertension.

Table 15.1 **Sex-specific echocardiographic cut-off pint values of LVH and its severity**

Parameter	Reference range	Mild LVH	Moderate LVH	Severe LVH
Women				
LVM/BSA (g/m^2)	43–95	96–108	109–121	≥122
LVM/height (g/m)	41–99	100–115	116–128	≥129
LVM/height$^{2.7}$ (g/m$^{2.7}$)	18–44	45–51	52–58	≥59
Men				
LVM/BSA (g/m^2)	49–115	116–131	132–148	≥149
LVM/height (g/m)	52–126	127–144	145–162	≥163
LVM/height$^{2.7}$ (g/m$^{2.7}$)	20–48	49–55	56–63	≥64

BSA = body surface area; LVM = left ventricular mass.
Modified from Lang et al. [5].

however, does not add prognostic information to the assessment of LVM, at least in the context of a normal LV systolic function [21].

The progression of hypertensive heart towards heart failure includes serial LV structural and geometric abnormalities (mainly myocardial fibrosis) [22] corresponding to LV concentric remodelling and LVH. In presence of these abnormalities, parallel alterations in LV diastolic properties occur and are globally defined as LV

DD. DD includes alterations of both relaxation and filling [23], precede LV chamber systolic dysfunction, and can *per se* induce symptoms/signs of heart failure even when EF is still normal (heart failure with normal EF). In this context, the simple Doppler transmitral inflow pattern is not sufficient to stratify the hypertensive prognosis and should be combined with further manoeuvers (Valsalva) applied to the assessment of LV filling and/or additional Doppler parameters (i.e., difference between pulmonary flow atrial reverse and mitral inflow A velocity, ratio between mitral inflow *E* velocity and early relaxation velocity of the mitral annulus on pulsed tissue Doppler [*E/e'* ratio] and left atrial volume index) [24]. *E/e'* ratio is highly feasible and accurate in the clinical setting [25] (Figure 15.2) and its value is highlighted in the recent ESC/ESH guidelines on arterial hypertension to detect early cardiac organ damage of hypertensive patients [26] (Table 15.2). The prognostic value of *e'* is recognized in the hypertensive setting [27]. Recently, the ASCOT Study highlighted the prognostic value of *E/e'* ratio, independent on traditional echocardiographic measurements (including LVM index and RWT) during a mean follow-up of 4.2 years of 980 hypertensive patients [28].

Among the advanced echocardiographic techniques, important insights can be gained by 2-D speckle tracking echocardiography, which allows the quantifying of the regional and global longitudinal strain (GLS) of subendocardial fibres with good accuracy [29]. An early impairment of GLS has been observed in pre-hypertensive stages [30] and in firstly diagnosed hypertensives [31] when EF is still normal (Figure 15.3). GLS progressively deteriorates in hypertensive heart disease, passing from NYHA I

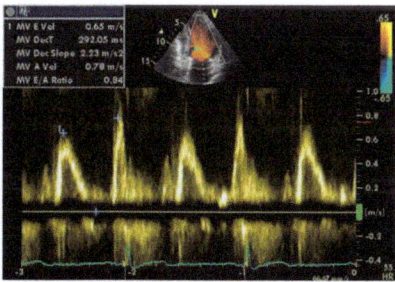

E/A ratio = 0.84

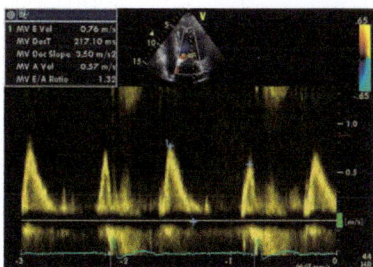

E/A ratio = 1.32

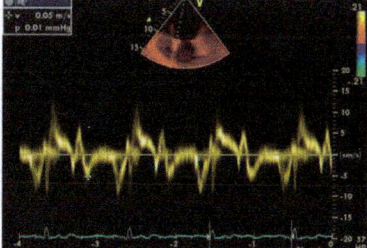

E/e' ratio = 15.2

Figure 15.2 Methodology for calculating *E/e'* ratio. Inb the upper panel transmitral flow, in the lower panel pulsed tissue Doppler of the mitral annulus.

Table 15.2 **Normal range and cut-off values for parameters used in the assessment of LV remodelling in patients with hypertension**

Parameter	Upper cut-off value
LV mass index (g/m^2)	>95 (women)
	>115 (men)
Relative wall thickness (RWT)	≥0.42
Diastolic function	
Septal e' (cm/s)	<8
Lateral e' (cm/s)	<10
LA volume index (ml/m^2)	≥34
LV filling pressures	
E/e' (averaged) ratio	≥13

Modified from 2013 ESC/ESH guidelines on diagnosis and management of arterial hypertension.

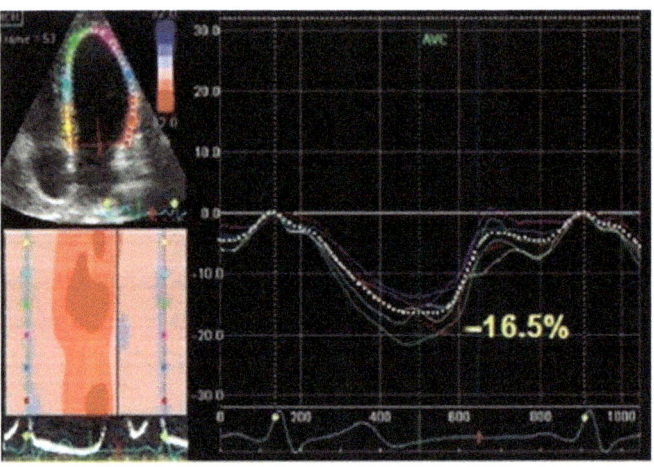

Figure 15.3 Methodology for calculating longitudinal strain. The white dotted line is the average longitudinal strain.

to IV class while LV circumferential systolic reduction becomes overt only in NYHA III and IV classes [32].

All LVM algorithms (M-mode, 2-D, 3-D) are based upon the subtraction of LV cavity volume from the volume enclosed by LV epicardium ("shell" volume) to obtain a myocardial volume, which is then multiplied by the specific weight of the myocardium (1.055 g/ml). The original ASE formula, which is based on M-mode linear measurements [33], is still currently used for the estimation of LVM. It may be considered appropriate for evaluating patients with normal LV geometry, but its accuracy is suboptimal (standard error of estimate from 29 to 97 g, 95% confidence interval [CI] 57–190 g) in comparison with post-mortem LVM [25,33]. The calculation of LVM from real-time three-dimensional

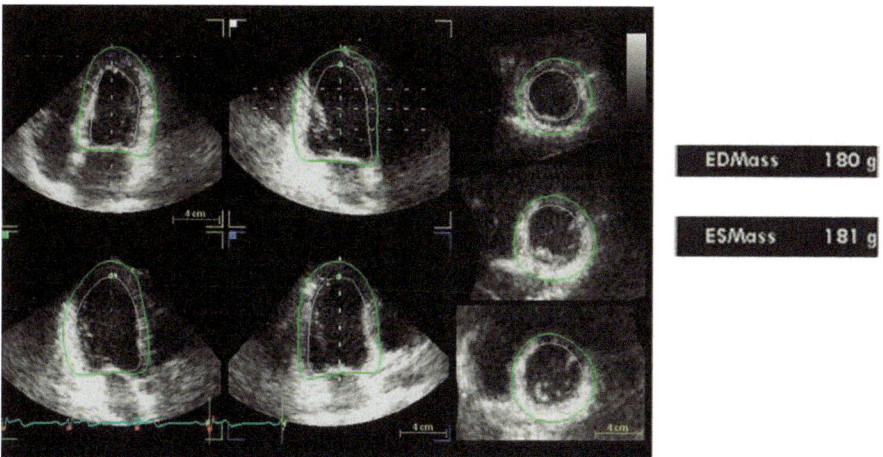

Figure 15.4 Methodology for obtaining left ventricular mass by 3D echocardiography. In agreement with the conservation of the mass, end-diastolic (ED) and end-systolic (ES) values shall be equal or, at least, very similar.

echocardiography (RT3DE) removes geometric assumptions of LV shape and reduces errors due to foreshortened views [34,35] (Figure 15.4). RT3DE-derived LVM has been validated against post-mortem measurement and cardiac magnetic resonance ($K = 0.92$ and 0.91, respectively) [34]. A much lower LVM underestimation versus cardiac magnetic resonance has been found using RT3DE rather than 2D echocardiography [34]. The very good reproducibility of LVM with RT3DE (intra-observer variability = 7–12.5%) [34,35] could significantly reduce sample size to assess LVM changes as compared to M-mode/and 2-D echocardiography [36]. However, nowadays, due to the superior inter- and intra-observer repeatability cardiac magnetic resonance is considered the gold standard in the assessment of LVM and is used to this purpose in modern clinical trials to evaluate the drug capability in reducing LVM [37].

Another possible application of cardiac magnetic resonance (CMR) is the evaluation of RV free wall mass, as the right sections can also be involved in the hypertrophic process. In fact, systemic hypertension might be associated with concentric right ventricular remodelling independently from the haemodynamic stress. Structural and functional right ventricular adaptation to systemic hypertension tends to parallel the homologous modifications induced by systemic haemodynamic overload on the left ventricle [38].

Specific procedures are reserved for the diagnosis of myocardial ischemia in hypertensive patients [39]. This is very challenging because hypertension strongly lowers the specificity of exercise ECG and perfusion scintigraphy. When exercise-ECG is positive (or ambiguous), an imaging test of inducible ischemia [40,41] is requested for a reliable identification of epicardial coronary artery stenosis. Stress echocardiography has higher specificity than exercise ECG or perfusion scintigraphy, with a similar sensitivity. Among the different types of stress, pharmacological stressors (dobutamine, dipyridamole, and adenosine) have higher feasibility than exercise testing, especially vasodilator testing. Stress-induced wall motion abnormalities are highly specific for the diagnosis of epicardial coronary artery stenosis, whereas myocardial perfusion abnormalities are frequently found also in presence of angiographically normal coronary arteries. This can occur in patients with LVH because of coronary microvascular disease [39]. Recent recommendations suggest the use of dual echo imaging of regional wall motion and CFR on left anterior descending artery to differentiate obstructive CAD (reduced coronary reserve + inducible wall motion abnormalities) from isolated coronary microcirculatory damage (reduced coronary reserve without wall motion abnormalities) [41]. While the use of stress cardiac magnetic resonance (dobutamine, adenosine, and dipyridamole) has been proven to be very accurate in ischemic heart disease, it is still under development in non-ischemic heart diseases. However, it might be already considered as a possible alternative to echocardiography and nuclear medicine.

Positron emission tomography (PET) offers the unique capability of measuring absolute myocardial flow (flow per unit of mass) *in vivo* by means of a regional, tridimensional, non-invasive approach. Using PET, myocardial perfusion abnormalities secondary to microvascular disorders have been investigated in arterial hypertension as well as in hypertrophic cardiomyopathy. In arterial hypertension, regional perfusion at rest is within the normal range, while the coronary reserve and flow response to increase in metabolic demand are blunted (Figure 15.5). These flow abnormalities are independent of the degree of cardiac hypertrophy and the severity of arterial

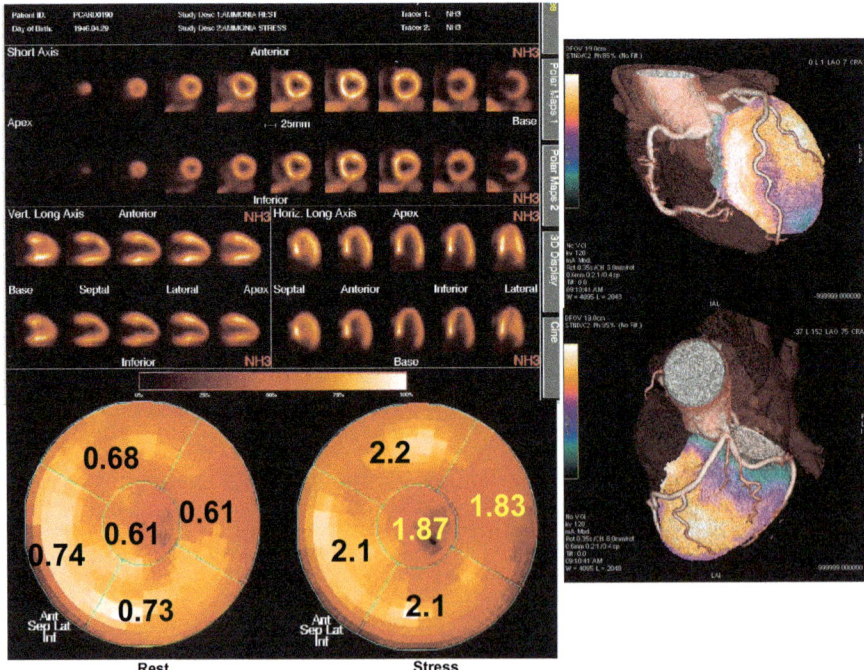

Figure 15.5 Coronary flow reserve determined by PET in a patient with normal epicardial coronary arteries.

hypertension; appropriate anti-hypertensive therapy is able to improve the perfusion abnormalities after long-term treatment, independently of the effect on myocardial hypertrophy. Hypertrophic cardiomyopathy demonstrates abnormal vasodilating capability, which has been shown to be present in the subclinical form of dilated cardiomyopathy; the reduction of coronary reserve is not related to the presence and extent of the haemodynamic impairment, and involves also non-hypertrophied myocardium in asymmetric hypertrophic cardiomyopathy. These findings indicate a primary involvement of coronary microcirculation in non-advanced forms of dilated and hypertrophic cardiomyopathy [42].

15.2 Diabetic cardiomyopathy

The first demonstration of a distinct diabetic cardiomyopathy occurred in the early 1990s, when the Framingham Study demonstrated an increase of LVM in diabetic women, independent of the effects of other common risk factors [43]. Subsequent studies confirmed these results in both genders, pointing out associations of both type 2 diabetes mellitus (DM2) and glucose intolerance (GI) with LV structure abnormalities (LV concentric remodelling/hypertrophy), independent of the influence of relevant covariates [44–47]. GI and DM2 were also found to negatively affect midwall systolic mechanics [46] and LV diastolic filling [48], even in the presence of normal chamber function [46], with an impact amplified by the coexistence of hypertension [48]. These findings have now been complemented by the ability of echo-Doppler techniques to identify, categorize, and quantify alteration of LV function and CFR.

15.2.1 Diabetes and LV diastolic dysfunction

A Doppler pattern of impaired LV relaxation is an early sign of DD (grade I) while more advanced grades (predominant early diastolic filling and rapid velocity deceleration, i.e., restrictive filling patterns) are associated with the most severe LV decompensation [49]. The crucial point of this grading is the intermediary, pseudonormal pattern, which occurs when LV filling pressure (LVFP) rises to keep cardiac output in the normal range and increases the early filling caused by impaired relaxation. Pseudonormal and normal patterns cannot be distinguished by transmitral inflow because of its preload dependence [49]. Accordingly, transmitral E/A ratio was found to exhibit 'U shape' prognostic behaviour in the Strong Heart Study (high prevalence of DM): subjects with values <0.6 (abnormal relaxation) and >1.5 (likely restrictive pattern) were both associated with increased mortality, but the intermediate range (0.6–1.5), encompassing patients with normal or unidentified, pseudonormal patterns, had no significant prognostic impact [50].

These dynamics are of great importance in DM2 without CAD, when abnormal LV relaxation is manifest but systolic function is still normal. When dyspnoea becomes overt, these abnormalities characterize "isolated" diastolic heart failure. Myocardial fibrosis and apoptosis [51] are likely the basis of these changes. Over time, diabetics may transition to a pseudonormal pattern. At this stage, accurate evaluation of DD requires additional analysis of Valsalva manoeuver, pulmonary venous flow, and/or left atrial volume determination [52]. A pseudonormal pattern was unmasked in 28% of diabetics by Valsalva manoeuver (*E/A* ratio decrease ≥25%) and/or pulmonary venous flow (atrial reverse velocity duration longer than mitral A duration) [53]. In this context, the combination of pulsed tissue Doppler with transmitral inflow may be very useful to characterize DD and elevated LVFP since early diastolic peak velocity (*E'*) of the mitral annulus reflects the rate of myocardial relaxation and is relatively insensitive to preload effects [54]. The ratio *E/e'* has been validated as reliable index of LVFP [27]. A reduction of annular *e'* was demonstrated in recent onset DM2 [55]. In 25 type 1 diabetics, increased *E/e'* ratio was associated with left atrial enlargement and correlated independently with glycosylated haemoglobin [56], thus confirming the association between level of glycemic control and DD [48]. *E/E'* ratio may be, therefore, used to detect and follow the progression of DD in DM.

15.2.2 Diabetes and coronary microvascular dysfunction

Alterations of myocardial composition and, thus, of diastolic properties and LVFP might be mediated by changes in the coronary microcirculation. Microvascular damage of DM2 [57] may lead to myocardial cell injury and reactive fibrosis/hypertrophy. Although focal microvascular alterations have not appeared sufficient to account for diffuse interstitial fibrosis [58], these observations looked at structure but not dynamics of coronary microvessels. Today, the function of coronary circulation may be evaluated by transthoracic echocardiography, by visualizing the distal left anterior descending artery [59,60], and measuring CFR as hyperemic to resting velocities ratio [59,60]. CFR has excellent concordance with intracoronary Doppler flow wire-derived CFR, high feasibility, and reproducibility [59]. In the absence of epicardial coronary stenosis, impaired CFR indicates coronary microvascular dysfunction [60]. A reduction of CFR has been documented in both type 1 and 2 DM (Figure 15.6) and appears as a direct consequence of elevated glycemia, as demonstrated by PET [61]. An alternative explanation is insulin resistance, which alters CFR during cold pressure test, a completely endothelium-dependent stimulus [62]. Endothelial function, another possible determinant of CFR, is impaired in early DM [63]. Also, increased cardiac sympathetic activity may account for abnormal CFR in diabetics [64].

15.2.3 The link of coronary microvascular and diastolic dysfunction in diabetes

DD is evident in type 1 diabetics free of CAD when CFR impairment is also detectable [64]. Similar relation between magnitude of CFR reduction and degree of myocardial DD was found also in uncomplicated hypertension without significant CAD [65], This association is not surprising, since coronary flow occurs predominantly during diastole. Both reduced CFR and DD are associated with insulin resistance [63,66], LV concentric geometry [4,48], sympathetic nervous system disorders [64], abnormalities of angiotensin–renin system [67], and endothelial dysfunction [68]. Therefore, coronary microvascular damage could play a mechanistic role for DD [69] or even vice versa, considering DD as a main expression of myocardial fibrosis. Determinants

Systemic diseases

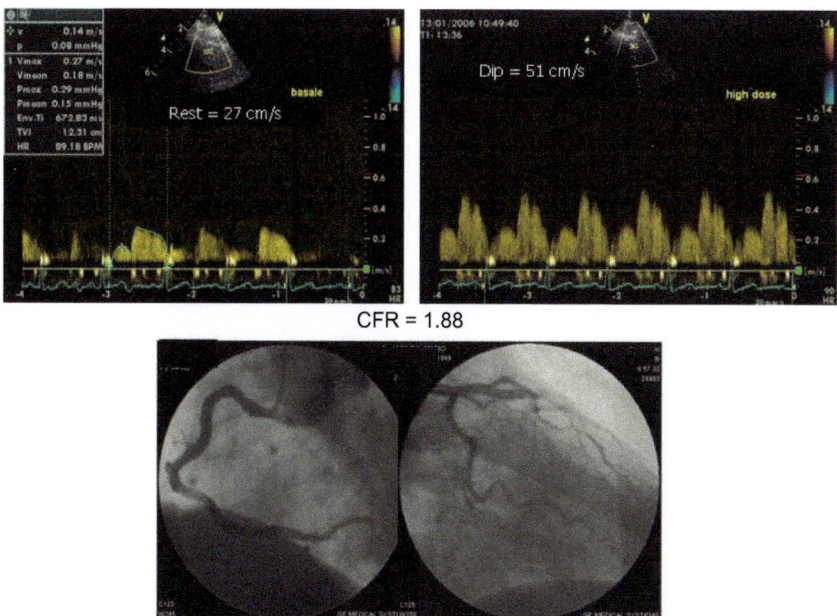

Figure 15.6 Reduced transthoracic Doppler-derived coronary flow reserve in diabetic patient with normal coronary angiography.

of microvascular dysfunction in DM, such as hyperglycemia and insulin resistance, and factors including sympathetic overdrive, endothelial dysfunction, and LV concentric remodelling, also contribute to the development of DD. Systolic contractile failure may be a further consequence, due to impairment of both diastolic properties and coronary microcirculation (Figure 15.7). A comprehensive transthoracic Doppler evaluation of diabetics should include, therefore, the assessment of diastolic function with estimation of LVFP by tissue Doppler, and of coronary microvascular function by CFR test. Analysis of the regional wall motion during stress would be required in patients with suspected CAD, another cause of DD.

15.3 Inotropic reserve in diabetic patients

Further documentation of diabetic cardiomyopathy can be obtained by assessing the inotropic response to physical or pharmacological stress in uncomplicated diabetic patients. This issue has been investigated by using Doppler-derived strain rate (SR) imaging, a technique able to produce indexes strongly related to invasively determined myocardial elastance and, therefore, to inform on the real LV inotropic state [70]. By using colour tissue Doppler, Fang and coworkers, 2003, demonstrated reduction at rest of longitudinal myocardial systolic velocities, and systolic SR [71,72] in multiple wall regions, in a sample of DM2 patients with normal EF and no evidence of CAD. The reduction of SR paralleled increased myocardial density derived by integrated backscatter, indicating interstitial fibrosis. The reduced increment of SR (and strain)

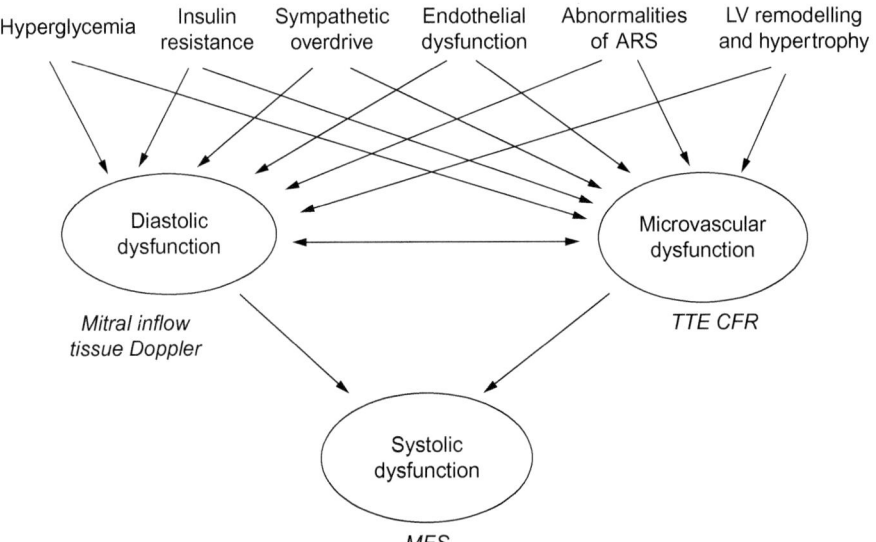

Figure 15.7 Suggested mechanisms underlying the relationships of coronary microvessel dysfunction and left ventricular function in diabetes mellitus. ARS = Angiotensin Renin System, CFR = Coronary Flow Reserve, MFS = Midwall Fractional Shortening, TTE = Trans-Thoracic Echocardiography.

at increasing dobutamine stage indicates altered myocardial inotropic reserve in diabetics free of CAD.

Myocardial contractility can be studied also by assessing variations of pressure/volume relation at increasing heart beating, i.e., the force–frequency relation [73]. This "force–frequency relation" has been shown to be blunted in isolated myocardial strips of DM2 patients [74]. In a study of [75], "regional" (septal) strain–frequency relation, built by plotting all together individuals values of heart rate (HR) and strain both at rest and during dobutamine (low and high doses), simulated a "global" force–frequency relation: HR and strain were closely related in diabetics as in controls, but the slope of the relation was significantly blunted in diabetics, demonstrating that HR increase is unable to track a normal increment of contractility in the diabetic heart (Figure 15.8). It is conceivable that underlying alterations of coronary microvessels, recognized in diabetic patients, might be responsible for their reduced inotropic response to stress [69].

The incidence of CAD in patients with diabetes is known to be higher than in non-diabetic patients. While the systematic evaluation of these patients is performed by echocardiography, CMR has been proven to have adjunctive value as it allows the detection of unexpected areas of myocardial necrosis by LE technique. The presence of unknown and clinically silent myocardial infarction heavily influences the prognosis of these patients and justifies a more aggressive diagnostic and therapeutic approach.

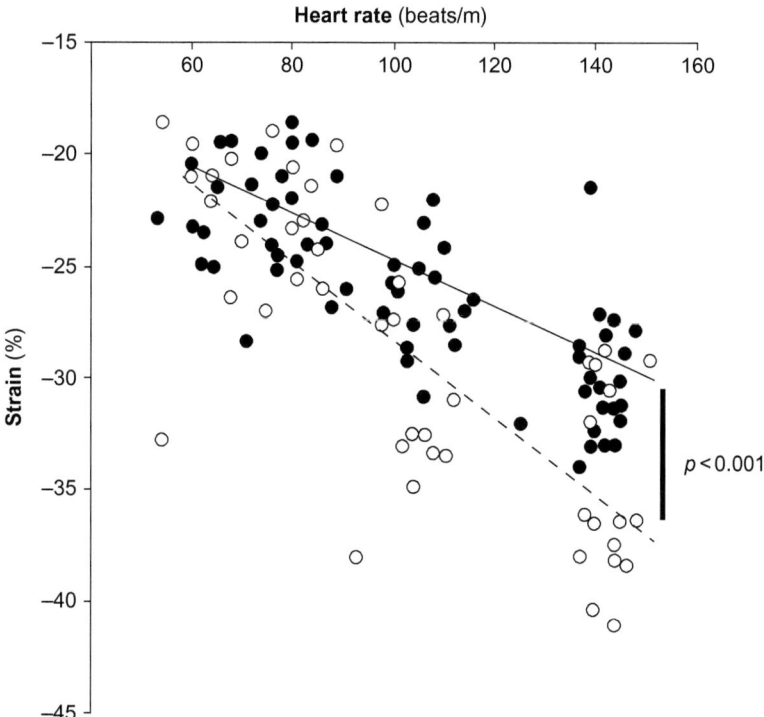

Figure 15.8 Scatter plot and regression line of individual values of heart rate (x-axis) and corresponding values of longitudinal strain (y-axis) in diabetic patients (= filled circles) and normal controls (= open circles) at any level of dobutamine test (rest, low-dose and high-dose dobutamine). Solid line = slope of the relation in diabetic, dotted line = slope of relation in normal controls (Ref. [75]).

Diabetic patients are more prone to atherosclerosis and have more CAD, which may stay subclinical longer due to blunted symptomatology. Accordingly, Cardiac CT could be used for early detection of CAD in the absence of symptoms.

15.4 Metabolic syndrome

Obesity, insulin resistance, GI/type 2 diabetes, hypertension, pro-inflammatory state, and prothrombotic state are clustered in the metabolic syndrome (MS), representing critical risk factors for increased incidence of cardio–cerebro-vascular diseases [76]. Abdominal obesity is the form of obesity most strongly associated with the MS. Insulin correlates univariately with the risk of developing cardiovascular diseases (CVD). Patients with longstanding insulin resistance frequently manifest GI, which might evolve into diabetes-level hyperglycemia. Elevated blood pressure strongly associates with obesity and commonly occurs in insulin-resistant persons. Hypertension thus commonly is listed among metabolic risk factors, even if it is multifactorial in origin.

The presence of dyslipidemia, such as raised triglycerides, low concentrations of HDL cholesterol, increased remnant lipoproteins, elevated apolipoprotein B, small LDL particles, and small HDL particles can also be found.

Finally, a pro-inflammatory state, represented by elevated serum C-reactive protein, is commonly present in persons with MS. Obesity itself is supposed to play a determinant role as excess adipose tissue releases inflammatory cytokines that may elicit higher serum C-reactive protein levels. Some patients manifested a pro-thrombotic state, characterized by increased plasma plasminogen activator inhibitor-1 and fibrinogen. Fibrinogen rises in response to a high-cytokine state.

MS is associated with a 2-fold increase in the relative risk of coronary heart disease and stroke events [77]. Recently, MS has also been linked to increased prevalence of aortic valve calcification [78,79], faster progression of calcific aortic stenosis [80], increased arterial stiffness [81], and faster degeneration of aortic bioprosthetic valves [82]. Moreover, recent experimental studies [83,84] reveal that, among animals with sustained pressure overload, those with insulin resistance induced by a high carbohydrate/high-fat diet have more severe LVH and dysfunction compared with animals fed with a standard diet. These findings suggest that not only valvular lesion, but also LV remodelling and function might be negatively influenced by the MS.

With regard to echocardiographic parameters, hypertensive patients with MS exhibited higher LVM (even normalized by BSA), RWT, left atrial size, and greater prevalence of LVH, lower mid-wall fractional shortening, and a longer E-wave deceleration time than subjects without MS. These results were independent from other variables such as age, gender distribution, severity and duration of hypertension, and previous anti-hypertensive therapy. In particular, after adjustment for these covariates, the likelihood of LVH was 2.89-fold higher in subjects with MS than in those without it, when LVM was indexed by height 2.7. Moreover, it is noteworthy that the relationship between MS and LVM was confirmed in multivariate regression models including MS together with its individual components, as independent variables; this suggests that MS may have a deleterious effect on cardiac structure over and above the potential contribution of each single component of this syndrome, and that the confluence of abnormalities that comprise MS may have a synergistic negative impact on LVM independently from patients with or without hypertension are considered [85,86]. In the Strong Heart Study, a longitudinal investigation conducted in American-Indian communities, a subset of the study population, including 1436 non-diabetic participants without prevalent CVD (61.2% of which had high BP), was examined to analyse the impact of the MS on cardiac structure and function. Subjects with MS showed greater LV dimension, mass and RWT, and left atrial diameter, and a higher prevalence of LVH, with lower mid-wall shortening than those who did not have MS [85]. Cuspidi et al. [86], in untreated middle-aged hypertensives, found that patients with MS had a more pronounced cardiac and extra-cardiac involvement than those without it. For example, the latter might be explained by insulin resistance and the accompanying compensatory hyperinsulinaemia, which are regarded as the patho-physiological key features underlying the MS [76]. Despite conflicting results [47], it is believed that the trophic effects of insulin on myocardial could be mediated, at least in part, by the insulin-like growth factor-1 receptors [87]. It has also to be considered that insulin may affect LVM indirectly by increasing sodium retention [88] or endothelin-1 levels

[89] or by inducing sympathetic activation [90] or by biological mediators of LVH, such as angiotensin II secreted from white adipose tissue, a potent growth factor in myocardial tissue [91], and leptin, whose mitogenic effect in cardiomyocytes has been recently evaluated with discrepant conclusions [92].

Considering these pathologic aspects, there are several findings, which are currently investigated by imaging techniques such as cardiac volumes, mass, systolic and diastolic function, arterial intima thickness, etc. While echocardiography is routinely used to evaluate these aspects, it is notable that some other measurements are noteworthy for a better comprehension of the disease itself. Namely, the measurement of epicardial and pericardial fat by echo or more efficiently by MRI suggests new insights on the disease and its intrinsic mechanisms [93–95] (Figure 15.9).

In patients with high likelihood of CAD, myocardial perfusion abnormalities at gated single-photon emission computed tomography (g-SPECT) are associated with a poor prognosis [96]. In fact, the annual risk of cardiac death or non-fatal myocardial infarction is <1% in the case of a normal stress g-SPECT, whereas the risk increases up to 8% with an increasing degree of perfusion abnormalities. Furthermore, the magnitude of perfusion abnormalities is the single most important indicator of an unfavourable outcome and provides independent and incremental information within respect to clinical, stress electrocardiographic, and coronary angiographic findings [97]. In this scenario, and in the view of using SPECT to predict CAD, reversible myocardial perfusion defects in patients without significant coronary stenoses are regarded as a "false-positive" result. Although these false-positive defects occur in a low number of patients studied by g-SPECT [98,99], their physiological meaning and prognostic implication are very important.

A functional and/or structural impairment in coronary microcirculation is a possible interpretation of these findings. Zeiher et al. [100] showed that an endothelial dysfunction of coronary microcirculation is associated with a high incidence of reversible defects at stress myocardial perfusion imaging in the absence of coronary stenosis. According to these authors, this feature may represent a stenosis-independent abnormality in blood flow distribution rather than the effect of technical artefacts. An abnormal flow reserve has been documented using PET in the myocardium of hypertensive patients in the absence of coronary stenosis [101] and has been attributed to the

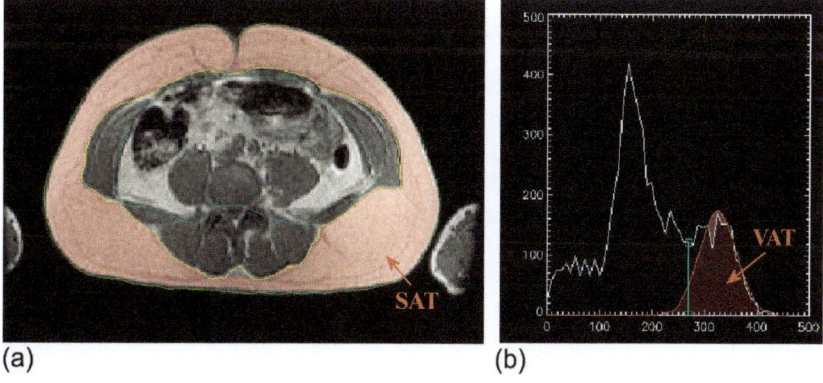

Figure 15.9 Measurements of epicardial and pericardial fat by CMR.

hypertrophy of the tunica media of small resistance vessels. Abnormalities in coronary blood flow and reserve have also been observed using PET in the myocardium perfused by normal coronary arteries of patients with coronary stenoses in remote vessels [102]. Furthermore, a reduction in coronary blood flow reserve has been documented in diabetic patients with angiographically normal coronary arteries by intra-coronary Doppler [103], trans-esophageal Doppler echocardiography [104], and PET [105]. In addition, the angiography was normal in 11–63% of diabetics with positive perfusion studies [106]. Abnormal values of myocardial blood flow have also been found in patients with dilated cardiomyopathy [107]. Finally, patients with chest pain and reversible myocardial perfusion defects at stress SPECT, but without obstructive CAD, have lower flow-mediated dilation, that is indicative of endothelial dysfunction, as compared with the patients with normal myocardial perfusion findings [108]. In agreement with the above studies, stress-induced myocardial perfusion abnormalities observed by g-SPECT in patients with normal or near normal coronary arteries can reflect a functional and/or structural impairment in coronary microcirculation. As a matter of fact, the correlation between CV risk factors and the extent of perfusion defects was very close. In this view, exposition to multiple risk factors could favour the development of coronary microvascular alterations that would be at the basis of "false" myocardial perfusion scans, as showed by a previous study [109] in which coronary blood flow and reserve were quantified in patients with normal epicardial coronary arteries by myocardial contrast echocardiography and by intra-coronary Doppler.

Finally, the "real" nature of myocardial perfusion defects in the absence of coronary stenoses is suggested by the effect of perfusion abnormalities on event-free survival. Although the prognosis of patients with normal coronary arteries is good, an extensive myocardial perfusion abnormality after stress was indicative of a slightly worsened outcome. A further suggestion of the "real" nature of perfusion abnormalities is the substantial concordance of the site of coronary lesions in the follow-up with respect to the location of early perfusion defects [110]. Finally, similar results were obtained by stress echocardiography in a group of 457 patients with angiographically non-significant stenoses and preserved LV function [111]: the 7-year survival was worse in those patients with "false" positive test compared to those with a true negative test.

15.5 Autoimmune connective tissue disorders

In patients with rheumatic diseases (RD), CV involvement is common, may have serious consequences, and can contribute to worsening of patients' outcome [112]. Incidence and prevalence of CVD in RD have recently been largely increased due to both the improved biochemical and cardiac imaging diagnostic techniques. CVD can be diagnosed in more than 50% of the patients with systemic lupus erythematosus (SLE) [113] and is the cause of nearly 40% of deaths in rheumatoid arthritis (RA) patients [114].

In particular, RA is a multi-organ inflammatory disorder affecting approximately 1% of the adult general population. A reduction in life expectancy in RA patients is primarily due to an increase of CV events [115] associated with both ischemic heart disease and congestive heart failure [116]. Importantly, myocardial disease is typically clinically silent [115], only manifesting as myocardial dysfunction after an extended preclinical phase. Myocardial dysfunction may arise from a number of distinct processes, including micro- and macrovascular coronary ischemia, myocardial inflammation (myocarditis), and/or myocardial fibrosis [117], any of which may be active in RA. Finally, systemic sclerosis is frequently associated with pulmonary hypertension and/or systemic hypertension, which can lead to subsequent complications.

The most common features of these pathologies are pericardial effusion, pericardial thickening, and valvular involvement. As a matter of fact, in RA, pericardial effusion is seen in 2–10% of the patients as chronic, asymptomatic pericardial effusion, while tamponade and constrictive pericarditis are rare (0.5%). In patients with SLE, symptomatic pericardial effusion has been reported in 6–50% (Figure 15.10), clinically significant pericarditis and pericardial thickening are described in <30%, while post-mortem pericardial lesions range from 60% to 80%.

Due to screening with high-efficiency technology, an increasing evidence of myocardial involvement is emerging. The myocardium is frequently affected in RD by means of different immunological mechanisms. In RA, myocardium was involved in 19% of the cases on post-mortem study [118]. Although myocarditis is not usually associated with RA, secondary amyloidosis could cause cardiomyopathy and atrioventricular conduction abnormalities [119]. Acute myocarditis has been reported in 8–25% of SLE patients, but due to introduction of steroid therapy, this decreased to 5%. In systemic sclerosis, myocardial involvement can manifest as incipient cardiomyopathy that could progress to ventricular dysfunction and heart failure.

Finally, in SLE, risk of developing CAD is 4–8 times higher than in controls, while in the middle-aged women with long-standing disease and a long period of corticosteroid intake, the risk is increased 50-fold than in the matching age group. In patients

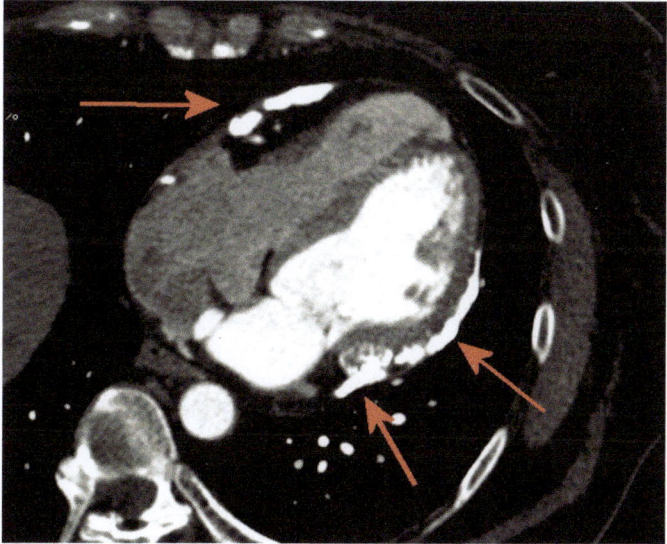

Figure 15.10 Pericardial effusion in a SLE patient.

with RA, risk of CAD is increased 2–3-fold in comparison with the general population. In addition, silent ischaemia and sudden cardiac death are more likely to be experienced by RA patients. Nowadays, the use of cardiac MR is highly suggested in order to obtain modality relevant information on cardiac morphology and function. Furthermore, images obtained late after paramagnetic contrast injection (late gadolinium enhancement) are crucial to assess the presence of myocardial fibrosis as well as intramyocardial permanent lesions [120].

Imaging techniques, for example, PET scanning and CT angiography, should clearly be reserved for patients with known CVD or very high CVD risk (based on traditional risk factors as well as the presence of SLE, for example). Others techniques, such as echocardiography and carotid ultrasound, are convenient and non-invasive and could be used as screening tools in asymptomatic patients, though it is still unclear how best to manage patients who have abnormalities on these tests. Perhaps the best way to use these imaging methods should be in combination with assessment of traditional risk factors, disease activity measurements, and blood tests relevant to CVD.

15.6 Thyroid disease

Thyroid disease is quite common. Current estimates suggest that it affects as many as 9–15% of the adult female population and a smaller percentage of adult males even if, beyond the eighth decade of life, the incidence of disease in men rises to be equal to that of women [121]. Some of the common signs and symptoms of thyroid disease are those that result from the effects of thyroid hormone on the heart and CV system [122].

The precise cellular and molecular mechanisms by which thyroid exerts its action on almost every cell and organ in the body have been well worked out [123].

As a matter of fact, thyroid hormone effects on the cardiac myocyte are intimately associated with cardiac function via regulation of the expression of key structural and regulatory genes as well as with extranuclear non-genomic effects on the cardiac myocyte and on the systemic vasculature.

Effects of thyroid hormone on CV haemodynamics: The effects of thyroid hormone on the heart and peripheral vasculature include decreased systemic vascular resistance and increased resting heart rate, LV contractility, and blood volume. Thyroid hormone causes decreased resistance in peripheral arterioles through a direct effect on vascular smooth muscle cells (VSM) and decreased mean arterial pressure, which, when sensed in the kidneys, activates the renin–angiotensin–aldosterone system and increases renal sodium absorption. T3 also increases erythropoietin synthesis, which leads to an increase in red cell mass. These changes combine to promote an increase in blood volume and preload. Relaxation of VSM leads to decreased arterial resistance and pressure, which thereby increases cardiac output. Moreover, whereas thyroid hormone decreases SVR and afterload, it increases renin and aldosterone secretion while increasing blood volume and preload and contributes to the characteristic increase in cardiac output [124]. Finally, expression of the pro-hormone genes for each natriuretic peptide is regulated by thyroid hormone and is altered with changes in blood pressure and disease states that affect cardiac function [125].

Direct effects of thyroid hormone on the heart: Hyperthyroidism in both humans and experimental animals leads to cardiac hypertrophy [126]. This cardiac growth is primarily the result of increased work imposed on the heart through increases in haemodynamic load. Thyroid hormone affects the action potential duration and repolarization currents in cardiac myocytes through both genomic and non-genomic mechanisms, as previously described [127]. Despite these well-characterized mechanisms, it is not clear how hyperthyroidism predisposes to atrial fibrillation. It may be that a combination of genomic and non-genomic actions on atrial ion channels plus the enlargement of the atrium as a result of the expanded blood volume are the underlying causes [128]. Treatment of hyperthyroidism with beta-adrenergic blockade improves many, if not all, of the CV signs and symptoms associated with hyperthyroidism. Heart rate is slowed, but the enhanced diastolic performance is not altered after treatment, which indicates that T3 acts directly on the heart to increase calcium cycling [129].

All these haemodynamic changes are assumed to be associated with alterations of oxygen consumption and metabolic performance of heart muscle. In a model of short-term hypothyroidism, we have previously used PET with [^{11}C] acetate for non-invasive quantification of changes of myocardial oxidative metabolism [130]. PET was combined with measurements of ventricular function by MRI, and the relation between cardiac work and oxygen consumption as an estimate of efficiency was investigated. The authors observed a reduction of myocardial oxygen consumption in the hypothyroid state that was associated with reduced metabolic efficiency. In the euthyroid state, oxidative metabolism as well as efficiency increased significantly.

On the contrary, hyperthyroidism is assumed to result in an increase of cardiac oxygen consumption [131], but it remains unclear whether cardiac efficiency will increase in parallel with thyroid hormone levels as suggested by our previous results in hypothyroidism, or whether it will decrease again (e.g., because of oxygen wastage as a result of the hyper-metabolic state). Bengel et al. [132]) suggested a non-linear relationship between thyroid function and myocardial metabolic performance. While efficiency is reduced in the hypothyroid state and can be enhanced by establishing euthyroid conditions, the sum of effects of thyroid hormone seems not to allow for a further increase when thyroid hormone levels are mildly elevated. Neither, however, does hyperthyroidism cause a decrease of metabolic efficiency under these circumstances. Alterations in more severe thyrotoxicosis cannot be determined from the published data, but are worth future study.

15.7 Systemic vasculitis

15.7.1 Kawasaki disease and coronary microcirculation: the role of cardiac imaging

Kawasaki disease (KD), first described by Tomisaku Kawasaki in 1967, is an acute systemic vasculitis of the small- and medium-sized arteries [133]. Also called mucocutaneous lymph node syndrome, approximately 90% of patients have mucocutaneous manifestations, leading to an important role in early diagnosis by dermatologists. KD is the second commonest vasculitic illness of childhood after Henoch Schönlein purpura and is the commonest cause of acquired heart disease in children in developed countries [134].

The aetiology of KD remains unknown. KD probably represents an aberrant inflammatory host response to one or more as yet unidentified pathogens, occurring in genetically predisposed individuals. KD is associated with systemic vasculitis particularly affecting the coronary arteries, causing coronary artery aneurism (CAA) in 15–25% of untreated patients, while 2–3% of untreated cases die as a result of coronary vasculitis [135].

The main sites of clinically important vascular involvement are the coronary arteries, although other vessels such as the axillary arteries can be involved. CAA occur in 15–25% of untreated cases, with additional cardiac features in a significant proportion of these including pericardial effusion, electrocardiographic abnormalities, pericarditis, myocarditis, valvular incompetence, cardiac failure, and myocardial infarction [135].

The most common complication of KD relates to coronary artery vasculitis, leading to coronary ectasia and aneurysms in 15–25% of untreated patients.

Other complications include decreased coronary arterial compliance, myopericarditis, arrhythmias, ischemic heart disease, pericardial effusion, valvular regurgitation, myocardial infarction, and/or sudden cardiac death. The myocardium can be affected in the absence of coronary artery lesions [136]. Peripheral arteries can also be involved, most often in those who also have giant coronary aneurysms.

Cardiac imaging is essential early in the disease course to seek coronary abnormalities; echocardiography is the preferred modality, but conventional coronary angiography, magnetic resonance angiography, and cardiac computed tomographic angiography may also be used when appropriate. In general, myocardial infarction is the most common cause of death in patients with KD and may present with symptoms of unrest, vomiting, and abdominal pain.

In general, echocardiography is the first choice technique for fast, accurate diagnosis, and follow-up of aneurysms in KD [137] although in some centres CT and/or MRI are currently used. Concerning the diagnosis of coronary artery stenosis, a study comparing transthoracic echocardiography and coronary angiography found that echo had a sensitivity of only 85% (right coronary artery) and 80% (left coronary artery) for detection of stenotic lesions in KD [138]. Dobutamine-stress echocardiography (DSE) has been recently used to detect perfusion abnormalities in KD, but the positive result was depending on the degree of both coronary obstruction and collateralization [139]. According to these data, no patients in American Heart Association (AHA) risk levels less than V category had positive DSE, whereas 2/4 of the risk level V category had positive DSE, with coronary occlusion >50% confirmed by angiography. Transthoracic Doppler assessment of coronary flow velocity reserve in the posterior descending and left anterior descending artery predicted the presence of significant coronary stenosis of either right or left coronary artery. These findings were in agreement with perfusion defects on Tl-201 SPECT [140]. Abnormal myocardial perfusion is present long term after complicated KD, and the worst anomalies accompany persistent giant aneurysms. However, there is a poor agreement between coronary angiography and myocardial perfusion SPECT findings and between dipyridamole Tc^{99m}-sestamibi myocardial perfusion and 2D echocardiography [141].

MRI has been successfully used in the diagnosis of KD [142]. The gadolinium-based contrast agent has already been used for myocardial infarction detection in patients with Kawasaki syndrome [143]. Prakash et al. [144] demonstrated that stress–rest perfusion and myocardial viability can reliably detect perfusion defects in patients with Kawasaki syndrome. Finally, due to its ability to diagnose accurately the presence of inflammation, MRI can be of value to detect subclinical myocardial inflammation during the acute phase of the disease, which is missed by other imaging techniques. Also, cardiac CT very effectively images the full extent of the aneurysms, both in terms of thrombotic aneurysms, which will not be seen on ICA, as well as coronary stenosis

15.7.2 Hypereosinophilia and Churg–Strauss

Eosinophilic granulomatosis with polyangiitis (Churg–Strauss, EGPA) is a systemic small-vessel vasculitis associated with asthma and eosinophilia. The pathogenesis of EGPA is multifactorial: the disease can be triggered by exposure to allergens or drugs, but a genetic background has also been recognized. EGPA is traditionally described to evolve through a prodromic, allergic phase characterized by asthma and rhino-sinusitis, an eosinophilic phase hallmarked by peripheral eosinophilia and organ involvement, and a vasculitic phase with clinical manifestations due to small-vessel vasculitis [145]. Heart involvement, particularly when clinically evident, is a well-known adverse prognostic factor. Peripheral eosinophilia is more pronounced in patients with cardiac damage: early lesions, dominated by eosinophilic infiltration, likely progress to fibrotic changes with consequent restrictive cardiomyopathy. Although endomyocardial infiltration is the dominant picture, coronary vasculitis, pericarditis, and valvular defects may also occur.

15.7.3 Sarcoidosis

Sarcoidosis is defined by the American Thoracic Society, European Respiratory Society, and World Association of Sarcoidosis and Other Granulomatous Disorders as "a multisystem disorder of unknown cause(s)" [146]. Some factors have been linked with sarcoidosis, such as environmental or occupational sources, infectious causes, and genetic predisposition, but the aetiology remains unclear. Clinical manifestations of sarcoidosis are dependent on both the profusion and location of granulomas. Cardiac sarcoidosis (CS) is associated with non-caseating granulomas which may involve the LV free wall, basal ventricular septum, right ventricle, papillary muscles, right atrium, and left atrium [147]. The clinical manifestation of CS ranges from asymptomatic to sudden cardiac death. It is determined by localization and severity of disease. The myocardium is most frequently affected [148], but granuloma may also affect the endocardium and pericardium [149]. Inflammatory granulomas or post-inflammatory scarring may lead to conduction abnormalities, arrhythmias, sudden cardiac death, and congestive heart failure. Banba et al. [150] reported that atrioventricular block develops mainly during the inflammatory phase. Ventricular tachycardia occurs in up to 23% of CS patients and represents the second most frequent clinical finding [150]. In addition to arrhythmic complications, congestive heart failure is frequent, being observed in up to 73% of patients dying from CS. Heart failure may be secondary to left-sided cardiac involvement with either systolic or DD and can occur when there is extensive infiltration of the myocardium by non-caseating granulomas. Small pericardial effusions detected by echocardiography were found in 19% of patients with sarcoidosis [151]. Valvular incompetence secondary to papillary muscle dysfunction can be seen in approximately 68% of patients [152]. Myocardial aneurysms may be associated with frequent and complex ventricular arrhythmias. Finally, pulmonary hypertension is a predictor of poor outcome in sarcoidosis. Similarly to other diseases involving the myocardium, CMR can be used to assess the presence of oedema, myocardial fibrosis, and intra-myocardial permanent lesions [153].

Nuclear medicine imaging is an important tool in the diagnosis of CS. The fibrogranulomatous lesions in the myocardium display segmental areas of decreased uptake in nuclear imaging. The most useful studies are performed with Tl-201 and Tc^{99m} sestamibi [154]. Gallium is highly sensitive for CS because it accumulates in the inflamed areas and is useful in judging the response of the disease to steroid therapy. Unfortunately, myocardial gallium SPECT images are not sufficiently clear in distinguishing gallium uptake in the myocardium from that in the lung or mediastinum. Therefore, the clinical usefulness of gallium SPECT scanning has not been adequately established [155]. PET can also identify sarcoid cardiac involvement and assess severity. The PET scan may be useful in patients with a pacemaker or cardioverter-defibrillator implanted who are unable to undergo MRI because of the safety concerns related to potential adverse effects on the device arising from the strong magnetic and radiofrequency forces generated by MRI. These include the possibility of erratic and inappropriate device functioning during or after the scan, over-sensing that can cause high rate pacing or thermal damage to the device, and induced voltages on leads that can cause over- and under-sensing. Moreover, combined effects can cause component failures, mechanical vibration, and device damage [156].

References

[1] Levy D, Larson MG, Vasan RS, Kannel WB, Ho KK. The progression from hypertension to congestive heart failure. JAMA 1996;275:1557–762.
[2] Levy D, Garrison RJ, Savage DD, Kannel WB, Castelli WP. Prognostic implications of echocardiographically determined left ventricular mass in the Framingham Heart Study. N Engl J Med 1990;322:1561–6.
[3] Froelich ED. Local hemodynamic changes in hypertension: insights for therapeutic preservation of target organs. Hypertension 2001;38:1388–94.
[4] Schäfer S, Kelm M, Mingers S, Strauer BE. Left ventricular remodeling impairs coronary flow reserve in hypertensive patients. J Hypertens 2002;20:1431–7.
[5] Lang RM, Bierig M, Devereux RB, Flachskampf FA, Foster E, Pellikka PA, et al. American Society of Echocardiography's Nomenclature and Standards Committee; Task Force on Chamber Quantification; American College of Cardiology Echocardiography Committee; American Heart Association; European Association of Echocardiography, European Society of Cardiology. Eur J Echocardiogr 2006;7:79–108.

[6] Galderisi M. Diagnosis and management of diastolic dysfunction in the hypertensive patient. Am J Hypertens 2011;24:507–17.
[7] Cicala S, de Simone G, Roman MJ, Best LG, Lee ET, Wang W, et al. Prevalence and prognostic significance of wall-motion abnormalities in adults without clinically recognized cardiovascular disease: the Strong Heart Study. Circulation 2007;116:143–50.
[8] de Simone G, Devereux RB, Roman MJ, Alderman MH, Laragh JH. Relation of obesity and gender to left ventricular hypertrophy in normotensive and hypertensive adults. Hypertension 1994;23:600–6.
[9] Devereux RB, Pickering TG, Harshfield GA, Kleinert HD, Denby L, Clark L, et al. Left ventricular hypertrophy in patients with hypertension: importance of blood pressure response to regularly recurring stress. Circulation 1983;69:470–4.
[10] Ganau A, Devereux RB, Roman MJ, de Simone G, Pickering TG, Saba PS, et al. Patterns of left ventricular hypertrophy and geometric remodeling in essential hypertension. J Am Coll Cardiol 1992;19:1550–8.
[11] Ghali JK, Liao Y, Simmons B, Castaner A, Cao G, Cooper RS. The prognostic role of left ventricular hypertrophy in patients with or without coronary artery disease. Ann Intern Med 1992;117:831–6.
[12] Verdecchia P, Schillaci G, Borgioni C, Ciucci A, Battistelli M, Bartoccini C, et al. Adverse prognostic significance of concentric remodeling of the left ventricle in hypertensive patients with normal left ventricular mass. J Am Coll Cardiol 1995;25:871–8.
[13] Klingbell AU, Schneider M, Martus P, Messerli FH, Schmieder RE. A meta-analysis of the effects of treatment on left ventricular mass in essential hypertension. Am J Med 2003;115:41–6.
[14] Schmieder RE, Schlaich MP. Comparison of therapeutic studies on regression of left ventricular hypertrophy. Adv Exp Med Biol 1997;432:191–8.
[15] Devereux RB, Wachtell K, Gerdts E, Boman K, Nieminen MS, Papademetriou V, et al. Prognostic significance of left ventricular mass change during treatment of hypertension. JAMA 2004;292:2350–6.
[16] Koren MJ, Ulin RJ, Koren AT, Laragh JH, Devereux RB. Left ventricular mass change during treatment and outcome in patients with essential hypertension. Am J Hypertens 2002;15:1021–8.
[17] Verdecchia P, Angeli F, Borgioni C, Gattobigio R, de Simone G, Devereux RB, et al. Changes in cardiovascular risk by reduction of left ventricular mass in hypertension: a meta-analysis. Am J Hypertens 2003;16:895–9.
[18] de Simone G, Devereux RB, Roman MJ, Ganau A, Saba PS, Alderman MH, et al. Assessment of left ventricular function by the midwall fractional shortening/end-systolic stress relation in human hypertension. J Am Coll Cardiol 1994;23:1444–51.
[19] de Simone G, Devereux RB, Koren MJ, Mensah GA, Casale PN, Laragh JH. Midwall left ventricular mechanics. An independent predictor of cardiovascular risk in arterial hypertension. Circulation 1996;93:259–65.
[20] Wachtell K, Gerdts E, Palmieri V, Olsen MH, Nieminen MS, Papademetriou V, et al. In-treatment midwall and endocardial fractional shortening predict cardiovascular outcome in hypertensive patients with preserved baseline systolic ventricular function: the Losartan Intervention For Endpoint reduction study. J Hypertens 2010;28:1541–6.
[21] de Simone G, Izzo R, Chinali M, De Marco M, Casalnuovo G, Rozza F, et al. Does information on systolic and diastolic function improve prediction of a cardiovascular event by left ventricular hypertrophy in arterial hypertension? Hypertension 2010;56:99–104.

[22] Takeda Y, Zhu A, Yoneda T, Usukura M, Takata H, Yamagishi M. Effects of aldosterone and angiotensin II receptor blockade on cardiac angiotensinogen and angiotensin-converting enzyme 2 expression in Dahl salt-sensitive hypertensive rats. Am J Hypertens 2007;20:1119–24.

[23] Aeschbacher BC, Hutter D, Fuhrer J, Weidmann P, Delacrétaz E, Allemann Y. Diastolic dysfunction precedes myocardial hypertrophy in the development of hypertension. Am J Hypertens 2001;14:106–13.

[24] Nagueh SF, Appleton CP, Gillebert TC, Marino PN, Oh JK, Smiseth OA, et al. Recommendations for the evaluation of left ventricular diastolic function by echocardiography. Eur J Echocardiogr 2009;10:165–93.

[25] Devereux RB, Alonso DR, Lutas EM, Gottlieb GJ, Campo E, Sachs I, et al. Echocardiographic assessment of left ventricular hypertrophy: comparison to necropsy findings. Am J Cardiol 1986;57:450–8.

[26] Mancia G, Fagard R, Redon J, Zanchetti A, Böhm M, et al. ESH/ESC guidelines for the management of arterial hypertension: the Task Force for the Management of Arterial Hypertension of the European Society of Hypertension (ESH) and of the European Society of Cardiology (ESC). Eur Heart J 2013;34:2159–219.

[27] Ommen SR, Nishimura RA, Appleton CP, Miller FA, Oh JK, Redfield MM, et al. Clinical utility of Doppler echocardiography and tissue Doppler imaging in the estimation of left ventricular filling pressures: a comparative simultaneous Doppler catheterization study. Circulation 2000;102:1788–94.

[28] Sharp AS, Tapp RJ, Thom SA, Francis DP, Hughes AD, Stanton AV, et al. ASCOT investigators. Tissue Doppler E/E' ratio is a powerful predictor of primary cardiac events in a hypertensive population: an ASCOT substudy. Eur Heart J 2010;31:747–52.

[29] Mor-Avi V, Lang RM, Badano LP, Belohlavek M, Cardim NM, Derumeaux G. Current and evolving echocardiographic techniques for the quantitative evaluation of cardiac mechanics: ASE/EAE consensus statement on methodology and indications endorsed by the Japanese Society of Echocardiography. Eur J Echocardiogr 2011;12:167–205.

[30] Di Bello V, Talini E, Dell'Omo G, Giannini C, Delle Donne MG, Canale ML, et al. Early left ventricular mechanics abnormalities in prehypertension: a two-dimensional strain echocardiography study. Am J Hypertens 2010;23:405–12.

[31] Galderisi M, Schiano Lomoriello V, Santoro A, Esposito R, Olibet M, Raia R, et al. Differences of myocardial systolic deformation and correlates of diastolic function in competitive rowers and young hypertensives: a Speckle Tracking Echocardiography Study. J Am Soc Echocardiogr 2010;23:1190–8.

[32] Kosmala W, Plaksej R, Strotmann JM, Weigel C, Herrmann S, Niemann M, et al. Progression of left ventricular functional abnormalities in hypertensive patients with heart failure: an ultrasonic two-dimensional speckle tracking study. J Am Soc Echocardiogr 2008;21:1309–17.

[33] Devereux RB, Reichek N. Echocardiographic determination of left ventricular mass in man. Anatomic validation of the method. Circulation 1977;55:613–8.

[34] Caiani EG, Corsi C, Sugeng L, Mac Eneaney P, Weinert L, Mor-Avi V, et al. Improved quantification of left ventricular mass based on endocardial and epicardial surface detection with real time three dimensional echocardiography. Heart 2006;92:213–9.

[35] Mor-Avi V, Sugeng L, Weinert L, Mac Eneaney P, Caiani EG, Koch R, et al. Fast measurement of left ventricular mass with real-time three-dimensional echocardiography: comparison with magnetic resonance imaging. Circulation 2004;110:1814–8.

[36] Van den Bosch AE, Robbers-Visser D, Krenning BJ, McGhie JS, Helbing WA, Meijboom FJ, et al. Comparison of real-time three-dimensional echocardiography to magnetic resonance imaging for assessment of left ventricular mass. Am J Cardiol 2006;97:113–7.

[37] Grothues F, Moon JC, Bellenger NG, Smith GS, Klein HU, Pennell DJ. Interstudy reproducibility of right ventricular volumes, function, and mass with cardiovascular magnetic resonance. Am Heart J 2004;147:218–23.

[38] Todiere GC, Neglia D, Ghione S, Fommei E, Capozza P, Guarini G, et al. Right ventricular remodelling in systemic hypertension: a cardiac MRI study. Heart 2011;97:1257–61.

[39] Picano E, Palinkas A, Amyot R. Diagnosis of myocardial ischemia in hypertensive patients. J Hypertens 2001;19:1177–83.

[40] Schulman DS, Francis CK, Black HR, Wackers FJ. Thallium-201 stress imaging in hypertensive patients. Hypertension 1987;10:16–21.

[41] Sicari R, Nihoyannopoulos P, Evangelista A, Kasprzak J, Lancellotti P, Poldermans D, et al. Stress echocardiography expert consensus statement—executive summary: European Association of Echocardiography (EAE) (a registered branch of the ESC). Eur Heart J 2009;30:278–89.

[42] Parodi O, Sambuceti G. The role of coronary microvascular dysfunction in the genesis of cardiovascular diseases. Q J Nucl Med 1996;40:9–16.

[43] Galderisi M, Anderson KM, Wilson PW, Levy D. Echocardiographic evidence for the existence of a distinct diabetic cardiomyopathy (the Framingham Heart Study). Am J Cardiol 1991;68:85–9.

[44] Ilercil A, Devereux RB, Roman MJ, Paranicas M, O'grady MJ, Welty TK, et al. Relationships of impaired glucose tolerance to left ventricular structure and function: the Strong Heart Study. Am Heart J 2001;14:992–8.

[45] Lee M, Gardin JM, Lynch JC, Smith VE, Tracy RP, Savage PJ, et al. Diabetes mellitus and echocardiographic left ventricular function in free-living elderly men and women. The Cardiovascular Health Study. Am Heart J 1997;133:36–43.

[46] Palmieri V, Bella JN, Arnett DK, Liu JE, Oberman A, Schuck MY, et al. Effect of type 2 diabetes mellitus on left ventricular geometry and systolic function in hypertensive subjects. Hypertension Genetic Epidemioloy Network (HyperGEN) study. Circulation 2001;103:102–7.

[47] Rutter MK, Parise H, Benjamin EJ, Levy D, Larson MG, Meigs JB, et al. Impact of glucose intolerance and insulin resistance on cardiac structure and function: sex-related differences in the Framingham Heart Study. Circulation 2003;107:448–54.

[48] Liu JE, Palmieri V, Roman MJ, Bella JN, Fabsitz R, Howard BV, et al. The impact of diabetes on left ventricular filling pattern in normotensive and hypertensive adults: the Strong Heart Study. J Am Coll Cardiol 2001;37:1943–9.

[49] Nishimura RA, Tajik J. Evaluation of diastolic filling of left ventricle in health and disease: Doppler echocardiography is the clinician's Rosetta Stone. J Am Coll Cardiol 1997;30:8–18.

[50] Bella JN, Palmieri V, Roman MJ, Liu JE, Welty TK, Lee ET, et al. Mitral ratio of peak early to late diastolic filling velocity as a predictor of mortality in middle-aged and elderly adults. The Strong Heart Study. Circulation 2002;105:1928–33.

[51] Frustaci A, Kajstura J, Chimenti C, Jakoniuk I, Leri A, Maseri A, et al. Myocardial cell death in human diabetes. Circ Res 2000;87:1123–32.

[52] Tsang TSM, Barnes ME, Gersh BJ, Bailey KR, Seward JB. Left atrial volume as a morphophysiologic expression of left ventricular diastolic dysfunction and relation to cardiovascular risk burden. Am J Cardiol 2002;90:1284–9.

[53] Poirier P, Bogaty P, Garneau C, Marois L, Dumensnil JC. Diastolic dysfunction in normotensive men with well controlled type 2 diabetes 2. Diabetes Care 2001;24:5–10.

[54] Sohn DW, Chai IH, Lee DJ, Kim HC, Kim HS, Oh BH, et al. Assessment of mitral annulus velocity by Doppler tissue imaging in the evaluation of left ventricular diastolic function. J Am Coll Cardiol 1997;30:474–80.
[55] Boyer JK, Thanigaraj S, Schechtman KB, Perez JE. Prevalence of ventricular diastolic dysfunction in asymptomatic, normotensive patients with diabetes mellitus. Am J Cardiol 2004;93:870–5.
[56] Shishehbor MH, Hoogwerf BJ, Schoenhagen P, Marso SP, Sun JP, Li J, et al. Relation of hemoglobin A1C to left ventricular relaxation in patients with type 1 diabetes mellitus and without overt heart disease. Am J Cardiol 2003;91:1514–7.
[57] Kawaguchi M, Techigawara M, Ishihata T, Asakura T, Saito F, Maehara K, et al. A comparison of ultrastructural changes on endomyocardial biopsy specimens obtained from patients with diabetes mellitus with and without hypertension. Heart Vessels 1997;12:267–74.
[58] Sunni S, Bishop SP, Kent SP, Geer JC. Diabetic cardiomyopathy. A morphological study of intramyocardial arteries. Arch Pathol Lab Med 1986;110:375–81.
[59] Pizzuto F, Voci P, Mariano E, Puddu PE, Sardella G, Nigri A. Assessment of flow velocity reserve by transthoracic Doppler echocardiography and venous adenosine infusion before and after left anterior descending coronary artery stenting. J Am Coll Cardiol 2001;38:155–62.
[60] Rigo F, Richieri E, Pasanisi E, Cutaia V, Zanella C, Della Valentina P, et al. Usefulness of coronary flow reserve over regional wall motion when added to dual-imaging dipyridamole echocardiography. Am J Cardiol 2003;91:269–73.
[61] Srinivasan M, Herrero P, McGill JB, et al. The effects of plasma insulin and glucose on myocardial blood flow in patients with type 1 diabetes mellitus. J Am Coll Cardiol 2005;46:42–8.
[62] Quinones MJ, Hernandez-Pampaloni M, Schelbert H, et al. Coronary vasomotor abnormalities in insulin-resistant individuals. Ann Intern Med 2004;140:700–8.
[63] Schalkwijk CG, Stehouwer CD. Vascular complications in diabetes mellitus: the role of endothelial dysfunction. Clin Sci 2005;109:143–59.
[64] Pop-Busui R, Kirkwood I, Schmid H, Marinescu V, Schroeder J, Larkin D, et al. Sympathetic dysfunction in type 1 diabetes: association with impaired myocardial blood flow reserve and diastolic dysfunction. J Am Coll Cardiol 2005;44:2368–74.
[65] Galderisi M, Cicala S, Caso P, De Simone L, D'Errico A, Petrocelli A, et al. Coronary flow reserve and myocardial diastolic dysfunction in arterial hypertension. Am J Cardiol 2002;90:860–4.
[66] Wisniacki N, Taylor W, Lye M, Wilding JP. Insulin resistance and inflammatory activation in older patients with systolic and diastolic heart failure. Heart 2005;91:32–7.
[67] Fiordaliso F, Leri A, Cesselli D, Limana F, Safai B, Nadal-Ginard B, et al. Hyperglycemia activates p53 and p53-regulated genes leading to myocyte cell death. Diabetes 2001;50:2363–675.
[68] Paulus WJ, Shah AM. NO and cardiac diastolic function. Cardiovasc Res 1999;43:595–606.
[69] Strauer BE, Motz W, Vogt M, Schwartzkopff B. Impaired coronary flow reserve in NIDDM: a possible role for diabetic cardiomyopathy in humans. Diabetes 1997;46:S119–24.
[70] Greenberg NL, Firstenberg MS, Castro PL, Main M, Travaglini A, Odabashian JA, et al. Doppler-derived myocardial systolic strain rate is a strong index of left ventricular contractility. Circulation 2002;105:99–105.
[71] Fang ZY, Yuda S, Anderson V, Short L, Case C, Marwick TH. Echocardiographic detection of early diabetic myocardial disease. J Am Coll Cardiol 2003;41:611–7.

[72] Fang ZY, Najos-Valencia O, Leano R, Marwick TH. Patients with early diabetic heart disease demonstrate a normal myocardial response to dobutamine. J Am Coll Cardiol 2003;42:446–53.
[73] Bowditch HP. Über die Eigenthümlichkeiten der Reizbarkeit, welche die Muskelfasern des Herzens zeigen. Ber Sachs Akad Wiss 1971;23:652–89.
[74] Mulieri LA, Hasenfuss G, Leavitt B, Allen PD, Alpert NR. Altered myocardial force–frequency relation in human heart failure. Circulation 1992;86:2017–8.
[75] Galderisi M, de Simone G, Innelli P, Turco A, Turco S, Capaldo B, et al. Impaired inotropic response in type 2 diabetes mellitus: a strain rate imaging study. Am J Hypertens 2007;5:548–55.
[76] Grundy SM, Brewer Jr. HB, Cleeman JI, Smith Jr. SC, Lenfant C. Definition of metabolic syndrome: Report of the National Heart, Lung and Blood Institute/American Heart Association Conference on Scientific Issues related to definition. American Heart Association; National Heart, Lung, and Blood Institute. Circulation 2004;109:433–8.
[77] Gami AS, Witt BJ, Howard DE, et al. Metabolic syndrome and risk of incident cardiovascular events and death: a systematic review and meta-analysis of longitudinal studies. J Am Coll Cardiol 2007;49:403–14.
[78] Katz R, Wong ND, Kronmal R, Takasu J, Shavelle DM, Probstfield JL, et al. Features of the metabolic syndrome and diabetes mellitus as predictors of aortic valve calcification in the Multi-Ethnic Study of Atherosclerosis. Circulation 2006;113:2113–9.
[79] Katz R, Budoff MJ, Takasu J, Shavelle DM, Bertoni A, Blumenthal RS, et al. Relationship of metabolic syndrome to incident aortic valve calcium and aortic valve calcium progression: the Multi-Ethnic Study of Atherosclerosis. Diabetes 2009;58:813–9.
[80] Briand M, Lemieux I, Dumesnil JG, Mathieu P, Cartier A, Després JP, et al. Metabolic syndrome negatively influences disease progression and prognosis in aortic stenosis. J Am Coll Cardiol 2006;47:2229–37.
[81] Safar ME, Thomas F, Blacher J, Nzietchueng R, Bureau JM, Pannier B, et al. Metabolic syndrome and age-related progression of aortic stiffness. J Am Coll Cardiol 2006;47:72–5.
[82] Briand M, Pibarot P, Despres JP, Voisine P, Dumesnil JG, Dagenais F, et al. Metabolic syndrome is associated with faster degeneration of bioprosthetic valves. Circulation 2006;114:I512–7.
[83] Akki A, Seymour AM. Western diet impairs metabolic remodelling and contractile efficiency in cardiac hypertrophy. Cardiovasc Res 2009;3:610–7.
[84] Raher MJ, Thibault HB, Buys ES, Kuruppu D, Shimizu N, Brownell AL, et al. A short duration of high-fat diet induces insulin resistance and predisposes to adverse left ventricular ventricular remodeling after pressure overload. Am J Physiol Heart Circ Physiol 2008;295:H2495–502.
[85] Chinali M, Devereux RB, Howard BW, Roman MJ, Bella JN, Liu JE, et al. Comparison of cardiac structure and function in American Indians with and without the metabolic syndrome (the Strong Heart Study). Am J Cardiol 2004;93:40–4.
[86] Cuspidi C, Meani S, Fusi V, Valerio C, Sala C, Zanchetti A, et al. Metabolic syndrome and target organ damage in untreated essential hypertensives. J Hypertens 2004;22:1991–8.
[87] Andronico G, Mangano M-T, Mule G, Mulè G, Piazza G, Cerasola G. Insulin-like growth factor 1 and sodium–lithium countertransport in essential hypertension and in hypertensive left ventricular hypertrophy. J Hypertens 1993;11:1097–101.
[88] de Simone G, Devereux RB, Camargo MJ, Wallerson DC, Laragh JH. Influence of sodium intake on in vivo left ventricular anatomy in experimental renovascular hypertension. Am J Physiol 1993;264:H2103–10.

[89] Sugden PH. An overview of endothelin signaling in the cardiac myocyte. J Mol Cell Cardiol 2003;35:871–86.
[90] Schlaich MP, Kaye DM, Lambert E, Sommerville M, Socratous F, Esler MD. Relation between cardiac sympathetic activity and hypertensive left ventricular hypertrophy. Circulation 2003;108:560–5.
[91] Engeli S, Negrel R, Sharma AM. Physiology and pathophysiology of the adipose tissue renin–angiotensin system. Hypertension 2000;35:1270–7.
[92] Rajapurohitam V, Gan XT, Kirshenbaum LA, Karmazyn M. The obesity associated peptide leptin induces hypertrophy in neonatal rat ventricular myocytes. Circ Res 2003;93:277–9.
[93] Positano V, Cusi K, Santarelli MF, Sironi A, Petz R, DeFronzo R, et al. Automatic correction of intensity inhomogeneities improves unsupervised assessment of abdominal fat by MRI. J Magn Reson Imaging 2008;28:403–10.
[94] Sironi AM, Gastaldelli A, Mari A, Ciociaro D, Positano V, Buzzigoli E, et al. Visceral fat in hypertension: influence on insulin resistance and beta-cell function. Hypertension 2004;44:127–33.
[95] Sironi AM, Pingitore A, Ghione S, De Marchi D, Scattini B, Positano V, et al. Early hypertension is associated with reduced regional cardiac function, insulin resistance, epicardial, and visceral fat. Hypertension 2008;51:282–8.
[96] Hachamovitch R, Hayes SW, Friedman JD, Cohen I, Berman DS. Stress myocardial perfusion single-photon emission computed tomography is clinically effective and cost effective in risk stratification of patients with a high likelihood of coronary artery disease (CAD) but no known CAD. J Am Coll Cardiol 2004;43:200–8.
[97] Iskandrian AS, Chae SC, Heo J, Stanberry CD, Wasserleben V, Cave V. Independent and incremental prognostic value of exercise single-photon emission computed tomographic (SPECT) thallium imaging in coronary artery disease. J Am Coll Cardiol 1993;22:665–70.
[98] Elhendy A, van Domburg RT, Sozzi FB, Poldermans D, Bax JJ, Roelandt JR. Impact of hypertension on the accuracy of exercise stress myocardial perfusion imaging for the diagnosis of coronary artery disease. Heart 2001;85:655–61.
[99] Smart SC, Bhatia A, Hellman R, Stoiber T, Krasnow A, Collier BD, et al. Dobutamine–atropine stress echocardiography and dipyridamole sestamibi scintigraphy for the detection of coronary artery disease: limitations and concordance. J Am Coll Cardiol 2000;36:1265–73.
[100] Zeiher AM, Krause T, Schächinger V, Minners J, Moser E. Impaired endothelium-dependent vasodilation of coronary resistance vessels is associated with exercise-induced myocardial ischemia. Circulation 1995;91:2345–52.
[101] Parodi O, Neglia D, Palombo C, et al. Comparative effects of enalapril and verapamil on myocardial blood flow in systemic hypertension. Circulation 1997;96:864–73.
[102] Sambuceti G, Marzullo P, Giorgetti A, Neglia D, Marzilli M, Salvadori P, et al. Global alteration in perfusion response to increasing oxygen consumption in patients with single vessel coronary artery disease. Circulation 1994;90:1696–705.
[103] Le Feuvre C, Raoux F, Beygui F, Helft G, Mogenet A, Dubois-Laforgue D, et al. Cumulative adverse effects of diabetes mellitus and hypertension on coronary flow velocity reserve. Arch Mal Coeur Vaiss 2004;97:849–54.
[104] Kranidis A, Zamanis N, Mitrakou A, Patsilinakos S, Bouki T, Tountas N, et al. Coronary microcirculation evaluation with transesophageal echocardiography Doppler in type II diabetics. Int J Cardiol 1997;59:119–24.

[105] Di Carli F, Janisse J, Grunberger G, Ager J. Role of chronic hyperglicemia in the pathogenesis of coronary microvascular dysfunction in diabetes. J Am Coll Cardiol 2003;41:1387–93.

[106] Wackers FJTh, Young LH, Inucchi SE, Chyun DA, Davey JA, Barrett EJ, et al. For the detection of Ischemia in asymptomatic diabetic Investigators. Detection of silent myocardial ischemia in asymptomatic diabetic subjects: the DIAD study. Diabetes Care 2004;27:1957–61.

[107] Neglia D, Parodi O, Gallopin M, Sambuceti G, Giorgetti A, Pratali L, et al. Myocardial blood flow response to pacing tachycardia and to dipyridamole infusion in patients with dilated cardiomyopathy without overt heart failure. A quantitative assessment by positron emission tomography. Circulation 1995;92:796–804.

[108] Soman P, Dave DM, Udelson JE, Han H, Ouda HZ, Patel AR, et al. Vascular endothelial dysfunction is associated with reversible myocardial perfusion defects in the absence of obstructive coronary artery disease. J Nucl Cardiol 2006;13:756–60.

[109] Wei K, Ragosta M, Thorpe J, Coggins M, Moos S, Kaul S. Noninvasive quantification of coronary blood flow reserve in humans using myocardial contrast echocardiography. Circulation 2001;29:2560–5.

[110] Saihara K, Hamasaki S, Okui H, Biro S, Ishida S, Yoshikawa A, et al. Association of coronary shear stress with endothelial function and vascular remodeling in patients with normal or mildly diseased coronary arteries. Coron Artery Dis 2006;17:401–7.

[111] Sicari R, Palinkas A, Pasanisi EG, Venneri L, Picano E. Long-term survival of patients with chest pain syndrome and angiographically normal or near-normal coronary arteries: the additional prognostic value of dipyridamole echocardiography test (DET). Eur Heart J 2005;26:2136–41.

[112] Mandell FB, Hoffman SG. Rheumatic diseases and the cardiovascular system. In: Zippes PD, Libby P, Bonow OR, Braunwald E, editors. Heart disease: a textbook of cardiovascular medicine, international. 7th ed. Elsevier Saunders; 2005. p. 2101–16.

[113] Doria A, Iaccarino L, Sarzi-Puttini P, Atzeni F, Turriel M, Petri M. Cardiac involvement in systemic lupus erythematosus. Lupus 2005;14:683–6.

[114] Gerli R, Goodson NJ. Cardiovascular involvement in rheumatoid arteritis. Lupus 2005;14:679–82.

[115] Maradit-Kremers H, Nicola PJ, Crowson CS, Ballman KV, Gabriel SE. Cardiovascular death in rheumatoid arthritis. Arthritis Rheum 2005;52:722–32.

[116] Nicola P, Crowson CS, Maradit-Kremers H, Gabriel SE. Contribution of congestive heart failure and ischemic heart disease to excess mortality in rheumatoid arthritis. Arthritis Rheum 2006;54:60–7.

[117] Giles JT, Fernandes V, Lima JA, Bathon JM. Myocardial dysfunction in rheumatoid arthritis: epidemiology and pathogenesis. Arthritis Res Ther 2005;7:195–207.

[118] Lebowitz WB. The heart in rheumatoid arthritis (rheumatoid disease): a clinical and pathological study of 62 cases. Ann Intern Med 1963;58:102–23.

[119] Riboldi P, Gerosa M, Luzzana C, Catelli L. Cardiac involvement in systemic autoimmune diseases. Clin Rev Allergy Immunol 2002;23:247–61.

[120] Marmursztejn J, Guillevin L, Trebossen R, Cohen P, Guilpain P, Pagnoux C, et al. Churg–Strauss syndrome cardiac involvement evaluated by cardiac magnetic resonance imaging and positron-emission tomography: a prospective study on 20 patients. Rheumatology 2013;52:642–50.

[121] Canaris GJ, Manowitz NR, Mayor G, Ridgway EC. The Colorado thyroid disease prevalence study. Arch Intern Med 2000;160:526–30.

[122] Klein I, Ojamaa K. Thyroid hormone and the cardiovascular system. N Engl J Med 2001;344:501–9.
[123] Brent G. The molecular basis of thyroid hormone action. N Engl J Med 1994;331: 847–53.
[124] Biondi B, Palmieri EA, Lombardi G, Fazio S. Effects of thyroid hormone on cardiac function: the relative importance of heart rate, loading conditions, and myocardial contractility in the regulation of cardiac performance in human hyperthyroidism. J Clin Endocrinol Metab 2002;87:968–74.
[125] Lewicki JA, Protter AA. Physiological studies of the natriuretic peptide family. In: Laragh JH, Brenner BM, editors. Hypertension: pathophysiology, diagnosis and management. New York: Raven Press; 1995. p. 1029–53.
[126] Dorr M, Wolff B, Robinson DM, John U, Ludemann J, Meng W, et al. The association of thyroid function with cardiac mass and left ventricular hypertrophy. J Clin Endocrinol Metab 2005;90:673–7.
[127] Sun Z, Ojamaa K, Coetzee WA, Artman M, Klein I. Effects of thyroid hormone on action potential and repolarization currents in rat ventricular myocytes. Am J Physiol Endocrinol Metab 2000;278:E302–7.
[128] Klein I. Endocrine disorders and cardiovascular disease. In: Zipes DP, Libby P, Bonow R, Braunwald E, editors. Braunwald's heart disease: a textbook of cardiovascular medicine. 7th ed. Philadelphia, PA: W.B. Saunders; 2005. p. 2051–65.
[129] Mintz G, Pizzarello R, Klein I. Enhanced left ventricular diastolic function in hyperthyroidism: noninvasive assessment and response to treatment. J Clin Endocrinol Metab 1991;73:146–50.
[130] Bengel FM, Nekolla SG, Ibrahim T, Weniger C, Ziegler SI, Schwaiger M. Effect of thyroid hormones on cardiac function, geometry and oxidative metabolism assessed noninvasively by positron emission tomography and magnetic resonance imaging. J Clin Endocrinol Metab 2000;85:1822–7.
[131] Torizuka T, Tamaki N, Kasagi K, Misaki T, Kawamoto M, Tadamura E, et al. Myocardial oxidative metabolism in hyperthyroid patients assessed by PET with carbon-11-acetate. J Nucl Med 1995;36:1981–6.
[132] Bengel FM, Lehnert J, Ibrahim T, Klein C, Bulow HP, Nekolla SG, et al. Cardiac oxidative metabolism, function, and metabolic performance in mild hyperthyroidism: a noninvasive study using positron emission tomography and magnetic resonance imaging. Thyroid 2003;13:471–6.
[133] Burns JC. Commentary: translation of Dr. Tomisaku Kawasaki's original report of fifty patients in 1967. Pediatr Infect Dis J 2002;21:993–5.
[134] Dillon MJ, Eleftheriou D, Brogan PA. Medium-size-vessel vasculitis. Pediatr Nephrol 2010;25:1641–52.
[135] Newburger JW, Takahashi M, Gerber MA, Gewitz MH, Tani LY, Burns JC, et al. Diagnosis, treatment, and long-term management of Kawasaki disease: a statement for health professionals from the Committee on Rheumatic Fever, Endocarditis and Kawasaki Disease, Council on Cardiovascular Disease in the Young, American Heart Association. Circulation 2004;110:2747–71.
[136] Brogan PA, Bose A, Burgner D, Shingadia D, Tulloh R, Michie C, et al. Kawasaki disease: an evidence based approach to diagnosis, treatment, and proposals for future research. Arch Dis Child 2002;86:286–90.
[137] Baer AZ, Rubin LG, Shapiro CA, Sood SK, Rajan S, Shapir Y, et al. Prevalence of coronary artery lesions on the initial echocardiogram in Kawasaki syndrome. Arch Pediatr Adolesc Med 2006;160:686–90.

[138] Hiraishi S, Misawa H, Takeda N, Horiguchi Y, Fujino N, Ogawa N, et al. Transthoracic ultrasonic visualization of coronary aneurysm, stenosis, and occlusion in Kawasaki disease. Heart 2000;83:400–5.
[139] Zilberman MV, Goya G, Glascock B, Kimball TR. Dobutamine stress echocardiography in the evaluation of young patients with Kawasaki disease. Pediatr Cardiol 2003;24:338–43.
[140] Hiraishi S, Hirota H, Horiguchi Y, Takeda N, Fujino N, Ogawa N, et al. Transthoracic Doppler assessment of coronary flow reserve children with Kawasaki disease: comparison with coronary angiography and thallium-201 imaging. J Am Coll Cardiol 2002;40:1816–24.
[141] Fu YC, Shiau YC, Tsai SC, Kao A, Hwang B, Chi CS. Discordance between dipyridamole stress technetium-99m tetrofosmin single photon emission computed tomography and coronary angiography in patients with Kawasaki disease. Int J Cardiovasc Imaging 2002;18:357–62.
[142] Mavrogeni S, Papadopoulos G, Douskou M, Kaklis S, Seimenis I, Baras P, et al. Magnetic resonance angiography is equivalent to X-ray coronary angiography for the evaluation of the coronary arteries in Kawasaki disease. J Am Coll Cardiol 2004;43:649–52.
[143] Fujiwara M, Yamada TN, Ono Y, Yoshibayashi M, Kamiya T, Furukawa S. Magnetic resonance imaging of old myocardial infarction in young patients with a history of Kawasaki disease. Clin Cardiol 2001;24:247–52.
[144] Prakash Powell R, Krishnamurthy R, Geva T. Magnetic resonance imaging evaluation of myocardial perfusion and viability in congenital and acquired pediatric heart disease. Am J Cardiol 2004;93:657–61.
[145] Vaglio A, Casazza I, Grasselli C, Corradi D, Sinico RA, Buzio C. Churg–Strauss syndrome. Kidney Int 2009;76:1006–11.
[146] Joint Statement of the American Thoracic Society (ATS), the European Respiratory Society (ERS) and the World Association of Sarcoidosis and Other Granulomatous Disorders (WASOG) adopted by the ATS Board of Directors and by the ERS Executive Committee. Statement on sarcoidosis. Am J Respir Crit Care Med 1999;160:736–55.
[147] Roberts WC, McAllister HA, Ferrans VJ. Sarcoidosis of the heart A clinicopathologic study of 35 necropsy patients (group I) and review of 78 previously described necropsy patients (group II). Am J Med 1977;63:86–108.
[148] Doughan AR, Williams BR. Cardiac sarcoidosis. Heart 2006;92:282–8.
[149] Tavora F, Cresswell N, Li L, Ripple M, Solomon C, Burke A. Comparison of necropsy findings in patients with sarcoidosis dying suddenly from cardiac sarcoidosis versus dying suddenly from other causes. Am J Cardiol 2009;104:571–7.
[150] Banba K, Kusano KF, Nakamura K, Morita H, Ogawa A, Ohtsuka F, et al. Relationship between arrhythmogenesis and disease activity in cardiac sarcoidosis. Heart Rhythm 2007;4:1292–9.
[151] Soejima K, Yada H. The work-up and management of patients with apparent or subclinical cardiac sarcoidosis: with emphasis on the associated heart rhythm abnormalities. J Cardiovasc Electrophysiol 2009;20:578–83.
[152] Okura Y, Dec GW, Hare JM, Kodama M, Berry GJ, Tazelaar HD, et al. A clinical and histopathologic comparison of cardiac sarcoidosis and idiopathic giant cell myocarditis. J Am Coll Cardiol 2003;41:322–9.
[153] Mavrogeni S, Sfikakis PP, Karabela G, Stavropoulos E, Spiliotis G, Gialafos E, et al. Cardiovascular magnetic resonance imaging in asymptomatic patients with connective tissue disease and recent onset left bundle branch block. Int J Cardiol 2014;171:82–7.

[154] Okayama K, Kurata C, Tawarahara K, Wakabayashi Y, Chida K, Sato A. Diagnostic and prognostic value of myocardial scintigraphy with thallium 201 and gallium 67 in cardiac sarcoidosis. Chest 1995;107:330–4.

[155] Nakazawa A, Ikeda K, Ito Y, Iwase M, Sato K, Ueda R, et al. Usefulness of dual 67Ga and 99mTc-sestamibi single- photon-emission CT scanning in the diagnosis of cardiac sarcoidosis. Chest 2004;26:1372–6.

[156] Kalin R, Stanton MS. Current clinical issues for MRI scanning of pacemaker and defibrillator patients. Pacing Clin Electrophysiol 2005;28:322–8.

Acquired valvular heart disease 16

Aortic root

V. Polsani*, X. Zhou†, M. Vannan*
*Marcus Heart Valve Center, Piedmont Heart Institute, Atlanta, GA, USA; †Chinese PLA General Hospital

Echocardiography has an established role in the morphological and hemodynamic assessment of the disorders of aortic root; hence, this section will focus on the essentials of advanced, integrated quantitative imaging of the aortic root to guide interventions. The annulus, the aortic valve (AV) leaflets, the sinuses of Valsalva (SoV), and the sino-tubular junction (STJ) are the anatomical components that constitute the aortic root. The functional anatomy of the aortic root involves imaging the geometric relationship of each of these components to delineate pathophysiology of the disease and to guide interventions. This is best achieved by a combination of echocardiography and another modality, the latter being dependent on the target anatomy and the planned intervention.

16.1 Annulus size and calcification

From the imaging perspective, the annulus is the virtual ring formed by the lowest point of the scalloped attachments of the crescent-shaped AV leaflets in left ventricular outflow tract (LVOT). This ring is below a true ring formed by the atrio-ventricular junction where the myocardium gives way to the aortic sleeve. This true ring is below the hinges of the leaflets, the so-called surgical annulus, which is below another true ring, the STJ junction [1,2]. Accurate measurement of the annulus (virtual ring) dimensions has become increasingly important with the advent of trans-catheter-based AV replacement (TAVR). It has also become evident that a single-dimensional 2-D measurement by 2-D echocardiography (2-DE) is anatomically incorrect because the virtual ring is, in fact, not circular, and like the LVOT, there is a minimum and maximum diameter. Thus, at least a mean diameter derived from the bi-plane measurement of the annulus is mandatory to accurately size the annulus. However, even this does not entirely account for the shape of the annulus. The latter is clinically relevant given that the prosthetic valves have a circular design and need to be placed within a noncircular annulus to prevent para-valvular leak (PVL) after TAVR. Thus, it appears that area-based or perimeter-based annulus diameters that account for the shape of the annulus seem to be a better predictor of optimal prosthesis size for TAVR [3–5]. Computed tomography (CT) has emerged as the most widely used method to size the annulus for TAVR, although 3-DE is equally good for this purpose [6–8]. Recent developments in automated quantitative modeling of the aortic root have in fact further

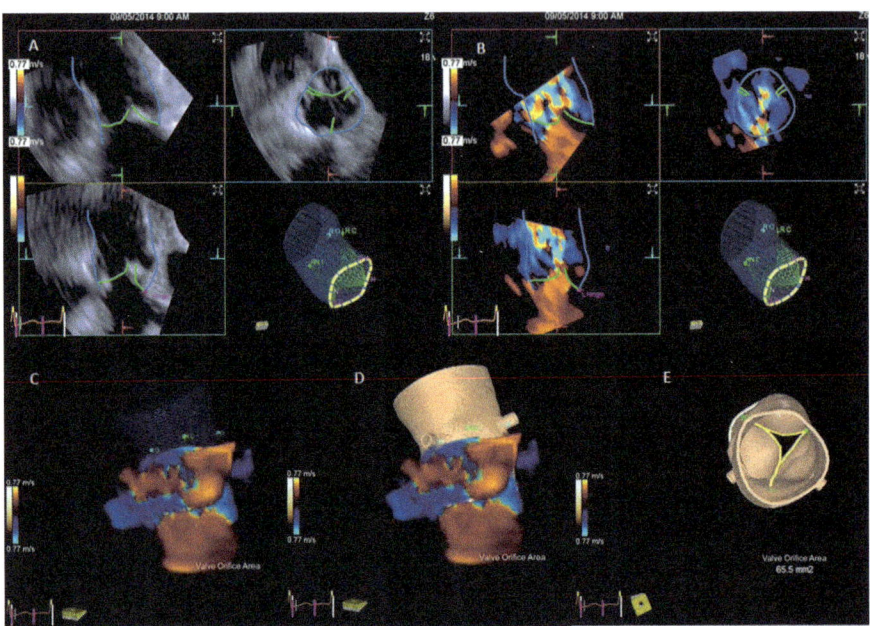

Figure 16.1 Example of automated aortic root modeling from 3-D TEE. A shows automated tracking from which the model is obtained with and without volume color Doppler. C and D show 2 displays of the model with color flow Doppler and E shows automated 3-D AV area measurement.

enhanced the reproducibility and workflow of CT and 3-DE (Figure 16.1) for the measurement of annulus size [9]. When contrast CT is hazardous, as in chronic kidney disease, or contraindicated, sizing the annulus using automated modeling from 3-DE is perhaps the best approach. Balloon sizing is an alternative in this situation, but it still requires contrast injection to ensure that there is no AR when the balloon is fully inflated [10]. Preliminary data indicate that 3-DE may be at least as good as balloon sizing in the choice of optimal prosthesis size for TAVR. Figure 16.2 shows an example of automated 3-D TEE and correlation to CT in TAVR planning.

Sizing the aortic graft during aortic valve-sparing (AVS) surgery in patients with AR due to dilatation of the ascending aorta (AA) or the aortic root can also be done using the geometric relationship between the annulus and the STJ junction. The diameter of the latter is usually 10–20% smaller than that of the annulus, about 15–20% is children, and 10–15% in adults. In AA aneurysm seen typically in the patients upwards of the fifth decade, the dilatation begins in the AA and extends proximally into the STJ and SOV and distally into the arch. The annulus is usually spared, therefore using the principle that the ideal graft size to remodel the STJ will be ~10% less than the annulus diameter holds true. While 2-DE diameter has been used for this purpose it is conceivable that the area or perimeter-based annulus diameter may be more accurate predictors of the graft size [11]. In aneurysms of the aortic root, typically seen in younger population,

Acquired valvular heart disease

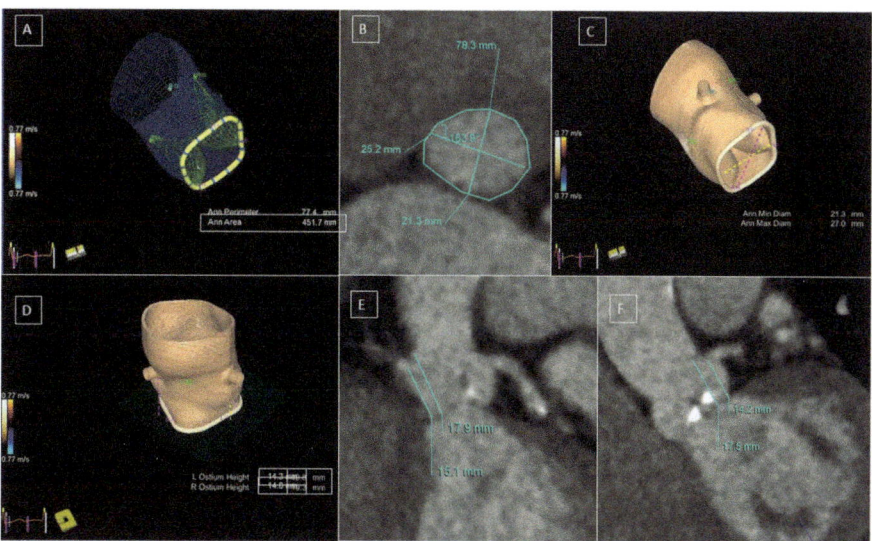

Figure 16.2 3-D TEE and CT aortic annulus sizing for TAVR planning. The annulus perimeter/area, and minimum/maximum diameters (A and C) by automated 3-D TEE modeling and CT are similar. D shows coronary ostia-annulus distance by 3-D TEE and these are similar to CT measurements in E and F.

the dilatation begins in the sinuses and extends proximally to the annulus and distally to the STJ and AA; using the annulus size to size the graft is not correct [11].

Annular calcification is both a friend and foe in TAVR. While the presence of calcification ensures stability of the implanted valve, it can interfere with the optimal seating of the fully deployed, appropriately sized valve. Bulky calcification of the annulus at the non-coronary cusp, especially those which extend into the LVOT, are predictors of significant PVL post-TAVR. CT is uniquely suited to assess the distribution and quantify the volume of annular calcification [12,13]. 2-DE and 3-DE can be used to visualize calcification, and the latter can be used to assess the distribution of annular calcium. However, both techniques are inferior to CT for this purpose.

16.2 Aortic valve leaflets

The aortic leaflets are semilunar shaped to conform to the scalloped curvature of each annular segment. The bases of the aortic leaflets are longer than the free edge length (~1.5 times), and the latter is 1.6–2.2 times the height of the leaflets. The normal leaflet edge lengths range from 26 to 35 (average ~31 mm) mm and height from 12 to 19 mm (average ~14.5 mm). The NCC tends be the largest (because most of the systolic flow occurs over this leaflet) followed by the RCC and LCC. The cusps form the belly of the leaflets, and the latter forms a sphere with their respective SOV. The thin fibrous coapting surfaces of the adjacent leaflets called the lunulae are about 2–4 mm in height, and the nodular thickening at the center of the free edge called the nodule of Arantius aids in the competence of the closed AV. About 50% of the leaflet height and 30% of the leaflet surface area are used for effective sealing of the valve orifice in diastole. The effective leaflet height is the vertical distance between the annular plane and the tips, which is usually 7–12 mm. The length of the cusp apposition during closure is called the coaptation length, which is 5–6 mm, and the closure point does not necessarily correspond to the geometric center of the AV orifice. The highest point of attachment of the leaflets to the aorta are the commissures which are just below the STJ. Beneath the commissures of the leaflets there are 3 triangular spaces at the junction of the scalloped annulus and the LVOT. The subcommissural segment between the NCC and RCC is fibrous and includes the membranous interventricular septum, the triangular space between the NCC and LCC is the fibrous aorto-mitral curtain, and the space between the RCC and LCC is the muscular interventricular septum. The two subcommissural spaces of the NCC constitute 55% of the circumference of the attachment of the annulus to the LVOT, the subaortic space between LCC, and RCC occupies the other 45% of the circumference. Dilatation of the annulus causes the two subcommissural triangular spaces beneath the NCC to become more obtuse, which reduces leaflet coaptation length and results in AR [11].

Echocardiography is the key imaging modality to assess the AV leaflets. CT and CMR provide limited information in this regard. While trans-thoracic echocardiography (TTE) can provide visualization of the morphology of the leaflets, measurement of leaflet parameters is best done by 2-D/3-DTEE. Real-time volume TEE of the aortic root is now an established clinical tool, and automated algorithms can be applied to measure leaflet free edge length, height, and coaptation height [9]. CT can also be used for this purpose but the leaflets can be difficult to identify for automated 3-D quantification. Dilatation of the STJ causes the commissures to be pulled outwards increasing the inter-commissural distance (ICD), which in turn causes AR both due to non-coaptation of the leaflets and downward displacement of the coaptation height relative to the annulus. However, often the aortic leaflets lengthen and become taller to compensate for the dilatation of the STJ and maintain competency of AV closure with no or minimal AR. However, this proportionate leaflet remodeling is offset by a limited increase in the height so that with progressive dilatation of the STJ, the leaflets continue to lengthen but the increase in height is blunted. This results in leaflets that are disproportionately longer than they are taller, at which point a regurgitant orifice and AR develop. This usually occurs when the leaflet length to the height ratio exceeds 2:1, which can be measured by automated modeling of the leaflets from 3-D TEE or CT data (Figure 16.3) [9,14].

The leaflet free-edge length and height are useful in estimating the size of the graft during AVS surgery. Generally, the optimal graft size is about 10% less than the average free-edge length but the considerable leaflet remodeling that occurs in AR associated with aortic root aneurysms renders this index less useful. However, the leaflet height is relatively fixed so that two-thirds of the average heights of the leaflets, plus 3–4 mm since the graft is sutured outside of the annulus, is a reliable predictor of the optimal graft size [11]. A number of other indices such 90% of the average free edge leaflet length, diameter of the best fit circle of the ICD, and commissural height have all been used for predicting graft size but all of these are affected by leaflet remodeling in aortic root aneurysms and do not provide a reliable estimate of the best-fit graft size. In older

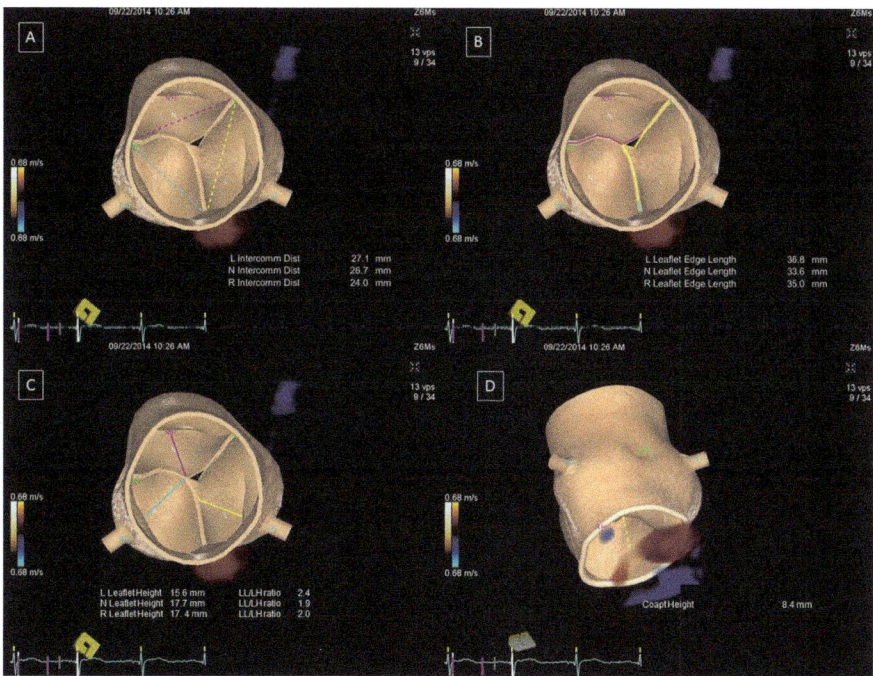

Figure 16.3 Automated quantitative modeling of the aortic root in aortic regurgitation. inter-commissural distance (A), leaflet free-edge length (b) and height (c) and their ratio, and co-aptation height can all measured.

patients with aortic aneurysm with STJ dilatation and normal annulus, sinuses and leaflets AVS surgery can be performed using a graft size estimated by the diameter of the imaginary best fit circle, which includes the ICD between the cusps when the cusps and pulled upwards to create an optimal coaptation after surgical exposure of the STJ. This is an alternative/additional approach to using the annulus diameter to predict the graft size during STJ remodeling operation, and a height <8 mm is predictive of recurrent AR after AVS surgery.

16.3 Sinus of Valsalva and sinotubular junction

The 3 sinuses can be considered as horizontal outpouchings from the annulus extending to the STJ. The shape of the normal sinuses can show individual variations with the height of the right SOV usually being the biggest followed by the non-SOV and the left SOV, respectively. The sinuses do not have a role in maintaining valve competency in diastole but play an important role in reducing the mechanical stress on the leaflets during closure. The eddy currents that form in the sinuses during systole allow the belly of the leaflets to approximate before the free edges of the leaflets during cosure, thereby reducing the trauma on the thin lunulae. The walls of the sinuses are thinner closer to annulus than the STJ, and circumference of the aortic root at the mid-point of the SOV is about 50% larger than the STJ. The origin of the coronary ostia is also distinctive, with the right arising higher (closer to the STJ) than the left, which arises almost from the mid-portion of the SOV. The STJ is a ridge of collagen and elastic fibers at the summit of the SOV just above the commissures. The circumference of the STJ in children (~15%) and younger adults (~10%) is less than that of the annulus; aging-related replacement fibrosis causes the STJ diameter to become equal to or exceed the diameter of the annulus.

Both echocardiography and CT are useful in the assessment of the SOV. Sinus height, width, and volume can be measured. Reduced sinus height, and perhaps volume can predict challenges during TAVR both with respect to optimal landing of the prosthetic valve and risk of rupture. Similarly, dilated sinuses may result in PVL due to improper landing of the valve during TAVR. During AVS surgery, using grafts that include sinuses have been advocated as beneficial in reducing closing stress on the native leaflets and ensuring durability of the repair. However, this has not been necessarily borne out in the long-term outcome data of AVS surgery, which may have to do with the design of these grafts rather than the concept that the preservation of the natural geometry of the SOV is a desirable goal. In the future, imaging flow patterns in SOV by phase contrast CMR may help design these grafts to have the intended benefits.

References

[1] Ho SY. Structure and anatomy of the aortic root. Eur J Echocardiogr 2009;10:i3–10.
[2] David TE. Surgical treatment of aortic valve disease. Nat Rev Cardiol 2013;10:375–86.
[3] Piazza N, de Jaegere P, Schultz C, Becker AE, Serruys PW, Anderson RH. Anatomy of the aortic valvar complex and its implications for transcatheter implantation of the aortic valve. Circ Cardiovasc Interv 2008;1:74–81.
[4] Hahn RT, Khalique O, Williams MR, Koss E, Paradis JM, Daneault B, et al. Predicting paravalvular regurgitation following transcatheter valve replacement: utility of a novel method for three-dimensional echocardiographic measurements of the aortic annulus. J Am Soc Echocardiogr 2013;26:1043–52.
[5] Hansson NC, Thuesen L, Hjortdal VE, Leipsic J, Andersen HR, Poulsen SH, et al. Three-dimensional multidetector computed tomography versus conventional 2-dimensional transesophageal echocardiography for annular sizing in transcatheter aortic valve replacement: influence on postprocedural paravalvular aortic regurgitation. Catheter Cardiovasc Interv 2013;82:977–86.
[6] Jilaihawi H, Doctor N, Kashif M, Chakravarty T, Rafique A, Makar M, et al. Aortic annular sizing for transcatheter aortic valve replacement using cross-sectional 3-dimensional transesophageal echocardiography. J Am Coll Cardiol 2013;61:908–16.
[7] Vaitkus PT, Wang DD, Greenbaum A, Guerrero M, O'Neill W. Assessment of a novel software tool in the selection of aortic valve prosthesis size for transcatheteraortic valve replacement. J Invasive Cardiol 2014;26:328–32.
[8] Stortecky S, Heg D, Gloekler S, Wenaweser P, Windecker S, Buellesfeld L. Accuracy and reproducibility of aortic annulus sizing using a dedicated three-dimensional

computed tomography reconstruction tool in patients evaluated for transcatheter aortic valve replacement. EuroIntervention 2014;10:339–46.
[9] Calleja A, Thavendiranathan P, Ionasec RI, Houle H, Liu S, Voigt I, et al. Automated quantitative 3-dimensional modeling of the aortic valve and root by 3-dimensional transesophageal echocardiography in normals, aortic regurgitation, and aortic stenosis: comparison to computed tomography in normals and clinical implications. Circ Cardiovasc Imaging 2013;6:99–108.
[10] O'Dea J, Nolan DJ. Assessment of annular distensibility in the aortic valve. Interact Cardiovasc Thorac Surg 2012;15:361–3.
[11] David TE, Feindel CM, David CM, Manlhiot C. A quarter of a century of experience with aortic valve-sparing operations. J Thorac Cardiovasc Surg 2014;148:872–9.
[12] Jilaihawi H, Makkar RR, Kashif M, Okuyama K, Chakravarty T, Shiota T, et al. A revised methodology for **aortic**-valvar complex calcium quantification for transcatheter **aortic**-valve implantation. Eur Heart J Cardiovasc Imaging 2014;15(12):1324–32.
[13] Khalique OK, Hahn RT, Gada H, Nazif TM, Vahl TP, George I, et al. Quantity and location of **aortic** valve complex calcification predicts severity and location of paravalvular regurgitation and frequency of post-dilation after balloon-expandable transcatheter aortic valve replacement. JACC Cardiovasc Interv 2014;8:885–94.
[14] Kim DH, Handschumacher MD, Levine RA, Sun BJ, Jang JY, Yang DH, et al. Aortic valve adaptation to aortic root dilatation: insights into the mechanism of functional aortic regurgitation from 3-dimensional cardiac computed tomography. Circ Cardiovasc Imaging 2014;7:828–35.
[15] Azzalini L, Ghoshhajra BB, Elmariah S, Passeri JJ, Inglessis I, Palacios IF, et al. The aortic valve calcium nodule score (AVCNS) independently predicts paravalvular regurgitation after transcatheter aortic valve replacement (TAVR). J Cardiovasc Comput Tomogr 2014;2:131–40.

Aortic stenosis

V. Polsani*, X. Zhou†, M. Vannan*
*Marcus Heart Valve Center, Piedmont Heart Institute, Atlanta, GA, USA; †Chinese PLA General Hospital

16.4 Aortic valve/root morphology

2-D trans-thoracic (TTE) usually suffices to image the etiology of aortic stenosis (AS) because calcific AS is the most common cause. If TTE is suboptimal, and it is necessary to visualize the valve anatomy, trans-esophageal echocardiography (TEE) is helpful for this purpose (Figure 16.4). Additionally, TEE can be useful to image the LVOT and the supra-valvular aorta if there is suspicion of associated abnormalities. For both of these, CMR is also a valuable additional or alternative imaging modality (Figures 16.4 and 16.5). CT is the modality of choice for the assessment of the aortic root in calcific AS for TAVR planning, and when contrast CT is contraindicated 3-D TEE is a useful alternative for TAVR planning (Figure 16.6) [1–7].

16.5 Severity of aortic stenosis

Doppler echocardiography is the cornerstone for hemodynamic evaluation of AS. It is now the established modality to assess the severity of AS in both normal and reduced stroke volume with preserved or reduced EF [8]. Measurement of

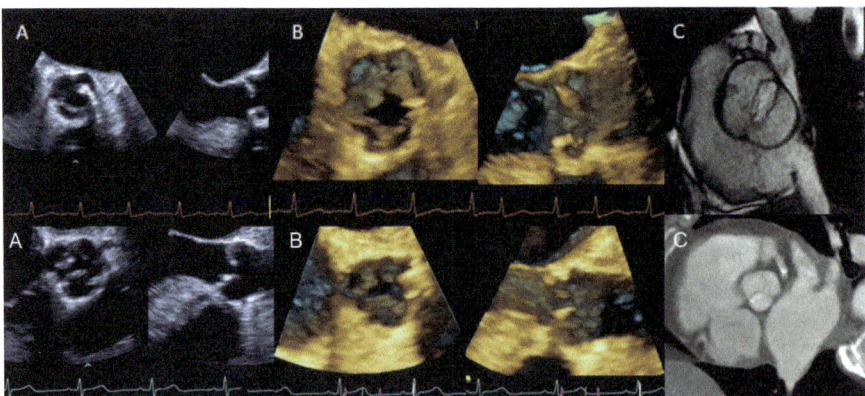

Figure 16.4 Illustrative examples of visualization of aortic valve (AV) morphology by 2-D TEE of mildly calcified AV (a, top) above and of significantly calcified AV (a, below). The corresponding 3-D TEE of the AV is shown in (b); note the dropouts in the leaflets in the example shown below. CMR shows the bicuspid valve morphology in (c) (top) without any calcium artifacts; the example below in (c), CT shows a 3-cuspid AV morphology. CT may be useful when it is performed primarily for CTA in AS to evaluate native or graft coronary anatomy.

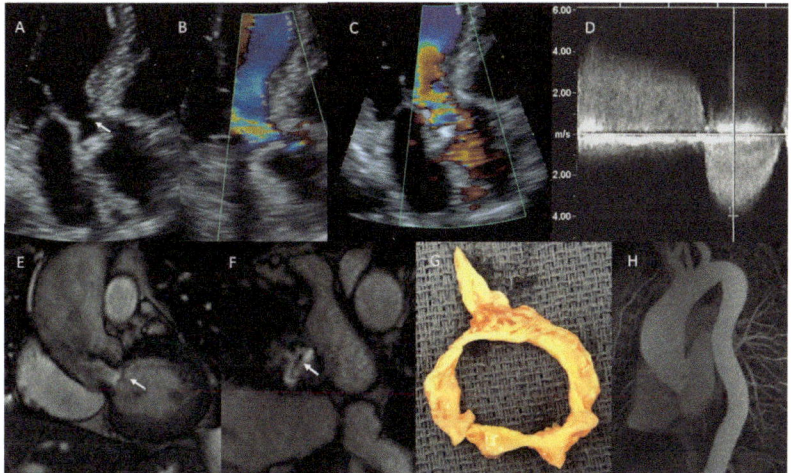

Figure 16.5 The role of CMR for sub-valvular AS. 2-D TTE (a–d) shows a linear echo-density on the LVOT (arrow) suggestive of a membrane, AR by color Doppler, and flow aliasing in the LVOT and across the AV in systole and a peak Doppler velocity of 4 m/s and AR. CMR shows the sub-aortic membrane in (e and f) in the long-axis and short-axis views of the LVOT and the AV. Furthermore, marked dilatation of the ascending aorta is seen in (h). In fact, the entire thoracic aorta can be evaluated (h), which is an important advantage of CMR. The pathologic specimen of the sub-aortic membrane removed during surgery is shown in (g).

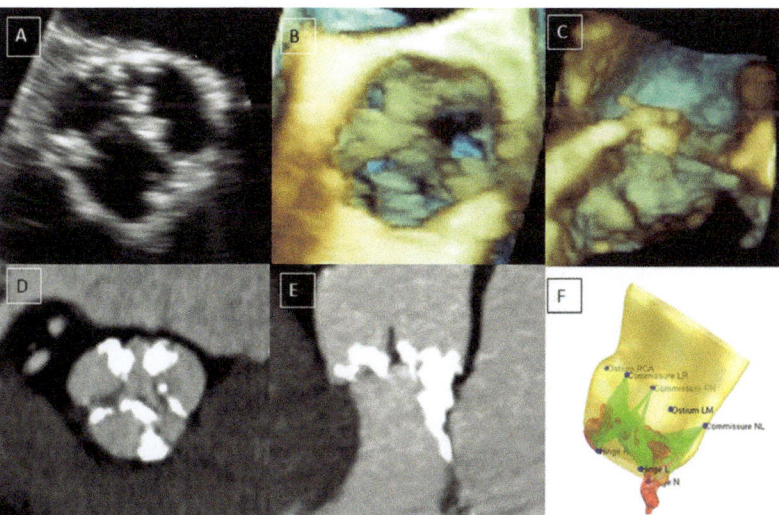

Figure 16.6 Echocardiography and CT of AV calcification in AS. In (a), 2-D TEE of calcium distribution in AS is shown in the short-axis view of the AV. 3-D TEE may be useful to examine the bulk of calcium (b and c), but significant calcification can cause dropouts in the image, and there is no method to quantify the calcium. Calcium amount and distribution is clearly depicted by CT in (c and d). This is valuable both to aid in the diagnosis of severe AS when hemodynamic data is uncertain or in cases of decision making for intervention in the setting of moderate–severe AS. Additionally, the pattern of distribution shown in D where the calcium protrudes into the LVOT is predictive of suboptimal positioning of the prosthesis during TAVR and consequent paravalvular leak.

instantaneous peak and mean gradient from aortic valve (AV) Doppler velocity and the calculation of the AVA using the continuity equation are the two most commonly used methods to assess the hemodynamic severity of AS. In most instances, these two indices provide a reliable assessment of the degree of valvular obstruction. In specific instances, the ratio of the peak LVOT velocity to that of the AV velocity (the so-called dimensionless index) and calculation of the arterial impedance (ZVa score) is helpful in making the diagnosis of severe AS (Figure 16.7). Not only is Doppler echocardiography essential in the diagnostic evaluation of AS, it has become the basis for prognostic assessment too, especially in the setting of asymptomatic severe AS. Very severe AS, low-flow low-gradient normal and reduced EF (LFLG-nEF, LFLG-rEF) severe AS are examples that are now recognized as groups with higher risk when not treated or may have variable response to valve replacement

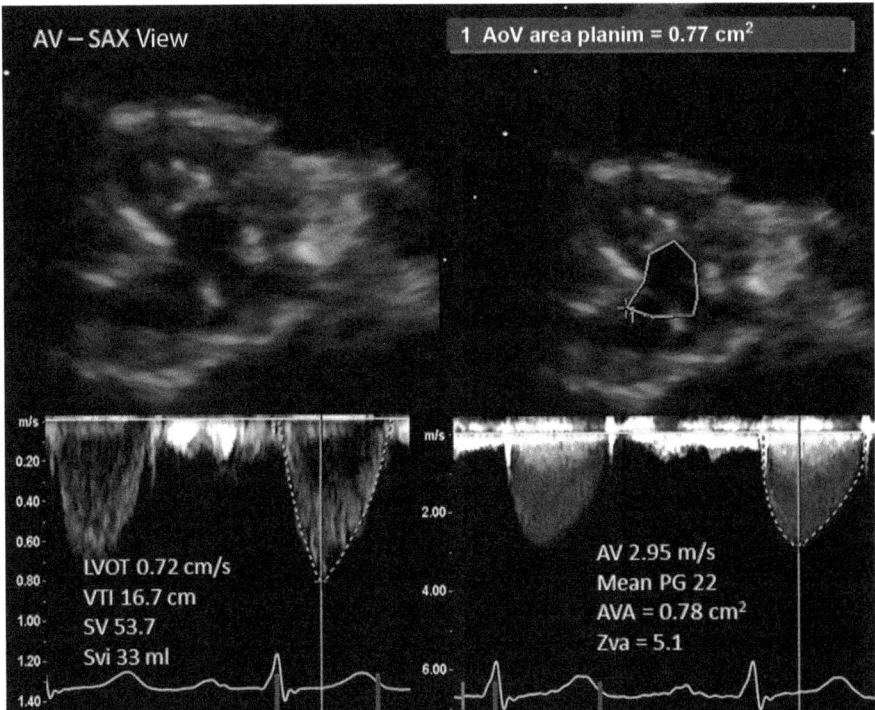

Figure 16.7 A 2-D Echo/Doppler echo of low-flow, low gradient, normal EF severe AS. The measured biplane EF was 61.2%, and there was moderate concentric LVH (wall thickness, 1.3 cm). The AVA by planimetry shown in the top panel was 0.77 cm^2. The peak AV Doppler velocity and the mean gradient suggest only mild–moderate AS. The stroke volume index based on LVOT spectral Doppler and LVOT diameter was 33 ml, and the calculated ZVa was 5.1 indicative of severe AS. The calculated AVA by continuity equation was 0.78 cm^2 consistent with severe AS.

(AVR) based on other factors [9–12]. Reduced global longitudinal strain measured by speckle-tracking echocardiography in very severe AS or LFLG-rEF or LFLG-nEF is an additional marker of adverse outcomes or suboptimal response to AVR [13,14]. Similarly, myocardial scar burden and extent of fibrosis on T1 mapping by CMR are evolving as powerful predictors of outcomes in these selected subgroups of severe AS [15]. When Doppler hemodynamics are equivocal in the evaluation of severity of AS, direct planimetry of the AV area (anatomic AVA) may be useful. It is often difficult if not impossible to obtain anatomic AVA by TTE, especially when there is significant calcification of the annulus and leaflets. Hence, 2-D TEE and 3-D TEE are preferred for this purpose, the latter being superior to the former (Figure 16.8). Both TEE techniques may be limited by bulky calcification for anatomic AVA, in which case CMR offers an alternative. Velocity-encoded CMR may also provide hemodynamic assessment of AS by measurement of peak velocity and gradient (Figure 16.9) [16]. It is also possible to use the amount of calcification of the AV as an index of the severity of AS in addition to hemodynamic assessment especially when the Doppler data is uncertain. Also, the extent of calcification of the AV may be used to predict progression to severe AS and used for decision making about the timing of intervention in specific circumstances [17,18]. The extent of calcification of the AV is best imaged and quantified by CT (Figure 16.6). Anatomic AVA may also be obtained by CT when it is done for assessment of coronary anatomy in patients with AS. Lastly, exercise hemodynamics of the AV using Doppler echocardiography and peak-exercise myocardial strain imaging are valuable when resting data do not resolve the issue of severity of AS, when symptoms are either apparently absent in the setting of severe AS, or when symptoms are out of proportion to the severity of AS [19].

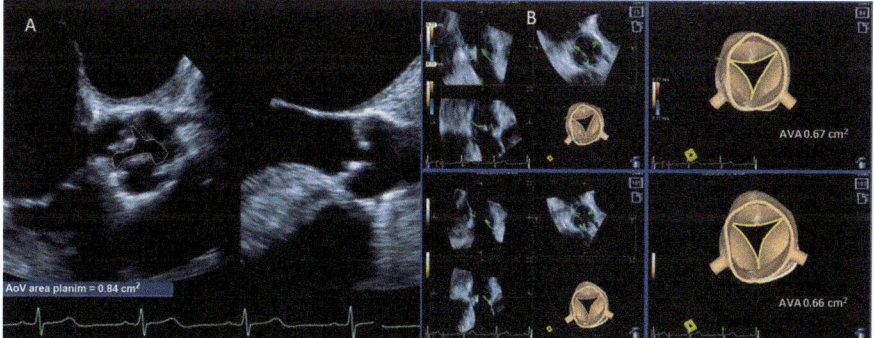

Figure 16.8 Planimetry of AV area by 2-D TEE (a) and 3-D TEE (b). In 3-D TEE, the anatomic landmarks of the aortic root are automatically identified from which a quantitative 3-D model is obtained. The automated 3-D AV area from two cardiac cycles are shown, and they are similar at 0.67 and 0.66 cm². Note that the 2-D planimetry shows a larger AV area, which may be due to not using the 2-D plane at the tips of the aortic leaflets.

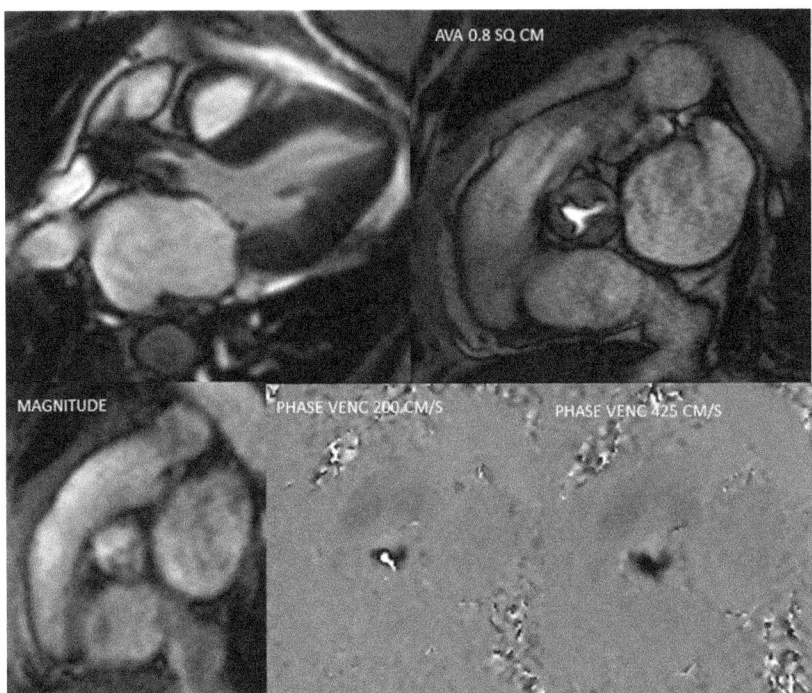

Figure 16.9 An example of phase contrast CMR for AS. Magnitude and phase images are shown in the panel below. When maximum velocity is set at 200 cm/s, the phase images show aliasing, whereas when it is set at 425 cm/s, there is no aliasing. The peak velocity was 4.1 m/s, and the AVA by planimetry was 0.8 cm^2.

16.6 Synthesis

Resting and exercise 2-D and Doppler echocardiography are the key techniques to assess the hemodynamic severity of AS. When the data from echocardiography is ambiguous or when additional data on the morphology of the AV is may provide additional insights, TEE or CMR may be used to obtain additional information. CT is particularly useful when the degree of AV calcification is needed for diagnostic or prognostic evaluation of AS, and is the modality of choice for evaluation of the aortic root for TAVR planning.

References

[1] Piazza N, de Jaegere P, Schultz C, Becker AE, Serruys PW, Anderson RH. Anatomy of the aortic valvar complex and its implications for transcatheter implantation of the aortic valve. Circ Cardiovasc Interv 2008;1:74–81.
[2] Hahn RT, Khalique O, Williams MR, Koss E, Paradis JM, Daneault B, et al. Predicting paravalvular regurgitation following transcatheter valve replacement: utility of a novel method for three-dimensional echocardiographic measurements of the aortic annulus. J Am Soc Echocardiogr 2013;26:1043–52.

[3] Hansson NC, Thuesen L, Hjortdal VE, Leipsic J, Andersen HR, Poulsen SH, et al. Three-dimensional multidetector computed tomography versus conventional 2-dimensional transesophageal echocardiography for annular sizing in transcatheter aortic valve replacement: influence on postprocedural paravalvular aortic regurgitation. Catheter Cardiovasc Interv 2013;82:977–86.
[4] Jilaihawi H, Doctor N, Kashif M, Chakravarty T, Rafique A, Makar M, et al. Aortic annular sizing for transcatheter aortic valve replacement using cross-sectional 3-dimensional transesophageal echocardiography. J Am Coll Cardiol 2013;61:908–16.
[5] Vaitkus PT, Wang DD, Greenbaum A, Guerrero M, O'Neill W. Assessment of a novel software tool in the selection of aortic valve prosthesis size for transcatheteraortic valve replacement. J Invasive Cardiol 2014;26:328–32.
[6] Stortecky S, Heg D, Gloekler S, Wenaweser P, Windecker S, Buellesfeld L. Accuracy and reproducibility of aortic annulus sizing using a dedicated three-dimensional computed tomography reconstruction tool in patients evaluated for transcatheter aortic valve replacement. EuroIntervention 2014;10:339–46.
[7] Calleja A, Thavendiranathan P, Ionasec RI, Houle H, Liu S, Voigt I, et al. Automated quantitative 3-dimensional modeling of the aortic valve and root by 3-dimensional transesophageal echocardiography in normals, aortic regurgitation, and aortic stenosis: comparison to computed tomography in normals and clinical implications. Circ Cardiovasc Imaging 2013;6:99–108.
[8] Baumgartner H, Hung J, Bermejo J, Chambers JB, Evangelista A, Griffin BP, et al. Echocardiographic assessment of valve stenosis: EAE/ASE recommendations for clinical practice. Eur J Echocardiogr 2009;10:1–25.
[9] Lancellotti P. Grading aortic stenosis severity when the flow modifies the gradient valve area correlation. Cardiovasc Diagn Ther 2012;2:6–9.
[10] Lancellotti P, Magne J, Donal E, Davin L, O'Connor K, Rosca M, et al. Clinical outcome in asymptomatic severe aortic stenosis: insights from the new proposed aortic stenosis grading classification. J Am Coll Cardiol 2012;59:235–43.
[11] Nguyen V, Cimadevilla C, Estellat C, Codogno I, Huart V, Benessiano J, et al. Haemodynamic and anatomic progression of aortic stenosis. Heart 2015;101:943–7.
[12] Clavel MA, Berthelot-Richer M, Le Ven F, Capoulade R, Dahou A, Dumesnil JG, et al. Impact of classic and paradoxical low flow on survival after aortic valve replacement for severe aortic stenosis. J Am Coll Cardiol 2015;65:645–53.
[13] Dahou A, Bartko PE, Capoulade R, Clavel MA, Mundigler G, Grondin SL, et al. Usefulness of global left ventricular longitudinal strain for risk stratification in low ejection fraction, low-gradient aortic stenosis: results from the multicenter true or pseudo-severe aortic stenosis study. Circ Cardiovasc Imaging 2015;8(3):e002117.
[14] Adda J, Mielot C, Giorgi R, Cransac F, Zirphile X, Donal E, et al. Low-flow, low-gradient severe aortic stenosis despite normal ejection fraction is associated with severe left ventricular dysfunction as assessed by speckle-tracking echocardiography: a multicenter study. Circ Cardiovasc Imaging 2012;5:27–35.
[15] Singh A, Horsfield MA, Bekele S, Khan J, Greiser A, McCann GP. Myocardial T1 and extracellular volume fraction measurement in asymptomatic patients with aortic stenosis: reproducibility and comparison with age-matched controls. Eur Heart J Cardiovasc Imaging 2015;16:763–70.
[16] Caruthers SD, Lin SJ, Brown P, Watkins MP, Williams TA, Lehr KA, et al. Practical value of cardiac magnetic resonance imaging for clinical quantification of aortic valve stenosis: comparison with echocardiography. Circulation 2003;108:2236–43.
[17] Chitsaz S, Gundiah N, Blackshear C, Tegegn N, Yan KS, Azadani AN, et al. Correlation of calcification on excised aortic valves by micro-computed tomography with severity of aortic stenosis. J Heart Valve Dis 2012;21:320–7.

[18] Aksoy O, Cam A, Agarwal S, Ige M, Yousefzai R, Singh D, et al. Significance of aortic valve calcification in patients with low-gradient low-flow aortic stenosis. Clin Cardiol 2014;37:26–31.

[19] Henri C, Piérard LA, Lancellotti P, Mongeon FP, Pibarot P, Basmadjian AJ. Exercise testing and stress imaging in valvular heart disease. Can J Cardiol 2014;30:1012–26.

Aortic regurgitation

V. Polsani*, X. Zhou[†], M. Vannan*
*Marcus Heart Valve Center, Piedmont Heart Institute, Atlanta, GA, USA; [†]Chinese PLA General Hospital

16.7 Aortic valve/root morphology

The combination of 2-D trans-thoracic and trans-esophageal echocardiography (TTE, TEE) usually suffices to image mechanism of aortic regurgitation (AR). Additionally, 3-D TEE provides additional insights into the aortic valve and root for a comprehensive assessment of the underlying mechanism of AR in most instances. CMR and CT may be helpful in specific circumstances to complement echocardiography in the assessment of the aortic root. For example, in bicuspid AV, the leaflet morphology and the associated aortic abnormalities can be accurately imaged by CMR. Similarly, CT may be useful to assess the aortic root when the cause of AR is aortic dissection/hematoma (Figure 16.10).

16.8 Severity of aortic regurgitation

While symptomatic severe aortic regurgitation (AR) is Class I indication for surgical intervention, symptoms are often non-specific or unreliable. Hence, quantitative imaging data is important in clinical decision-making and has been included in guidelines in the management of AR. In fact, among the objective parameters that influence the current clinical practice for intervention in chronic AR, almost all of these can be obtained by non-invasive imaging [1,2].

Current quantitative assessment of the AR is done by three principal approaches: measuring the effective regurgitant orifice area (EROA), the width of the vena contract (VC), and the regurgitant volume and fraction (RV, RF). The first two approaches are done by color flow Doppler (CFD) imaging, and the RV and RF can be measured by both echocardiography and CMR. Measurement of EROA and RV using the 2-D flow convergence radius (PISA method) is both validated and recommended to quantify AR [3,4]. But the PISA method in AR is technically demanding and often not possible, especially in eccentric and multiple jets. The measurement of VC width by 2-D CFD imaging (Figure 16.11) is more practical than the PISA method but it is a semi-quantitative measure of the regurgitant orifice size, unlike the PISA method. Also, the 2-D VC width is limited by the lateral resolution of the CFD, is not valid in multiple jets, and small technical errors in measurement can lead to misclassifying the degree of AR. Whether 3-D echo can improve the accuracy of the PISA method and the VC (area) to quantify AR remains to be seen but has shown promise in preliminary

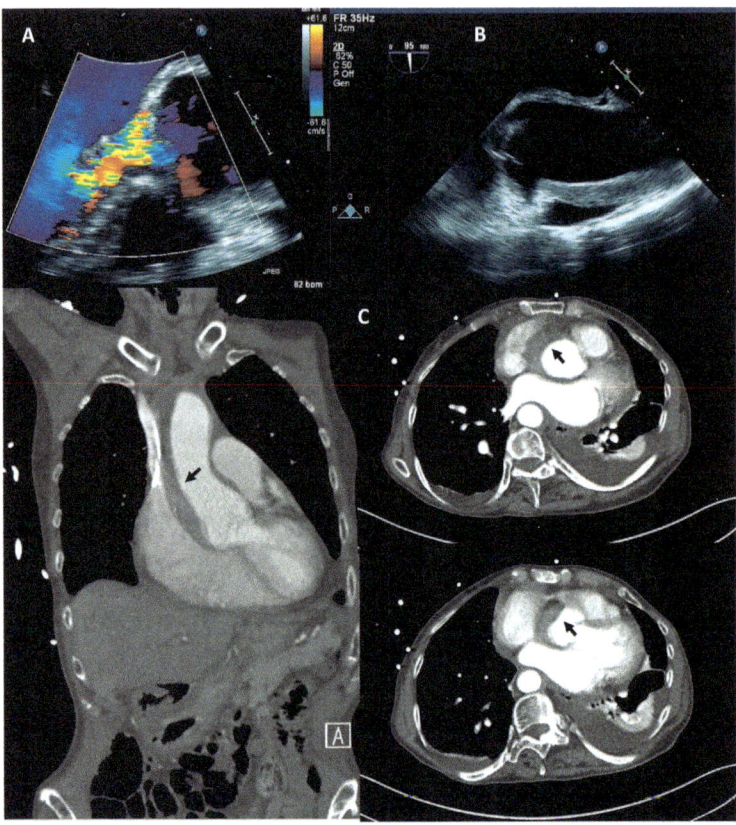

Figure 16.10 An example of AR secondary due to aortic root and ascending aorta hematoma. The upper panel (a) shows 2-D TEE CFD of AR, and hematoma (b). The extent of hematoma is better visualized by CT, extending from the root to the arch (black arrows in c).

studies [5]. Another potential quantitative measure of AR is the direct measurement of the anatomic orifice area using 3-D TEE, the so-called anatomic orifice area (AOA, Figure 16.12). This is less validated in AR compared to mitral regurgitation but may offer an additional or alternative approach where other quantitative measures are equivocal or not possible.

Measurement of RV and RF is the most optimal way to quantify AR and in this regard CMR clearly is the preferred technique. While RV and RF can be measured by Doppler echocardiography, it is both impractical and fraught with technical challenges where small errors can lead to big inaccuracies, hence it is largely abandoned in routine clinical practice [6]. The PISA method does yield RV/RF but in addition to the limitations of the PISA method mentioned above, the spectral Doppler of AR is often incomplete especially in eccentric jets making it an unreliable index. Hence, CMR is the preferred method to measure RV and RF. Using both magnitude and phase-contrast (PC) images from velocity-encoded CMR imaging, instantaneous flow volume can be obtained by measuring the flow velocities of each pixel within a

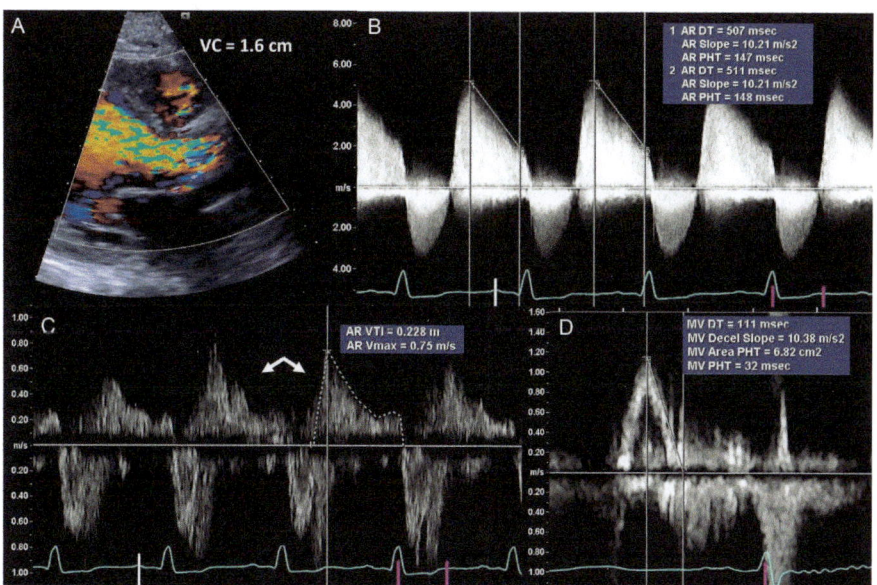

Figure 16.11 Elements of quantitative trans-thoracic echocardiography for AR. In (a) a wide jet of AR is seen with VC measuring 1.6 cm, in (b) dense spectral Doppler of AR is seen with a pressure-HT of ~140 ms, in (c) holo-diastolic flow reversal is seen with a VTI of ~23 cm, and a shortened mitral-inflow Doppler deceleration time of 111 ms is seen in (d).

region of interest (lumen of the aorta) (Figure 16.13). Integrating the flow volume in each frame over the entire cardiac cycle generates forward and regurgitant flow volumes from which RF can be calculated (Figure 16.14) [7,8]. When velocity-encoded PC-CMR is unreliable as when the area of interest is obscured by hardware artifacts and or when flow is complex in a markedly dilated aortic root, PC-CMR of the descending thoracic aorta may be used to demonstrate holo-diastolic flow reversal similar to flow reversal seen in the distal aortic arch or the abdominal aorta by Doppler echocardiography (Figure 16.11) [7,9]. Alternatively, holo-diastolic flow reversal may be used for additional evidence of severe AR during CMR imaging, albeit this is a semi-quantitative measure of severity of AR. Similarly, Doppler echocardiography provides a number of semi-quantitative measures of severe AR, such as the dense envelope (when optimally aligned with the direction of the AR jet), a short pressure half-time (typically <250 ms), deceleration time <150 ms of the mitral-inflow Doppler, and the time-velocity integral of the flow reversal in the distal aortic arch >15 cm (Figure 16.11) [3].

Another advantage of CMR over echocardiography is for accurate measurement of LV volumes and EF [7]. Both of these parameters are necessary for determining the need to intervene in AR. Both, 2-D and M –Mode echo are excellent for measurement of single-plane LV dimension, but accurate measurement of EF is often not reliable or limited by sub-optimal acoustic windows. Contrast echocardiography improves the feasibility and accuracy of EF measurements and may also aid in

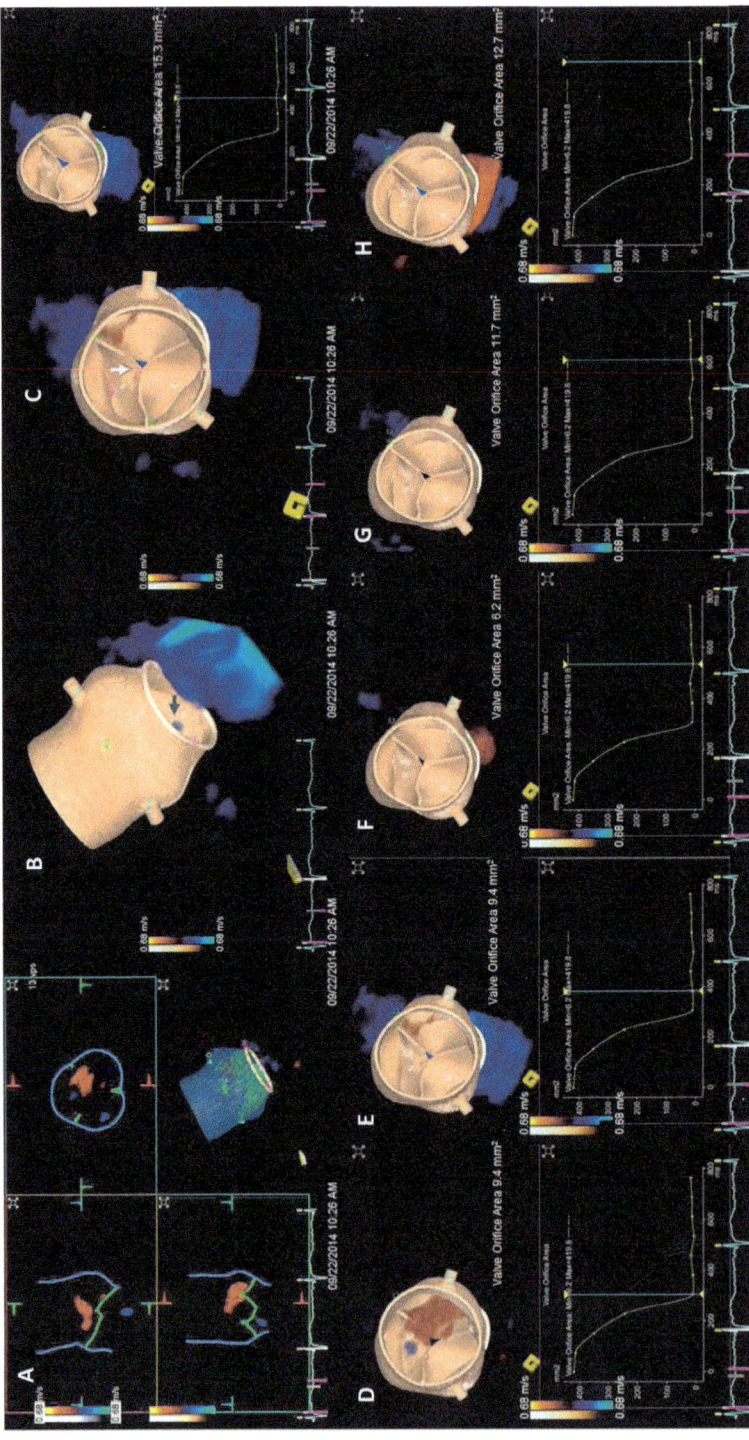

Figure 16.12 An example of anatomic 3-D AROA measured automated modeling of the aortic root by real-time volume color Doppler TEE. The landmarks of the aortic root can be automatically detected and tracked to model the aortic root (a), and mild AR (white arrow in b) can be seen, in (c) the largest 3-D AROA of 15 mm^2 is shown, and in (d–h) the variation in 3-D AROA throughout diastole is seen (9.4–12.7 mm^2).

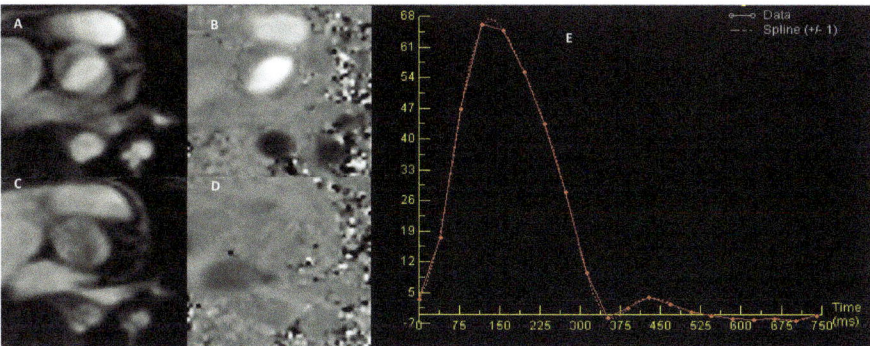

Figure 16.13 Quantification of flow using phase-contrast CMR. (a and b) Show magnitude and phase images of bicuspid aortic valve is systole, and (c and d) show the same in diastole. There is not phase-shift seen in diastole (no AR). The velocity–time curve in (e) shows no reversed flow (below baseline in diastole) and the AUC during systole yields aortic forward flow (stroke volume).

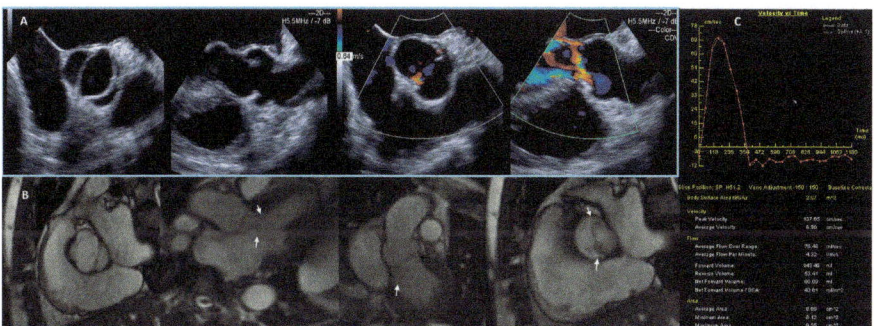

Figure 16.14 An example of eccentric AR in bicuspid aortic valve. (a) (in the blue box) From left to right shows 2-D TEE of the AV morphology and the eccentric AR by CFD. (b) Shows CMR from the patient, from left to right showing AV morphology in systole, two long-axis views showing two jets of AR (arrows), a short-axis of the AV and the two commissural jest of AR (arrows). In (c) quantification of AR is shown using phase-contrast velocity-encoded CMR. Total forward flow was 143.49 ml and the regurgitant volume (reverse flow below baseline in the curve) was 53.41 ml indicative of moderate AR. The regurgitant fraction is 37%.

the measurement of LV dimensions in the setting of sub-optimal acoustic windows. Whether 3-D echocardiography can provide improved quantification of LV size and EF specifically in AR remains to be seen [10]. However, at the present time, if accurate LV size and EF are needed either to confirm the degree of AR or for clinical decision-making CMR is the preferred method. Also, the extent of myocardial fibrosis measured by CMR may be another break-point for intervention in severe AR even in the absence of symptoms in the future [11].

Table 16.1 summarizes the parameters used to measure severity of AR and the applicable imaging techniques.

Table 16.1 **Imaging severity of aortic regurgitation**

	Echocardiography	CMR
Semi-quantitative parameters		
Density of spectral Doppler	++	–
Spectral Doppler pressure HT	++	–
Aortic HDFR	+++	++
Color-Doppler VC	+++	–
Quantitative parameters		
EROA	++	-
Anatomic ROA	++	-
RV/RF	+	+++
LV dimension	+++	++
LV volume/EF	+	+++

HT = half-time; HDFR = holo-diastolic flow reversal; VC = vena contracta; EROA = effective regurgitant orifice area; RV/RF = regurgitant volume and fraction; LV = left ventricle; EF = ejection fraction; – = not applicable; + = possible, not recommended or not done; ++ = useful or non-standard; +++ = useful, practical and recommended modality.

References

[1] Nishimura RA, Otto CM, Bonow RO, Carabello BA, Erwin 3rd. JP, Guyton RA, et al. American College of Cardiology/American Heart Association Task Force on Practice Guidelines. 2014 AHA/ACC guideline for the management of patients with valvular heart disease: a report of the American College of Cardiology/American Heart Association Task Force on Practice Guidelines. J Am Coll Cardiol 2014;63:2438–88.
[2] Vahanian A, Alfieri O, Andreotti F, Antunes MJ, Barón-Esquivias G, Baumgartner H, et al. Guidelines on the management of valvular heart disease (version 2012). Joint Task Force on the Management of Valvular Heart Disease of the European Society of Cardiology (ESC); European Association for Cardio-Thoracic Surgery (EACTS). Eur Heart J 2012;33:2451–96.
[3] Lancellotti P, Tribouilloy C, Hagendorff A, Moura L, Popescu BA, Agricola E, et al. European Association of Echocardiography. European Association of Echocardiography Recommendations for the Assessment of Valvular Regurgitation. Part 1: aortic and pulmonary regurgitation (native valve disease). Eur J Echocardiogr 2010;11:223–44.
[4] Zoghbi WA, Enriquez-Sarano M, Foster E, Grayburn PA, Kraft CD, Levine RA, et al. Recommendations for evaluation of the severity of native valvular regurgitation with two-dimensional and Doppler echocardiography. J Am Soc Echocardiogr 2003;16:777–802.
[5] Perez de Isla L, Zamorano J, Fernandez-Golfin C, Ciocarelli S, Corros C, Sanchez T, et al. 3D color-Doppler echocardiography and chronic aortic regurgitation: a novel approach for severity assessment. Int J Cardiol 2013;166:640–5.
[6] Thomas JD. Doppler echocardiographic assessment of valvar regurgitation. Heart 2002;88:651–7.
[7] Cawley PJ, Maki JH, Otto CM. Cardiovascular magnetic resonance imaging for valvular heart disease: technique and validation. Circulation 2009;119:468–78.

[8] Cawley PJ, Hamilton-Craig C, Owens DS, Krieger EV, Strugnell WE, Mitsumori L, et al. Prospective comparison of valve regurgitation quantitation by cardiac magnetic resonance imaging and transthoracic echocardiography. Circ Cardiovasc Imaging 2013;6:48–57.

[9] Bolen MA, Popovic ZB, Rajiah P, Gabriel RS, Zurick AO, Lieber ML, et al. Cardiac MR assessment of aortic regurgitation: holodiastolic flow reversal in the descending aorta helps stratify severity. Radiology 2011;260:98–104.

[10] Thavendiranathan P, Liu S, Verhaert D, Calleja A, Nitinunu A, Van Houten T, et al. Feasibility, accuracy, and reproducibility of real-time full-volume 3D transthoracic echocardiography to measure LV volumes and systolic function: a fully automated endocardial contouring algorithm in sinus rhythm and atrial fibrillation. JACC Cardiovasc Imaging 2012;5:239–51.

[11] Zendaoui A, Lachance D, Roussel E, Couet J, Arsenault M. Effects of spironolactone treatment on an experimental model of chronic aortic valve regurgitation. J Heart Valve Dis 2012;21:478–86.

Mitral regurgitation

P. Lancellotti[*,†]
*University of Liège Hospital, CHU Sart Tilman, Liège, Belgium
†GVM Care and Research, E.S. Health Science Foundation, Lugo (RA), Italy

16.9 Introduction

Mitral regurgitation (MR) is the second most frequent valve disease in Europe after aortic stenosis [1]. MR consists of abnormal systolic regurgitation of blood from the left ventricle (LV) to the left atrium (LA). Imaging plays a major role in assessing the aetiology, mechanisms and severity of MR [2–4].

16.10 Aetiology and mechanisms

Assessment of MR by imaging involves comprehensive evaluation of the aetiology (cause of the valve disease) and mechanism (lesion/deformation resulting in valve dysfunction), including the dysfunction type (leaflet motion abnormality). The cause of MR is classified as either primary (i.e., organic/structural) or secondary (i.e., functional/non-structural), whereas the mechanism is based on Carpentier's classification of leaflet motion: Type I: normal leaflet motion, Type II: excessive motion, or Type III: restrictive motion (A: diastolic (e.g., rheumatic disease) and B: systolic (e.g., ischaemic or non-ischaemic LV remodeling with leaflet tethering due to local or diffuse ventricular dilatation)). The same aetiology can cause different MR mechanisms (e.g., endocarditis causing perforation-Type I or ruptured chordae-Type II) [1,2].

Normal mitral valve function depends on coordinated interaction between the annulus, leaflets, sub-valvular apparatus (chordae tendineae and papillary muscles) and the LV (Figure 16.15). Dysfunction of any component can cause MR. The location of the involved leaflets (A: anterior; P: posterior) and scallops (numbered 1–3 for anterolateral, middle, and posteromedial, respectively), the calcification location (limited to annulus or extending to leaflets, commissures or sub-valvular apparatus), and the extent (localized or diffuse) determine the feasibility of valve repair.

Degenerative disease, the most common surgical MR cause, involves mitral valve prolapse (type II) and covers a large spectrum of lesions, such as (1) isolated billowing with the leaflet tips remaining intra-ventricular to flail leaflet with valvular eversion, (2) isolated scallop to multi-segment (or generalized) prolapse and (3) thin/non-redundant leaflets to thick/excess tissue (Barlow's disease). Prolapse location, valvular/annular calcifications and the severity of the annulus dilatation may affect the feasibility and choice of surgical/percutaneous repair techniques.

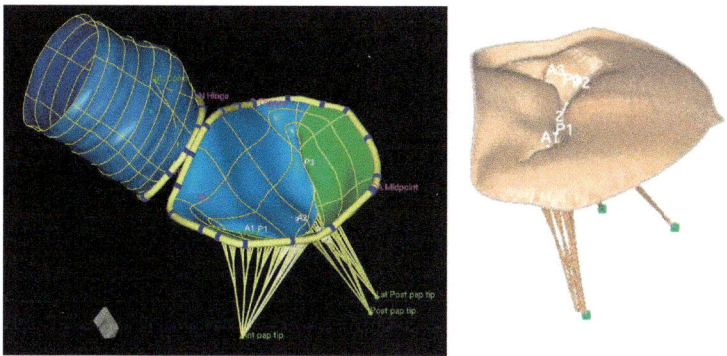

Figure 16.15 Mitral valve complex showing the mitral leaflets and the valve apparatus.

Secondary (functional) MR develops despite a structurally normal mitral valve due to mitral tethering secondary to ventricular deformation/remodeling, annular dilatation/dysfunction and insufficient LV-generated closing forces. Assessing ventricular global (diameters, volumes, sphericity, mass) and local remodeling (displacement of papillary muscles) and mitral valve deformation (coaptation depth, tenting area and volume in 3D) is of paramount importance in evaluating repairability and results of treatment [3].

16.11 2D/3D echocardiographic evaluation

Two-dimensional (2D) TTE is critical to initial and longitudinal assessment of patients with MR [3]. However, TOE plays a major role when TTE is non-diagnostic, when further diagnostic refinement is required or when mitral valve surgery is contemplated. Use of 3D echocardiography, especially 3D TOE, for mitral morphology and function evaluation is growing. A 3D display of complex mitral pathology or cardiac structures not well visualized by 2D echo (mitral annulus, papillary muscles) enhances pathophysiologic insight and communication.

- Mitral valve analysis

The assessment of the different components of the mitral valve apparatus requires multiple views. The **short-axis view** can be obtained by TTE or TOE, using the classical parasternal short-axis view and the transgastric view at 0°. This view permits, in diastole, the assessment of the six scallops and the two commissures. In systole, the localization of prolapse may be identified by the localization of the origin of the regurgitant jet. With TTE, a classical **apical 4-chamber view** is obtained and explores the anterior leaflet; the segments A3 and A2 and the posterior leaflet in its external scallop P1 can be visualized (Figure 16.16). With TOE, different valvular segments are observed, which depend on the position of the probe in the oesophagus when progressing from up to down. This allows successive observation of A1 and P1 close to the anterolateral commissure, A2 and P2 and finally A3 and P3 close to

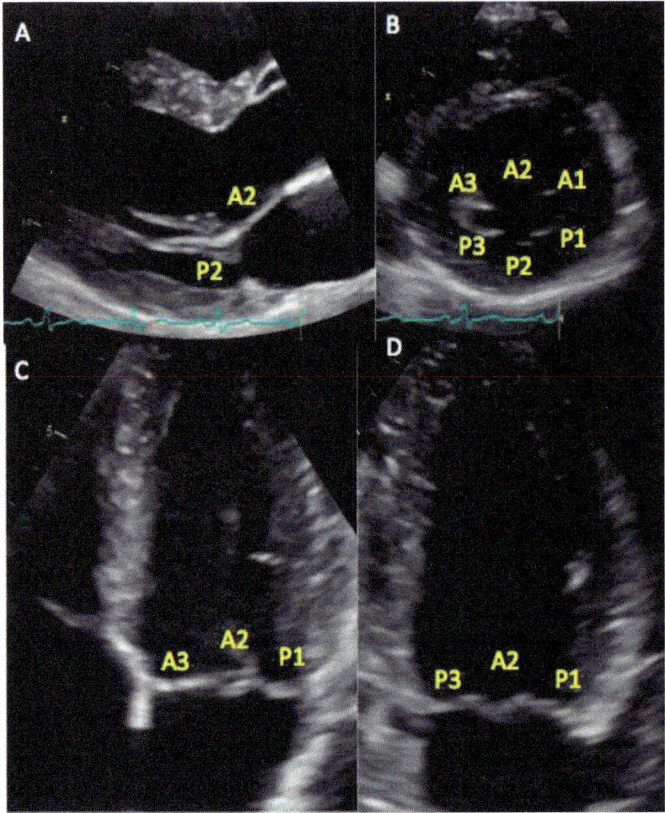

Figure 16.16 Mitral valve segmentation analysis with TTE.

the posteromedial commissure (at 40–60°). The **parasternal long-axis view** with TTE and the sagittal view at 120° with TEE show the medium portions of the leaflets (A2 and P2). A bi-commissural view can be obtained in the apical 2-chamber view with TTE, and a view at 40–60° with TOE shows the two commissural regions and, from left to right, P3, A2 and P1. A 2-chamber view from the transgastric position, perpendicular to the sub-valvular apparatus, allows measurement of the length of the chordae and the distances between the head of the papillary muscle and the mitral annulus. With the use of **real-time 3D imaging**, the mitral valve is best imaged when obtained in zoom mode to avoid stitch artefacts that may occur in a wide-angled acquisition. With both TTE and TOE, the unique 'en face' view, which is similar to the surgical view after left atriotomy, can be displayed (Figure 16.17) [5]. To simulate the surgeon's view of the valve, the 3D images are reoriented to exhibit the aortic valve at the 11 o'clock position. The sub-valvular apparatus is, on the opposite, best imaged from the LV perspective. To note, the gated full volume modality (wide-angled acquisition of 4 ECG gated pyramidal volumes) is the ideal way to obtain imaging of the entire mitral valve apparatus (chordae, papillary muscles, LV). Recently, new dedicated software for advanced 3D analysis of the mitral valve has been developed

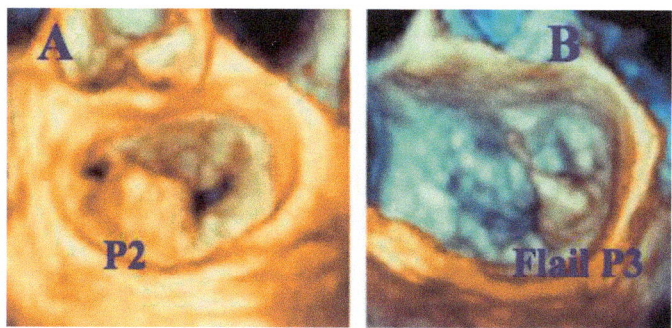

Figure 16.17 3D volume rendering of the mitral valve. (a) P2 prolapse, (b) Flail of P3.

to be incorporated into clinical practice [6]. It provides a realistic 3D model of the mitral valve and allows the calculation of a wide range of potentially useful parameters (annulus, anterior and posterior leaflet, leaflet segmentation, coaptation line and potential coaptation defects, mitral valve spatial relationship with the papillary muscles and aortic valve). The possibility of measuring the surface of the anterior leaflet to estimate, in a beating heart, the size of the annular ring ranks among the software's most interesting features. The added value of these parameters still needs to be defined.

- Repairability

Repairability prediction requires a systematic approach to describe the combination of lesions contributing to mitral dysfunction that all require specific correction (Table 16.2). Surgical mitral valve repair can be compromised in the presence of a large central regurgitant jet, severe annular dilatation (>50 mm), involvement of 3 or more scallops (especially if the anterior leaflet is involved) and extensive valve calcifications or calcified rheumatic valve disease. Additionally, in secondary MR, extensive LV remodeling (end-systolic diameter >51 mm), severely altered geometry of the mitral valve apparatus (systolic tenting area >2.5 cm^2 and coaptation distance >1 cm) and extensive basal LV necrosis have been shown to increase the risk of unsuccessful mitral valve repair [3,7].

- Assessment of MR severity

Comprehensive MR severity assessment is mandatory, using an integration of qualitative findings (e.g., mitral valve morphology, color flow and continuous wave signal of MR jet), semi-quantitative findings (e.g., vena contracta width, pulmonary vein flow, mitral inflow) and quantitative findings (regurgitant volume (RVol) and effective regurgitant orifice area (EROA)), as well as supportive findings (enlarged LV and/or LA, increased pulmonary arterial pressure) [3]. MR can easily be diagnosed with color-flow imaging, but this technique should not be used for grading MR severity. Localization, duration, timing and direction of regurgitant jet into the LA should be evaluated. Only holosystolic MR jets are typically associated with significant regurgitation. When feasible, measurements of vena contracta width and flow convergence are recommended

Table 16.2 Probability of successful mitral valve repair in MR based on echo findings

Aetiology	Dysfunction	Calcification	Mitral annulus dilatation	Probability of repair
Degenerative	II: Localized prolapse (P2 and/or A2)	No/Localized	Mild/Moderate	Feasible
Secondary	I or IIIb	No	Moderate	Feasible
Barlow	II: Extensive prolapse (3 or more scallops, posterior commissure)	Localized (annulus)	Moderate	Difficult
Rheumatic	IIIa but pliable anterior leaflet	Localized	Moderate	Difficult
Severe Barlow	II: Extensive prolapse (3 or more scallops, anterior commissure)	Extensive (annulus + leaflets)	Severe	Unlikely
Endocarditis	II: Prolapse but destructive lesions	No	No/Mild	Unlikely
Rheumatic	IIIa but stiff anterior leaflet	Extensive (annulus + leaflets)	Moderate/Severe	Unlikely
Secondary	IIIb but severe valvular deformation	No	No or Severe	Unlikely

Adapted from Lancellotti et al. [3] (Eur Heart J Cardiovasc Imaging 2013).

when more than a small central jet is observed. The width of the vena contracta – the narrowest part of the jet – correlates with quantitative measurements of MR. Using a Nyquist limit of 40–70 cm/s, a vena contracta width <3 mm correlates with mild MR, whereas a width ≥7 mm indicates severe MR (Table 16.3; Figure 16.18). Intermediate values are not accurate at distinguishing moderate from mild or severe MR (large overlap); they require the use of another method for confirmation. The moderate lateral resolution is a limitation. In the absence of mitral stenosis, a peak mitral E wave velocity >1.5 m/s suggests severe MR. A pulsed Doppler mitral (at the mitral leaflet tips) to aortic velocity time integral (VTI) ratio >1.4 also strongly suggests severe MR, whereas a VTI ratio <1 is in favor of mild MR. In severe MR, the S wave component of pulsed Doppler pulmonary venous flow becomes frankly reversed if the jet is directed into the sampled vein. A dense MR continuous wave Doppler signal with a full envelope indicates more severe MR than a faint signal. When truncated (notch) with a triangular contour and an

Table 16.3 Grading the severity of primary MR

Parameters	Mild	Moderate	Severe
Qualitative			
MV morphology Color flow MR jet	Normal/Abnormal Small, central	Normal/Abnormal Intermediate	Flail leaflet/Ruptured PMs Very large central jet or eccentric jet adhering, swirling and reaching the posterior wall of the LA
Flow convergence zone	None or small	Intermediate	Large
CW signal of MR jet	Faint/Parabolic	Dense/Parabolic	Dense/Triangular
Semi-quantitative			
VC width (mm)	<3	Intermediate	≥7 (>8 for biplane)[a]
Pulmonary vein flow	Systolic dominance	Systolic blunting	Systolic flow reversal
Mitral inflow	A wave dominant	Variable	E wave dominant (>1.5 m/s)
VTI mit/VTI Ao	<1	Intermediate	>1.4
Quantitative			
EROA (mm^2)	<20	20–29; 30–39[b]	≥40
RVol (ml)	<30	30–44; 45–59[b]	≥60

+ LV and LA size and the systolic pulmonary pressure.
[a] Average between apical 4- and 2-chamber views.
[b] Grading of severity of organic MR classifies regurgitation as mild, moderate or severe, and sub-classifies the moderate regurgitation group into 'mild-to-moderate' (EROA of 20–29 mm^2 or a RVol of 30–44 ml) and 'moderate-to-severe' (EROA of 30–39 mm^2 or a RVol of 45–59 ml). In secondary MR, the thresholds of severity, which are of prognostic value, are 20 mm^2 and 30 ml, respectively.
Adapted from Lancellotti et al. [3] (Eur Heart J Cardiovasc Imaging 2013).

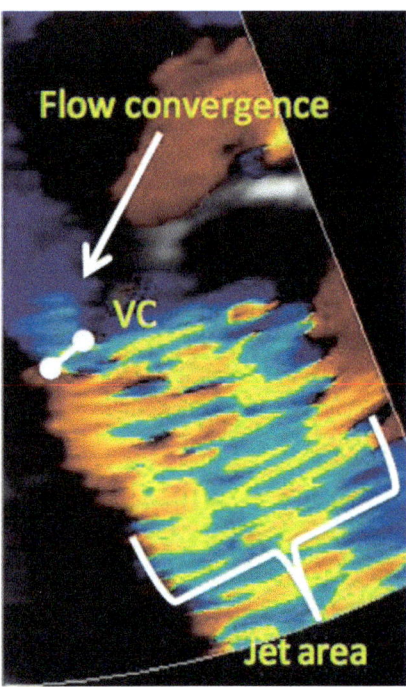

Figure 16.18 A semi-quantitative assessment of MR severity using the vena contracta width. The three components of the regurgitant jet (flow convergence zone, vena contracta, jet turbulence) are shown.

early peak velocity (blunt), it indicates elevated LA pressure or a prominent regurgitant pressure wave into the LA due to severe MR. Quantitation of MR severity is essential for MR grading and clinical decision-making. Quantitatively defined severe MR portends a poor prognosis regardless of the aetiology. Quality control of the flow convergence method (proximal isovelocity surface area (PISA)), particularly important with eccentric jets, dynamic MR throughout systole and the proximal flow convergence shape, is essential in practice as this method has demonstrated links to outcome (Figure 16.19). The use of 3D color flow volumetric imaging allows direct assessment of the size and shape of the regurgitant orifice, preventing the geometric assumptions applied by 2D imaging. With manual cropping of the image plane perpendicularly orientated to the jet direction, the narrowest cross-sectional area of the MR jet can be obtained in an 'en face' view and measured by planimetry in systole (Figure 16.20). In primary MR, the shape of the regurgitant orifice has been shown to be relatively rounder. Several studies using 3D TOE for planimetry of the anatomical regurgitant orifice (the vena contracta area) have found a high correlation with the 2D vena contracta and the PISA method [8,9]. A recent study showed its superiority over the PISA method in eccentric jets [10]. Of note, new 3D/4D ultrasound probe generations will allow automatic visualization of the 3D PISA surface and anatomic orifice area, with expected higher accuracy of the subsequent RVol calculation.

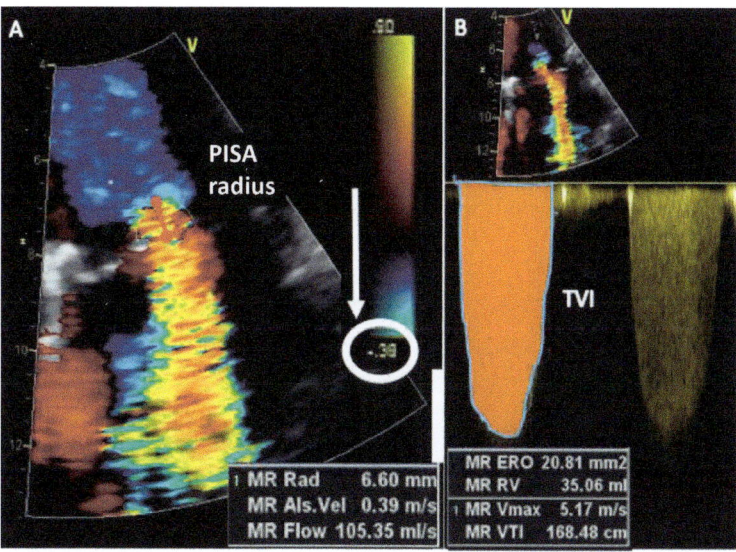

Figure 16.19 Quantitative assessment of MR severity using the PISA method. Stepwise analysis of MR: (a) Apical 4-chamber view, color-flow display, zoom of the selected zone, downward shift of zero baseline to obtain an hemispheric PISA; measurement of the PISA radius using the first aliasing; (b) Continuous wave Doppler of MR jet allowing calculation of the effective regurgitant orifice area (EROA) and regurgitant volume (RVol).

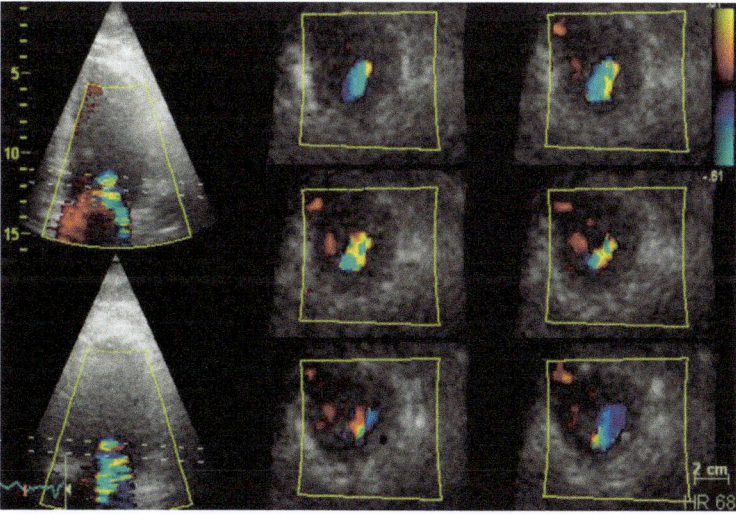

Figure 16.20 Vena contracta area as assessed by 3D echocardiography showing that the vena contracta of the regurgitant jet can be elliptic. 3D echocardiography allows correct alignment perpendicular to the jet direction and accurate measurement of the vena contracta area.

Severe MR is defined according to current recommendations with different criteria for primary/organic MR (severe: RVol ≥60 ml, EROA ≥40 mm^2) and for secondary/functional MR (severe: RVol ≥30 ml, EROA ≥20 mm^2) based on outcome studies. Exercise echocardiography can also be useful to evaluate the changes in EROA and RVol during stress; an increase by one MR grade is indicative of higher cardiovascular risk [11–15].

- Consequences of MR

MR hemodynamic consequences on LV, LA and pulmonary pressure should be evaluated. LV enlargement is measured by LV diameters and/or volumes (2D method of discs or 3D echo when imaging is of high quality). LV dysfunction is evaluated by either ejection fraction or end-systolic LV size. Of note, LV ejection fraction is load dependent and often overestimates LV systolic performance. An increased LV end-systolic diameter (>40–45 mm) and an LV ejection fraction <60% are indicators of LV systolic dysfunction, portend poor long-term prognosis and generally are accepted as indications for surgery even in the absence of symptoms [16]. A systolic tissue Doppler velocity measured at the lateral annulus <10.5 cm/s has been shown to identify subclinical LV dysfunction and to predict post-operative LV dysfunction in patients with asymptomatic primary MR [17]. Similarly, a global longitudinal strain <18% (2D-speckle tracking) has been associated with post-operative LV dysfunction [18]. More recently, LV global longitudinal strain <20% was associated with reduced cardiac event-free survival in asymptomatic patients with primary MR and no LV dysfunction/dilatation [19]. The response to exercise stress echocardiography can be used to identify the presence of contractile reserve (viability) in patients with secondary MR. In primary MR, it is defined as a <4% increase in LV ejection fraction or exercise-induced <2% changes in longitudinal strain [19]. The LA dilates in response to chronic volume and pressure overload. A normal-sized LA is not normally associated with significant MR unless it is acute, in which case the valve appearance is likely to be grossly abnormal. An enlarged LA (LA volume index >60 ml/m^2) predicts poor prognosis in patients with primary MR [20]. A systolic pulmonary arterial pressure >50 mm Hg at rest or >60 mm Hg (obtained by summing the transtricuspid pressure gradient and the estimated right atrial pressure) at exercise markedly affects the outcome of patients with primary MR [21]. A tricuspid annulus dilatation (≥40 mm or >21 mm/m^2) contributes to recurrent tricuspid regurgitation after mitral valve surgery [21].

16.12 Cardiac magnetic resonance

In patients with inadequate or discrepant echocardiography, cardiac magnetic resonance (CMR) permits quantification of MR severity and evaluation of LV anatomy and function. CMR is the most accurate and reproducible non-invasive method for assessing LV volumes, the LV ejection fraction and remodeling findings [22] (Figure 16.21). For instance, the extent of LV remodeling is often undervalued in patients with degenerative MR, especially when localized at the LV apical region [23,24]. It has been

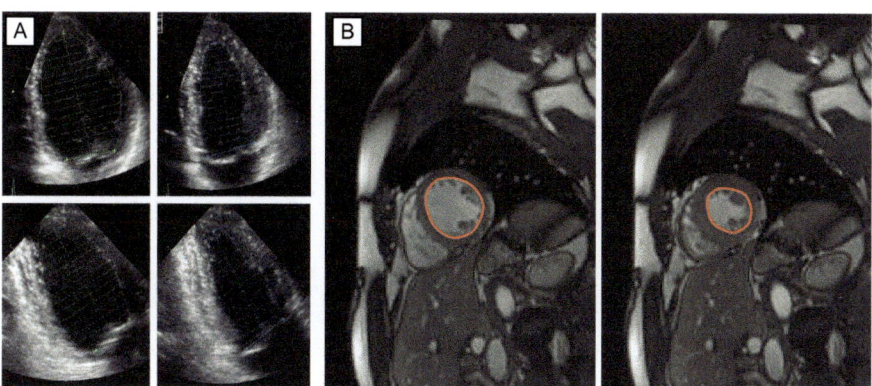

Figure 16.21 (a) The LV ejection fraction by 2D TTE was obtained by the modified Simpson's method in the apical 4- and 2-chamber view.(b) The LV ejection fraction by CMR was calculated by assessment of end-diastolic and end-systolic LV volumes in multiple parallel short-axis slices.
Permission from Van De Heyning CM. Cardiovasc Ultrasound 2013 Dec 27;11:46. doi:10.1186/1476-7120-11-46.

recently shown that in patients with moderate to severe primary MR without overt LV dysfunction, 2D TTE may significantly underestimate LV remodeling in comparison to CMR [25].

CMR can also be used for valve analysis using steady-state free precession (SSFP) sequences, which precisely discriminate blood from tissue [26]. Turbulent flow through the mitral regurgitant orifice is easily visible with SSFP (visualization of signal voids due to spin dephasing in moving protons). Mitral valve anatomy can be imaged by acquisition of standard short-axis, 2-, 3- and 4-chamber long-axis views in combination with oblique long-axis cines orthogonal to the line of coaptation [27]. CMR has comparable diagnostic value to echocardiography for identification of prolapsing scallops, but it is inferior for imaging the sub-valvular apparatus (torn chordae) due to its lower spatial and temporal resolution.

Only a few studies have used SSFP CMR for assessing the EROA by planimetry of the regurgitant orifice in a slice parallel to the valvular plane and perpendicular to the regurgitant jet at mid-systole. Quantification of EROA seems to be correlated well with angiographic and echocardiographic data [28]. There is also a good agreement with the PISA method by 2D or 3D echo and CMR planimetry of the regurgitant orifice [29–31] (Figure 16.22). To note, CMR planimetry defines the anatomic regurgitant lesion, whereas the area of EROA by PISA yields the narrowest flow stream, which tends to be smaller than the anatomic orifice area. It should also be emphasized that the regurgitant orifice is frequently inconstant throughout systole in primary MR. This can potentially affect the estimation of the regurgitant severity. Lastly, planimetry of the MR regurgitant orifice is time consuming and remains challenging because appropriate plane alignment and angulation may be more difficult

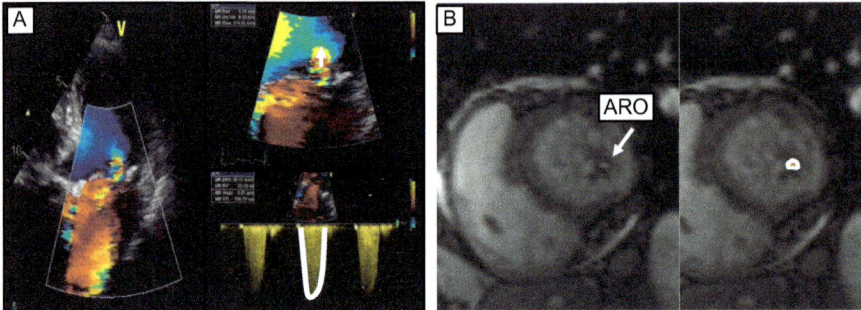

Figure 16.22 Measurement of the regurgitant orifice by 2D TTE and CMR. (a) Acquisition of PISA radius and continuous wave Doppler of the MR jet allows calculation of the effective regurgitant orifice. The PISA radius is measured at mid-systole using the first aliasing with a reduced Nyquist limit (15–40 m/s). (b) The anatomic regurgitant orifice can be measured by planimetry on a slice parallel to the valvular plane obtained by cardiovascular magnetic resonance.
Permission from Van De Heyning CM. Cardiovasc Ultrasound 2013 Dec 27;11:46. doi:10.1186/1476-7120-11-46.

due to the longitudinal movement of the mitral annulus and, in some cases, of the irregular shapes of the regurgitant orifice. Furthermore, with CMR, blood flow and velocity can be accurately obtained by phase-contrast velocity mapping. Hence, RVol can be measured indirectly as the difference between the total stroke volume and the aortic flow (forward stroke volume), as well as directly as the regurgitant flow across the mitral valve. This latter measurement, however, requires a specialized imaging sequence that tracks the motion of the mitral valve annulus during the cardiac cycle. Lastly, it should be noted that all measurements with velocity imaging might be inaccurate in patients with high heart rate variability. In the absence of other regurgitant lesions, a rare situation in primary MR, RVol can also be calculated by subtracting the right ventricular stroke volume from the LV stroke volume. However, the calculation of the right ventricular stroke volume is less reproducible due to the extensive trabeculation of the right ventricle.

Late gadolinium enhancement CMR (images obtained 10–20 min after injection of contrast) is widely used to assess cardiac fibrosis in various cardiomyopathies. In contrast, very few studies have investigated cardiac fibrosis by CMR in primary MR. For instance, Han et al., using 3D high-resolution late gadolinium enhancement CMR imaging, showed the presence of focal myocardial fibrosis in the papillary muscles in some patients with mitral valve prolapse and complex ventricular arrhythmias [27]. Also, the presence of LV remodeling seems to be associated with the presence of myocardial fibrosis in primary MR [29] (Figure 16.23). In addition, the blood-to-leaflet contrast ratio was also increased in these patients, which might reflect the significantly expanded spongia layer with proteoglycans in the myxomatous valve. In secondary MR, CMR can play a major role in the evaluation of the extent of myocardial necrosis, which may limit the extent of functional recovery after revascularization or of functional recruitment in resynchronized patients [7].

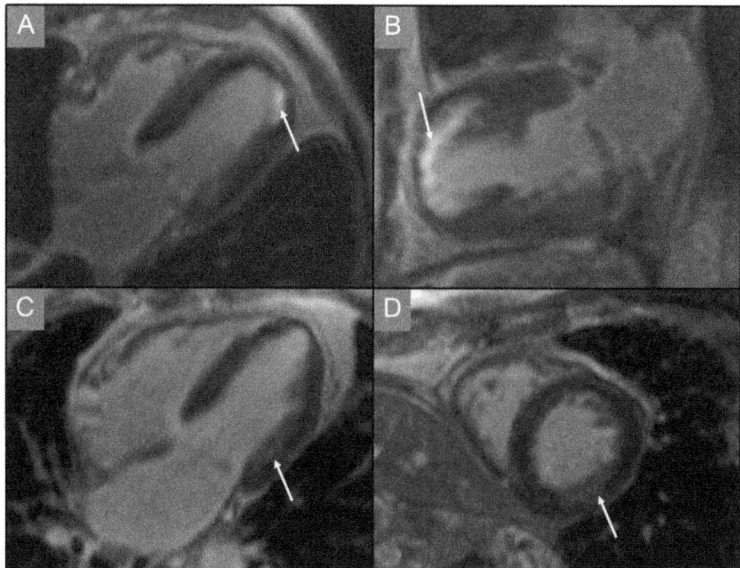

Figure 16.23 Different patterns of fibrosis on late enhancement (LE) CMR in primary mitral regurgitation. Arrows point at zones of late contrast enhancement on CMR, indicating the presence of fibrosis. (a and b) Infarct-like pattern in a 71-year-old male with moderate-to-severe MR due to prolapse of P2. This patient had normal coronary arteries on coronary angiography. (c and d) Late contrast enhancement in the lateral wall of a 72-year-old male with severe MR due to prolapse of P2.
Permission from Van De Heyning CM. Eur J Clin Invest 2014;44:840-7.

16.13 Multislice cardiac computed tomography

Experience with multislice cardiac computed tomography (MSCT) in MR is still limited but may be considered for quantifying mitral and coronary calcification or to assess coronary artery disease preoperatively [32] (Figure 16.24). Given its high spatial resolution, MSCT can accurately delineate MV anatomy, and it is uniquely useful in demonstrating the size and course of the coronary sinus in relation to the mitral annulus and circumflex coronary artery, an important consideration for some transcatheter mitral valve devices [7,33,34].

MSCT, from thin-section reconstructions, allows direct visualization of the thickening and calcification of the leaflets, mitral annulus, chordae and papillary muscles. A recent study showed good correlation with 3D TOE concerning measurements of mitral valve geometry and leaflet lengths and angles. The extent of calcification of the mitral annulus might even be better demonstrated than by echo or CMR [32,33].

The inner contour of the regurgitant orifice can be manually outlined on reconstructed cross-sectional images of the mitral valve in oblique short-axis. Two studies have demonstrated that the MSCT-derived anatomical regurgitant orifice area correlates well with EROA measured by echocardiography [35,36]. Chamber dimensions can be obtained after post-processing of the images with a contour-detection algorithm

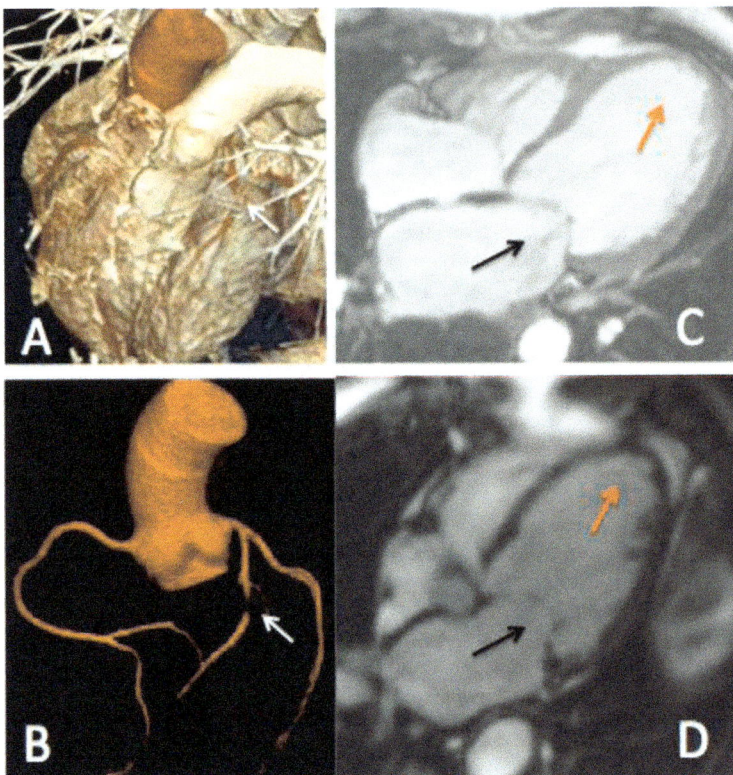

Figure 16.24 Patient with a history of anterior myocardial infarction, secondary MR and severe left ventricular remodeling. Three-dimensional (3D) cardiac computed tomography showing a significant left anterior descending artery stenosis (a and b, white arrows). Cardiac magnetic resonance demonstrated the presence of significant mitral valve deformation with a severe tenting (black arrows) and a large zone of myocardial scar tissue (orange arrows) (c and d). Permission from Lancellotti P et al. Circ Cardiovasc Imaging 2014;7:735-46.

and manual correction, if not satisfactory. The RVol can be generated as the difference between the calculated stroke volume of the left and the right ventricle and has recently been shown to have a good correlation with the RVol obtained by CMR. Although MSCT might be particularly useful in the preoperative setting because it provides complementary information on the coronary arteries (high negative predictive value in patients who are at low risk of atherosclerosis), a routine clinical implementation is not yet recommended.

16.14 Conclusion

For assessment of MR, 2D/3D TTE and TOE remain the first-line imaging modalities. In patients with poor echogenicity, CMR is the imaging modality of choice for assessment of MR. Routine assessment with cardiac CT is not yet recommended, but its use is steadily increasing. In the future, it is likely that CMR and MSCT will be increasingly used for pre-procedure assessment and planning of intervention procedures in patients with MR.

References

[1] Iung B, Baron G, Butchart EG, Delahaye F, Gohlke-Barwolf C, Levang OW, et al. A prospective survey of patients with valvular heart disease in Europe: The Euro Heart Survey on Valvular Heart Disease. Eur Heart J 2003;24:1231–43.
[2] Van de Heyning CM, Magne J, Vrints CJ, Piérard L, Lancellotti P. The role of multi-imaging modality in primary mitral regurgitation. Eur Heart J Cardiovasc Imaging 2012;13:139–51.
[3] Lancellotti P, Tribouilloy C, Hagendorff A, Popescu BA, Edvardsen T, Pierard LA, et al. Recommendations for the echocardiographic assessment of native valvular regurgitation: an executive summary from the European Association of Cardiovascular Imaging. Eur Heart J Cardiovasc Imaging 2013;14:611–44.
[4] Grayburn PA, Weissman NJ, Zamorano JL. Quantitation of mitral regurgitation. Circulation 2012;126:2005–17.
[5] Pepi M, Tamborini G, Maltagliati A, Galli CA, Sisillo E, Salvi L, et al. Head-to-head comparison of two- and three-dimensional transthoracic and transesophageal echocardiography in the localization of mitral valve prolapse. J Am Coll Cardiol 2006;48:2524–30.
[6] Fattouch K, Castrovinci S, Murana G, Novo G, Caccamo G, Bertolino EC, et al. Multiplane two-dimensional versus real time three-dimensional transesophageal echocardiography in ischemic mitral regurgitation. Echocardiography 2011;28:1125–32.
[7] Lancellotti P, Zamorano JL, Vannan MA. Imaging challenges in secondary mitral regurgitation: unsolved issues and perspectives. Circ Cardiovasc Imaging 2014;7:735–46.
[8] Schmidt FP, Gniewosz T, Jabs A, Münzel T, Hink U, Lancellotti P, et al. Usefulness of 3D-PISA as compared to guideline endorsed parameters for mitral regurgitation quantification. Int J Cardiovasc Imaging 2014;30:1501–8.
[9] Plicht B, Kahlert P, Goldwasser R, Janosi RA, Hunold P, Erbel R, et al. Direct quantification of mitral regurgitant flow volume by real-time three-dimensional echocardiography using dealiasing of color Doppler flow at the vena contracta. J Am Soc Echocardiogr 2008;21:1337–46.
[10] Zeng X, Levine RA, Hua L, Morris EL, Kang Y, Flaherty M, et al. Diagnostic value of vena contracta area in the quantification of mitral regurgitation severity by color Doppler 3D echocardiography. Circ Cardiovasc Imaging 2011;4:506–13.
[11] Lancellotti P, Troisfontaines P, Toussaint A-C, Piérard LA. Prognostic importance of exercise-induced changes in mitral regurgitation in patients with chronic ischemic left ventricular dysfunction. Circulation 2003;108:1713–7.
[12] Lancellotti P, Magne J, Dulgheru R, Ancion A, Martinez C, Piérard LA. Clinical significance of exercise pulmonary hypertension in secondary mitral regurgitation. Am J Cardiol 2015;115:1454–61.
[13] Lancellotti P, Fattouch K, La Canna G. Therapeutic decision-making for patients with fluctuating mitral regurgitation. Nat Rev Cardiol 2015;12:212–9. http://dx.doi.org/10.1038/nrcardio.2015.16, Epub 2015 Feb 10.
[14] Magne J, Donal E, Mahjoub H, Miltner B, Dulgheru R, Thebault C, et al. Impact of exercise pulmonary hypertension on postoperative outcome in primary mitral regurgitation. Heart 2015;101:391–6.

[15] Lancellotti P, Magne J. Stress echocardiography in regurgitant valve disease. Circ Cardiovasc Imaging 2013;6:840–9.
[16] Tribouilloy C, Rusinaru D, Grigioni F, Michelena HI, Vanoverschelde JL, Avierinos JF, et al. Long-term mortality associated with left ventricular dysfunction in mitral regurgitation due to flail leaflets: a multicenter analysis. Circ Cardiovasc Imaging 2014;7:363–70.
[17] Agricola E, Galderisi M, Oppizzi M, Schinkel AF, Maisano F, De BM, et al. Pulsed tissue Doppler imaging detects early myocardial dysfunction in asymptomatic patients with severe mitral regurgitation. Heart 2004;90:406–10.
[18] Lancellotti P, Cosyns B, Zacharakis D, Attena E, Van Camp G, Gach O, et al. Importance of left ventricular longitudinal function and functional reserve in patients with degenerative mitral regurgitation: assessment by two-dimensional speckle tracking. J Am Soc Echocardiogr 2008;21:1331–6.
[19] Magne J, Mahjoub H, Dulgheru R, Pibarot P, Pierard LA, Lancellotti P. Left ventricular contractile reserve in asymptomatic primary mitral regurgitation. Eur Heart J 2014;35:1608–16.
[20] Le Tourneau T, Messika-Zeitoun D, Russo A, Detaint D, Topilsky Y, Mahoney DW, et al. Impact of left atrial volume on clinical outcome in organic mitral regurgitation. J Am Coll Cardiol 2010;56:570–8.
[21] Van de Veire NR, Braun J, Delgado V, Versteegh MI, Dion RA, Klautz RJ, et al. Tricuspid annuloplasty prevents right ventricular dilatation and progression of tricuspid regurgitation in patients with tricuspid annular dilatation undergoing mitral valve repair. J Thorac Cardiovasc Surg 2011;141:1431–9.
[22] Mogelvang J, Stokholm KH, Saunamaki K, Reimer A, Stubgaard M, Thomsen C, et al. Assessment of left ventricular volumes by magnetic resonance in comparison with radionuclide angiography, contrast angiography and echocardiography. Eur Heart J 1992;13:1677–83.
[23] Schiros CG, Dell'Italia LJ, Gladden JD, Clark D, Aban I, Gupta H, et al. Magnetic resonance imaging with 3-dimensional analysis of left ventricular remodeling in isolated mitral regurgitation: implications beyond dimensions. Circulation 2012;125:2334–42.
[24] Ozdogan O, Yuksel A, Gurgun C, Kayikcioglu M, Yavuzgil O, Cinar CS. Assessment of cardiac remodeling in asymptomatic mitral regurgitation for surgery timing: a comparative study of echocardiography and magnetic resonance imaging. Cardiovasc Ultrasound 2010;8:32.
[25] Van De Heyning CM, Magne J, Piérard LA, Bruyère PJ, Davin L, De Maeyer C, et al. Assessment of left ventricular volumes and primary mitral regurgitation severity by 2D echocardiography and cardiovascular magnetic resonance. Cardiovasc Ultrasound 2013;11:46. http://dx.doi.org/10.1186/1476-7120-11-46.
[26] Fujita N, Chazouilleres AF, Hartiala JJ, O'Sullivan M, Heidenreich P, Kaplan JD, et al. Quantification of mitral regurgitation by velocity-encoded cine nuclear magnetic resonance imaging. J Am Coll Cardiol 1994;23:951–8.
[27] Han Y, Peters DC, Salton CJ, Bzymek D, Nezafat R, Goddu B, et al. Cardiovascular magnetic resonance characterization of mitral valve prolapse. JACC Cardiovasc Imaging 2008;1:294–303.
[28] Buchner S, Debl K, Poschenrieder F, Feuerbach S, Riegger GA, Luchner A, et al. Cardiovascular magnetic resonance for direct assessment of anatomic regurgitant orifice in mitral regurgitation. Circ Cardiovasc Imaging 2008;1:148–55.
[29] Van De Heyning CM, Magne J, Piérard LA, Bruyère PJ, Davin L, De Maeyer C, et al. Late gadolinium enhancement CMR in primary mitral regurgitation. Eur J Clin Invest 2014;44:840–7.

[30] Hamada S, Altiok E, Frick M, Almalla M, Becker M, Marx N, et al. Comparison of accuracy of mitral valve regurgitation volume determined by three-dimensional transesophageal echocardiography versus cardiac magnetic resonance imaging. Am J Cardiol 2012;110:1015–20.

[31] Shanks M, Siebelink HM, Delgado V, van de Veire NR, Ng AC, Sieders A, et al. Quantitative assessment of mitral regurgitation: comparison between three-dimensional transesophageal echocardiography and magnetic resonance imaging. Circ Cardiovasc Imaging 2010;3:694–700.

[32] Pontone G, Andreini D, Bertella E, Cortinovis S, Mushtaq S, Foti C, et al. Pre-operative CT coronary angiography in patients with mitral valve prolapse referred for surgical repair: comparison of accuracy, radiation dose and cost versus invasive coronary angiography. Int J Cardiol 2013;167:2889–94.

[33] Delgado V, Tops LF, Schuijf JD, de Roos A, Brugada J, Schalij MJ, et al. Assessment of mitral valve anatomy and geometry with multislice computed tomography. JACC Cardiovasc Imaging 2009;2:556–65.

[34] Tops LF, Van de Veire NR, Schuijf JD, de Roos A, van der Wall EE, Schalij MJ, et al. Noninvasive evaluation of coronary sinus anatomy and its relation to the mitral valve annulus: Implications for percutaneous mitral annuloplasty. Circulation 2007;115:1426–32.

[35] Guo YK, Yang ZG, Ning G, Rao L, Dong L, Pen Y, et al. Isolated mitral regurgitation: quantitative assessment with 64-section multidetector CT-comparison with MR imaging and echocardiography. Radiology 2009;252:369–76.

[36] Vural M, Ucar O, Celebi OO, Cicekcioglu H, Durmaz HA, Selvi NA, et al. Evaluation of effective regurgitant orifice area of mitral valvular regurgitation by multislice cardiac computed tomography. J Cardiol 2010;56:236–9.

[37] Le Tourneau T, Richardson M, Juthier F, Modine T, Fayad G, Polge AS, et al. Echocardiography predictors and prognostic value of pulmonary artery systolic pressure in chronic organic mitral regurgitation. Heart 2010;96:1311–7.

Tricuspid and pulmonary valves

D. Muraru, M.P. Marra, L.P. Badano
University of Padua, Padua, Italy

Echocardiography is the primary imaging modality for initial and longitudinal evaluation of patients with right-sided valvular heart disease. Cardiovascular magnetic resonance (CMR) has emerged as an additional or alternative modality for providing information not only about the valve itself, but also about the pulmonary artery (PA) and the consequences on the right ventricle (RV), including myocardial scar or fibrosis. This chapter highlights the use of current imaging modalities in state-of-the-art assessment of right-sided valvular heart diseases, with emphasis on indications as well as on strengths and limitations of each technique.

16.15 Tricuspid valve

TV disease commonly occurs in combination with left-sided heart disease. Despite its former neglect, TV has recently gained more consideration as physicians become aware of the detrimental consequences of severe TV regurgitation on patient survival, functional capacity, and surgical risk [1].

16.15.1 Anatomy

TV is the largest and most caudally located among the four cardiac valves. Classically, TV is described as having three leaflets (Figure 16.25), however a great variability in the number of leaflets (from 2 to 4) has been described in autopsy studies [2,3]. Normal TV is thinner than the mitral valve due to lower right-sided pressures. Tricuspid annulus (TA) has an elliptical saddle-shape and is a highly dynamic structure, with up to 40% of area decrease during systole. Effective TV function depends on the structural

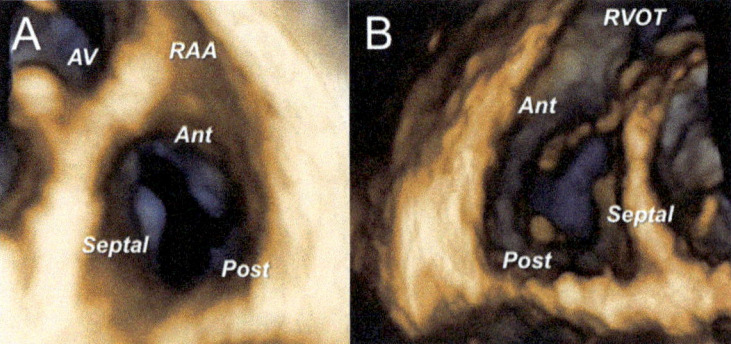

Figure 16.25 *En face* views of normal tricuspid valve anatomy by transthoracic three-dimensional echocardiography: atrial or surgical view (a); ventricular view (b). AV, aortic valve; RAA, right atrial appendage; RVOT, right ventricular outflow tract.

integrity and functional coordination of all components of TV apparatus, which include leaflets, TA, chordae tendineae, papillary muscles, and ventricular myocardium [4].

16.15.2 Pathology

The etiology of TV diseases is generally divided into **organic** (having intrinsic structural changes of TV leaflets) and **functional** (no structural leaflet abnormalities). While tricuspid stenosis due to rheumatic, carcinoid, or congenital diseases is rather uncommon nowadays, tricuspid regurgitation (TR) is a relatively frequent finding in adult patients. Trivial or mild functional TR without any detectable abnormality of the TV is seen in 65–75% of healthy subjects and is considered benign, while significant functional TR is associated with poor prognosis. Only a minority of severe TR (8–10%) is organic, and due to various etiologies: prolapse (myxomatous disease), endocarditis, rheumatic, traumatic, carcinoid, tumors, congenital, induced by leads/catheters, or drug etc. [5]

In most instances, TR is functional in nature and develops as a consequence of deformation of the TV apparatus, such as dilation and abnormal shape of TA, leaflet tenting, and RV dilatation with papillary muscle displacement [6]. Common conditions evolving with functional TR are left-sided heart valve diseases, pulmonary hypertension, congenital heart defects, and cardiomyopathies [7].

16.15.3 Imaging

16.15.3.1 2D Echocardiography (2DE)

2DE is the current imaging gold standard for assessing TV disease and is often sufficient for diagnosis. Doppler echocardiography detects the presence of regurgitation, but also enables the understanding of the mechanisms of TR and quantitation of its severity and consequences (Table 16.4) [8]. However, several views are required to assess TV during a 2DE study, and poor acoustic windows and suboptimal patient

Table 16.4 Echocardiographic indices for severe tricuspid regurgitation

Parameters	Imaging	Severe TR, if:
Qualitative		
TV morphology	*Septal leaflet flail*	Abnormal/Flail/Large coaptation defect

Continued

Table 16.4 Continued

Parameters	Imaging	Severe TR, if:
Color Doppler flow		Very large central jet or eccentric wall impinging jet
CW signal of TR jet		Dense/Triangular with early peaking (peak <2 m/s in massive TR)
Semi-quantitative		
Vena contracta width (mm)		>7
PISA radius (mm)		>9

Table 16.4 **Continued**

Parameters	Imaging	Severe TR, if:
Hepatic vein flow		Systolic flow reversal
Tricuspid inflow		E wave dominant (≥1 cm/s)
Quantitative		
EROA (mm²) R Vol (ml)		≥40 ≥45
Supportive		
RV/RA/IVC size		Abnormal

Adapted from Lancellotti et al. [8].

body habitus can compromise image quality. Transoesophageal echocardiography is performed when further diagnostic refinement is required, but may result less satisfactory than for left-sided valves, since TV is located farther from the transducer and obliquely oriented with respect to the Doppler beam.

16.15.3.2 3D Echocardiography

3DE provides realistic and intuitive anatomic images of TV apparatus, important functional insights, and unique quantitation opportunities for a better understanding of TV pathophysiology (Figure 16.26). 3DE has the unique capability to provide *en face* visualizations of the anatomy and dynamics of TV leaflets and TA in the beating heart. The designation of individual leaflets is therefore more reliable by 3DE, unless a satisfactory short-axis view of TV can be rarely obtained by 2DE. However, TV prolapse/flail is best delineated from TV "surgical" view, which is impossible to obtain by 2DE (Figure 16.26a). A limitation of 2DE in assessing TR severity by vena contracta width is the fact that regurgitant orifice geometry is complex and not necessarily circular, particularly in functional TR [7] (Figure 16.26d). 3DE allows the area of vena contracta to be quantitated without any erroneous geometric assumptions, as well as the dynamics of effective regurgitant orifice and regurgitant volume (Figure 16.26f). Routine 2DE assessment of TA size in four-chamber view by a single linear dimension is representative of neither the maximal, nor the minimal TA diameter (Figure 16.26e). 3DE brings

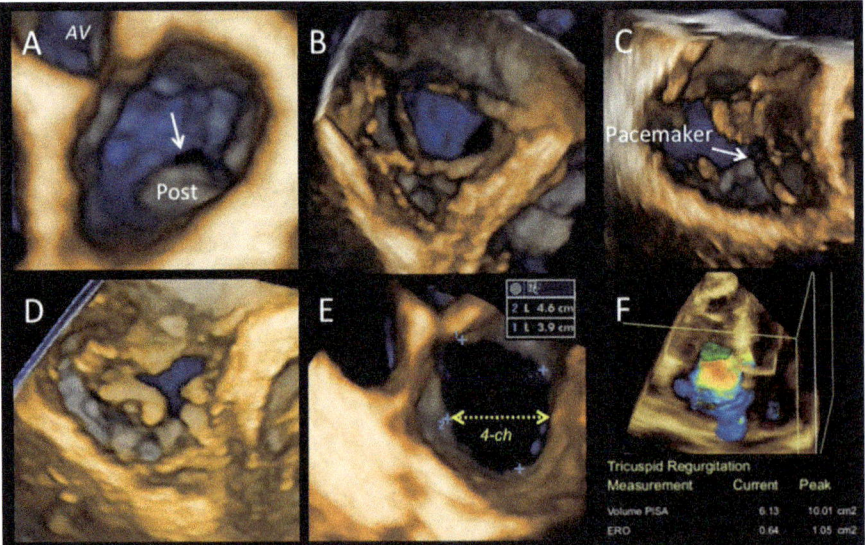

Figure 16.26 Added value of three-dimensional echocardiography for assessing various tricuspid valve pathologies: detection of posterior leaflet flail (a, arrow); identification of typical morphologic changes with valvular steno-insufficiency in carcinoid disease (b); assessing the spatial relationship of pacemaker leads with tricuspid leaflets (c, arrow); depicting the irregular shape of regurgitant orifice in functional regurgitation (d); more anatomically sound and reproducible sizing of tricuspid annulus (e); quantitation of tricuspid regurgitation severity and dynamics without geometric assumptions by 3D PISA (f). AV, aortic valve.

unique opportunities for a sound quantitation of the complex three-dimensional shape of TV (e.g., TA area and perimeter, TA height, leaflet tenting volume, etc.) which will hopefully improve our capabilities to guide the management of patients with functional TR. Finally, 3DE is more accurate and reproducible than 2DE for quantitating the hemodynamic consequences of the TR on RV [9]. Poor acoustic window and irregular rhythms are currently limiting the application of 3DE for TV assessment.

16.15.3.3 Cardiac magnetic resonance (CMR)

Morphologic assessment of TV anatomy by CMR is commonly performed by using balanced steady-state free-precession (SSFP) sequences, which offer an optimal blood-to-myocardium contrast with high signal-to-noise ratio. Cine SSPF imaging may reveal anatomic leaflet abnormalities, such as Ebstein anomaly (Figure 16.27), leaflet thickening (e.g., in rheumatic or carcinoid disease), abnormal movement, or loss of coaptation. Rather than calculated, TV area can be directly planimetered on the slice passing through the TV tips in diastole in stenotic valves. TR jet can be qualitatively evaluated in a long-axis right ventricular view by in-plane velocity mapping. The "signal void" phenomenon (corresponding to the turbulent regurgitant flow, Figure 16.28) and its extension into the right atrium can be used as a semi-quantitative parameter of TR severity by CMR. However, similarly to color Doppler jet area, this method is also influenced by right atrial pressure and by imaging parameters (i.e., echo time, flip angle, alignment with jet direction). In case of isolated TR, TV regurgitation volume can be calculated as the difference between the RV and left ventricular stroke volumes. The assessment of TR with phase-contrast CMR imaging (PC) is more difficult than of pulmonary regurgitation, because of the larger excursion of TA during systole. The consequences of TV disease on right ventricular (RV) volumes and systolic function can be accurately evaluated by cine SSFP CMR imaging [10] and represent the current gold standard for RV assessment. Finally, CMR has the unique capability of enabling *in vivo* tissue characterization (i.e., fibrosis). In pulmonary hypertension, late gadolinium enhancement is typically located at the septal junction (Figure 16.29) and may be used in the prognostic stratification of these patients.

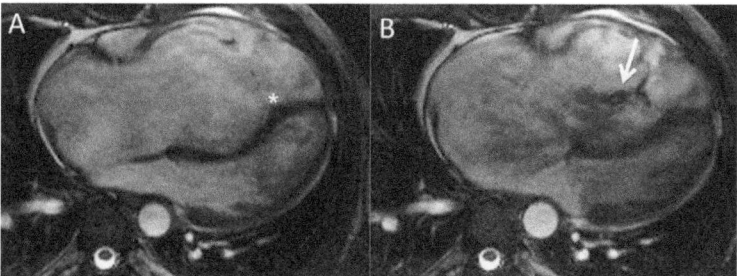

Figure 16.27 Cardiac magnetic resonance imaging in Ebstein's anomaly. (a) (diastolic frame of cine SSFP 4-chamber view) shows severe enlargement of right chambers with the characteristic apical displacement of septal tricuspid valve (asterisk). (b) (systolic frame of same view) shows the signal void in the atrialized portion of the right ventricle, corresponding to the turbulent tricuspid regurgitant flow (arrow).

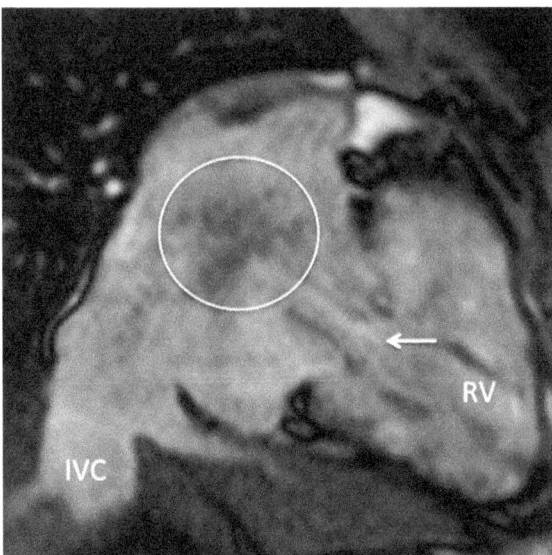

Figure 16.28 Cardiac magnetic resonance imaging of tricuspid regurgitation. Two-chamber view of right ventricle (RV, systolic frame of cine SSFP) showing the lack of coaptation of tricuspid leaflets (arrow) and the valvular regurgitation demonstrated as "signal void" in the right atrium (white circle). IVC = inferior vena cava.

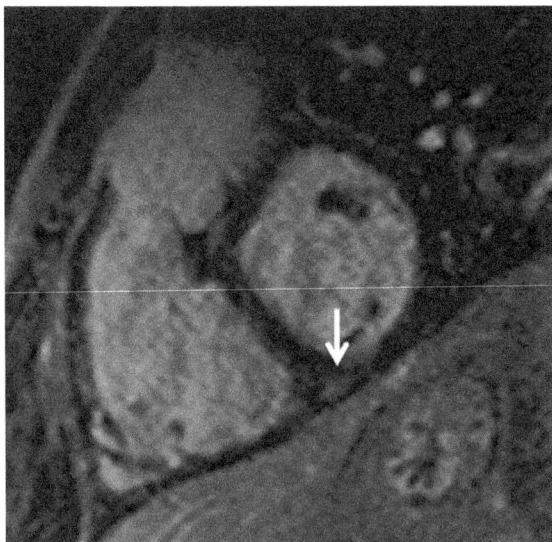

Figure 16.29 Cardiac magnetic resonance imaging (right ventricular outflow short-axis view) of a patient with pulmonary hypertension, showing the marked dilatation and hypertrophy of the right ventricle, as well as the typical late gadolinium enhancement noticeable at the inferior septal junction (arrow).

Patients with very irregular heart rhythms (e.g., uncontrolled atrial fibrillation, frequent ventricular ectopy), can present a challenge for CMR, particularly to acquiring accurate flow data.

16.15.3.4 Computerized tomography

Multi-detector row cardiac CT imaging (MDCT) may demonstrate clinical usefulness in TV disease—especially when echo and CMR are either suboptimal or contraindicated—with information about TV morphology and right chambers size and function. MDCT is faster and less hampered by metal artifacts than CMR, and can be particularly helpful for assessing patients with pacemakers/defibrillators. However, visualization of right-sided valves is less reliable than for the left-sided valves, due to their thinner structure and the fact that contrast injection protocols are not timed to enable visualization of the right heart. [11] Protocols for right heart enhancement prolong the duration of contrast injection in comparison to a coronary CT study [12]. Radiation exposure, the lower temporal resolution, and the inability to assess transvalvular flow and pressure gradients, as well as leaflet morphology, are important drawbacks, favoring the use of echo (± CMR) for the routine TV workup.

16.16 Pulmonary valve

Pulmonary valve (PV) disease is relatively less frequent and more challenging to image in comparison with the other valvular pathologies.

16.16.1 Anatomy

PV is a three-cusped structure, anatomically similar with the aortic valve. However, the PV is separated from the TV by crista supraventricularis and is thinner than aortic valve because of lower right-sided pressures.

16.16.2 Pathology

PV stenosis is a rare condition, primarily congenital and only rarely acquired in the setting of carcinoid disease, or large vegetations and tumors causing PV obstruction. PV regurgitation (PR) is far more frequent than stenosis and can be classified as either organic (abnormal cusps) or functional (normal cusps with pulmonary annulus and PA dilation due to pulmonary hypertension or idiopathic). Common causes of organic PR are: post-valvulotomy/ valvuloplasty, carcinoid, rheumatic, endocarditis, myxomatous degeneration, and tumors. Trivial or mild PR is seen in a large proportion of healthy subjects (60–70%) and is considered benign. In contrast, severe PR is relatively infrequent, usually organic, and associated in the long term with reduced exercise capacity, arrhythmias, and sudden cardiac death.

16.16.3 Imaging
16.16.3.1 2D Echocardiography

Echocardiographic assessment of PV requires integration of data from 2DE imaging of PV, PA, and RV, with Doppler parameters used to estimate the severity of PV disease.

PV morphology (thickening, calcifications), mobility and coaptation, annulus, and PA size can be evaluated by 2DE. However, among all cardiac valves, the anatomy of PV is the most challenging to image by ultrasound, being limited by poor acoustic access. With 2DE, typically only two cusps can be simultaneously visualized, while short-axis PV views can be obtained only exceptionally. Useful approaches for PV are from parasternal, subcostal, or, less frequently, modified four-chamber views. Doppler echocardiography can help to assess the severity and localization of stenosis (valvular, sub- or supravalvular). PR severity grading remains difficult, since standards for the quantification of PR are less robust than for aortic regurgitation and less valid, when compared with CMR (Table 16.5) [8].

Table 16.5 **Echocardiographic indices for severe pulmonary regurgitation**

Parameters	Imaging	Severe PR, if:
Qualitative		
PV morphology		Abnormal/Flail/Large coaptation defect
Color Doppler flow jet width		Large with a wide origin; may be brief in duration
Reversal flow in pulmonary artery		Present

Table 16.5 **Continued**

Parameters	Imaging	Severe PR, if:
CW signal of PR jet		Dense/steep deceleration, early termination of diastolic flow
Parameters	Imaging	Severe PR, if:
Pulmonic vs. aortic flow by PW		Greatly increased
Semi-quantitative		
Vena contracta width (mm)		Not defined

Continued

Table 16.5 **Continued**

Pressure half-time (ms)	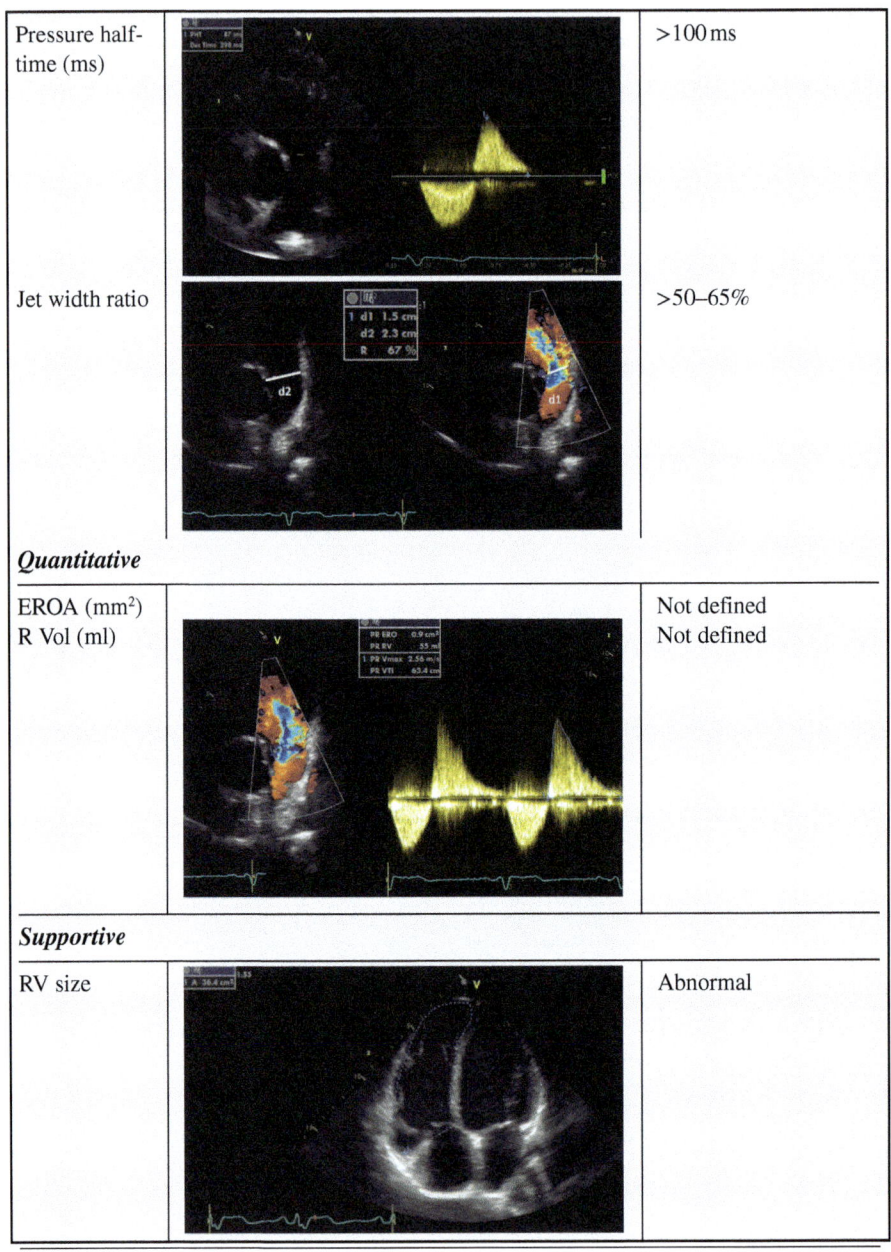	>100 ms
Jet width ratio		>50–65%
Quantitative		
EROA (mm²) R Vol (ml)		Not defined Not defined
Supportive		
RV size		Abnormal

Adapted from Lancellotti et al. [8].

16.16.3.2 3D Echocardiography

The usefulness of 3DE for assessing PV is limited, due to its poor acoustic access and thin cusps affected by dropouts. When feasible, 3DE provides *en face* images of PV, which enable to appreciate the number and integrity of cusps, their mobility, and coaptation (Figure 16.30). 3DE color allows the cropping plane to be positioned exactly parallel to the vena contracta (Figure 16.31), which can be planimetered accurately for estimating PR severity [13]. The 3D assessment of vena contracta area relies on no geometric assumptions regarding the shape of regurgitant orifice and may potentially improve the quantitation of PR severity in comparison with vena contracta diameter by 2DE.

16.16.3.3 Cardiac magnetic resonance

CMR offers an excellent visualization of the RV outflow tract, therefore being a highly attractive alternative to echo in assessing PV pathology. The qualitative assessment of PV anatomy is done on cine SSFP sequences, which enable also the differential diagnosis with subvalvular and supravalvular stenoses and the direct planimetry of valvular orifice in PV stenosis. In PV stenosis, the peak systolic velocity can be measured on PC images, but the artifacts related to the high-velocity turbulent flow may limit its reliability (Figure 16.32). As for aortic regurgitation, PR can be quantified on in-plane PC velocity mapping sequences. PV forward flow measurement is combined with RV stroke volume from SSFP cine images for calculating the PR regurgitant volume and PR regurgitant fraction. PR regurgitant fraction of 40% or more is considered severe [14]. For optimal visualization of flow velocities in PC it is important that the scaling of velocity map is adapted to the velocity observed in the region of interest and that the predicted peak velocity should cover approximately two-thirds of the interval set by the encoding velocity (Table 16.6) [15].

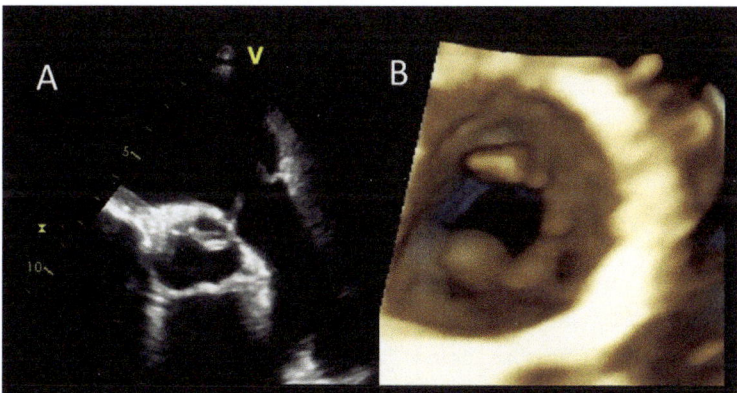

Figure 16.30 Echocardiographic assessment of pulmonary valve morphology in a patient with severe organic pulmonary regurgitation, demonstrating a flail valve with lack of coaptation: two-dimensional long-axis view (a); three-dimensional *en face* view of all three leaflets from the right ventricular outflow perspective (b).

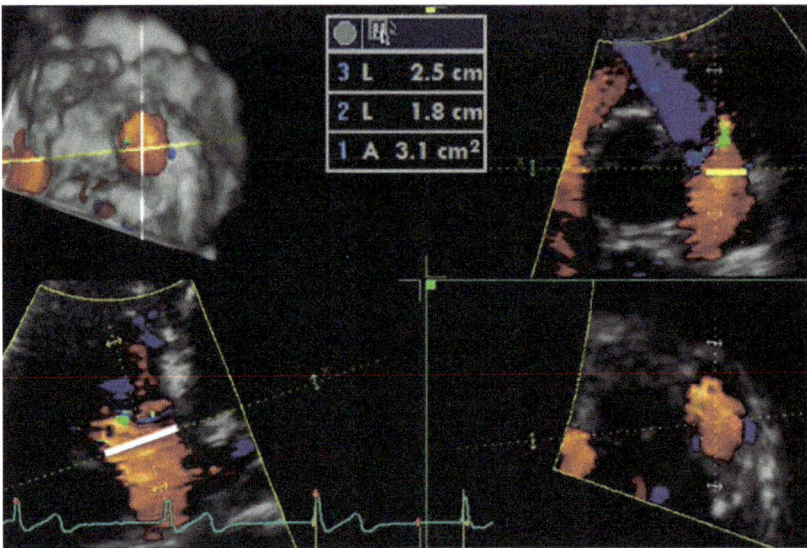

Figure 16.31 Assessment of pulmonary regurgitation severity by 3D color flow imaging. Left upper panel shows the elliptical shape of the vena contracta, which can be quantified as linear dimensions in orthogonal 2D views (white and yellow lines), but also in terms of vena contracta area, which can be performed by planimetering the color jet on a short-axis plane exactly aligned at the vena contracta level (right lower panel).

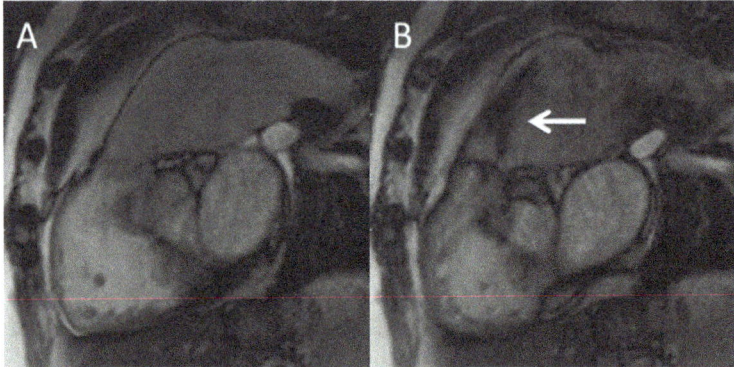

Figure 16.32 Right ventricular outflow tract imaging by cardiac magnetic resonance in a patient with pulmonary valve stenosis. (a) (diastolic frame of cine SSFP) shows the marked post-stenotic pulmonary artery enlargement. (b) (systolic frame of cine SSFP) shows the turbulent flow across the pulmonary valve as a supravalvular signal void (arrow).

After right-sided surgery, CMR is useful for the evaluation of the RV outflow tract, RV-PA conduits (stenosis or aneurysm), and branch pulmonary arteries [16]. Gadolinium-enhanced 3D MR angiography (MRA) offers a better delineation of great vessels and of possible stenoses (Figure 16.33). MRA is highly accurate to depict all sources of pulmonary blood supply in patients with complex pulmonary stenosis or atresia. Presence of

Table 16.6 Imaging sequences and indications for cardiac magnetic resonance (CMR) imaging in right-sided valvular diseases

CMR sequences	Indications
SSFP cine images	• Tricuspid valve anatomy: leaflets insertion, motion, coaptation
• Pulmonary valve anatomy: number of leaflets, calcifications, motion
• Right-ventricular volumes, ejection fraction and mass
Gradient echo images
Phase contrast	• Visualization of turbulent flow
• Velocity mapping
• Flow quantification: velocity encoding (VENC) for main pulmonary artery 120 cm/s, for right/left pulmonary artery 150 cm/s
3D MR angiography
Post-contrast T1 inversion recovery images	• Evaluation of great vessels, including stents and conduits
• Myocardial fibrosis

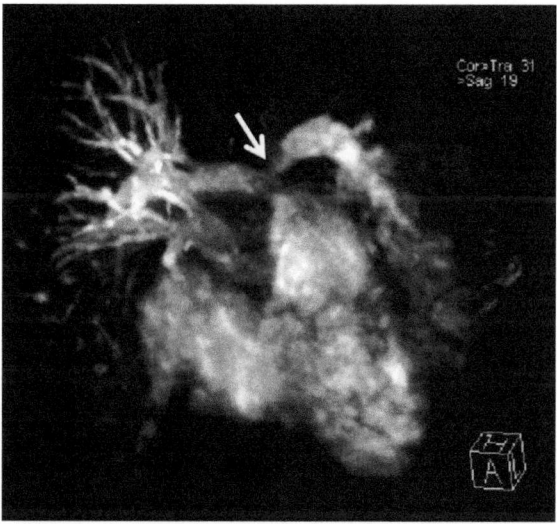

Figure 16.33 Gadolinium-enhanced three-dimensional (3D) magnetic resonance angiography, showing dilatation of the main pulmonary artery and stenosis of the left branch of pulmonary artery (arrow).

late gadolinium enhancement after surgical repair for tetralogy of Fallot or other congenital right-sided diseases seems to be related with arrhythmic risk [16].

16.16.3.4 Computerized tomography

MDCT has limited utility to assess PV anatomy, substantially for the same reasons as for TV (see Section 16.15.3.4). CT angiography can provide an accurate quantitation of PV annulus, PA, and RV remodeling, when echo and CMR are either unfeasible or unsatisfactory.

References

[1] Mascherbauer J, Maurer G. The forgotten valve: lessons to be learned in tricuspid regurgitation. Eur Heart J 2010;31:2841–3.
[2] Sutton 3rd. JP, Ho SY, Vogel M, Anderson RH. Is the morphologically right atrioventricular valve tricuspid? J Heart Valve Dis 1995;4:571–5.
[3] Victor S, Nayak VM. The tricuspid valve is bicuspid. J Heart Valve Dis 1994;3:27–36.
[4] Basso C, Muraru D, Badano LP, Thiene G. Anatomy and pathology of right-sided atrio-ventricular and semilunar valves. In: Rajamannan N, editor. Cardiac valvular medicine. London: Springer-Verlag London Ltd.; 2013.
[5] Muraru D, Badano LP, Sarais C, Solda E, Iliceto S. Evaluation of tricuspid valve morphology and function by transthoracic three-dimensional echocardiography. Curr Cardiol Rep 2011;13:242–9.
[6] Sagie A, Schwammenthal E, Padial LR, et al. Determinants of functional tricuspid regurgitation in incomplete tricuspid valve closure: Doppler color flow study of 109 patients. J Am Coll Cardiol 1994;24:446–53.
[7] Badano LP, Muraru D, Enriquez-Sarano M. Assessment of functional tricuspid regurgitation. Eur Heart J 2013;34:1875–85.
[8] Lancellotti P, Tribouilloy C, Hagendorff A, et al. Recommendations for the echocardiographic assessment of native valvular regurgitation: an executive summary from the European association of cardiovascular imaging. Eur Heart J Cardiovasc Imaging 2013;14:611–44.
[9] Lang RM, Badano LP, Tsang W, et al. EAE/ASE recommendations for image acquisition and display using three-dimensional echocardiography. Eur Heart J Cardiovasc Imaging 2012;13:1–46.
[10] Sommer G, Bremerich J, Lund G. Magnetic resonance imaging in valvular heart disease: clinical application and current role for patient management. J Magn Reson Imaging 2012;35:1241–52.
[11] Nasis A, Mottram PM, Cameron JD, Seneviratne SK. Current and evolving clinical applications of multidetector cardiac ct in assessment of structural heart disease. Radiology 2013;267:11–25.
[12] Tops LF, Krishnan SC, Schuijf JD, Schalij MJ, Bax JJ. Noncoronary applications of cardiac multidetector row computed tomography. JACC Cardiovasc Imaging 2008;1:94–106.
[13] Lang RM, Tsang W, Weinert L, Mor-Avi V, Chandra S. Valvular heart disease. The value of 3-dimensional echocardiography. J Am Coll Cardiol 2011;58:1933–44.
[14] Cawley PJ, Maki JH, Otto CM. Cardiovascular magnetic resonance imaging for valvular heart disease: technique and validation. Circulation 2009;119:468–78.
[15] Karamitsos TD, Myerson SG. The role of cardiovascular magnetic resonance in the evaluation of valve disease. Prog Cardiovasc Dis 2011;54:276–86.
[16] Kilner PJ, Geva T, Kaemmerer H, et al. Recommendations for cardiovascular magnetic resonance in adults with congenital heart disease from the respective working groups of the European Society of Cardiology. Eur Heart J 2010;31:794–805.

Prosthetic valves

H. Mahjoub, P. Pibarot
Université Laval/Laval University, Québec, QC, Canada

Abbreviations

CT	computed tomography
CW	continuous wave
DVI	Doppler velocity index
EOA	effective orifice area
MDCT	multidetector computed tomography
PET	positron emission tomography
PHV	prosthetic heart valve
PPM	prosthesis–patient mismatch
PW	pulse-wave
SD	standard deviation
SPECT	Single photon emission computed tomography
TEE	transesophageal echocardiography
TTE	transthoracic echocardiography

16.17 Introduction

Valve replacement has dramatically improved the outcome of patients with valvular heart diseases over the past decades. Approximately 85,000 prosthetic valves are implanted each year in the United States and 300,000 worldwide, of which approximately 20% are mechanical valves and 80% are bioprosthetic valves [1,2]. However, valve replacement does not provide a definite cure to the patient, instead native valve disease is traded for "prosthetic valve disease" and the outcomes of patients undergoing valve replacement is affected by prosthetic valve hemodynamics, durability, and thrombogenicity. Many of the prosthesis-related complications can be prevented or their impact minimized through optimal prosthesis selection in the individual patient, careful medical management, and close follow-up of prosthetic valve function after implantation. Doppler echocardiography is the primary imaging modality for the evaluation and the management of patients with prosthetic heart valves. Other imaging modalities such as cinefluoroscopy and multidetector computed tomography (MDCT) are also often used to confirm or expand the information obtained by echocardiography, particularly in patients with mechanical prostheses. Furthermore, cardiac magnetic resonance and nuclear imaging, which have been shown to provide incremental value in the diagnosis and management of native valve diseases, have also recently been used for the evaluation of prosthetic valves with promising results. The purpose of this chapter is to review the different imaging modalities in the evaluation and management of patients with prosthetic valves and to present the new directions for future research and clinical applications.

16.18 Echocardiography

Owing to its versatile, non-invasive, radiation-free, and low-cost nature, Doppler echocardiography is undoubtedly the method of choice to evaluate prosthetic valve structure and function (Figure 16.34). This evaluation follows the same principles used for the evaluation of native valves with some specifics and caveats that make echocardiography of prosthetic valves more demanding both to perform and to interpret compared to the assessment of native valves. A complete echocardiography includes two-dimensional imaging of the prosthetic valve, evaluation of the valve leaflet/occluder morphology and mobility, measurement of the transprosthetic gradients and valve effective orifice area (EOA), estimation of the degree of regurgitation, evaluation of left ventricular size, and systolic function and calculation of systolic pulmonary arterial pressure (Figure 16.34). Transesophageal echocardiography (TEE) is more likely to be needed for native valves than for the evaluation of prosthetic valve structure and associated complications.

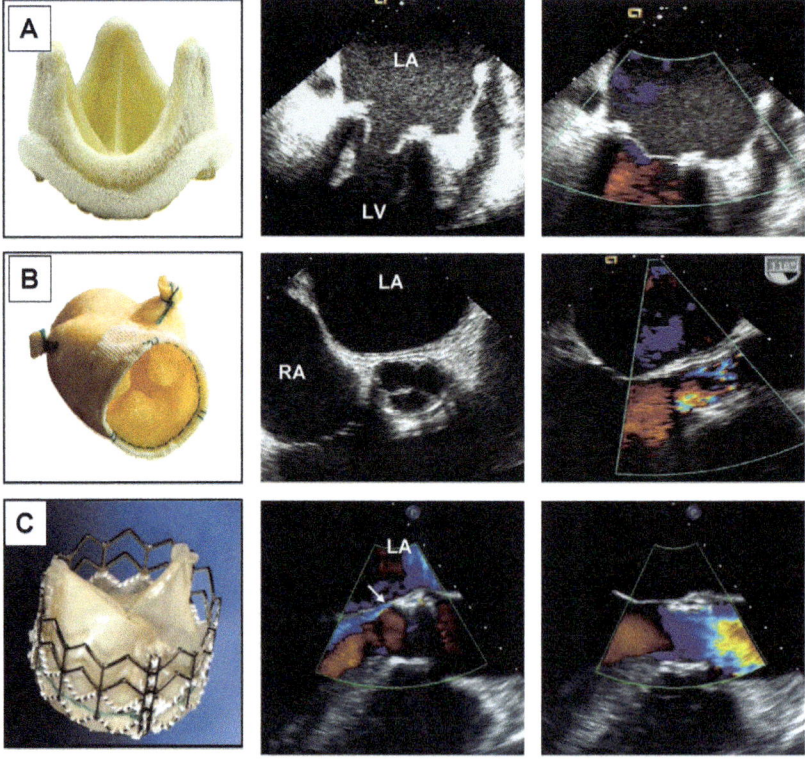

Figure 16.34 Examples of prosthetic valves and their transesophageal echocardiographic characteristics. Stented (a), stentless (b), and transcatheter (c) bioprosthetic valves, and bileaflet

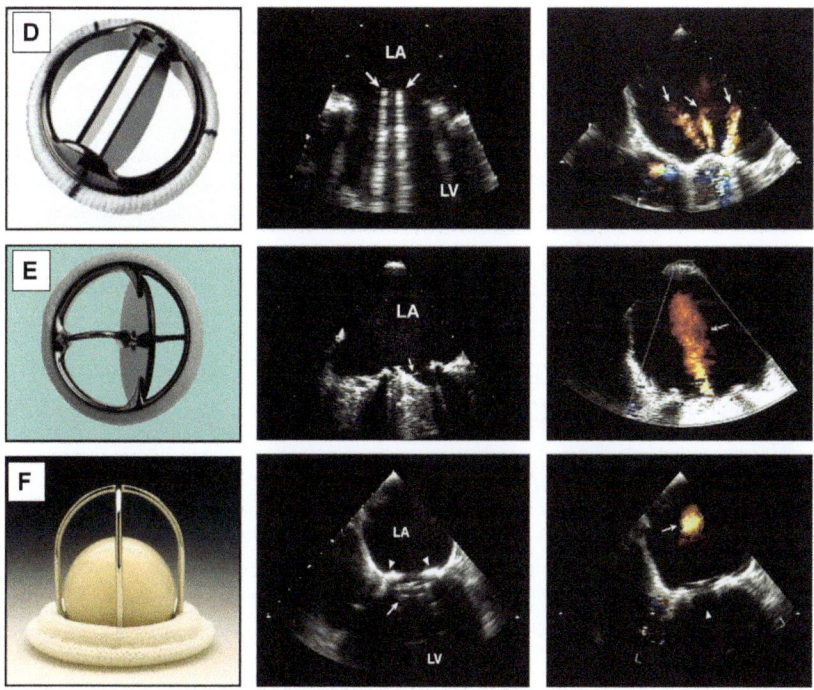

Figure 16.34 Continued (d), monoleaflet (e), and caged-ball (f) mechanical valves in diastole (middle) and in systole (right) as seen by TEE. The stentless valve is inserted by the root inclusion technique. Mild paravalvular aortic regurgitation in the transcatheter valve is shown by arrow (c). The arrows in diastole point to the occluder mechanism of the mechanical valves and in systole to the characteristic physiologic regurgitation observed with each valve (d–f).
Reproduced with permission of the American Society of Echocardiography [3].

The hemodynamic performance of most prosthetic valves is inferior to that of the normal native valve. Hence, owing to their "imperfect" design, prosthetic valves often cause some degree of obstruction to blood flow, which may vary depending on the model and size of prosthesis as well as the patient's body size. It may be difficult to differentiate inherent obstructive hemodynamics due to prosthesis design and ensuing prosthesis–patient mismatch (PPM) from those related to acquired pathological obstructive processes (i.e., thrombus, pannus, calcific degeneration).

16.18.1 Prosthesis–patient mismatch

PPM occurs when the valve EOA of a normally functioning prosthesis is too small in relation to the patient's body size (and thus cardiac output requirements), resulting in abnormally high postoperative velocities and gradients. The most widely accepted and validated parameter for identifying PPM is the indexed EOA, i.e., the EOA of the prosthesis divided by the patient's body surface area [4].

Table 16.7 **Criteria of indexed prosthetic valve effective orifice area (in cm^2/m^2) for the identification and quantitation of prosthesis–patient mismatch**

	Mild or not clinically significant	Moderate	Severe
Aortic position	>0.85 (0.8–0.9)	≤0.85 (0.7–0.8)	≤0.65 (0.6–0.7)
Mitral position	>1.2 (1.2–1.3)	≤1.2 (0.9–1.2)	≤0.9(0.9)

Numbers in parentheses represent the range of threshold values that have been used in the literature.
Reproduced with permission from Ref. [4].

Table 16.7 shows the cut-off values of indexed EOA generally used to identify PPM and quantify its severity.

16.18.2 Acquired prosthetic valve stenosis

Pathologic obstruction of the prosthetic valve may be caused by an acute process such a thrombosis, a subacute process such as endocarditis or a chronic process such as pannus formation or calcific degeneration of bioprosthetic valve leaflets (Figure 16.35). The suspicion of prosthesis stenosis may be the appearance of a new murmur or symptom in a patient with a prosthetic valve or the incidental finding of abnormally high flow velocities and gradients detected during a routine examination. Tables 16.8 and 16.9 present the Doppler-echocardiographic parameters and criteria for the detection and quantification of aortic and mitral prosthetic valve stenosis, respectively.

16.18.2.1 Valve structure and motion

Prosthetic valve stenosis is often associated with abnormal valve leaflet morphology and/or mobility (Figure 16.35). Transthoracic echocardiography (TTE) imaging of the valve occluder is often difficult to obtain because of reverberations and shadowing caused by the prosthetic valve components. TEE can provide improved image quality and thereby detection of leaflet calcification and thickening, valvular vegetations due to endocarditis, thrombus or pannus, and reduced leaflet/disc/ball mobility [5]. Three-dimensional echocardiography (TEE or TTE) can also help to obtain a more complete visualization of the different aspects of the prosthesis and therefore enhance the detection and description of prosthesis dehiscence, vegetations, abscesses, pannus, and thrombi (Figure 16.36) [7].

After exclusion of PPM, the most probable cause of acquired mechanical prosthetic valve obstruction is thrombosis or pannus formation. One of the therapeutic options for obstructive thrombosis is fibrinolysis, whereas in obstructive pannus this treatment is contraindicated [8,9]. It is thus important to differentiate thrombi from a fibrous pannus. The latter is usually annular in location and typically appears as a very dense immobile echo (Figure 16.35).

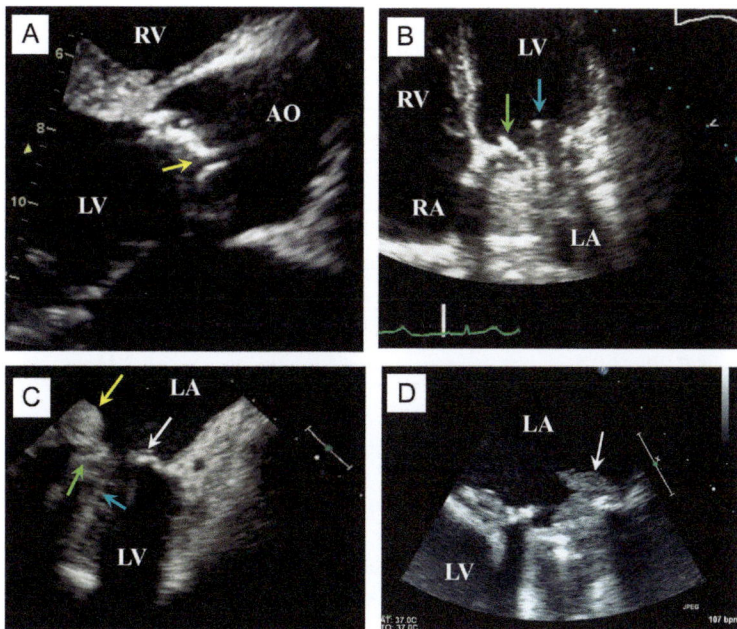

Figure 16.35 Echocardiographic evaluation of prosthetic valve leaflet morphology and mobility. (a) TTE systolic image of a patient with thickening and reduced mobility of aortic bioprosthetic valve cusps (yellow arrow). (b) TTE view of mitral bileaflet mechanical prosthesis in diastole with a fixed leaflet (green arrow), the other leaflet is still mobile (blue arrow). (c) TEE diastolic image of a patient with obstructed mitral bileaflet mechanical valve (yellow arrow: large-size thrombus, white arrow: pannus; blue arrow: mobile leaflet; green arrow: immobile leaflet). (d) large vegetation attached to a mitral bioprosthetic valve cusp and prolapsing in the left atrium during systole. AO: aorta; LA: left atrium; LV: left ventricle; RV: right ventricle; RA: right atrium.
Courtesy of Dr. John Chambers, Guy's and St Thomas Hospitals, London, UK (a), Dr. Steven A Goldstein, Washington Hospital Center (c), and Dr. Gilbert Habib, Hôpital La Timone, Marseille, France.

16.18.2.2 Quantitative parameters

Quantitative parameters of prosthetic valve function include transprosthetic flow velocity and pressure gradients, valve EOA, and Doppler velocity index (DVI). The principles of interrogation and recording of flow velocity through prosthetic valves are similar to those used in evaluating native valve stenosis, but because the direction of the transprosthetic jet may be eccentric, multi-windows examination should be carefully performed to detect the highest velocity signal in prosthetic valves [3,10,11]. Occasionally, an abnormally high jet gradient corresponding to a localized high velocity may be recorded by continuous wave (CW) Doppler interrogation through the smaller central orifice of the bileaflet mechanical prostheses in the aortic or mitral

Table 16.8 **Doppler-echocardiographic criteria for detection and quantitation of aortic prosthetic valve stenosis**

	Normal	Possible stenosis	Significant stenosis
Valve structure and motion			
Mechanical or bioprosthesis	Normal	Often abnormal[a]	Abnormal[a]
Doppler quantitative parameters			
Peak velocity (m/s)[b,c]	<3	3–4	≥4
Mean gradient (mmHg)[b,c]	<20	20–35	≥35
Doppler velocity index[b]	≥0.30	0.25–0.29	<0.25
Effective orifice area (cm^2)[b,d]	>1.2	0.8–1.2	<0.8
Measured EOA versus normal reference value[b]	Reference ±1SD	< Reference −1SD	< Reference −2SD
Difference (measured EOA—reference EOA) (cm^2)[b]	<0.25	≥0.25	≥0.37
Contour of the transprosthetic jet[e]	Triangular, early peaking	Triangular to intermediate	Rounded, symmetrical
Acceleration time (ms)[e]	<80	80–100	>100
Acceleration time/LV ejection time ratio	<0.32	0.32–0.37	>0.37

See Table 16.10 to obtain the normal reference values of effective orifice area for the different models and sizes of prostheses.
SD: standard deviation.
[a] Abnormal mechanical valves: occluder that is immobile or with restricted mobility, thrombus or pannus; abnormal biologic valves: leaflet thickening/calcification, thrombus or pannus.
[b] The criteria proposed for these parameters are valid for near normal or normal stroke volume (50–90 ml) and flow rate (200–300 ml/s).
[c] These parameters are more affected by low or high flow states including low LV output and concomitant aortic regurgitation.
[d] This parameter is dependent on the size of the LV outflow tract.
[e] These parameters are affected by LV function and chronotropy.
Adapted in part from Ref. [3] with permission of American Society of Echocardiography.

position [3]. This phenomenon may lead to an overestimation of gradient and a false suspicion of prosthesis stenosis. Hence, a high transprosthetic velocity or gradient alone is not a proof of intrinsic prosthetic obstruction and may be secondary to PPM, high flow conditions, prosthetic valve regurgitation, or localized high central jet velocity in bileaflet mechanical valves.

The prosthetic valve EOA is less flow dependent than the transprosthetic velocity or gradient, and is thus often a better index of intrinsic valve hemodynamic performance. However the cut-off values of EOA proposed in the 2009 ASE/EAE guidelines to identify prosthetic valve stenosis (Tables 16.8 and 16.9) [3] have an important limitation, given that they overlap substantially with the normal reference values of EOA of several prostheses models. The recognition of prosthetic valve stenosis is generally better achieved by comparing the measured EOA to the normal

Table 16.9 Doppler-echocardiographic criteria for detection and quantitation of mitral prosthetic valve stenosis

	Normal	Possible stenosis	Significant stenosis
Valve structure and motion			
Mechanical or bioprosthesis	Normal	Often abnormal[a]	Abnormal[a]
Doppler quantitative parameters			
Peak velocity (m/s)[b,c,d]	<1.9	1.9–2.5	≥2.5
Mean gradient (mmHg)[b,c,d]	≤5	6–10	≥10
Doppler velocity index[b,d,e]	<2.2	2.2–2.5	>2.5
Effective orifice area (cm^2)[b,f]	≥2	1–2	<1
Effective orifice area versus normal reference value[b,f]	Reference ±1SD	<Reference −1SD	<Reference −2SD
Pressure half time (ms)[g]	<130	130–200	>200

See Table 16.11 to obtain the normal reference values of effective orifice area for the different models and sizes of prostheses.
PHT: pressure half time; SD: standard deviation.
[a] Abnormal mechanical valves: occluder that is immobile or with restricted mobility, thrombus or pannus; abnormal biologic valves: leaflet thickening/calcification, thrombus or pannus.
[b] The criteria proposed for these parameters are valid for near normal or normal diastolic volume (i.e., stroke volume: 50–90 ml) and heart rate (50–80 bpm).
[c] These parameters are more affected by flow and chronotropy.
[d] These parameters are also abnormal in presence of significant mitral prosthesis regurgitation.
[e] This parameter is dependent on the size of the LV outflow tract.
[f] These parameters are not valid when > mild concomitant aortic or mitral regurgitation is present.
[g] This parameter is influenced by chronotropy, left atrial compliance, and left ventricular compliance.
Adapted in part from Ref. [3] with permission of American Society of Echocardiography.

reference value of EOA for the model and size of prosthesis implanted in the patient (Tables 16.10 and 16.11), rather than applying fixed cut-off values to all patients regardless of the characteristics of their prosthesis [10]. If the measured EOA is less than the reference EOA-1SD (standard deviation) one should suspect possible stenosis (Tables 16.10 and 16.11). If the measured EOA is less than reference EOA-2SD, there is a high likelihood of significant stenosis. Recent studies [12] in patients with aortic prostheses suggested that a difference between reference EOA and measured EOA >0.37 cm^2 is suggestive of significant stenosis (Table 16.10). For aortic prostheses, the DVI is calculated as the ratio of the proximal flow velocity (peak velocity or Time-Velocity Integral) in the LVOT to the transprosthetic flow velocity (or Time-Velocity Integral). For mitral prostheses, this is the inverse: ratio of transprosthetic flow velocity to LVOT flow velocity. This parameter can be helpful to screen for valve stenosis, particularly when the cross-sectional area of the LVOT cannot be obtained to calculate the EOA by the continuity equation method (Tables 16.8 and 16.9). Parameters of flow ejection dynamics, and particularly the ratio of the acceleration time to the LV ejection time measured on the continuous-wave Doppler signal of the transprosthetic flow velocity (Figure 16.37), are reliable angle-independent parameters that can also help to distinguish between

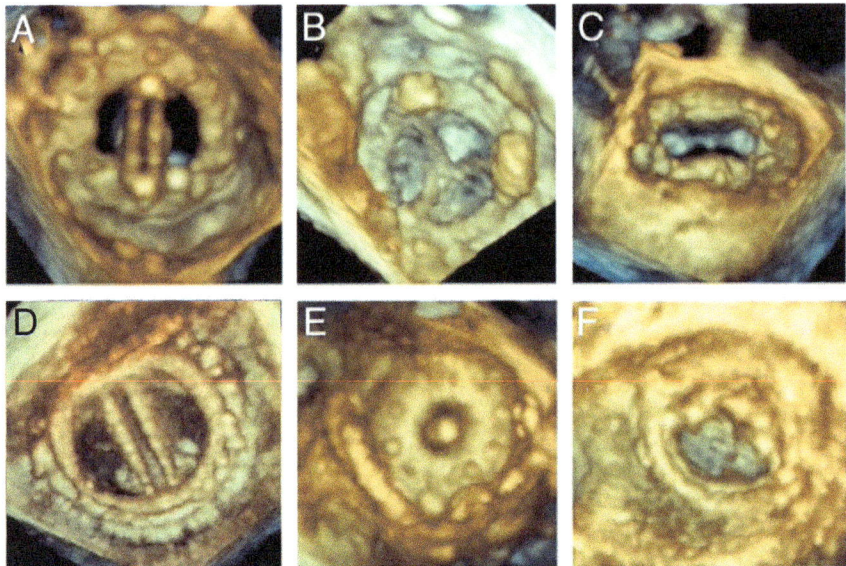

Figure 16.36 Three-dimensional transesophageal views of prosthetic valves and rings. Zoomed 3D TEE images of prosthetic valves. (a) Bileaflet, mechanical mitral valve as viewed from the left atrium. (b) Bioprosthetic mitral valve as viewed from the left ventricle. (c) Mitral annuloplasty ring from the left atrium. (d) Mitral bileaflet mechanical valve from the left atrium: this image shows thrombi (black arrows) attached to the hinge mechanism of the valve; the motion of the leaflets is not impaired. (e) *En face* view from the left atrium of a ball-and-cage valve implanted in the mitral annulus. (f) Single tilting-disk valve in the mitral position as viewed from the left atrium.
Adapted with permission from Ref. [6].

normal prosthetic valve function (with or without PPM) versus acquired prosthetic valve stenosis (Tables 16.8 and 16.9) [12,13].

16.18.2.3 Stress echocardiography

Stress echocardiography is a valuable tool for the evaluation of prosthetic valve hemodynamic function especially when there is discordance between the patient's symptomatic status and the prosthetic valve hemodynamics. Indeed normally and abnormally functioning prostheses can produce similar estimated gradients at rest, in contrast, during exercise a stenotic prosthetic valve or PPM is generally associated with a marked increase in gradient often with pulmonary arterial hypertension and a subsequent impaired exercise capacity. A disproportionate increase in transvalvular gradient (>20 mmHg for aortic prostheses or >12 mmHg for mitral prostheses) generally indicates severe prosthesis dysfunction or PPM [14]. High resting and stress gradients occur more often with smaller (≤21 mm for aortic and ≤25 for mitral) rather than larger-sized prostheses, and mismatched rather than non-mismatched prostheses.

Table 16.10 Normal reference values of effective orifice areas for the aortic prosthetic valves

Prosthetic valve size (mm)	19	21	23	25	27	29
Stented bioprosthetic valves						
Mosaic	1.1±0.2	1.2±0.3	1.4±0.3	1.7±0.4	1.8±0.4	2.0±0.4
Hancock II	–	1.2±0.2	1.3±0.2	1.5±0.2	1.6±0.2	1.6±0.2
Carpentier-Edwards Perimount	1.1±0.3	1.3±0.4	1.50±0.4	1.80±0.4	2.1±0.4	2.2±0.4
Carpentier-Edwards Magna	1.3±0.3	1.5±0.3	1.8±0.4	2.1±0.5	–	–
Biocor (Epic)	1.0±0.3	1.3±0.5	1.4±0.5	1.9±0.7	–	–
Mitroflow	1.1±0.2	1.2±0.3	1.4±0.3	1.6±0.3	1.8±0.3	–
Trifecta[a]	1.41	1.63	1.8	2.02	2.20	2.35
Stentless bioprosthetic valves						
Medtronic Freestyle	1.2±0.2	1.4±0.2	1.5±0.3	2.0±0.4	2.3±0.5	–
St. Jude Medical Toronto SPV	–	1.3±0.3	1.5±0.5	1.7±0.8	2.1±0.7	2.7±1.0
Prima Edwards	–	1.3±0.3	1.6±0.3	1.9±0.4	–	–
Mechanical valves						
Medtronic-Hall	1.2±0.2	1.3±0.2	–	–	–	–
St. Jude Medical Standard	1.0±0.2	1.4±0.2	1.5±0.5	2.1±0.4	2.7±0.6	3.2±0.3
St. Jude Medical Regent	1.6±0.4	2.0±0.7	2.2±0.9	2.5±0.9	3.6±1.3	4.4±0.6
MCRI On-X	1.5±0.2	1.7±0.4	2.0±0.6	2.4±0.8	3.2±0.6	3.2±0.6
Carbomedics Standard and Top Hat	1.0±0.4	1.5±0.3	1.7±0.3	2.0±0.4	2.5±0.4	2.6±0.4
ATS Medical[b]	1.1±0.3	1.6±0.4	1.8±0.5	1.9±0.3	2.3±0.8	–

Effective orifice area is expressed as mean values available in the literature. Further studies are needed to validate these reference values.
[a] In particular, for the newer models such as, for example, the Trifecta.
[b] For the ATS medical valve, the label valve sizes are: 18, 20, 22, 24, 26 mm.
Adapted with permission from American Heart Association [4].

Table 16.11 **Normal reference values of effective orifice areas for the prosthetic mitral valves**

Prosthetic valve size (mm)	25	27	29	31	33
Stented bioprosthetic valves					
Medtronic Mosaic	1.5±0.4	1.7±0.5	1.9±0.5	1.9±0.5	–
Hancock II	1.5±0.4	1.8±0.5	1.9±0.5	2.6±0.5	2.6±0.7
Carpentier-Edwards Perimount	1.6±0.4	1.8±0.4	2.1±0.5	–	–
Mechanical valves					
St. Jude Medical Standard	1.5±0.3	1.7±0.4	1.8±0.4	2.0±0.5	2.0±0.5
[a]MCRI On-X	2.2±0.9	2.2±0.9	2.2±0.9	2.2±0.9	2.2±0.9

Effective orifice area is expressed as mean values available in the literature. Further studies are needed to validate these reference values.
[a] The On-X valve has just 1 size for 27–29 and 31–33 mm prostheses. In addition, the strut and leaflets are identical for all sizes (25–33 mm); only the size of the sewing cuff is different.
Adapted with permission of American Heart Association [4].

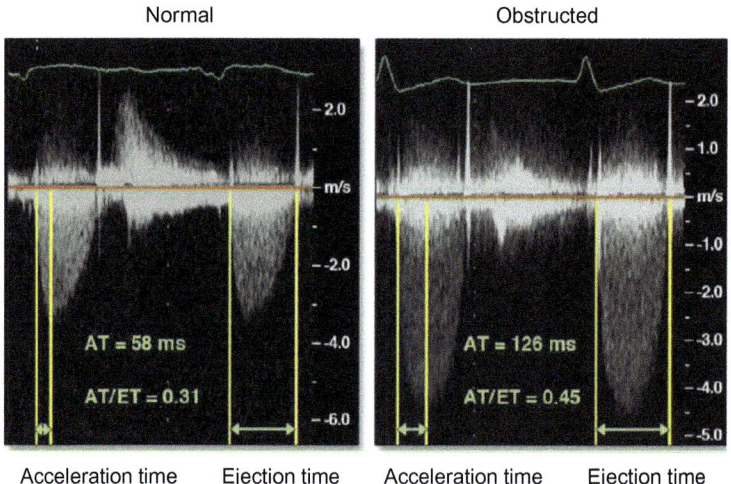

Figure 16.37 Parameters of flow ejection dynamics to detect prosthetic valve stenosis. Note the rounded flow velocity curve for the obstructed valve (right) and the early peaking of the velocity in the normal valve (left). AT: acceleration time; ET: ejection time; PAV: prosthetic aortic valve. Reproduced with permission from Ref. [13].

16.18.3 Prosthetic valve regurgitation

Assessment of severity of prosthetic aortic valve regurgitation is generally much more complex than in native valves because of the high prevalence of paravalvular regurgitation and eccentric jets. Mechanical prostheses have a normal regurgitant volume known as leakage backflow. As opposed to the pathologic regurgitant jets, the normal leakage backflow jets are characterized by being short in duration, narrow, and symmetrical (Figure 16.38).

TTE generally provides a good visualization of the LVOT and of prosthetic aortic regurgitation. TEE may be useful to identify the origin of the regurgitant jets in technically difficult TTE studies and to identify the mechanism of regurgitation and the associated complications such as flail bioprosthetic cusp, presence of pannus, thrombus, vegetations, masses, or chordae interacting with occluder closure, abscess formation, or prosthesis dehiscence [5]. Assessment of prosthetic mitral regurgitation by TTE is problematic because the left atrium is largely occulted by the acoustic shadowing due to the metallic components of the prosthesis (Figure 16.39) [3]. This problem is more frequent in mechanical valves than in bioprosthetic valves. TEE is superior to TTE in detecting prosthetic mitral regurgitation and determining its localization and mechanism [15,16].

The same principles and methods used for grading severity of native valve regurgitation may be used for grading severity of prosthetic valve regurgitation (Tables 16.12 and 16.13). However, quantitative methods such as the proximal isovelocity surface area (PISA) are often not feasible in the context of prosthetic valves, and limited data are available about their accuracy [17]. Hence, a comprehensive multi-parametric approach is highly recommended (Tables 16.12 and 16.13) [9].

16.18.3.1 Aortic prosthetic valve regurgitation

The ratio of regurgitant jet diameter/LVOT diameter may be overestimated in the case of eccentric jets and underestimated in the case of jets impinging the wall of the LVOT or the anterior mitral valve (Table 16.12). In contrast to native valves, the width of the vena contracta may be difficult to measure accurately in the long-axis view due to the shadowing caused by the prosthesis ring or stent. The PISA method is generally not feasible or may be inaccurate for the quantitation of aortic prosthetic valve regurgitation. However, the Doppler method may be used to estimate the regurgitant volume by calculating the difference between the stroke volume measured in the LVOT and the stroke volume measured in the right ventricular outflow tract or at the mitral annulus (Table 16.12).

16.18.3.2 Mitral prosthetic valve regurgitation

At TTE examination, the presence of occult mitral prosthesis regurgitation should be suspected when the following signs are present: presence of flow convergence on the LV side of the prosthesis during systole; increased mitral peak E wave velocity, gradient, and/or DVI; unexplained or new worsening of pulmonary arterial hypertension; and a dilated and hyperkinetic left ventricle (Table 16.13) [3]. TEE should be systematically performed when there is a clinical or TTE suspicion of occult mitral regurgitation (Figures 16.38 and 16.39). As for aortic prostheses, the volumetric method is often preferred to the PISA method for quantification of mitral prosthesis regurgitation.

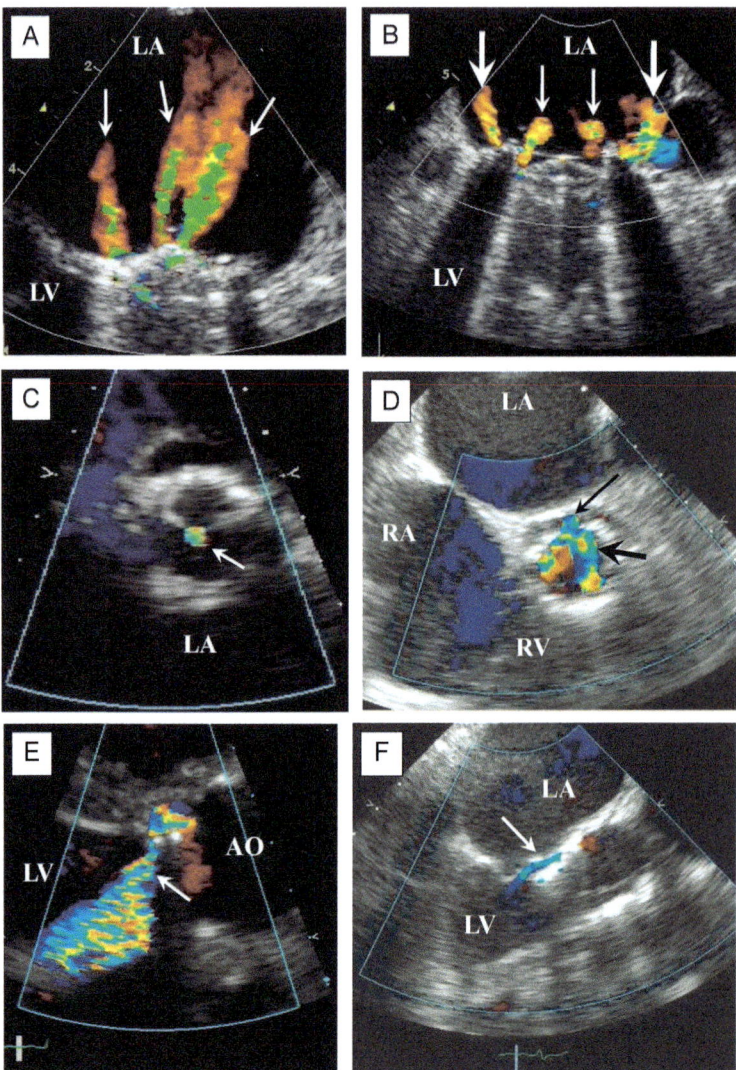

Figure 16.38 Color-Doppler images of transvalvular and paravalvular prosthetic valve regurgitation. The white or black arrows indicate the regurgitant jet(s). (a and b) TEE views of normal physiological regurgitant jets (thin white arrows; a and b) and paravalvular regurgitant jets (thick white arrows; b) in mitral bileaflet mechanical valves. (c) TTE short-axis view of mild transvalvular regurgitation in a stented bioprosthetic aortic valve. (d) TEE short-axis view of severe transvalvular regurgitation (thick black arrow; one of the cusps is blocked in open position) and mild paravalvular regurgitation (thin black arrow) in a transcatheter bioprosthetic aortic valve. (e) TTE long-axis view of moderate paravalvular eccentric regurgitant jet in a stented bioprosthetic aortic valve. (f) TEE long-axis view of a mild paravalvular regurgitation in a transcatheter bioprosthetic aortic valve.

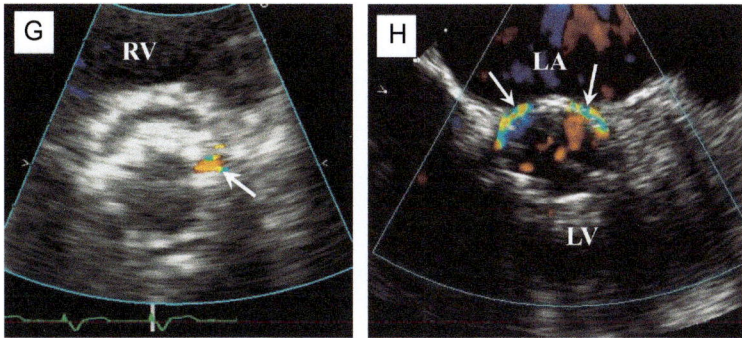

Figure 16.38 Continued. (g) TTE short-axis view of a mild paravalvular regurgitation (one single jet occupying <10% of circumference) in a stented aortic bioprosthetic valve. (h) TEE short-axis view of a severe paravalvular regurgitation (two jets occupying >20% of circumference) in a transcatheter bioprosthetic aortic valve. AO: aorta; LA: left atrium; LV: left ventricle; RV: right ventricle; RA: right atrium.
Courtesy of Dr. John Chambers, Guy's and St Thomas Hospitals, London (a, e) and Dr. Arsène Basmadjian, Montreal Heart Institute (b). Reproduced with permission from Ref. [10].

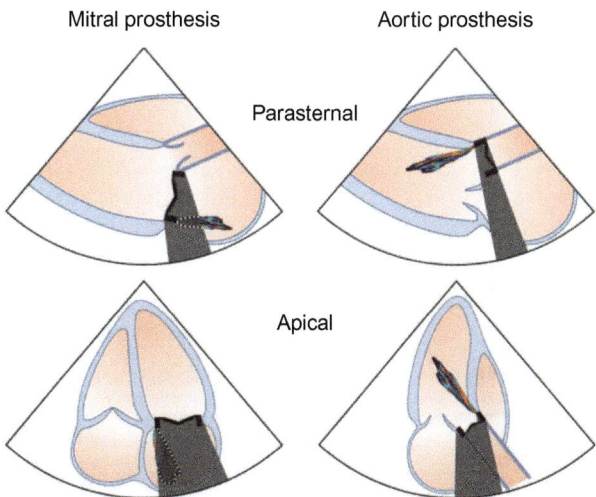

Figure 16.39 Effect of the position of the mechanical prosthetic valve and the echocardiographic imaging view on shadowing and masking of a regurgitation jet by Doppler. A higher effect from transthoracic imaging is seen on prostheses in the mitral position compared to the aortic position.
Reproduced with permission of the American Society of Echocardiography [3].

Table 16.12 **Doppler-echocardiographic criteria for severity of aortic prosthetic valve regurgitation (central and paravalvular)**

	Mild	Moderate	Severe
Valve structure and motion			
Mechanical or bioprosthesis	Usually normal	Usually abnormal[a]	Usually abnormal[a]
Doppler parameters (qualitative or semi-quantitative)			
Jet width in central jets (%LVOT diameter): color Doppler[b]	Narrow (≤25)	Intermediate (26–64)	Large (>65)
Jet density: CW Doppler	Incomplete or faint	Dense	Dense
Jet deceleration rate (PHT, ms): CW Doppler[c]	Slow (>500)	Variable (200–500)	Steep (>200)
Diastolic flow reversal in the ascending aorta: PW Doppler	Absent or brief early diastolic	Intermediate	Prominent holodiastolic (end-diastolic velocity >20 cm/s)
Circumferential extent of paravalvular regurgitation (%)[d]	<10	10–29	≥30
Doppler parameters (quantitative)			
Vena contracta width (mm)[b][e]	<3	3–6	>6
Regurgitant volume (ml/beat)[e]	<30	30–59	>60
Regurgitant fraction (%)	<30	30–50	>50
Indirect signs			
LV size[f]	Normal	Normal/mildly dilated	Dilated

PHT: pressure half time.
[a] Abnormal mechanical valves: immobile occluder, dehiscence or rocking (paravalvular regurgitation); abnormal biologic valves: leaflet thickening/calcification or prolapse, dehiscence or rocking (paravalvular regurgitation).
[b] Parameter applicable to central jets and is less accurate in eccentric jets.
[c] This parameter is influenced by left ventricular compliance.
[d] Applies only to paravalvular regurgitation.
[e] Can be estimated by the difference of stroke volume in LVOT minus stroke volume in RV outflow tract (if no > mild pulmonary regurgitation) or at the mitral annulus (if no > mild mitral regurgitation).
[f] Applies to chronic, late postoperative prosthetic aortic valve regurgitation in the absence of other etiologies.
Adapted in part from Ref. [3] with permission of American Society of Echocardiography.

16.18.4 Specifics for assessment of transcatheter aortic valve function

The flow pattern of transcatheter aortic valves differs from that of surgical bioprostheses in the sense that there are two levels of flow acceleration at the inflow aspect of the valve: a first level when the flow enters into the apical portion of the stent, and a second level when the flow passes through the prosthetic valve

Table 16.13 Doppler-echocardiographic criteria for severity of mitral prosthetic valve regurgitation (central and paravalvular)

	Mild	Moderate	Severe
Valve structure and motion			
Mechanical or bioprosthesis	Usually normal	Usually abnormal[a]	Usually abnormal[a]
Doppler parameters (qualitative or semi-quantitative)			
Color flow jet area	Small, central jet (usually <4 cm² or <20% of LA area)	Variable	Large central jet (usually >8 cm² or >40% of LA area) or variable size wall impinging jet swirling in LA
Flow convergence	None or minimal	Intermediate	Large
Jet density: CW Doppler	Incomplete or faint	Dense	Dense
Jet contour: CW Doppler[b]	Parabolic	Usually parabolic	Early peaking, triangular
Pulmonary venous flow: PW Doppler	Systolic dominance	Systolic blunting	Systolic flow reversal
Doppler velocity index: PW Doppler	<2.2	2.2–2.5	>2.5
Doppler parameters (quantitative)			
Vena contracta width (mm)	<3	3–5.9	≥6
Regurgitant volume (ml/beat)	<30	30–59	>60
Regurgitant fraction (%)	<30	30–50	>50
Effective regurgitant orifice area (mm²)	<20	20–39	≥40
Indirect signs			
LV size[c]	Normal	Normal/mildly dilated	Dilated
LA size	Normal	Normal/mildly dilated	Dilated
Pulmonary hypertension			
(SPAP ≥50 mmHg at rest and ≥60 mmHg at exercise)	Generally absent	Variable	Generally present

[a] Abnormal mechanical valves: immobile occluder, dehiscence or rocking (paravalvular regurgitation); abnormal biologic valves: leaflet thickening/calcification or prolapse, dehiscence or rocking (paravalvular regurgitation).
[b] This parameter is influenced by left ventricular compliance. Measured at the mitral annulus and stroke volume measured in the LVOT (if no > mild aortic regurgitation).
[c] Applies to chronic, late postoperative prosthetic aortic valve regurgitation in the absence of other etiologies.
Adapted in part from Ref. [3] with permission of American Society of Echocardiography.

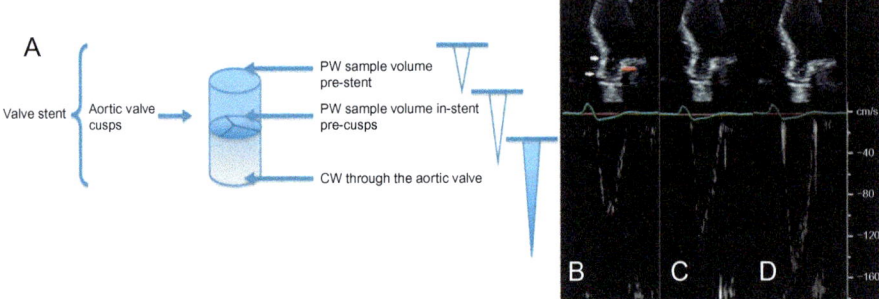

Figure 16.40 Schematic and examples of spectral Doppler flow acceleration in a transcatheter aortic valve. (a) Schematic presentation of echocardiographic pulse-wave (PW) Doppler patterns when the sample volume is placed pre-stent, in-stent but pre-cusps, and CW through the transcatheter aortic valve (SAPIEN). Due to flow acceleration, it is generally recommended that the subvalvular velocities used in either Doppler velocity index or effective orifice area be sampled proximal to the stent. (b) The PW Doppler pattern of a sample volume placed before stent. White arrows show the extent of the transcatheter heart valve in the aortic root. Red arrow shows the level of the prosthetic aortic cusps. (c) The PW Doppler pattern of sample volume placed within the stent but before cusps. (d) The PW Doppler pattern of a sample volume placed at the level of the cusps.
Reproduced with permission from Ref. [18].

leaflets (Figure 16.40). For that reason, it is generally recommended to measure the LVOT diameter and velocity immediately proximal to the apical end of the stent when measuring the stroke volume and EOA of transcatheter valves [19,20]. However, if the stent sits low in the LVOT, which may occur more frequently with the self-expandable prostheses, it may be preferable to measure the LVOT diameter and velocity within the proximal portion of the stent below the bioprosthetic leaflets.

Paravalvular regurgitation is more common following transcatheter aortic valve implantation (TAVI) than after surgical aortic valve replacement (Figures 16.38 and 16.41). A recent meta-analysis reports that moderate-severe paravalvular regurgitation occurs in 5–20% of patients undergoing TAVI and is associated with a 2.0–2.5fold increase in mortality [22]. Semi quantitative evaluation of the severity of paravalvular regurgitation can be achieved by careful imaging of the neck of the jet(s) in the short axis view cross-secting the lower (i.e., apical) portion of the stent and by estimating the circumferential extent of the regurgitation (Table 16.12) [3,20]. However, this parameter has not been well validated and is subject to many pitfalls. It is thus important to also assess the other views (parasternal long-axis, apical five- and three-chamber; Figure 16.41) and the other parameters (width of the jet at its origin, flow reversal in the descending aorta etc., estimation of regurgitant volume by difference of LVOT stroke volume minus RV outflow stroke volume etc. (Table 16.12). Some paravalvular regurgitant jets may only be visible on the short-axis view but, vice versa, other

Acquired valvular heart disease

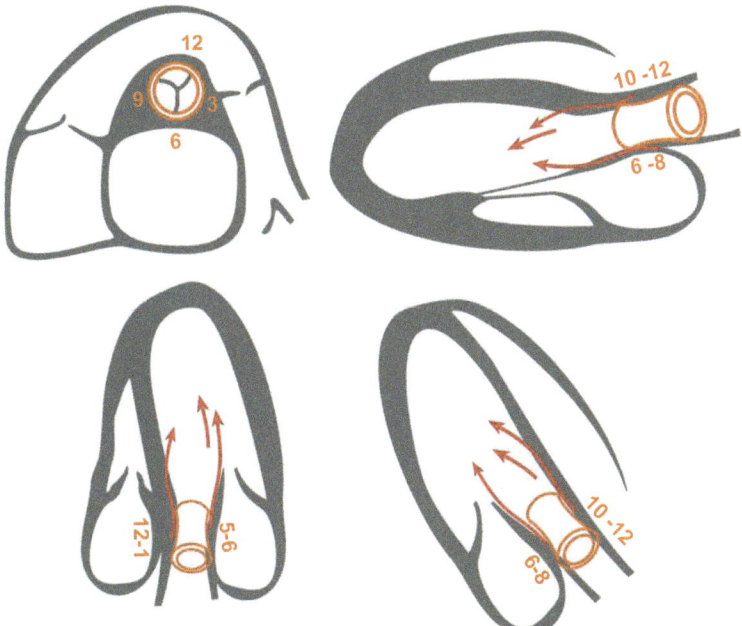

Figure 16.41 Representation of paravalvular aortic regurgitation jets location according to the face of a clock. Conventional 2D transthoracic echocardiographic views are represented.
(a) Parasternal short-axis view. (b) Parasternal long-axis view. (c) Apical five-chamber view.
(d) Apical three-chamber view.
Reproduced with permission from Ref. [21].

jets may be detected only in the apical views (Figure 16.41). Hence, multi-window and multi-parametric approach is mandatory to properly identify and quantitate paravalvular regurgitation following TAVI [11,20]. The role of 3D color-Doppler echocardiography and magnetic resonance imaging in quantitating paravalvular prosthetic regurgitation is promising and needs further investigation.

16.19 Cinefluoroscopy

The evaluation of valve occluder mobility is key to identify the presence of intrinsic dysfunction of the prosthesis and differentiate this condition from normal valve function or PPM. In the case of mechanical prostheses, this can be attempted with some degree of success by TTE or TEE but valve cinefluoroscopy is certainly the most accurate, economical, and least invasive technique that can be used for this purpose [12,23]. Cinefluoroscopy indeed provides accurate information on the mobility and the opening/closing angles of the leaflets of mechanical prostheses (Table 16.14). For orientations such as an anatomically placed mitral bileaflet

Table 16.14 **Normal reference opening and closing angles for mechanical prosthetic valves**

Valve model	Valve type	Leaflet opening angle (°)	Leaflet closing angle (°)
Aortic prostheses			
ATS open pivot	Bileaflet	85	25
Carbomedics	Bileaflet	78	25
Duromedics	Bileaflet	78	20
On-X	Bileaflet	90	40
Sorin Bicarbon	Bileaflet	80	20
St Jude Medical	Bileaflet	85 (19–25 mm)	30 (19–25 mm)
		85 (27–31 mm)	25 (27–31 mm)
Björk-Shiley spherical	Tilting disc	60[a]	0[a]
Medtronic-Hall	Tilting disc	75	0
Omniscience	Tilting disc	60	0
Sorin Allcarbon	Tilting disc	60	0
Aortic prostheses			
Carbomedics	Bileaflet	78	25
Duromedics	Bileaflet	73	20
On-X	Bileaflet	90	40
Sorin® Bicarbon	Bileaflet	80	20
St Jude Medical	Bileaflet	85 (19–25 mm)	30 (19–25 mm)
		85 (27–31 mm)	25 (27–31 mm)
Björk-Shiley spherical	Tilting disc	60[a]	0[a]
		70[b]¶	0[b]
Sorin® Allcarbon	Tilting disc	60	0

This table presents the normal opening and closing angles as provided by the manufacturer.
[a] Before 1981.
[b] After 1981.
Adapted with permission from Ref. [24].

mechanical valves positioned in the anatomical position or for aortic bileaflet valves positioned with leaflets parallel to the septum, it may not be possible to obtain a good perpendicular view of the leaflets [23]. In a recent review of 11 studies reporting on mechanical valve obstruction, all prosthetic valves obstructed by thrombus showed leaflet restriction on cinefluoroscopy, and when leaflet restriction was absent despite significant increase in Doppler transprosthetic gradients (5% of the cases), no thrombus was found in these prostheses at surgical examination: pannus or LVOT obstruction was the underlying cause [25]. Hence, cinefluoroscopy is likely the best imaging modality to assess restriction of leaflet mobility in patients with mechanical valves, but TEE or computed tomography (CT) are often useful to identify the underlying cause (thrombus vs. pannus vs. other) of the leaflet restriction and/or valve obstruction.

16.20 Computed tomography

MDCT is a promising complementary technique for evaluation of prosthetic valves, especially in patients with suspected obstruction and also in patients with suspected endocarditis (see subchapter 16.34 on infective endocarditis). The image quality obtained by MDCT is adequate for most prosthetic valves except those containing cobalt-chrome alloy rings (e.g., Björk-Shiley and Allcarbon tilting-disk prostheses), which cause severe prosthesis-related artifacts [26,27].

MDCT is useful: (i) to assess the mobility of the occluder in patients with mechanical valves (Figure 16.42 and Table 16.14), (ii) to detect the underlying cause of valve obstruction (Figure 16.43); and (iii) to differentiate thrombus versus pannus (Figure 16.43). Pannus is visualized as a hypodense mass with a semi-circular

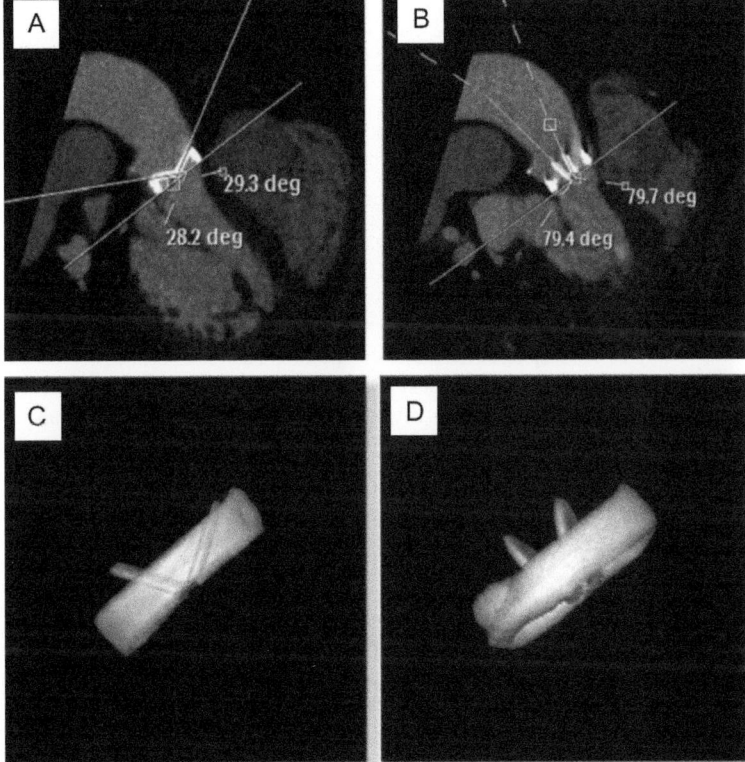

Figure 16.42 Utility of multidetector CT to assess leaflet mobility in bileaflet mechanical valves. (a and b) Measurement of closing (a) and opening (b) angles of a normally functioning bileaflet mechanical valve by MDCT. (c and d) 3D volume rendered MDCT images showing asymmetric leaflet restriction in a thrombosed bileaflet mechanical valve (c). After 2 months of additional anticoagulation therapy (warfarin plus low-molecular weight heparins) and antiplatelet therapy (aspirin), MDCT shows normal opening of both leaflets (d).
(a and b) Reproduced with permission from Ref. [28]; (c and d) Reproduced with permission from Ref. [29].

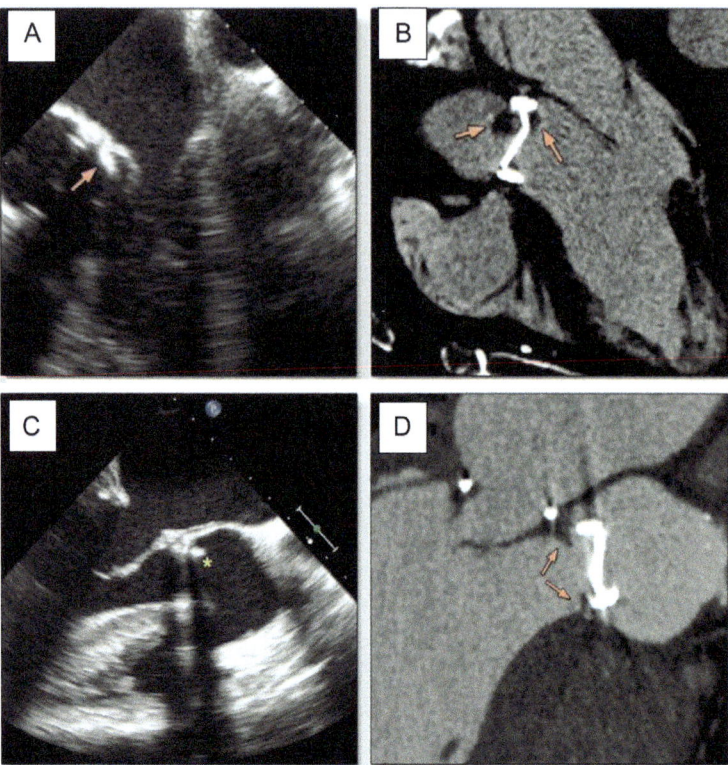

Figure 16.43 Utility of multidetector CT to differentiate thrombus versus pannus in prosthetic valves. (a) In this patient with increased gradient across a Carbomedics mechanical valve, TEE shows a subvalvular echodense mass located between the septal side of the prosthetic valve and the anterior mitral valve leaflet (arrow). (b) MDCT confirmed the presence of this mass on the ventricular side of the prosthesis. Moreover, an additional hypodense mass was seen on the aortic side of the valve (arrows). The irregular shape and the location on both the aortic and ventricular side of the prosthetic valve favors the diagnosis of valve thrombosis over pannus formation. (c) In this other patient, TTE revealed an increased pressure gradient across a Carbomedics valve but could not determine its exact cause. On TEE (c), the assessment of the prosthesis, especially its subvalvular aspect, was hampered by acoustic shadowing. No echodense masses were seen on the subvalvular side, but a possible supravalvular echodense mass (*) was identified. (d) MDCT did not show any supravalvular mass. However, MDCT identified a semi-circular hypodense mass on the ventricular side of the prosthetic valve ring (arrows), which is compatible with pannus formation.
Adapted with permission from Ref. [29].

anatomical configuration curved along and subvalvular to the valve ring. In contrast, obstructive thrombi are imaged as supra- and subvalvular hypodense masses with irregular anatomy directly attached to the leaflets and hingepoints causing mechanical obstruction by leaflet restriction (Figure 16.43) [25,30,31].

In patients with bioprosthetic valves, MDCT may also be helpful: (i) to assess leaflet mobility, (ii) detect and quantitate leaflet calcification, which is the predominant mechanism leading to structural valve failure [32,33] and (iii) detect and differentiate thrombus versus pannus (Figure 16.44).

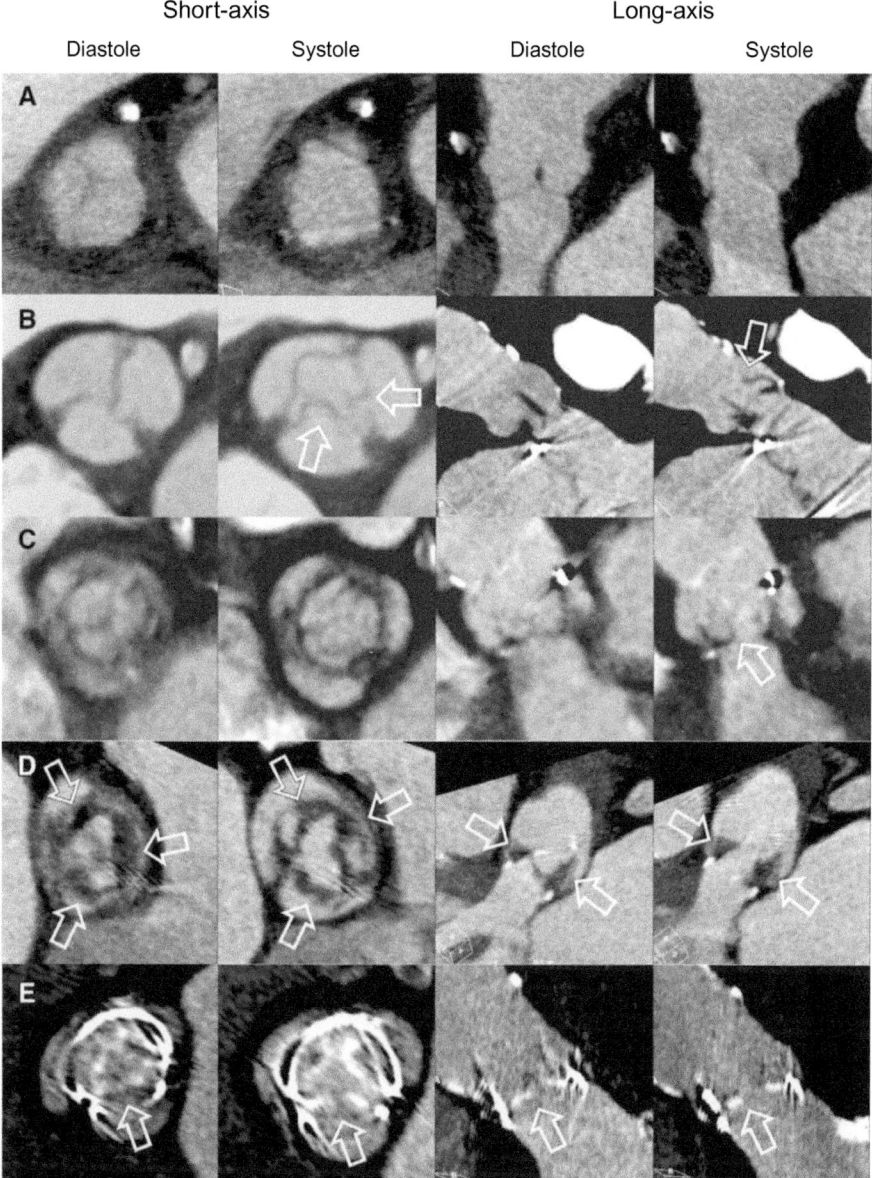

Figure 16.44 Multidetector CT images of morphologic features in normal and dysfunctional aortic bioprostheses. This figure shows short-axis views at the level of leaflet tips and long-axis views during systole and diastole. (a) Stentless bioprosthesis with normal opening and morphology. (b) Stentless bioprosthesis with restrictive motion of two leaflets (arrows), one of them opening with folding (arrow in right column). The insertion margins of those leaflets appear thickened. (c) Stented bioprosthesis with restrictive leaflet motion opening in a comma-shaped (arrow) folding pattern with restricted motion at the base. (d) Stented bioprosthesis with diffuse thickening and reduced opening of the leaflets as well as additional hypo-attenuating structures at the leaflet base (arrows), suspected to represent thrombus. (e) Stented bioprosthesis with severe and diffuse calcification of the three leaflets (arrows) associated with severely reduced opening.
Reproduced with permission from Ref. [32].

16.21 Nuclear imaging

Nuclear imaging may be useful to detect prosthetic valve endocarditis and associated septic embolism (see subchapter 16.34 on infective endocarditis) [34,35]. Because the prosthetic valves are relatively small structures, fusion of the molecular imaging technique (positron emission tomography, PET), or single-photon emission computed tomography (SPECT) with a robust anatomical imaging technique (MDCT) is necessary. In a large contemporary cohort of patients with presumed prosthetic valve endocarditis, Saby et al. found that the sensitivity and specificity of ^{18}F-PET/CT (^{18}Fluorodeoxyglucose PET/CT) were 73% and 80%, respectively [35] (see subchapter 16.34 on infective endocarditis for more details).

Some recent studies suggest that ^{18}F-sodium fluoride PET/CT is able to identify active tissue calcification and predict disease progression in patients with native aortic stenosis [36]. Further studies are needed to determine if this technique would be able to identify active mineralization of bioprosthetic valve tissues and thereby predict the risk of structural valve degeneration.

16.22 Magnetic resonance imaging

Magnetic resonance imaging (MRI) with magnetic fields of 1.5 or 3.0 T has been shown to be safe in patients with bioprosthetic or mechanical prosthetic valves. MRI can be used to measure: (i) the geometric orifice area of bioprosthetic valves by cine MRI and planimetry [37,38] or (ii) the EOA of all types of prosthetic valves by phase-contrast MRI using the continuity equation principle or direct measurement of the vena contracta [39,40]. These techniques may be helpful, particularly when the transprosthetic gradient is increased at Doppler-echocardiographic exam but the measurement of valve EOA is not feasible or is discordant with that of gradient. Recent developments in 4D flow velocity mapping by MRI now enable the visualization and characterization of the flow patterns upstream and downstream of prosthetic valves [41,42].

As described above, quantification of paravalvular regurgitation by Doppler echocardiography remains a difficult challenge following TAVI. MRI may help to corroborate the severity of paravalvular regurgitation when Doppler echocardiography remains inconclusive or if there is a discordance between the regurgitation grading by echocardiography and the patient's symptomatic status. For this purpose, phase-contrast imaging is obtained in a short-axis plane cutting the aorta just above the transcatheter valve stent to measure the antegrade and retrograde aortic flows and then to calculate the regurgitant volume and fraction (Figure 16.45) [43,44]. Recent studies in patients with native aortic valve regurgitation suggest that MRI-derived regurgitant fractions <10% corresponds to mild, 10–29% to moderate, and ≥30% to severe aortic regurgitation [45,46]. The repercussion of the paravalvular regurgitation on LV volumes and function can also be assessed using standard cine MRI sequences. Further studies are needed to establish the diagnostic and prognostic values of MRI for the assessment of paravalvular regurgitation following TAVI.

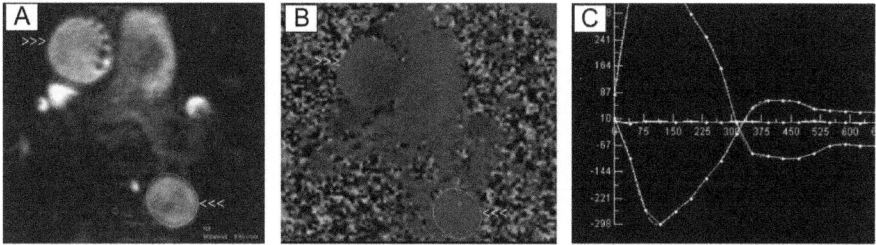

Figure 16.45 Magnetic resonance imaging for the assessment of paravalvular regurgitation following transcatheter aortic valve implantation. (a) Magnitude phase-contrast MR image used for anatomic correlation. (b) Velocity MR image: upper arrowheads show ascending aorta at the level of the pulmonary artery bifurcation, the lower show the descending aorta. (c) Profile of aortic flow rate during cardiac cycle in a patient with paravalvular aortic regurgitation following TAVI. Areas under the positive and negative parts of the curve represent forward and regurgitant flow, respectively. The upper curve corresponds to flow in the ascending aorta, while the lower curve corresponds to flow in the descending aorta. Quantification with MR velocity mapping yields to a regurgitant fraction of 31% corresponding to moderate-to-severe regurgitation.
Adapted with permission from Ref. [43].

16.23 Conclusion

The particular context of prosthetic valves poses major challenges in terms of imaging and flow dynamics that push Doppler echocardiography to its limits. A comprehensive approach that integrates several parameters of valve function measured by TTE, TEE, and 3D echocardiography is key to appropriately detect and quantitate prosthetic valve dysfunction. Other imaging modalities such as cinefluoroscopy, MDCT, MRI, and nuclear imaging are valuable additional tools in the diagnosis and management of prosthetic valve complications, especially in cases of inconclusive echocardiography as well as in the detection of periprosthetic abnormalities. Discrimination between thrombus, pannus and vegetation, or hematoma and abscess may be difficult when based only on morphological findings obtained by echocardiography and an approach based on multimodality imaging is essential to accurately identify the causal mechanism of prosthetic valve dysfunction and provide additional relevant anatomic information that can have an impact on patient care.

References

[1] Dunning J, Gao H, Chambers J, Moat N, Murphy G, Pagano D, et al. Aortic valve surgery: marked increases in volume and significant decreases in mechanical valve use–an analysis of 41,227 patients over 5 years from the Society for Cardiothoracic Surgery in Great Britain and Ireland National database. J Thorac Cardiovasc Surg 2011;142(4):776–82, 4.

[2] Brown JM, O'Brien SM, Wu C, Sikora JA, Griffith BP, Gammie JS. Isolated aortic valve replacement in North America comprising 108,687 patients in 10 years: changes in risks, valve types, and outcomes in the Society of Thoracic Surgeons National Database. J Thorac Cardiovasc Surg 2009;137(1):82–90.

[3] Zoghbi WA, Chambers JB, Dumesnil JG, Foster E, Gottdiener JS, Grayburn PA, et al. Recommendations for evaluation of prosthetic valves with echocardiography and Doppler ultrasound: a report From the American Society of Echocardiography's Guidelines and Standards Committee and the Task Force on Prosthetic Valves, developed in conjunction with the American College of Cardiology Cardiovascular Imaging Committee, Cardiac Imaging Committee of the American Heart Association, the European Association of Echocardiography, a registered branch of the European Society of Cardiology, the Japanese Society of Echocardiography and the Canadian Society of Echocardiography, endorsed by the American College of Cardiology Foundation, American Heart Association, European Association of Echocardiography, a registered branch of the European Society of Cardiology, the Japanese Society of Echocardiography, and Canadian Society of Echocardiography. J Am Soc Echocardiogr 2009;22(9):975–1014, quiz 1082–4.
[4] Pibarot P, Dumesnil JG. Prosthetic heart valves: selection of the optimal prosthesis and long-term management. Circulation 2009;119(7):1034–48.
[5] Bach DS. Transesophageal echocardiographic (TEE) evaluation of prosthetic valves. Cardiol Clin 2000;18(4):751–71.
[6] Lang RM, Tsang W, Weinert L, Mor-Avi V, Chandra S. Valvular heart disease. The value of 3-dimensional echocardiography. J Am Coll Cardiol 2011;58(19):1933–44.
[7] Singh P, Inamdar V, Hage FG, Kodali V, Karakus G, Suwanjutah T, et al. Usefulness of live/real time three-dimensional transthoracic echocardiography in evaluation of prosthetic valve function. Echocardiography 2009;26(10):1236–49.
[8] Roudaut R, Serri K, Lafitte S. Thrombosis of prosthetic heart valves: diagnosis and therapeutic considerations. Heart 2007;93(1):137–42.
[9] Vahanian A, Alfieri O, Andreotti F, Antunes MJ, Baron-Esquivias G, Baumgartner H, et al. Guidelines on the management of valvular heart disease (version 2012). Eur Heart J 2012;33(19):2451–96.
[10] Pibarot P, Dumesnil JG. Doppler echocardiographic evaluation of prosthetic valve function. Heart 2012;98(1):69–78.
[11] Zamorano JL, Badano LP, Bruce C, Chan KL, Goncalves A, Hahn RT, et al. EAE/ASE recommendations for the use of echocardiography in new transcatheter interventions for valvular heart disease. Eur Heart J 2011;32(17):2189–214.
[12] Muratori M, Montorsi P, Maffessanti F, Teruzzi G, Zoghbi WA, Gripari P, et al. Dysfunction of bileaflet aortic prosthesis: accuracy of echocardiography versus fluoroscopy. JACC Cardiovasc Imaging 2013;6(2):196–205.
[13] Ben Zekry S, Saad RM, Ozkan M, Al Shahid MS, Pepi M, Muratori M, et al. Flow acceleration time and ratio of acceleration time to ejection time for prosthetic aortic valve function. JACC Cardiovasc Imaging 2011;4(11):1161–70.
[14] Picano E, Pibarot P, Lancellotti P, Monin JL, Bonow RO. The emerging role of exercise testing and stress echocardiography in valvular heart disease. J Am Coll Cardiol 2009;54(24):2251–60.
[15] Alton ME, Pasierski TJ, Orsinelli DA, Eaton GM, Pearson AC. Comparison of transthoracic and transesophageal echocardiography in evaluation of 47 Starr-Edwards prosthetic valves. J Am Coll Cardiol 1992;20(7):1503–11.
[16] Daniel LB, Grigg LE, Weisel RD, Rakowski H. Comparison of transthoracic and transesophageal assessment of prosthetic valve dysfunction. Echocardiography 1990;7(2):83–95.
[17] Vitarelli A, Conde Y, Cimino E, Leone T, D'Angeli I, D'Orazio S, et al. Assessment of severity of mechanical prosthetic mitral regurgitation by transoesophageal echocardiography. Heart 2004;90(5):539–44.

[18] Bloomfield GS, Gillam LD, Hahn RT, Kapadia S, Leipsic J, Lerakis S, et al. A practical guide to multimodality imaging of transcatheter aortic valve replacement. JACC Cardiovasc Imaging 2012;5(4):441–55.
[19] Clavel MA, Rodes-Cabau J, Dumont E, Bagur R, Bergeron S, De Larochelliere R, et al. Validation and characterization of transcatheter aortic valve effective orifice area measured by Doppler echocardiography. JACC Cardiovasc Imaging 2011;4(10):1053–62.
[20] Kappetein AP, Head SJ, Genereux P, Piazza N, van Mieghem NM, Blackstone EH, et al. Updated standardized endpoint definitions for transcatheter aortic valve implantation: the Valve Academic Research Consortium-2 consensus document. J Thorac Cardiovasc Surg 2013;145(1):6–23.
[21] Goncalves A, Almeria C, Marcos-Alberca P, Feltes G, Hernandez-Antolin R, Rodriguez E, et al. Three-dimensional echocardiography in paravalvular aortic regurgitation assessment after transcatheter aortic valve implantation. J Am Soc Echocardiogr 2012;25(1):47–55.
[22] Athappan G, Patvardhan E, Tuzcu EM, Svensson LG, Lemos PA, Fraccaro C, et al. Incidence, predictors, and outcomes of aortic regurgitation after transcatheter aortic valve replacement: meta-analysis and systematic review of literature. J Am Coll Cardiol 2013;61(15):1585–95.
[23] Montorsi P, De Bernardi F, Muratori M, Cavoretto D, Pepi M. Role of cine-fluoroscopy, transthoracic, and transesophageal echocardiography in patients with suspected prosthetic heart valve thrombosis. Am J Cardiol 2000;85(1):58–64.
[24] Habets J, Budde RP, Symersky P, van den Brink RB, de Mol BA, Mali WP, et al. Diagnostic evaluation of left-sided prosthetic heart valve dysfunction. Nat Rev Cardiol 2011;8(8):466–78.
[25] Tanis W, Habets J, van den Brink RB, Symersky P, Budde RP, Chamuleau SA. Differentiation of thrombus from pannus as the cause of acquired mechanical prosthetic heart valve obstruction by non-invasive imaging: a review of the literature. Eur Heart J Cardiovasc Imaging 2014;15(2):119–29.
[26] Habets J, Symersky P, van Herwerden LA, de Mol BA, Spijkerboer AM, Mali WP, et al. Prosthetic heart valve assessment with multidetector-row CT: imaging characteristics of 91 valves in 83 patients. Eur Radiol 2011;21(7):1390–6.
[27] Konen E, Goitein O, Feinberg MS, Eshet Y, Raanani E, Rimon U, et al. The role of ECG-gated MDCT in the evaluation of aortic and mitral mechanical valves: initial experience. AJR Am J Roentgenol 2008;191(1):26–31.
[28] Habets J, Mali WP, Budde RP. Multidetector CT angiography in evaluation of prosthetic heart valve dysfunction. Radiographics 2012;32(7):1893–905.
[29] Habets J, Tanis W, Mali WP, Chamuleau SA, Budde RP. Imaging of prosthetic heart valve dysfunction: complementary diagnostic value of TEE and MDCT? JACC Cardiovasc Imaging 2012;5(9):956–61.
[30] Girard SE, Miller Jr. FA, Orszulak TA, Mullany CJ, Montgomery S, Edwards WD, et al. Reoperation for prosthetic aortic valve obstruction in the era of echocardiography: trends in diagnostic testing and comparison with surgical findings. J Am Coll Cardiol 2001;37(2):579–84.
[31] Ueda T, Teshima H, Fukunaga S, Aoyagi S, Tanaka H. Evaluation of prosthetic valve obstruction on electrocardiographically gated multidetector-row computed tomography—identification of subprosthetic pannus in the aortic position. Circ J 2013;77(2):418–23.
[32] Chenot F, Montant P, Goffinet C, Pasquet A, Vancraeynest D, Coche E, et al. Evaluation of anatomic valve opening and leaflet morphology in aortic valve bioprosthesis by using multidetector CT: comparison with transthoracic echocardiography. Radiology 2010;255(2):377–85.

[33] Mahjoub H, Mathieu P, Senechal M, Larose E, Dumesnil J, Despres JP, et al. ApoB/ApoA-I ratio is associated with increased risk of bioprosthetic valve degeneration. J Am Coll Cardiol 2013;61(7):752–61.

[34] Hyafil F, Rouzet F, Lepage L, Benali K, Raffoul R, Duval X, et al. Role of radiolabelled leukocyte scintigraphy in patients with a suspicion of prosthetic valve endocarditis and inconclusive echocardiography. Eur Heart J Cardiovasc Imaging 2013;14(6):586–94.

[35] Saby L, Laas O, Habib G, Cammilleri S, Mancini J, Tessonnier L, et al. Positron emission tomography/computed tomography for diagnosis of prosthetic valve endocarditis: increased valvular ^{18}F-fluorodeoxyglucose uptake as a novel major criterion. J Am Coll Cardiol 2013;61(23):2374–82.

[36] Dweck MR, Jones C, Joshi NV, Fletcher AM, Richardson H, White A, et al. Assessment of valvular calcification and inflammation by positron emission tomography in patients with aortic stenosis. Circulation 2012;125(1):76–86.

[37] von Knobelsdorff-Brenkenhoff F, Rudolph A, Wassmuth R, Bohl S, Buschmann EE, Abdel-Aty H, et al. Feasibility of cardiovascular magnetic resonance to assess the orifice area of aortic bioprostheses. Circ Cardiovasc Imaging 2009;2(5):397–404, 2 p following 404.

[38] von Knobelsdorff-Brenkenhoff F, Rudolph A, Wassmuth R, Schulz-Menger J. Assessment of mitral bioprostheses using cardiovascular magnetic resonance. J Cardiovasc Magn Reson 2010;12:36.

[39] Garcia J, Marrufo OR, Rodriguez AO, Larose E, Pibarot P, Kadem L. Cardiovascular magnetic resonance evaluation of aortic stenosis severity using single plane measurement of effective orifice area. J Cardiovasc Magn Reson 2012;14:23.

[40] Caruthers SD, Lin SJ, Brown P, Watkins MP, Williams TA, Lehr KA, et al. Practical value of cardiac magnetic resonance imaging for clinical quantification of aortic valve stenosis: comparison with echocardiography. Circulation 2003;108(18):2236–43.

[41] Kozerke S, Hasenkam JM, Pedersen EM, Boesiger P. Visualization of flow patterns distal to aortic valve prostheses in humans using a fast approach for cine 3D velocity mapping. J Magn Reson Imaging 2001;13(5):690–8.

[42] Markl M, Kilner PJ, Ebbers T. Comprehensive 4D velocity mapping of the heart and great vessels by cardiovascular magnetic resonance. J Cardiovasc Magn Reson 2011;13:7.

[43] Sherif MA, Abdel-Wahab M, Beurich HW, Stocker B, Zachow D, Geist V, et al. Haemodynamic evaluation of aortic regurgitation after transcatheter aortic valve implantation using cardiovascular magnetic resonance. EuroIntervention 2011;7(1):57–63.

[44] Merten C, Beurich HW, Zachow D, Mostafa AE, Geist V, Toelg R, et al. Aortic regurgitation and left ventricular remodeling after transcatheter aortic valve implantation: a serial cardiac magnetic resonance imaging study. Circ Cardiovasc Interv 2013;6(4):476–83.

[45] Myerson SG, d'Arcy J, Mohiaddin R, Greenwood JP, Karamitsos TD, Francis JM, et al. Aortic regurgitation quantification using cardiovascular magnetic resonance: association with clinical outcome. Circulation 2012;126(12):1452–60.

[46] Gabriel RS, Renapurkar R, Bolen MA, Verhaert D, Leiber M, Flamm SD, et al. Comparison of severity of aortic regurgitation by cardiovascular magnetic resonance versus transthoracic echocardiography. Am J Cardiol 2011;108(7):1014–20.

Interventional imaging for transcatheter valve procedures

J. Zamorano, C. Fernández-Golfín
University Hospital Ramon y Cajal, Madrid, Spain

Invasive therapies have presented remarkable growth in the last decade. Echocardiography has the advantage of create images in real time, being available before, during, and immediately after invasive procedures. This updated review provides a summary of the use of echocardiography to guide interventions from patient selection to the assessment of results in the most recent cardiac intervention settings.

16.24 Transcatheter aortic valve implantation

Transcatheter aortic valve implantation (TAVI) by percutaneous or transapical approach has emerged as an alternative treatment for patients with severe symptomatic aortic stenosis and high risk for conventional open-heart surgery [1]. Different types of percutaneous valves are currently available: the balloon expandable, such as the Edwards Sapiens™ prosthesis, and the self-expanding, such as the CoreValve™ system. Echocardiography plays a key role in selecting patients and may be used for guiding the procedure and evaluating the results and possible complications. New types of prosthesis are also available; even if the implantation is easier, there is still a need for careful monitoring with the imaging of the procedure.

16.25 Transoesophageal echocardiography approach before TAVI

Transesophageal echocardiography (TEE) can be performed as part of the screening of patients for TAVI or as the initial step of intraprocedure monitoring. The number, mobility, and thickness of the aortic valve cusps, as well as the extension and location of cusps calcification, must be accurately described, as it has implications for proper prosthesis sizing and deployment [2]. Bicuspid aorta is a relative contra-indication for TAVI with the risk of incorrect prosthesis deployment. However, in cases of tricuspid aortic valves with highly asymmetric calcification, the differences in the tension force can cause prosthesis asymmetric deployment and increase the risk of compression of the coronary arteries. The distance between coronary ostia and the aortic annulus has been recommended to be at a minimum of 14 mm from the leaflets insertion for the CoreValve™ and 11 mm for the Edwards Sapiens™ prosthesis. The annulus distance to the left coronary ostia, may

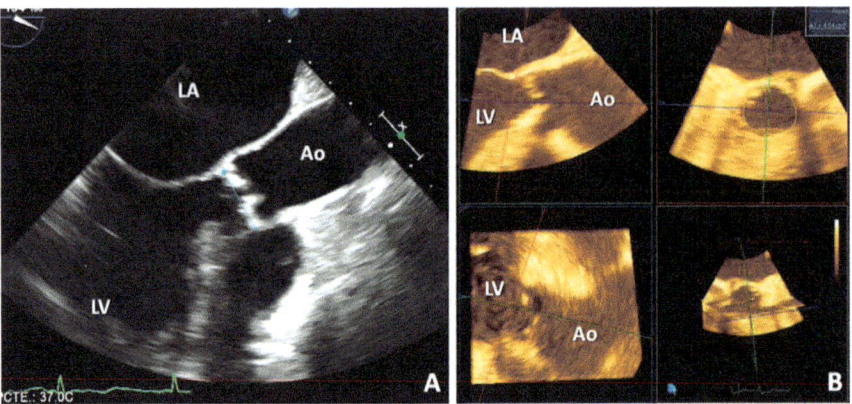

Figure 16.46 (a) Annular sizing with 2D transoesophageal echocardiography; (b) annular sizing with 3D transoesophageal echocardiography with the image aligned in order to avoid oblique measurements. Ao: Aorta; LA: left atrium; LV: left ventricle.

be measured by 3D TEE, although multislice computed tomography (MDCT) is the most accurate method. Moreover, an extended valve calcification may influence the decision of the prosthesis size to a smaller one than the aortic annulus measurement would suggest.

The aortic annular dimension guides the selection of the type and size of the prosthesis. It is measured in the systole long-axis view and corresponds to the distance between the insertion of the non-coronary cusp to the insertion of the right coronary cusp (Figure 16.46a). The evaluation of the aortic annulus with 2D echocardiography presupposes a circular shape, which leads to erroneous measurements in patients with an oval-shaped annulus. 3D TEE has the capability of presenting a real short-axis view of the annulus; consequently, the larger and shorter diameter as well as the planimetry can be performed (Figure 16.46b). However, in spite of the tendency toward underestimation of the aortic annulus when compared with MDCT, 2D TEE measurement has been associated with good clinical results and is now the recommended approach [3].

16.26 Transoesophageal echocardiography during prosthesis implantation

TEE is not mandatory at the time of prosthesis implantation, as it usually requires general anesthesia. However, it is useful to guide balloon valvuloplasty, to confirm prosthesis location and function, and to detect early complications. The aortic rim should be positioned above the native aortic leaflets and below the level of the coronary ostia. An excessively low location may affect the mitral valve (MV) apparatus, causing mitral regurgitation, or destabilize a patient with marked sub aortic septal hypertrophy. If the valve is implanted too high, the risks are migration of the prosthesis, occlusion of the coronary ostia, or significant aortic regurgitation (AR). The latter can occur in consequence of prosthesis incomplete expansion, incorrect positioning, restrict cusp motion, or inappropriate prosthetic size [4]. To estimate AR severity, the guidelines suggest criteria based on the percentage occupied on the left ventricle outflow tract (LVOT) ($\leq 25\%$ mild, 26–64% moderate, $\geq 65\%$ severe) [5]. However, this method presents constrains in eccentric and in paravalvular AR jets, which are the most common after TAVI. 3D TEE can provide additional data for the complete visualization of the paravalvular AR jets and for the assessment of aortic regurgitant volume; however, the best method for accurate quantification is still a matter of debate. An added potential problem that must be considered is the appearance of central AR due to hypotension immediately after the procedure. Patient's hemodynamic stabilization is required before assessing the severity of AR. Moreover, during the procedure, TEE may identify severe life-threatening complications as cardiac tamponade, by right ventricle or left ventricle perforation or new wall motion abnormalities as a result of sudden coronary ostium occlusion [4].

16.27 Percutaneous transcatheter repair of paravalvular regurgitation

Paravalvular dehiscence is a complication occurring after surgical valve replacement as a cause of infection, annular calcification, or friable tissue at the site of suturing or for technical factors. Percutaneous transcatheter repair of paravalvular regurgitation (PVR) is a treatment proposed to patients with high risk for re-operation. It is a technically challenging process in which TEE plays a decisive part for proper diagnosis and procedure guidance.

16.28 TEE before transcatheter repair of paravalvular regurgitation

PVR may be located in aortic or mitral prosthesis and, if hemodynamically significant, it may cause heart failure and/or hemolysis. The assessment of aortic PVR can be performed by transthoracic echocardiography (TTE) and complemented with TEE, but TEE may be less effective for mechanical aortic valves, due to the distortion of the valve plane. Conversely, PVR in the presence of mechanical prosthesis is technically more demanding and limited by artifacts, being TEE mandatory. The area of dehiscence is detected by TEE as an echo drop-out outside the sewing ring, either by 2D or 3D, which must be confirmed by color Doppler (Figure 16.47). The 3D TEE face view/"surgeon view" of the mitral prosthesis, acquired by *3D Zoom*, allows the precise determination of the number and location of the areas of dehiscence, which is essential for procedure planning. It is the preferred imaging modality because of its ability to identify the real shape and the existence of multiple defects and for its facility in

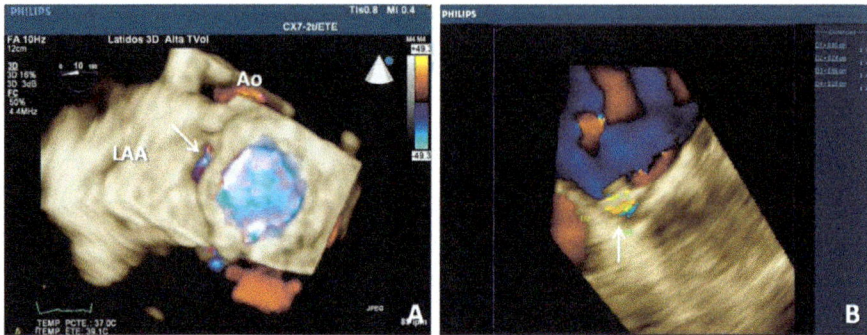

Figure 16.47 3D Transoesophageal echocardiography (*en face* view) showing a paravalvular mitral leak with color-flow imaging confirming the origin of the mitral regurgitation (a). 3D measurements of the paravalvular leak before percutaneous repair (b). AV: aortic valve; LAA: left atrial appendence.

providing sizing estimation through planimetry of the regurgitant orifice. However, for accurate measurements, the resolution may be limited, particularly when the areas of dehiscence are slit-like [2].

When using 2D TEE, the entire sewing ring should be observed, from 0° to 180° and the circumferential extent of the dehiscence may be estimated from the point of first detection, until its disappearance. The transgastric view with color-flow showing the short-axis view of the valve provides a face view of the entire circumference and it is a valuable incidence for proper location of the dehiscence, specially in absence of 3D TEE. The description of the PVR location with the use of main references as aorta and left atrial appendage simplifies communication between the echocardiographer and the interventionist. Additional care must be taken when the defect is larger than 25% of the circumference, as prosthesis rocking may be observed and transcatheter closure should not be performed because of the high risk of device embolization.

Considering aortic prosthetic valves, the location of the coronary arteries must be routinely assessed, as a coronary ostium close to the valve ring may convey a significant technical problem for the leak closure and affect the choice of device [2].

16.29 TEE during percutaneous transcatheter repair of paravalvular regurgitation

When the procedure is performed by antegrade approach, TEE may be used to guide the transseptal puncture. Real-time 3D TEE images are especially useful for the visualization of the wires and catheters extension [6]. This facilitates the assessment of the anatomical relations between the catheter tips and the surrounding anatomical structures. The chosen device is also visualized and its exact location evaluated at time of deployment. At this time, TEE is used for the evaluation of residual PVR and possible device interference with the prosthetic function. Only after these parameters are considered is the device is released and the catheters removed. If significant residual regurgitation persists, an additional device can be contemplated.

16.30 Percutaneous mitral valve intervention by edge-to-edge repair

A variety of approaches can be used for percutaneous valve repair (leaflet repair, direct or indirect annuloplasty, and ventricular remodeling); however, MitraClip™ is the most studied device and the only with CE mark, that has completed pivotal trial evaluation and is available for compassionate use in the United States for patients with either degenerative or functional severe MR.

This method replicates the surgical technique introduced by Alfieri, approximating the middle scallops of the MV and creating a double orifice. It is an alternative solution for patients with severe mitral regurgitation to whom surgery is denied because of excessive surgical risk. TEE is essential for patient selection and for guiding the procedure.

16.31 TEE for patients selection for edge-to-edge repair

The appropriate patients proposed for MitralClip™ closure should present MR 3-4+ with predominant mechanism from the central mitral scallops, A2 and P2 (type II or IIIB of Carpentier classification). Up to now, the guidelines for patient selection reflected the selection criteria used in the two Everest trials [7]. Patients with functional MR, must present a coapting surface length ≥2 mm and a coaptation depth of ≤11 mm, assessed by TEE four-chamber view. In patients with degenerative MR, the maximum acceptable flail height is <10 mm and the flail width <15 mm, measured by TEE aligned to demonstrate the maximal excursion of the flail segment. Patients with rheumatic disease, endocarditis, severe leaflet thickness or calcification, or with MV area of less than 4 cm^2 are excluded from the procedure. 3D TEE approach provides a better visualization of the MV and interpretation of MR mechanism than 2D TEE, by best assessment of the scallops involved, commissures, and chordae anatomy [2].

16.32 TEE during edge-to-edge repair

The MitraClip™ is easily imaged with TEE permitting reliable step-by-step guidance. The procedure starts with *a posterior* and superior transseptal puncture, 3.5–4.0 cm above the leaflets, in order to align the device at the A2P2 interface perpendicular to the commissure. The point for puncturing is chosen by assessing the tenting it creates on the adjacent septum. The best alignment can be achieved by the use of simultaneously displayed biplane imaging or by *Live 3D* mode, using TEE 3D probes. Afterward, the delivery system angles for the mitral leaflets for A2P2 gasping. In degenerative MR, the percutaneous clip has to anchor the flail and/or prolapsed leaflet, whereas in patients with functional

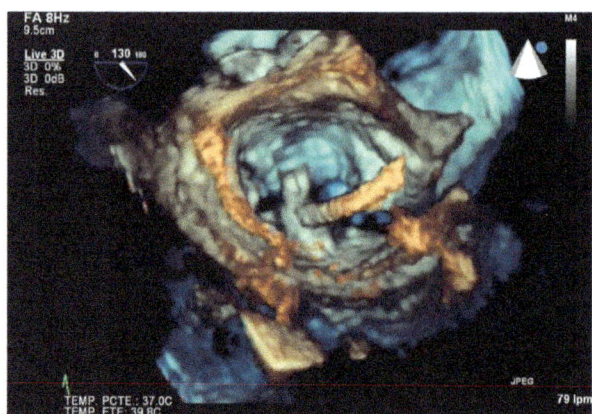

Figure 16.48 3D Transoesophageal echocardiography showing MitralClip™ deployment by face view of the mitral valve.

mitral regurgitation, attaching A2-P2 leaflets improves coaptation and decreases tethering. The correct position can be confirmed from the different 2D TEE views of the MV and preferably by TEE 3D *Zoom* with en face view of the MV, which considerably simplifies this part of the procedure (Figure 16.48). The regurgitant orifice must be identified by the maximal PISA effect and the delivery system positioned above. The clip is oriented perpendicular to the commissure, entering with arms closed through the MV to LV. Afterward, it is pulled back toward the left atrium, simultaneously grasping both leaflets. Then, the capture of both leaflets must be verified and the clip closed. Subsequently, it is fundamental to evaluate the severity of MR and to exclude mitral stenosis by transvalvular continuous wave Doppler and planimetry of both orifices. If MR reduction is reasonable and the degree of stenosis is acceptable (mean gradient ≤ 5 mmHg), the clip may be fully deployed. If significant MR persists, an additional clip may be needed [8]. Using 3D TEE, it is possible to view the repaired valve en face from both atrial and ventricular perspectives, documenting the eventual eccentricity of the dual orifices created by the device.

During the procedure TEE may detect potential complications, including perforation of the atrial wall, partial detachment of the clip and leaflet, or chordal tears caused by repeated attempts to leaflets grasping [8].

16.33 Conclusion

Echocardiography has become an essential tool for new valvular invasive procedure guidance in this new era of minimal invasive therapies. The new advances of the echocardiography as 3D capabilities have improved the understanding of heart interventions through real-time visualization for the heart team. This concept seems to be the key for the success of procedures.

References

[1] Smith CR, Leon MB, Mack MJ, et al. Transcatheter versus surgical aortic-valve replacement in high-risk patients. N Engl J Med 2011;364(23):2187–98.
[2] Zamorano JL, Badano LP, Bruce C, et al. EAE/ASE recommendations for the use of echocardiography in new transcatheter interventions for valvular heart disease. Eur Heart J Sep 2011;32(17):2189–214.
[3] Messika-Zeitoun D, Serfaty JM, Brochet E, et al. Multimodal assessment of the aortic annulus diameter: implications for transcatheter aortic valve implantation. J Am Coll Cardiol 2010;55(3):186–94.
[4] Goncalves A, Marcos-Alberca P, Zamorano JL. Echocardiography: guidance during valve implantation. EuroIntervention 2010;6(Suppl G):G14–9.
[5] Zoghbi WA, Chambers JB, Dumesnil JG, et al. Recommendations for evaluation of prosthetic valves with echocardiography and Doppler ultrasound: a report From the American Society of Echocardiography's Guidelines and Standards Committee and the Task Force on Prosthetic Valves, developed in conjunction with the American College of Cardiology Cardiovascular Imaging Committee, Cardiac Imaging Committee of the American Heart Association, the European Association of Echocardiography, a registered branch of the European Society of Cardiology, the Japanese Society of Echocardiography and the Canadian Society of Echocardiography, endorsed by the American College of Cardiology Foundation, American Heart Association, European Association of Echocardiography, a registered branch of the European Society of Cardiology, the Japanese Society of Echocardiography, and Canadian Society of Echocardiography. J Am Soc Echocardiogr 2009;22(9):975–1014, quiz 1082–1014.
[6] Becerra JM, Almeria C, de Isla LP, Zamorano J. Usefulness of 3D transoesophageal echocardiography for guiding wires and closure devices in mitral perivalvular leaks. Eur J Echocardiogr Dec 2009;10(8):979–81.
[7] Feldman T, Foster E, Glower DD, et al. Percutaneous repair or surgery for mitral regurgitation. N Engl J Med 2011;364(15):1395–406.
[8] Franzen O, Baldus S, Rudolph V, et al. Acute outcomes of MitraClip therapy for mitral regurgitation in high-surgical-risk patients: emphasis on adverse valve morphology and severe left ventricular dysfunction. Eur Heart J Jun 2010;31(11):1373–81.

Endocarditis

G. Habib, S. Camilleri, J.-Y. Gaubert
Hôpital de la Timone, Marseille, France

16.34 Introduction

Infective endocarditis (IE) is a life-threatening disease associated with a high mortality rate, difficult diagnosis, and controversial management [1,2]. Several complications may occur, causing high morbidity and mortality [3], and justifying early surgery in more than half of the patients [4].

Imaging is of major value in the assessment of IE. If echocardiography, particularly transesophageal echocardiography (TEE), is still the first-line evaluation, other imaging techniques, including magnetic resonance imaging (MRI), multislice computed tomography (MSCT), and nuclear imaging, are also useful in the diagnosis and management of endocarditis [5].

16.35 Echocardiography

Recent guidelines [6,7] emphasized the value and limitations of echocardiography in IE and gave recommendations for the optimal use of both transthoracic echocardiography (TTE) and TEE in IE. Echocardiography is useful for the diagnosis of endocarditis, the assessment of the severity of the disease, the prediction of short-term and long-term prognosis, the prediction of embolic risk, the management of its complications, and the follow-up of patients under therapy.

16.35.1 Diagnostic value of echocardiography

Echocardiography is the method of choice for the diagnosis of the two major criteria of IE, that is, vegetation and abscess [8]. Vegetation usually presents as an oscillating mass attached to a valvular structure (Figure 16.49), with a sensitivity of 75% for TTE and 85–90% for TEE [7]. However, atypical findings are frequent, and echocardiography may be falsely negative in about 15% of IE [9], particularly in cases of pre-existing severe lesions (mitral valve prolapse, degenerative lesions, and prosthetic valves), and echocardiography must be repeated 7–10 days after the first examination when the clinical level of suspicion is still high [6].

Abscesses typically present as perivalvular zones of reduced echo density, without color flow detected inside (Figure 16.50), and this condition may be complicated by pseudoaneurysm or fistulization [10]. The sensitivity of TTE is about 50%, and that of TEE 90%. Diagnosis of an abscess may be difficult in case of a small abscess, in the

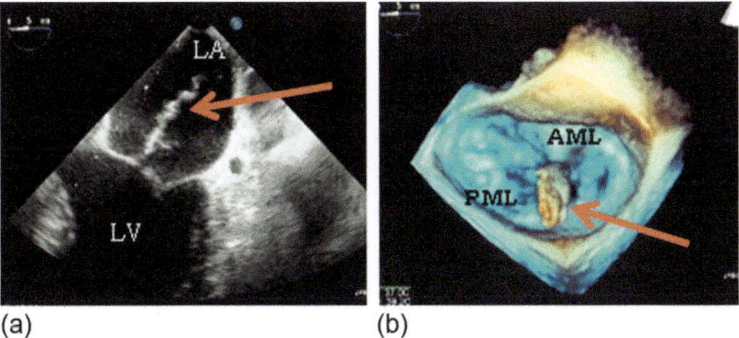

Figure 16.49 Mitral valve endocarditis. Mitral valve infective endocarditis with a huge vegetation attached to the anterior mitral leaflet (arrows) by 2D-TEE (a) and 3D-TEE (b). LA: left atrium, LV: left ventricle, AML: anterior mitral leaflet, PML: posterior mitral leaflet.

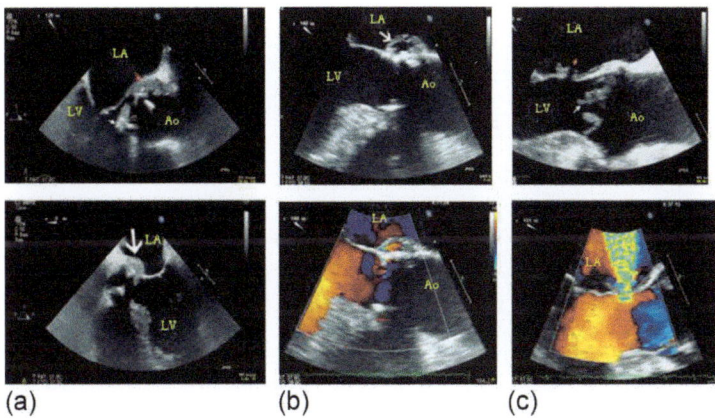

Figure 16.50 Perivalvular lesions in infective endocarditis. Role of TEE: (a) Abscess: Thickened nonhomogeneous perivalvular area with echodense or echolucent aspect. (b) Pseudo-aneurysm: Pulsatile perivalvular echo-free space with color-Doppler flow detected. (c) Mitral aneurysm with anterior mitral valve perforation into the left atrium. LA: left atrium, LV: left ventricle, Ao: aorta.

presence of prosthetic material, and in patients who have an abscess localized around calcification in the posterior mitral annulus [7].

Other echocardiographic features suggestive of IE include valve destruction and prolapse as well as aneurysm and/or perforation of a valve (Figure 16.51).

Figure 16.52 summarizes the respective indications of TTE and TEE in IE as proposed by the European Society of Cardiology (ESC) recommendations. Finally, 3D echocardiography gives additional information about the extent of valvular and perivalvular lesions and appears useful for the assessment of patients who have IE (Figures 16.49, 16.51, and 16.53).

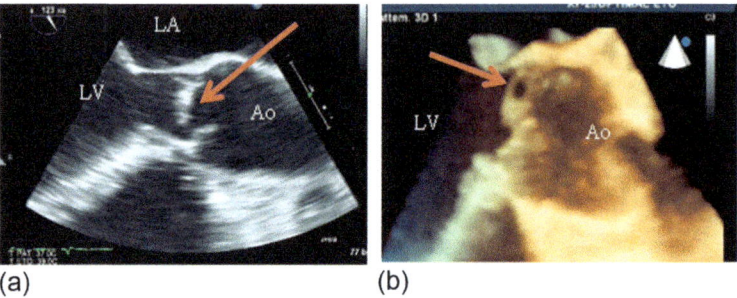

Figure 16.51 Aortic valve infective endocarditis. Case illustrating the additional role of 3D TEE: (a) 2D TEE showing a prolapse of the left coronary aortic leaflet. (b) 3D TEE: long-axis view revealing a perforation of the left coronary aortic leaflet (arrows). LA: left atrium, LV: left ventricle, Ao: aorta.

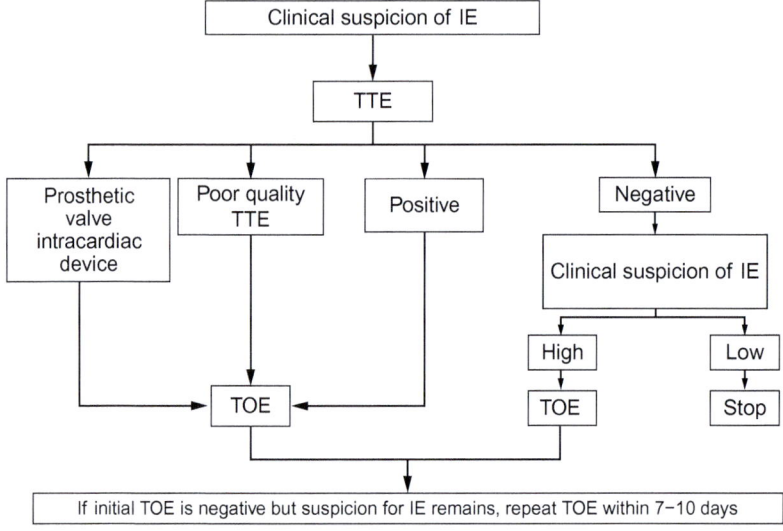

Figure 16.52 Algorithm showing the role of echocardiography in the diagnosis and assessment of IE (adapted from reference [6]). IE: infective endocarditis, TTE: transthoracic echocardiography, TEE: transesophageal echocardiography.

16.35.2 Prognostic value of echocardiography

Echocardiography also plays an important role both in the short-term and the long-term prognostic assessment of patients who have IE [11], for the decision to operate or not and for the choice of the optimal time of the surgery [6]. Several echocardiographic features have been associated with a worse prognosis, including periannular complications, severe valve regurgitation or obstruction, low LV ejection fraction, pulmonary hypertension, and premature mitral valve closure [12]. The presence of vegetation, its size, and its multivalvular location have been associated with a worse prognosis. In a recent series [13], large vegetations (>15 mm length) were associated with a worse prognosis.

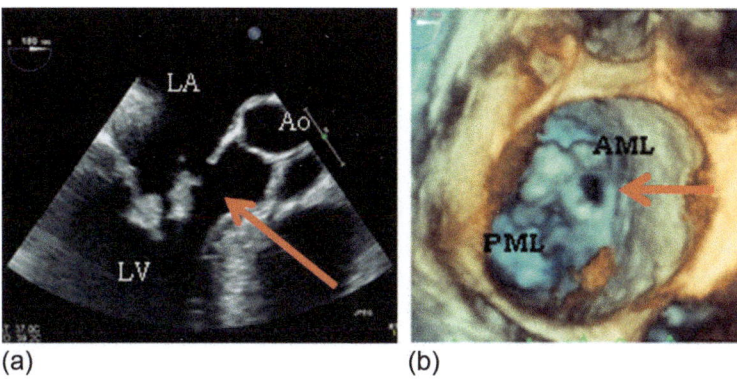

Figure 16.53 Mitral valve infective endocarditis with a large vegetation and mitral perforation (arrows) by 2D TEE (a) and 3D TEE (b). LA: left atrium, LV: left ventricle, Ao: aorta, AML: anterior mitral leaflet, PML: posterior mitral leaflet.

Embolic events are a frequent and life-threatening complication of IE, and they are associated with increased morbidity and mortality [14]. Echocardiography plays a key role in predicting embolic events. Several factors have been associated with an increased risk of embolism [1]. We recently found that six variables were associated with the risk of embolism, including age, diabetes, atrial fibrillation, embolism before antibiotics, vegetation length, and *Staphylococcus aureus* infection [15]. Among them, the size and mobility of the vegetations are the most potent independent predictors of new embolic event in patients who have IE [13–17]. In summary, a careful measurement of the maximal vegetation size is crucial in IE because this parameter is clearly related to the risk of a new embolic event. A recent randomized trial demonstrated that early surgery in patients who have large vegetations significantly reduced the risk of death and embolic events as compared with conventional therapy [18]. The ESC guidelines [6] recommend surgical therapy in case of large (>10 mm) vegetations following one or more embolic episodes, as well as when the large vegetation is associated with other predictors of a complicated course.

Finally, echocardiography is also useful during surgery to assess the immediate operative result [19] and, after surgery, for the subsequent follow-up of these patients.

16.36 Molecular imaging

The clinical performance of the Duke criteria to establish the diagnosis of infective endocarditis (IE) can be improved through functional imaging procedures such as metabolic imaging from FDG-PET [20–22] or ^{99m}Tc-HMPAO-labeled leukocyte SPECT/CT [22]. FDG-PET has become an established diagnostic tool in oncology, and evidence is also increasing regarding its value for assessing infectious and inflammatory diseases. FDG uptake in infection is based on the fact that mononuclear cells and granulocytes use large quantities of glucose by way of the hexose monophosphate shunts.

Using ^{18}F-FDG, a PET-CT imaging scan can be obtained within 1 h of injection. SPECT/CT-^{99m}Tc-HMPAO-labeled leukocyte imaging uses more acquisition time with whole-body and planar spot 30 mn post-injection time of 4–6 h (early imaging) and 20–24 h (delayed imaging) [22]. ^{18}F-FDG PET-CT is the most promising approach for the diagnosis of IE. Recent case reports first observed that this technique would be useful for the diagnosis of pacemaker and prosthetic valve IE [23–25]. More recently, we found PET-CT was particularly useful for the diagnosis of prosthetic valve IE [26]. In 76 consecutive patients suspected of having PVE [26], the sensitivity, specificity, positive predictive value (PPV), negative predictive value (NPV), and global accuracy of ^{18}F-FDG PET/CT were 76%, 80%, 86%, 67%, and 77%, respectively. Adding abnormal FDG uptake as a new major criterion significantly increased the sensitivity of the modified Duke criteria at admission (70% vs. 97%, $p=0.004$), without a significant decrease in specificity. The results of this study support the addition of abnormal FDG uptake as a novel major criterion for PVE (Figure 16.54).

In addition, ^{18}F-FDG PET/CT can detect hypermetabolic activity in peripheral embolic sites and metastatic infections, having a potential role in the discovery of neoplastic lesions as colonic tumors, which may cause IE (Figure 16.55). Splenic or osteomedullar diffuse hyperactivity may also be observed in relation with the septic status of the patient.

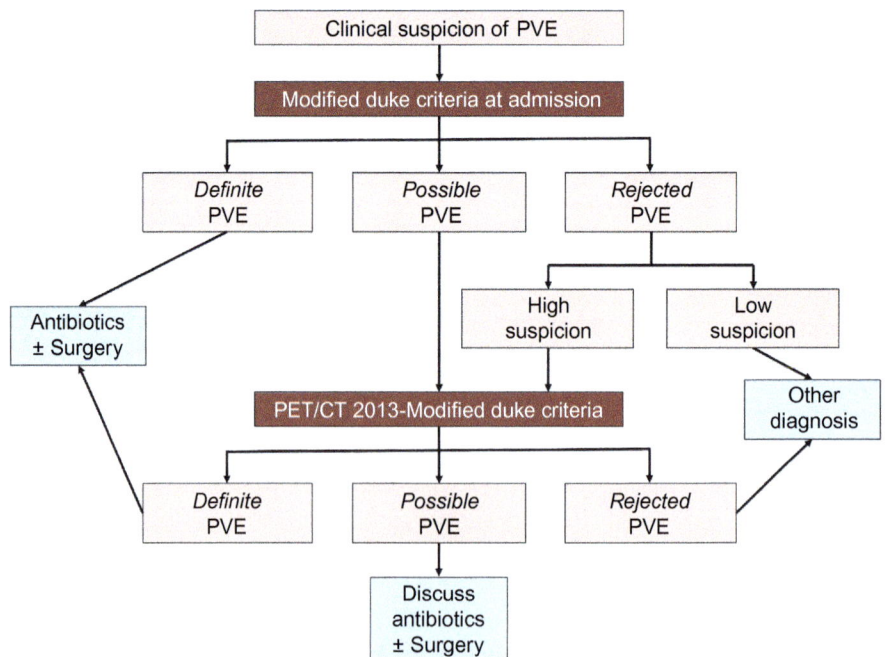

Figure 16.54 Proposed algorithm for evaluating patients with suspected PVE. From reference [26], with permission.

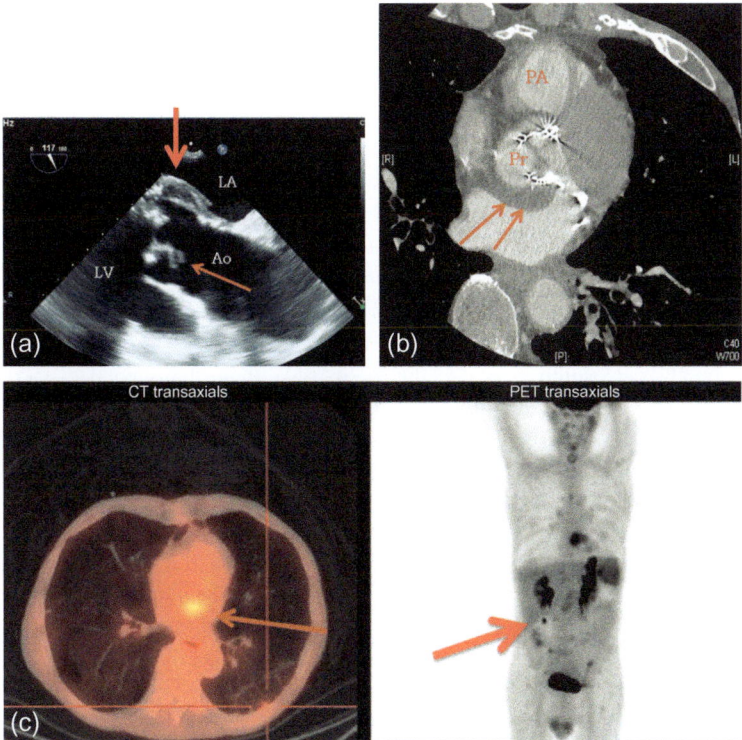

Figure 16.55 Multimodality imaging in a patient with bioprosthetic aortic valve endocarditis. (a) TEE: small vegetation (thin arrow) and posterior abscess (thick arrow) on the bioprosthetic leaflet. (b) CT scan: posterior abscess behind the aorta (arrows). (c) ^{18}F-fluorodeoxyglucose positron emission tomography-computed tomography showing intensive uptake on both the bioprosthesis (thin arrow) and the abdominal area (thick arrow), revealing a colonic tumor. LA: left atrium, LV: left ventricle, Ao: aorta, Pr: prosthesis, PA: pulmonary artery.

However, PET/CT may be limited by its low availability, the need for rigorous patient preparation, and its limited value in patients who have native valve endocarditis and during the immediate postoperative period [22]. The value of 99mTc-HMPAO-labeled leukocyte SPECT/CT in this setting needs to be assessed by further studies.

16.37 Multislice computed tomography

Although echocardiography remains the first-line examination in clinically suspected IE, ECG-gated MSCT has proved to be a reliable tool in cardiac imaging. Besides the evaluation of coronary arteries, some studies reported the ability of MSCT to analyze valvular diseases such as aortic valve stenosis [27] and, more recently, IE [28,29].

These new indications of cardiac MSCT are based on major recent advances in temporal resolution combined with high spatial resolution.

In a series of 37 patients, Feuchtner et al. compared results of MSCT to TEE and surgery [28], and they observed convincing results in the detection of valvular lesions and perivalvular damage related to IE with MSCT. In a per-patient based analysis, sensitivity and specificity were 97% and 88%, respectively, with a PPV and a NPV of 97% and 88%, respectively. No significant difference was found when MSCT results were compared to TEE. MSCT provided more precise anatomic evaluation of the extent of perivalvular damage (abscess or pseudoaneurysms) than TEE, but some small leaflet perforations were not detected. Gahide et al. reported similar results in patients who have aortic valve IE [30].

More recently, Fagman et al. conducted a study in 27 patients who have aortic prosthetic valve IE. They compared MSCT results to TEE and found a good strength of agreement for the diagnosis of abscess or dehiscence; it was moderate for the diagnosis of vegetation. When compared with operative data, MSCT identified three more pseudoaneurysms that were not detected by TEE. Two of the three were located close to the right coronary cusp, an anatomic topography difficult to investigate with TEE [29]. Other reports confirm that MSCT is accurate in describing perivalvular abnormalities related to IE (Figure 16.55) [31,32].

In addition to its value in demonstrating cardiac endocarditic damage, MSCT provides a fast and high-resolution examination of extra-cardiac organs. It can be used as a "one-shot" evaluation in patients who have proved or highly suspected IE to diagnose cardiac lesions and distant complications such as embolic events, hemorrhagic and septic complications, and infectious aneurysms. All these findings can induce a modification of the therapeutic strategy. In patients referred for surgery, MSCT offers a safe and accurate evaluation of the coronary arteries [28], especially in patients who have aortic valve vegetations, which represent a real risk of embolic event after coronary catheterization.

To evaluate patients referred for clinically suspected IE, MSCT should be used when echocardiography is negative or inconclusive. However, MSCT requires iodine contrast injection and therefore needs careful pre-procedure evaluation in patients presenting with renal insufficiency or hemodynamic impairment, especially when they are treated with nephrotoxic antibiotics [33]. In the near future, routine use of MSCT in IE will require the definition of dedicated specific recommendations.

16.38 Magnetic resonance imaging

Although less frequently used in IE, MRI, as a non-ionizing imaging technique, is particularly useful for the diagnosis and management of cerebral complications of IE. MRI may be used in cases of suspected arterial mycotic aneurysm and is particularly useful for the identification of silent cerebral complications of IE. Recent studies found that systematic MRI could detect subclinical cerebrovascular complications in about 50% of patients who have IE [34–36], that MRI improves the diagnosis of IE, and that MRI may affect therapeutic strategies.

16.39 Conclusion

Imaging plays a key role in IE, in its diagnosis, the diagnosis of its complications, its follow-up under therapy, and its prognostic assessment. Echocardiography is particularly useful for the initial assessment of embolic risk and in decision making in IE. TEE plays a major role both before surgery and during surgery (intraoperative echocardiography). Other imaging techniques are complementary with echocardiography for the evaluation of patients who have IE. Among them, FDG PET/CT imaging seems the most promising new imaging technique, particularly for the diagnosis of prosthetic valve endocarditis. Finally, echocardiography and other imaging techniques must not be considered as competitive but rather as complementary. All these techniques can be used in patients who have suspected or confirmed PVE, depending on the clinical presentation and on the results of initial echographic evaluation, in the new era of multimodality imaging.

References

[1] Habib G. Embolic risk in subacute bacterial endocarditis: role of transesophageal echocardiography. Curr Cardiol Rep 2003;5:129–36.
[2] Hoen B, Alla F, Selton-Suty C, Beguinot I, Bouvet A, Briancon S, et al. Changing profile of infective endocarditis: results of a 1-year survey in France. JAMA 2002;288:75–81.
[3] Hasbun R, Vikram HR, Barakat LA, Buenconsejo J, Quagliarello VJ. Complicated left-sided native valve endocarditis in adults: risk classification for mortality. JAMA 2003;289(15):1933–40.
[4] Tornos P, Iung B, Permanyer-Miralda G, Baron G, Delahaye F, Gohlke-Barwolf C, et al. Infective endocarditis in Europe: lessons from the Euro heart survey. Heart 2005;91:571–5.
[5] Bruun NE, Habib G, Thuny F, Sogaard P. Cardiac imaging in infectious endocarditis. Eur Heart J. 2014;35:624–32.
[6] Habib G, Hoen B, Tornos P, Thuny F, Prendergast B, Vilacosta I, et al. Guidelines on the prevention, diagnosis, and treatment of infective endocarditis (new version 2009): The Task Force on the Prevention, Diagnosis, and Treatment of Infective Endocarditis of the European Society of Cardiology (ESC). Eur Heart J 2009;30:2369–413.
[7] Habib G, Badano L, Tribouilloy C, Vilacosta I, Zamorano JL, Galderisi M, et al. Recommendations for the practice of echocardiography in infective endocarditis. Eur J Echocardiogr 2010;11:202–19.
[8] Durack DT, Lukes AS, Bright DK. New criteria for diagnosis of infective endocarditis: utilization of specific echocardiographic findings. Duke Endocarditis Service. Am J Med 1994;96:200–9.
[9] Habib G, Derumeaux G, Avierinos JF, Casalta JP, Jamal F, Volot F, et al. Value and limitations of the Duke criteria for the diagnosis of infective endocarditis. J Am Coll Cardiol 1999;33(7):2023–9.
[10] Karalis DG, Bansal RC, Hauck AJ, Ross Jr. JJ, Applegate PM, Jutzy KR, et al. Transesophageal echocardiographic recognition of subaortic complications in aortic valve endocarditis. Clinical and surgical implications. Circulation 1992;86:353–62.
[11] San Román JA, López J, Vilacosta I, Luaces M, Sarriá C, Revilla A, et al. Prognostic stratification of patients with left-sided endocarditis determined at admission. Am J Med 2007;120(4):369.e1–7.

[12] San Roman JA, Lopez J, Vilacosta I, Luaces M, Sarria C, Revilla A, et al. Prognostic stratification of patients with left-sided endocarditis determined at admission. Am J Med 2007;120:369.e1–7.
[13] Thuny F, Di Salvo G, Belliard O, Avierinos JF, Pergola V, Rosenberg V, et al. Risk of embolism and death in infective endocarditis: prognostic value of echocardiography: a prospective multicenter study. Circulation 2005;112:69–75.
[14] Di Salvo G, Habib G, Pergola V, Avierinos JF, Philip E, Casalta JP, et al. Echocardiography predicts embolic events in infective endocarditis. J Am Coll Cardiol 2001;37:1069–76.
[15] Hubert S, Thuny F, Resseguier N, Giorgi R, Tribouilloy C, Le Dolley Y, et al. Prediction of symptomatic embolism in infective endocarditis: construction and validation of a risk calculator in a multicenter cohort. J Am Coll Cardiol 2013;62:1384–92.
[16] Steckelberg JM, Murphy JG, Ballard D, Bailey K, Tajik AJ, Taliercio CP, et al. Emboli in infective endocarditis: the prognostic value of echocardiography. Ann Intern Med 1991;114:635–40.
[17] Vilacosta I, Graupner C, San Roman JA, Sarria C, Ronderos R, Fernandez C, et al. Risk of embolization after institution of antibiotic therapy for infective endocarditis. J Am Coll Cardiol 2002;39:1489–95.
[18] Kang D-H, Kim Y-J, Kim S-H, Sun BJ, Kim D-H, Yun S-C, et al. Early surgery versus conventional treatment for infective endocarditis. N Engl J Med 2012;366(26):2466–73.
[19] Shapira Y, Weisenberg DE, Vaturi M, Sharoni E, Raanani E, Sahar G, et al. The impact of intraoperative transesophageal echocardiography in infective endocarditis. Isr Med Assoc J 2007;9:299–302.
[20] Erba PA, Sollini M, Lazzeri E, Mariani G. FDG-PET in cardiac infections. Semin Nucl Med 2013;43:377–95.
[21] Bensimhon L, Lavergne T, Hugonnet F, et al. Whole body [(18) F]fluorodeoxyglucose positron emission tomography imaging for the diagnosis of pacemaker or implantable cardioverter defibrillator infection: a preliminary prospective study. Clin Microbiol Infect 2010;17:836–44.
[22] Erba PA, Conti U, Lazzeri E, Sollini M, Doria R, De Tommasi SM, et al. Added value of ^{99m}Tc-HMPAO-labeled leukocyte SPECT/CT in the characterization and management of patients with infectious endocarditis. J Nucl Med 2012;53(8):1235–43.
[23] Bertagna F, Bisleri G, Motta F, et al. Possible role of F18-FDG-PET/CT in the diagnosis of endocarditis: preliminary evidence from a review of the literature. Int J Cardiovasc Imaging 2012;28:1417–25.
[24] Cautela J, Alessandrini S, Cammilleri S, Giorgi R, Richet H, Casalta JP, et al. Diagnostic yield of FDG positron-emission tomography/computed tomography in patients with CEID infection: a pilot study. Europace 2013;15(2):252–7.
[25] Saby L, Le Dolley Y, Laas O, et al. Early diagnosis of abscess in aortic bioprosthetic valve by 18F-fluorodeoxyglucose positron emission tomography-computed tomography. Circulation 2012;126:e217–20.
[26] Saby L, Laas O, Habib G, et al. Positron emission tomography-computed tomography for diagnosis of prosthetic valve endocarditis: increased valvular (18)F-fluorodeoxyglucose uptake as a novel major criterion. J Am Coll Cardiol 2013;61:2374–82.
[27] Piazza N, Lange R, Martucci G, Serruys PW. Patient selection for transcatheter aortic valve implantation: patient risk profile and anatomical selection criteria. Arch Cardiovasc Dis 2012;105:165–73.

[28] Feuchtner GM, Stolzmann P, Dichtl W, et al. Multislice computed tomography in infective endocarditis: comparison with transesophageal echocardiography and intraoperative findings. J Am Coll Cardiol 2009;53:436–44.
[29] Fagman E, Perrotta S, Bech-Hanssen O, et al. ECG-gated computed tomography: a new role for patients with suspected aortic prosthetic valve endocarditis. Eur Radiol 2012;22:2407–14.
[30] Gahide G, Bommart S, Demaria R, et al. Preoperative evaluation in aortic endocarditis: findings on cardiac CT. AJR Am J Roentgeno 2010;194:574–8.
[31] Matsuo Y, Kimura F, Inoue K, Ogawa H, Tabata M, Uwabe K, et al. Evaluation of perivalvular infectious ventricular pseudoaneurysm by ECG-gated cardiac computed tomography: 2 case reports. J Thorac Imaging 2012;27(6):165–7.
[32] Budde RP, Kluin J, Symersky P, Chamuleau SA, van Herwerden LA, Prokop M. Visualization by 256-slice computed tomography of mycotic aortic root aneurysms in infective endocarditis. J Heart Valve Dis 2010;19(5):623–5.
[33] Thuny F, Gaubert JY, Jacquier A, Tessonnier L, Cammilleri S, Raoult D, et al. Imaging investigations in infective endocarditis: current approach and perspectives. Arch Cardiovasc Dis 2013;106(1):52–62.
[34] Cooper HA, Thompson EC, Laureno R, et al. Subclinical brain embolization in left-sided infective endocarditis: results from the evaluation by MRI of the brains of patients with left-sided intracardiac solid masses (EMBOLISM) pilot study. Circulation 2009;120:585–91.
[35] Duval X, Iung B, Klein I, et al. Effect of early cerebral magnetic resonance imaging on clinical decisions in infective endocarditis: a prospective study. Ann Intern Med 2010;152:497–504.
[36] Snygg-Martin U, Gustafsson L, Rosengren L, et al. Cerebrovascular complications in patients with left-sided infective endocarditis are common: a prospective study using magnetic resonance imaging and neurochemical brain damage markers. Clin Infect Dis 2008;47:23–30.

Cardiac tumours

17

J.P. Greenwood*, M. Motwani*, A.M. Crean†
*University of Leeds, Leeds, UK; †Peter Munk Cardiac Centre, Toronto, ON, Canada

17.1 Introduction

Cardiac tumours are a rare finding, with an autopsy prevalence of less than 0.5% [1,2]. However, even when pathologically benign, they can fatally compromise cardiac haemodynamics or lead to serious complications such as embolism or arrhythmia [3]. Approximately 75% of all primary cardiac tumours are benign, and the most common in adults are myxomas (50%), papillary elastomas (20%), lipomas (15–20%), and haemangiomas (5%) [4,5]. The remaining 25% of primary cardiac tumours are malignant; ~95% of these are sarcomas and ~5% are lymphomas (Table 17.1 and Figure 17.1) [5,7]. Secondary cardiac tumours, i.e. metastases, are 20–40 times more common than primary cardiac tumours [3,8]. However, the differential diagnosis for a cardiac mass extends beyond cardiac tumours, and more common diagnoses are intra-cardiac thrombus or misinterpreted normal anatomical variants [9]. Multimodality knowledge regarding the imaging features of cardiac neoplasms and other masses is therefore important for establishing an accurate diagnosis, avoiding misinterpretation of normal variants and for guiding treatment and staging in confirmed tumours. In this chapter, we review the role of echocardiography, cardiovascular magnetic resonance (CMR), cardiac computed tomography (CCT), and nuclear imaging techniques in the assessment of a suspected cardiac mass.

17.2 Echocardiography

Transthoracic echocardiography (TTE) is the most readily available noninvasive imaging technique and thus remains the first-line diagnostic test when a cardiac tumour is suspected (Figure 17.2). Moreover, many cardiac masses are detected incidentally during routine echocardiographic studies for other indications. In many cases, echocardiography demonstrates characteristic anatomical and functional features that already permit a differential diagnosis of a cardiac mass. 3D echocardiography has further enhanced the role of echocardiography in the assessment of cardiac masses particularly in terms of anatomical location, morphology, and functional impact [10,11] (see Chapter 2).

Although the widespread availability of echocardiography is a major advantage, there are also several limitations, including operator dependence/experience, a restricted field of view (particularly in patients with pulmonary disease or a large body habitus), and limited imaging of the right heart and mediastinal structures.

Table 17.1 **Approximate relative incidence of primary cardiac tumours**

Benign		Malignant	
Myxoma	30%	Angiosarcoma	9%
Lipoma	10%	Rhabdomyosarcoma	6%
Fibroelastoma	10%	Mesothelioma	4%
Rhabdomyoma	8%	Fibrosarcoma	3%
Fibroma	4%	Lymphoma	2%
Hemangioma	3%	Other sarcomas	3%
Teratoma	3%	Teratoma	<1%
Others	5%	Others	<1%
Total	70–75%	Total	25–30%

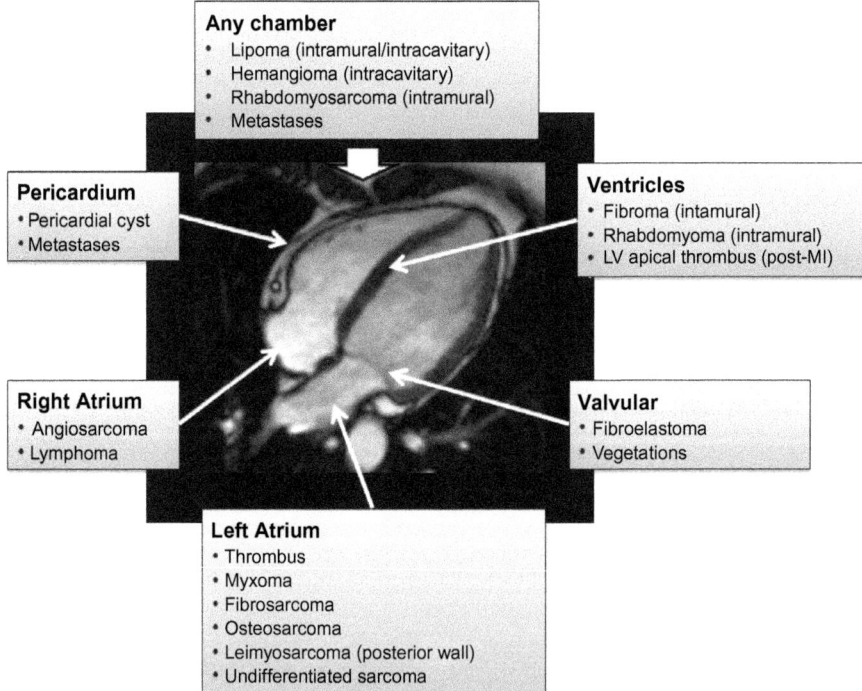

Figure 17.1 The Typical Location of Common Cardiac Masses. The typical locations of the most common masses are illustrated. Please note, however, that the location of the various pathologies can vary and many cardiac tumours can occur in any chamber.
Reproduced with permission from Motwani et al. [6].

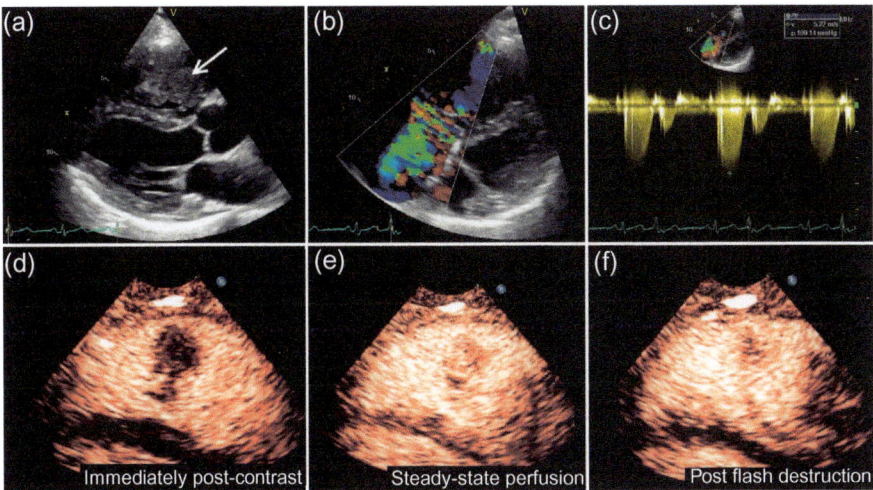

Figure 17.2 Right Ventricular Mass assessed with Echocardiography. A 40-year-old female presented with signs of right-sided heart failure. Transthoracic echocardiography showed a large, mobile, irregular mass within the RV chamber which prolapsed into the right atrium (a). The tricuspid valve was disrupted and there was severe tricuspid regurgitation seen on colour flow (b) and continuous wave Doppler (c). This case illustrates the ability of echocardiography to readily identify a cardiac mass and its functional consequences. Although tissue characterisation is generally best assessed with CMR, contrast echocardiography with power modulation imaging can also be used to assess vascularity (dependent on local expertise) (d–f): Panel D shows intravenous contrast agent (microbubbles) outlining the mass in the RV soon after administration; Panel E shows contrast uptake in the myocardium (steady-state perfusion) and in the RV mass suggesting it has high vascularity; Panel F shows that after a high-power impulse is used to destroy the contrast bubbles, there is early replenishment within the mass even before the septal myocardium, confirming significant vascularity. A large intravascular mass extending from the pelvic veins and inferior vena cava was found at surgery. Histopathology confirmed a rare case of intravascular leiomyoma.

Although TTE is usually sufficient to identify a cardiac mass, transoesophageal echocardiography (TOE) can sometimes be more informative due to the higher spatial resolution afforded by high-frequency transducers, better acoustic windows, and the feasibility of additional imaging planes. Whilst some tissue characterisation is possible with echocardiography (particularly assessment of calcification) and some masses show specific echogenic properties, it is generally limited outside of advanced research techniques such as ultrasonic back scatter, strain rate analysis, or contrast-enhanced power modulation for perfusion imaging (Figure 17.2) [12–14] (see Chapter 2).

17.3 Cardiovascular magnetic resonance

Whilst most cardiac masses are first detected by echocardiography, patients commonly undergo further advanced cross-sectional imaging with either CMR or CCT to characterise the lesion and inform management [6,12,15,16]. In this context, CMR is particularly attractive because it offers a multi-plane assessment, high spatial resolution, and an unrestricted field of view, without the use of ionising radiation [17–19]. This usually allows a definitive anatomical assessment of lesion size, location, functional impact, and relationship to other cardiac structures, which is vital for any proposed surgical intervention or biopsy. Furthermore, CMR has the unique ability to characterise the tissue composition of a mass based on differing signal patterns with T1- and T2-weighted techniques according to relative water and fat content of the tissue [12,20,21]. Neoplastic cells tend to be larger than normal cells and contain more free intracellular water; in addition, they are usually associated with an inflammatory reaction and more interstitial fluid. As a result, malignant tissue has higher free water content than normal tissue and thus longer T1/T2 relaxation times, creating an inherent signal intensity difference between tumours and normal tissue [16,22]. Differences between the individual T1 and T2 signal patterns which depend on the exact tissue composition are exploited for further tissue characterisation. With contrast-enhanced pulse sequences, additional tissue properties such as vascularity and fibrosis can also be demonstrated [23–25] (Table 17.2).

CMR tissue characterisation can be used to predict the likelihood of malignancy of a cardiac mass [20,24] (Table 17.3). Hoffman et al. used a multi-parametric CMR imaging protocol to evaluate the signal properties, morphological characteristics (location, size, infiltrative nature, presence of pleural/pericardial effusions) and contrast enhancement of cardiac tumours in 55 patients [24]. An overall interpretation of the CMR imaging features was found to have a diagnostic accuracy of 0.92 (area under the curve) for predicting the histological malignancy of a cardiac mass.

In general, lesions are identified and localised with a black-blood (BB) T1-weighted (T1w) transaxial stack covering the entire thorax, and then further examined with cine imaging in multiple planes for morphology and functional consequences such as contractile impairment or obstruction to flow [26] (Figure 17.3). Myocardial tissue tagging (see Chapter 6) can sometimes be useful to detect more subtle regions of contractile dysfunction due to tissue infiltration (Figure 17.3) or for assessing pericardial involvement. Further tissue characterisation is then possible with a number of different pulse sequence acquisitions as described below.

In recognition of its diagnostic capabilities, several consensus statements now position CMR imaging as the primary imaging technique in the work-up of cardiac tumours [19,27]. More realistically, the conjugate use of echocardiography and CMR provides a pathway for rapid initial diagnosis (TTE or TOE), subsequent detailed assessment (CMR), and the option of surveillance with either modality.

Table 17.2 CMR tissue characteristics of common cardiac masses

Cardiac mass	T1-w imaging[a]	T2-w imaging[a]	Post-contrast (LGE)
Pseudotumours			
Thrombus	Low (high if recent)	Low (high if recent)	No uptake[b]
Pericardial cyst	Low	High	No uptake
Benign			
Myxoma	Isointense	High	Heterogeneous
Lipoma	High[c]	High[c]	No uptake
Fibroma	Isointense	Low	Hyperenhancement [d]
Rhabdomyoma	Isointense	Isointense/high	No/minimal uptake
Malignant			
Angiosarcoma	Heterogenous	Heterogenous	Heterogeneous
Rhabdomyosarcoma	Isointense	Hyperintense	Homogeneous
Undifferentiated sarcoma	Isointense	Hyperintense	Heterogeneous/Variable
Lymphoma	Isointense	Isointense	No/minimal uptake
Metastasis[e]	Low	High	Heterogeneous

Note: Typical characteristics are presented in table, but all tumours can have atypical appearances due to altered tissue composition. T1-w = T1-weighted; T2-w = T2-weighted; LGE = late gadolinium enhancement.
[a]T1-w and T2-w imaging signal is given relative to myocardium.
[b]Best seen on early gadolinium enhancement imaging (no uptake) 2 min after contrast (Figure 17.1).
[c]Similar to surrounding fat signal and characterized by marked suppression with fat-saturation pre-pulse.
[d]However, fibromas are non-enhancing on perfusion-imaging due to avascularity.
[e]The exception is metastatic melanoma which has a high T1-w and a low T2-w signal.
Reproduced with permission from Motwani et al. [6].

Table 17.3 Imaging features suggestive of malignancy

Tumour location and morphology
Large size – especially if >5 cm
Irregular, ill-defined borders
Direct invasion through tissue planes
Most cardiac tumours involving the right heart are suspicious for malignancy
Pericardial or pleural involvement – effusions and nodular masses
Multiple lesions
Tissue characterisation with CMR – features suggestive of malignancy
Tissue heterogeneity on T1-w and T2-w imaging (haemorrhage and necrosis within mass)
Haemorrhagic pericardial effusion (high T1-w signal)
Contrast enhancement
A high T1-w with low T2-w signal is suggestive of metastatic malignant melanoma

T1-w = T1-weighted; T2-w = T2-weighted.
Reproduced with permission from Motwani et al. [6].

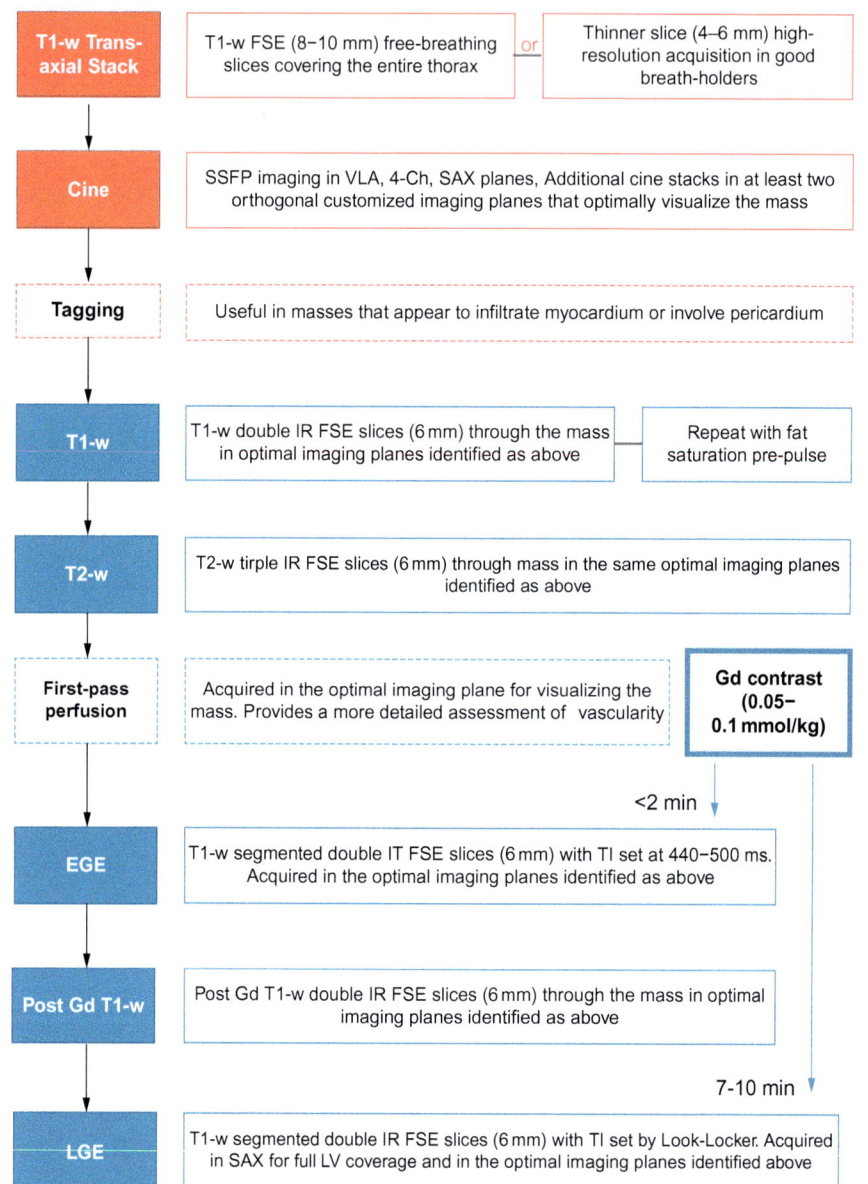

Figure 17.3 Core Protocol for CMR Imaging of Cardiac Masses. Sequences in red are used for 'localisation' of the mass. Sequences in blue are used for 'tissue characterisation'. Tagging and first-pass perfusion sequences are optional sequences that can supplement the core dataset. The second bolus of gadolinium (Gd) contrast is given with the first-pass perfusion sequence if performed – or alternatively as a 'top-up dose' prior to EGE imaging. T1-w = T1-weighted imaging; FSE = fast spin echo; SSFP = steady-state free precession; VLA = vertical long axis; 4-Ch = 4-Chamber; SAX = short-axis; IR = inversion recovery; SPIR = selective partial inversion recovery; T2-w = T2-weighted imaging; EGE = early-gadolinium enhancement; LGE = late-gadolinium enhancement.
Reproduced with permission from Motwani et al. [6].

17.4 Cardiac computed tomography

Where echocardiography alone has not been sufficient to fully assess a mass, or where CMR is not available or is contraindicated, CCT is a commonly used second-line diagnostic modality [28,29]. In addition, incidental findings of cardiac masses are becoming more common as CCT is increasingly used to evaluate coronary artery disease [30,31]. Several technological advances in computed tomography (CT) including sub-millimetre detector arrays, increased rows of detectors, half-scan post-processing algorithms, and ECG synchronisation have resulted in improved imaging of cardiac structures [32,33] (see Chapter 5).

Although less versatile than CMR, CCT is able to provide some degree of tissue characterisation, discriminating fat, soft tissues and calcium particularly well. Although dynamic perfusion is possible it is rarely done since – even with dose restraints applied – the return of information is often marginal compared to the higher radiation dose required. However, tumour vascularity can be assessed indirectly by acquiring a low-dose set of images up to 5 min after contrast injection. This technique of 'late iodine enhancement', which has been demonstrated for ischaemic scar is analogous in principal to the late gadolinium enhancement technique in CMR, although the contrast-to-noise ratio is substantially lower in CCT because of an inability to null remote normal myocardium [34].

One benefit of CCT over both echocardiography and CMR is its flexibility. A rapid acquisition in 10 s or less not only minimises the problems associated with scanning unstable or uncooperative patients for more prolonged periods, but also provides a large field of view 3D data set which may be post-processed at leisure in order to assess the mass in any plane desired. This can be extremely useful with more diffuse or infiltrating mass lesions, in communicating the extent of the lesion to surgical colleagues. If CT coronary angiography is performed as part of the scanning protocol, it can also provide information on concomitant coronary artery disease which may be important if surgical removal of the cardiac mass is considered. Finally, the ability to interrogate the lungs and bones by CCT allows for assessment of metastatic spread or indeed identification of the primary malignancy if the cardiac mass is a secondary metastasis.

17.5 Nuclear imaging techniques

Nuclear imaging techniques have traditionally held a rather restricted role in the imaging of intra-cardiac masses. High radiation doses and limited spatial resolution are the major disadvantages, whilst lack of availability of machinery and radiotracers continue to hamper the development of positron emission tomography (PET) as a diagnostic tool in many countries (see Chapters 3 and 4). Single-photon emission computed tomography (SPECT) is occasionally used in the investigation of carcinoid tumours, with the tracer octreotide showing avidity for both the primary tumour and even relatively small metastases, but there is no other significant role of SPECT in the diagnostic work up of a cardiac mass.

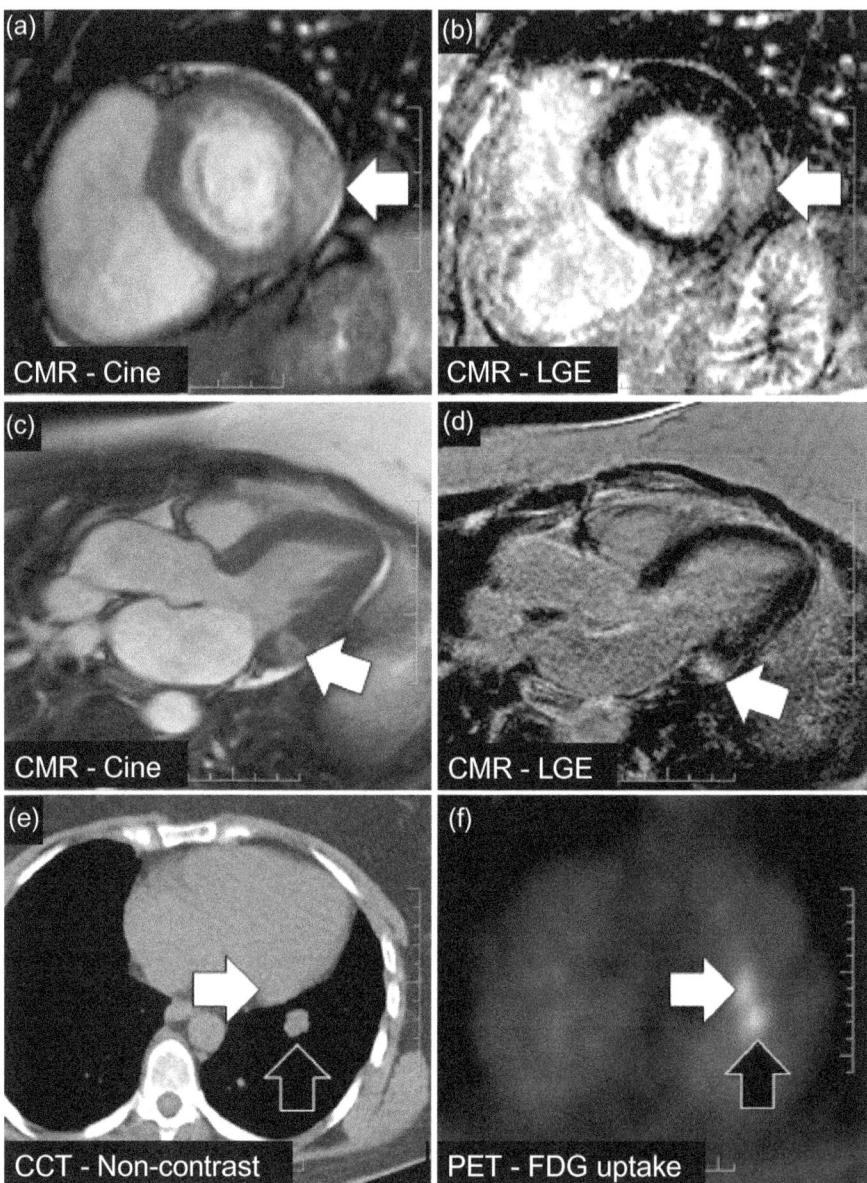

Figure 17.4 Metastatic Melanoma. A patient with previously excised malignant melanoma underwent CMR for suspected cardiac metastases. Short-axis images show an expansile hyperenhancing mass in the lateral LV wall on post-contrast cine imaging (arrow a) and LGE imaging (arrow, b). Corresponding 3-chamber post-contrast cine and LGE images also confirm the presence of a hyperenhancing lateral wall mass (arrows, c,d). The patient was scheduled for a PET-FDG/CT scan for functional assessment of the mass. The contrast axial CCT images (e) acquired as part of the PET/CT study do not clearly show a significant myocardial lesion at the expected location in the lateral LV wall (white arrow, e) – but an adjacent lung metastasis is seen (black arrow, e). Matched FDG uptake images clearly demonstrate uptake not only in the lung metastasis (black arrow, e) but also in the previously occult myocardial metastasis (white arrow, e). Note that the appearances are not specific to melanoma but could be seen in many forms of malignant secondary tumour.

PET with ^{18}F-fluorodexyglucose (18 F-FDG) is considered the gold standard technique for assessing staging and evaluating metabolic response to therapy for a large variety of systemic malignancies (including extracardiac primaries with cardiac metastases). 18 F-FDG uptake can be quantified using standardised uptake values (SUV), which represent the ratio of mean tissue radioactivity concentration in a given region of interest (in MBq/kg = kBq/g) over injected dose (MBq) per body weight (kg).

Generally, PET signal is fused with anatomical information from CT (using a PET/CT hybrid scanner) to co-localise 18 F-FDG signal with anatomical structures. In primary cardiac tumours, however, the evidence of PET/CT is limited to small series in which metabolic activity of large cardiac masses can be assessed and used to distinguish between malignant and benign and to detect extracardiac manifestations [35–37]. Rahbar and colleagues analysed 18 F-FDG PET/CT scans (whole-body imaging with low-dose CT) in 24 consecutive patients with newly diagnosed cardiac tumours (7 benign, 17 malignant [8 primary, 9 metastases]) and measured the maximum standardised uptake values (SUV_{max}) in each tumour [38]. Mean SUV_{max} was 2.8 ± 0.6 in benign cardiac tumours and significantly higher in both primary and secondary malignant cardiac tumours (8.0 ± 2.1 and 10.8 ± 4.9, $P < 0.01$). Malignancy was determined with a sensitivity of 100% and specificity of 86% (accuracy, 96%) using a cut-off SUV_{max} value of 3.5. In addition, extra-cardiac tumour manifestations were detected in four patients by whole-body 18 F-FDG PET/CT. These findings suggest that quantification of 18 F-FDG uptake with PET/CT may support the non-invasive, pre-treatment differentiation between benign and malignant cardiac tumours and be helpful in detecting metastases of malignant cardiac tumours (Figure 17.4).

A limitation of 18 F-FDG PET is the high and often inhomogeneous baseline myocardial 18 F-FDG uptake which may obscure weak pathological uptake from malignancy. Very recently, several vendors have developed integrated PET/MR scanners which might be expected to provide additional benefit in terms of cardiac mass characterisation over PET alone (Chapter 4). The validity of this approach is currently untested, however.

17.6 Cardiac masses

17.6.1 Pseudotumours

17.6.1.1 Thrombus

Thrombus is one of the commonest causes of an intra-cardiac mass and is a frequent differential diagnosis for suspected cardiac tumours. Thrombus is typically found in the left atrium (LA) or atrial appendage in association with atrial fibrillation or mitral valve disease, or in a severely dysfunctional left ventricle following MI (Figure 17.5). Right-sided thrombi are sometimes seen in association with veno-thromboembolism, and more rarely, thrombi can be found in any cardiac chamber due to systemic conditions such as Churg-Strauss syndrome (Figure 17.5).

It can be difficult to reliably distinguish thrombus from tumour with echocardiography alone as the imaging appearance can vary. In particular, thrombi show a different echodensity depending on their age and degree of thrombus organisation

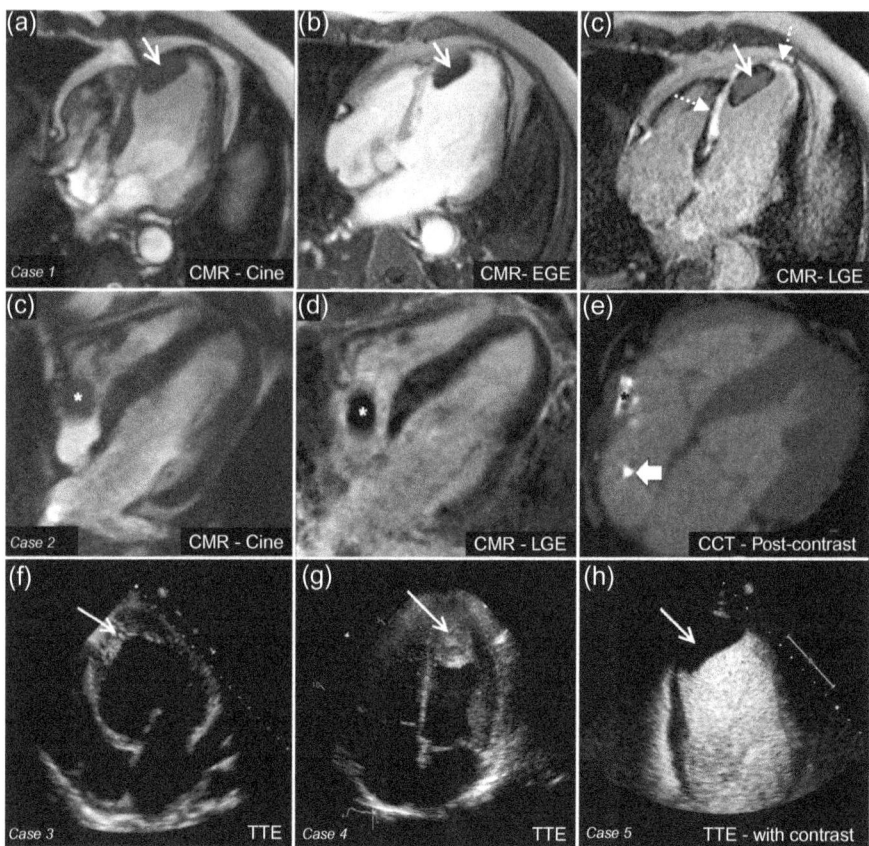

Figure 17.5 Intra-cardiac Thrombus. Case 1 – Post-MI LV thrombus: A 55-year-old man with a history of MI underwent CMR. A mass is clearly seen in the LV on cine imaging (arrow, a) and is adherent to a severely hypokinetic mid to apical antero-septum. There is no uptake of contrast in the mass on EGE imaging (arrow, b) which suggests it is avascular. LGE imaging demonstrates hyperenhancement (dashed arrows, c) in the mid to apical antero-septum consistent with a left anterior descending territory MI, and the adjacent mass lesion is non-enhancing. The combination of an avascular mass, overlying a regional wall motion abnormality with demonstrable infarction confirms the diagnosis of LV thrombus. Case 2 – Calcified RA thrombus: A heart donor underwent pre-operative CMR. Cine imaging demonstrated a rounded mass (white asterisk, c) lying in the right atrium. Post-contrast LGE imaging failed to show any evidence of contrast uptake in the mass suggesting it is avascular (white asterisk, d). The mass was removed at the time of heart transplantation and histopathology confirmed it to be a calcified thrombus. Post-operative contrast-enhanced CCT demonstrated some persistent calcification in the region of the right atrioventricular groove representing adherent thrombus that could not be removed at the time of surgery (black asterisk, e). An indwelling venous catheter is also seen on CCT (white arrow, e) and this was present prior to transplantation and likely acted as the nidus for thrombus formation. Case 3 – Mural thrombus: apical LV mural thrombus is seen with TTE in a patient with dilated cardiomyopathy (arrow f). Case 4 – Eosinophilic thrombus: very echo-bright thrombus is seen with TTE consistent with eosinophilic thrombus in a patient with Churg-Strauss syndrome (arrow, g). Case 5 – Contrast echocardiography: the use of contrast clearly outlines an apical LV thrombus in this patient with previous MI (arrow, h).

(Figure 17.5). Often, it is the presence of risk factors for thrombus formation, such as adjacent regional wall motion abnormalities, chamber dilatation, or slow flow with spontaneous echo-contrast that allows some differentiation from cardiac tumours. With regards to thrombus in the LA or left atrial appendage (LAA), this is best assessed by TOE in order to achieve the optimal imaging plane. Atrial fibrillation, LA dilatation, low filling/emptying velocities (<40 cm/s with pulsed wave Doppler placed 1 cm into the LAA), and smoke-like spontaneous contrast due to sludging of red blood cells are all associated with an increased risk of atrial thrombus. With regards to LV thrombus detection, TTE provides high sensitivity (95%) and specificity (85–90%), provided the thoracic anatomy of the patient allows sufficient visualisation [39,40]. However, in reality, the LV apex is frequently poorly defined, leading to an estimated 10–46% of echocardiograms that are inconclusive [39]. Although the use of intravenous echocardiography contrast during TTE improves the diagnostic assessment of LV thrombus, non-protruding and small mural LV thrombi may still go undetected [41] (Figure 17.5). A tangentially cut or foreshortened LV can also lead to a false positive study; therefore, it is important to vary the depth of field settings and to acquire images in multiple views. Additionally, care must be taken to exclude false tendons and trabeculae and to rule out artefacts (reverberations, side lobe or near field artefacts), which constitute the most common cause for a false diagnosis with echocardiography [39].

CMR features also vary depending on the age of a thrombus and its state of degradation or organisation, but in a more predictable fashion than with echocardiography. An acute thrombus can have high or intermediate signal intensity on both T1- and T2-weighted images depending on how much of the haemoglobin content remains in the oxygenated state. In sub-acute thrombus, the haemoglobin has been metabolised to methaemoglobin, which has a different paramagnetic effect leading to a higher T1-weighted signal intensity and lower T2-weighted signal intensity (Table 17.4) [42]. Over time, a chronic organised thrombus becomes heavily water-depleted and therefore has low signal intensity on both T1- and T2-weighted images (Table 17.2). Contrast-enhanced CMR with first pass perfusion, EGE, or LGE imaging reliably differentiates thrombus from surrounding myocardium because thrombus is avascular and hence characterised by an absence of contrast uptake; rarely, very chronic, organised thrombus may enhance peripherally due to its fibrous content [42].

Table 17.4 **CMR imaging signal characteristics for thrombus**

Age of thrombus	T1-w Signal	T2-w Signal	EGE imaging	LGE imaging
Acute	High	High	No uptake	No uptake
Subacute	High	Low	No uptake	No uptake
Chronic	Low	Low	No uptake	No uptake[a]

T1-w = T1-weighted imaging; T2-w = T2-weighted imaging; EGE = early-gadolinium enhancement; LGE = late-gadolinium enhancement.
[a]Organised chronic thrombus may show peripheral enhancement on LGE imaging due to fibrous content.

CMR with EGE or LGE imaging has significantly better accuracy than TTE and TOE for the diagnosis of LV thrombus [39]. In 24 patients with known or suspected thrombus, Barkhausen et al detected 15 thrombi with EGE imaging compared to only 12 by a combination of TTE and TOE [43]. Another study by Srichai et al. compared CMR and LGE with echocardiography in a cohort of patients undergoing LV reconstruction surgery in whom surgical and/or post-mortem verification of thrombus was performed [40]. This study reported that the sensitivity of CMR was 88% compared to only 40% with TTE (patients with suboptimal imaging were not excluded unlike in previous studies).

CCT is generally not regarded as a first-line technique for the identification or exclusion of thrombus. Nonetheless, it has been shown to perform well compared to TOE in screening for LA/LAA thrombus prior to cardioversion – particularly if a delayed imaging protoctol 2–5 min post-contrast injection is used [44,45]. Thrombus is readily identifiable on contrast-enhanced CCT as a uniformly low attenuation mass compared to adjacent (enhanced) myocardium; and if delayed imaging is used, thrombus will show a Hounsfield attenuation identical to the pre-contrast scan.

17.6.1.2 Pericardial cysts

Pericardial cysts are benign congenital fluid-filled structures usually located in the right pericardiophrenic angle [5,46]. In most cases, they are incidental findings detected on chest radiography or an echocardiogram. However, if they are very large, as in the example in Figure 17.6, they can cause symptoms due to compression of adjacent structures.

Echocardiography is useful in differentiating a pericardial cyst from other solid structures because a cyst is filled with clear fluid and therefore appears as an echolucent structure [47]. With CMR, pericardial cysts have a well-demarcated and homogenous appearance with low or iso-intense signal on T1-weighted imaging (unless the content of the cyst is proteinaceous) and very high signal intensity on T2-weighted imaging [48]. There is no contrast uptake on LGE imaging (Figure 17.6). Similarly, with CCT, pericardial cysts typically appear as thin-walled, unilocular non-enhancing structures, with attenuation values similar to water.

17.6.1.3 Normal intra-cardiac structures

Normal intra-cardiac structures or embryological remnants can sometimes be mistaken for tumours or thrombus. For example, the 'coumadin ridge' is a normal rim of tissue between the left upper pulmonary vein and left atrial appendage that can sometimes be misinterpreted as thrombus, especially if prominent or viewed in cross-section. Although it can be difficult to discriminate from thrombus with TTE, versatile imaging planes with TOE, CMR, or CCT usually allow full visualisation of its characteristic elongated structure with clubbed head and continuity with the left atrial wall [9]. The Eustachian valve, Chiari network, and crista terminalis are other normal structures that sometimes raise suspicion during routine echocardiography but are generally easily characterised by more advanced imaging with TOE, CMR, or CCT.

Cardiac tumours

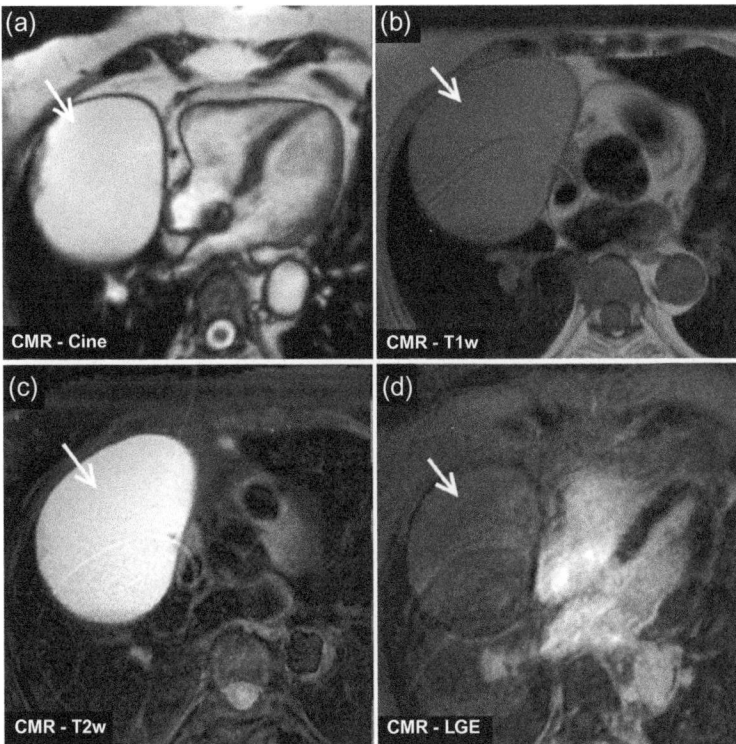

Figure 17.6 Pericardial Cyst. A 70-year-old female presented with dyspnea; although a large mass could be seen on her echocardiogram, its exact nature and anatomical origin was not clear. With CMR, a mass located in the right pericardiophrenic angle (arrow, a) was seen. Pericardial cysts have a well-demarcated and homogenous appearance with low or isointense signal on T1-weighted imaging (arrow, b) and very high signal intensity on T2-weighted imaging (arrow, b). There is no contrast uptake on LGE imaging (arrow d). Pericardial cysts are benign fluid-filled structures. In most cases, they are incidental findings, but, if very large, as in this example, can cause symptoms due to compression of adjacent structures. Reproduced with permission from Motwani et al. [6].

17.6.2 Benign tumours

17.6.2.1 Myxoma

Myxomas are the commonest type of primary cardiac tumour (~30%) and usually occur in the fourth to seventh decade [5,49] (Table 17.1). They are typically solitary, vary in size from 1 to 15 cm and have a predilection for the inter-atrial septum near the fossa ovalis [3]. Approximately 75% occur in the left atrium, 20% in the right atrium, and 5% in either ventricle [49] (Figure 17.1).

With echocardiography, myxomas are generally well-defined, smooth, globular, and relatively mobile [47] (Figure 17.7). They are typically isodense to the myocardium and often have a pedunculated attachment to the inter-atrial septum which is best visualised in the apical and subcostal views. Thrombi on the other hand tend to be more

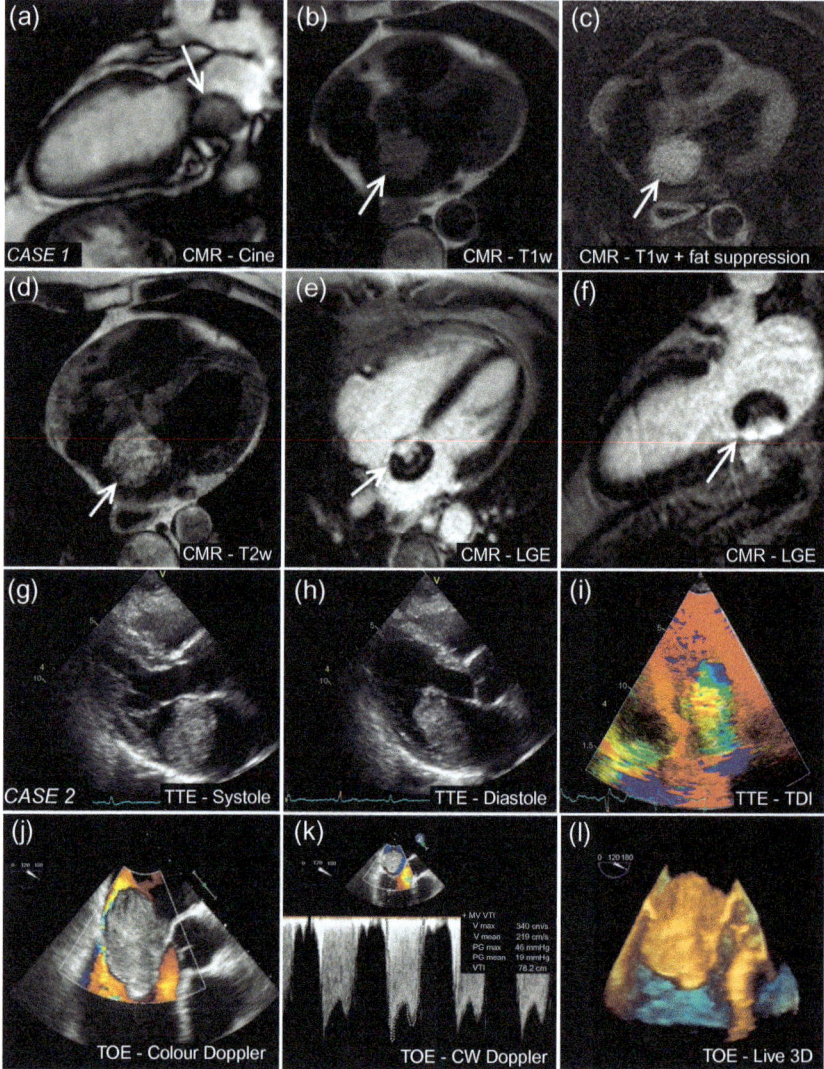

Figure 17.7 Myxoma. Case 1 – CMR: A 75-year-old female with a suspected myxoma underwent CMR. Cine imaging shows a solitary, well-defined, spherical mass in the left atrium (arrow, a) which arises from the inter-atrial septum near the fossa ovalis (the location seen in 75% of myxomas). As in this example, myxomas are typically isointense on T1-weighted imaging (arrow,b); and because they do not contain fatty tissue, they do not suppress when a fat saturation pre-pulse is used (arrow,c). As in this example, they are frequently hyperintense on T2-weighted imaging (arrow, d). One of the cardinal features on CMR is a heterogeneous pattern of late gadolinium enhancement due to areas of cystic degeneration, necrosis, haemorrhage, calcification, and sometimes surface thrombus (arrows, e and f). Case 2 – Echocardiography: A 55-year-old male underwent TTE after complaining of syncope. A large heterogeneous mass consistent with a myxoma was seen in the left atrium (g). The mass was highly mobile and prolapsed into the LV during diastole causing significant inflow obstruction (h). Tissue Doppler imaging (TDI) shows the mass (yellow) moves independently and incoherently from the myocardium. TOE was also performed for further assessment (j-l). Colour flow (j) and continuous Wave (CW) Doppler (k) illustrate the significant LV inflow obstruction (pseudo-mitral stenosis) caused by the mass and accounting for the syncope. Panel l shows live 3D TOE as the mass prolapses into the LV.

immobile, irregular, broad-based, and accompanied by chronic atrial fibrillation, atrial dilatation, or spontaneous echo-contrast. Nonetheless, reliable differentiation between myxoma and thrombus remains difficult with echocardiography alone. Furthermore, although myxomas are usually relatively homogenous or finely speckled on echocardiography, they can also appear as inhomogenous masses due to intra-tumoural haemorrhage, necrosis, and calcification. Surface thrombus on myxomas can also add to the diagnostic challenge with echocardiography. However, compared to other modalities, echocardiography offers the best assessment of their dynamic effects such as prolapse into the left ventricle, and also allows detailed mitral valve assessment with quantification of any associated mitral regurgitation or effective stenosis (Figure 17.7). TOE can offer a more detailed assessment than TTE, especially in the case of small myxomas, and offers the additional benefit of excluding alternative sources of systemic embolism [50]. With CMR, myxomas appear isointense on T1-weighted imaging with a higher signal on T2-weighted imaging due to the high extracellular water content (Figure 17.7). Areas of acute haemorrhage within myxomas appear hypointense on both T1 and T2, and older areas appear hyperintense as the haemoglobin becomes oxidised to methaemoglobin [25,51–53] (Figure 17.7 and Table 17.2). Cine imaging is very useful in the work-up of myxomas, as they are highly mobile, occasionally prolapsing through the mitral valve causing obstruction. With SSFP cine techniques, myxomas appear hyperintense relative to the myocardium but hypointense relative to the blood pool. Internally, myxomas may contain cysts, areas of necrosis, fibrosis, haemorrhage, and calcification leading to a typically heterogenous appearance on contrast enhancement [3,54,55]. Compared to echocardiography, surface thrombus on myxomas is easily distinguished as a layer of low signal tissue on LGE images [56].

Myxomas cannot usually be confidently identified as such by CCT, as they often have rather bland attenuation characteristics shared by many similar mass lesions. An exception can be made for those with a typical point of attachment to the inter-atrial septum where statistical probability favours myxoma. It is useful to perform delayed imaging if a myxoma is suspected as the majority will demonstrate heterogenous increase in contrast density. A rare exception is the gelatinous form of myxoma which is relatively avascular and may be confused with thrombus by CCT.

The majority of myxomas occur sporadically, but approximately 7% constitute part of an autosomal dominant syndrome known as Carney complex associated with skin lentigines, endocrine tumours, fibroadenomas, and melanotic schwannnomas [57]. They can be asymptomatic if small, but most patients present with symptoms due to mass effect (e.g. inflow/outflow obstruction), embolisation, or constitutional symptoms (due to release of IL-6) [58]. The treatment is surgical resection with a margin of normal tissue and is considered curative. The overall risk of recurrence after resection is 13% and is much more common with familial myxomas [4].

17.6.2.2 Lipoma

Lipomas are a common benign tumour, accounting for ~10% of all primary cardiac tumours [5] (Table 17.1). They are well-defined, homogenous, encapsulated tumours containing neoplastic adipose cells. The majority arise from the epicardial surface and can extend into the pericardial space; subendocardial lipomas are less common and tend to be smaller and sessile [59]. Many lipomas are discovered incidentally during routine echocardiography and patients typically remain asymptomatic without the need for surgical intervention.

On echocardiography, lipomas are generally well demarcated, homogeneous, broad-based masses but have no specific diagnostic features and can occur in any chamber. Their appearance varies with location: in the pericardial space they arise from the epicardium and are hypoechogenic, while intra-cavity lipomas are hyperechogenic [3]. CCT and CMR are, however, the best imaging tools for confirmatory diagnosis, as they identify fat with high specificity. Once a diagnosis of lipoma is suspected, periodic imaging should be performed, as they have a tendency to grow; rarely, very large lipomas can lead to symptomatic obstruction, especially if they involve the pericardial space [60,61]. The key diagnostic finding on CMR is a homogenous high signal (relative to myocardium) on T1-weighted imaging which markedly suppresses with the application of additional fat-saturation pre-pulses (SPIR) (Figure 17.8). An additional useful clue is the similar signal intensity of surrounding chest wall fat on T1- and T2-weighted imaging [59]. Lipomas are avascular and do not enhance with

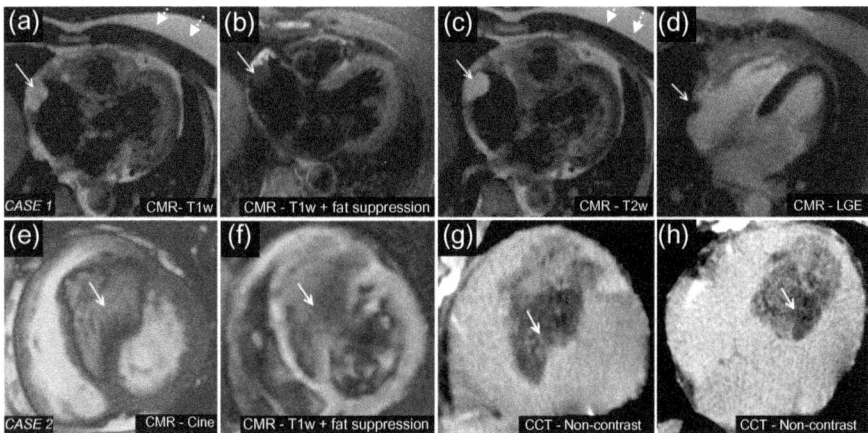

Figure 17.8 Lipoma. Case 1 – Lipomas are usually solitary, well circumscribed and encapsulated (solid arrow, a). The key diagnostic finding on CMR is homogenous high signal (relative to myocardium) on T1-weighted imaging which markedly suppresses with the application of additional fat-saturation pre-pulses (solid arrows, b). An additional useful clue is the similar signal intensity of surrounding chest wall fat on T1- and T2-weighted imaging (dashed arrows, a and c). Lipomas are avascular and do not enhance with contrast (d). Case 2 – CMR cine imaging in the short axis orientation demonstrates a large apparently encapsulated lesion within the interventricular septum (arrow, e) where it is causing focal expansion. Note the black outline around the mass, which is characteristic of the chemical shift artefact seen in the presence of fat. Signal drop out on fat suppressed T1-weighted images (arrow, f) suggests this is likely to be an inter-ventricular lipoma. Short axis (g) and 4 chamber (h) reconstructions of a non-contrast CCT show a large, mainly low-attenuation lesion, with negative Hounsfield values also consistent with fatty content.

gadolinium contrast (Table 17.2). With CCT, lipomas appear as homogenous, low attenuation masses (−100 to −20 Hounsfield units) [62] (Figure 17.8).

Lipomatous hypertrophy can sometimes be confused with lipomas, as both have similar signal characteristics due to their fat content [3,63]. However, lipomatous hypertrophy is a benign, non-encapsulated, non-neoplastic condition characterised by adipose cell hyperplasia and associated with older age and obesity [20]. It can usually be distinguished from true encapsulated lipomas by its morphological features – the fatty mass in lipomatous hypertrophy is by definition greater than 2 cm in transverse diameter and classically involves the limbus of the fossa ovalis, sparing the fossa ovalis membrane, giving rise to a bilobed dumbbell or hour-glass shape [16,63,64].

17.6.2.3 Fibroelastoma

Papillary fibroelastomas are small (usually <1.5 cm) benign endocardial papillomas that predominantly affect the cardiac valves (90%), accounting for 75% of all valvular neoplasms [15,65] (Figure 17.1). In surgical series, they account for approximately 10% of primary cardiac tumours but their prevalence in the general population is uncertain as they are often asymptomatic and discovered incidentally [66,67] (Table 17.1). Macroscopically, they have a papillary, frond-like structure; microscopically, they consist of avascular connective tissue lined by endothelium [68]. Due to their small size and high mobility, they are usually best diagnosed with echocardiography rather than CMR or CCT, which are rarely helpful, except in atypical large cases [69] (Figure 17.9).

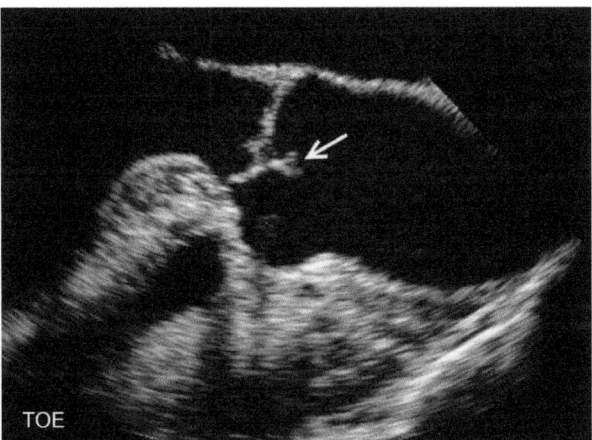

Figure 17.9 Papillary fibroelastoma. A 57-year-old female underwent a TOE following a stroke. Multiple frond-like masses with high-frequency oscillations were seen attached to the downstream side of the aortic valve leaflets (arrow). The masses were suspected to be a source of systemic embolism accounting for the stroke at a young age and were therefore excised. Subsequent histopathology confirmed the masses to be papillary fibroelastomas. The small size and rapid mobility of papillary fibroelastomas means they are best detected with TOE due to the high spatial and temporal resolution. They are often missed with CMR and CCT techniques.

With TTE, papillary fibroelastomas are typically seen as small (<1 cm), highly mobile, pedunculated structures. They usually occur on the aortic and mitral valves and less frequently on tricuspid and pulmonary valves or the mural endocardium. Given their small size, TOE is often required (greater spatial resolution than TTE) to aid differentiation from vegetations, thrombi, valvular calcifications, or Lambl's excrescences (Figure 17.9). Similarly, typical CMR features are of small, highly mobile homogenous masses usually attached to valvular leaflets with a small pedicle; hypointense signal and surrounding turbulent flow on cine imaging, and isointense T1 and hyperintense T2 signal [70,71] (Table 17.2). They are occasionally seen with CCT, and Lembcke et al. reported an example using contrast-enhanced ECG-gated 64-slice spiral CT depicting a well-defined, pedunculated, mobile, spherical lesion (density 69 ± 21 Hounsfield units) attached to the commissure of the left coronary and noncoronary aortic valve leaflet [72].

The main differentials include vegetations and thrombus. Thrombus is usually easily discriminated by the echocardiographic or CMR features of thrombus previously discussed. Vegetations are usually present in the clinical context of suspected infected endocarditis and cause destruction of valvular leaflets, whereas fibroelastomas are rarely associated with a functional impact on the valve. Additionally, in contrast to vegetations, papillary fibroelastomas are usually located on the downstream side of the valve. Clinically fibroelastomas can be asymptomatic or sometimes associated with systemic embolisation from attached thrombi or fragmentation [68]. Surgical excision is only recommended in symptomatic patients or in those with larger (>1 cm), highly mobile, left-sided tumours [3].

17.6.2.4 Fibroma

Cardiac fibromas are the second-most common congenital tumour and typically present in paediatric or young adult life. They are usually solitary tumours (unlike rhabdomyomas), most often located intramurally in the ventricles involving the interventricular septum or LV lateral wall [73] (Figure 17.1). Those associated with polyposis syndromes (e.g. familial adenomatous polyposis or Gardner's syndrome) occur more commonly in the atria [3,74]. Clinically, they can present with syncope, palpitations, sudden cardiac death, chest pain, or cardiac failure as sequelae of mass effects, outflow-tract obstruction, or arrhythmias. Macroscopically, they are solitary, well-defined masses within the myocardium; microscopically they are composed of neoplastic fibroblasts without cystic change, haemorrhage, or necrosis – but frequently have central calcification which can help differentiate them from rhabdomyomas.

With echocardiography, fibromas appear as highly echogenic, well-circumscribed, non-contractile, solid masses [3]. Their predilection for the septal wall means they can sometimes mimic hypertrophic cardiomyopathy [75]. Typically, they range from 1 to 10 cm, sometimes extending into the LV cavity and often have central calcification [76]. With CMR imaging, fibromas are iso-intense relative to normal myocardium on T1-weighted imaging and characteristically hypointense on T2-weighted imaging (unlike other masses) [24,25] (Figure 17.10 and Table 17.2). They are generally homogenous unless there is central calcification which may be seen as patchy central hypointensity. With gadolinium administration, fibromas generally show non-enhancement during

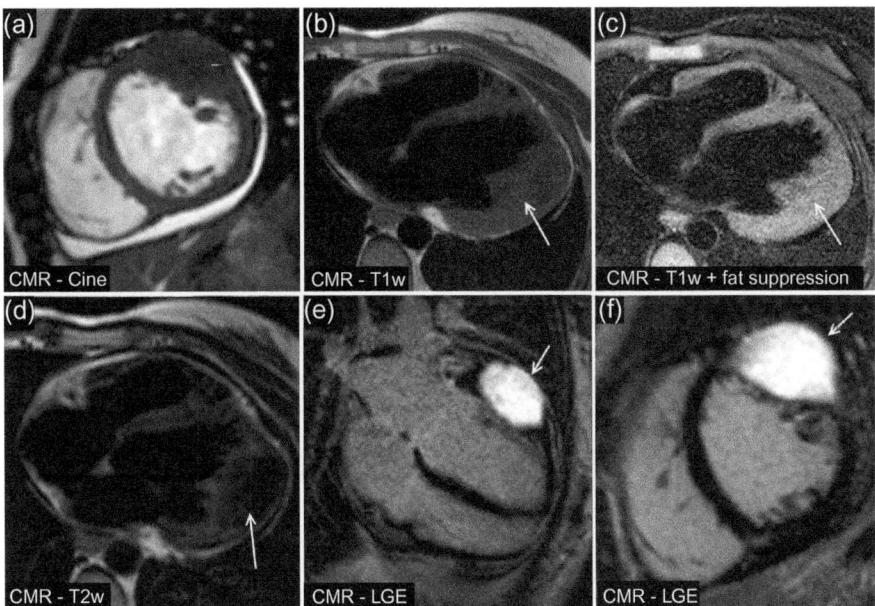

Figure 17.10 Fibroma. A 30-year-old female with unexplained syncope underwent CMR. As seen on cine imaging in this example, fibromas are usually intra-myocardial, and can exert a local mass effect (arrow, a). Fibromas typically appear isointense (relative to myocardium) on T1-weighted imaging (arrow, b and c) and hypointense on T2-weighted imaging (arrow, d). The most characteristic feature on CMR imaging is diffuse homogenous enhancement of the mass on LGE imaging (arrow, e and f) – consistent with its composition of fibroblasts and loose collagen fibres with large extracellular spaces for contrast uptake.
Reproduced with permission from Motwani et al. [6].

perfusion imaging, due to their avascularity. However, 7–10 min later they classically show intense hyperenhancement on LGE imaging. The explanation of this late hyperenhancement pattern is that microscopically fibromas are a collection of fibroblasts interspersed with large amounts of collagen and therefore have a very large extracellular space compartment. Gadolinium diffuses into interstitial spaces but not across cell membranes, and this phenomenon results in a delayed and persistently higher concentration of gadolinium in the fibroma (Figure 17.10) [16,18,77]. With CCT, a fibroma appears as a homogenous mural mass with sharply demarcated or infiltrative soft-tissue attenuation, and any areas of calcification are readily detected [15]. Late iodine enhancement is present on CCT for the same reason that late gadolinium enhancement is seen on CMR; as such, a late phase CT scan may be very revealing.

17.6.2.5 Rhabdomyoma

Rhabdomyomas are the most common primary cardiac tumours in infants and children. They typically present in the first year of life, and more than 50% are associated with tuberous sclerosis. They arise intra-murally in the ventricular myocardium; however, unlike fibromas, they are multiple in 90% of cases (Figure 17.1). Microscopically, they are hamartomas, and macroscopically they are well circumscribed and vary from a few millimetres to a few centimetres in size. Although rhabdomyomas can protrude into the ventricular chambers causing obstruction, the majority remain asymptomatic and spontaneously regress before the age of 4 years without the need for surgical intervention.

On echocardiography, they appear as multiple, homogeneous, and hyperechogenic tumours located intra-murally or pedunculated, protruding into the ventricular cavity. With CMR, they appear isointense to normal myocardium on T1-weighted imaging and hyperintense on T2-weighted imaging (in contrast to fibromas) (Table 17.2) [77,78]. They typically show minimal or no enhancement with a gadolinium-based contrast agent consistent with their hamartomatous composition [77]. Rhabdomyomas are rare in adult practice, and CCT is not usually the diagnostic modality of choice, although focal distortions of endo and epicardial contour by larger lesions can be readily appreciated. Tuberous sclerosis may also be associated with intra-myocardial lipomata – these are very easily picked up by CCT, even if relatively small, due to their fatty constituency.

17.6.2.6 Haemangioma

Cardiac haemangiomas are vascular tumours accounting for 5–10% of all primary benign cardiac tumours [5] (Table 17.1). They are typically solitary and found in either ventricle, but can be located in any cardiac chamber (Figure 17.1). Histologically, they can be capillary, cavernous, or arteriovenous in nature. Associated symptoms depend upon their location and include conduction disturbances, arrhythmias, pericardial effusions, and angina – but they are often clinically insignificant and diagnosed incidentally. Notably, they are sometimes first detected on coronary angiography, which produces a 'tumour blush' and delineates its vascular supply [79].

On echocardiography, they appear as hyperechogenic, well-demarcated masses, ranging from 1 to 8 cm in size [79,80]. Myocardial contrast echocardiography can also be used to confirm their vascularity [13,81]. On CMR, haemangiomas are typically heterogeneous and hyperintense on T1- and T2-weighted imaging due to slow blood flow (Table 17.2) [77,82]. During and after contrast administration they intensely hyperenhance due to their vascular content – but there may be areas of inhomogeneity due to calcification or fibrous septa (Figure 17.11). Similarly, with CCT they are also seen as heterogeneous masses on unenhanced imaging, which intensely enhance after contrast administration [82] (Figure 17.11). Larger haemangiomas may insinuate around the coronary vessels and CCT and CMR are useful in this situation, since it often renders the tumour inoperable (Figure 17.11).

17.6.3 Malignant tumours

Malignant primary cardiac tumours are rare, constituting only 25% of all primary cardiac tumours (Table 17.1) [8]. The majority (95%) of malignant primary cardiac tumours are sarcomas, and the remainder are lymphomas or pericardial mesotheliomas [5]. Metastatic cardiac malignancy on the other hand is much more common.

Cardiac tumours

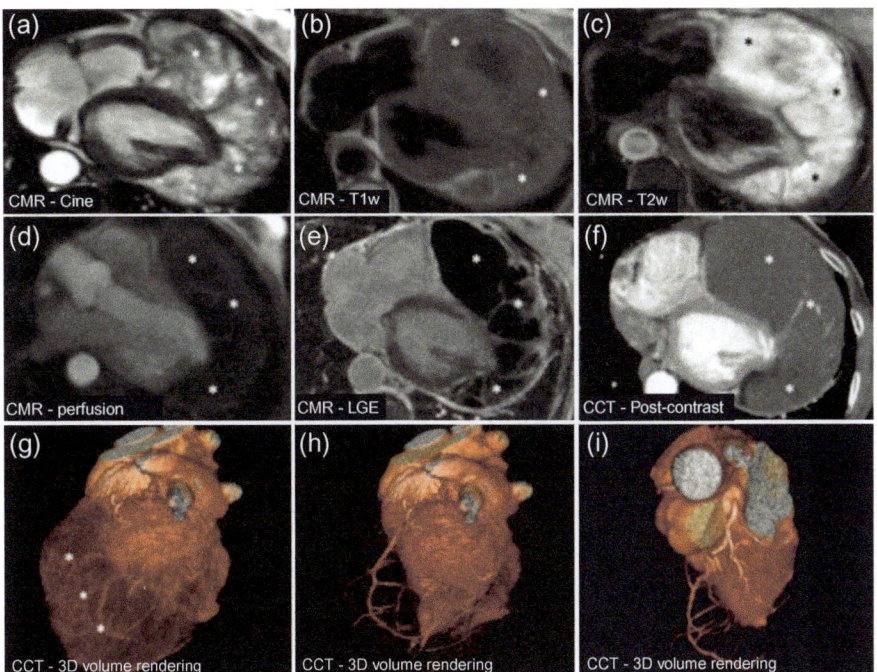

Figure 17.11 Haemangioma. This patient was found to have a large intra-cardiac mass on echocardiography, prompting further evaluation with CMR and CCT. CMR cine imaging demonstrated a large septated mass enveloping the apex of the heart (asterisks, a). This mass appears isointense to myocardium on T1-weighted imaging (b) but near-uniformly bright on T2-weighted images (c) with low signal internal septations (asterisks) running through the mass. First-pass perfusion (d) demonstrates minimal enhancement in the body of the mass, although some of the septations do appear to perfuse. Late enhancement imaging (e) shows uptake of contrast confined to the septations alone. Axial post-contrast CCT (f) suggests that some of these septations have a contrast density similar to that of the aorta and are in fact coronary arterial branches engulfed by the low attenuation mass. CCT derived 3D volume rendered images of the heart with the mass (asterisks, g) and without the mass (h, i) demonstrate the extent to which the coronary arterial tree has been engulfed by the tumour. Biopsy was performed and histopathology revealed a benign pericardial haemangioma. The extent of coronary involvement was such that it was felt to be inoperable.

17.6.3.1 Sarcoma

Sarcomas occur mainly in adulthood, usually between the third and fifth decades, and carry an extremely poor prognosis [3]. Survival after diagnosis rarely exceeds 6 months due to rapid progression, widespread local infiltration, intra-cavity obstruction, or metastases which are often already present by the time of diagnosis [83]. Primary cardiac sarcomas most commonly metastasize to the lungs but also to the lymph nodes, bone, brain, bowel, liver, spleen, and adrenals, kidneys, thyroid, and skin. There are various histological subtypes, of which angiosarcomas are the most common (~40%) [5,84]. Angiosarcomas are the commonest primary cardiac

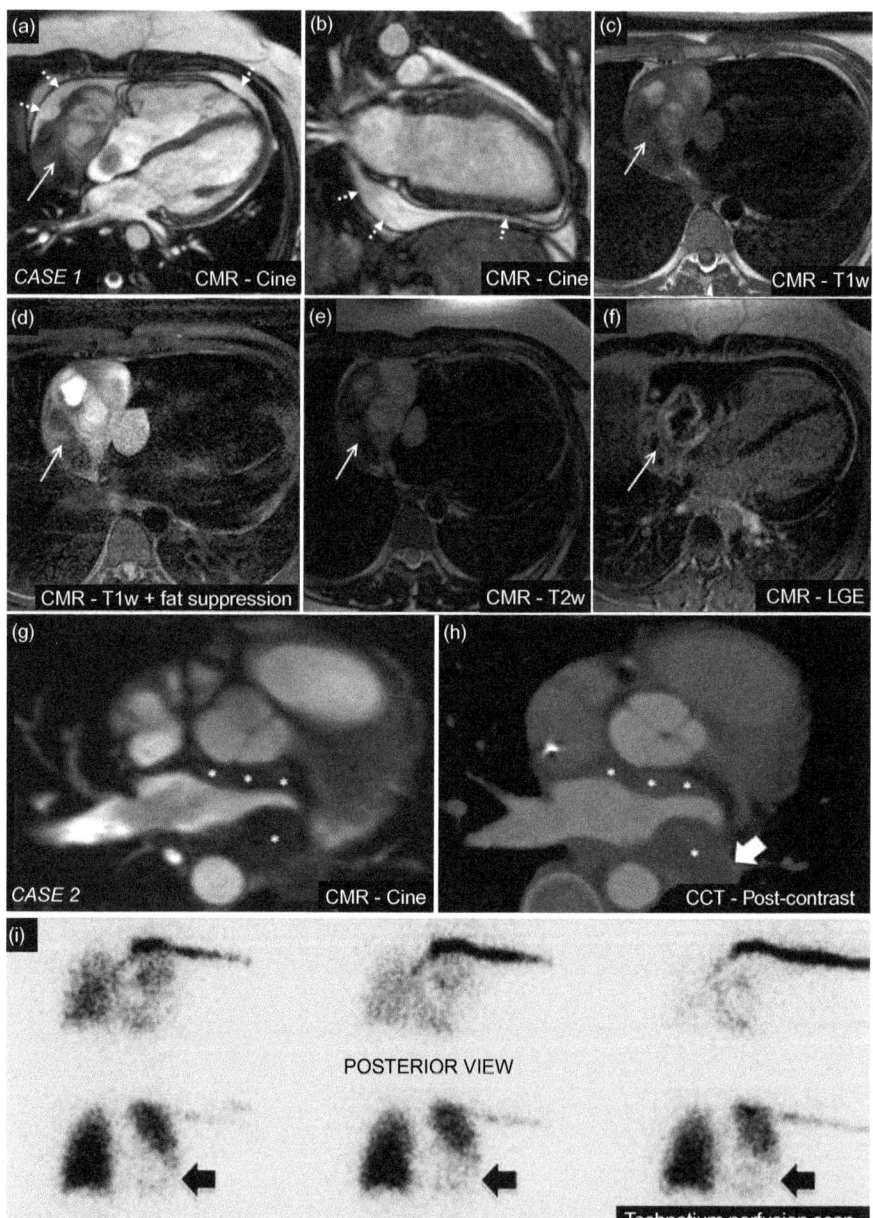

Figure 17.12 Angiosarcoma. Case 1 – Focal type: Angiosarcomas typically involve the right atrium and may directly invade into the pericardial space (solid arrow, a). This 20-year-old man presented with cardiac tamponade due to the compressive effects of the mass and associated haemorrhagic effusion (dashed arrows, a and b). As in this example, angiosarcomas typically have heterogeneous signal uptake on both T1- and T2-weighted imaging due to areas of haemorrhage, ischemia, and necrosis (arrows, c, d, and e). On first-pass perfusion imaging (not shown),

malignancy in adulthood, and rhabdomyosarcomas are the commonest in childhood [5,85]. With echocardiography, sarcomas are visualised as large, mobile, and inhomogenous masses. Although they are readily detected and distinguished from benign tumours with echocardiography, it is generally not possible to differentiate between the various histological subtypes with echocardiography alone. The exception is osteosarcomas, which may show areas of calcification. Generally, however, only more advanced imaging with CMR or CCT is able to offer further insight before tissue biopsy/surgery (Figure 17.12).

Unlike other sarcomas, angiosarcomas typically begin in the right atrium and usually present with right-heart failure, haemorrhagic pericardial effusions, or metastases (Figures 17.1 and 17.12) [3]. Microscopically, angiosarcomas consist of rapidly proliferating, extensively infiltrating anaplastic cells derived from blood vessels and lining irregular blood-filled spaces, and there are usually large areas of haemorrhage and necrosis within the tumour [84]. Macroscopically, there are two morphological variants: the 'focal' variety is typically a well-defined mass, protruding into the right atrium causing serious intra-cavity obstruction; the 'diffuse' variety is a more extensive mass that rapidly infiltrates the right ventricle and pericardium presenting with right-sided heart failure or tamponade. These features are reflected on CMR imaging, which typically demonstrates a large heterogeneous right atrial mass with or without pericardial involvement (thickening, effusion, nodularity, frank disruption of fat planes) (Figure 17.12). They appear heterogeneous on T1- and T2-weighted imaging, reflecting tumour tissue, necrosis, and haemorrhage and demonstrate arterial phase enhancement on first-pass perfusion imaging due to their vascularity. On LGE imaging they appear to have heterogeneous enhancement due to peripheral fibrosis (surface hyperenhancement) and focal hypoenhancement due to central necrosis (Figure 17.12 and Table 17.2) [15,16,86].

Rhabdomyosarcomas account for approximately 20% of sarcomas and occur most frequently in infants and children [5]. They often involve multiple sites within the heart including the valves unlike other sarcomas [87]. With CMR, they are isointense on T1-weighted imaging, hyperintense on T2-weighted imaging and generally demonstrate

---

Figure 17.12 Continued. the mass in this example heterogeneously enhanced, especially in the periphery, consistent with a degree of tissue vascularity. Typical of angiosarcomas, LGE revealed heterogeneous enhancement with areas of central necrosis (hypoenhancement) and surrounding fibrosis (hyperenhancement) (arrow, f). Post-operative histology confirmed a highly invasive, poorly differentiated focal angiosarcoma. Case 2 – Diffuse type: Infiltrating soft tissue is seen along both front and back walls of the left atrium extending towards the left lower pulmonary vein on axial CMR cine imaging (asterisks, g). This is more clearly seen on the corresponding slice of a post-contrast CCT (asterisks, h), where the orifice of the pulmonary vein is noted to be expanded and occluded by tumour (arrow, h). Technetium perfusion images acquired dynamically from the patient's back, reveal the physiological consequences of this pulmonary vein obstruction with a substantial fixed perfusion defect in the left lower lobe (black arrows, i). Histopathology revealed a highly invasive diffuse angiosarcoma.

homogenous enhancement after contrast – occasionally with areas of hypoenhancement due to central necrosis [49,77].

A cardiac sarcoma with no specific histologic pattern is classified as undifferentiated. Undifferentiated sarcomas account for approximately one-third of all cardiac sarcomas and are therefore the second most common primary cardiac malignancy. Similar to angiosarcomas, they may appear as focal or infiltrative masses with necrosis and haemorrhage and thus have similar CMR imaging features. However, unlike angiosarcomas, which are usually found in the right atrium, undifferentiated sarcomas have a predilection for the left atrium (81%) [88]. The remaining histological subtypes of sarcomas, including fibrosarcomas, osteosarcomas, leiomyosarcomas, and liposarcomas, are extremely rare; as a result, there are insufficient data to permit reliable non-invasive distinction between them. However, even histological distinction has not been shown to alter their course of treatment or outcome [89]. Like the other sarcomas, they generally appear isointense on T1-weighted imaging, hyperintense on T2-weighted imaging and show varying degrees of non-homogenous contrast enhancement depending on their exact composition and presence of necrosis or haemorrhage [15].

The role of CCT in sarcoma diagnosis/management is relatively limited to the assessment of tumour invasion in cases where the histology has already been established. The higher spatial resolution of CCT sometimes makes it easier to identify breach of fat planes and local invasion of adjacent structures than on CMR, as does the ability to view the dataset from any perspective (Figure 17.12). In general however, CMR is usually better suited for overall assessment of a mass suspected to be sarcomatous in nature. PET imaging usually shows a highly FDG-avid mass and has the advantage of revealing potentially occult metastases elsewhere in the thorax and axial skeleton at the same examination.

17.6.3.2 Primary cardiac lymphoma

Primary cardiac lymphomas are a rare entity, and cardiac metastases from extracardiac forms of lymphoma are far more common (~25% of patients with lymphoma have cardiac involvement) [7]. Nearly all primary cardiac lymphomas are aggressive B-cell lymphomas and they predominantly occur in immunocompromised patients, especially those with HIV infection (Figure 17.13) [90]. They most commonly involve the right side of the heart, particularly the right atrium, but any chamber can be involved and there are frequently multiple lesions (Figures 17.1 and 17.13). There is often pericardial invasion accompanied by a large pericardial effusion. Presentation is with rapidly progressive cardiac failure, obstructive symptoms, arrhythmias, or tamponade. By the time of presentation, they are usually large with extensive nodular infiltration of the myocardium [91]. Prognosis is invariably poor, although there have been reported remissions with early diagnosis and chemotherapy [92].

There are no specific echocardiographic features, but lymphomas are usually seen as immobile polypoid masses in the right atrium associated with a pericardial effusion. Unlike other malignant tumours such as sarcomas, lymphomas generally lack areas

Cardiac tumours

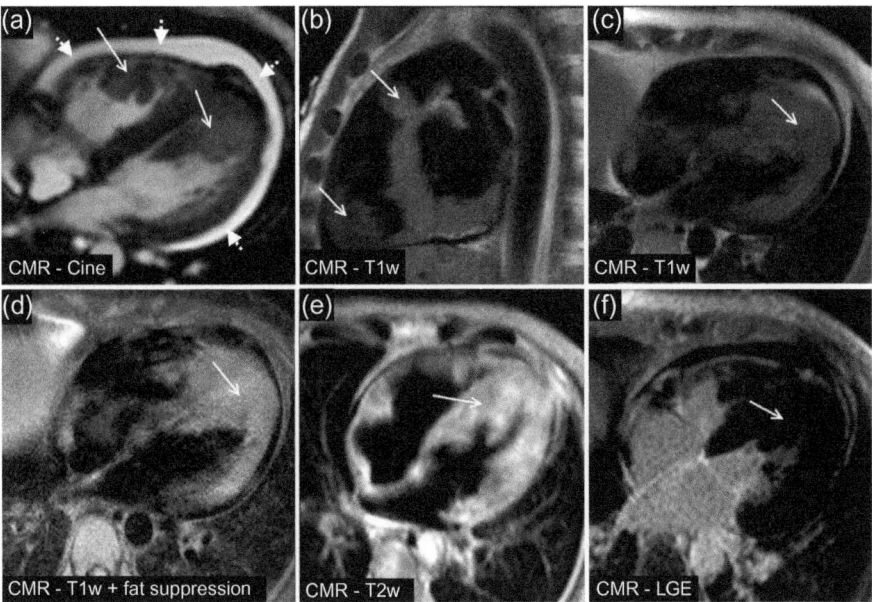

Figure 17.13 Primary Cardiac Lymphoma. A 25-year-old HIV positive male underwent CMR. A mass was seen in both the left and right ventricles on cine imaging (arrows, a). The presence of more than one mass, their irregular outline, large size, and associated pericardial effusion (dashed arrows, a) all suggest malignancy. Unlike other malignant tumours such as sarcomas, lymphomas generally lack areas of central necrosis and haemorrhage. As a result, lymphomas are typically homogenous and isointense on T1 and T2-weighted imaging, which can be a useful discriminating feature (c, d, and e). Similarly, unlike other malignant tumours, there is generally minimal contrast uptake on LGE (arrow, f).
Reproduced with permission from Motwani et al. [6].

of central necrosis and haemorrhage. Therefore, with CMR, lymphomas are typically homogenous and isointense on T1- and T2-weighted imaging, which can be a useful discriminating feature (Figure 17.13 and Table 17.2) [93,94]. Unlike other malignant tumours, there is generally minimal contrast uptake on LGE [16,18]. With CCT, primary cardiac lymphomas are hypo-attenuating or iso-attenuating relative to the myocardium and demonstrate heterogeneous enhancement after contrast administration [92]. The transaxial anatomy stacks on CMR and CCT should be carefully examined for mediastinal lymphadenopathy to identify extra-cardiac involvement and for the purpose of biopsy targets.

17.6.3.3 Cardiac metastasis

Cardiac metastases are 20–40 times more common than primary cardiac tumours [8]. Most patients have no cardiac symptoms and the metastases are discovered at post-mortem. In autopsy series, 10–12% of patients with a primary neoplasm are found to have cardiac metastases [95,96]. The most common malignancies to spread to the heart are lung and breast cancers, lymphoma, and malignant melanoma. Metastatic spread to the heart can occur by direct invasion (lung, breast, oesophagus), haematogenous (melanoma, lymphoma, leukaemia), transvenous via the great veins (renal cell carcinoma, hepatoma), or via mediastinal lymphatics. The most common site of involvement is the pericardium (usually from direct invasion or lymphatic spread) and malignant pericardial effusions are the commonest consequence of cardiac metastasis [96]. Intramural myocardial metastases tend to be the result of haematogenous spread from melanoma, lymphoma, or rarely carcinoid tumours (Figures 17.5 and 17.14). Transvenous spread leads to intra-cavity metastases, typically in the right atrium, e.g., from renal cell carcinoma via the IVC.

There are no specific echocardiographic features for metastases, but they are usually seen as wall thickening or infiltration with an associated pericardial effusion. Sometimes, metastatic masses are seen within the pericardial effusion itself. Similarly, there are no specific CMR features, but cardiac metastases generally have low signal intensity on T1-weighted and high signal intensity on T2-weighted imaging (Figure 17.15 and Table 17.2) – with the exception of melanoma which appear bright on T1-weighted imaging due to the paramagnetic properties of melanin pigment [97,98]. Haemorrhagic and exudative pericardial effusions have a high signal on T1-weighted imaging, whereas benign transudates have a low signal. The uptake of contrast in metastases is usually heterogeneous (Figure 17.15). CCT, like CMR, is usually unable to identify the point of origin of a cardiac metastasis unless the primary tumour happens to lie within the imaged field of view. This is occasionally seen for example in lung cancer and breast cancer or renal cell cancer, where tumour growing into the right atrium from the IVC and renal vein may be evident.

17.7 Conclusions

Although cardiac tumours are rare, they can lead to serious complications, such as intra-cardiac obstruction and fatal arrhythmias, even when benign. All the major imaging modalities have a role to play in their assessment. Most cardiac masses are initially detected with echocardiography; this remains the most widely accessible form of imaging. Recent advances, such as 3D echocardiography offer increasingly detailed and sophisticated imaging. However, CMR has become the most established method for further detailed assessment and tissue characterisation, which cannot be achieved with routine echocardiography alone. A core protocol of CMR pulse sequences can provide information on the anatomy, morphology, tissue characteristics, malignant potential, and the functional impact of a suspected tumour, all within a single examination. When CMR is not possible, CCT is a useful second-line option for detailed cross-sectional imaging, but with inferior soft-tissue characterisation. Finally, although PET is well-established in general oncology, its role in cardiac tumour assessment is currently far less well defined.

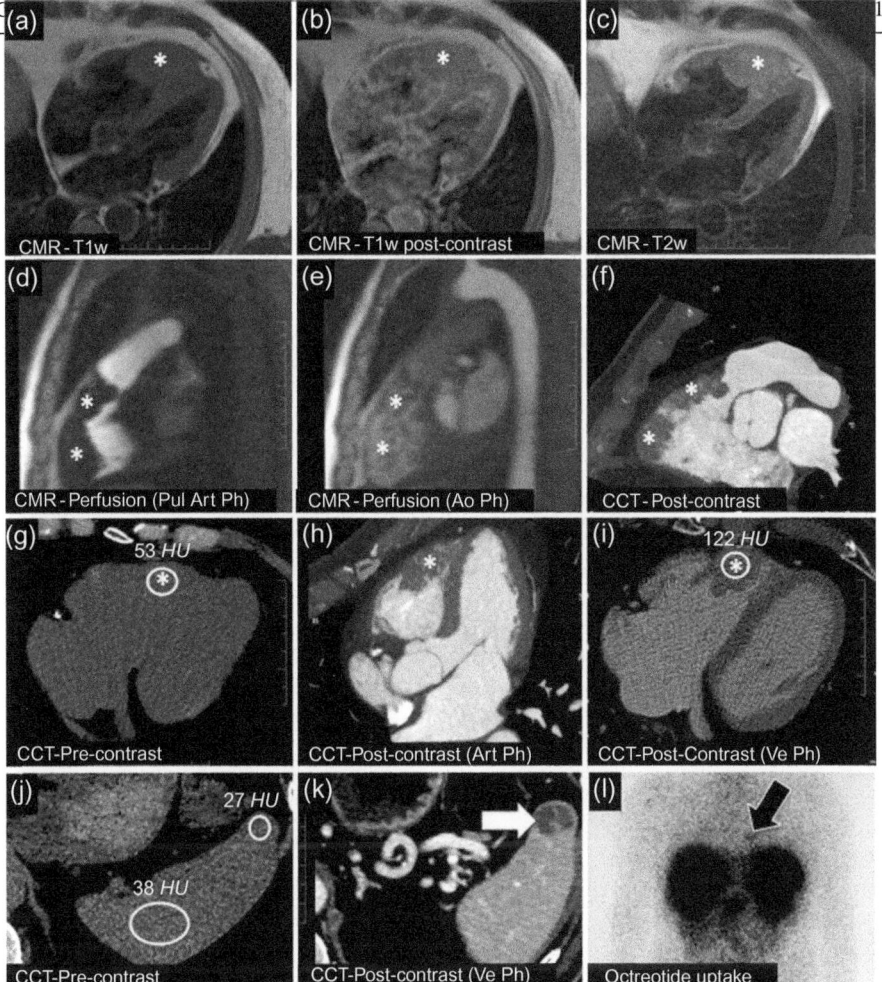

Figure 17.14 Metastatic Carcinoid. A large mass lesion at the apex of the right ventricle (asterisk) appears relatively iso-intense to myocardium on both pre- and post-contrast T1-weighted imaging (a and b) and on T2-weighted imaging (c). Dynamic perfusion imaging confirms that the mass is highly vascular with very rapid enhancement of the mass occurring between the pulmonary arterial phase (d) and the aortic phase (e) of contrast passage. Reconstructed RVOT views from post-contrast CCT demonstrate the relationship of the mass to the outflow tract and pulmonary valve, which may be useful information for surgical planning (f). Multiphase CCT imaging demonstrates an increase in Hounsfield attenuation value from 53 HU in the pre-contrast phase (g), increasing after the arterial phase (h) to a value of 122 HU in the early venous phase (i). Similarly, pre-contrast CT tissue characterisation of the spleen demonstrates a subtle area of hypointensity anteriorly (small ROI, j) with a value of 27 HU, which is lower than normal tissue measuring 38 HU (large ROI, j) and therefore suggests underlying tissue abnormality. This is confirmed on the venous phase scan where an obvious lesion becomes visible (arrow, k) due to differential wash in/wash out characteristics compared to normal splenic tissue. Octreotide uptake imaging demonstrates heavy uptake in liver and spleen but focal increased tracer activity is also evident at the site of RV metastasis (black arrow, l). HU = Hounsfield Units; ROI = region of interest.

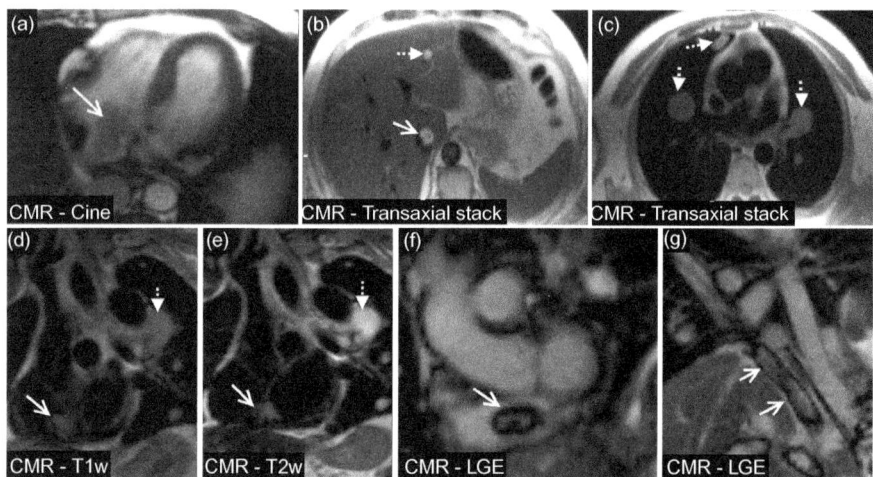

Figure 17.15 Cardiac Metastases. A 64-year-old male patient with cachexia underwent CMR. Cine imaging shows an irregular mass in the right atrium (arrow, a). In transaxial slices, the right atrial mass is seen to extend up from the inferior vena cava (solid arrow, b); and additional metastases are seen in the liver and lungs (dashed arrows, b and c). Although cardiac metastases do not have any specific appearances, they generally have low signal intensity on T1 and high signal intensity on T2-weighted imaging (arrow, d, e). In this example, the cardiac mass (solid arrows, d and e) shares the same T1/T2 signal pattern as the pulmonary metastases (dashed arrows, d and e) in keeping with them having the same underlying pathology. The uptake of contrast in metastases is usually heterogeneous, and here we see a centrally-enhancing core with a peripheral capsule on LGE imaging (arrow f). In this example, the contrast uptake also delineates the extent of the mass in the inferior vena cava (arrows, g). Post-mortem examination confirmed advanced colorectal adenocarcinoma with pulmonary, hepatic and cardiac metastases.
Reproduced with permission from Motwani et al. [6].

References

[1] Lam KY, Dickens P, Chan AC. Tumors of the heart. A 20-year experience with a review of 12,485 consecutive autopsies. Arch Pathol Lab Med 1993;117:1027–31.
[2] Sütsch G, et al. Heart tumors: incidence, distribution, diagnosis. Exemplified by 20,305 echocardiographies. Schweiz Med Wochenschr 1991;121:621–9.
[3] Bruce CJ. Cardiac tumours: diagnosis and management. Heart 2011;97:151–60.
[4] ElBardissi AW, et al. Survival after resection of primary cardiac tumors. Circulation 2008;118:S7–15.
[5] McAllister HA. Primary tumors and cysts of the heart and pericardium. Curr Probl Cardiol 1979;4:1–51.
[6] Motwani M, et al. MR imaging of cardiac tumors and masses: a review of methods and clinical applications. Radiology 2013;268:26–43.
[7] Roberts WC. Primary and secondary neoplasms of the heart. Am J Cardiol 1997;80:671–82.
[8] Butany J, et al. Cardiac tumours: diagnosis and management. Lancet Oncol 2005;6:219–28.

[9] Gupta S, Plein S, Greenwood JP. The coumadin ridge: an important example of a left atrial pseudotumour demonstrated by cardiovascular magnetic resonance imaging. J Radiol Case Rep 2009;3:1–5.
[10] Plana JC. Added value of real-time three-dimensional echocardiography in assessing cardiac masses. Curr Cardiol Rep 2009;11:205–9.
[11] Zaragosa-Macias E, Chen MA, Gill EA. Real time three-dimensional echocardiography evaluation of intracardiac masses. Echocardiography 2012;29:207–19.
[12] Altbach MI, et al. Cardiac MRI is complementary to echocardiography in the assessment of cardiac masses. Echocardiography 2007;24:286–300.
[13] Kirkpatrick JN, et al. Differential diagnosis of cardiac masses using contrast echocardiographic perfusion imaging. J Am Coll Cardiol 2004;43:1412–9.
[14] Pauliks LB, Miller S, Banerjee A. Intracardiac fibroma in nevoid-basal cell carcinoma (Gorlin) syndrome: tissue characterization by strain rate imaging. Echocardiography 2006;23:79–80.
[15] Araoz PA, et al. CT and MR imaging of benign primary cardiac neoplasms with echocardiographic correlation. Radiographics 2000;20:1303–19.
[16] Sparrow P, Kurian J, Jones T. MR imaging of cardiac tumors. Radiographics 2005;25:1255–76.
[17] Finn JP, et al. Cardiac MR imaging: state of the technology1. Radiology 2006;241: 338–54.
[18] O'Donnell DH, et al. Cardiac tumors: optimal cardiac MR sequences and spectrum of imaging appearances. AJR Am J Roentgenol 2009;193:377–87.
[19] Pennell DJ, et al. Clinical indications for cardiovascular magnetic resonance (CMR): Consensus Panel report. Eur Heart J 2004;25:1940–65.
[20] Restrepo CS, et al. CT and MR imaging findings of benign cardiac tumors. Curr Probl Diagn Radiol 2005;34:12–21.
[21] Restrepo CS, et al. CT and MR imaging findings of malignant cardiac tumors. Curr Probl Diagn Radiol 2005;34:1–11.
[22] Mitchell DG, et al. The biophysical basis of tissue contrast in extracranial MR imaging. Am J Roentgenol 1987;149:831–7.
[23] Funari M, et al. Cardiac tumors: assessment with Gd-DTPA enhanced MR imaging. J Comput Assist Tomogr 1991;15:953–8.
[24] Hoffmann U. Usefulness of magnetic resonance imaging of cardiac and paracardiac masses. Am J Cardiol 2003;92:890–5.
[25] Luna A, et al. Evaluation of cardiac tumors with magnetic resonance imaging. Eur Radiol 2005;15:1446–55.
[26] Kramer CM, et al. Standardized cardiovascular magnetic resonance imaging (CMR) protocols, society for cardiovascular magnetic resonance: board of trustees task force on standardized protocols. J Cardiovasc Magn Reson 2008;10:35.
[27] Hundley WG, et al. ACCF/ACR/AHA/NASCI/SCMR 2010 expert consensus document on cardiovascular magnetic resonance: a report of the American College of Cardiology Foundation Task Force on Expert Consensus Documents. J Am Coll Cardiol 2010;55:2614–62.
[28] Hendel RC, et al. ACCF/ACR/SCCT/SCMR/ASNC/NASCI/SCAI/SIR 2006 appropriateness criteria for cardiac computed tomography and cardiac magnetic resonance imaging: a report of the American College of Cardiology Foundation Quality Strategic Directions Committee Appropriateness Criteria Working Group. J Am Coll Cardiol 2006;48:1475–97.
[29] Kakouros N, et al. The utility of cardiac CT beyond the assessment of suspected coronary artery disease. Clin Radiol 2012;67:695–708.

[30] Budoff MJ, et al. Assessment of coronary artery disease by cardiac computed tomography. Circulation 2006;114:1761–91.
[31] Mueller J, et al. Cardiac CT angiography after coronary bypass surgery: prevalence of incidental findings. AJR Am J Roentgenol 2007;189:414–9.
[32] Achenbach S, Kondo T. Technical advances in cardiac CT. Cardiol Clin 2012;30:1–8.
[33] Cody DD, Mahesh M. Technologic advances in multidetector CT with a focus on cardiac imaging1. Radiographics 2007;27:1829–37.
[34] Crean AM, et al. High-resolution 3D scar imaging using a novel late iodine enhancement multidetector CT protocol to guide ventricular tachycardia catheter ablation. J Cardiovasc Electrophysiol 2013;24:708–10.
[35] Agostini D, et al. Detection of cardiac myxoma by F-18 FDG PET. Clin Nucl Med 1999;24:159–60.
[36] Buchmann I, et al. FDG PET for imaging pericardial manifestations of Hodgkin lymphoma. Clin Nucl Med 2003;28:760–1.
[37] Gates GF, Aronsky A, Ozgur H. Intracardiac extension of lung cancer demonstrated on PET scanning. Clin Nucl Med 2006;31:68–70.
[38] Rahbar K, et al. Differentiation of malignant and benign cardiac tumors using 18 F-FDG PET/CT. J Nucl Med 2012;53:856–63.
[39] Delewi R, Zijlstra F, Piek JJ. Left ventricular thrombus formation after acute myocardial infarction. Heart 2012;98:1743–9.
[40] Srichai MB, et al. Clinical, imaging, and pathological characteristics of left ventricular thrombus: a comparison of contrast-enhanced magnetic resonance imaging, transthoracic echocardiography, and transesophageal echocardiography with surgical or pathological validation. Am Heart J 2006;152:75–84.
[41] Weinsaft JW, et al. Contrast-enhanced anatomic imaging as compared to contrast-enhanced tissue characterization for detection of left ventricular thrombus. JACC Cardiovasc Imaging 2009;2:969–79.
[42] Paydarfar D, et al. In vivo magnetic resonance imaging and surgical histopathology of intracardiac masses: distinct features of subacute thrombi. Cardiology 2001;95:40–7.
[43] Barkhausen J, et al. Detection and characterization of intracardiac thrombi on MR imaging. Am J Roentgenol 2002;179:1539–44.
[44] Romero J, et al. Detection of left atrial appendage thrombus by cardiac computed tomography in patients with atrial fibrillation a meta-analysis. Circ Cardiovasc Imaging 2013;6:185–94.
[45] Wada H, et al. Contrast echocardiography for the diagnosis of left ventricular thrombus in anterior myocardial infarction. Heart Vessels 2013;29(3):308–12.
[46] Wang ZJ, et al. CT and MR imaging of pericardial disease. Radiographics 2003;23:S167–80.
[47] Peters PJ, Reinhardt S. The echocardiographic evaluation of intracardiac masses: a review. J Am Soc Echocardiogr 2006;19:230–40.
[48] White CS. MR evaluation of the pericardium. Top Magn Reson Imaging 1995;7:258–66.
[49] Grebenc ML, et al. Primary cardiac and pericardial neoplasms: radiologic-pathologic correlation1. Radiographics 2000;20:1073–103.
[50] Lee RJ, et al. Enhanced detection of intracardiac sources of cerebral emboli by transesophageal echocardiography. Stroke 1991;22:734–9.
[51] Masui T, et al. Cardiac myxoma: identification of intratumoral hemorrhage and calcification on MR images. Am J Roentgenol 1995;164:850–2.

[52] Matsuoka H, et al. Morphologic and histologic characterization of cardiac myxomas by magnetic resonance imaging. Angiology 1996;47:693–8.
[53] De Roos A, et al. Calcified right atrial myxoma demonstrated by magnetic resonance imaging. Chest 1989;95:478–9.
[54] Schvartzman PR, White RD. Imaging of cardiac and paracardiac masses. J Thorac Imaging 2000;15:265–73.
[55] Singh SD, Lansing AM. Familial cardiac myxoma – a comprehensive review of reported cases. J Ky Med Assoc 1996;94:96–104.
[56] Basso C, et al. Surgical pathology of primary cardiac and pericardial tumors. Eur J Cardiothorac Surg 1997;12:730–8.
[57] Carney JA, et al. The complex of myxomas, spotty pigmentation, and endocrine overactivity. Medicine (Baltimore) 1985;64:270–83.
[58] Kanda T, et al. Interleukin-6 and cardiac myxoma. Am J Cardiol 1994;74:965–7.
[59] Hananouchi GI, Goff II WB. Cardiac lipoma: six-year follow-up with MRI characteristics, and a review of the literature. Magn Reson Imaging 1990;8:825–8.
[60] Lang-Lazdunski L, et al. Successful resection of giant intrapericardial lipoma. Ann Thorac Surg 1994;58:238–41.
[61] Puvaneswary M, et al. Pericardial lipoma: ultrasound, computed tomography and magnetic resonance imaging findings. Australas Radiol 2000;44:321–4.
[62] Kamiya H, et al. Cardiac lipoma in the interventricular septum: evaluation by computed tomography and magnetic resonance imaging. Am Heart J 1990;119:1215–7.
[63] Heyer CM, et al. Lipomatous hypertrophy of the interatrial septum. Chest 2003;124:2068–73.
[64] Suarez-Mier MP, Fernandez-Simón L, Gawallo C. Pathologic changes of the cardiac conduction tissue in sudden cardiac death. Am J Forensic Med Pathol 1995;16:193–202.
[65] Edwards FH, et al. Primary cardiac valve tumors. Ann Thorac Surg 1991;52:1127–31.
[66] Burke A. Tumors of the heart and great vessels. Atlas tumor Pathol 1996;16:171–9.
[67] Tazelaar HD, Locke TJ, McGregor CG, 957–965. Pathology of surgically excised primary cardiac tumors. Mayo Clin Proc 1992;67:957–65.
[68] Sun JP, et al. Clinical and echocardiographic characteristics of papillary fibroelastomas: a retrospective and prospective study in 162 patients. Circulation 2001;103:2687–93.
[69] Sengupta PP, Khandheria BK. Transoesophageal echocardiography. Heart 2005;91:541–7.
[70] Klarich MD, et al. Papillary fibroelastoma: echocardiographic characteristics for diagnosis and pathologic correlation. J Am Coll Cardiol 1997;30:784–90.
[71] Wintersperger BJ, et al. Tumors of the cardiac valves: imaging findings in magnetic resonance imaging, electron beam computed tomography, and echocardiography. Eur Radiol 2000;10:443–9.
[72] Lembcke A, et al. Papillary fibroelastoma of the aortic valve appearance in 64-slice spiral computed tomography, magnetic resonance imaging, and echocardiography. Circulation 2007;115:e3–6.
[73] Cho JM, et al. Surgical resection of ventricular cardiac fibromas: early and late results. Ann Thorac Surg 2003;76:1929–34.
[74] Yang HS, et al. Left atrial fibroma in Gardner Syndrome. Circulation 2008;118:e692–6.
[75] Veinot JP, et al. Cardiac fibroma mimicking apical hypertrophic cardiomyopathy: a case report and differential diagnosis. J Am Soc Echocardiogr 1996;9:94–9.
[76] Burke AP, et al. Cardiac fibroma: clinicopathologic correlates and surgical treatment. J Thorac Cardiovasc Surg 1994;108:862–70.

[77] Kiaffas MG, Powell AJ, Geva T. Magnetic resonance imaging evaluation of cardiac tumor characteristics in infants and children. Am J Cardiol 2002;89:1229–33.
[78] Berkenblit R, et al. MRI in the evaluation and management of a newborn infant with cardiac rhabdomyoma. Ann Thorac Surg 1997;63:1475–7.
[79] Brizard C, et al. Cardiac hemangiomas. Ann Thorac Surg 1993;56:390–4.
[80] Kojima S, et al. Cardiac hemangioma: a report of two cases and review of the literature. Heart Vessels 2003;18:153–6.
[81] Lepper W, et al. Assessment of the vascularity of a left ventricular mass using myocardial contrast echocardiography. J Am Soc Echocardiogr 2002;15:1419–22.
[82] Oshima H, et al. Cardiac hemangioma of the left atrial appendage: CT and MR findings. J Thorac Imaging 2003;18:204–6.
[83] Hamidi M, et al. Primary cardiac sarcoma. Ann Thorac Surg 2010;90:176–81.
[84] Donsbeck A, et al. Primary cardiac sarcomas: an immunohistochemical and grading study with long-term follow-up of 24 cases. Histopathology 1999;34:295–304.
[85] Beghetti M, et al. Pediatric primary benign cardiac tumors: a 15-year review. Am Heart J 1997;134:1107–14.
[86] Bruna J, Lockwood M. Primary heart angiosarcoma detected by computed tomography and magnetic resonance imaging. Eur Radiol 1998;8:66–8.
[87] Shapiro LM. Cardiac tumours: diagnosis and management. Heart 2001;85:218–22.
[88] Perchinsky MJ, Lichtenstein SV, Tyers GFO. Primary cardiac tumors. Cancer 1997;79:1809–15.
[89] Burke AP, Cowan D, Virmani R. Primary sarcomas of the heart. Cancer 1992;69:387–95.
[90] Holladay AO, Siegel RJ, Schwarfz DA. Cardiac malignant lymphoma in acquired immune deficiency syndrome. Cancer 1992;70:2203–7.
[91] Petrich A, Cho SI, Billett H. Primary cardiac lymphoma. Cancer 2011;117:581–9.
[92] Ceresoli GL, et al. Primary cardiac lymphoma in immunocompetent patients. Cancer 1997;80:1497–506.
[93] Dorsay TA, et al. Primary cardiac lymphoma: CT and MR findings. J Comput Assist Tomogr 1993;17:978–81.
[94] Tada H, et al. Primary cardiac B-cell lymphoma. Circulation 1998;97:220–1.
[95] Abraham KP, Reddy V, Gattuso P. Neoplasms metastatic to the heart: review of 3314 consecutive autopsies. Am J Cardiovasc Pathol 1990;3:195–8.
[96] Klatt EC, Heitz DR. Cardiac metastases. Cancer 1990;65:1456–9.
[97] Crean AM, Juli C. Diagnosis of metastatic melanoma to the heart with an intrinsic contrast approach using melanin inversion recovery imaging. J Comput Assist Tomogr 2007;31:924–30.
[98] Mousseaux E, et al. Cardiac metastatic melanoma investigated by magnetic resonance imaging. Magn Reson Imaging 1998;16:91–5.

Pericardial diseases

B. Cosyns*, B. Paelinck†, O. Cappeliez‡
*Universitair Ziekenhuis Brussel, Brussels, Belgium; †Antwerp University Hospital, Edegem, Belgium; ‡CHIREC, Brussels, Belgium

18.1 Introduction

Pericardial diseases represent a broad range of clinical syndromes and may be present in various associated diseases conveying significant morbidity and mortality [1,2]. The evaluation of pericardial conditions can be complex, and imaging techniques play a key role for an appropriate clinical approach. Although echocardiography is the first-line imaging technique for the diagnosis and the follow-up of pericardial disease, computed tomography (CT), and cardiac magnetic resonance (CMR) imaging offer many advantages in providing complementary information to echocardiography [3]. This chapter will illustrate the ability of different noninvasive imaging techniques in the diagnosis and the management of pericardial diseases in various clinical scenarios.

18.2 Technical aspects

The main strengths of CT and CMR as compared with echocardiography are superior anatomic visualization and tissue characterization. Different modalities may be used with each technique and may have various advantages and limitations as summarized in Table 18.1.

Bi-dimensional echocardiography is the examination of choice for the evaluation of pericardial effusion, and allows the assessment of the hemodynamic and functional consequences of pericardial disease. 2D echocardiography's image quality has enhanced dramatically with improved technology, including new probes with better crystals, better spatial resolution, and signal-noise ratio. An additional transesophageal approach may be useful in particular cases. The use of tissue harmonic imaging has also improved the field of view, reducing inadequate examinations to 5–10%. Contrast echocardiography may improve the detection of pericardial effusion, especially in the acute setting of myocardial infarction with pseudoaneurysm and free-wall rupture [4]. M-mode can play a complementary role for demonstrating a flattening of the posterior wall during diastole or the respiratory variation of ventricular size. Doppler allows the evaluation of restrictive inflow and the reciprocal respiratory changes of mitral and tricuspid inflow. Tissue Doppler imaging velocity analysis is now part of all echocardiographic examinations in patients with pericardial disease to help to make the difference between constrictive pericarditis and restrictive cardiomyopathy with an

Table 18.1 **Imaging the pericard: advantages and limitations of each modality**

Echocardiography	Cardiac CT	CMR
Advantages		
First line for diagnosis and follow-up	Anatomic assessment	Anatomic assessment
Widely available	Evaluation of associated/extracardiac disease	Evaluation of associated/extracardiac disease
Low cost	Preoperative planning	Preoperative planning
Safe and repeatable	Detection of pericardial calcification	Safe and repeatable
Bedside (critically ill and pericardiocentesis)		Functional assessment
Hemodynamics		
Functional assessment		
Modalities		
M-mode	Axial imaging	Cine SSFP
2D echocardiography	Multiplanar reconstruction	Black blood spin-echo (+STIR)
Doppler	Volume rendered imaging	Tagging
Tissue Doppler	Cine-imaging	
Deformation Imaging including twist and rotation		Late gadolinium enhancement
3D echocardiography		Real-time gradient-echo cine
Contrast echocardiography		
Limitations		
Echogenicity	Ionizing radiation	Time-consuming
Acoustic windows	Iodinated contrast	Difficult in case of arrhythmias
Operator dependency	Functional evaluation only possible with retrospective gated studies	Contraindications (e.g. pacemakers, AICD,...)
Limited tissue characterization	Difficult in case of arrhythmias	Calcifications not well visualized
	Patient cooperation (breath-holding)	Gadolinium not recommended if glomeral filtration rate <30 ml/min)
	Hemodynamically stable patients only	Patient cooperation (breath-holding)
		Hemodynamically stable patients only

E' cut-off proposed at <7 cm/s favoring the diagnosis of restrictive cardiomyopathy. Deformation imaging has entered the clinical arena mainly to assess the impact of various pathological conditions on ventricular function. Strain is a measure of how much an object has been deformed, and several formulas can be used to calculate different types of strain. The preferred modality is speckle-tracking echocardiography (STE) [5,6]. In addition, left ventricular (LV) rotation can be measured clinically by STE and twist and torsion can be calculated [7,8]. In a normal individual, the heart slides and twists easily within the parietal pericardium, which is lubricated by a small amount of fluid. The importance of this motion has been illustrated in experiments in which the epicardium has been fixed to the pericardium [9]. Pericardial adhesions reduced LV twist by limiting the free motion of the heart inside the pericardium. In patients with congenital absence of the pericardium, a reduction in LV twist has been reported [10]. Finally, three-dimensional echocardiography has the potential to provide a complete evaluation of the entire pericardium in any anatomical plane, and therefore detect loculated effusions. New software programs to accurately quantify the volume of liquid in the pericardium are under evaluation.

CT is a widely available technique with a short acquisition time of a few seconds. Modern CT scanners have a spatial resolution well below 1.0 mm. High temporal resolution and dedicated image acquisition techniques, which either trigger prospective image acquisition to the patient's electrocardiogram or retrospectively select raw data acquired during suitable segments of the cardiac cycle for image reconstruction, provide motion artifact free data sets [11]. The pericardium can be visualized both in noncontrast and contrast-enhanced CT data sets. Following the administration of intravenous contrast, enhancement of thickened pericardium can be observed in case of suspected pericarditis or tumor infiltration [3,12–14]. Iodinated contrast administration is contraindicated in advanced renal failure. Furthermore, CT is highly sensitive for identifying calcification, and volume-rendered imaging allows a precise evaluation of the extent and distribution of pericardial calcification.

Multiplanar reconstruction CT can provide secondary functional information, such as enlargement of the atria and venae cavae in cases of pericardial constriction, but cine imaging ventricular functional parameters can be acquired only with retrospective ECG-gated acquisitions, requiring an increased radiation dose.

CMR imaging is performed by using magnetic gradient field switches and radiofrequency waves. Improvements in scanner hardware (powerful gradients and coils for parallel imaging) and software (new sequences) have resulted in improved image quality and shortened scan time [15]. CMR requires a stable heart rhythm and respiratory cooperation (breath-hold sequences). Therefore, CMR imaging is feasible in hemodynamic stable patients only. Due to the absence of signal from calcium, CMR cannot directly prove the presence of calcification. The use of gadolinium intravenous contrast is contraindicated in advanced renal insufficiency (glomerular filtration rate <30 ml/min). Largely, CMR is contraindicated in patients with a pacemaker or defibrillator. The imaging protocol may differ depending on the diagnostic question [3,16]. Imaging sequences are triggered by ECG. One scan protocol consists of dark-blood morphological images (fast spin-echo or newer half-Fourier acquisition turbo spin-echo = HASTE) for tissue characterization, detection of effusion, and assessment of pericardial thickening, respectively. Cine images (steady-state free precession = SSFP) in the short-axis and long-axis planes are used to evaluate atrial and ventricular size, shape, and function, but also pericardial thickening or effusion. Real-time cine images allow assessment of exaggerated ventricular interdependence. Late gadolinium enhancement of the pericardium indicates inflammation [17].

18.3   The pericardium: normal findings

The pericardium is a fibrous sac surrounding the heart. It consists of two layers: the visceral (serous) pericardium, which folds back to form the parietal (fibrous) pericardium at the base of the heart forming the pericardial space. The pericardial space normally contains a trace of pericardial fluid (<15–35 ml). There are two blind ending pockets or recesses: the sinus tranversus (behind the big arteries) and the sinus obliquus (behind the left atrium).

The normal pericardium is not easily visualized by echocardiography (Figure 18.1).

On CT, the pericardium is seen as a thin, intermediate density linear structure (against the surrounding fat, which displays low attenuation) (Figure 18.2). The normal pericardium is best seen anterior to the right ventricle and at the apex of the heart as opposed to the left lateral and left posterior wall because of the scarcity of pericardial fat.

The normal fibrous pericardium is visible as a thin (<4 mm) low-intensity line on morphologic T1- and T2-weighted spin-echo images and on gradient echo cine images, surrounded by high-intensity pericardial fat [5,6] (Figure 18.3).

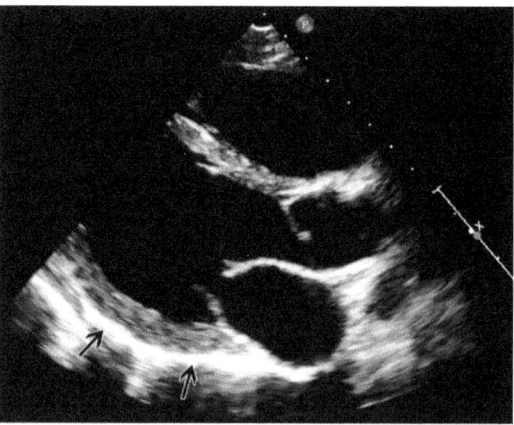

Figure 18.1 Parasternal long-axis view showing a normal pericardium (arrows).

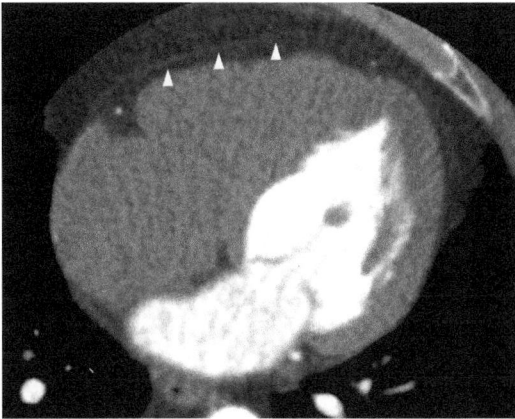

Figure 18.2 Computed tomography showing a normal pericardium (arrows).

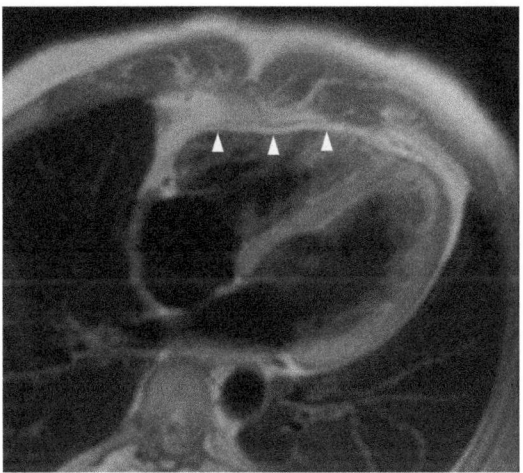

Figure 18.3 MRI showing a normal pericardium (arrows).

18.4 Clinical scenarios

18.4.1 Acute pericarditis

18.4.1.1 Definition and etiologies

It is a clinical syndrome characterized by typical chest pain eventually accompanied by friction rub and/or characteristic ECG changes or an elevation of inflammatory markers in relation with pericardial inflammation. Most of the cases are of idiopathic or viral etiology, but systemic illnesses, malignancies, or acute ischemic cardiac disease are other potential etiologies. An imaging test should be performed within the first 24 h of presentation to search for pericardial effusion, its characteristics, etiology, and its hemodynamic consequences. Echocardiography is the first-line examination.

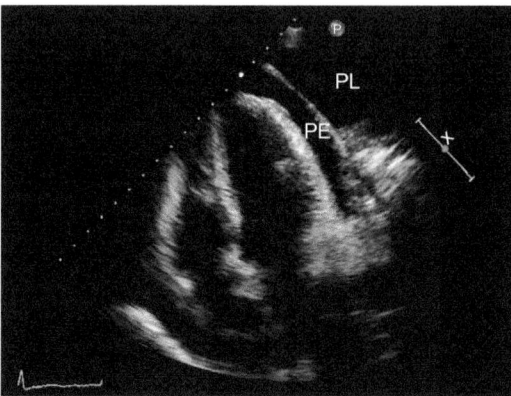

Figure 18.4 Apical four-chamber view showing acute pericardial effusion (PE) and concomitant pleural effusion (PL).

Echocardiography is useful to rule out ischemic heart disease. In acute pericarditis, echocardiography may appear normal. The amount of pericardial fluid can be variable, large, or localized (Figure 18.4). Bright or thickened pericardium is a less specific feature that can also be observed. Echogenic material within the pericardial effusion suggests clotted blood usually, primary or secondary tumors, or inflammatory origin. Tamponade physiology needs to be evaluated. It is important to note that in patients with large effusion, pericardiocentesis has to be considered even in the absence of typical features of tamponade. CMR has the ability to visualize pericardial inflammation (T2-weighted spin-echo STIR to visualize edema and late gadolinium enhancement to detect inflammation [17,18]), thickening and fluid. In addition, late gadolinium enhancement allows diagnosis of associated myocarditis [19–21] (Figure 18.5). CMR should be considered to confirm the diagnosis of pericarditis, to detect small effusions,

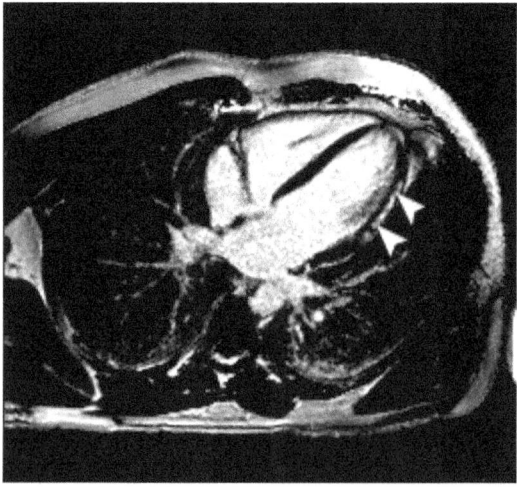

Figure 18.5 Acute pericarditis with subepicardial late gadolinium enhancement of the left ventricular myocardial wall in acute myocarditis (arrowheads).

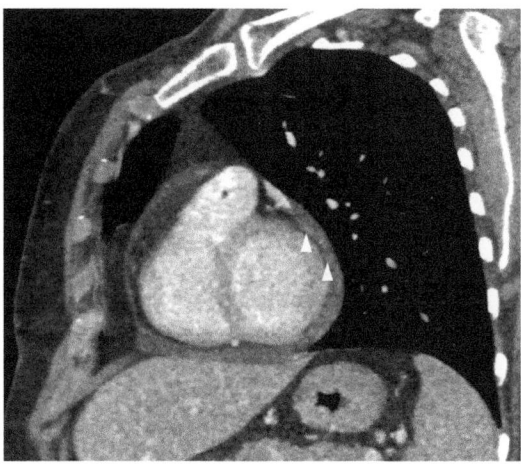

Figure 18.6 Effusion showed by CT during acute pericarditis.

and to investigate a complicated course. Noninvasive assessment of hemodynamics is done by echo, but CMR can also provide similar information. Uncomplicated/simple effusions usually have low signal intensity on T1-weighted images. Pericardial effusions demonstrate high signal intensity on cine gradient SSFP images. Hemorrhage can be suspected when the effusion is complex and contains regions of different signal intensity. CT has the ability to diagnose pericardial effusion (Figure 18.6). It is particularly suited to diagnose localized pericardial effusion. CT provides limited characterization of pericardial fluid by attenuation values (Hounsfield units=HU). Generally, 30 HU is a useful cutoff between simple effusions and bloody or exudative effusions. The more HU corresponds to the more protein content. A noncalcified thickening of the pericardium with or without effusion can be suggestive of acute pericarditis. Enhancement of the pericardium with the administration of iodinated contrast suggests an active inflammation process [12,13].

18.4.2 Subacute pericarditis and chronic pericarditis without constriction

18.4.2.1 Definition and etiologies

Subacute or recurrent pericarditis should be considered when pericarditis lasts longer than 3 months or when episodes of pericarditis are reoccurring after a latent or asymptomatic period of >6 weeks. Most of the time, it is related to autoimmune inflammation, neoplasm, viral reactivation, or tuberculosis. Echocardiographic findings are similar to the findings observed in acute pericarditis. In addition, constrictive physiology has to be assessed. Although cardiac CT and CMR are usually not indicated as a first-line examination in this setting, these modalities may be helpful if echocardiography is inconclusive, when malignancy is suspected, to show the presence of blood, or to assess the inflammatory changes of the pericardium during treatment course (Figures 18.7 and 18.8).

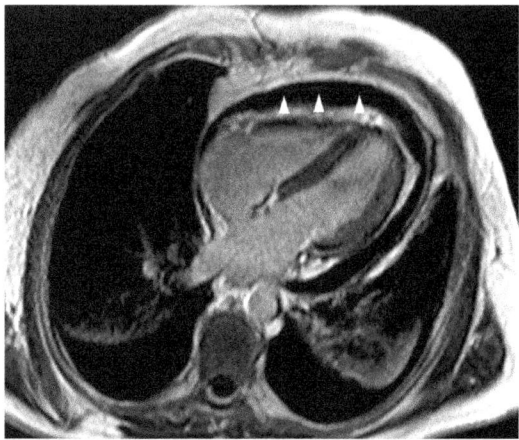

Figure 18.7 Example of chronic pericarditis without constriction (arrows).

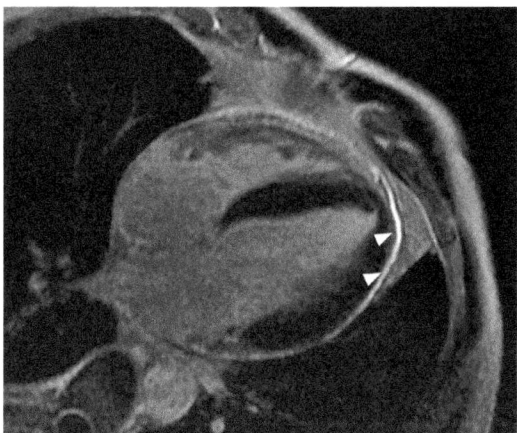

Figure 18.8 Late gadolinium enhancement of inflammation in chronic pericarditis (arrows).

18.4.3 Cardiac tamponade and pericardiocentesis

18.4.3.1 Definition and etiologies

Tamponade is a critical clinical condition related to the presence of pericardial fluid under pressure limiting cardiac filling. The severity of symptoms is depending on the amount, the localization, and the rate of fluid accumulation. Main etiologies are similar to acute pericarditis. Bedside echocardiography should be performed urgently in case of initial suspicion. Cardiac CT and CMR are usually not required, but may be useful to in case of less typical hemodynamics, especially and if tamponade is not clear [22]. When the imaging quality is poor, transesophageal echocardiography will help to confirm the diagnosis even in case of postsurgical hematomas or of loculated effusions [23]. Imaging findings in cardiac tamponade are summarized in Table 18.2.

Table 18.2 Imaging findings pericardial tamponade

Echocardiography	CT	CMR

M-mode:
- Effusion
- Echogenic effusion = usually haemorrhagic effusion/clots
- Respiratory, reciprocal changes RV and LV size
- Respiratory changes interventricular septum (septal bounce)
- Inferior vena cava and hepatic vein dilatation + blunted respiratory changes
 	
2D:
- Effusion
- Localization of effusion
- Echogenic effusion = usually haemorrhagic effusion/clots
- Respiratory, reciprocal changes RV and LV size
- Respiratory changes interventricular septum (septal bounce)
- Collapse cavity (-ies): RV diastolic collapse, RA systolic collapse/inversion (duration>1/3 systole)
- Swinging motion (in large circumferential effusion)
- Inferior vena cava and hepatic vein dilatation + blunted respiratory changes
 	
Doppler:
- Respiratory, reciprocal changes RV and LV filling:
- Inspiratory increase (>25%) and exspiratory decrease of forward flow right; inspiratory decrease (>25%) and expiratory increase of forward flow left
	Static and dynamic:
	- Effusion
	- Localization effusion
	- Characterization fluid:
	  <30HU: simple effusion
	  ≥30HU: usually hemorrhagic/protein rich effusion
	
	Static:
	- Angulation or bowing of the interventricular septum
	- Flattened heart
	- Inferior vena cava and hepatic vein dilatation
	
	Dynamic:
	- Collapse cavity (-ies)
	- Inferior vena cava and hepatic vein dilatation
		All sequences:
		- Effusion
		- Localization of effusion
		- Characterization fluid:
		  Low T1: simple effusion
		  High T1 or complex: hemorrhagic effusion
		
		Real-time cine:
		- Respiratory, reciprocal changes RV and LV size
		- Respiratory changes interventricular septum (septal bounce)
		- Inferior vena cava and hepatic vein dilatation + blunted respiratory changes
		
		Cine SSFP:
		- Collapse cavity (-ies): RV diastolic collapse, RA systolic collapse/inversion (duration>1/3 systole)
		- Swinging motion (in large circumferential effusion)
		- Inferior vena cava and hepatic vein dilatation

CMR, cardiovascular magnetic resonance; CT, computed tomography; HU, Hounsfield Unit; LV, left ventricle; RV, right ventricle; SSFP, steady-state free precession.

Echocardiography (with or without contrast injection) is the tool of choice for guiding pericardiocentesis and to assess the immediate hemodynamic effect of fluid removal.

18.4.4 Chronic constrictive pericarditis

18.4.4.1 Definition and etiologies

It occurs when the diseased pericardium limits the filling of the ventricles because of decrease in its compliance. It is a difficult clinical diagnosis. The most common etiologies are postcardiac surgery, viral infections, radiation, tuberculosis, and idiopathic depending on the regions. Echocardiography with respirometry plays a key role for establishing the diagnosis of constriction in most of the patients based on M-mode, 2D echocardiography, Doppler, Doppler flow velocity imaging, and Strain imaging observations. It allows the differential diagnosis with alternative pathologies, such as restrictive cardiomyopathy, right ventricular dysfunction, or severe tricuspid regurgitation. Additional imaging testing (cardiac CT or CMR) is required in patients with inconclusive echocardiography but is often necessary for subsequent management. These two techniques evaluate the pericardium anatomy more precisely, and allow the presence of coexistent myocardial or pulmonary disease. CT is the best technique to detect and localize pericardial calcifications, especially when a pericardiotomy is planned (Figure 18.9). The different technical modalities of examination and typical findings obtained in this setting with CT and CMR are summarized in Table 18.3.

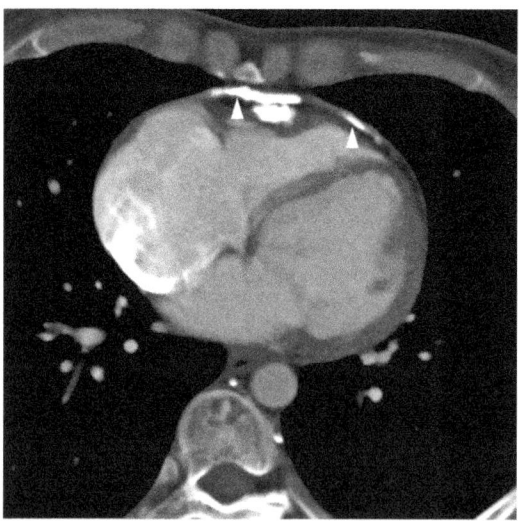

Figure 18.9 CT is the best technique to localize and to evaluate the extent of pericardial calcifications (arrows).

Table 18.3 Imaging findings constrictive pericarditis

Echocardiography	CT	CMR
M-mode: • Thickened pericardium and increased echogenicity of the pericardium • Flattened motion of the posterior wall in diastole • Inspiratory shift of the interventricular septum to the left septal bounce • Inferior vena cava and hepatic vein dilatation + blunted respiratory changes	**Static and dynamic:** • Pericardial thickness ≥0.4 cm localization pericardial thickening	**T1 and T2 spin-echo:** **SSFP:** • Pericardial thickness ≥0.4 cm localization pericardial thickening
2D: • Inspiratory shift of the interventricular septum to the left (septal bounce) • Early diastolic LV and RV diastolic filling halt (diastolic checking) • Inferior vena cava and hepatic vein dilatation + blunted respiratory changes	**Static and dynamic:** • Pericardial calcification	Late gadolinium enhancement and **T2-STIR:** • Pericardial inflammation and edema
Doppler: • Restrictive filling left and right ventricle • Reciprocal respiratory changes in E-wave velocity: Transmitral ≥25% increase at exspiration and transtricuspid ≥40% increase at inspiration • Hepatic vein forward flow markedly increases with inspiration and decreases with exspiration, together with prominent holodiastolic flow rersersal	**Static:** • Narrowing and tubular deformation of the right or left ventricle, normal or small ventricular size, and straightening of the interventricular septum	**Tagging:** • Pericardial-myocardial adherence

Continued

Table 18.3 Continued

Echocardiography	CT	CMR
Tissue Doppler: • E' <7 cm/s (septal annulus) • E/E' low, despite high ventricular filling pressures (annulus paradoxus)		Real-time cine: • Inspiratory shift of the interventricular septum to the left (septal bounce) • Abrupt cessation of diastolic filling
Color M-mode: • Normal or increased propagation velocity of early diastolic transmitral flow	Static and dynamic: • Vena cava inferior and hepatic vein dilatation	Cine SSFP: • Vena cava inferior and hepatic vein dilatation
Speckle tracking: • Reduced LV twist		Velocity encoded CMR (phase-contrast): • Restrictive filling left and right ventricle

CMR, cardiovascular magnetic resonance; CT, computed tomography; E, early diastolic transmitral flow velocity; E', early diastolic septal mitral annulus velocity; LV, left ventricle; RV, right ventricle; SSFP, steady-state free precession.

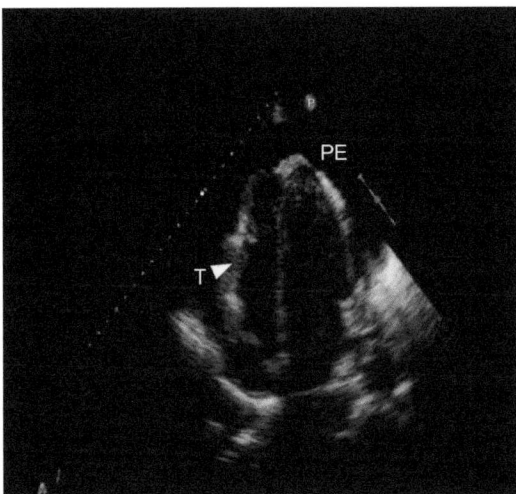

Figure 18.10 Echo apical four-chamber view showing a large pericardial effusion (PE) with thickened or fibrous pericardium (T). Effusive constrictive pericarditis should be suspected when the clincal state does not improve after pericardiocentesis and the clinical features are those of constrictive pericarditis.

18.4.5 Effusive constrictive pericarditis

18.4.5.1 Definition and etiologies

It is a rare clinical entity characterized by the hemodynamic occurrence of an elevated RA pressure, elevated RV and LV pressures with a respiratory interventricular dependence occurring after pericardiocentesis, typically when pericardial fluid accumulates between a thickened or fibrous parietal and visceral pericardium (Figure 18.10). In this condition, the clinical state of the patient doesn't improve after the pericardiocentesis, and the clinical features are those of CP. It may also be considered in case of patients with a clinical presentation of right heart failure and chronic effusion. Most of the time, effusive constrictive pericarditis is idiopathic, induced by radiation or related to malignancy. Early stage echocardiography features are typically those of pericardial effusion with tamponade, while late stage features are those of CP. Irregularities of the visceral pericardium can be observed, and intrapericardial material is also suggestive of CP. The role of cardiac CT is limited, and CMR can be complementary to echocardiography in cases of poor quality images or in cases of loculated effusion.

18.5 Cardiac masses (cysts, diverticula, hematoma, tumors)

Pericardial cyst and diverticula are uncommon benign lesions and usually incidental findings. Pericardial cysts originate from a part of the pericardium cut from the remainder pericardium during embryologic development. Typically, pericardial cysts are located near the heart in the right anterior cardiophrenic angle (70%). Diverticula can change in size overtime, with the body position, and communicate with the pericardial space. Although echocardiography is the first-line examination, cysts and diverticula appearing as a well-contoured echo-free space to the heart border, CT, and CMR provide better characterization and are usually required to guide management in symptomatic patients. CMR diagnoses pericardial cysts displaying typical tissue characteristics: delineated homogeneous paracardiac structures (most commonly in the right cardiophrenic angle) without septations and with low- to intermediate signal intensity on T1 and high-signal intensity on T2-weighted images [24,25] (Figure 18.11). Cardiac CT can identify pericardial cysts or diverticula in the entire mediastinum as thin-walled, unilocular near-water-attenuation fluid collection. An open communication with the pericardial space can be seen with CT in case of diverticula.

Pericardial hematoma usually occurs following surgery or trauma (Figure 18.12). It may be difficult to diagnose with echocardiography, and transesophageal approach may be required in some acute cases. Their appearance using CT or CMR depends on their age. On CT, they are usually seen as a nonenhancing mass displaying increased attenuation initially but decreasing in density with time [13]. Focal calcifications can be seen in chronic hematomas. On CMR, acute hematomas usually show high signal on T1 as opposed to chronic hematomas, which display a low signal rim on T1 imaging with further low signal foci within the lesion (often related to calcification) (Figure 18.13). Primary pericardial tumors are rare and mesothelioma is the most common. Other primary malignant tumors include sarcomas, lymphomas, and malignant teratomas. These tend to present as large masses with a blood-stained pericardial effusion or as a CP when the thickening of the pericardium is the dominant process. Metastatic pericardial disease is significantly

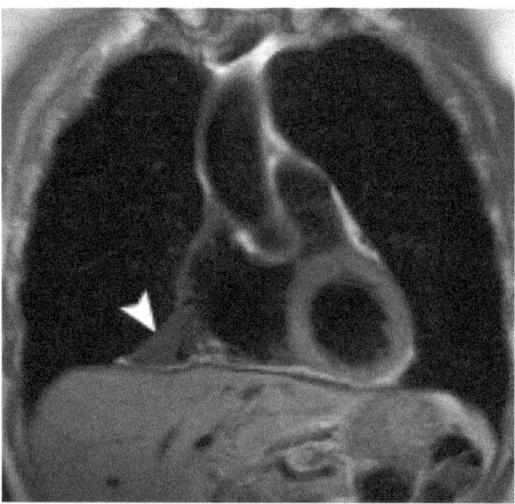

Figure 18.11 Frontal image of a pericardial cyst in the right cardiophrenic angle showing low signal intensity on T1 spin-echo image.

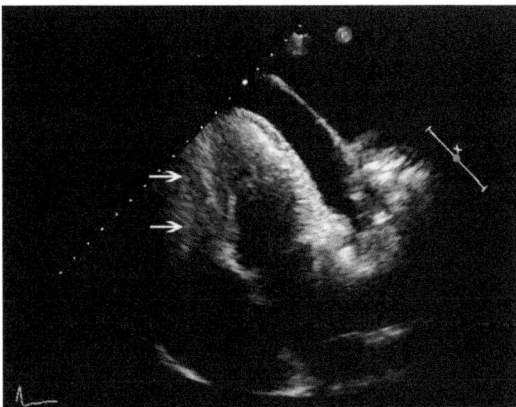

Figure 18.12 Pericardial hematoma after a trauma (arrows), similar density to the myocardium can make it difficult to diagnose.

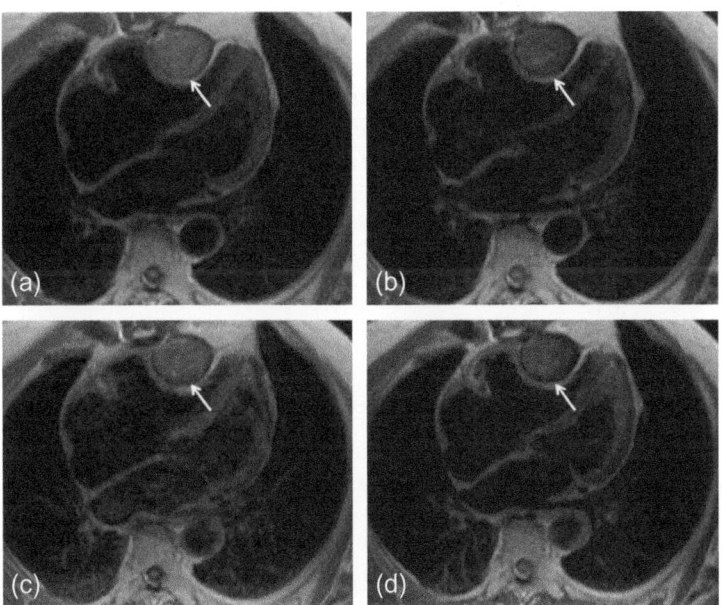

Figure 18.13 Encapsulated pericardial hematoma with compression of the right ventricular free wall after coronary bypass surgery. T1- and T2-weighted images (panels A and B) before and after (panels C and D) gadolinium infusion showing no enhancement.

more common (breast, lung, melanoma, and hematological). Echocardiography is usually the initial investigation. Secondary pericardial tumors are most often diagnosed as pericardial effusion, which tend to be hemorrhagic. CT and CMR allow a better characterization of the lesions and a more precise evaluation of the extension of the tumor (Figure 18.14). Furthermore, these two techniques are more appropriate for identifying other thoracic lesions. Encapsulated and well-defined

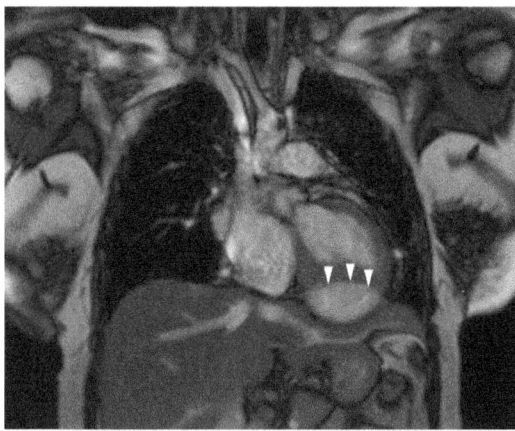

Figure 18.14 Coronal bSSFP image of a malignant synoviosarcoma (arrows).

margins are suggestive of a benign pericardial tumor, while invasion of the great vessels and tethering of surrounding tissue are suggestive of a malign pericardial tumor. Although both techniques may indicate the nature of the tumor by analyzing the densities and morphologic appearance (i.e., liposarcomas will present as a low attenuation tumor on CT with central solid elements, high signal on T1 and low signal on fat-saturation CMR sequences), the imaging features remain rather nonspecific and pericardiocentesis or biopsy is usually required [12]. Tumors frequently display contrast enhancement and delayed contrast wash-out (Figure 18.7).

18.6 Congenital absence of pericardium

Congenital absence of the pericardium is uncommon and is an incidental finding mostly. Partial (usually at the lateral side of the left ventricle) or total agenesis of the pericardium is suspected in extreme levorotation and leftward displacement of the heart or cardiac indentation at the site of the defect (Figure 18.15) [26,27]. Defects of the pericardium are rare (0.002–0.004%) and usually involve the left side. Echocardiographic presentation is variable and can be characterized by an enlarged right ventricle, heart hypermobility in all views, abnormal inter-ventricular motion (mimicking right ventricle overload) and may be associated with other congenital abnormalities or tricuspid chordae rupture associated with severe tricuspid regurgitation. The absence of pericardial layer with CT or CMR is challenging because of the difficulty to differentiate from the adjacent myocardium or epicardial fat. Indirect signs like levorotation of the heart may suggest the diagnosis. The most specific sign is interposition of lung tissue between the aorta and the pulmonary artery or between the diaphragm and the base of the heart (Figure 18.5).

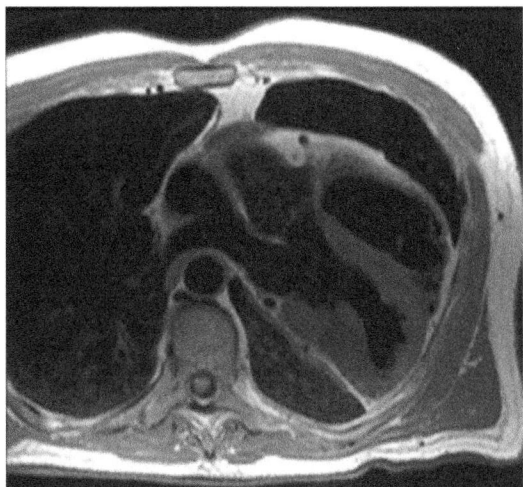

Figure 18.15 T1-weighted four chamber image showing extreme levorotation in agenesis of the pericardium.

References

[1] Khandaker MH, Espinosa RE, Nishimura RA, Sinak LJ, Hayes SN, Melduni RM, et al. Pericardial disease: diagnosis and management. Mayo Clin Proc 2010;85(6):572–93.
[2] Troughton RW, Asher CR, Klein AL. Pericarditis. Lancet 2004;363(9410):717–27.
[3] Verhaert D, Gabriel RS, Johnston D, Lytle BW, Desai MY, Klein AL. The role of multimodality imaging in the management of pericardial disease. Circ Cardiovasc Imaging 2010;3(3):333–43.
[4] Main ML, Ryan AC, Davis TE, Albano MP, Kusnetzky LL, Hibberd M. Acute mortality in hospitalized patients undergoing echocardiography with and without an ultrasound contrast agent (multicenter registry results in 4,300,966 consecutive patients). Am J Cardiol 2008;102(12):1742–6.
[5] Amundsen BH, Helle-Valle T, Edvardsen T, Torp H, Crosby J, Lyseggen E, et al. Noninvasive myocardial strain measurement by speckle tracking echocardiography: validation against sonomicrometry and tagged magnetic resonance imaging. J Am Coll Cardiol 2006;47(4):789–93.
[6] Mor-Avi V, Lang RM, Badano LP, Belohlavek M, Cardim NM, Derumeaux G, et al. Current and evolving echocardiographic techniques for the quantitative evaluation of cardiac mechanics: ASE/EAE consensus statement on methodology and indications endorsed by the Japanese Society of Echocardiography. Eur J Echocardiogr 2011;12(3): 167–205.
[7] Notomi Y, Setser RM, Shiota T, Martin-Miklovic MG, Weaver JA, Popovic ZB, et al. Assessment of left ventricular torsional deformation by Doppler tissue imaging: validation study with tagged magnetic resonance imaging. Circulation 2005;111(9): 1141–7.
[8] Helle-Valle T, Crosby J, Edvardsen T, Lyseggen E, Amundsen BH, Smith HJ, et al. New noninvasive method for assessment of left ventricular rotation: speckle tracking echocardiography. Circulation 2005;112(20):3149–56.

[9] Alharthi MS, Jiamsripong P, Calleja A, Sengupta PP, McMahon EM, Khandheria B, et al. Selective echocardiographic analysis of epicardial and endocardial left ventricular rotational mechanics in an animal model of pericardial adhesions. Eur J Echocardiogr 2009;10(3):357–62.

[10] Tanaka H, Oishi Y, Mizuguchi Y, Miyoshi H, Ishimoto T, Nagase N, et al. Contribution of the pericardium to left ventricular torsion and regional myocardial function in patients with total absence of the left pericardium. J Am Soc Echocardiogr 2008;21(3):268–74.

[11] Halliburton SS. Recent technologic advances in multi-detector row cardiac CT. Cardiol Clin 2009;27(4):655–64.

[12] Wang ZJ, Reddy GP, Gotway MB, Yeh BM, Hetts SW, Higgins CB. CT and MR imaging of pericardial disease. Radiographics 2003; 23(1):167–80.

[13] O'Leary SM, Williams PL, Williams MP, Edwards AJ, Roobottom CA, Morgan-Hughes GJ, et al. Imaging the pericardium: appearances on ECG-gated 64-detector row cardiac computed tomography. Br J Radiol 2010;83(987):194–205.

[14] Rajiah P, Kanne JP. Computed tomography of the pericardium and pericardial disease. J Cardiovasc Comput Tomogr 2010;4(1):3–18.

[15] Fuster V, Kim RJ. Frontiers in cardiovascular magnetic resonance. Circulation 2005;112(1):135–44.

[16] Bogaert J, Francone M. Cardiovascular magnetic resonance in pericardial diseases. J Cardiovasc Magn Reson 2009;11:14.

[17] Zurick AO, Bolen MA, Kwon DH, Tan CD, Popovic ZB, Rajeswaran J, et al. Pericardial delayed hyperenhancement with CMR imaging in patients with constrictive pericarditis undergoing surgical pericardiectomy: a case series with histopathological correlation. JACC Cardiovasc Imaging 2011;4(11):1180–91.

[18] Taylor AM, Dymarkowski S, Verbeken EK, Bogaert J. Detection of pericardial inflammation with late-enhancement cardiac magnetic resonance imaging: initial results. Eur Radiol 2006;16(3):569–74.

[19] Friedrich MG, Strohm O, Schulz-Menger J, Marciniak H, Luft FC, Dietz R. Contrast media-enhanced magnetic resonance imaging visualizes myocardial changes in the course of viral myocarditis. Circulation 1998;97(18):1802–9.

[20] Abdel-Aty H, Boye P, Zagrosek A, Wassmuth R, Kumar A, Messroghli D, et al. Diagnostic performance of cardiovascular magnetic resonance in patients with suspected acute myocarditis: comparison of different approaches. J Am Coll Cardiol 2005;45(11):1815–22.

[21] Mahrholdt H, Wagner A, Judd RM, Sechtem U, Kim RJ. Delayed enhancement cardiovascular magnetic resonance assessment of non-ischaemic cardiomyopathies. Eur Heart J 2005;26(15):1461–74.

[22] Mulvagh SL, Rokey R, Vick III GW, Johnston DL. Usefulness of nuclear magnetic resonance imaging for evaluation of pericardial effusions, and comparison with two-dimensional echocardiography. Am J Cardiol 1989;64(16):1002–9.

[23] Berge KH, Lanier WL, Reeder GS. Occult cardiac tamponade detected by transesophageal echocardiography. Mayo Clin Proc 1992;67(7):667–70.

[24] Sechtem U, Tscholakoff D, Higgins CB. MRI of the abnormal pericardium. Am J Roentgenol 1986;147(2):245–52.

[25] Breen JF. Imaging of the pericardium. J Thorac Imaging 2001;16(1):47–54.

[26] Gutierrez FR, Shackelford GD, McKnight RC, Levitt RG, Hartmann A. Diagnosis of congenital absence of left pericardium by MR imaging. J Comput Assist Tomogr 1985;9(3):551–3.

[27] Psychidis-Papakyritsis P, de Roos A, Kroft LJ. Functional MRI of congenital absence of the pericardium. Am J Roentgenol 2007;189(6):W312–4.

Congenital heart disease

19

A.A. Pasquet, B.L. Gerber
Cliniques Universitaires St. Luc Université Catholique de Louvain, Brussels, Belgium

Abbreviations and acronyms

3D	three-dimensional
4 CV	apical 4-chamber view
AICD	automatic implantable cardiac defibrillator
ASD	atrial septal defect
ccTGA	congenitally corrected transposition of the great arteries
CHD	congenital heart disease
CoA	coarctation of the aorta
CMR	cardiac magnetic resonance
CT	computed tomography
LV	left ventricle
LVOT	left ventricular outflow tract
RV	right ventricle
RVOT	right ventricular outflow tract
SPECT	single photon emission computed tomography
TAPSE	tricuspid annular plane systolic excursion
TDI	tissue Doppler imaging
TGA	transposition of the great arteries
TEE	transesophageal echocardiography
TOF	tetralogy of Fallot
TTE	transthoracic echocardiography
VSD	ventricular septal defect

19.1 Introduction

The past 30 years have seen tremendous improvements in diagnosis and treatment of congenital heart disease (CHD). This allows more than 90% of babies born with heart malformation today to reach adulthood. This new population of adults who have CHD brings new problems and diagnostic challenges. Apart from the small number of adult patients who have previously undiagnosed CHD, it is important to recognize surgical corrections, residual lesions, and new complications in previously treated patients. In this setting, cardiac imaging plays an important role in the understanding of cardiac anatomy and physiology, helps to ensure a correct diagnosis of the lesion, and sometimes plays a role in treatment. Recent years have seen a shift from diagnosis by cardiac catheterization to echocardiography and more recently to tomographic techniques such as cardiac magnetic resonance and computed tomography (CT) [1]. In the first part of this chapter, we will review the different imaging modalities available, their advantages and limitations, and then, in the second part of this chapter, we will analyze the role of the different imaging modalities in specific lesions.

19.2 Imaging modalities

Several imaging modalities are currently available to assess patients with CHD. Cardiac catheterization was for a long time the reference technique for diagnosis.

19.2.1 Echocardiography

Echocardiography is and remains the first-line technique in patients who have CHD. It must be performed in every patient who has or is suspected to have CHD. It has the advantage of being a widely available, low cost, portable, and radiation-free technique, and it provides information on both anatomy and physiology (see Chapter 2). CHD may cover a very wide range of lesions, from a simple "hole" such as an atrial septal defect (ASD) or a ventricular septal defect (VSD) to very complex anatomy such as transposition of the great arteries (TGA) corrected by atrial switch. Because the initial anatomy may have been modified by surgical intervention (baffle, conduit, and so on), it is important to precisely know not only the malformation but also all the surgical interventions that have been performed. Therefore, it is important to use a segmental approach when performing an echo on a patient with CHD [2,3]. The first step is to know the position of the heart (*dextro* or *levo* position). This step is best achieved using the subcostal view, which also allows for assessment of the position of the liver. The second step is to recognize the cardiac chambers and their relative positions. For example, the morphological right ventricle has coarse trabeculations and a moderator band, and the tricuspid valve is the only atrioventricular valve with three leaflets and septal attachments (the mitral valve is a two-leaflet valve with attachments on papillary muscles normally located in the anterolateral or posteromedial position). The third step is to look at the arrangement of the great vessels: the aorta and the pulmonary artery. Finally, surgical "modifications" will be investigated.

In addition to this important anatomical knowledge, echocardiography allows assessment of ventricular function and volume or pressure overload. Doppler techniques play a determinant role in the assessment of intracardiac shunts (ASD, VSD, and so on), valvular function (regurgitation or stenosis), right ventricular or left ventricular outflow tract obstruction, surgical conduit or baffle obstruction, and pulmonary pressure using the velocity of tricuspid regurgitant jet.

Despite numerous strengths, echocardiography has some limitations due to poor acoustic windows after surgery or due to unusual heart positions. Some structures, including the pulmonary veins, the great arteries, and the pulmonary artery branches, are difficult to assess. Because of the heart's particular structure, right ventricular function and volumes may be poorly assessed by echocardiography, especially in the case of a systemic ventricle or tetralogy of fallot (TOF) [4–6]. This is also the case for univentricular hearts. Doppler measurements also have limitations and may lead to misinterpretation of the severity of lesions: This is particularly true in aortic coarctation, right ventricular outflow tact obstruction, and serial stenosis [7].

In some cases, transesophageal echocardiography (TEE) may provide additional information. The main indications accepted for TEE are [8,9]:

1. Diagnostic indications:
   - inconclusive transthoracic echocardiography (TTE) in suspected or known CHD (poor TTE acoustic windows)
   - evaluation of intracardiac or extracardiac baffles following Fontan or atrial switch repair operation
2. General indications: infective endocarditis, prosthetic valve function, before cardioversion
3. Perioperative indication
4. For percutaneous procedure guidance: e.g., ASD closure

Tissue Doppler imaging (TDI) was proposed to assess right ventricular function and circumvent one of the limitations of conventional 2D echocardiography [10]. Because of all the limitations related to the technique, it was never widely used.

Real-time three-dimensional (3D) echocardiography could also provide useful information. In patients who have heart defects (e.g., ASDs), it allows for precise location and measurement of the defect's dimensions to guide therapeutic decisions. In complex CHD, 3D echocardiography shows the relative position of each structure. It also represents a valuable tool for assessing RV and LV ventricular function and valve disease [11,12].

Deformation imaging, one of the most recent developments in the field of echocardiography, was also used to assess CHD patients. It seems particularly useful to assess ventricular function and detect subclinical impairment [13,14]. In the future, use of 3D speckle tracking echocardiography will certainly open new opportunities to understand ventricular mechanics in CHD [15].

Stress echocardiography has little indication in CHD except to detect ischemia in coronary abnormalities. Only a few studies have proposed the use of stress echo to assess right ventricular function after atrial switch surgery [16].

19.2.2 Cardiac magnetic resonance imaging

In the past decade, cardiac magnetic resonance imaging (CMR) has gained a particular place in CHD imaging. This technique has several advantages over echocardiography, including the ability to use unrestricted image planes to assess the different cardiac structures or vessels, and the ability to perform tissue characterization without exposing the patient to any radiation, which is particularly relevant for young patients who may require multiple investigations during their lifetimes. CMR allows evaluation of anatomy of native or post-surgery CHD, in particular ventricular function (right and left), measurement of systemic or pulmonary blood flow, quantification of valvular regurgitation, and identification of myocardial fibrosis.

When using echocardiography, it is important to have a good understanding of the underlying CHD and of the previous surgery or surgeries to obtain the most clinically useful information from CMR imaging. A standard approach should be applied to CHD patients to ensure reproducibility and accuracy of measurements [17].

Recently, the European Society of Cardiology published standardized CMR protocols to be used for CHD. Most of the studies realized were performed with 1.5 Tesla CMR; today 3.0 Tesla magnets are used more and more frequently. This may permit not only a shorter examination time but also better spatial and temporal definition of the acquired images [18].

A typical CMR approach to a patient who has CHD is:

- *Morphological (T1-weighted) imaging* typically generates a stack of axial images, which provides an anatomical overview.
- *Steady-state free precession* imaging allows for anatomical assessment and evaluation of right and left ventricular volume and function. Two-dimensional stacks of cine images will be acquired in several orientations, allowing visualization of different cardiac structures:
  - vertical long axis, horizontal, and left ventricular short-axis planes,
  - 4-chamber and 3-chamber planes,
  - a coronal, LVOT plane orthogonal to the first, aligned with the flow through the LVOT and aortic valve,
  - aortic arch cine aligned with the arch and proximal descending aorta,
  - RVOT cine(s) aligned with the RVOT and proximal MPA,
  - a contiguous stack of transaxial cines, from the lower heart border up to the aortic arch,
  - a contiguous stack of straight coronal cine images, from the front of the heart to the descending aorta,
  - a stack centered on a particular structure, according to the clinical situation; for example, the atrium, mitral valve, aortic valve.
- *Cine images with tissue tagging* may be acquired to permit assessment of regional deformation or strain of the myocardium [19].
- *Phase contrast sequences* are used to assess flow dynamics. Velocity-encoded images allow measurement of the through phase flow in the aortic and pulmonary arteries, permitting calculation of valve regurgitant volume and fraction and shunt quantification (flow estimate through the pulmonary and the aortic valves). A pitfall of the technique is aliasing; to avoid it, the velocity of encoding should be slightly above the expected peak velocity and increased if necessary. Also, there may be some phase offset that, to be minimized, requires centering the patient in the magnet or a phantom correction [20].
- *Contrast-enhanced magnetic resonance angiography* (CEMRA) is used in CHD to visualize anomalous pulmonary or systemic venous return, and aortic pathology, such as coarctation and associated collaterals.
- *Late gadolinium-enhanced CMR* may be used to view a suspected infarction, infiltration, or scarring [21].

The main indications for using CMR in CHD include:

- as an adjunct to echocardiography, when additional information is necessary to fully assess the clinical problem;
- to confirm echocardiographic findings in valvular disease, ventricular function and volume, and shunt;
- as a first line tool for assessment of RV function and volumes and aortic coarctation.

Particular challenges of using CMR in CHD include the need for sedation or anesthesia in infants, the faster heart rate in children, occasional claustrophobia, and non-MR compatible implants.

19.2.3 Computed tomography

With the arrival of multidetector systems, CT has improved in performance (shortened acquisition times) and precision (spatial resolution) and is now a well-established tool used to analyze cardiac and pulmonary structures [22] (see Chapter 5). CT is the preferred technique to noninvasively assess the coronary artery anatomy, and it is also well suited to analyze prosthetic valves and large stents (e.g., after treatment of aortic coarctation) [23–25]. Additionally, the entire aorta and pulmonary artery can easily be investigated using CT.

ECG-gated CT can be used to obtain volume datasets and calculate left and right ventricular volume and ejection fraction and thus represents an alternative to echocardiography and CMR [26]. Due to the high spatial and temporal resolution of the latest-generation scanners, CT can analyze intracardiac structures, such as valves, like echocardiography or CMR [27]. However, the significant radiation exposure patients receive from CT is an important deterrent for wider use of the technique as a first-line test or for repeat imaging studies, particularly in younger patients.

Most CT examinations require injection of a contrast iodine agent. This is contraindicated in cases of allergy to iodine products, hyperthyroidism, and renal failure.

In addition to cardiac and great vessel anatomy, CT gives also information regarding tracheobronchial anatomy, lung parenchyma, and thoracic bone structures, which may be of interest for particular congenital conditions. Use of radiation represents a major drawback of CT, especially when multiple follow-up studies are contemplated or for younger people. Recently, new acquisition protocols have been developed to minimize the dose of radiation, which will potentially help to promote the use of CT in younger patients who have CHD.

19.2.4 Chest X-ray

Chest X-ray can be used for longitudinal assessment of heart size and could be useful for the assessment of pulmonary vascularization. Nevertheless, its routine use is no longer recommended [1].

19.2.5 Radionuclide imaging

Right or left ventricular ejection fraction and volumes can be calculated by radionuclide angiography using multiple gated acquisitions (MUGAs) obtained after equilibration of ^{99m}Tc-labeled imaging agents. This technique is no longer considered to be a first-line technique because of the lack of other information conveyed about cardiac structure and function and the use of radiation. It must be considered a valuable alternative to assess ventricular function and volume when echocardiography cannot answer the question and when CMR is contraindicated.

In some rare cases of coronary abnormalities or coronary reimplantation, myocardial ischemia could be identified by stress single photon emission computed tomography (SPECT) (see Chapter 3).

Lung perfusion scintigraphy using ^{99m}Tc-macroaggregated albumin may be used to determine perfusion in each lung, which could help to determine the physiological repercussions of pulmonary artery or vein stenosis.

19.2.6 Cardiac catheterization

Developments in echocardiography and tomographic techniques have contributed to the drastic decrease in the use of cardiac catheterization for diagnostic purposes. This technique is currently used to solve specific questions that are not answered by other noninvasive techniques or for hemodynamic assessment rather than for imaging. The remaining indications are measurement of pulmonary vascular resistance and reversibility of pulmonary hypertension; and assessment of coronary arteries, collateral vessels, the pulmonary artery, and, in some cases, surgical shunts (e.g., Glenn shunt, Fontan).

Invasive measurement of systolic and end-diastolic ventricular function, pressure gradients, or shunts should be proposed for patients in whom noninvasive evaluation cannot solve the clinical problem, especially in very complex cases of CHD when the information is required for clinical decision making.

In shunt lesions, if pulmonary hypertension is suspected after echocardiography, confirmation of elevated pulmonary pressure and resistance and vasoreactivity testing using oxygen or nitric oxide are important before making the decision to close the shunt.

However, today, the main use of cardiac catheterization in CHD is for an interventional procedure.

19.2.7 When to use specific imaging

As outlined above, a wide range of imaging techniques is available to assess CHD, often with overlapping indications. Nevertheless, particular techniques are more suited to answer specific questions. Recently, Orwat et al. presented a proposal to appropriately use the different imaging modalities based on the recommendations of the European Society of Cardiology [1,7,18]. An adapted version is listed here:

- Echocardiography is preferred as the first imaging modality to evaluate a patient who has CHD and to try to solve the clinical problem.
- Echocardiography is superior to other imaging techniques for assessment of vegetation or small mobile structures.
- CMR or CT can be used as an alternative technique to echocardiography if reliable information to make a clinical decision cannot be obtained by echocardiography due to poor echocardiographic image quality.
- CMR can be used a second choice when echocardiographic measurements are borderline or need to be confirmed, for example, for ventricular function and volumes (regurgitant and shunt lesion) or assessment of the severity of shunt or regurgitant lesions.
- For some indications, CMR or CT is considered to be superior to echocardiography and bring more valuable information for management of CHD patients. These are:
  - quantification of RV volumes and ejection fraction (TOF, systemic RV, and tricuspid regurgitation) (CMR),

- evaluation of the RV outflow tract and RV-PA conduits (CMR and CT),
- quantification of pulmonary regurgitation (PR) (CMR),
- evaluation of pulmonary arteries (stenoses and aneurysms) and the entire aorta (aneurysm, dissection, coarctation) (CMR and CT) and stents (CT),
- evaluation of systemic and pulmonary veins (anomalous connection, obstruction, and so on) (CMR and CT),
- collaterals and arteriovenous malformations (CT is preferred over CMR),
- coronary anomalies and coronary artery disease (CT is preferred over CMR),
- evaluation of intra- and extracardiac masses (CMR and CT),
- quantification of myocardial masses (CMR and CT),
- detection and quantification of myocardial fibrosis/scar (gadolinium late enhancement) (CMR),
- tissue characterization (fibrosis, fat, iron loading, and so on) (CMR).

When both CMR and CT could be used, the choice between these techniques must take into account the local expertise, the presence of any allergy to the iodine component, the repeated use of radiation, and the presence of a pacemaker or automatic implantable cardioverter-defibrillator (AICD).

19.3 Specific lesions

19.3.1 Atrial septal defect

ASD is the most frequently encountered CHD that goes undiagnosed until adulthood. Indeed, ASD can remain asymptomatic until an advanced age. Several types of ASD can be differentiated:

- The ASD ostium secundum is the most frequent form of ASD, representing 80% of the lesions. It is located in the region of the fossa ovalis, and it is the most frequent form diagnosed in adults.
- The ASD ostium primum is located near the crux of the heart and accounts for approximately 15% of ASDs. It is frequently associated with mitral or tricuspid valve malformation or with VSD, forming a partial or complete atrioventricular canal. Most of the time it will be cured during childhood.
- The sinus venosus ASD is located at the mouths of the caval veins (inferior and superior vena cava) and is frequently associated with partial abnormal venous return.
- Unroofed coronary sinus is a very rare form of ASD characterized by a communication between the coronary sinus and the left atrium. It is associated with a persistent left superior caval vein.

Imaging plays a crucial role in the management of ASD. First, imaging confirms the diagnosis of ASD and its location. Second, imaging is used to quantify the severity of the interatrial shunt and the repercussions of the ASD (e.g., RV dilatation, pulmonary hypertension). Finally, if percutaneous closure is considered, imaging confirms the feasibility and guides the procedure.

Echocardiography is the key examination in a case of suspected ASD. TTE examination must assess the interatrial septum from the parasternal modified long axis,

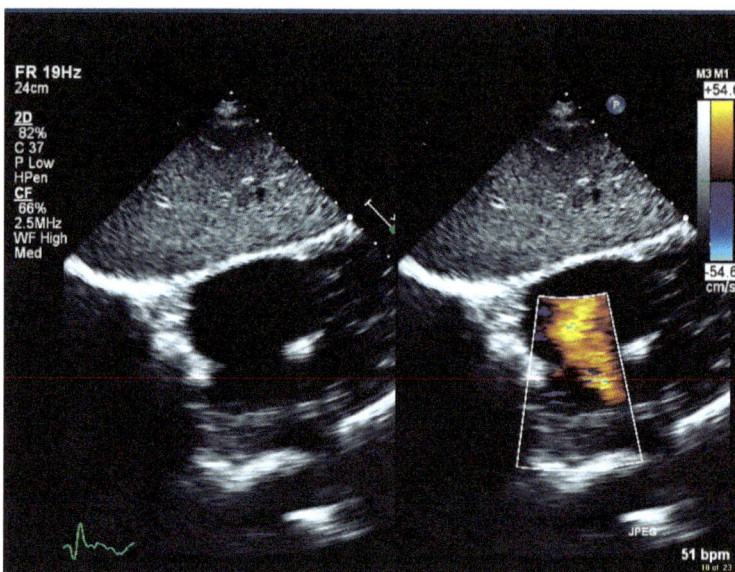

Figure 19.1 TTE subcostal view showing a ASD ostium secundum.

short axis, apical, and subcostal views (Figure 19.1). Color Doppler is used to confirm the shunting. The RV size and volume overload will also be determined using the same views. When an unexplained RV enlargement is discovered, an atrial shunting should always be examined. The severity of the shunt is calculated by the ratio of blood flow in the systemic and pulmonary circulation (Qp/Qs). The calculation requires the measurement of the diameter of the RVOT and LVOT, and the time velocity integral of pulmonary and aortic flow obtained by pulsed Doppler. Unfortunately, measurement is hampered by several potential errors, mainly in the RVOT measurement. Therefore, the clinical use is limited, and international recommendations rely more on RV dilatation to prove the hemodynamic burden of ASD [1,28].

Pulmonary pressures are assessed by continuous wave Doppler using the tricuspid regurgitation.

In the case of ostium primum ASD, mitral and tricuspid valve anatomy and the severity of regurgitation must be assessed before surgical correction (Figure 19.2).

TEE will generally be proposed to confirm defect localization, especially for sinus venosus ASD and pulmonary vein position. Abnormal pulmonary venous drainage is rare in ostium secundum defects, but it may be more often encountered with sinus venosus defects. Moreover, TEE can provide measurements of the size of the ASD, assessment of the remaining septum (search for multiple ASD), and a measurement of the rim if a percutaneous procedure is proposed. If involved, mitral and tricuspid anatomy should be precisely examined by TEE. Three-dimensional TEE has been proposed to assess the size of the defect [29]. As with TEE, 3D TEE can also be used to guide a percutaneous closure [30].

CMR is used as a complement to echocardiography to confirm RV dilatation and volume overload, if echocardiography could not answer the question, or to assess pulmonary vein position. CMR can overcome some limitations of echocardiography

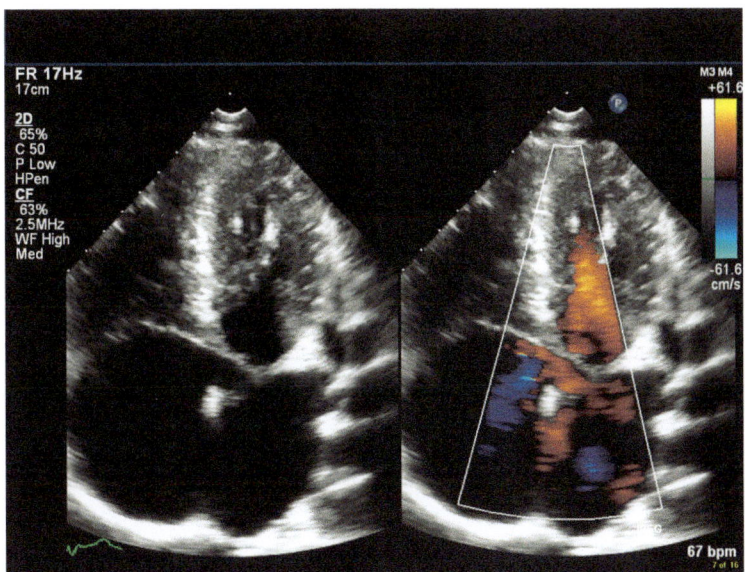

Figure 19.2 TTE apical 4 CV showing ASD ostium primum with color Doppler showing the flow through the ASD.

for Qp/Qs measurement and may be used for this purpose with more accuracy and reproducibility [31]. CT could be an alternative to CMR for RV volume measurement and to search for abnormal pulmonary venous drainage, but it is rarely used for this purpose.

First-pass radionuclide ventriculography is an alternative technique used to measure shunt severity (using first-pass stroke counts for the left and right ventricle) and right ventricular function, but currently it is reserved for patients in whom both echocardiography and CMR were inconclusive or contraindicated.

Finally, cardiac catheterization is used in the case of elevated pulmonary pressure to determine pulmonary vascular resistance and systemic vascular resistance and guide the treatment or to perform a test of reversibility using nitric oxide. ASD closure is contraindicated if pulmonary resistances are >5 Wood units with elevated pulmonary pressure (>2/3 systemic pressure) [1]. A trial of balloon occlusion with a standard sizing balloon can reveal increases in LV or RV filling pressures and/or pulmonary pressures, which preclude percutaneous closure with a nonfenestrated device.

19.3.2 Ventricular septal defect

VSD is the most frequent type of CHD. It may be isolated or associated with other lesions (e.g., TOF, complete atrioventricular canal). Several forms of VSD are described (Figure 19.3).

- A perimembranous/paramembranous/conoventricular VSD located in the membranous septum represents the most common form, accounting for 80% of VSDs.

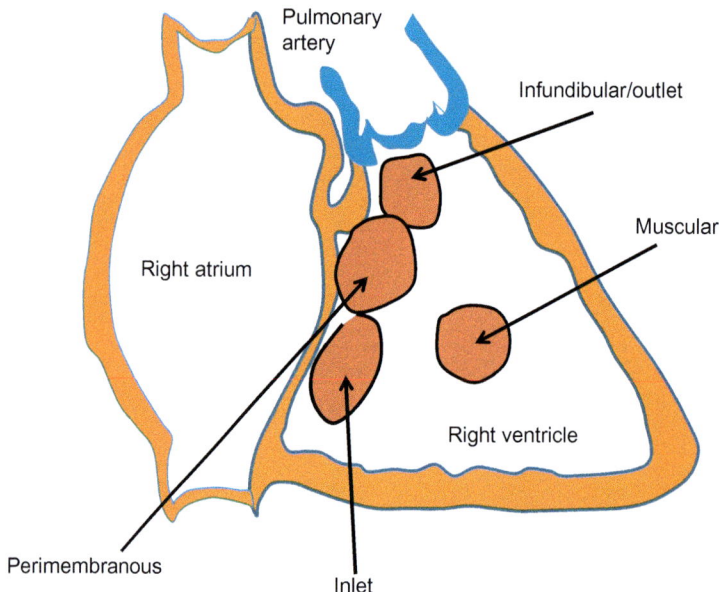

Figure 19.3 Schematic representation of the location of the different types of VSD.

- Muscular VSDs are totally surrounded by myocardial muscle and represent between 15% and 20% of all VSDs.
- Outlet supracristal/subarterial/subpulmonary/infundibular/supracristal/conal/doubly committed juxta-arterial VSDs make up <5% of VSDs. This type is located just below the semilunar valve and is frequently associated with progressive aortic regurgitation due to prolapse of the aortic cusp.
- The inlet/AV canal/AVSD type is the least common (inlet of the ventricular septum inferior to the atrioventricular valve typically occurring in Down syndrome).

Large VSDs cause symptoms and are treated during childhood. Some VSDs will spontaneously close and leave only some aneurysms visible at the level of the membranous septum. Most VSDs are single defects, but some are multiple; thus, a careful examination must always be performed to exclude this possibility.

As with ASD, echocardiography is the cornerstone of diagnosis and hemodynamic assessment of VSD. The whole interventricular septum is assessed using several TTE views to provide the number, location, and size of the VSD (Figure 19.4). The shunt is confirmed by color Doppler. The hemodynamic burden of the VSD is assessed by the severity of LV overload (due to the shunt or to aortic regurgitation). Pulmonary pressure can be estimated from the tricuspid regurgitant jet velocity measured by continuous Doppler. Care must be taken to avoid the VSD jet, which may interfere with the tricuspid regurgitant jet and lead to overestimation of the pulmonary pressure. A turbulent jet through the VSD measured by color Doppler is indicative of a restrictive VSD, but this diagnosis must be confirmed by a continuous Doppler measurement through the jet. A velocity >4 m/s confirms a restrictive VSD. The severity of the shunt can also be evaluated by echocardiography but with the same limitations as for

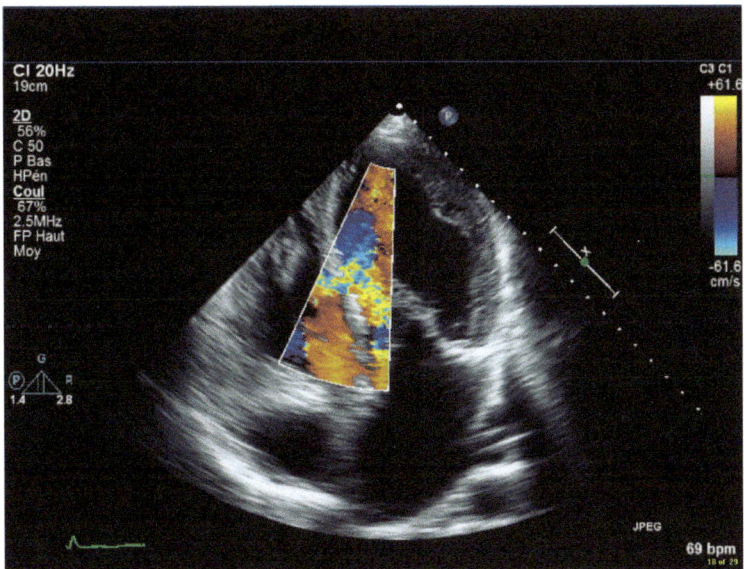

Figure 19.4 TTE apical 44 CV showing a muscular VSD with color Doppler flow.

ASD. Aortic regurgitation may occur with certain types of VSD and can be detected and quantified by echocardiography (see Chapter 16).

TEE is indicated to confirm the location of the VSD, rule out vegetation in the case of suspected endocarditis, and assess aortic valve anatomy in the case of regurgitation. The associated aortic regurgitation is frequently due to prolapse of the right cusp caused by the Venturi effect of the high-velocity jet through the VSD. Three-dimensional echocardiography can also be used to precisely visualize the anatomy of the VSD [32].

CMR can be used as an alternative to echocardiography to assess LV volume and function as well as the severity of aortic regurgitation using a combination of cine and phase velocity-encoded images. In borderline cases, when a surgical intervention is contemplated, pulmonary resistance must be measured by cardiac catheterization.

ASD and VSD may be found on cardiac CT scans performed for other reasons on adult patients. Shunting may be visible if the contrast medium concentration is different between the left and right side.

19.3.3 Tetralogy of Fallot

Patients operated on for a TOF have excellent long-term survival, with more than 85% surviving more than 30 years post-operation [33,34]. Nevertheless, lifelong follow-up is mandatory for these patients because of the occurrence of late complications:

- PR is a frequent long-term complication in patients who have repaired TOF, especially in patients in whom a transannular patch was used for TOF repair. Severe chronic PR induces RV dilatation and, finally, RV dysfunction, leading to heart failure.

- Right ventricular outflow tract obstruction: residual obstruction can occur at the level of the infundibulum, the valve, the main pulmonary trunk, or the pulmonary branch.
- RV dilatation and dysfunction, mainly due to severe PR, may cause tricuspid annulus enlargement and secondary tricuspid regurgitation, which may worsen ventricular dilatation.
- Residual VSD due to patch dehiscence or incomplete closure during repair may lead to LV overload and dilatation.
- LV dysfunction occurs most of the time as a consequence of RV dysfunction due to ventriculoventricular interaction.
- Aortic root dilatation and aortic regurgitation are related to intrinsic aortic abnormalities seen in TOF patients and are present in about 15% of these patients.
- Arrhythmia and sudden death; both ventricular and supraventricular arrhythmia account for significant morbidity and mortality in TOF patients. They are related to poor hemodynamic conditions, surgical scars, and fibrosis.

Pulmonary valve replacement using open heart surgery or, more recently, using percutaneous valves is the treatment for PR. The question of the optimal timing for intervention remains open. Some studies have demonstrated that an enlarged RV (volume $>160\,\text{ml/m}^2$ body surface area) will not recover normal volume after pulmonary valve replacement [35]. In other studies, this threshold is about $150\,\text{ml/m}^2$ [36,37]. Moreover, normalization of the size of the RV does not imply *per se* a normalization of the RV function or an improvement in the patient's physical capacity. Thus, actual guidelines do not recommend any threshold for intervention but rather careful consideration and monitoring of changes in RV volume and a decrease in RV function [1,28].

A complete TTE examination needs to be performed at each follow-up visit for TOF patients [38]. The main points of interest are RV and LV size and function, presence and severity of pulmonary or aortic regurgitation, RVOT obstruction, size of the aortic root, tricuspid valve regurgitation, presence of a residual VSD, and function of the pulmonary homograft or conduit if the patient has a history of previous surgery.

Precise assessment of RV ventricular volume and function using TTE remains challenging due to the complex anatomy and location of the RV [4,39] (Figures 19.5 and 19.6). Some authors have suggested that an apical 4-chamber view RV end-diastolic cross-sectional area $<20\,\text{cm}^2/\text{m}^2$ body surface area has been associated with a CMR-measured RV end-diastolic volume $<170\,\text{ml/m}^2$ [40].

The tricuspid annular plane systolic excursion (TAPSE) was proposed as a method to assess longitudinal RV function and as an index of global RV function. In TOF patients, the correlation between TAPSE and the RV ejection fraction (EF) determined by CMR is weak, and, thus, these indices are not clinically useful [39,41].

Residual RVOT obstruction is assessed using several echo views (parasternal short axis, modified long axis, modified apical 4 CV, subcostal view). Color Doppler will help to localize the level of the obstruction: subvalvular, valvular, or supravalvular. A peak velocity measured by continuous wave Doppler of $>4\,\text{m/s}$ (or $64\,\text{mmHg}$) indicates a severe stenosis, $3-4\,\text{m/s}$ a moderate stenosis, and $<3\,\text{m/s}$ a mild stenosis [42]. The obstruction can also be located at the level of the branches. An obstruction at any level should be considered if the velocities of the tricuspid jet are elevated.

PR is an important factor in the prognosis of TOF patients, but the assessment of PR severity by echocardiography remains difficult [43]. Some patients present with

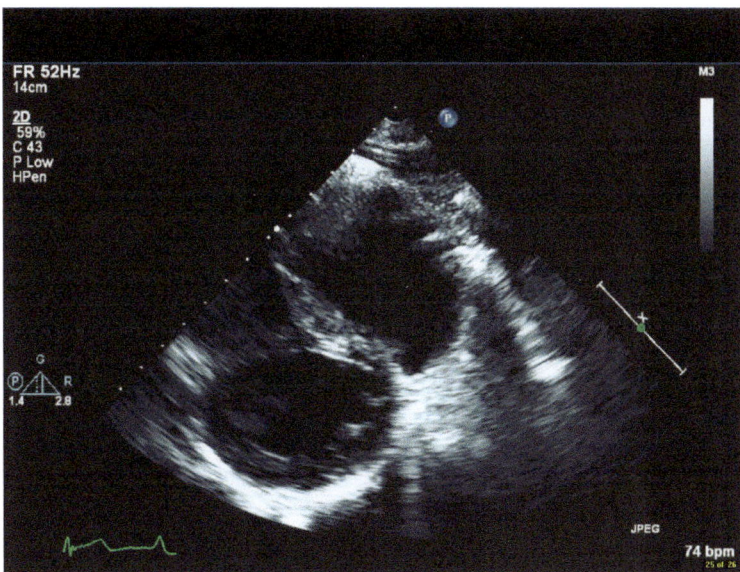

Figure 19.5 TTE sax view in patient with TOF and enlarged RV.

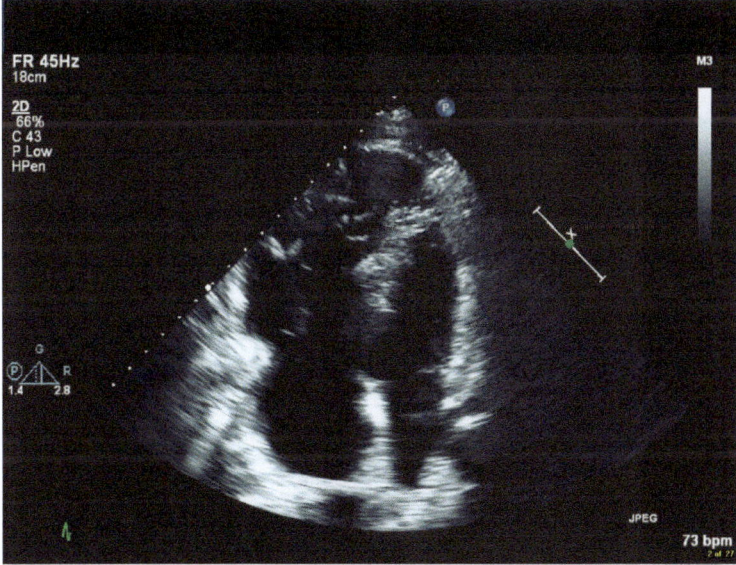

Figure 19.6 TTE apical 4 CV in patient with TOF showing enlarged RV.

a "restrictive" physiology. In other words, the RV dilatation is less despite a severe regurgitation, and, thus, clinical tolerance is better (Figure 19.4). This pattern can be recognized by the presence of a diastolic forward flow in the pulmonary artery during atrial contraction [44].

The examination must be completed by assessment of the tricuspid valve and tricuspid regurgitation, the aortic root and aortic regurgitation, and the search for residual VSD.

The main use of TEE is to more precisely evaluate intracardiac structures, especially in preoperative period.

Three-dimensional echocardiography has been proposed to measure RV volumes more accurately than 2D echocardiography. Nevertheless, a meta-analysis demonstrates that 3D echocardiography tends to underestimate RV volumes and function [45].

Deformation imaging can be useful for detecting subclinical myocardial dysfunction, but this role needs to be defined in the future [15,46].

With its ability to quantify RV volumes and function as well as PR, CMR is a key tool for assessing patient who have TOF, and it should be part of routine follow-up visits [1,18,47]. CMR is the recommended technique for assessment of RV volumes and function and has the advantage of high reproducibility [48] (Figure 19.7). In the same way, CMR is also used to assess LV function.

CMR is largely preferred over echocardiography to quantify PR [49]. Using phase contrast CMR, it is possible to quantify the severity of PR. Measurements are obtained by the difference between the right and left stroke volume or directly by measuring the flow in the main pulmonary artery. PR can be quantified by providing the regurgitant volume and regurgitant fraction. A free PR corresponding to a nonfunctional pulmonary valve corresponds to a 35–45% regurgitant fraction that may also be presented as an indexed regurgitant volume [50,51].

CMR is also useful to assess RVOT obstruction, to assess the size of pulmonary arteries, and to rule out stenosis. Aortic regurgitation, LV volume and function, and the ascending aorta can also be investigated. Moreover, CMR has the advantage of being able to visualize extracardiac structures inside the thorax and to show, for example, the

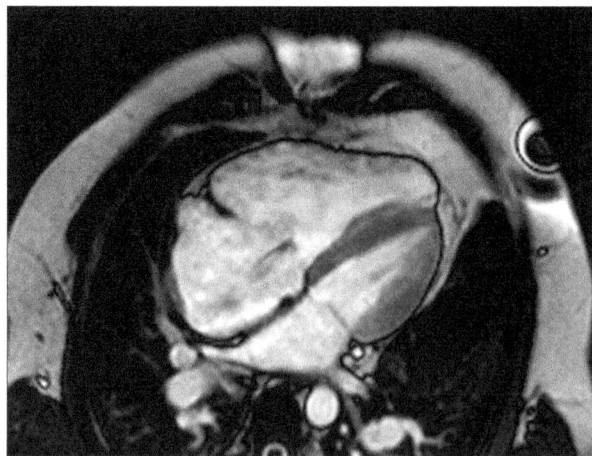

Figure 19.7 MRI apical 4 CV showing in patient with TOF showing enlarged RV.

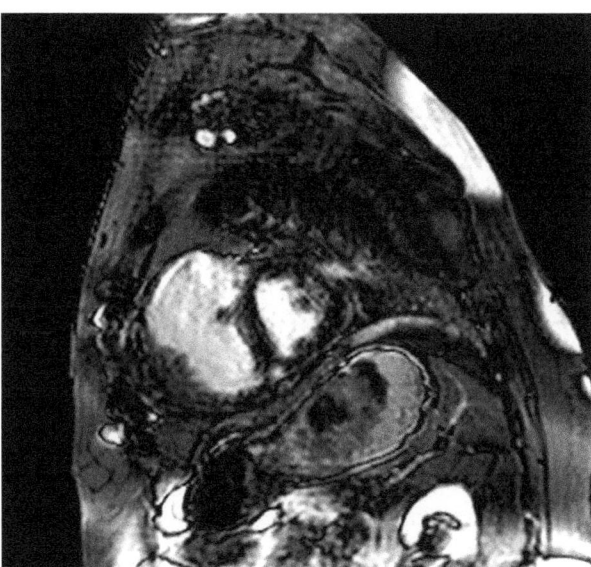

Figure 19.8 MRI sequence showing fibrosis at the level of the RV and lower part of the interventricular septum.

relative positions of the great vessels and the sternum, which may be of interest in case surgery is needed. Myocardial fibrosis detected by late gadolinium-enhanced CMR is a marker of arrhythmia and poor clinical outcomes [52] (Figure 19.8).

CT is a valuable alternative to CMR for assessment of RV function in patients who have pacemakers or other contraindications to CMR. CT is particularly useful to assess the extent of calcification of the conduits and the position of the coronary arteries, which plays an important role when a percutaneous valve implantation is considered. In addition, CT permits visualization of the lungs and the relationship between the great vessels and extracardiac structures such as the sternum.

Cardiac catheterization is reserved to interventional procedures such as stent implantation for pulmonary artery stenosis, percutaneous valve implantation, or in the rare case where noninvasive imaging cannot solve the clinical question.

19.3.4 Transposition of the great arteries

TGA is characterized by ventriculo-arterial discordance (i.e., the pulmonary artery is connected to the left ventricle, and the aorta is connected to the right ventricle) and atrioventricular concordance. The malformation exists as an isolated form or is associated with other malformations such as VSD, aortic coarctation, and so on. TGA is not compatible with long-term survival. The first correction proposed was to switch the pulmonary and systemic circulation at the level of the atrium with the creation of a baffle (with the atrial septum (Senning surgery) or with pericardium (Mustard surgery)) to separate both circulations. This correction is called atrial switch.

TGA are corrected by arterial switch: the aorta (with the coronary arteries) and the pulmonary artery are switched together, restoring the normal ventricular arterial sequence.

19.3.4.1 Atrial switch surgery

The most frequent complications related to the atrial correction are:
- Arrhythmia: brady- or tachyarrhythmia related to atrial damage due to switch surgery.
- RV dysfunction. The atrial correction has the disadvantage of using the RV as the systemic ventricle. Thus, tricuspid regurgitation and heart failure are frequent complications in such patients. The prognosis of the patient largely depends on the ability of the right ventricle to adapt to the high-pressure environment of systemic circulation.
- Baffle stenosis or leakage.

Echocardiography remains the first-line examination to assess TGA atrial switch patients. It is used to assess the size and function of the systemic (RV) and subpulmonary (LV) ventricles. Atrioventricular valve regurgitation, or subpulmonary or aortic obstruction, can also be analyzed.

As in TOF patients, precise assessment of RV function by echo is difficult, and CMR is considered the gold standard [18]. Tricuspid regurgitation can also be measured by CMR.

Correct imaging of the atrial baffle is of the utmost importance in TGA atrial switch patients; leakage may explain shunt and ventricular surcharge or poor exercise capacity and stenosis may favor arrhythmias. Echocardiography using 2D imaging with color Doppler or continuous and pulsed Doppler can demonstrate leakage or stenosis (Figures 19.9 and 19.10). Vena cava stenoses are sometimes more difficult to diagnose by echocardiography. Contrast echo is indicated to bring out the baffle leakage. TEE can be useful in some cases. Three-dimensional echocardiography allows for better visualization of the baffle, and volume acquisition can be cropped according to various planes to better visualize the different parts of the baffle (Figure 19.11). Furthermore, CMR with angiography permits high resolution and dynamic imaging of the baffle [53] (Figure 19.12). Vena caval and pulmonary veins are more adequately visualized by CMR.

As for other CHD, CT represents an alternative when CMR cannot be performed. CT can further be performed to assess coronary artery anatomy, which can be abnormal in patients who have TGA. Significant baffle obstruction can result in enlargement of the azygos venous system or other venous colaterals, which can be appreciated on CT or MR.

19.3.4.2 Arterial switch surgery

The most frequent complications occurring late after arterial switch surgery are pulmonary artery subvalvular stenosis and pulmonary branch stenosis mainly due to stretching of the artery during the surgical correction, dilatation with aortic regurgitation of the neo-aortic root (former pulmonary root), and coronary artery pathology (coronary arteries were reimplanted during corrective surgery) [54].

For this congenital condition, echocardiography is the first among the imaging techniques. Echocardiography enables evaluation of global and regional LV function,

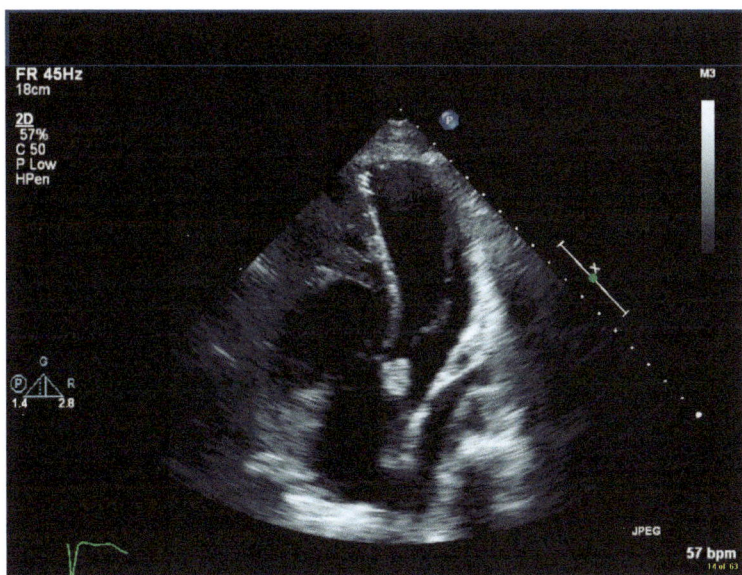

Figure 19.9 TTE apical 4 CV in a patient with atrial switch surgery showing the baffle.

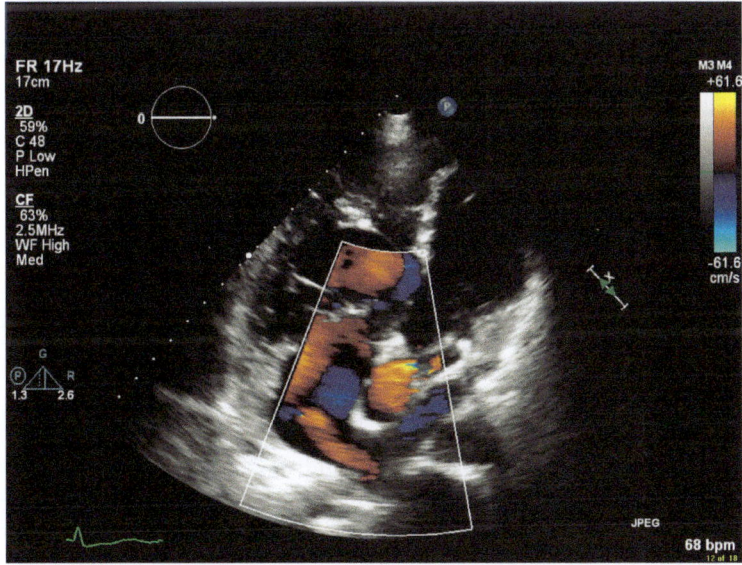

Figure 19.10 TTE apical 4 CV in a patient with atrial switch surgery showing the baffle, color Doppler allows visualization of the flow through the baffle.

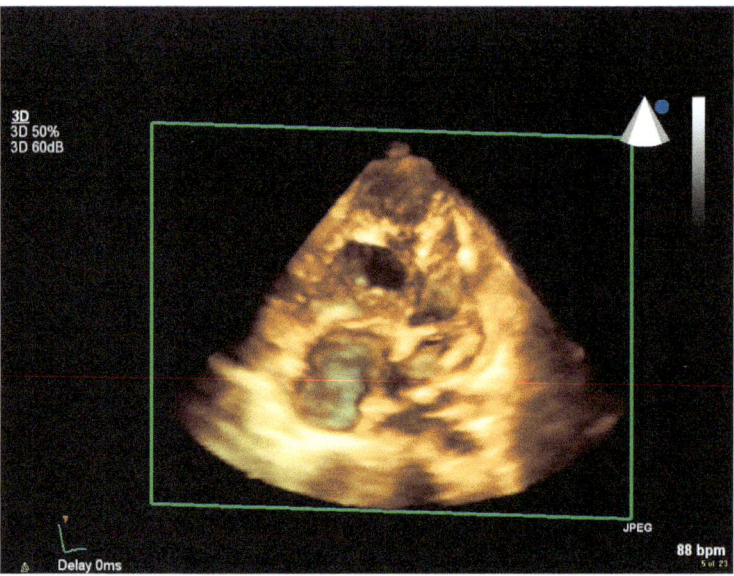

Figure 19.11 3D TTE apical view in a patient with atrial switch surgery showing the baffle.

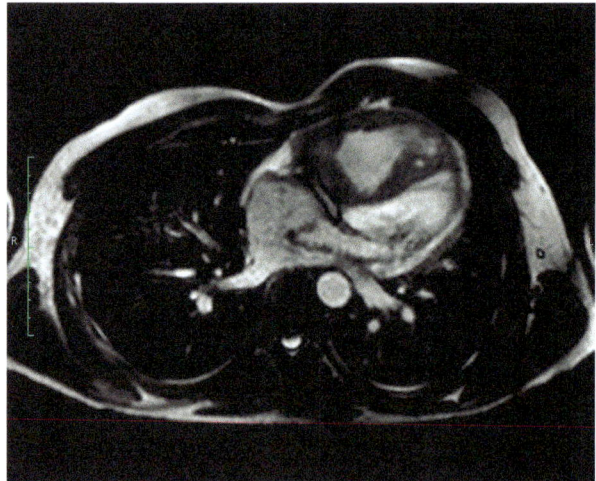

Figure 19.12 MRI view in a patient with atrial switch surgery showing the baffle.

stenosis at the level of arterial anastomosis (mainly pulmonary anastomosis), and aortic root dilatation and aortic regurgitation. If there are no complications, echocardiography in a TGA arterial switch patient may look like a normal examination. TEE can be used to assess the aortic root and potentially aortic regurgitation. Stress echocardiography may be used to unmask myocardial ischemia.

CMR is reserved to answer questions left unresolved by echocardiography. CMR is also used to assess the pulmonary artery and branch as well as the aorta.

CT is specifically indicated to assess the coronary ostia and the anatomy of the coronary artery. It may also be used as alternative to CMR for pulmonary artery and aorta imaging.

Radionuclide imaging can be used to demonstrate myocardial ischemia or to assess regional pulmonary perfusion in the case of pulmonary stenosis (relative distribution of the flow between the right and left lungs).

19.3.4.3 Congenitally corrected transposition of the great artery

Congenitally corrected transposition of the great artery (ccTGA) accounts for <1% of the CHD and may remain undiagnosed until late adulthood. ccTGA is characterized by ventriculo-arterial discordance and atrio-ventricular discordance, or, more simply, the position of the RV and LV are inverted compared with a normal heart.

Echocardiography plays an important role in the initial diagnosis of ccTGA, revealing the discordance. The ventricles are identified by specific morphologic features: The RV has more trabeculations, a moderator band, and a more apically inserted tricuspid valve, whereas the LV has more smooth muscle and a continuity between the mitral and arterial valves. A complete examination should be performed to assess ventricular and valvular function. As for other cases of systemic RV failure, CMR can be used to assess RV function and volume. CT can be proposed as an alternative to CMR or to analyze the coronary artery anatomy.

19.3.5 Univentricular heart and Fontan circulation

The term *univentricular heart* encompasses a wide range of malformations where either the RV or the LV is missing or hypoplastic and cannot serve as a separate ventricle. Fontan surgery was introduced as palliative surgery in cases of univentricular hearts, by connecting the superior and inferior vena cava to the pulmonary artery, thereby bypassing the nonfunctional right ventricle [57].

The major complications after this surgery are related to the dysfunction of the Fontan tunnel or to ventricular or atrioventricular valve dysfunction. Some patients have a "fenestration" (or hole) on the Fontan pathway. This represents a shunt between the venous circulation and systemic circulation and may play a role in oxygen desaturation during exercise as well as in embolic events.

Echocardiography can be used to assess the function of the ventricle and of the atrioventricular valve. A fenestration must be searched out, but Fontan pathways are frequently difficult to image by TTE and require TEE. In the future, 3D echocardiography will certainly play an important role in examining patients who have univentricular hearts.

CMR is the method of choice to assess ventricular function [55]. It may also be used to identify intra-atrial thrombus or patency or the stenosis of the cavopulmonary connection [18].

CT can also be used to assess the patency of the Fontan connections. For this purpose, both CT and CMR require angiographic contrast injections. Adequate opacification can be obtained by combining injections in the arm and the leg (the inferior and superior vena cava).

19.3.6 Coarctation of the aorta

Coarctation of the aorta (CoA) is a narrowing of the aorta in the region of the insertion of the arterial ductus. The more severe cases are diagnosed and treated during childhood, but the presence of CoA must always be suspected in the work-up of young people who have hypertension. Treatment options include open heart surgery or dilatation with stenting. Late complications of CoA include recoarctation or aneurysm at the site of surgery or previous dilatation.

Echocardiography is mainly used to assess the repercussions of CoA such as LV hypertrophy and LV dysfunction. Suprasternal views can be used to assess the aortic arch, but the site of coarctation or recoarctation escapes echocardiographic visualization. Measurement of high velocities by continuous Doppler is not always a sign of obstruction; this may simply be due to the form of the arch. In contrast, high velocities that continue throughout diastole (diastolic tail) indicate a significant coarctation.

A bicuspid aortic valve is frequently found in patients who have CoA. The anatomy and the function of the aortic valve must be verified by echocardiography as the aortic root may be dilated [58].

CMR and CT are the preferred noninvasive methods to assess the entire aorta and potential complications related to CoA [56]. CMR has the advantage over CT because it provides better visualization of the collaterals and can be performed repeatedly without the use of radiation. In contrast, CT is the method of choice after stenting of the CoA (Figure 19.13) [59].

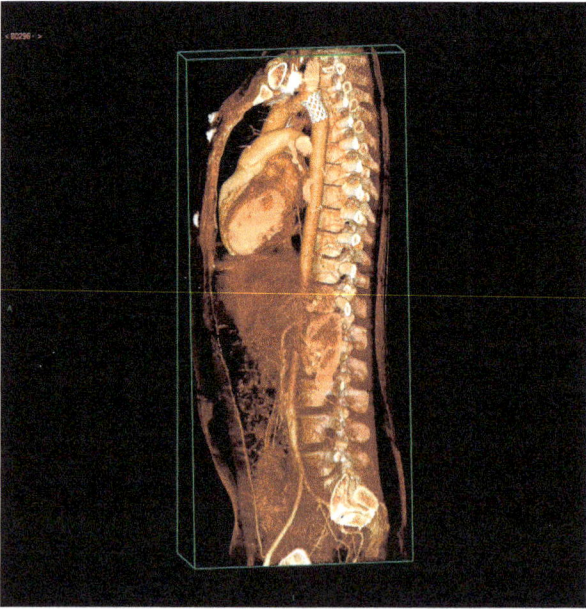

Figure 19.13 CT showing the result of a stenting for aortic coarctation.

19.4 Summary

Adults who have CHD are a growing population with new diagnostic challenges. Today, a wide range of imaging techniques is available to address clinical questions in this population. While echocardiography remains the cornerstone of multiple diagnoses, CMR and CT have additional value, especially when the right ventricle or the great arteries are involved. A good knowledge of the remaining lesion and the limitations of all imaging techniques is mandatory to choose the most appropriate imaging modalities, taking into account resources and local expertise.

References

[1] Baumgartner H, Bonhoeffer P, De Groot NMS, de Haan F, Deanfield JE, Galie N, et al. ESC Guidelines for the management of grown-up congenital heart disease (new version 2010). Eur Heart J 2010;31:2915–57.

[2] Gurvit M. General approach to the adult patients with suspected congenital heart disease. In: Otto CM, editor. Practice of Clinical Echocardiography. 4th ed. Philadelphia: Saunders: 2012 [Chapter 43]. ISBN: 978-1-4377-2765-4.

[3] Anderson RH, Becker AE, Freedom RM, Macartney FJ, Quero-Jimenez M, Shinebourne EA, et al. Sequential segmental analysis of congenital heart disease. Pediatr Cardiol 1984;5:281–7.

[4] Rudski LG, Lai WW, Afilalo J, Hua L, Handschumacher MD, Chandrasekaran K, et al. Guidelines for the echocardiographic assessment of the right heart in adults: a report from the American Society of Echocardiography endorsed by the European Association of Echocardiography, a registered branch of the European Society of Cardiology, and the Canadian Society of Echocardiography. J Am Soc Echocardiogr 2010;23:685–713.

[5] Lai WW, Gauvreau K, Rivera ES, Saleeb S, Powell AJ, Geva T. Accuracy of guideline recommendations for two-dimensional quantification of the right ventricle by echocardiography. Int J Cardiovasc Imaging 2008;24:691–8.

[6] Khattab K, Schmidheiny P, Wustmann K, Wahl A, Seiler C, Schwerzmann M. Echocardiogram versus cardiac magnetic resonance imaging for assessing systolic function of subaortic right ventricle in adults with complete transposition of great arteries and previous atrial switch operation. Am J Cardiol 2013;111:908–13.

[7] Orwat S, Diller GP, Baumgartner H. Imaging of congenital heart disease in adults: choice of modalities. Eur Heart J Cardiovasc Imaging 2014;15(1):6–17.

[8] Ayres N, Miller-Hance W, Fyfe D, Stevenson JG, Sahn DJ, Young LT, et al. Indications and guidelines for performance of transesophageal echocardiograpy in the patient with pediatric or congenital heart disease. J Am Soc Echocardiogr 2005;18:91–8.

[9] Flachskampf FA, Wouters PF, Edvardsen T, Evangelista A, Habib G, Hoffman P, et al. Recommendations for transoesophageal echocardiography: EACVI update. Eur Heart J Cardiovasc Imaging 2014;15(4):353–65.

[10] Lytrivi ID, Lai WW, Ko HH, Nielsen JC, Parness IA, Srivastava S. Color Doppler tissue imaging for evaluation of right ventricular systolic function in patients with congenital heart disease. J Am Soc Echocardiogr 2005;18(10):1099–104.

[11] Vettukattil JJ. Three dimensional echocardiography in congenital heart disease. Heart 2012;98:79–88.

[12] Grewal J, Majdalany D, Syed I, Pellikka P, Warnes CA. Three-dimensional echocardiographic assessment of right ventricular volume and function in adult patients with congenital heart disease: comparison with magnetic resonance imaging. J Am Soc Echocardiogr 2010;23:127–33.
[13] Friedberg MK, Mertens L. Deformation imaging in selected congenital heart disease: is it evolving to clinical use? J Am Soc Echocardiogr 2012;25:919–31.
[14] Moiduddin N, Asoh K, Slorach C, Benson LN, Friedberg MK. Effect of transcatheter pulmonary valve implantation on short-term right ventricular function as determined by two-dimensional speckle tracking strain and strain rate imaging. Am J Cardiol 2009;104:862–7.
[15] Yu HK, Li SJ, Ip JJ, Lam WW, Wong SJ, Cheung YF. Right ventricular mechanics in adults after surgical repair of tetralogy of fallot: insights from three-dimensional speckle-tracking echocardiography. J Am Soc Echocardiogr 2014;27(4):423–9.
[16] Li W, Hornung TS, Francis DP, OSullivan C, Duncan A, Gatzoulis M, et al. Relation of biventricular function quantified by stress echocardiography to cardiopulmonary exercise capacity in adults with Mustard (atrial switch) procedure for transposition of the great arteries. Circulation 2004;110:1380–6.
[17] Kramer CM, Barkhausen J, Flamm SD, Kim RJ, Nagel E. Society for Cardiovascular Magnetic Resonance Board of Trustees Task Force on Standardized Protocols. Standardized cardiovascular magnetic resonance imaging (CMR) protocols, Society for Cardiovascular Magnetic Resonance: board of trustees task force on standardized protocols. J Cardiovasc Magn Reson 2008;10:35.
[18] Kilner PJ, Geva T, Kaemmerer H, Trindade PT, Schwitter J, Webb GD. Recommendations for cardiovascular magnetic resonance in adults with congenital heart disease from the respective working groups of the European Society of Cardiology. Eur Heart J 2010;31:794–805.
[19] Ibrahim El-Sayed H. Myocardial tagging by cardiovascular magnetic resonance: evolution of techniques–pulse sequences, analysis algorithms, and applications. J Cardiovasc Magn Reson 2011;13:36.
[20] Markl M, Kilner Ph J, Tino Ebbers T. Comprehensive 4D velocity mapping of the heart and great vessels by cardiovascular magnetic resonance. J Cardiovasc Magn Reson 2011;13:7.
[21] Broberg CS, Chugh SS, Conklin C, Sahn DJ, Jerosch-Herold M. Quantification of diffuse myocardial fibrosis and its association with myocardial dysfunction in congenital heart disease. Circ Cardiovasc Imaging 2010;3:727–34.
[22] Ghoshhajra BB, Sidhu MS, El-Sherief A, Rojas C, Yeh DD, Engel LC, et al. Adult congenital heart disease imaging with second-generation dual-source computed tomography: initial experiences and findings. Congenit Heart Dis 2012;7(6):516–25.
[23] Fujimoto S, Kondo T, Orihara T, Sugiyama J, Kondo M, Kodama T, et al. Prevalence of anomalous origin of coronary artery detected by multi-detector computed tomography at one center. J Cardiol 2011;57(1):69–76.
[24] Budoff MJ, Shittu A, Roy S. Use of cardiovascular computed tomography in the diagnosis and management of coarctation of the aorta. J Thorac Cardiovasc Surg 2013;146(1):229–32.
[25] American College of Cardiology Foundation Task Force on Expert Consensus Documents, Mark DB, Berman DS, Budoff MJ, Carr JJ, Gerber TC, et al. ACCF/ACR/AHA/NASCI/SAIP/SCAI/SCCT 2010 expert consensus document oncoronary computed tomographic angiography: a report of the American College of Cardiology Foundation Task Force on Expert Consensus Documents. J Am Coll Cardiol 2010;55:2663–99.

[26] Lin FY, Devereux RB, Roman MJ, Meng J, Jow VM, Jacobs A, et al. Cardiac chamber volumes, function, and mass as determined by 64-multidetector row computed tomography: mean values among healthy adults free of hypertension and obesity. J Am Coll Cardiol Img 2008;1:782–6.
[27] Delgado V, Tops LF, Schuijf JD, de Roos A, Brugada J, Schalij MJ, et al. Assessment of mitral valve anatomy and geometry with multislice computed tomography. J Am Coll Cardiol Img 2009;2:556–65.
[28] Warnes CA, Williams RG, Bashore ThM, Child JS, Connolly HM, Dearani JA, et al. ACC/AHA 2008 guidelines for the management of adults with congenital heart disease: a report of the American College of Cardiology/American Heart Association Task Force on Practice Guidelines (Writing Committee to Develop Guidelines on the Management of Adults With Congenital Heart Disease). Developed in Collaboration with the American Society of Echocardiography, Heart Rhythm Society, International Society for Adult Congenital Heart Disease, Society for Cardiovascular Angiography and Interventions, and Society of Thoracic Surgeons. J Am Coll Cardiol 2008;2008(52):e143–263.
[29] Saric M, Perk G, Purgess JR, Kronzon I. Imaging atrial septal defects by real-time three-dimensional transesophageal echocardiography: step-by-step approach. J Am Soc Echocardiogr 2010;23:1128–35.
[30] Faletra FF, Pedrazzini G, Pasotti E, Muzzarelli S, Dequarti MC, Murzilli R, et al. 3D TEE during catheter-based interventions. J Am Coll Cardiol Img 2014;7:292–308.
[31] Powell AJ, Tsai-Goodman B, Prakash A, Greil GF, Geva T. Comparison between phase-velocity cine magnetic resonance imaging and invasive oximetry for quantification of atrial shunts. Am J Cardiol 2003;91:1523–5.
[32] Cheng OT, Xie M-X, Wang X-F, Wang Y, Lu Q. Real-time 3-dimensional echocardiography in assessing atrial and ventricular septal defects: an echocardiographic-surgical correlative study. Am Heart J 2004;148:1091–5.
[33] Murphy JG, Gersh BJ, Mair DD, Fuster V, McGoon MD, Ilstrup DM, et al. Long-term outcome in patients undergoing surgical repair of tetralogy of Fallot. N Engl J Med 1993;329:593–9.
[34] Nollert G, Fischlein T, Bouterwek S, Böhmer C, Klinner W, Reichart B. Longterm survival in patients with repair of tetralogy of Fallot: 36-year follow-up of 490 survivors of the first year after surgical repair. J Am Coll Cardiol 1997;30:1374–83.
[35] Oosterhof T, van Straten A, Vliegen HW, Meijboom FJ, van Dijk APJ, Spijkerboer AM, et al. Preoperative thresholds for pulmonary valve replacement in patients with corrected tetralogy of Fallot using cardiovascular magnetic resonance. Circulation 2007;116:545–51.
[36] Buechel ERV, Dave HH, Kellenberger CJ, Dodge-Khatami A, Pretre R, Berger F, et al. Remodelling of the right ventricle after early pulmonary valve replacement in children with repaired tetralogy of Fallot: assessment by cardiovascular magnetic resonance. Eur Heart J 2005;26:2721–7.
[37] Frigiola A, Tsang V, Bull C, Coats L, Khambadkone S, Derrick G, et al. Biventricular response after pulmonary valve replacement for right ventricular outflowtract dysfunction: is age a predictor of outcome? Circulation 2008;118:S182–90.
[38] Valente AM, Cook S, Festa P, Ko HH, Krishnamurthy R, Taylor AM, et al. Multimodality imaging guidelines for patients with repaired tetralogy of fallot: a report from the American Society of Echocardiography. J Am Soc Echocardiogr 2014;27:111–41.
[39] Srinivasan C, Sachdeva R, Morrow WR, Greenberg SB, Vyas HV. Limitations of standard echocardiographic methods for quantification of right ventricular size and function in children and young adults. J Ultrasound Med 2011;30:487–93.

[40] Alghamdi MH, Grosse-Wortmann L, Ahmad N, Mertens L, Friedberg MK. Can simple echocardiographic measures reduce the number of cardiac magnetic resonance imaging studies to diagnose right ventricular enlargement in congenital heart disease? J Am Soc Echocardiogr 2012;25:518–23.

[41] Morcos P, Vick III GW, Sahn DJ, Jerosch-Herold M, Shurman A, Sheehan FH. Correlation of right ventricular ejection fraction and tricuspid annular plane systolic excursion in tetralogy of Fallot by magnetic resonance imaging. Int J Cardiovasc Imaging 2009;25:263–70.

[42] Baumgartner H, Hung J, Bermejo J, Chambers JB, Evangelista A, Griffin BP, et al. Echocardiographic assessment of valve stenosis: EAE/ASE recommendations for clinical practice. J Am Soc Echocardiogr 2009;22:1–23.

[43] Redington AN. Determinants and assessment of pulmonary regurgitation in tetralogy of Fallot: practice and pitfalls. Cardiol Clin 2006;24:631–9.

[44] Cullen S, Shore D, Redington A. Characterization of right ventricular diastolic performance after complete repair of tetralogy of Fallot. Restrictive physiology predicts slow postoperative recovery. Circulation 1995;91:1782–9.

[45] Shimada YJ, Shiota M, Siegel RJ, Shiota T. Accuracy of right ventricular volumes and function determined by three-dimensional echocardiographyin comparison with magnetic resonance imaging: a meta-analysis study. J Am Soc Echocardiogr 2010;23:943–53.

[46] Scherptong RWC, Mollema SA, Blom NA, Kroft LJM, Roos A, Vliegen HW, et al. Right ventricular peak systolic longitudinal strain is a sensitive marker for right ventricular deterioration in adult patients with tetralogy of Fallot. Int J Cardiovasc Imaging 2009;25:669–76.

[47] Oosterhof T, Mulder BJM, Vliegen HW, de Roos A. Cardiovascular magnetic resonance in the follow-up of patients with corrected tetralogy of Fallot: a review. Am Heart J 2006;151:265–72.

[48] Geva T. Repaired tetralogy of Fallot: the roles of cardiovascular magnetic resonance in evaluating pathophysiology and for pulmonary valve replacement decision support. J Cardiovasc Magn Reson 2011;13:9.

[49] Mercer-Rosa L, Yang W, Kutty S, Rychik J, Fogel M, Goldmuntz E. Quantifying pulmonary regurgitation and right ventricular function in surgically repaired tetralogy of Fallot: a comparative analysis of echocardiography and magnetic resonance imaging. Circ Cardiovasc Imaging 2012;5:637–43.

[50] Samyn MM, Powell AJ, Garg R, Sena L, Geva T. Range of ventricular dimensions and function by steady-state free precession cine MRI in repaired tetralogy of Fallot: right ventricular outflow tract patch vs. conduit repair. J Magn Reson Imaging 2007;26:934–40.

[51] Wald RM, Redington AN, Pereira A, Provost YL, Paul NS, Oechslin EN, et al. Refining the assessment of pulmonary regurgitation in adults after tetralogy of Fallot repair: should we be measuring regurgitant fraction or regurgitant volume? Eur Heart J 2009;30:356–61.

[52] Babu-Narayan SV, Kilner PJ, Li W, Moon JC, Goktekin O, Davlouros PA, et al. Ventricular fibrosis suggested by cardiovascular magnetic resonance in adults with repaired tetralogy of Fallot and its relationship to adverse markers of clinical outcome. Circulation 2006;113:405–13.

[53] Dorfman AL, Geva T. Magnetic resonance imaging evaluation of congenital heart disease: conotruncal anomalies. J Cardiovasc Magn Reson 2006;8:645–59.

[54] Losay J, Touchot A, Serraf A, Litvinova A, Lambert V, Piot JD, et al. Late outcome after arterial switch operation for transposition of the great arteries. Circulation 2001;104(12 Suppl. 1):I121–6.

[55] Eicken A, Fratz S, Gutfried Ch, Balling G, Schwaiger M, Lange R, et al. Hearts late after fontan operation have normal mass, normal volume, and reduced systolic function: a magnetic resonance imaging study. J Am Coll Cardiol 2003;42:1061–5.
[56] Parks WJ, Ngo TD, Plauth WH, Bank ER, Sheppard SK, Pettigrew RI, et al. Incidence of aneurysm formation after Dacron patch aortoplasty repair for coarctation of the aorta: long-term results and assessment utilizing magnetic resonance angiography with three-dimensional surface rendering. J Am Coll Cardiol 1995;26:266–71.
[57] Khairy P, Poirier N, Mercier L-A. Univentricular heart. Circulation 2007;115:800–12.
[58] Tan J-L, Babu-Narayan SV, Henein MY, Mullen M, Li W. Doppler echocardiographic profile and indexes in the evaluation of aortic coarctation in patients before and after stenting. J Am Coll Cardiol 2005;46:1045–53.
[59] Rosenthal E, Bell A. Optimal imaging after coarctation stenting. Heart 2010;96:1169–71.

Diseases of the thoracic aorta and pulmonary arteries

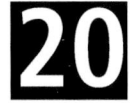

R. Salgado*, J. Habets†, R.P.J. Budde‡, T. Leiner†
*Antwerp University Hospital, Antwerp, Belgium; †University Medical Center Utrecht, Utrecht, The Netherlands; ‡Erasmus Medical Center, Rotterdam, The Netherlands

20.1 Introduction

A wide variety of diseases can affect the great thoracic arteries. They include entities resulting from long-standing atherosclerotic degeneration (e.g., aortic aneurysms) that as such can go undetected for a prolonged time, as well as diseases presenting with acute severe and potentially life-threatening symptoms, like pulmonary embolism and acute aortic dissection. As clinical signs and other preliminary tests are often unreliable to establish a correct diagnosis, patients suspected of having thoracic vascular disease are in general promptly referred for imaging examinations to establish presence and extent of disease. In clinical practice, a wide variety of modern imaging techniques are generally available, including echocardiography, computed tomography (CT), magnetic resonance imaging (MRI), and positron emission tomography (PET), the latter sometimes combined with computed tomography (PET-CT).

Given the amount of morphological and functional information that can be derived from these imaging modalities, the acquired data imaging is increasingly not only used for diagnostic purposes, but forms also an important cornerstone in the pre-procedural planning of a variety of interventional procedures. In this chapter, we will provide an overview of the most important diseases of the thoracic great vessels and discuss the specific contributions of different imaging modalities.

20.2 Acute aortic syndrome

20.2.1 Introduction

The term "acute aortic syndrome" (AAS) is often used to refer to a number of potentially life-threatening diseases, which can all present with acute chest pain [1]. Traditionally, AAS encompasses three entities: classic aortic dissection (AD), intramural hematoma (IMH), and penetrating atherosclerotic ulcer (PAU). While these components of AAS have historically been considered separate entities, this view has been recently challenged. Improvements in CT imaging, including the introduction of ECG-triggered acquisitions, have increased the available imaging detail of the aortic wall leading to a better understanding of the underlying pathophysiological mechanism [2]. It has also been demonstrated that the different AAS entities have both discriminating and overlapping features, which can dynamically evolve over time [3]. This is especially true for classic aortic dissection and intramural hematoma, which can be considered two different presentations of the same pathologic process arising from the aortic media. Conversely, a PAU has a completely different etiology, as it is the consequence of an atherosclerotic degeneration of the intimal layer.

20.2.2 Clinical presentation

The clinical presentation of AAS is often non-specific, with a common denominator of severe chest pain. In acute aortic dissection this pain is often described as intense, acute, shearing/tearing, throbbing, or sometimes migratory. When the ascending aorta is involved, pain can be referred to the anterior chest, throat, neck, and jaw. When the abdominal aorta is also affected, patients can have back and abdominal pain. Furthermore, patients can develop ischemic symptoms due to stenosis and occlusion of side branches of the aorta by the dissection flap.

Given the myriad of potential clinical complaints, clinical features are as such unreliable to differentiate between the different etiologies of AAS and other important entities such as myocardial infarction and pulmonary embolism [4]. Additional non-invasive imaging is therefore needed to establish the correct diagnosis and initiate the appropriate treatment.

20.2.3 Classification

Two classifications of aortic dissection exist: the DeBakey classification and the Stanford classification [5,6]. The DeBakey classification distinguishes three different types of dissection. Type I involves the ascending aorta, the arch, and a variable length of the thoracic and abdominal aorta. Type II is restricted to the ascending aorta. Type IIIA is confined to the descending thoracic aorta and type IIIB extends in the abdominal aorta to the bifurcation/iliac vessels.

The Stanford classification only distinguishes between two types: type A and B aortic dissection. Type-A is defined as involving the ascending aorta, regardless of further involvement of the aortic arch and descending aorta. A Stanford type-B dissection includes every dissection in which the ascending aorta is not involved.

Many centers routinely use the Stanford classification as the distinction between a dissection with its origin proximal or distal from the ostium of the left subclavian artery to quickly differentiate between different treatment strategies (in general urgent surgery for type-A dissection vs. strict hypertension control and follow-up for uncomplicated type-B dissections).

20.2.4 Classic aortic dissection—Intramural hematoma

An aortic dissection is caused by a primary intimal tear. While the exact etiology of this entry tear is often unknown, several predisposing conditions exist which can affect the integrity of the media (Table 20.1). One of the most common risk

Table 20.1 Risk factors for acute aortic dissection

Acquired
Arterial hypertension
Pregnancy
Inflammatory disease (Giant cell aortitis, Takayashu, SLE)
Syphilitic aortitis
Traumatic deceleration injury
Cocaine abuse
Iatrogenic (i.e., percutaneous coronary angiography)
Inherited
Marfan syndrome
Ehlers-Danlos syndrome
Adult polycystic disease
Turner syndrome
Noonan syndrome
Osteogenesis imperfecta
Polycystic kidney disease
Congenital
Bicuspid aortic valve
Aortic coarcation

factors is long-standing arterial hypertension, which increases shearing forces on and augments stiffness of the aortic wall. Other causes include connective tissue disorders like Marfan and Ehlers-Danlos syndrome, and traumatic aortic deceleration injuries.

Once an intimal tear has developed, this acquired entry point allows blood from the aorta to disseminate in the media layer and extend both proximally and distally with inward displacement of the intima (Figure 20.1). The entry tear is typically located at the site of highest wall tension, most often a few centimeters above the aortic valve or at the attachment site of the ligamentum arteriosum just distally from the left subclavian artery origin (Figure 20.1).

This intramural blood flow and the consequent dissection of the aortic wall commonly lead to a double-barrel lumen consisting of two channels: a true and a false lumen. The false lumen is completely contained within the aortic media, and divided from the true lumen by a dissection flap consisting of intima and a portion of the media layer.

In a *classic dissection*, both an entry and exit site exists for the intramural flowing blood. Consequently, both true and false lumina contain flowing blood, with faster flow in the true lumen. As pressure builds in the false lumen, the cross-sectional diameter of the false lumen decreases and often becomes the smallest channel (Figure 20.2).

Conversely, an *intramural hematoma* is best understood as a dissection in which there is a clear intramural entry site, but no clear or adequate exit site for the blood back in the true lumen. As such, the false lumen contains thrombosed blood, and

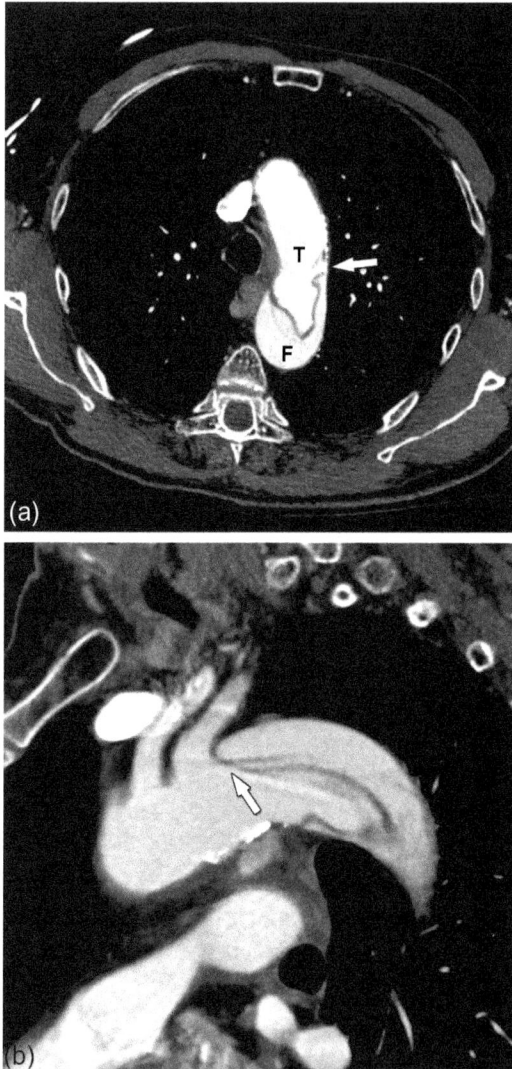

Figure 20.1 Contrast-enhanced CT-scan of a Stanford Type-B aortic dissection. The axial image (a) clearly shows a defect in the intima wall (arrow), allowing blood to flow from the original true lumen (T) into the vessel wall, as such, creating a second false (F) lumen. A second oblique sagittal reformatted image of the same patient (b) shows that the resulting dissection flap (arrow) has its origin just distally from the ostium of the unaffected left subclavian artery, a typical location for a classic Stanford type-B dissection.

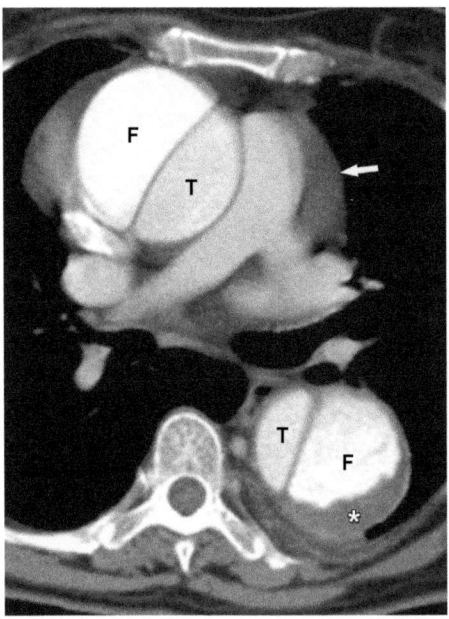

Figure 20.2 Contrast-enhanced CT-scan of a Stanford type-A aortic dissection. The axial CT image shows a double-barreled aortic lumen, consisting of a small true lumen (T) and a larger false (F) lumen. Note the difference in contrast enhancement between these two channels, reflecting a different flow speed. The slower flow in the false lumen further contributes to the forming of thrombus material adjacent to the posterior aortic wall (*). Also, there is an overall increase in diameter of the affected aorta as a post-dissection aortic dilatation settles in secondary to decreased wall strength. Finally, a pericardial effusion can also be appreciated (arrow), a common finding in Stanford Type-A aortic dissections.

remains the smallest channel next to a larger true lumen (Figure 20.3). It is important to realize that over time, an exit site can develop, allowing an intramural hematoma to transgress into a channel with flowing blood and reaching the configuration of a classic dissection (Figure 20.4).

20.2.5 Imaging techniques

Many imaging techniques can be used to visualize an aortic dissection, each with their specific strengths and weaknesses. An overview is given in Table 20.2.

20.2.5.1 Radiography

While a chest radiograph is often the first imaging examination performed on a patient with acute chest pain, its value in the evaluation of a potential acute aortic event is very limited. Several signs, including widening of the mediastinum and aortic contour,

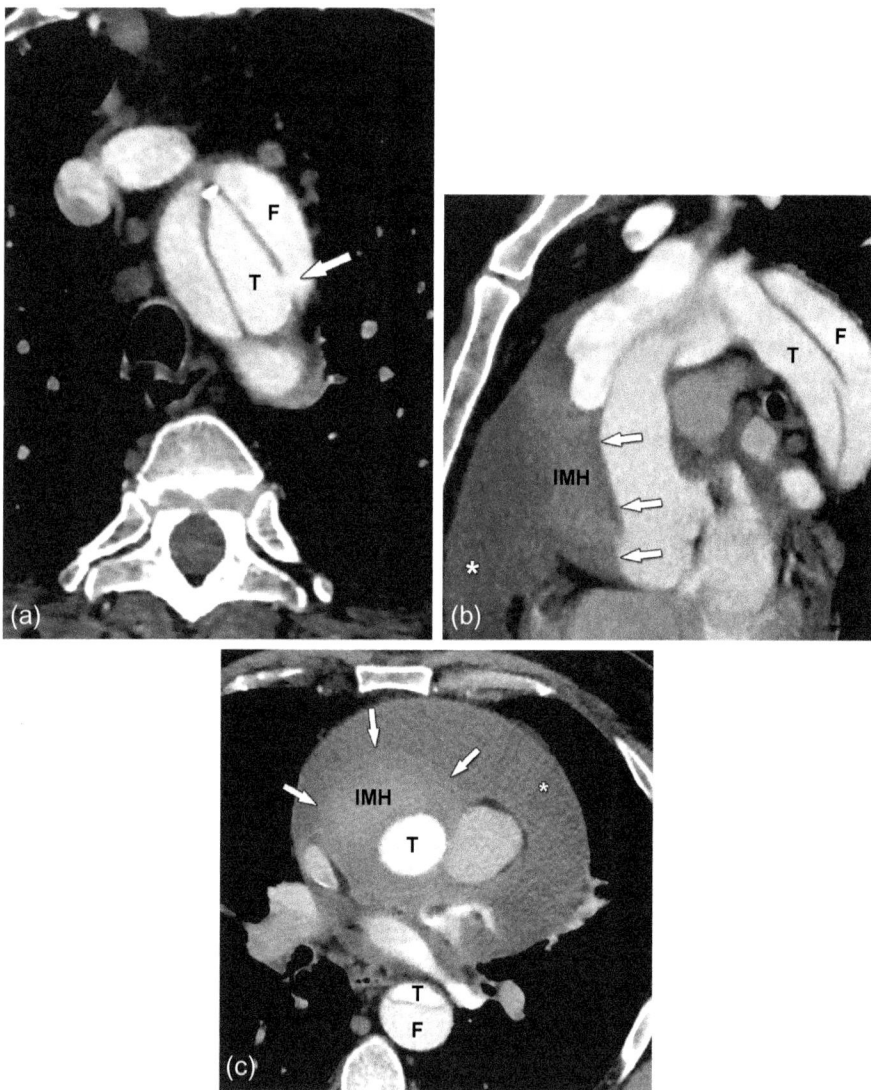

Figure 20.3 Contrast-enhanced CT-scan of an aortic dissection initially originating in the proximal descending aorta, but with retrograde extension into the ascending aorta. The axial image (a) shows a clear defect in the aortic wall (arrow), as entry site for a classic Stanford type-B aortic dissection with two channels of flowing blood: the true (T) and false (F) lumen. The sagittal reformatted image (b) shows retrograde extension of this dissection into the aortic arch and ascending aorta. However, in contrast to the initial rupture in the descending aorta, the dissection flap (arrows in b) does not have a re-entry site. As a consequence, in the ascending aorta the false lumen contains stagnant blood, with thrombus from the aortic sinus upwards, as such forming an intramural hematoma (IMH in b, c). An axial image at a mid-level of the ascending aorta (c) shows that the intramural hematoma (arrows) has a slight hyperdense appearance, and can be distinguished from a large pericardial effusion (asterisk). These images show an initially Stanford type-B dissection with a secondary retrograde acquired Stanford type-A dissection, in which both intramural hematoma and classic dissection are simultaneously present in the same patient.

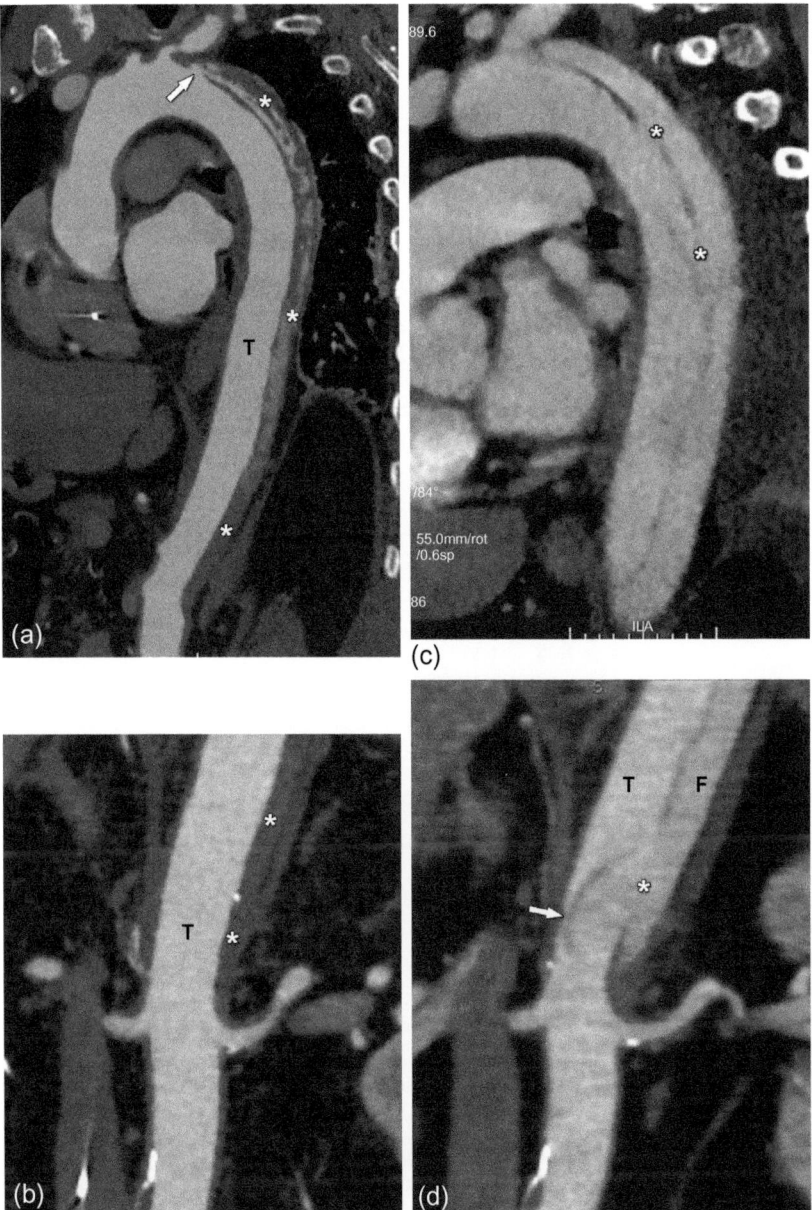

Figure 20.4 Contrast-enhanced CT examinations of the same patient within a time span of a week, initially presenting with acute chest pain. The first CT examination (a, b) shows a Stanford type-B dissection starting just distally from the ostium of the left subclavian artery and ending just above the renal arteries. However, while the entry site is clearly visible (arrow in a), there is no identifiable exit site. As such, the false lumen if formed by an intramural hematoma consisting of mostly stagnant blood (asterisk in a, b). Six days later, the patient was re-evaluated on clinical grounds. The second CT examination (c, d) now shows multiple new defects in the dissection flap (asterisks in c, d). With the development of these multiple entry and exit sites, the false lumen contains now flowing blood. The now increased pressure in the false lumen pushes the dissection flap inwards (arrow in d), with true and false lumen now having similar dimensions.

Table 20.2 Comparison of imaging modalities

Imaging modality	Sensitivity	Specificity	Availability	Examination time	Evaluation of aortic sinus & ascending aorta	Evaluation of aortic arch and more distal aorta segments	Evaluation of aortic side branch involvement	Overall benefits	Overall disadvantages
Chest radiography	−	−	+++	Short	−	−	−	Quick initial chest review	Very non-specific
Transthoracic echocardiography	+/−	+/−	+++	Variable	++	−	−	Good evaluation possible of aortic root & ascending aorta, bedside examination possible, hemodynamic evaluation of aortic valve	Operator-dependent, no complete aorta evaluation possible
Transesophageal echocardiography	+/−	+/−	++	Variable	+++	−	+		
CT	+++	+++	+++	Short	+++	+++	+++	Modality of choice for acute initial evaluation, detection & follow-up of complications	Use of iodinated-contrast material, radiation exposure

								Can be used when iodinated contrast agents are contra-indicated, or in patients with impaired renal function	Longer examination time, more patient cooperation required, more sensitive to artifacts in critically ill patients
MR	+++	+++	+	Long	+++	+++	+++		
Angiography	++	++	–	Long	+++	+++	+++	Intervention possible (endografts) in specific cases	Less suitable for evaluation of intramural hematoma, operator-dependent technique, more prone to procedure-related complications, use of iodinated contrast-agent, radiation exposure

disparity in size between the ascending and descending aorta, changes in aortic configuration on serial examinations, and displacement of aortic calcification by at least 10 mm, have been described but remain non-specific.

20.2.5.2 Ultrasound

Ultrasound techniques available for the detection of AAS include transthoracic and transoesophageal echocardiography (TTE/TOE).

Both TOE and TTE are non-invasive, widely available, and relatively inexpensive imaging modalities. They can also be performed bedside in a critically ill patient.

TTE is a valid imaging choice to detect complications involving the aortic valve, for example, aortic regurgitation. However, a large part of the ascending aorta and aortic arch are often not visualized with TTE due to poor acoustic window. TOE is superior in depicting the ascending aorta and therefore useful in the further evaluation of a potential type-A dissection (Figure 20.5). Also, it can simultaneously visualize complications such as aortic regurgitation (in a dissection involving the aortic sinus), pericardial effusion, coronary artery involvement, and left ventricular function. It is less suitable for evaluation of the distal ascending aorta and proximal aortic arch. TOE can also detect localized wall thickening in patients with intramural hematoma.

Nevertheless, both TTE and TOE are operator-dependent techniques, which are unable to visualize the complete thoracic aorta, and can produce false-positive results due to reverberation artifacts. As such, they are rarely relied upon as the sole diagnostic imaging modality in patients with suspected acute aortic syndrome and have a more complementary function.

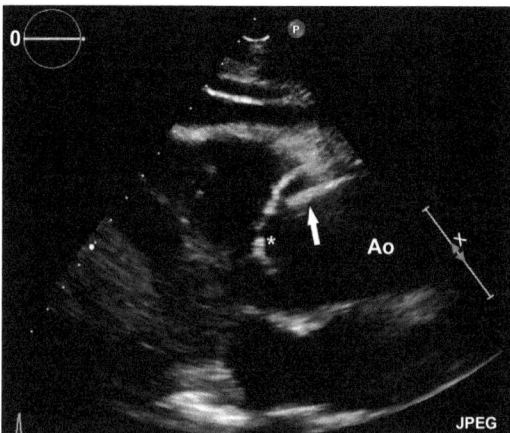

Figure 20.5 Parasternal long-axis transthoracic echocardiographic image demonstrating a Stanford type-A dissection with a hyperechogenic dissection flap (arrow). Ao: aorta, asterisk: aortic valve.

20.2.5.3 Computed tomography

Computed tomography angiography (CTA) is the imaging technique of first choice in patients with acute aortic syndrome. CTA is the only imaging modality that can provide an accurate and complete assessment of the whole thoraco-abdominal aorta and side-branches in a very short examination time, with a reported sensitivity and specificity for aortic dissection of more than 95%. Furthermore, it can simultaneously evaluate all other non-vascular structures (such as the pulmonary parenchyma and visceral abdominal organs), thus allowing detection of an alternative etiology for the acute clinical presentation.

In practice, all CTA examinations are invariably performed with the use of intravenous contrast administration for optimal vascular enhancement and evaluation. However, an initially performed non-enhanced CT-scan can have incremental value in patients with suspected aortic dissection, as it can depict a hyperdense acute intramural hematoma (Figure 20.6), that may not otherwise be seen. Our recommendation is to add an unenhanced examination to your institutional CT protocol for evaluation of patients with suspected aortic dissection.

Despite all the clear advantages of CTA over other imaging modalities, its use of an iodinated contrast agent and associated radiation exposure limits its application in patients with impaired renal function and known intolerance to iodinated dye. Radiation exposure is especially an important issue, as patients with a stable type-B dissection require follow-up imaging over years to monitor for the development of (among others) a post-dissection aneurysmal dilatation of the affected aortic segments. Consequently, and especially in young patients, many centers often use MRI for follow-up of stable patients with a type-B dissection. However, the recent introduction of iterative reconstruction techniques has made radiation dose less of a concern [7,8].

20.2.5.4 Magnetic resonance imaging

Both non-contrast (phase-contrast and time-of-flight techniques) and contrast-enhanced acquisitions are available to visualize the thoracic aorta with MRI. However, non-contrast techniques have significant drawbacks, including a longer examination time, a shorter anatomic coverage, and greater difficulty in differentiating between slow-flow effects and the presence of thrombus. Consequently, contrast-enhanced MR angiography (MRA) is the method of choice to evaluate the thoracic aorta for the presence and extent of dissection.

MRA has similar advantages over echocardiography as CT, including a comparable high sensitivity and specificity (>95%) to diagnose aortic dissection, a large anatomic coverage, and the evaluation of the relation of the dissection flap with aortic side branches. Additionally, given the lack of radiation exposure, multiple acquisitions are possible to visualize the dynamics of contrast enhancement of the true and false lumen with no compromise to the patient's safety (Figure 20.7). The use of Gadolinium-chelates as a contrast agent makes MRA also the technique of choice in patients with impaired renal function. It is also a good choice for repeated follow-up of patients with a known and stable (type-B) dissection to monitor for the presence and evolution of

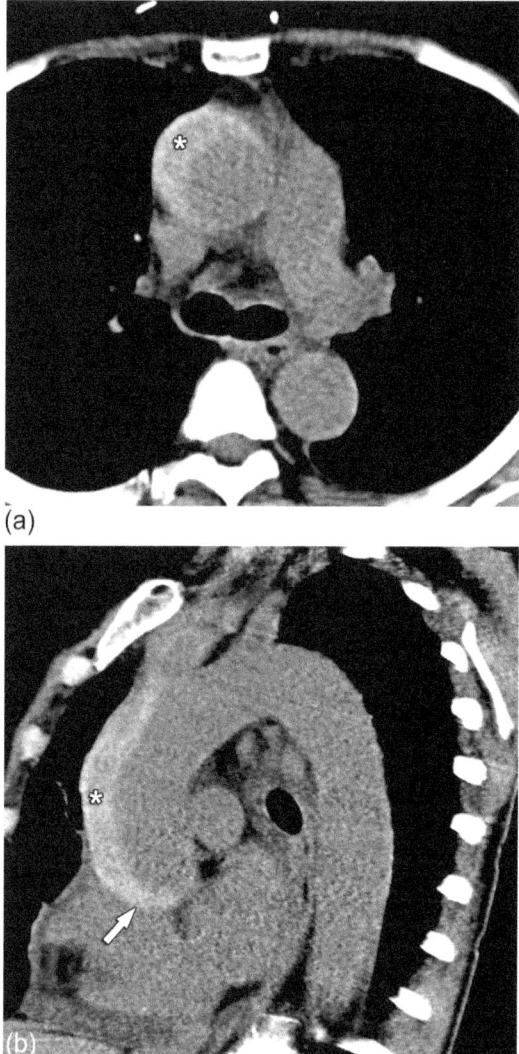

Figure 20.6 CT examination of a type-A dissection presenting as an intramural hematoma. Axial (a) and sagittal (b) unenhanced CT images. The spontaneous hyperdense acute intramural hematoma (asterisks) is clearly seen on these unenhanced CT images. Note the typical semicircular crescent-like shape of the hematoma, and the extension into the aortic sinus (arrow in b).

a post-dissection aortic aneurysm. Finally, it has increased sensitivity compared with CT to detect an intramural hematoma, providing as such additional value to CT in equivocal cases.

However, it is a technically more complex study with a longer examination time, requiring a higher level of patient cooperation compared with CT. Therefore, it is less suitable for critically ill patients. Also, while the anatomic coverage acquired during a single study is generally large enough to cover the thoracic and supra-renal aorta,

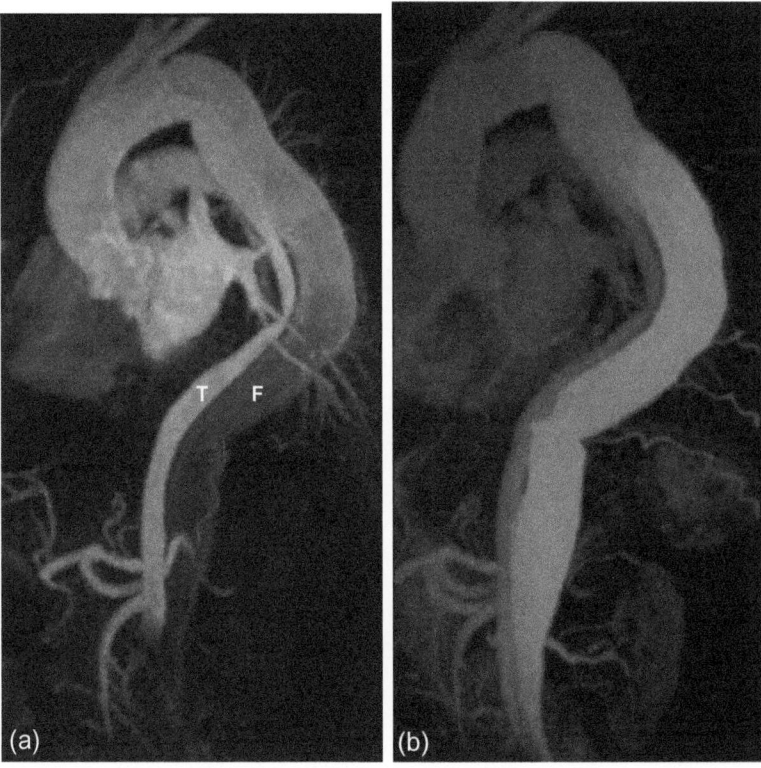

Figure 20.7 Follow-up of a Stanford type-B aortic dissection in a 52-year-old man. Sagittal reformatted T1-weighted images after intravenous contrast administration, acquired in arterial (a) and venous (b) phase. These MR angiography images demonstrate the presence of a double-barreled aortic lumen, consisting of a true (T) and false (F) lumen. In the first-pass arterial images (a) the true lumen is nicely enhanced with almost no opacification of the false lumen. The image acquired 60 s (b) later now shows the delayed enhancement of the false lumen, compatible with slower flow. In this contrast phase, the contrast in the true lumen has almost completely washed out. This example shows the dynamics on contrast-enhancement of the different lumina within an aortic dissection.

contrary to CT, most MR systems cannot cover the whole aorta and iliac arteries in a single examination. These disadvantages make MRA rarely the first imaging choice in a patient with a suspected aortic dissection.

20.2.5.5 Angiography

In every mainstream radiology practice, the excellent sensitivity and specificity of CT and MRI for diagnosing acute aortic dissection have completely obliterated the need for invasive angiography for this indication. While both direct and indirect signs of aortic dissection can be distinguished using angiography (including visualization of the intima and lumina, inward displacement of the true lumen by the intima flap, and the presence of aortic valve regurgitation), it has virtually no place in the initial evaluation. Furthermore, and despite the high sensitivity and specificity for the detection of dissection, it only visualizes the lumen and is not suitable for detection of an intramural hematoma, peri-aortic complications, and total size of the aorta.

However, the continuous development of percutaneous intervention techniques has increased their potential application in the treatment of selected patients with type-B dissection, in recent years reflected as an increased number of endovascular stenting procedures in specialized centers. While not commonplace, highly specialized imaging techniques like cine-angiography of different segments of the aorta and intravascular or phased-array linear ultrasound may additionally provide a supporting role during these aortic interventions. These adjuvant techniques may as such further contribute to a better distinction between true from false lumen, detect side branch compromise, and further facilitate interventions such as flap-fenestration.

20.2.6 Structured reporting

Communication of the imaging findings to the surgeon and clinician is facilitated when using a logically structured report. A summary of the most important points to evaluate can be found in Table 20.3.

Table 20.3 Structured reporting

The following items should be looked for and discussed in the different imaging reports.
Echocardiography (TTE & TEE)   • Presence and extension of an acute aortic dissection in the ascending aorta and root   • Involvement of the aortic valve and degree of aortic valve insufficiency   • General functional cardiac assessment   • Evaluation of potential complication: pericardial effusion, peri-aortic hematoma
Unenhanced CT examination   • The presence and extension of an intramural hematoma   • Displacement of intima calcifications suggestive for dissection
Contrast-enhanced CT and MR examinations   • The presence of an aortic dissection   • Classification of the dissection according to the Stanford classification   • The extension of the dissection into the splanchnic and supra-aortic arteries   • The presence of concomitant aortic aneurysms with double oblique measurements of their size   • Complication: pericardial effusion, extension into the aortic sinus, aortic valve and coronary arteries, imminent aortic rupture/hemothorax, signs of ischemia (brain, cardiac, and abdominal organs)   • Eligibility for endovascular repair in case of a Stanford type-B dissection. Look for suitable proximal and distal sealing zones   • Iliac and femoral vessels (diameters, calcifications, elongation)   • Aorta (diameter, calcification, angulation)
Conclusion   1. The presence, extension, and classification of the aortic dissection   2. The presence of complications   3. Suitability for endovascular repair in case of Stanford type-B aortic dissection

Generally, echocardiography will be used to evaluate the presence and extent of a dissection in the aortic root and ascending aorta. It also provides excellent assessment of the functional cardiac repercussions in general, and more specifically at the level of the aortic valve.

A more complete and accurate evaluation of an aortic dissection can be delivered with contrast-enhanced CT or MR. Here, the presence and extent of the dissection must be accurately evaluated, as well as the involvement of the supra-aortic and splanchnic side branches.

Finally, the possibility of treatment using an endovascular approach in type-B dissection can be evaluated, discussing entry and exit sites and potential sealing locations.

20.3 Vasculitis

20.3.1 Introduction

A broad variety of diseases can lead to symptomatic inflammatory changes in the arterial wall. In clinical practice, the distinction is made between large vessel vasculitis (i.e., giant cell arteritis and Takayasu arteritis), and medium vessel and small vessel vasculitis [9]. In this chapter, we will focus on thoracic aortitis, which can have different infectious and non-infectious causes (Table 20.4).

20.3.2 Clinical presentation

The initial clinical presentation of aortitis is often characterized by non-specific symptoms like persistent fever without a clear origin, malaise, night sweating, and arthralgia. In patients with a late clinical presentation symptoms related to complications (stroke, myocardial infarction, heart failure, aortic rupture, and ischemia distal to a stenosis) can often be observed [9]. In patients with giant cell arteritis, a minority (15%) show involvement of extracranial vessels. In this subgroup of patients, amaurosis fugax may be the presenting symptom if the ophthalmic artery is involved. In contrast, Takayasu arteritis develops characteristically in the thoracic aorta with involvement of the subclavian arteries. It can extend into the abdominal aorta/iliac and

Table 20.4 **Classification of thoracic aortitis**

Non-infectious	Infectious
Takayasu arteritis	Pyogenic infection
Giant cell arteritis	Tuberculous aortitis
Behçet's disease	Syphilitic aortitis
Ankylosing spondylitis	
Relapsing polychondritis	
Rheumatoid arthritis	
Idiopathic isolated aortitis	

Table 20.5 **Differentiation between Takayasu arteritis and giant-cell arteritis**

Giant cell arteritis	Takayasu arteritis
Age at onset of disease >50 years	Age at onset of disease <40 years
New headache	Claudication of an extremity
Associated with stiffness and pain of the joints (polymyalgia rheumatica)	Decreased brachial artery pulse
Temporal artery abnormality	Difference in systolic blood pressure between arms
Elevated erythrocyte sedimentation rate	A bruit over the subclavian arteries or the aorta
Abnormal findings on biopsy of temporal artery	Imaging criteria: – Evidence of narrowing or occlusion of the entire aorta

femoral vessels and cause hypertension due to occlusion/stenosis of the renal arteries (Table 20.5).

20.3.3 Imaging techniques

Several imaging modalities are used and suitable for evaluation of patients with (suspected) thoracic aortitis. The advantages and disadvantages of the different techniques are listed in Table 20.6.

20.3.3.1 Radiography

Radiography can demonstrate very non-specific findings such as a dilated aorta or mediastinal widening due to dilatation of aortic branch vessels. In the late phase, calcifications can be present in the aortic arch and the descending aorta. Radiography can be of value in ruling out alternative explanations of non-specific vascular complaints such as cervical ribs in patients with thoracic outlet syndrome.

20.3.3.2 Ultrasound

In patients with aortitis, ultrasound can demonstrate a hypoechogenic halo around the arterial lumen, stenosis, and occlusions in 93% of the cases [10]. Differentiation between arterial wall inflammation and atherosclerosis is crucial and clinically very relevant. Several echographic characteristics are associated with arterial wall inflammation: concentric and long segment involvement, the presence of minimal amount of plaque content, and the location of the lesion (atherosclerosis has typical preferential locations) [11]. Furthermore, a luminal halo is 100% specific for wall inflammation and is absent in patients with atherosclerosis [10]. TTE can be useful to evaluate the ascending aorta and the presence of aortic regurgitation. TOE can evaluate a larger section of the thoracic aorta.

Table 20.6 **Comparison of imaging modalities in large vessel vasculitis**

Imaging modality	Advantages	Disadvantages
Ultrasound	• High spatial resolution (0.1 mm) • Wall elasticity measures • Calcium/plaque imaging • Directional blood flow • Non-invasive • Portable • Relatively cheap	• Not all vessels are accessible (aorta/subclavian) • Operator-dependent • No measurement of disease activity
MRI/MRA	• Moderate resolution of wall (1 mm) • Good lumen visualization • Suitable for measurement for disease activity (edema/DCE) • Wide coverage	• Expensive • Relative long acquisition times • Moderate plaque/calcium imaging
CTA	• Moderate resolution of wall (1 mm) • Good lumen visualization • Suitable for measurement of disease activity (DCE) • Wide coverage • Plaque/calcium imaging	• Radiation exposure • Iodinated contrast
^{18}FDG PET-CT	• Disease activity measured by SUV quantification • Early detection • Wide coverage	• Limited information on arterial wall morphology • Expensive • Limited access

20.3.3.3 Computed tomography

Computed tomography (CT) is often the preferred initial imaging modality. Unenhanced CT images can demonstrate mural calcifications. CT angiography can demonstrate vessel wall thickening, representing vessel wall inflammation. Typically a double-ring pattern is present with a poor enhancing ring centrally and well-enhancing ring peripherally. Furthermore, a hypodense ring around the vessel wall (vessel wall thickening) representing peri-vasculitis can be visualized as well. Besides this vessel wall thickening, peri-vascular infiltration can be a presenting sign in patients with vasculitis. Moreover, CTA can reveal the presence of mural thrombi. Furthermore, CTA can very accurately (sensitivity 93% and specificity 98%) demonstrate findings typical for the late phase of the disease: arterial stenosis, occlusions, dilatations, and aneurysm formation [11,12] (Figure 20.8).

20.3.3.4 Magnetic resonance imaging

MRI is a superior imaging technique compared to CTA and ultrasound in evaluating early and late arterial wall inflammation. MRI has additional value in evaluating the large arteries in patients with large vessel arteritis, especially Takayasu arteritis [10,13,14]. However, in patients with giant-cell arteritis, the role for MRI is limited. MRI can accurately depict vessel wall inflammation and mural thickening. Furthermore, MRI

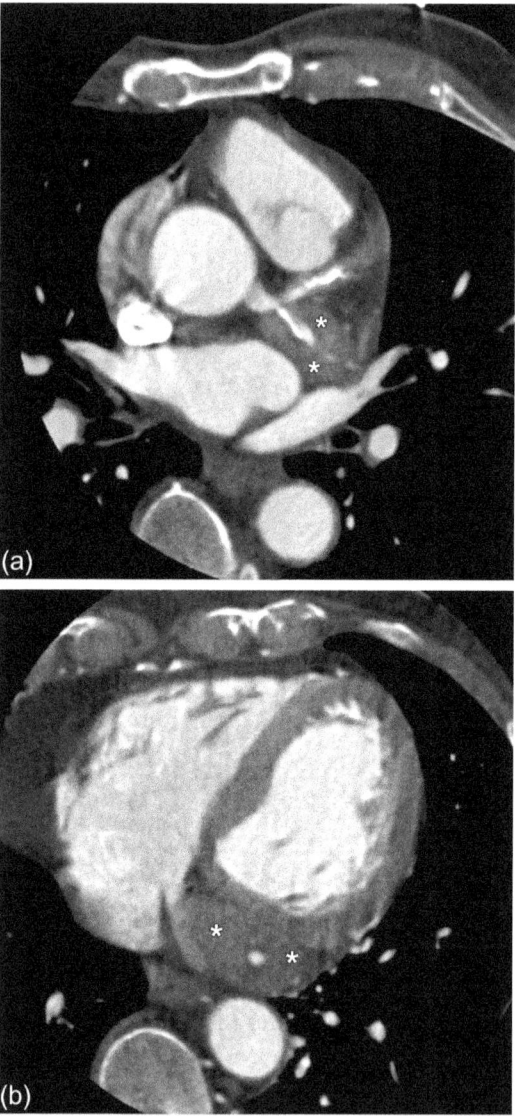

Figure 20.8 A 72-year-old of Southeast Asian origin with complaints of chest pain. Note two partially thrombosed aneurysms (asterisk) with a diameter of approximately 3 cm of the left circumflex coronary artery. The patient reported having been diagnosed with Kawasaki disease as a child.

can also demonstrate peri-vasculitis as soft tissue around the vessel wall. T2 inversion recovery weighted images can depict mural oedema as hyperintense signal, which correlates to active early disease [13]. Although experimental, diffusion-weighted MRI has shown promise to detect inflammatory changes in the thoracic aorta. MR angiography is suitable for the detection of late findings in aortitis such as stenosis, dilatations and aneurysms (Figures 20.9 and 20.10). Furthermore, MRI can reveal involvement of

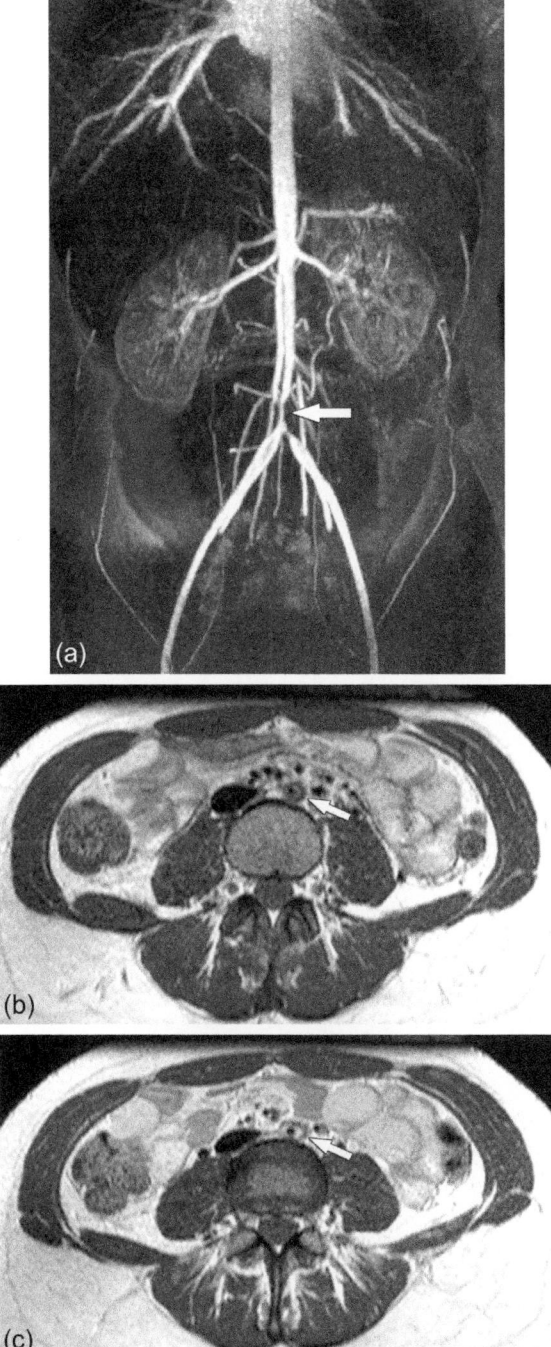

Figure 20.9 Takayasu disease in a 25-year-old female with intermittent claudication. In the maximum intensity projection image of the first-pass MR angiography (a) a smoothly delineated stenosis in the distal aorta with a typical "hour-glass" morphology (arrow) is seen. Corresponding axial T1-weighted images performed before (b) and after (c) intravenous contrast administration show concentric wall thickening with intense enhancement after contrast (arrow).

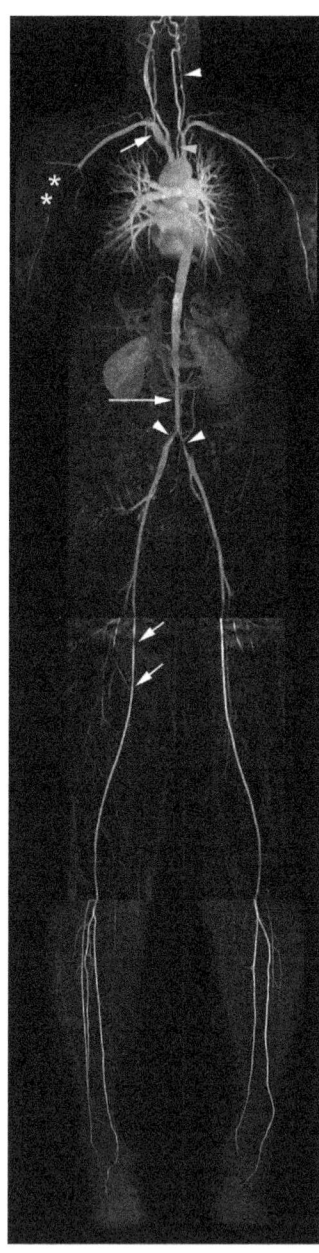

Figure 20.10 A 29-year-old female with long-standing complaints of lower and upper extremity intermittent claudication due to Takayasu disease. Note the multiple smooth, short segmental stenoses (arrowheads), as well as aneurysmal dilatation of the proximal right subclavian artery (short, upper arrow) and a somewhat longer segmented stenoses in the distal abdominal aorta (long arrow) and common iliac arteries (short, lower arrows). These findings are characteristic of circumferential vessel wall thickening due to inflammation. The right brachial artery is nearly occluded (asterisks).

the aortic valve and quantify concomitant aortic valve regurgitation or stenosis. Edema imaging is very sensitive (sensitivity up to 94%) in detection of large-vessel vasculitis [11]. Furthermore, dynamic contrast-enhanced (DCE) MRI can accurately (sensitivity up to 86%) monitor inflammation activity with a comparable accuracy to FDG-PET examinations [11,15]. Enhancement of the vessel wall decreases in case of lower disease activity.

20.3.3.5 PET-CT

F-18-fluorodeoxyglucose (FDG)-PET-CT is an imaging technique that is able to visualize vessel wall metabolism. In patients with aortitis, vessel wall inflammation metabolic rate will increase, resulting in a higher uptake and accumulation of FDG in inflammatory cells. In the literature, PET-CT has a varying sensitivity (77–92%) and specificity (77–100%) for diagnosing arteritis [10,13,16].

PET-CT is not able to detect arteritis in small arteries (<4mm) [17], because of limited spatial resolution. Besides disease detection, PET-CT is suitable for disease monitoring and to evaluate the metabolic response to treatment [15].

20.3.3.6 Angiography

Prior to the widespread use of CT and MRI, angiography was considered the standard of reference for evaluation of aortitis. However, it has been virtually abandoned for this indication because early signs of aortitis such as vessel wall thickening and perivasculitis are not visualized. In the late phase, angiography can nicely evaluate smooth long segments stenosis, dilatations, and aneurysms. Furthermore, angiography can demonstrate collaterals in patients with stenosis. Angiography is an invasive technique and has no role in the diagnostic algorithm today. It is used to perform interventional procedures such as percutaneous angioplasty and stent insertions in patients with long-standing arterial stenosis due to aortitis.

20.3.4 Structured reporting

A proposal for structured reporting is given in Table 20.7.

20.4 Imaging of the postoperative aorta

20.4.1 Introduction

Post-operative imaging of the aorta has become increasingly popular over the last decade, due to continuous and significant development of the surgical and endovascular treatment options of a variety of diseases affecting the aortic root and thoraco-abdominal aorta. Broadly, non-invasive imaging focuses on the evaluation of surgical vascular reconstructions and the assessment of endovascular endoprostheses.

Table 20.7 **Structured reporting of aortitis**

The following items should be looked for and discussed in the different imaging report:
Ultrasound
- Presence of a hypoechogenic halo around the arterial lumen
- The extent and the length of the segment suspected of arterial wall inflammation
- Differentiation from atherosclerosis

Contrast-enhanced CT and MR examinations
- The presence of vessel wall thickening and peri-vasculitis
- The extension and the involvement of the specific vessels
- The presence of late signs of aortitis such as stenosis, dilatations, occlusions, aneurysms
- Disease activity determined with dynamic contrast-enhanced MRA and IR T2 edema imaging

PET-CT examinations
- The presence and extent of aortitis
- Disease activity determined with quantification of FDG uptake and comparison with previous examinations

Conclusions
1. The presence, extension of aortitis
2. The presence of late complications
3. Disease activity

20.4.2 Thoracic aorta: Surgical interventions and endografts

Surgery on the thoracic aorta is generally performed for aneurysmatic dilatation or dissection. Common surgical interventions include replacement of the ascending aorta up to the aortic arch by prosthetic graft material. These are very invasive procedures, potentially requiring circulatory arrest under deep hypothermia if the arch vessels are involved. Combined replacement of the aortic valve and ascending aorta is called a Bentall procedure. Aneurysmatic dilatation of the entire thoracic aorta can also be managed in a two-stage approach. First, the ascending aorta and arch are replaced surgically with a prosthetic graft vessel. At the anastomosis with the descending aorta, the graft is inverted and extends for several centimeters in the lumen (the so-called elephant trunk) (Figure 20.11). Subsequently, a stented graft is placed in the descending aorta with the proximal landing zone in the distal free end of the graft. This free end of the graft should not be mistaken for a dissection on CT. Thoracic endovascular aneurysm repair (TEVAR) using stent grafts similar to those used in abdominal EVAR are used to treat descending aortic aneurysms, aortic ulcers, traumatic aortic injury, and in some centers even dissection. Overstenting of the aortic arch vessels is preferentially avoided, unless the arteries at risk can be bypassed. Complications include endoleaks, pseudoaneurysm formation, stent migration, kinking, and rupture.

20.4.3 Imaging modalities

Several imaging modalities are used in the evaluation after aortic surgery and endovascular procedures. While echocardiography is usually limited in its anatomic scope, it traditionally provides important functional information after

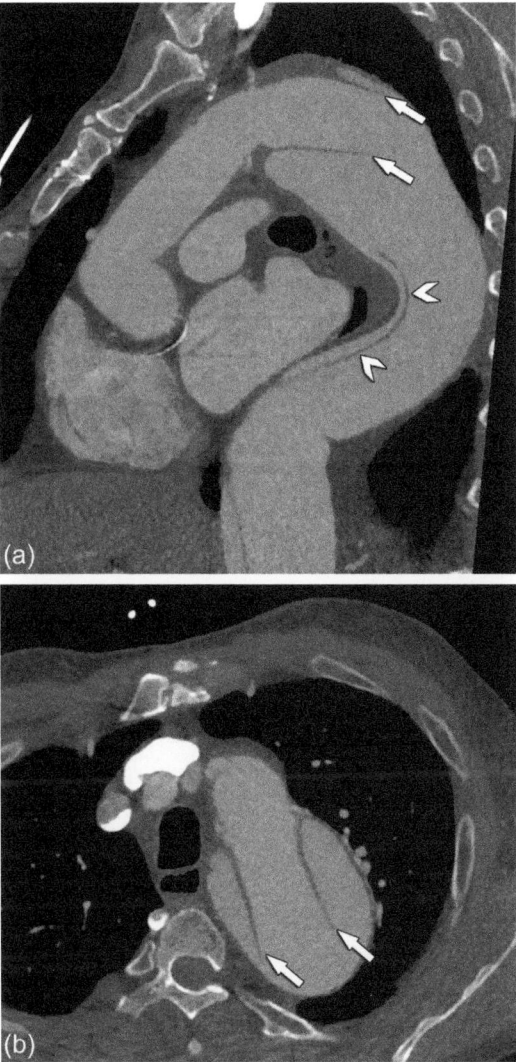

Figure 20.11 Sagittal oblique (a) and axial oblique (b) CT reconstruction of the aorta in a patient who underwent replacement of the ascending aorta and arch with a graft. The distal end of the graft extends into the lumen of the descending aorta, the so-called elephant trunk (arrows). This should not be mistaken for an aortic dissection, which is also present in this patient and can be seen in the descending aorta (arrowheads).

aortic valve replacement. However, recent advances in MR and especially CT technology have increasing added functional information to the excellent morphological evaluation provided by these modalities. As such, MR may play an important role in the evaluation of patients after valve replacement with non-stented biological valves.

20.4.3.1 Ultrasound

TTE and TOE can image only a small part of the thoracic aorta and as such their use is very limited, except for assessment of the aortic valve in case of Bentall or TAVR procedures.

20.4.3.2 Computed tomography

CT with intravenous contrast material is the preferred technique for assessment and follow-up of the thoracic aorta after surgery due to its availability, speed, and high spatial resolution. Acquisition is timed at maximal contrast enhancement in the aorta. To reduce or eliminate motion artifacts of the aortic root and ascending aorta, ECG-gated acquisitions that may be combined with a high pitch are recommended [18].

Anastomoses are predilection sites for false aneurysm formation and should be carefully evaluated. Kinking of the graft material is seen quite regularly and usually does not cause hemodynamically significant stenosis (Figure 20.12). Aortic surgery performed using cardiopulmonary bypass and cannulation sites may present with characteristic findings on CT [19]. As with prosthetic heart valves (PHV) implantation, polytetrafluoroethylene (PTFE) material is also used to reinforce the suture lines at anastomoses of interposition grafts of the aorta. Since PTFE is hyperdense on CT it should not be mistaken for contrast extravasation. Its location and appearance (at suture lines and often as a circular strip) are clues used for identification (Figure 20.13). Checking with the surgical report may be helpful in case of doubt.

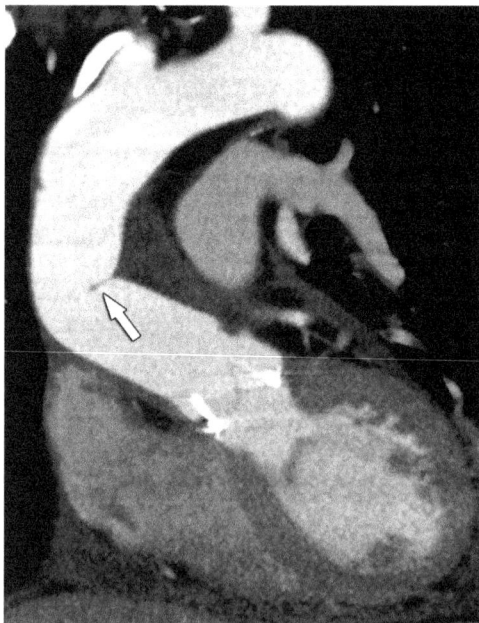

Figure 20.12 Coronal oblique CT image of a patient after replacement of the ascending aorta with an interposition graft. Notice the kinking of the graft in the lesser curvature of the graft, causing part of the graft wall to fold into the lumen (arrow).

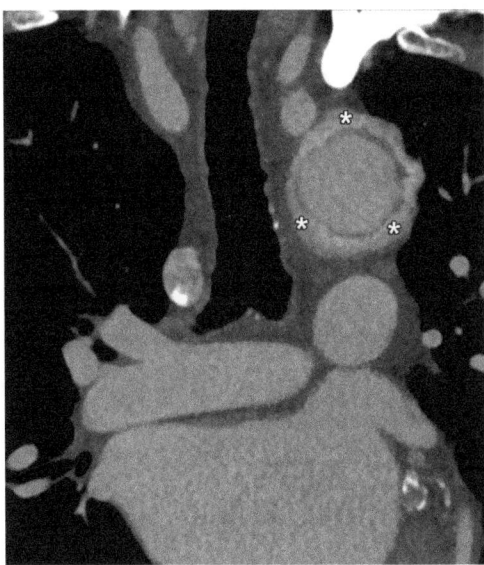

Figure 20.13 Same patient as in Figure 20.11. Multiplanar reconstruction perpendicular to the aorta showing the hyperdense circular PTFE material around the aorta at the distal anastomosis (asterisks).

TEVAR graft stent material generally does not cause artifacts that impair image assessment. 3D volume rendered images can be helpful in detecting stent fracture or bending. Using fixed anatomical landmarks, stent migration should be assessed.

20.4.3.3 Magnetic resonance imaging

MRI can be used to assess endovascular stent grafts. Most current stent grafts are MRI compatible but safety issues must always be addressed [20]. Specific MR-device compatibility should be checked with the relevant manufacturer and/or on the official site of the Institute for Magnetic Resonance Safety, Education, and Research (www.mrisafety.com). The stent itself generates signal voids due to the metal components [21]. The use of turbo spin-echo sequences can mitigate most artifacts except when stainless steel stents are used. Stent diameters measured on MRI are comparable to those measured on CT. Although MRI offers dynamic imaging, this advantage is offset by the lower spatial resolution compared to CT, the somewhat blurred appearance of the stent and the longer duration of the image acquisition. Therefore, MRI is not routinely used for TEVAR follow-up. Novel 4D flow imaging is likely to provide new insights into the dynamics of thoracic aorta disease but is still confined to a research setting in specialized centers [22]. Nevertheless, the potential of 4D MR imaging to simultaneously provide flow-sensitive hemodynamic, (semi-)quantitative, and operator-independent information additional to the already excellent morphological anatomy evaluation may prove an exciting new future investigation tool, both in the pre- and post-operative patient [23,24].

Table 20.8 Structured report

The following items should be looked for and discussed in the contrast enhanced CT report: Aorta: • diameter • calcification • anastomoses • false aneurysms • graft kinking • PTFE material TEVAR: • stent position • kinking/angulation • stent fracture • endoleaks

20.4.3.4 PET-CT

PET-CT has been used in patients with suspected aortic graft or stent infection. Although promising, normal reference values are lacking [25]. Furthermore, atherosclerotic plaques may show FDG uptake as well, making it difficult to discriminate between atherosclerosis and infection.

20.4.4 Structured reporting

A proposal for structured reporting is given in Table 20.8.

20.5 Pulmonary circulation

20.5.1 Introduction

Non-invasive imaging of the pulmonary circulation is a common task in every imaging department. In practice, most of the attention focuses on the evaluation of the pulmonary arteries and right heart when pulmonary embolism, a relatively common cardiovascular emergency, is suspected. Furthermore, imaging plays also an important role in the work-up of patients with pulmonary hypertension.

20.5.2 Clinical presentation

20.5.2.1 Acute pulmonary embolism

Acute pulmonary embolism (PE) is mostly a consequence of underlying deep venous thrombosis (DVT). As such, several predisposing factors exist, including prolonged immobilization due to surgery or major trauma, presence and manipulation of deep venous lines, chronic heart or respiratory failure, oral contraceptive therapy, smoking, pregnancy, and malignancy. Non-thrombotic emboli are rare.

The major clinical consequence of PE is primarily hemodynamic, with pulmonary artery clots leading to increased vascular resistance, syncope, and systemic hypotension. The clinical condition may then rapidly progress to shock and death due to acute right ventricular failure. The suspicion of PE is usually based on a combination of clinical findings (including dyspnea, non-specific chest pain, cough, hemoptysis, and syncope), laboratory findings like elevated plasma D-dimer (a non-specific marker for the presence of acute clot), and the patient's medical history (e.g., recent surgery or prolonged immobilization). However, despite the development of clinical scoring systems like the Wells score and the widespread availability of D-dimer tests, imaging (mostly CT) is nearly always requested to exclude or confirm the presence and extent of PE.

20.5.2.2 Pulmonary hypertension

Pulmonary hypertension (PHT) is defined as an abnormal elevated pressure of the pulmonary circulation due to a wide variety of diseases, with a mean resting pulmonary arterial pressure of 25 mm Hg or more [26]. The recently updated Dana Point classification of 2013 [27] recognizes five groups (Table 20.9), grouping different manifestations of the disease that share similar pathophysiological traits. The clinical course extends from an asymptomatic compensated status, over symptomatic episodes of decompensation, to finally advanced decompensated disease with right-sided heart failure.

When PHT is suspected, a multistep approach is usually needed to not only establish the diagnosis, but also to detect the specific cause, evaluate right ventricular functional and hemodynamic impact, and to establish a proper treatment course. Several imaging modalities have a specific contribution in this multifactorial process.

Table 20.9 **Dana Point classification of pulmonary hypertension**

Group	Description
1	Pulmonary arterial hypertension
1.1	Idiopathic pulmonary arterial hypertension
1.2	Heritable
1.3	Drug and toxin induced
1.4	Associated with connective tissue diseases, HIV infection, portal hypertension, congenital heart disease, and schistosomiasis
1'	Pulmonary veno-occlusive disease and/or pulmonary capillary hemangiomatosis
1''	Persistent pulmonary hypertension of the newborn
2	Pulmonary hypertension due to left heart disease
3	Pulmonary hypertension due to lung diseases and/or hypoxemia
4	Chronic thromboembolic pulmonary hypertension
5	Pulmonary hypertension with unclear or multifactorial mechanisms

20.5.3 Imaging techniques for acute pulmonary embolism

Of all available imaging techniques, CT is the most commonly used when acute PE is suspected. However, other imaging techniques can be valuable adjuncts.

20.5.3.1 Radiography

Chest radiography has little value in the diagnosis of acute PE. While it can show an alternate etiology in a patient with acute chest pain (e.g., infectious pneumonia), it has no place in confirming or excluding PE in modern medical practice.

20.5.3.2 Compression ultrasonography of the lower limbs

Because 90% of acute PE cases arise from a DVT of a lower limb [28], compression ultrasonography (CUS) has a clear role in establishing a primary etiology for acute PE. For proximal DVT, CUS has a sensitivity over 90%, with a specificity of about 95%, revealing a DVT in 30–50% of patients with PE [29,30]. It has also been reported that detecting a proximal DVT with CUS in a patient suspected with PE is enough to start anticoagulant therapy without further testing, which can be helpful in pregnant patients [31]. Nevertheless, given the widespread availability of CT, CUS has currently no role as a primary diagnostic tool for acute PE, as it does not directly visualize PE. It can rarely be used as a backup tool to reduce false-negative examinations when only single-detector CT equipment is available, or to avoid CT when positive in patients with contraindications for iodinated contrast medium [32].

20.5.3.3 Ventilation-perfusion scintigraphy

Ventilation-perfusion scintigraphy (V/Q scan) is a well-known, validated, and safe imaging tool for suspected PE, with only few allergic reactions described. A normal perfusion scan safely excludes PE. A non-diagnostic V/Q scan in a patient with low clinical probability for PE can also be acceptable for excluding PE [32]. A high-probability V/Q scan confirms PE with a high degree of probability. However, in patients with low clinical probability, a high-probability V/Q scan has a low positive predictive value, warranting further testing [32]. Similarly, all other combinations of V/Q scan results and clinical probability should be further investigated to confirm or exclude PE [32]. Finally, a V/Q scan has no use in detecting alternative etiologies for acute chest pain as it provides little anatomic detail. Consequently, it has been mostly replaced by CT as the initial imaging tool for detecting PE.

20.5.3.4 Computed tomography

Advances in CT technology and the widespread availability of multidetector CT systems, which are among others characterized by an isotropic submillimeter spatial resolution combined with an ever-increasing acquisition speed, have made CT the primary imaging tool for both detecting and excluding PE in an acute clinical setting (Figure 20.14). A properly executed contrast-enhanced CT examination can detect and exclude PE with a high sensitivity and specificity up to subsegmental arteries.

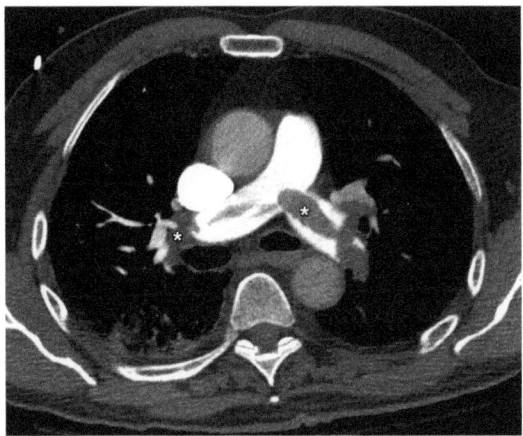

Figure 20.14 Contrast-enhanced axial CT image in a 72-year-old men complaining of shortness of breath after a recent surgical intervention. The image shows extensive and bilateral pulmonary emboli (asterisk). CT imaging is often the first choice in such an acute setting for the detection of pulmonary embolism.

Nevertheless, it remains unclear if further testing is needed when a patient with a high clinical probability has a negative CT examination [32].

Recent advances in CT technology have further introduced the application of dual-energy techniques for the evaluation of PE (see Chapter 5). In dual-energy acquisitions, images are acquired at two different tube potentials (usually 80 and 140kVp), either with one or two detector tubes (depending on the manufacturer). As such, the difference in attenuation of different structures at different energy levels allows for a better differentiation between tissues such as soft tissue, iodine, and air in the chest. In the setting of PE, this technique has shown promise for an improved detection of PE by quantification of lung perfusion by assessing the iodine concentration in the lung parenchyma in contrast-enhanced CT-scans [33] (Figure 20.15). Furthermore, some investigators are evaluating the application of dual-energy CT for the differentiation between acute and chronic PE [34]. However, technical challenges, lack of multicenter prospective trials, and the limited availability of dual-energy CT systems currently limit the application of this technique in mainstream radiology practices.

20.5.3.5 Magnetic resonance imaging

MRI is not often used for the detection of acute PE, as it is less readily available and is a technically more complex examination. Furthermore, while it can be used in selected patients with impaired renal function or a contra-indication for intravenous iodinated contrast administration, its ability to detect PE does not match the high sensitivity and specificity of CT. Despite reported excellent sensitivity and specificity for proximal PE, these values rapidly decline for more distally located clots with up to 30% inconclusive results [35].

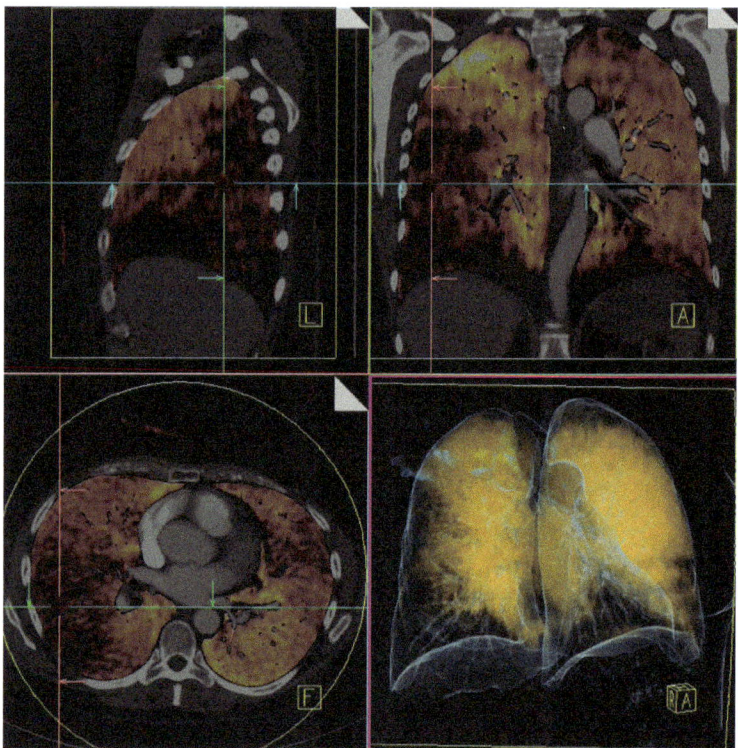

Figure 20.15 Contrast-enhanced dual-energy CT in a middle-aged woman suspected of having an acute pulmonary embolism. While the conventional CT images didn't reveal any segmental or subsegmental emboli in the pulmonary artery, the CT-derived perfusion images clearly show several perfusion defect in the right long, most prominent in the basal segment. Image courtesy of Dr. Daniel Devos, RUG Ghent University Hospital.

20.5.3.6 Pulmonary angiography

Historically, direct angiographic visualization of the pulmonary arteries has been the method of choice for the evaluation of suspected PE. However, advances in CT technology and the use of V/Q scans have largely replaced this imaging tool for this indication. Furthermore, it is associated with the known potential complications of a percutaneous vascular puncture, catheter manipulation, and technical complexity additionally to similar radiation exposure and iodinated contrast administration risks as CT. In practice, pulmonary angiography is now very rarely performed for this indication, except in cases where other non-invasive imaging tools are inconclusive [32]. In selected cases, it can be used for endovascular thrombectomy.

20.5.3.7 Echocardiography

Echocardiography is unable to directly visualize PE, unless located very centrally. However, it can accurately assess the hemodynamic impact of PE on right ventricular function. Also, it can be used at the bedside in a critically ill patient with shock or hypotension, where an echocardiographic absence of right ventricular overload and dysfunction virtually excludes PE as a cause of hemodynamic deterioration [32]. In non-critical non-high-risk patients, echocardiography is used to further stratify between the low- to intermediate-risk categories, and to follow-up right ventricular morphology and function.

20.5.4 Imaging techniques for pulmonary hypertension

20.5.4.1 Radiography

In practice, a chest radiography is one of the first imaging examination performed in a patient suspected of pulmonary hypertension. However, typical signs of PHT are only apparent late in the disease (Figure 20.16), limiting the diagnostic value of chest radiographs, especially in follow-up. Nevertheless, this simple examination can on occasion reveal an underlying etiology of PHT, including interstitial lung disease and emphysema.

20.5.4.2 Computed tomography

CT has an important role in the evaluation of patients with PHT, delivering information regarding vascular, parenchymal, and cardiac anatomy. The size of the main pulmonary artery is easily evaluated on contrast-enhanced CT examination, where a diameter of 29 mm or more has a positive predictive value of 97% for PHT (Figure 20.17). When dilated, a segmental artery-to-bronchus diameter ratio of 1:1 or more in three or four lobes has a reported specificity of 100% for PHT. However, a main pulmonary artery diameter of less than 29 mm does not necessarily exclude PHT.

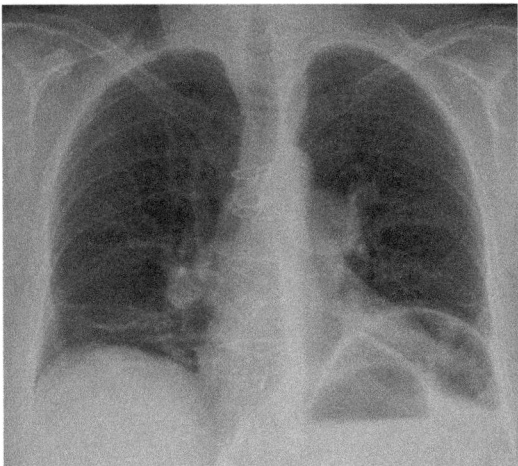

Figure 20.16 Conventional chest film reveals prominent bilateral pulmonary artery shadows. While this finding is suggestive of underlying pulmonary hypertension, its lack of specificity and sensitivity makes it of little use in clinical practice for this diagnosis.

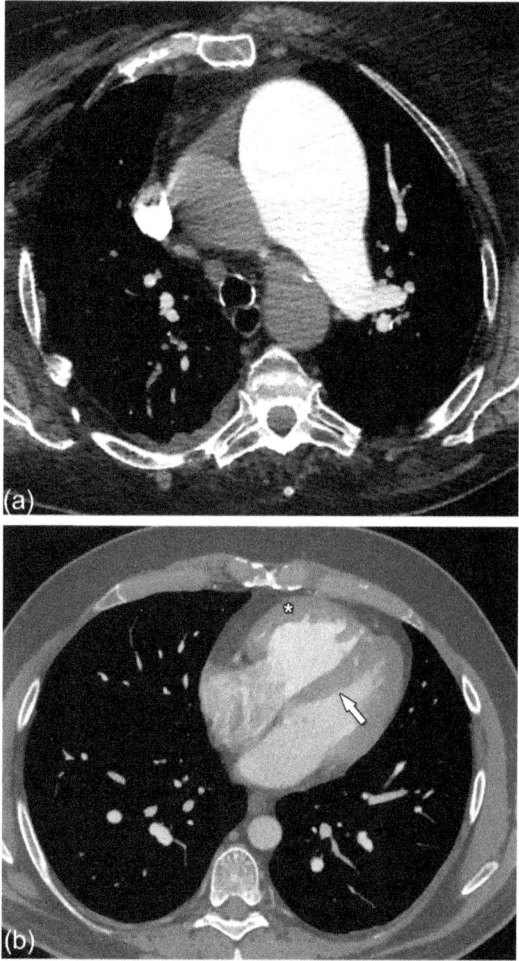

Figure 20.17 A 72-year-old man with long-standing pulmonary hypertension. A severely dilated pulmonary trunk can be seen (a), together with a dilated and hypertrophic right ventricular wall (asterisk in b), the latter consistent with a chronic condition. Note also the typical inward bowing of the ventricular septum (arrow in b).

The hemodynamic impact of increased pulmonary pressure on the right heart can also be seen on (especially ECG-gated) CT examinations, and includes right ventricular hypertrophy and dilatation, dilated inferior vena cava and hepatic veins, and a straightening or leftward bowing of the interventricular septum (Figure 20.17). Nevertheless, it has little added value over echocardiography and cardiac MRI in this respect.

Finally, every CT examination for PHT must include an assessment of the lung parenchyma, as it may harbor the underlying cause of PHT, including extensive interstitial lung disease (Figure 20.18) and signs of chronic thromboembolic disease. CT can also show intra- and extracardiac vascular shunts, which may be an underlying cause of PHT.

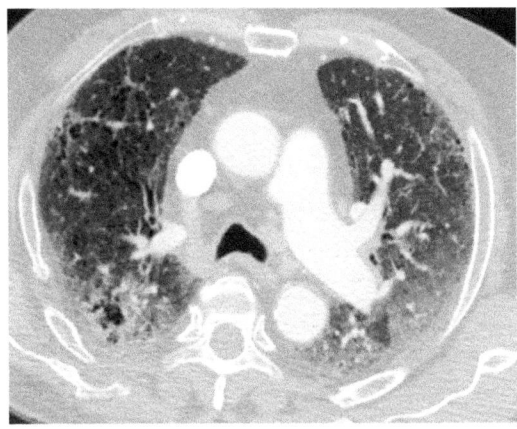

Figure 20.18 A 65-year-old woman with pulmonary hypertension due to severe interstitial lung disease. While CT is very sensitive in documenting the interstitial pathologic findings, it is, however, often not able to provide a specific diagnosis due to the amount of overlapping findings between different interstitial lung diseases.

20.5.4.3 Magnetic resonance imaging

Providing a combined morphological and functional evaluation of the heart, cardiac MRI can deliver valuable information regarding ventricular volume, mass, wall abnormalities/fibrosis, and function together with a morphological evaluation of the proximal pulmonary vasculature in one examination. Phase-contrast imaging can also provide flow velocity measurements in the main pulmonary artery, with decreasing flow velocity in patients with PHT. It can also detect and quantify intracardiac shunts as a cause for PHT.

In comparison with CT, cardiac MRI is nevertheless a more complex examination requiring more patient cooperation and expertise from the performing radiologist. As such, it application is generally decided on a case-by-case basis.

20.5.4.4 Echocardiography

Echocardiography is one of the most important imaging modalities in pulmonary hypertension, as it can reliably assess right ventricular function and morphology (Figure 20.19). It is a safe examination, which is routinely used to follow the effect of treatment. Despite these clear advantages over CT, it cannot provide any information regarding the status of the lung parenchyma. As such, both echocardiography and CT are complementary to each other and form the cornerstone for non-invasive imaging in the evaluation and follow-up of patients with PHT.

20.5.4.5 Right-heart catheterization

Right-heart catheterization is the only test that can directly measure the pressure and resistance in the pulmonary arteries, together with cardiac output. No angiography is usually performed. Therefore, and despite advances in non-invasive imaging techniques

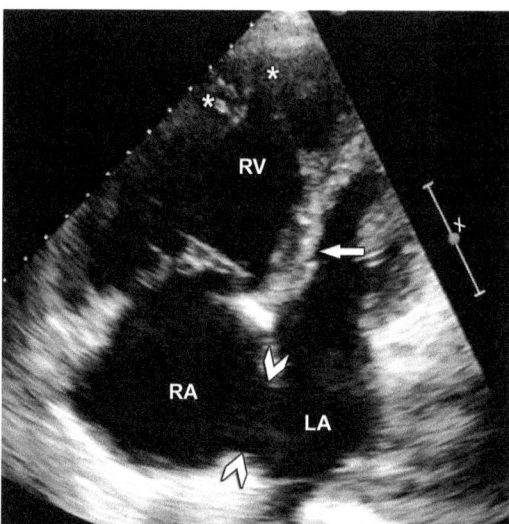

Figure 20.19 Echocardiography can quickly and reliably assess right ventricular function and morphology, revealing in this case typical findings of long-standing pulmonary hypertension with a hypertrophic right ventricular (RV) wall (asterisk) and inward bowing of the ventricular septum (arrow). RA: right atrium; LA: left atrium; LV: left ventricle; short arrows: aortic valve.

like CT and cardiac MR, it remains the reference standard for the diagnosis of pulmonary hypertension, further aiding in the differentiation between pulmonary hypertension and pulmonary *arterial* hypertension. As with every intervention, it suffers from the usual potential complications of a vascular percutaneous puncture, and it does not deliver morphological information.

20.5.5 Structured reporting

A proposal for structure reporting can be found in Table 20.10.

20.6 Aneurysmatic disease

20.6.1 Introduction

Imaging of atherosclerotic aortic disease forms an important part of the daily routine in every radiology department. This is to a great extent due to the increasing age of the general population and the associated greater prevalence of atherosclerotic disease. Furthermore, advances in endovascular treatment options have significantly reduced the need for open surgery in many cases of aneurysmal atherosclerotic disease, further emphasizing the role of non-invasive pre-operative imaging for optimal pre-interventional planning.

Table 20.10 Structured reporting

The following items should be looked for and discussed in the different imaging reports:

Echocardiography (TTE and TEE)
- Right ventricular function and morphology
- General functional cardiac assessment

Contrast-enhanced CT
- Presence and extent of pulmonary embolism
- Effect on right-heart morphology: ventricular dilatation and hypertrophy
- Diameter of the main pulmonary artery: > 29 mm is suggestive for pulmonary hypertension
- Complications of PE like lung infarction
- Status of lung parenchyma: e.g., presence of interstitial lung disease, emphysema, etc.
- Look for intra- and extracardiac shunts as a potential cause for pulmonary hypertension

Magnetic resonance imaging
- Detection of proximal PE, evaluation of main pulmonary artery dimension
- Morphological and functional evaluation of the right heart
- Evaluation and quantification of potential intracardiac shunts

V/Q scan
- Report on low, intermediate to high probability of the presence of PE
- Look for signs of chronic thromboembolic disease

Compression ultrasonography of the lower limbs
- Presence and extent of DVT

Right-heart catheterization
- Report pressure measurements for diagnosis and treatment monitoring of PHT

Conclusion
- Use CT for detection/exclusion of PE and complications, or to detect an alternate diagnosis
- Use echocardiography and to a lesser extent MR for further functional and morphological evaluation. MR can also be used for proximal PE when CT is contra-indicated
- Use V/Q scan for detection of PE when CT is contra-indicated or inconclusive, or when chronic thromboembolic disease is suspected
- Right-heart catheterization with pressure measurements is gold standard for diagnosis of pulmonary hypertension

20.6.2 Clinical presentation

Aneurysmatic disease remains often asymptomatic for a prolonged period of time, or presents with non-specific complaints, such as backache. As such, an atherosclerotic aortic aneurysm is often detected incidentally during imaging for unrelated reasons. When a patient has a known predisposition for vascular disease, e.g., in case of known valvular disease or pre-existing conditions like Marfan syndrome (often non-atherosclerotic), vascular disease can be detected in its initial stage during screening examinations, often performed with CT or MRI (Figure 20.20).

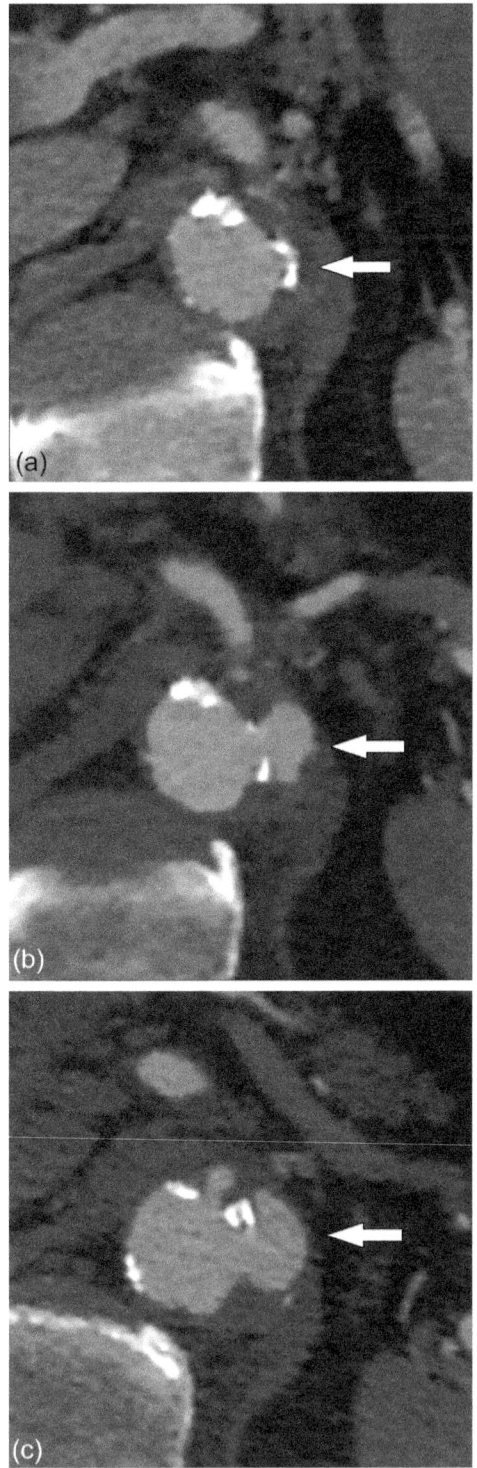

Figure 20.20 See figure Legend on Opposite page.

20.6.3 Aortic dimensions and the need for intervention

Although normal reference values for the ascending thoracic aortic diameter vary, the general opinion is to consider 4 cm the upper limit of normal. Aneurysmatic dilatation of the thoracic aorta has multiple etiologies, the most common being cystic media degeneration associated with normal aging processes and atherosclerotic disease. Other etiologies include connective tissue diseases such as Marfan syndrome, a bicuspid aortic valve, and aortic dissection. Operative repair of the aorta is considered if the diameter of the ascending aorta exceeds 5.5 cm, or 5.0 cm in case of connective tissue disease. An even lower threshold of 4.5 cm can be considered in case of planned aortic valve surgery, with additional risk factors, including family history of dissection, size increase of >3 mm/year (in repeated examinations using the same technique and confirmed by another technique), severe aortic regurgitation, or desire for pregnancy [36].

There is general agreement on the levels that are used to measure the diameter of the thoracic aorta: annulus, sinus of Valsalva, sinotubular junction, ascending aorta, arch, and descending aorta. Unfortunately, there is no binding consensus on the exact measurement procedure. This is partly due to the fact that some imaging modalities like ultrasound only allow diameter measurements in a single plane. Consequently, this measurement may be significantly affected by the chosen imaging plane as well as the used imaging technique and operator. Furthermore, the dynamic diameter changes present in a dilated thoracic aorta due to the pulsatile blood flow may be as much as 12%, and thus be significant especially when comparing follow-up examinations [37].

In practice, we promote the use of CT or MR-based double-oblique reconstructions perpendicular to the vessels' axis for diameter measurements (Figure 20.21). Furthermore, one must also consider that the aortic cross-sectional morphology is often not perfectly circular. In such instance, one can choose to report either the largest or both the maximal short- and long-axis diameter at each anatomic level. Irrespective of the chosen measurement technique, it is of the utmost importance to use it consistently because only then a reliable comparison in time is possible, as many patients undergo multiple examinations during follow-up.

If possible, the aortic valve should be assessed concomitantly with the used imaging technique. The presence of a bicuspid valve is associated with aortic dilatation and must be always considered when a dilated ascending aorta is found in a younger patient (Figure 20.22). Furthermore, aortic valve insufficiency may be associated with aortic root dilatation and should therefore be evaluated.

Figure 20.20 Axial contrast-enhanced CT image at the level of the diaphragm in a patient with an incidentally detected small pseudoaneurysm (arrow). On the initial CT examination, only a small outpouching of the left aortic wall is seen, with some surrounding soft tissue stranding. On subsequent follow-up examination performed after 2 (b) and 4 (c) weeks, a rapid growth of the pseudoaneurysm (arrow) is clearly seen, illustrating the utility of CT for follow-up of even small but suspected vascular lesions.

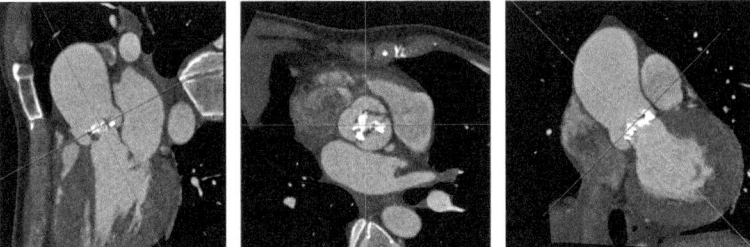

Figure 20.21 CT images of a patient with a bicuspid aortic valve and aneurysmatic dilatation of the ascending aorta. In order to measure the diameter of the sinus of Valsalva accurately in this patient, a double oblique reconstruction in plane with the sinus of Valsalva (middle panel) is mandatory. Using a multiplanar mode with three axes perpendicular to each other, a double oblique reconstruction is easily obtained. By adjusting the purple axis in the left and right panel perpendicular to the sinus of Valsalva, the in-plane reconstruction in the middle panel is obtained.

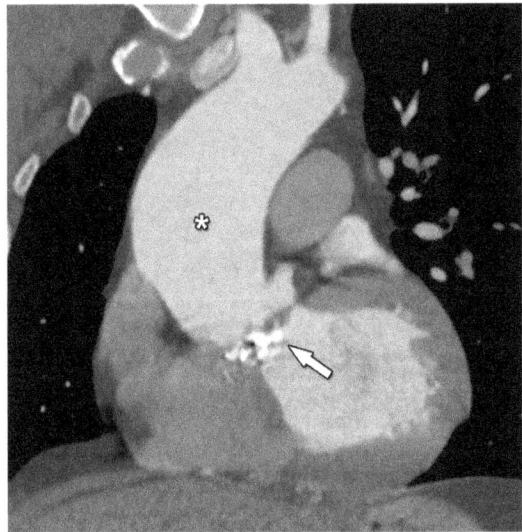

Figure 20.22 This contrast-enhanced coronal CT image illustrates a fusiform dilatation of the ascending aorta (asterisk) in a 38-year-old man. Note also the peculiarly advanced degeneration of the aortic valve (for his age), with thickened and heavily calcified leaflets (arrow). Closer examination with CT revealed a bicuspid aortic valve.

20.6.4 Imaging techniques

CT is the most commonly used imaging technique for initial assessment and follow-up of aneurysmatic disease of the thoracic aorta. However, other imaging techniques, especially MRI, can be used as an alternative in specific situations.

20.6.4.1 Radiography

Chest radiography has little value in the diagnosis of aneurysmatic disease of the thoracic aorta. It can provide a first clue to its presence by demonstrating a wide aortic shadow, but otherwise remains non-specific.

20.6.4.2 Echocardiography

Using echocardiography, only portions of the ascending aorta and arch can be visualized whereas the descending aorta cannot. The usual limitations of echocardiography (operator dependence, poor acoustic windows in certain patients (COPD, obesity)) also apply. Furthermore, for accurate measurement of the diameter, ideally a double-oblique orientation perpendicular to the aortic axis is used, which is difficult to obtain with echocardiography. However, echocardiography does provide valuable information on the morphology and function of the aortic valve, which is of value for reasons mentioned above.

20.6.4.3 Computed tomography

Contrast-enhanced CT is the most commonly used imaging technique for diagnosis and follow-up of aneurysmatic disease of the thoracic aorta. It provides high-resolution three-dimensional image datasets that can be reformatted in any desired imaging plane at every anatomic level of the aorta. This is especially helpful, as previously explained, for diameter measurement perpendicular to the vessel's long axis. Furthermore, three-dimensional volume rendering views enable clear visualization of the entire aorta, facilitating pre-operative planning in complex cases. Due to the motion of the ascending aorta, ECG-gated or triggered acquisitions are often used and prove especially helpful to assess the aortic root. Radiation exposure is currently less of an issue with modern scanners being able to image the entire thoracic aorta at around 2 mSv [38]. Besides morphological information on the aorta, CT can also demonstrate aortic valve insufficiency resulting from annulus dilatation by showing central noncoaptation of the aortic valve leaflets. However, outside selected cases, echocardiography and MRI are still being preferred in practice to assess the aortic valve, as they benefit from a longer experience and scientific validation for this indication and provide functional as well as anatomical information.

20.6.4.4 Magnetic resonance imaging

MRI provides an alternative to CT in selected cases, its main advantage being the lack of radiation and iodinated contrast exposure. The former advantage is particularly valuable in young patients with frequent follow-up examinations, the latter in elderly patients with decreased renal function. Contrast-enhanced MRI provides excellent anatomic detail of the ascending and descending aorta as well as the arch (Figure 20.23). Similar with CT, 3D contrast-enhanced MRI sequences allow image reformatting of the aorta in various planes after the acquisition providing as such a correct assessment of aortic cross-sectional dimensions. However, some techniques require the definition

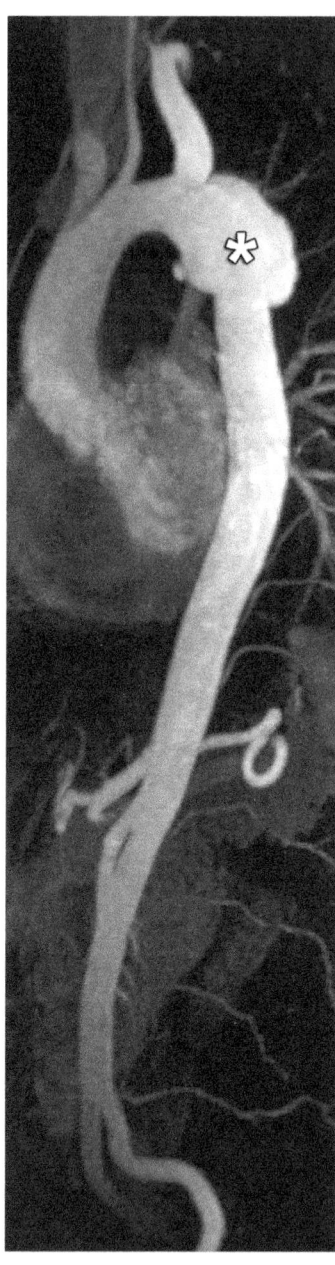

Figure 20.23 Contrast-enhanced MR angiography of the aorta in a 52-year-old man for follow-up of a known aneurysm at the aortic isthmus (asterisk). Long-term follow-up of such a findings is required for close monitoring of the aneurysms' dimensions. The use of MR angiography for this indication is very well suited, as it can provide the necessary information without the need of repeated radiation exposure and with a much better tolerated contrast agent compared with CT.

of the imaging plane before the actual acquisition, making it on occasion difficult to see whether one is truly perpendicular to the vessels' axis (especially in a tortuous thoracic aorta).

However, ECG gating is still needed if adequate visualization of the aortic root is required in order to eliminate motion artifacts and resultant blurring of the aortic borders, making this portion of the examination technically more complex. Other more advanced techniques, like ECG-gated steady-state free precession acquisitions, offer dynamic imaging of the aorta along the cardiac cycle, allowing diameter measurements to be performed in systole or diastole as desired. Finally, black-blood imaging usually offers the best contrast between the aortic lumen and wall, and is therefore often used in the investigation of possible infectious/inflammatory wall disease (Figure 20.24). Nevertheless, it suffers from long acquisition times as a breath-hold maneuver is required for each image, making it less applicable in older or less cooperative patients.

Also, MRI offers concomitant evaluation on the aortic valve for insufficiency, which may deliver a cause for premature aortic dilatation, especially in younger patients.

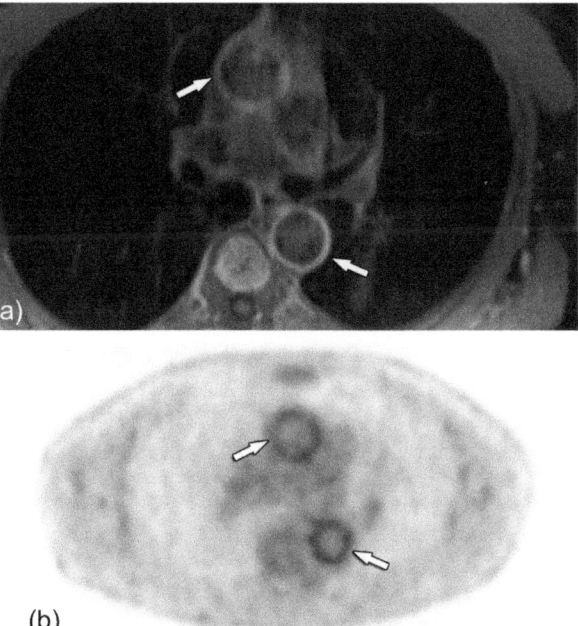

Figure 20.24 Black blood T1-weighted contrast-enhanced MR image (a) of a 65-year-old patient, initially referred for vascular thoracic screening with non-specific thoracic complaints. A black blood MR sequence allows an improved evaluation of possible enhancement of the aortic wall in contrast-enhanced MR examinations, as the contrast-enhancement of the vessel lumen is suppressed. In this case, the images showed normal aortic dimensions but a clear enhancement of the thoracic aortic wall (arrows in a), compatible with large vessel vasculitis. This was consequently further corroborated with a PET-examination (b), showing clear circumferential FDG-18 uptake in the vessel wall (arrows).

Table 20.11 **Structured reporting**

The following items should be looked for and discussed in the different imaging reports:
Echocardiography (TTE)   • Aorta (ascending and arch) diameter   • Aortic valve morphology (bi- vs. tricuspid) and insufficiency   • Left ventricular function
Contrast-enhanced CT   • Use of ECG-triggering or gating and phase (systole/diastole) used for diameter measurements   • Aortic diameter in double oblique reconstructions (levels see below)   • Aortic valve morphology (bi- vs. tricuspid) and insufficiency (central noncoaptation in diastole)
Magnetic resonance imaging   • Use of ECG gating and phase (systole/diastole) used for diameter measurements   • Acquisition sequence used for measurements   • Aortic diameter in double oblique reconstructions if possible (levels see below)   • Aortic valve morphology (bi- vs. tricuspid) and insufficiency (phase contrast imaging)   • Left ventricular function
Conclusion   • Use double oblique reconstructions for diameter measurement when possible   • Use specific anatomical sites for diameter measurement: annulus, sinus of Valsalva, sino-tubular junction, ascending aorta, arch, descending aorta.   • Always try to assess aortic valve morphology and function

20.6.4.5 Conventional catheter angiography

Invasive conventional catheter angiography has no place in the current era for diagnosis of thoracic aortic aneurysms but is of course an integral part of endovascular thoracic aneurysm repair.

20.6.5 Structured reporting

A proposal for structure reporting can be found in Table 20.11.

References

[1] Vilacosta I, Roman JA. Acute aortic syndrome. Heart 2001;85:365–8.
[2] Fleischmann D, Mitchell RS, Miller DC. Acute aortic syndromes: new insights from electrocardiographically gated computed tomography. Semin Thorac Cardiovasc Surg 2008;20:340–7.
[3] Ueda T, Chin A, Petrovitch I, Fleischmann D. A pictorial review of acute aortic syndrome: discriminating and overlapping features as revealed by ECG-gated multidetector-row CT angiography. Insights Imaging 2012;3:561–71.
[4] Hayter RG, Rhea JT, Small A, Tafazoli FS, Novelline RA. Suspected aortic dissection and other aortic disorders: multi-detector row CT in 373 cases in the emergency setting. Radiology 2006;238:841–52.

[5] Hagan PG, Nienaber CA, Isselbacher EM, Bruckman D, Karavite DJ, Russman PL, et al. The International Registry of Acute Aortic Dissection (IRAD): new insights into an old disease. JAMA 2000;283:897–903.
[6] Hiratzka LF, Bakris GL, Beckman JA, Bersin RM, Carr VF, Casey Jr DE, et al. 2010 ACCF/AHA/AATS/ACR/ASA/SCA/SCAI/SIR/STS/SVM guidelines for the diagnosis and management of patients with thoracic aortic disease: executive summary. A report of the American College of Cardiology Foundation/American Heart Association Task Force on Practice Guidelines, American Association for Thoracic Surgery, American College of Radiology, American Stroke Association, Society of Cardiovascular Anesthesiologists, Society for Cardiovascular Angiography and Interventions, Society of Interventional Radiology, Society of Thoracic Surgeons, and Society for Vascular Medicine. Catheter Cardiovasc Interv 2010;76:E43–86.
[7] Willemink MJ, de Jong PA, Leiner T, de Heer LM, Nievelstein RA, Budde RP, et al. Iterative reconstruction techniques for computed tomography Part 1: technical principles. Eur Radiol 2013;23:1623–31.
[8] Willemink MJ, Leiner T, de Jong PA, de Heer LM, Nievelstein RA, Schilham AM, et al. Iterative reconstruction techniques for computed tomography Part 2: initial results in dose reduction and image quality. Eur Radiol 2013;23:1632–42.
[9] Belhocine T, Blockmans D, Hustinx R, Vandevivere J, Mortelmans L. Imaging of large vessel vasculitis with (18) FDG PET: illusion or reality? A critical review of the literature data. Eur J Nucl Med Mol Imaging 2003;30:1305–13.
[10] Levine SM, Hellmann DB. Giant cell arteritis. Curr Opin Rheumatol 2002;14:3–10.
[11] Kissin EY, Merkel PA. Diagnostic imaging in Takayasu arteritis. Curr Opin Rheumatol 2004;16:31–7.
[12] Glaudemans AW, de Vries EF, Galli F, Dierckx RA, Slart RH, Signore A. The use of (18) F-FDG-PET/CT for diagnosis and treatment monitoring of inflammatory and infectious diseases. Clin Dev Immunol 2013;2013:623036.
[13] Bleeker-Rovers CP, Bredie SJ, van der Meer JW, Corstens FH, Oyen WJ. F-18-fluorodeoxyglucose positron emission tomography in diagnosis and follow-up of patients with different types of vasculitis. Neth J Med 2003;61:323–9.
[14] Nastri MV, Baptista LP, Baroni RH, Blasbalg R, de Avila LF, Leite CC, et al. Gadolinium-enhanced three-dimensional MR angiography of Takayasu arteritis. Radiographics 2004;24:773–86.
[15] Cyran CC, Sourbron S, Bochmann K, Habs M, Pfefferkorn T, Rominger A, et al. Quantification of supra-aortic arterial wall inflammation in patients with arteritis using high resolution dynamic contrast-enhanced magnetic resonance imaging: initial results in correlation to [18F]-FDG PET/CT. Invest Radiol 2011;46:594–9.
[16] Zerizer I, Tan K, Khan S, Barwick T, Marzola MC, Rubello D, et al. Role of FDG-PET and PET/CT in the diagnosis and management of vasculitis. Eur J Radiol 2010;73:504–9.
[17] Brodmann M, Lipp RW, Passath A, Seinost G, Pabst E, Pilger E. The role of 2-18F-fluoro-2-deoxy-D-glucose positron emission tomography in the diagnosis of giant cell arteritis of the temporal arteries. Rheumatology (Oxford) 2004;43:241–2.
[18] Christensen JD, Seaman DM, Lungren MP, Hurwitz LM, Boll DT. Assessment of vascular contrast and wall motion of the aortic root and ascending aorta on MDCT angiography: dual-source high-pitch vs non-gated single-source acquisition schemes. Eur Radiol 2014;24:990–7.
[19] El-Sherief AH, Wu CC, Schoenhagen P, Little BP, Cheng A, Abbara S, et al. Basics of cardiopulmonary bypass: normal and abnormal postoperative CT appearances. Radiographics 2013;33:63–72.

[20] Levine GN, Gomes AS, Arai AE, Bluemke DA, Flamm SD, Kanal E, et al. Safety of magnetic resonance imaging in patients with cardiovascular devices: an American Heart Association scientific statement from the Committee on Diagnostic and Interventional Cardiac Catheterization, Council on Clinical Cardiology, and the Council on Cardiovascular Radiology and Intervention: endorsed by the American College of Cardiology Foundation, the North American Society for Cardiac Imaging, and the Society for Cardiovascular Magnetic Resonance. Circulation 2007;116:2878–91.
[21] Rasche V, Oberhuber A, Trumpp S, Bornstedt A, Orend KH, Merkle N, et al. MRI assessment of thoracic stent grafts after emergency implantation in multi trauma patients: a feasibility study. Eur Radiol 2011;21:1397–405.
[22] Markl M, Frydrychowicz A, Kozerke S, Hope M, Wieben O. 4D flow MRI. J Magn Reson Imaging 2012;36:1015–36.
[23] Stankovic Z, Allen BD, Garcia J, Jarvis KB, Markl M. 4D flow imaging with MRI. Cardiovasc Diagn Ther 2014;4:173–92.
[24] van Bogerijen GH, van Herwaarden JA, Conti M, Auricchio F, Rampoldi V, Trimarchi S, et al. Importance of dynamic aortic evaluation in planning TEVAR. Ann Cardiothorac Surg 2014;3:300–6.
[25] Tokuda Y, Oshima H, Araki Y, Narita Y, Mutsuga M, Kato K, et al. Detection of thoracic aortic prosthetic graft infection with 18F-fluorodeoxyglucose positron emission tomography/computed tomography. Eur J Cardiothorac Surg 2013;43:1183–7.
[26] Rubin LJ. Primary pulmonary hypertension. N Engl J Med 1997;336:111–7.
[27] Simonneau G, Gatzoulis MA, Adatia I, Celermajer D, Denton C, Ghofrani A, et al. Updated clinical classification of pulmonary hypertension. J Am Coll Cardiol 2013;62:D34–41.
[28] Sevitt S, Gallagher N. Venous thrombosis and pulmonary embolism. A clinico-pathological study in injured and burned patients. Br J Surg 1961;48:475–89.
[29] Kearon C, Ginsberg JS, Hirsh J. The role of venous ultrasonography in the diagnosis of suspected deep venous thrombosis and pulmonary embolism. Ann Intern Med 1998;129:1044–9.
[30] Perrier A, Bounameaux H. Ultrasonography of leg veins in patients suspected of having pulmonary embolism. Ann Intern Med 1998;128:243, author reply 244–245.
[31] Le Gal G, Righini M, Sanchez O, Roy PM, Baba-Ahmed M, Perrier A, et al. A positive compression ultrasonography of the lower limb veins is highly predictive of pulmonary embolism on computed tomography in suspected patients. Thromb Haemost 2006;95:963–6.
[32] Torbicki A, Perrier A, Konstantinides S, Agnelli G, Galie N, Pruszczyk P, et al. Guidelines on the diagnosis and management of acute pulmonary embolism: the Task Force for the Diagnosis and Management of Acute Pulmonary Embolism of the European Society of Cardiology (ESC). Eur Heart J 2008;29:2276–315.
[33] Zhang LJ, Zhou CS, Schoepf UJ, Sheng HX, Wu SY, Krazinski AW, et al. Dual-energy CT lung ventilation/perfusion imaging for diagnosing pulmonary embolism. Eur Radiol 2013;23:2666–75.
[34] Kim SS, Hur J, Kim YJ, Lee HJ, Hong YJ, Choi BW. Dual-energy CT for differentiating acute and chronic pulmonary thromboembolism: an initial experience. Int J Cardiovasc Imaging 2014;30(Suppl. 2):113–20.
[35] Revel MP, Sanchez O, Couchon S, Planquette B, Hernigou A, Niarra R, et al. Diagnostic accuracy of magnetic resonance imaging for an acute pulmonary embolism: results of the 'IRM-EP' study. J Thromb Haemost 2012;10:743–50.
[36] Erbel R, Aboyans V, Boileau C, Bossone E, Bartolomeo RD, Eggebrecht H, et al. 2014 ESC Guidelines on the diagnosis and treatment of aortic diseases: Document covering acute and chronic aortic diseases of the thoracic and abdominal aorta of the adultThe Task

Force for the Diagnosis and Treatment of Aortic Diseases of the European Society of Cardiology (ESC). Eur Heart J 2014;35:2873–926.

[37] van Prehn J, Bartels LW, Mestres G, Vincken KL, Prokop M, Verhagen HJ, et al. Dynamic aortic changes in patients with thoracic aortic aneurysms evaluated with electrocardiography-triggered computed tomographic angiography before and after thoracic endovascular aneurysm repair: preliminary results. Ann Vasc Surg 2009;23:291–7.

[38] Goetti R, Baumuller S, Feuchtner G, Stolzmann P, Karlo C, Alkadhi H, et al. High-pitch dual-source CT angiography of the thoracic and abdominal aorta: is simultaneous coronary artery assessment possible? AJR Am J Roentgenol 2010;194:938–44.

Arrhythmia

S.C.A.M. Bekkers, B.L. Kietselaer, L. Pison
Maastricht University Medical Center, Maastricht, The Netherlands

21.1 Introduction

Electrophysiology comprises catheter ablations and cardiac implantable electrical devices (CIED) for malconduction and arrhythmia management, prevention of sudden cardiac death, or cardiac resynchronization, and is a rapidly growing field in cardiology. There is an increased clinical use of advanced cardiac imaging for pre-procedural assessment, procedure guidance, detection of complications, and follow-up in patients with arrhythmias or conduction disturbances (Table 21.1) [1]. The partly overlapping capabilities, differing diagnostic accuracies, and continuing technological developments require a thorough understanding of the indications, advantages, and disadvantages of different imaging technologies by both cardiac imaging specialists and electrophysiologists. In this chapter, the role of different imaging modalities is discussed focussed on common atrial and ventricular arrhythmias and cardiac resynchronization therapy (CRT).

21.2 Fluoroscopy

Catheter ablations are traditionally performed under X-ray fluoroscopic guidance. Rotational angiography is a new technique that enables the creation of real-time 3D images during the ablation procedure. The most important application of both classic X-ray fluoroscopy and rotational angiography is procedural guidance.

21.2.1 Routine fluoroscopy

21.2.1.1 Procedural guidance

The main role of X-ray fluoroscopy is the guidance of endocardial catheters during ablation procedures of supraventricular and ventricular arrhythmias (see Figure 21.1). X-ray fluoroscopy is also used to visualize pacemaker and implantable cardioverter-defibrillator (ICD) leads during implantation. A major concern in relation to radiation exposure is its deterministic and stochastic effects that may lead to observable skin injury [2] and irreversible radiation damage to DNA. The latter is associated with induction of cancer [3]. Because of this, several methods have been developed to minimize radiation dose during ablation procedures [4,5]. The use of newer technologies such as non-fluoroscopic three-dimensional navigation systems allow for minimal radiation exposure during catheter ablation [6].

Table 21.1 Non-invasive imaging in arrhythmia management

Technique	Supraventricular arrhythmias	Ventricular arrhythmias	CIED	Advantage	Limitation
Routine fluoroscopy	Procedural guidance			• Visualization of catheters and anatomical landmarks	• Ionizing radiation exposure • Iodine contrast
3D rotational angiography	Procedural guidance			• Improved anatomic definition • Diminished need for pre-procedural imaging (CT, CMR) • Avoidance of registration errors	• Ionizing radiation exposure (comparable to CT) • Iodine contrast
Ultrasound					
2D-TTE (3D-TTE and STE may give additional information)	• Pre-EP procedural assessment (anatomy, identification of underlying heart disease, patient selection) • Post EP-procedural assessment of complications • Follow-up (routine)			• Availability, safety, cost-effectiveness	• Operator dependency • Individual image quality • Incomplete anatomic definition
TOE (3D-TTE may give additional information)	• Pre-procedural assessment (anatomy, LAA thrombus, valvular disease, patient selection) • Procedural guidance • Post-/peri-procedural assessment of complications • Follow-up (not routine: alternative or additional to TTE)			• Availability, safety • Better resolution, image quality and identification relation of atria with surrounding structures (esophagus) than TTE	• Semi-invasive • Operator dependency • Individual image quality
ICE	• Procedural guidance • Peri-procedural assessment of complications			• Reduced fluoroscopic time • May abandon procedural TOE	• Costs

Modality	Indications	Advantages	Disadvantages
Computed tomography (CT)	• Pre-procedural assessment (anatomy, patient selection) • Post-procedural assessment of complications (PV stenosis, atrio-esophageal fistula, CIED placement)	• Good 3D anatomic definition • Short acquisition time • Availability	• Ionizing radiation exposure • Iodine contrast
Cardiovascular magnetic resonance (CMR)	• Pre-procedural assessment (anatomy, identification of underlying heart disease and substrate, patient selection) • Procedural guidance (using real-time CMR, magnetic catheter steering) • Post-procedural assessment of complications (PV stenosis) • Follow-up (completeness of ablation lesion)	• Absence of ionizing radiation • Identification of underlying heart disease • Substrate identification	• Relatively long acquisition time • Limited availability • Regular MRI contra-indications • Suboptimal image quality in irregular rhythms
Electroanatomic mapping (EAM)	• Procedural guidance	• Improved catheter positioning • Reduced fluoroscopic time • Increased procedural success rate	
^{123}I-mIBG—SPECT	• Pre-procedural assessment (patient selection)	• Possible improved patient selection	• Costs • Preparatory time • Ionizing radiation exposure • Limited scientific data
Image integration			
EAM with CT or CMR	• Procedural guidance	• Improved catheter positioning • Reduced fluoroscopic time • Better scar delineation	• Insufficient proof of usefulness
EAM with ICE	• Procedural guidance	• Improved catheter positioning • Reduced fluoroscopic time • Increased procedural success	• Insufficient proof of usefulness

CIED, cardiac implantable electronic device; CMR, cardiac magnetic resonance imaging; CT, computed tomography; EAM, electroanatomic mapping; EP, electrophysiological; ICE, intracardiac echocardiography; ^{123}I-mIBG-SPECT, Iodine-123-metaiodobenzylguanidine single-photon emission computed tomography; PV, pulmonary vein; STE, speckle tracking echocardiography; TOE, transesophageal echocardiography; TTE, transthoracic echocardiography; 2D, two-dimensional; 3D, three-dimensional.

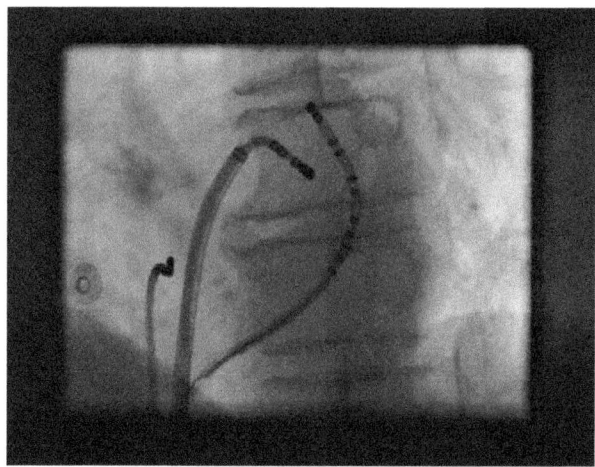

Figure 21.1 X-ray fluoroscopy image (left anterior oblique) showing the catheters during ablation of an accessory pathway at the left lateral aspect of the mitral valve annulus.

21.2.2 Rotational angiography

21.2.2.1 Procedural guidance

Three-dimensional rotational angiography (3DRA) was initially introduced as a new modality for 3D imaging of the left atrium (LA) during atrial fibrillation (AF) ablation procedures. To perform this, an X-ray tube mounted on a C-arm performs a 200–240° rotation around the patient while contrast medium is injected in the LA. A large number of 2D projections are acquired during rotation. Reconstruction algorithms transform these 2D images into a set of 3D-reconstructed computed-tomography (CT)-like images. Spatial resolution of 3DRA is comparable or even exceeds that of conventional cardiac CT [7]. 3DRA enhances lesion identification during AF ablation by improving visualization of the sometimes variable and complex left atrial–pulmonary venous anatomy. 3DRA also allows visualization of surrounding structures such as the esophagus in order to prevent ablation-related fistula formation [8]. 3DRA has the potential to eliminate the need for pre-procedural CT or cardiac magnetic resonance imaging (CMR). Another important advantage of 3DRA is that it is performed immediately prior to the procedure, thereby avoiding registration errors of the per-procedural catheter position. This may occur when the volume status or position of the patient differs between pre-acquired 3D-roadmap images and the ablation procedure. 3DRA can be performed with acceptable patient radiation dose (5–8 mSv), comparable to cardiac CT [9]. There is limited data about the use of 3DRA in patients with right ventricular outflow tract ventricular tachycardia (VT) [8]. ECG-gated rotational angiography is a valuable tool for visualizing coronary venous anatomy during left ventricular lead implantation procedures [10].

21.3 Ultrasound

21.3.1 Transthoracic echocardiography

Two-dimensional echocardiography (2DE) is widely available, safe, and cost-effective. It remains an important initial investigation, because arrhythmias are often associated with underlying heart disease and reduced left ventricular ejection fraction (LVEF). It is also useful to detect certain complications of electrophysiological procedures and as a tool for follow-up. Speckle tracking echocardiography (STE) is a novel technique that more accurately determines myocardial deformation (strain) than tissue Doppler methods. Three-dimensional echocardiography (3DE) overcomes the limitations of 2DE derived geometric assumptions, and has become an established method to determine chamber volumes and function [11].

21.3.1.1 Pre-procedural assessment

AF, atrial flutter, or atrial tachycardia, is often associated with hypertension (70%), valvular heart disease (36%), coronary artery disease (28%), and cardiomyopathy (10%) [12]. Catheter ablation with electro-isolation of pulmonary venous (PV) foci that frequently trigger AF is an effective treatment option for patients with symptomatic and drug-refractory AF [13]. Although less well suited than CT or CMR, 2DE can give pre-procedural information on atrial and PV anatomy and left atrial (LA) appendage thrombus.

2DE derived parameters predict the success of therapy, i.e., LA-size ≥ 50 mm (from M-mode) increases the risk of AF recurrence both after cardioversion and ablation [14] [15]. 3DE more accurately assesses LA volume than 2DE approaches, but cut-off values that predict procedural success after ablation are currently unknown [16]. Decreased STE-derived LA global and regional strain may become important pre-procedural determinants to predict AF recurrence after ablation. 2DE can also be used to risk stratify patients with AF, because LVEF $\leq 40\%$ is strongly associated with stroke [13,17].

Sudden cardiac death (SCD) remains a leading cause of death worldwide. All patients with serious ventricular arrhythmias should undergo 2DE because of the association with underlying cardiomyopathy. 2DE should also be performed in all patients scheduled for VT ablation to rule out intracardiac thrombus.

LVEF determination after myocardial infarction (MI) is important and incorporated in current international guidelines because echocardiography derived cut-off values are used for prophylactic CIED implantation (either CRT, and/or ICD) [18]. Despite this, considerable risk heterogeneity exists among patients with low LVEF, and a reduced LVEF is a non-specific predictor of future life-threatening arrhythmias. Less than 50% of patients with prior MI who die suddenly have LVEF $< 30\%$. This indicates that improved risk stratification to determine which patient is at greatest risk for SCD and which patient will likely not benefit form ICD therapy is urgently needed. Malignant arrhythmias are the result of a complex interaction between heterogeneity in scar tissue and regional electrophysiological properties. Mechanical dispersion of 70 ms using STE is a strong and independent predictor for identifying arrhythmic events (65% sensitivity and 92% specificity) [19]. The risk for arrhythmic events increases with more extensive wall motion abnormalities (HR 2.18, 95% CI 1.03–4.65, $P=0.04$, for every 1-point increase in wall motion score index), restrictive filling pattern, and inducible myocardial ischemia [20].

CRT is an effective therapy for patients with drug-refractory end-stage heart failure, low LVEF ($\leq$35%), and wide QRS complex ($\geq$120ms). Eligible patients should undergo careful pre-implantation imaging to evaluate cardiac anatomy, LV size, and function to predict long-term clinical outcome [21]. 2DE has an advantage over other diagnostic modalities that determine EF, because it is widely available and provides valuable information on concomitant valvular disease, diastolic function, and volume status. Preferentially, volumetric methods (Simpson's biplane or 3DE) instead of biplane methods should be used to assess LV volumes and EF [22]. Although 2DE quantification of mechanical dyssynchrony using tissue Doppler imaging emerged as a promising technique to predict the response of CRT, it failed to show a consistent benefit in larger prospective multicenter trials [23]. The systolic dyssynchrony index (SDI), a 3DE-derived parameter of dyssynchrony ($10.7\pm3.6\%$ in patients vs. $2.7\pm0.9\%$ in healthy volunteers; $P<0.001$; see Figure 21.2), or STE-derived delays

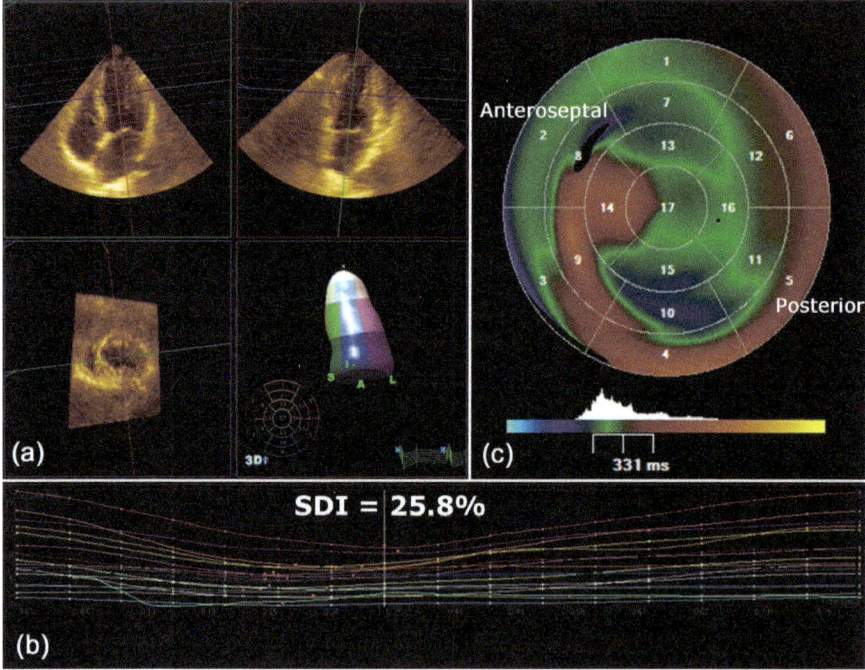

Figure 21.2 Patient example of mechanical dyssynchrony using transthoracic three-dimensional echocardiography (3DE). After acquisition of an apical 3DE dataset (full volume), designated software allows quantification of global and regional function (a). A regional time to minimal systolic volume (Tmsv) curve can be generated for all segments (b) that can be shown as a polar plot (c). The systolic dyssynchrony index (SDI) is a measure of mechanical dyssynchrony and expressed as the standard deviation of the Tmsv of all segments and as a percentage of the cardiac cycle (in this case 25.8%; normal $1.3\pm0.5\%$).

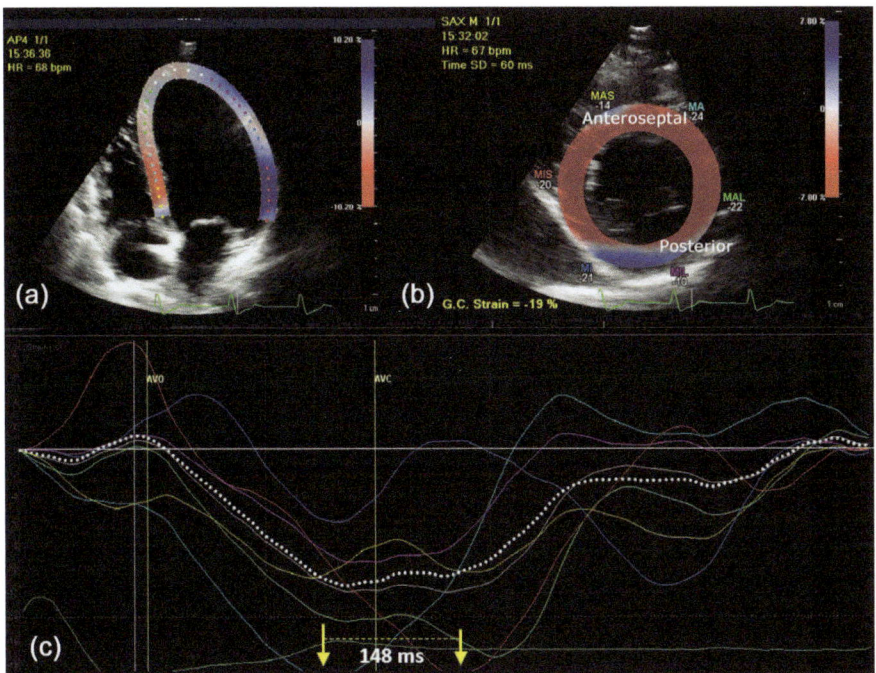

Figure 21.3 Speckle tracking echocardiography (STE). Patient example of STE analysis of apical four-chamber view (a) and mid-ventricular short-axis (b) for measuring longitudinal and radial strain, respectively. Specifically designed software measures the movement of natural acoustic markers (speckles) during the cardiac cycle. (c) A time difference between the anteroseptal and posterior wall segmental peak systolic strain of 148 ms (arrows) was found (≥130 ms is considered significant dyssynchrony).

(≥130 ms between anteroseptal and posterior wall using radial and transverse strains; see Figure 21.3) are novel methods to predict response to CRT but need further prospective multicenter investigation [24,25].

21.3.1.2 Procedural guidance

2DE has no role in the procedural guidance during ablation of (supra) ventricular arrhythmias or CIED implantation. However, tissue Doppler imaging of the atria using 2DE holds promise as a non-invasive tool to determine AF cycle length, allowing the effect of antiarrhythmic therapy to be monitored [26].

21.3.1.3 Complications

Pericardial effusion (PE) and cardiac tamponade may occur in up to 14% after CIED implantation and up to 6% of arrhythmia ablations, depending on technique used, and concomitant antiplatelet or anticoagulant therapy [27,28]. PE after ablation for AF may be related to the transseptal puncture, ablation-related damage to the LA or myocardial or coronary venous perforation during CIED implantation. 2DE is well suited to detect PE and cardiac tamponade and should be performed as soon as there is a suspicion (chest discomfort), even in the absence of hemodynamic abnormalities. Although these complications typically develop during the procedure, they may occur days later as well, particularly if anticoagulant therapy is restarted.

PV stenosis after AF catheter ablation is a rare complication, which is mostly mild and clinically silent. Although CT and CMR are the diagnostic modalities of choice, 2DE can detect increased flow velocities in the PV with color and pulsed wave Doppler. Tricuspid valve insufficiency after electrophysiological procedures and CIED implantation can be recognized early with transthoracic echocardiography (TTE). It carries an adverse prognosis and may be corrected by repositioning the lead. CIED-related endocarditis occurs in 0.3–0.4/1000 [29]. Although TEE is superior, 2DE can be helpful to diagnose right- (lead-related) and left-sided endocarditis. Importantly, a negative 2DE in the setting of high clinical suspicion and positive blood cultures necessitates further investigation.

21.3.1.4 Follow-up

Studies suggest that after successful ablation, LA enlargement reverses and contraction and reservoir function improve (reverse structural remodeling) in so-called responders (i.e. ≥15% decrease in maximum LA volume). Because responders suffer fewer AF recurrences, LA reverse remodeling may become a surrogate marker of successful AF ablation. In a study of 144 patients undergoing catheter ablation for AF, responders (63%) had a significant decrease in maximum LA volumes (from 31 ± 7 to $22 \pm 6 \, \text{ml/m}^2$), whereas non-responders showed an increase (29 ± 5 to $31 \pm 6 \, \text{ml/m}^2$) after 13.2 ± 6.7 months. Two-thirds of responders remained in sinus rhythm, whereas one-third had recurrent AF [30].

TTE plays a role in the serial follow-up of patients after CRT to assess ventricular function and remodeling, which is characterized by a reduction in LV volumes and improvement in LVEF after 3–6 months. However, only two-thirds of patients respond to CRT and improve in terms of heart failure symptoms, functional status, and cardiac function. Although individual optimization of atrioventricular (AV) and ventriculoventricular (VV) delays after CRT using Doppler techniques (mitral inflow, aortic velocity time integral) have shown to improve hemodynamic function acutely [31], the role of routine optimization in all patients is controversial. There are little to no data that support long-term clinical improvement after routine CRT optimization. In the SMART-AV trial, comparing a fixed nominal AV delay of 120 ms, CRT device-determined (SmartDelay), and echocardiography-determined AV optimization, no difference in improvement in LV end-systolic volume, LVEF, and functional measures was found after 6 months [32]. Despite the availability of numerous AV optimization methods, only the simple and iterative method of finding the optimal AV delay that optimizes diastolic filling is recommended in non-responders or in advanced diastolic dysfunction [21,33]. The role of VV optimization is even less clear.

21.3.2 Transesophageal echocardiography

Transesophageal echocardiography (TOE) is a widely available, safe, and reliable technique to evaluate cardiac chambers, major vessels, and cardiac and valvular function. When carried out by experienced operators, it is associated with a very low risk (below 0.05%) of complications [34,35]. TOE is mainly carried out after routine TTE and offers more detailed information of structures close to the esophagus than TTE. In recent years, three-dimensional TOE (3D-TOE) has become available by most vendors [35] and provides 3D overviews of cardiac structures. 3D-TOE is useful to visualize complex structures such as the inter-atrial septum during punctures, the left atrial appendage (LAA), and tracking of catheters.

21.3.2.1 Pre-procedural assessment

AF is associated with an increased risk of atrial thrombus formation. Presence of LA thrombus (see Figure 21.4) is considered a contraindication for performing (electrical) cardioversion or intracardiac ablation of atrial tachyarrhythmias. TTE offers information on risk factors associated with thrombus formation, such as LA size or depressed LV function, but lacks specificity and sensitivity for thrombus detection in comparison to TOE [36]. TOE is considered the gold standard to exclude LA thrombus prior to catheter ablation [37]. Spontaneous echo contrast on TOE is also considered a risk factor for embolic stroke in patients with AF. TOE prior to cardioversion may decrease the risk of hemorrhagic stroke when compared to a strategy using oral

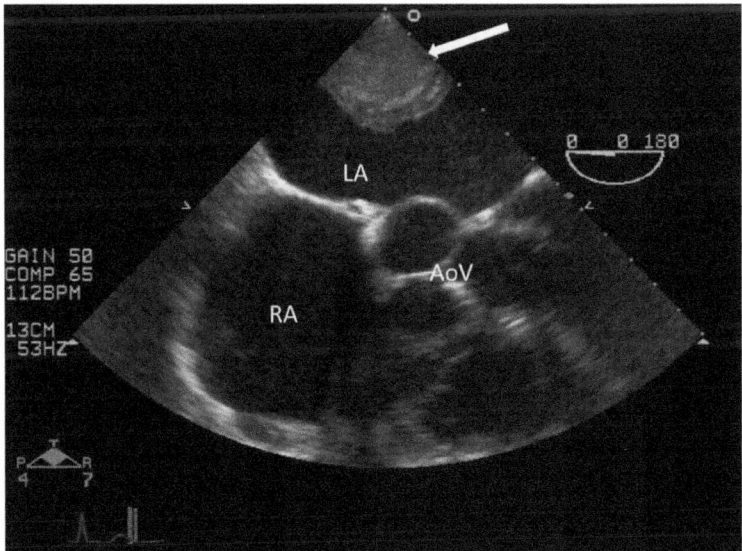

Figure 21.4 Transesophageal imaging of a large left atrial thrombus (arrow) in a patient with chronic atrial fibrillation and poor therapeutic adherence to anticoagulation. LA, left atrium; RA, right atrium; AOV, aortic valve.

anticoagulation alone [38]. In the workup of patients with ventricular arrhythmias, SCD prevention, or CRT, TOE can be useful in patients with LV dysfunction related to underlying valvular disease, with respect to mechanism and additional (surgical) treatment options [37].

21.3.2.2 Procedural guidance

Intraprocedural cardioversion can be safely performed while the TOE probe remains in place. TOE helps guide the puncture of the inter-atrial septum and tracking of catheters and safe guide wire placement in the pulmonary veins (PV), thereby avoiding unnecessary complications [39]. Peri-procedural guidance with TOE is advised in challenging cases, such as redo-procedures with increased septal thickness [40], after atrial septal closure device placement, or in grown-up congenital heart disease [41]. LAA closure devices (for instance WATCHMAN™) are being used to prevent thrombotic complications in patients with AF who have contraindication for anticoagulation therapy [42]. Placement of such devices is performed under TOE guidance to ensure correct sizing and placement and to identify early complications during or after device placement. Finally, recent literature suggests that 3D-TOE guided PV isolation without fluoroscopy is feasible [43].

Lead placement for CRT is routinely carried out under fluoroscopic guidance, although (3D) TOE may be useful in the localization of the coronary sinus. TOE guided transseptal puncture can help in endocardial left ventricular lead placement in patients with unfavorable venous anatomy or failed epicardial lead placement [44,45].

21.3.2.3 Complications

After transseptal puncture, TOE allows early intraprocedural detection of complications such as PE. When clinical suspicion of PE remains high, TOE should follow a negative TTE examination. With current ablation techniques such as cryoablation, PV stenosis is becoming increasingly rare. As with TTE, TOE may detect increased Doppler flow velocities, but CT and CMR remain the most appropriate techniques to detect this complication. CIED-associated infections have a poor prognosis, and prompt lead removal is generally advised [46]. TOE has superior sensitivity to TTE for detection of endocardial lead infection. Although a negative initial TOE does not rule out CIED infection, complications can readily be visualized [47]. A recent study showed that a lead-associated mass occurred in 14% of patients after CIED placement using TOE. However, 72% of these patients did not have any evidence of infective endocarditis. Thus, consideration should be given before routinely removing leads that have masses attached [48].

21.3.2.4 Follow-up

TOE may be considered for detecting late complications after electrophysiological procedures when TTE has substandard image quality, but does not play a role in routine follow-up.

21.3.3 Intracardiac echocardiography

21.3.3.1 Procedural guidance

In contrast to TEE, intracardiac echocardiography (ICE) represents a purely peri-procedural tool for guidance and safety of catheter-based procedures. ICE permits direct imaging of all structures relevant to a transseptal puncture. The individual components of the atrial septum—septum primum and septum secundum, the relationship of the fossa ovalis to the aortic valve and ascending aorta, and the posterior atrial wall—can all be readily visualized. ICE guided transseptal puncture may abandon the need for fluoroscopic guidance of catheters, thereby decreasing radiation burden associated with electrophysiological procedures [49]. In addition, ICE causes less patient discomfort as compared to TOE, decreasing the need for peri-procedural sedation. Newer generation phased array-ICE probes produce wedge-shaped images and even allow (color) Doppler imaging that can be post-processed on conventional echocardiographic workstations. PV dimensions and LAA thrombus can be detected reliably, especially when employing multiple ICE views [50]. These advantages and a low complication rate (3.3% in a single-center registry of 1192 ICE guided procedures) [51] have led to the widespread use of ICE during electrophysiological procedures.

Three-dimensional reconstruction of ICE images is feasible, and may be used for electroanatomical mapping studies (see also Section 21.6). Future developments in real-time 3D ICE may further assist complicated transseptal puncture and catheter guidance.

21.3.3.2 Complications

An important advantage of ICE during electrophysiological procedures is the continuous surveillance of complications. Early recognition of PE may lead to anticoagulation reversal and prevent cardiac tamponade. ICE also allows guiding subsequent pericardiocentesis. Future studies comparing accuracy, reproducibility, and clinical outcome of ICE guidance versus TOE versus isolated fluoroscopy is needed to adopt ICE imaging as a primary nonradiographic imaging tool during electrophysiological procedures [52].

21.4 Computed tomography

21.4.1 Pre-procedural assessment

CT angiography is commonly used to image LA and PV anatomy prior to catheter-based treatment of AF. Since PV anatomy can be variable and complex, suboptimal PV visualization may compromise procedural success. Pre-acquired CT images are routinely used for co-registration with electroanatomical mapping (see also Section 21.6). Novel CT scanning technology has drastically reduced the radiation dose associated with PV anatomy imaging. Current scanning protocols, such as high-pitch spiral CT scanning with second-/third-generation dual-source CT scanners

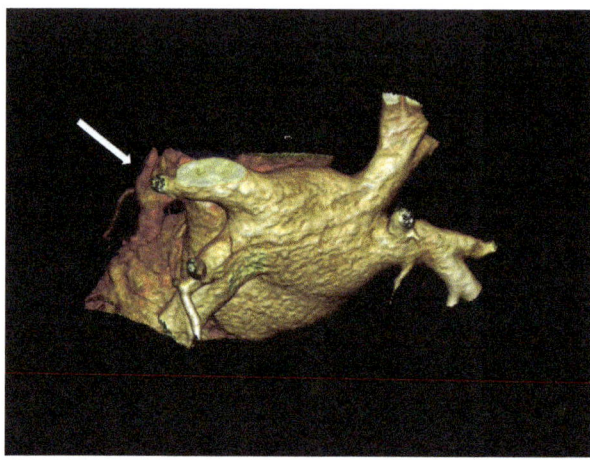

Figure 21.5 Multislice computed tomography imaging of pulmonary veins, left atrium, and left atrial appendage (arrow). CT image was acquired at a sub-millisievert dose using a second-generation dual-source CT scanner.

allow for sub-millisievert radiation exposure while maintaining high image quality. Using this acquisition protocol, investigators showed that 99% of scans were of good or excellent image quality, even in patients who had AF during image acquisition (see Figure 21.5) [53].

A large proportion of patients referred for PV ablation suffer from coronary artery disease (CAD), suggesting an association with AF. Patients who were diagnosed with lone AF more often have insidious coronary artery disease than matched controls (49% vs. 38%) [54]. The Framingham Heart Study, among others, has provided evidence that epicardial fat volume, as determined by CT, is an independent risk factor for occurrence of AF [55]. Nonetheless, AF with a significantly irregular ventricular response is considered a contraindication for CTCA due to poor image quality with a lack of reliable ECG-triggering. Although, in some patients with slow heart rates and relative constant beat-to-beat intervals acceptable image quality can be obtained on standard 64-slice CT scanners, the use of fast scanners with high temporal resolution (e.g., dual-source CT) and aggressive treatment with beta-blockers should be advocated whenever CTCA is considered despite permanent AF.

CT allows pre-procedural exclusion of LAA sludge or thrombus in patients referred for ablation for AF (Figure 21.6), which is vital for peri-procedural safety. A recent meta-analysis comprising 19 studies and over 2900 patients revealed that delayed LAA imaging by CT angiography, either employing a single or dual contrast bolus, can accurately detect LAA thrombus/LAA sludge and safely discriminate this from incomplete mixing of contrast [56]. This may abolish the need for preprocedural TOE. CT also allows for the determination of LAA anatomy prior to LAA occlusion and a better planning of the procedure. Di Biase divided LAAs into four distinct morphologies: windsock, chicken wing, cauliflower, and cactus. The chicken wing morphology was the most common (48%), followed by cactus (30%), windsock

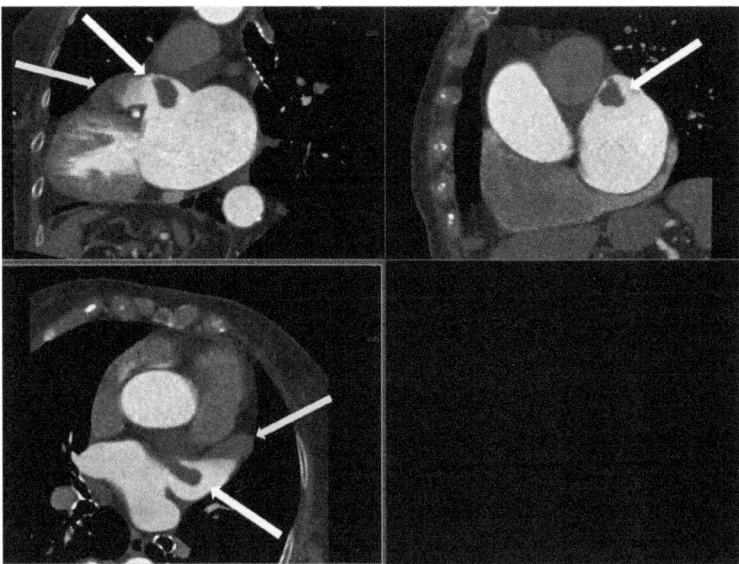

Figure 21.6 Multislice computed tomography imaging of a left atrial thrombus in an octogenarian with persistent atrial fibrillation. White arrows highlight a mobile thrombus in the left atrial appendage. In addition, poor contrast opacification of the tip of the LAA can be appreciated (grey arrows), either depicting LAA sludge or LAA slow flow.

(19%), and cauliflower (3%). Interestingly, the latter morphology carries the highest risk for stroke/TIA (odds ratio 8.0 compared to chicken wing), followed by cactus and windsock with ORs of 4.1 and 4.5, respectively [57].

TTE and CMR remain the most widely implemented techniques for determination of LV function and myocardial scar. In patients with a poor acoustic window and contra-indications for CMR, CT can be an acceptable alternative for determining LA, LV, and LV function. Automated assessment of functional CT imaging can be carried out reliably, and is in agreement with CMR determined chamber assessment [58]. Scar detection has shown to have prognostic implications in assessment of patients at risk for ventricular arrhythmias and SCD. Delayed clearance of contrast agent in myocardial tissue has been shown to correlate with myocardial scar. Although CMR is considered the gold standard of non-invasive myocardial scar detection (see also Section 21.5), scar detection using delayed enhancement CT (DE-CT) is feasible. Small series have demonstrated prediction of VT with DE-CT in hypertrophic cardiomyopathy and ischemic cardiomyopathy [59].

Interestingly, in an animal model of ischemic heart disease, DE-MDCT provided more detailed assessment of the peri-infarct zone than CMR and was less susceptible to partial volume effects [60]. Nevertheless, DE-CT for clinical myocardial scar detection should currently only be considered in patients with contra-indications for CMR.

Unfavorable cardiac venous anatomy may affect successful CRT therapy. Hence, imaging of the cardiac venous system prior to LV lead implantation can provide guidance for pre-procedural planning [61]. Finally, dyssynchrony imaging using CT has been clinically demonstrated [62], rendering CT to be a potentially alternative technique for patients with poor acoustic windows and relative contra-indications for CMR.

21.4.2 Complications

CT angiography is considered the gold standard for detecting PV stenosis. Due to the high spatial resolution in all imaging planes, it has a distinct advantage to reliably measure PV diameters, and compare these to pre-procedural values. Although comparative trials are lacking, the diagnostic performances of CT and CMR to detect PV stenosis are likely comparable. In the ROTEA trial, where TOE was compared with CT for PV imaging, CT was able to detect smaller PVs, but TOE was able to detect the hemodynamic consequences of PV stenosis. PV dimensions on TOE may be underestimated, especially the inferior PVs [63]. Selection of an imaging modality to detect PV stenosis should depend on patient characteristics and local expertise. A rare complication of catheter-based treatment of AF is the occurrence of an atrio-esophageal fistula (AEF) [64]. Because of a mortality rate of up to 80%, suspected AEF requires urgent CT imaging and should be treated as soon as possible [65].

21.5 Cardiac magnetic resonance imaging

The high contrast-to-noise ratio combined with good spatial and temporal resolution and multi-planar capabilities of CMR makes it a very accurate and reproducible technique to assess anatomy, measure volumes, global contractile function, and mass. Sustained monomorphic VT after MI is usually caused by myocardial re-entry in the borderzone of the infarct. Because LGE-CMR allows identification and characterization of the infarct zone, it may help to further unravel the underlying pathophysiological mechanisms of arrhythmias and complement traditional risk stratification approaches.

21.5.1 Pre-procedural assessment

Three-dimensional MR angiography (MRA) provides similar anatomic and quantitative information as multislice CT with respect to PV (number, branching pattern, ostial diameters, and abnormal venous drainage) and LA anatomy (dimensions, volumes, LA ridges, and relation of LA to esophagus, aorta, and coronary arteries). In 473 patients who underwent MRA, 40% had a typical PV branching pattern (two left and two right PVs), and variations were found in the majority (common left trunk, multiple right PVs, or other complex anatomic variations) [66]. Pre-procedural 3D reconstructed CMR datasets can also be merged with electroanatomic maps (EAM) during ablation. This reduces procedural time and radiation exposure, but whether it improves clinical outcomes remains controversial [67].

AF is associated with electrical, contractile, and structural remodeling (i.e. fibrosis). As with TTE, CMR determined LA volume is a predictor of recurrent AF after ablation but definite cut-off values have not yet been determined. Although challenging, late gadolinium enhanced (LGE) CMR is a promising technique to detect LA fibrosis and scar. In 81 patients with AF, LGE-CMR (using a 3D inversion-recovery-prepared, respiration-navigated, gradient-echo pulse sequence with fat saturation; voxel size $1.25 \times 1.25 \times 2.5$ mm) demonstrated mild ($8.0 \pm 4.2\%$), moderate ($21.3 \pm 5.8\%$), and extensive ($50.1 \pm 15.4\%$) LA fibrosis [68]. The extent of fibrosis was significantly related to LA-volume, correlated with low-voltage regions on EAM ($R^2 = 0.61$, $P < 0.05$; 95% CI 0.83–1.30), and predicted AF recurrence after ablation.

There are preliminary data to suggest that CMR can be used as an alternative to TEE to detect LA appendage thrombus. Pre-PV ablation TOE and contrast and non-contrast enhanced CMR in 97 consecutive patients with AF detected LAA thrombus in two patients (2%), with 100% concordance [69]. A recent study found LA fibrosis by LGE-CMR to be independently associated with stroke, but these data need prospective multicenter confirmation.

Patients with new ventricular arrhythmias should be screened for ischemia, structural, or functional myocardial disease. Although echocardiography provides important information on ventricular and valvular function, it is inferior to CMR for the detection of structural abnormalities. Although used for risk stratification, LVEF has limitations in predicting SCD and eligibility for an ICD. Scar-related re-entry is believed to be the major mechanism underlying most lethal ventricular arrhythmias in both ischemic and non-ischemic heart disease. Size, surface area, transmurality, and the borderzone of scar by LGE-CMR better identified patients at increased risk for SCD than LVEF. In a recent prospective study evaluating 137 patients for possible ICD placement, of all clinical and CMR characteristics (including LVEF), scar size >5% of LV mass best predicted mortality and appropriate ICD shocks (HR = 4.6 [1.8–11.8], $P = 0.002$) [70]. Importantly, patients with LVEF > 30% but scar size >5% had a similar adverse events rate to those with LVEF ≤ 30%, and patients with LVEF ≤ 30% and minimal-or-no scar had similar low risk to those with LVEF > 30%. Thus, LGE-CMR seems to be useful to better identify and characterize the arrhythmia substrate, which may lead to more efficient catheter ablation of incessant and recurrent monomorphic VT (see Figure 21.7). It is anticipated that the infarct gray zone by LGE-CMR represents a mixture of viable and necrotic tissue, particularly at the isthmus, that may serve as a substrate for ventricular arrhythmias (see Figure 21.8). This infarct tissue heterogeneity was shown to be a powerful predictor of inducible and spontaneous ventricular arrhythmias and mortality in patients after MI [71]. Prospective studies should address the potential of CMR to improve risk stratification in SCD and guide treatment of scar-related ventricular arrhythmias.

The main rationale for CRT is correction of AV, interventricular, and intraventricular mechanical dyssynchrony. Based on currently used criteria, up to 30–40% of patients do not respond significantly, suggesting that improved techniques to assess dyssynchrony are needed for effective patient selection. Myocardial tagging [72]

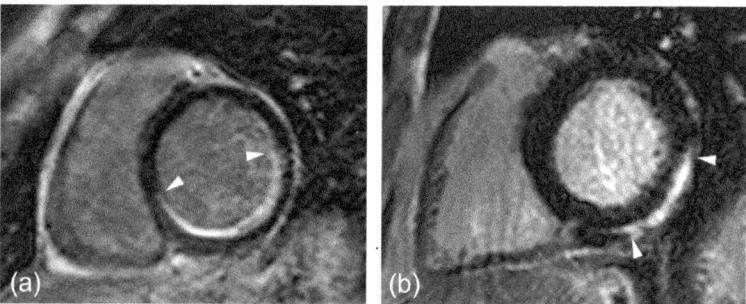

Figure 21.7 Localizing scar (arrowheads). Late gadolinium enhanced short-axis cardiac magnetic resonance images of two different patients. (a) subendocardial inferior-inferolateral scar (chronic myocardial infarction); (b) epicardial scar (myocarditis). The location of scar (endocardial, epicardial, left-sided, or right-sided) is useful to direct the ablation procedure. Patient (b) underwent successful epicardial ablation of a monomorphic ventricular tachycardia after initial subendocardial ablation failed.

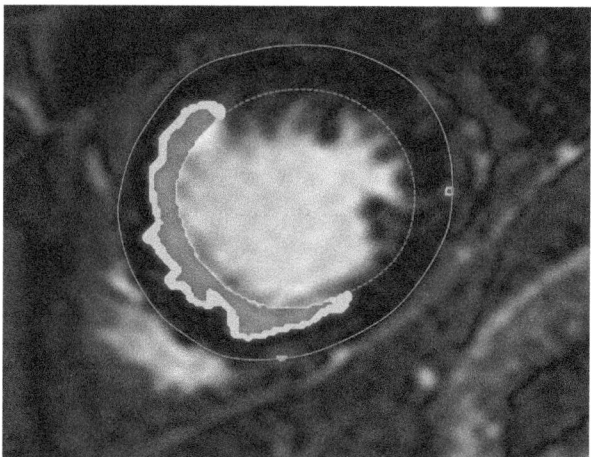

Figure 21.8 Infarct tissue heterogeneity and infarct gray zone determination. Late gadolinium enhanced short-axis cardiac magnetic resonance image of a patient with an anteroseptal myocardial infarction. Using specifically designed software, epicardial and endocardial borders were manually traced and the infarct core (dark gray area (15.2% of LV mass)) and infarct periphery i.e., gray zone (light gray area (7.2% of LV mass)) were determined.

(Figure 21.9), strain-encoded MRI (SENC), phase-contrast MRI, and displacement encoding with stimulated echoes (DENSE) can be used to assess intra- and interventricular dyssynchrony [73]. Observational studies suggest that response to CRT is related to absence of inferolateral scar, decreased scar extent, and transmurality as assessed with LGE-CMR. Whether these CMR-derived parameters provide more accurate CRT selection to reduce non-responsiveness needs to be investigated in clinical outcome studies.

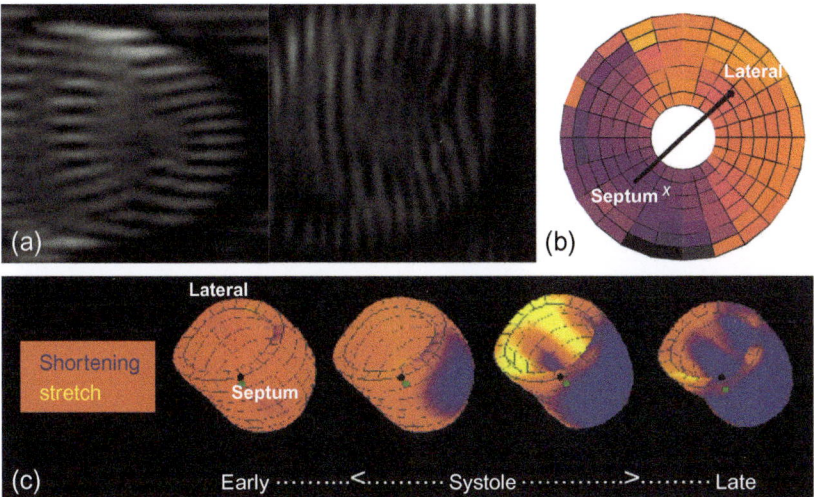

Figure 21.9 Short-axis tagging images (with taglines in horizontal and vertical direction) of a patient with mechanical dyssynchrony (a). Post-processing allows calculation of segmental circumferential strain and onset of shortening. Mechanical dyssynchrony can then be visualized with polar maps (b) and three-dimensional color rendering of strain (yellow, stretch; blue, shortening) (c).
Courtesy: Prof. Dr. F. W. Prinzen, Maastricht University, The Netherlands.

21.5.2 Procedural guidance

Catheter guidance in electrophysiology procedures is commonly performed via fluoroscopy. Reduced ablation efficacy may be related to lack of soft-tissue visualization and direct visualization of ablation lesions by fluoroscopy, and registration errors of catheter position using pre-acquired 3D-roadmap images. Real-time CMR offers a fluoroscopy-free environment, real-time visualization of the anatomic substrate, and direct visualization of ablation injuries (see Figure 21.10), to evaluate gaps in and need for additional ablation lines.

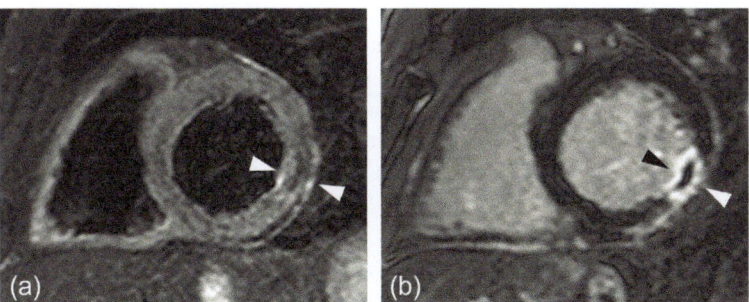

Figure 21.10 T2-weighted-turbo spin echo (a) and late gadolinium enhanced (b) short-axis magnetic resonance image of a radiofrequency ablation lesion (arrowheads) in the basal lateral segment of the left ventricle (arrowheads). The typical features of an ablation lesion can be seen: peripheral ring of increased signal intensity with a central dark core (hypoenhancement), reflecting intramyocardial hemorrhage (a) and microvascular obstruction (b).

Real-time CMR-guided catheter positioning has been shown to be accurate, feasible, and safe, and holds promise to improve success rates in the electrophysiological therapy of arrhythmias [74,75]. Robotic catheter and remote magnetic navigation systems have been successfully applied in ablation procedures for AF and VT, but larger prospective and randomized trials are needed to confirm these initial positive experiences. It is expected that faster CMR imaging techniques with improved coil and catheter tracking technology will take real-time CMR-guided interventions in efficient practice.

21.5.3 Complications

Although intracardiac echocardiographic guidance has reduced the rate of PV stenosis post ablation for AF, CMR can be used to screen for this complication. Detectable PV narrowing occurred in 38% of PVs following ablation, of which 3.2% were moderate and 0.6% severe [76]. The occurrence of this complication has significantly decreased since PV isolation is performed more and more often at the antrum rather than the ostium of the PVs.

21.5.4 Follow-up

Ablation relies on electrically isolating the LA from arrhythmogenic foci in the PV in AF and targeting the critical isthmus in monomorphic VT. Failure is thought to be due to incomplete ablation lesions. Ablation lesions can be visualized with non-contrast enhanced T1 and T2 weighted CMR, and LGE-CMR imaging (see Figure 21.10), and may be useful to determine the need for repeat procedures [77]. Compatibility of CMR is still an important consideration in patients with CIED and does not allow routine follow-up CMR investigations.

21.6 Electroanatomic mapping

The use of EAM systems in cardiac electrophysiological procedures was introduced more than 15 years ago [78]. These systems provide three different types of information: (1) non-fluoroscopic catheter localization; (2) 3D display of electrical activation sequences (activation maps) during sinus rhythm or arrhythmia and voltage information (voltage maps) within the cardiac cavity that is mapped; and (3) 3D display of the anatomy of the heart chambers, generated from catheter localization information. The two most frequently used, commercially available systems are EnSite™ NavX™ (St. Jude Medical, St. Paul, Minnesota, USA) and Carto® (Biosense Webster, Diamond Bar, California, USA).

The EnSite™ NavX™ functions with three pairs of skin patches on the patient's chest in x-axis, y-axis, and z-axis direction. The electrodes from standard electrophysiology catheters sense the electrical signals transmitted between the skin patches. The EnSite™ NavX™ system uses the electrical data from the catheters to visualize their movement, construct 3D models of the cardiac chambers, and create activation and voltage maps. The EnSite™ NavX™ system can be used with the EnSite™ Array™ non-contact mapping catheter: this is an ellipsoid balloon with a multi-electrode array counting 64 electrodes. These electrodes sense far-field electrograms that are used to create more than 3000 virtual endocardial surface electrograms (see Figure 21.11).

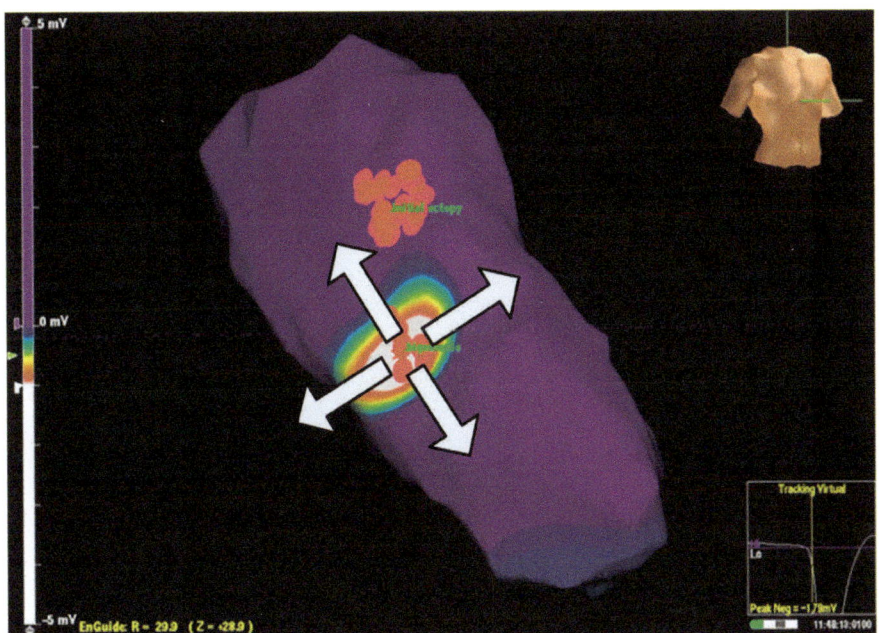

Figure 21.11 Activation map of the right ventricular outflow tract using the EnSite™ Array™ system, showing centrifugal spread (white arrow) of a non-sustained ventricular tachycardia at the free wall.

The EnSite™ Array™ is mainly used for mapping non-sustained or hemodynamically non-sustainable tachycardias.

The Carto® system localizes the electrodes of dedicated electrophysiology catheters equipped with a magneto-sensor, based on the information of three magnetic fields created by skin patches on the patient's chest and back. This technique allows 3D geometry reconstruction of the cardiac chambers and navigation within the mapped cavity. Activation and voltage maps can also be created.

The use of EAM systems results in a significant reduction in radiation exposure [79]. EAM systems are increasingly being used for procedural guidance during AF and VT ablation procedures. To overcome some of the limitations of currently available EAM systems (insufficient compensation for respiration, cardiac cycle, and patient movement), the MediGuide™ system was introduced. This system allows real-time and non-fluoroscopic tracking of sensor-equipped catheters by the electromagnetic sensor field in pre-recorded fluoroscopy cine loops.

21.6.1 Procedural guidance

To date, catheter ablation of AF is based on two fundamental principles: (1) PV isolation and eradication of focal triggers, and (2) atrial substrate modification consisting of linear lesions and/or ablation of sites demonstrating complex atrial fractionated electrograms. The latter approach at this time is usually reserved for patients with persistent AF. The use of EAM systems during AF ablation is useful in improving

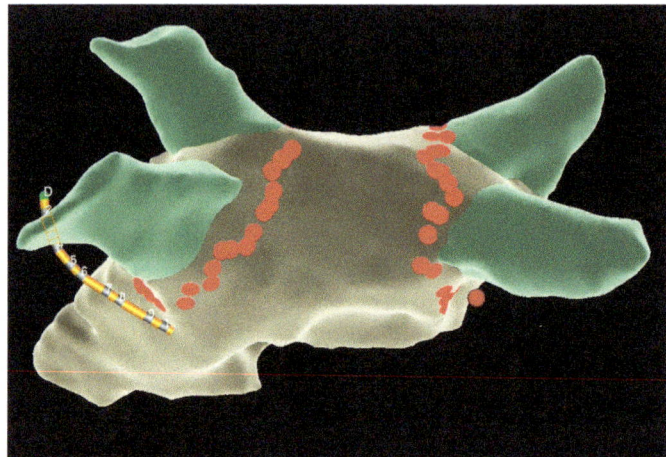

Figure 21.12 Postero-anterior view of the left atrium (in gray) using the EnSite™ system. The red dots indicate the ablation lesions resulting in complete electrical isolation of the pulmonary veins (in green).

the operator's understanding of the anatomy of the LA and the PV (see Figure 21.12). They enhance the accuracy of ablation lesion delivery, reduce fluoroscopy time and procedural duration, and improve clinical outcomes [80]. The additional anatomic information provided by EAM systems (e.g., relation of LA and PV with esophagus and aorta), is important to prevent ablation-related complications [81].

EAM technology is an important tool for mapping and ablation of focal VT, re-entrant VT utilizing the conduction system, and scar-related VT. In idiopathic and focal VT arising in structurally normal hearts, EAM is useful to display the site of earliest activation and sites of optimal pace-mapping. By identifying low-voltage regions in the right ventricle, EAM can also be useful to discriminate between idiopathic right ventricle outflow tract tachycardia and underlying subtle arrhythmogenic right ventricular cardiomyopathy [82]. In patients with re-entrant VT, EAM helps identify and characterize the substrate for the re-entrant circuit [83,84].

There is limited data concerning the use of EAM to identify the most optimal site of left ventricular lead implantation during CRT [85].

21.7 Radionuclide imaging

21.7.1 Pre-procedural assessment

Although systolic LV function is a powerful predictor to selection of patients at risk for SCD, it has several drawbacks. Most patients who suffer from SCD do not have characteristics that would qualify them for preventative ICD implantation. In addition, MADIT-II showed that two-thirds of patient with ICD did not receive therapy during the 2-year follow-up [86]. Imaging the autonomic nervous system in patients with heart failure using SPECT with the radiotracer ^{123}I-*m*IBG has been possible for several decades [87] (see Chapter 11). ^{123}I-*m*IBG is an analog of the neurotransmitter norepinephrine, and uses the same uptake and storage mechanisms. Neuronal ^{123}I-*m*IBG uptake from the synaptic cleft seems to be the predominant mechanism in the heart. This is illustrated by the fact that uptake is absent in denervated transplanted hearts [88]. The multicenter ADMIRE-HF included 995 patients, and demonstrated that the heart/mediastinal (h/m) ratio identifies patients at risk for major adverse cardiac events in patients with depressed LV function [89]. The largest prospective trial to examine the predictive value of ^{123}I-*m*IBG imaging showed that 52% of patients with a large ^{123}I-*m*IBG defect had appropriate ICD therapy, as opposed to 5% of patients who had a small ^{123}I-*m*IBG defect [90]. Despite these promising results, data supporting a decision algorithm including ^{123}I-*m*IBG imaging to select patients for ICD implantation have not been published yet.

Similar results were obtained with positron emission tomography (PET) using ^{11}C-labeled meta-hydroxyephedrine (^{11}C-MHED). ^{11}C-MHED is like *m*IBG, a radiolabeled analog of norepinephrine that is taken up by presynaptic sympathetic nerve endings. In the PAREPET study, 204 subjects with ischemic cardiomyopathy and LVEF <35% underwent ^{11}C-MHED PET. The amount of viable but denervated myocardium (with reduced ^{11}C-MHED uptake) was a significant and independent predictor of SCD or ICD discharge over a 4-year follow-up. Most importantly, the predictive power was independent of LVEF or end-systolic LV volumes.

Finally, the use of viability imaging may be useful to increase responder rates from CRT. Nonviable myocardial territories are likely to respond inappropriately to electrical stimulation. Van Campen and colleagues demonstrated larger extent of viable myocardium in patients with ischemic cardiomyopathy who responded to CRT [91]. Hybrid PET/CT approaches could obtain co-registered information on myocardial viability and coronary venous anatomy, and thereby determine suitability of a given patient for CRT. However, at present such approaches are still in an experimental phase and their appropriateness not yet confirmed by clinical studies.

21.8 Image integration

This concerns the integration of pre-procedural CMR or CT images within a 3D EAM system in order to better visualize and track catheters during the procedure. This technique has been developed to overcome two specific limitations of "classical" EAM systems. First, the ability to precisely reconstruct a specific cardiac chamber is heavily dependent on the operator's skills; second, EAM systems are not able to fully render the complex anatomy of the chamber being mapped. Image integration plays a significant role in procedural guidance. It is also possible to integrate ICE images into some EAM systems.

21.8.1 Procedural guidance

21.8.1.1 Integration of EAM and multislice CT or CMR

CartoMerge™ (Biosense Webster, Diamond Bar, California, USA) and NavX™ Fusion (St. Jude Medical, St. Paul, Minnesota, USA) allow integration of CT or

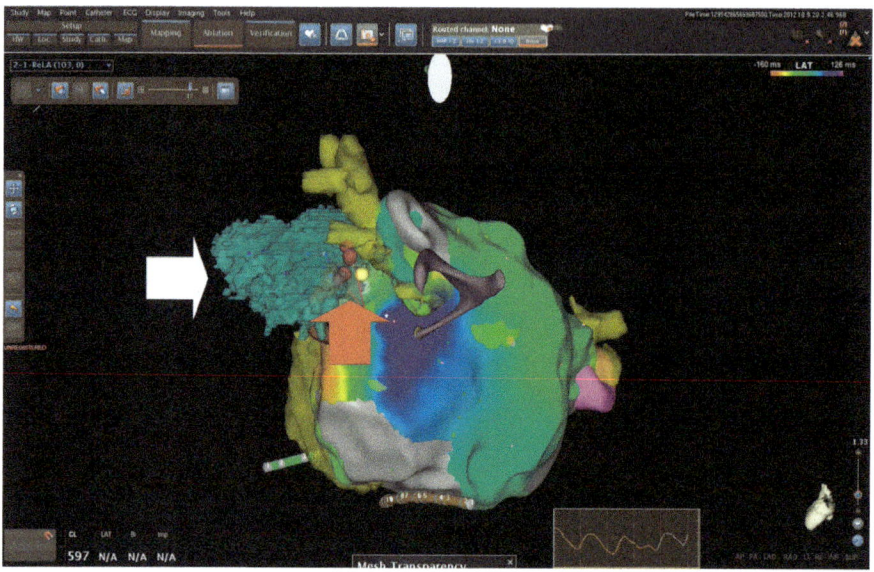

Figure 21.13 Left lateral view of the left atrium using the CartoMerge™ system. The computed tomography image clearly depicts the anatomy of the left atrial appendage (white arrow). The red dots (red arrow) show the successful ablation site of an atrial tachycardia with origin at the base of the left atrial appendage.

CMR images in EAM. Image integration greatly enhances the intraprocedural visualization of the PV and LA (see Figure 21.13). Nevertheless, the exact effects of this technique on fluoroscopy/procedure times and the outcome of the AF ablation procedure are still controversial due to the absence of prospective and randomized studies. Indeed, a recent study showed that (1) the use of CartoMerge™ did not result in an improved single-procedure success rate at 6 months; and (2) there was no difference in fluoroscopy and procedure duration, as compared with the conventional EAM group [92].

The integration of LGE-CMR into EAM during VT ablation in patients with a history of MI results in a more precise delineation of the post-infarct scar [93]. This should result in shorter mapping times, increase the success rate and reduce the complication rate.

21.8.1.2 Integration of EAM and ICE

The CartoSound® system (Biosense Webster, Diamond Bar, California, USA) allows the creation of 3D reconstructions of the cardiac chambers by tracing the endocardial surface contours on the imported ultrasound images. The CartoSound® system provides reliable guidance for PV isolation during AF ablation. It appears to be a safe and effective alternative to magnetic resonance and CT image data registration, although randomized comparisons are lacking [94]. Especially during VT ablation, the real-time assessment of LV wall motion abnormalities may be of great value [95].

References

[1] Pison L, et al. Imaging techniques in electrophysiology and implantable device procedures: results of the European Heart Rhythm Association survey. Europace 2013;15:1333–6.
[2] Mahesh M. Fluoroscopy: patient radiation exposure issues. RadioGraphics 2001;21:1033–45.
[3] Mcfadden SL, et al. X-ray dose and associated risks from radiofrequency catheter ablation procedures. Br J Radiol 2002;75:253–65.
[4] Davies AG, et al. X-ray dose reduction in fluoroscopically guided electrophysiology procedures. Pacing Clin Electrophysiol 2006;29:262–71.
[5] Kotre CJ, et al. Application of low dose rate pulsed fluoroscopy in cardiac pacing and electrophysiology: patient dose and image quality implications. Br J Radiol 2004;77:597–9.
[6] Scaglione M, et al. Visualization of multiple catheters with electroanatomical mapping reduces X-ray exposure during atrial fibrillation ablation. Europace 2011;13:955–62.
[7] Ector J, et al. Adenosine-induced ventricular asystole or rapid ventricular pacing to enhance three-dimensional rotational imaging during cardiac ablation procedures. Europace 2009;11:751–62.
[8] Orlov MV, et al. First experience with rotational angiography of the right ventricle to guide ventricular tachycardia ablation. Heart Rhythm 2011;8:207–11.
[9] Wielandts JY, et al. Three-dimensional cardiac rotational angiography: effective radiation dose and image quality implications. Europace 2010;12:194–201.
[10] Blendea D, et al. Variability of coronary venous anatomy in patients undergoing cardiac resynchronization therapy: a high-speed rotational venography study. Heart Rhythm 2007;4:1155–62.
[11] Lang RM, et al. EAE/ASE recommendations for image acquisition and display using three-dimensional echocardiography. J Am Soc Echocardiogr 2012;25:3–46.
[12] Nabauer M, et al. The Registry of the German Competence NETwork on Atrial Fibrillation: patient characteristics and initial management. Europace 2009;11:423–34.
[13] Camm AJ, et al. 2012 focused update of the ESC Guidelines for the management of atrial fibrillation: an update of the 2010 ESC Guidelines for the management of atrial fibrillation. Developed with the special contribution of the European Heart Rhythm Association. Eur Heart J 2012;33:2719–47.
[14] Zhuang J, et al. Association between left atrial size and atrial fibrillation recurrence after single circumferential pulmonary vein isolation: a systematic review and meta-analysis of observational studies. Europace 2012;14:638–45.
[15] Arya A, et al. Long-term results and the predictors of outcome of catheter ablation of atrial fibrillation using steerable sheath catheter navigation after single procedure in 674 patients. Europace 2010;12:173–80.
[16] Muller H, et al. Evaluation of left atrial size in patients with atrial arrhythmias: comparison of standard 2D versus real time 3D echocardiography. Echocardiography 2007;24:960–6.
[17] Ezekowitz M, et al. Echocardiographic predictors of stroke in patients with atrial fibrillation: a prospective study of 1066 patients from 3 clinical trials. Arch Intern Med 1998;158:1316–20.
[18] Tracy CM, et al. 2012 ACCF/AHA/HRS focused update of the 2008 guidelines for device-based therapy of cardiac rhythm abnormalities: a report of the American College of Cardiology Foundation/American Heart Association Task Force on Practice Guidelines. J Am Coll Cardiol 2012;60:1297–313.
[19] Haugaa KH, et al. Mechanical dispersion assessed by myocardial strain in patients after myocardial infarction for risk prediction of ventricular arrhythmia. JACC Cardiovasc Imaging 2010;3:247–56.

[20] Mahenthiran J, et al. Prognostic importance of wall motion abnormalities in patients with ischemic cardiomyopathy and an implantable cardioverter-defibrillator. Am J Cardiol 2006;98:1301–6.
[21] Daubert JC, et al. 2012 EHRA/HRS expert consensus statement on cardiac resynchronization therapy in heart failure: implant and follow-up recommendations and management. Europace 2012;14:1236–86.
[22] Chuang ML, et al. Importance of imaging method over imaging modality in noninvasive determination of left ventricular volumes and ejection fraction: assessment by two- and three-dimensional echocardiography and magnetic resonance imaging. J Am Coll Cardiol 2000;35:477–84.
[23] Chung ES, et al. Results of the predictors of response to CRT (PROSPECT) trial. Circulation 2008;117:2608–16.
[24] Kleijn SA, et al. A meta-analysis of left ventricular dyssynchrony assessment and prediction of response to cardiac resynchronization therapy by three-dimensional echocardiography. Eur Heart J Cardiovasc Imaging 2012;13:763–75.
[25] Tanaka H, et al. Dyssynchrony by speckle-tracking echocardiography and response to cardiac resynchronization therapy: results of the Speckle Tracking and Resynchronization (STAR) study. Eur Heart J 2010;31:1690–700.
[26] Duytschaever M, et al. Transthoracic tissue Doppler imaging of the atria: a novel method to determine the atrial fibrillation cycle length. J Cardiovasc Electrophysiol 2006;17:1202–9.
[27] Bernard ML, et al. Meta-analysis of bleeding complications associated with cardiac rhythm device implantation. Circ Arrhythm Electrophysiol 2012;5:468–74.
[28] Calkins H, et al. 2012 HRS/EHRA/ECAS Expert Consensus Statement on Catheter and Surgical Ablation of Atrial Fibrillation: recommendations for patient selection, procedural techniques, patient management and follow-up, definitions, endpoints, and research trial design. Europace 2012;14:528–606.
[29] Baddour LM, et al. Update on cardiovascular implantable electronic device infections and their management: a scientific statement from the American Heart Association. Circulation 2010;121:458–77.
[30] Tops LF, et al. Left atrial strain predicts reverse remodeling after catheter ablation for atrial fibrillation. J Am Coll Cardiol 2011;57:324–31.
[31] Auricchio A, et al. Effect of pacing chamber and atrioventricular delay on acute systolic function of paced patients with congestive heart failure. The Pacing Therapies for Congestive Heart Failure Study Group. The Guidant Congestive Heart Failure Research Group. Circulation 1999;99:2993–3001.
[32] Ellenbogen KA, et al. Primary results from the SmartDelay determined AV optimization: a comparison to other AV delay methods used in cardiac resynchronization therapy (SMART-AV) trial: a randomized trial comparing empirical, echocardiography-guided, and algorithmic atrioventricular delay programming in cardiac resynchronization therapy. Circulation 2010;122:2660–8.
[33] Gorcsan 3rd J, et al. Echocardiography for cardiac resynchronization therapy: recommendations for performance and reporting – a report from the American Society of Echocardiography Dyssynchrony Writing Group endorsed by the Heart Rhythm Society. J Am Soc Echocardiogr 2008;21:191–213.
[34] Cote G, et al. Transesophageal echocardiography-related complications. Can J Anaesth 2008;55:622–47.
[35] Flachskampf FA, et al. Recommendations for transoesophageal echocardiography: update 2010. Eur J Echocardiogr 2010;11:557–76.

[36] Omran H, et al. Imaging of thrombi and assessment of left atrial appendage function: a prospective study comparing transthoracic and transoesophageal echocardiography. Heart 1999;81:192–8.
[37] Douglas PS, et al. ACCF/ASE/AHA/ASNC/HFSA/HRS/SCAI/SCCM/SCCT/SCMR 2011 Appropriate Use Criteria for Echocardiography. A Report of the American College of Cardiology Foundation Appropriate Use Criteria Task Force, American Society of Echocardiography, American Heart Association, American Society of Nuclear Cardiology, Heart Failure Society of America, Heart Rhythm Society, Society for Cardiovascular Angiography and Interventions, Society of Critical Care Medicine, Society of Cardiovascular Computed Tomography, Society for Cardiovascular Magnetic Resonance American College of Chest Physicians. J Am Soc Echocardiogr 2011;24:229–67.
[38] Klein AL, et al. Use of transesophageal echocardiography to guide cardioversion in patients with atrial fibrillation. N Engl J Med 2001;344:1411–20.
[39] Bayrak F, et al. Added value of transesophageal echocardiography during transseptal puncture performed by inexperienced operators. Europace 2012;14:661–5.
[40] Tomlinson DR, et al. Interatrial septum thickness and difficulty with transseptal puncture during redo catheter ablation of atrial fibrillation. Pacing Clin Electrophysiol 2008;31:1606–11.
[41] Pedersen ME, et al. Successful transseptal puncture for radiofrequency ablation of left atrial tachycardia after closure of secundum atrial septal defect with Amplatzer septal occluder. Cardiol Young 2010;20:226–8.
[42] Reddy VY, et al. Left atrial appendage closure with the Watchman device in patients with a contraindication for oral anticoagulation: the ASAP study (ASA Plavix Feasibility Study With Watchman Left Atrial Appendage Closure Technology). J Am Coll Cardiol 2013;61:2551–6.
[43] Faletra FF, et al. Real-time, fluoroless, anatomic-guided catheter navigation by 3D TEE during ablation procedures. JACC Cardiovasc Imaging 2011;4:203–6.
[44] Morina-Vazquez P, et al. Direct left ventricular endocardial pacing: an alternative when traditional resynchronization via coronary sinus is not feasible or effective. Pacing Clin Electrophysiol 2013;36:699–706.
[45] Wright GA, et al. Transseptal left ventricular lead placement using snare technique. Pacing Clin Electrophysiol 2012;35:1248–52.
[46] Bongiorni MG, et al. How European centres diagnose, treat, and prevent CIED infections: results of an European Heart Rhythm Association survey. Europace 2012;14:1666–9.
[47] Victor F, et al. Pacemaker lead infection: echocardiographic features, management, and outcome. Heart 1999;81:82–7.
[48] Downey BC, et al. Incidence and significance of pacemaker and implantable cardioverter-defibrillator lead masses discovered during transesophageal echocardiography. Pacing Clin Electrophysiol 2011;34:679–83.
[49] Ruisi CP, et al. Use of intracardiac echocardiography during atrial fibrillation ablation. Pacing Clin Electrophysiol 2013;36:781–8.
[50] Ren JF, et al. Intracardiac echocardiographic diagnosis of thrombus formation in the left atrial appendage: a complementary role to transesophageal echocardiography. Echocardiography 2013;30:72–80.
[51] Aldhoon B, et al. Complications of catheter ablation for atrial fibrillation in a high-volume centre with the use of intracardiac echocardiography. Europace 2013;15:24–32.
[52] Bartel T, et al. Why is intracardiac echocardiography helpful? Benefits, costs, and how to learn. Eur Heart J 2013;35:69–76.

[53] Thai WE, et al. Pulmonary venous anatomy imaging with low-dose, prospectively ECG-triggered, high-pitch 128-slice dual-source computed tomography. Circ Arrhythm Electrophysiol 2012;5:521–30.

[54] Weijs B, et al. Patients originally diagnosed with idiopathic atrial fibrillation more often suffer from insidious coronary artery disease compared to healthy sinus rhythm controls. Heart Rhythm 2012;9:1923–9.

[55] Thanassoulis G, et al. Pericardial fat is associated with prevalent atrial fibrillation: the Framingham Heart Study. Circ Arrhythm Electrophysiol 2010;3:345–50.

[56] Romero J, et al. Detection of left atrial appendage thrombus by cardiac computed tomography in patients with atrial fibrillation: a meta-analysis, *Circulation*. Circ Cardiovasc Imaging 2013;6:185–94.

[57] Di Biase L, et al. Does the left atrial appendage morphology correlate with the risk of stroke in patients with atrial fibrillation? Results from a multicenter study. J Am Coll Cardiol 2012;60:531–8.

[58] Fuchs A, et al. Automated assessment of heart chamber volumes and function in patients with previous myocardial infarction using multidetector computed tomography. J Cardiovasc Comput Tomogr 2012;6:325–34.

[59] Shiozaki AA, et al. Myocardial fibrosis detected by cardiac CT predicts ventricular fibrillation/ventricular tachycardia events in patients with hypertrophic cardiomyopathy. J Cardiovasc Comput Tomogr 2013;7:173–81.

[60] Schuleri KH, et al. Characterization of peri-infarct zone heterogeneity by contrast-enhanced multidetector computed tomography: a comparison with magnetic resonance imaging. J Am Coll Cardiol 2009;18:1699–707.

[61] Jongbloed MR, et al. Noninvasive visualization of the cardiac venous system using multislice computed tomography. J Am Coll Cardiol 2005;45:749–53.

[62] Truong QA, et al. Quantitative analysis of intraventricular dyssynchrony using wall thickness by multidetector computed tomography. JACC Cardiovasc Imaging 2008;6:772–81.

[63] To AC, et al. Role of transesophageal echocardiography compared to computed tomography in evaluation of pulmonary vein ablation for atrial fibrillation (ROTEA study). J Am Soc Echocardiogr 2011;24:1046–55.

[64] Pappone C, et al. Atrio-esophageal fistula as a complication of percutaneous transcatheter ablation of atrial fibrillation. Circulation 2004;109:2724–6.

[65] Calkins H, et al. HRS/EHRA/ECAS expert consensus statement on catheter and surgical ablation of atrial fibrillation: recommendations for personnel, policy, procedures and follow-up. A report of the Heart Rhythm Society (HRS) Task Force on Catheter and Surgical Ablation of Atrial Fibrillation developed in partnership with the European Heart Rhythm Association (EHRA) and the European Cardiac Arrhythmia Society (ECAS); in collaboration with the American College of Cardiology (ACC), American Heart Association (AHA), and the Society of Thoracic Surgeons (STS). Endorsed and approved by the governing bodies of the American College of Cardiology, the American Heart Association, the European Cardiac Arrhythmia Society, the European Heart Rhythm Association, the Society of Thoracic Surgeons, and the Heart Rhythm Society. Europace 2007;9:335–79.

[66] Anselmino M, et al. Morphologic analysis of left atrial anatomy by magnetic resonance angiography in patients with atrial fibrillation: a large single center experience. J Cardiovasc Electrophysiol 2011;22:1–7.

[67] Caponi D, et al. Ablation of atrial fibrillation: does the addition of three-dimensional magnetic resonance imaging of the left atrium to electroanatomic mapping improve the clinical outcome?: a randomized comparison of Carto-Merge vs. Carto-XP three-dimensional mapping ablation in patients with paroxysmal and persistent atrial fibrillation. Europace 2010;12:1098–104.

[68] Oakes RS, et al. Detection and quantification of left atrial structural remodeling with delayed-enhancement magnetic resonance imaging in patients with atrial fibrillation. Circulation 2009;119:1758–67.
[69] Rathi VK, et al. Contrast-enhanced CMR is equally effective as TEE in the evaluation of left atrial appendage thrombus in patients with atrial fibrillation undergoing pulmonary vein isolation procedure. Heart Rhythm 2013;10:1021–7.
[70] Klem I, et al. Assessment of myocardial scarring improves risk stratification in patients evaluated for cardiac defibrillator implantation. J Am Coll Cardiol 2012;60:408–20.
[71] Roes SD, et al. Infarct tissue heterogeneity assessed with contrast-enhanced MRI predicts spontaneous ventricular arrhythmia in patients with ischemic cardiomyopathy and implantable cardioverter-defibrillator. Circ Cardiovasc Imaging 2009;2:183–90.
[72] Bilchick KC, et al. Cardiac magnetic resonance assessment of dyssynchrony and myocardial scar predicts function class improvement following cardiac resynchronization therapy. JACC Cardiovasc Imaging 2008;1:561–8.
[73] Heydari B, et al. Imaging for planning of cardiac resynchronization therapy. JACC Cardiovasc Imaging 2012;5:93–110.
[74] Eitel C, et al. Electrophysiology study guided by real-time magnetic resonance imaging. Eur Heart J 2012;33:1975.
[75] Nazarian S, et al. Feasibility of real-time magnetic resonance imaging for catheter guidance in electrophysiology studies. Circulation 2008;118:223–9.
[76] Dong J, et al. Incidence and predictors of pulmonary vein stenosis following catheter ablation of atrial fibrillation using the anatomic pulmonary vein ablation approach: results from paired magnetic resonance imaging. J Cardiovasc Electrophysiol 2005;16:845–52.
[77] Peters DC, et al. Detection of pulmonary vein and left atrial scar after catheter ablation with three-dimensional navigator-gated delayed enhancement MR imaging: initial experience. Radiology 2007;243:690–5.
[78] Gepstein L, et al. A novel method for nonfluoroscopic catheter-based electroanatomical mapping of the heart. In vitro and in vivo accuracy results. Circulation 1997;95:1611–22.
[79] Earley MJ, et al. Radiofrequency ablation of arrhythmias guided by non-fluoroscopic catheter location: a prospective randomized trial. Eur Heart J 2006;27:1223–9.
[80] Kabra R, et al. Recent trends in imaging for atrial fibrillation ablation. Indian Pacing Electrophysiol J 2010;10:215–27.
[81] Donaldson DM, et al. Relevance of imaging structures adjacent to the left atrium during catheter ablation for atrial fibrillation. Heart Rhythm 2010;7:269–75.
[82] Corrado D, et al. Three-dimensional electroanatomical voltage mapping and histologic evaluation of myocardial substrate in right ventricular outflow tract tachycardia. J Am Coll Cardiol 2008;51:731–9.
[83] Arenal A, et al. Tachycardia-related channel in the scar tissue in patients with sustained monomorphic ventricular tachycardias: influence of the voltage scar definition. Circulation 2004;110:2568–74.
[84] Ouyang F, et al. Electroanatomic substrate of idiopathic left ventricular tachycardia: unidirectional block and macroreentry within the purkinje network. Circulation 2002;105:462–9.
[85] Kautzner J, et al. Selecting CRT candidates: the value of intracardiac mapping. Europace 2008;10(Suppl. 3):iii106–9.
[86] Moss AJ, et al. Long-term clinical course of patients after termination of ventricular tachyarrhythmia by an implanted defibrillator. Circulation 2004;110:3760–5.
[87] Raffel DM, et al. Development of mIBG as a cardiac innervation imaging agent. JACC Cardiovasc Imaging 2010;3:111–6.

[88] Dae MW, et al. Scintigraphic assessment of MIBG uptake in globally denervated human and canine hearts – implications for clinical studies. J Nucl Med 1992;33:1444–50.
[89] Jacobson AF, et al. Myocardial iodine-123 meta-iodobenzylguanidine imaging and cardiac events in heart failure. Results of the prospective ADMIRE-HF (AdreView Myocardial Imaging for Risk Evaluation in Heart Failure) study. J Am Coll Cardiol 2010;55:2212–21.
[90] Boogers MJ, et al. Cardiac sympathetic denervation assessed with 123-iodine metaiodobenzylguanidine imaging predicts ventricular arrhythmias in implantable cardioverter-defibrillator patients. J Am Coll Cardiol 2010;55:2769–77.
[91] van Campen CM, et al. FDG PET as a predictor of response to resynchronisation therapy in patients with ischaemic cardiomyopathy. Eur J Nucl Med Mol Imaging 2007;34:309–15.
[92] Kistler PM, et al. The impact of image integration on catheter ablation of atrial fibrillation using electroanatomic mapping: a prospective randomized study. Eur Heart J 2008;29:3029–36.
[93] Codreanu A, et al. Electroanatomic characterization of post-infarct scars comparison with 3-dimensional myocardial scar reconstruction based on magnetic resonance imaging. J Am Coll Cardiol 2008;52:839–42.
[94] Deftereos S, et al. Integration of intracardiac echocardiographic imaging of the left atrium with electroanatomic mapping data for pulmonary vein isolation: first-in-Greece experience with the CartoSound system and brief literature review. Hellenic J Cardiol 2012;53:10–6.
[95] Khaykin Y, et al. Real-time integration of 2D intracardiac echocardiography and 3D electroanatomical mapping to guide ventricular tachycardia ablation. Heart Rhythm 2008;5:1396–402.

Imaging guided interventions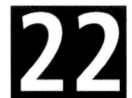

D. Braun, B. Bischoff, J. Hausleiter
Klinikum Großhadern der Ludwig-Maximilians-Universität München, Munich, Germany

22.1 Introduction

Recently, several minimally invasive approaches for interventional therapy of structural heart diseases have been developed. For example, transcatheter aortic valve implantation (TAVI) is an alternative therapeutic option for high-risk patients that serves as an alternative for surgical aortic valve replacement. Also, high-risk patients with mitral valve regurgitation may benefit from interventional mitral valve clipping. Furthermore, left atrial appendage (LAA) closure devices may reduce the risk for thromboembolic complications in patients with atrial fibrillation and a contraindication for oral anticoagulation. Lastly, selected patients may benefit from interventional closure of atrial septal defect (ASD) as well as persistent foramen ovale (PFO). For planning purposes prior to these interventions as well as for peri-interventional guidance, imaging techniques play an important role. Beyond the use of several imaging techniques for structural heart diseases, it has been shown that coronary CT angiography (CCTA) can improve success rates of percutaneous coronary revascularization of chronic total occlusions (CTOs).

22.2 Transcatheter aortic valve implantation

Over the past years, TAVI has been established as a minimally invasive treatment strategy in patients with severe aortic valve stenosis who are not considered suitable for conventional surgical valve replacement. While new devices are currently being introduced into the market, the most common valves currently used for TAVI are the Sapien® valve (Edwards Lifesciences) and the CoreValve® system (Medtronic, Inc.) (Figure 22.1). These devices are available only in certain sizes and thus are not suitable for all patients. The presence of device-aortic annular mismatch negatively impacts outcome due to the occurrence of aortic regurgitation after implantation, as well as peri-interventional annular rupture.

Furthermore, it is crucial to evaluate the most appropriate vascular access pathway (e.g., femoral, apical, or subclavian artery) prior to TAVI. Therefore, imaging techniques are essential for the planning of TAVI. Imaging may also be helpful during valve implantation and for follow-up. The specific imaging protocols are highly dependent on the experience and equipment of the individual institutions. Several centers are using echocardiography for the evaluation of the aortic annulus and root, and initial studies have been based on sizing by ultrasound. However, multidetector computed

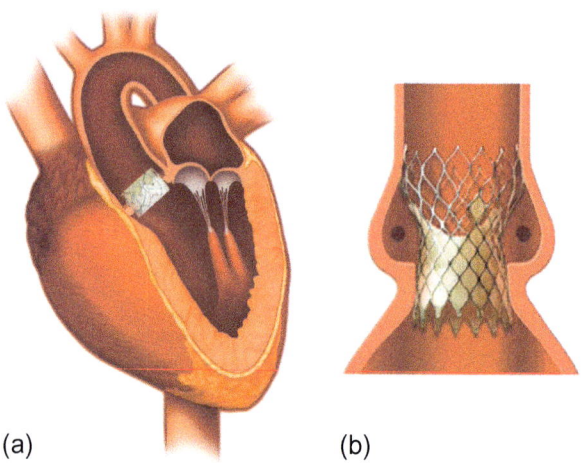

(a) (b)

Figure 22.1 (a) Edwards Sapien® prosthesis after implantation. Courtesy of Edwards Lifesciences; (b) Medtronic CoreValve® prosthesis after implantation. Courtesy of Medtronic.

tomography (MDCT) has become the standard for the evaluation prior to TAVI, especially in many high-volume centers, because the aortic annular shape, which is elliptical rather than circular, can be depicted best using this imaging modality.

Furthermore, tomographic imaging—especially MDCT—has been established for evaluation of the thoracoabdominal aorta and potential access vessels.

Table 22.1 summarizes and compares the importance of several screening CT and echo measurements as well as the principal techniques of preparation and implantation of the Sapien® valve and the CoreValve®.

22.2.1 Echocardiography

22.2.1.1 Screening transthoracic and transesophageal echocardiography

Transthoracic echocardiography is the gold standard for the evaluation of the severity of aortic stenosis. Besides aortic valve gradients, the aortic valve orifice area can reliably be determined using the continuity equation (see also Chapter 16).

An important challenge for successful trancatheter aortic valve implantation is the correct measurement of specific aortic valve dimensions. Initially these measurements, critical for selection of valve type and size, were performed using 2D transthoracic or transesophageal echocardiography. But because standard transesophageal echocardiography enables the acquisition of high-resolution images, this approach is considered superior to transthoracic echocardiography.

First, the determination of a set of qualitative and semi-quantitative parameters is of importance. These include the assessment of the severity of aortic stenosis as well as concomitant aortic regurgitation. Furthermore, the number, mobility, and structure

Table 22.1 Imaging guided interventions

	Medtronic CoreValve®	Edwards Sapien®
Screening CT/Echo Measurement		
LVOT diameter	+	–
Mean diameter of the aortic annulus (longitudinal/transverse)	++	++
Circumference of the aortic annulus	+	–
Area of the aortic annulus	–	+
Distance annulus - coronary ostia	(+)	+
Annulus/leaflet calcification	–	+
Sinus of valsalva width	–	+
Sinus of valsalva hight (annulus - sinutubular junction)	–	+
Diameter of the proximal ascending aorta	+	–
Peripheral access	++	++
Technique of preparation and implantation		
Balloon valvulopasty	+	+
Rapid pacing	–	+
Balloon-assisted expansion	–	+
Self-Expanding	+	–

LVOT: left ventricular outflow tract.
++: very important; +: important; (+): less important; –: not relevant.

of the aortic valve cusps, including the extent and location of calcifications are of importance. Currently, the presence of a bicuspid aortic valve is generally considered an exclusion criterion for TAVI because an increased risk for suboptimal valve deployment is assumed. Furthermore, bulky calcified aortic leaflets in close proximity to the coronary ostia might be associated with an increased risk of peri-procedural coronary occlusion, particularly with the use of the Sapien® valve.

Second, the determination of several quantitative parameters affects the selection of valve type and size (Figure 22.2, Table 22.1):

(1) **Left ventricular outflow tract (LVOT) diameter.**
The LVOT should be evaluated particularly if the CoreValve® is used since significant basal septal hypertrophy might lead to displacement of the prosthesis at the time or shortly after the implantation procedure.

(2) **Diameter of the aortic annulus.**
The most critical measurement for all available valve types is the determination of the diameter of the aortic annulus. The annular diameter predominantly determines the size and type of the prosthesis. An undersized prosthesis might eventually lead to mostly

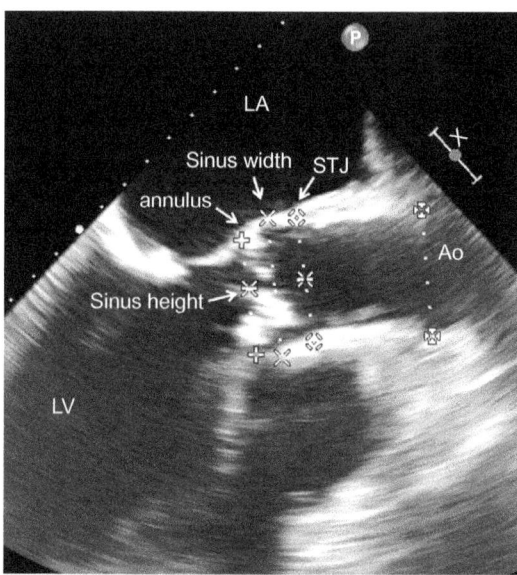

Figure 22.2 Aortic stenosis with 2D valve measurement in the LVOT view. LV, left ventricle; LA, left atrium; Ao, ascending aorta; Sinus, sinus of Valsalva; STJ, sinutubular junction.

paravalvular regurgitation as well as displacement of the device. An oversized prosthesis might lead to peri-interventional annular rupture. The diameter of the aortic annulus is typically measured at the beginning of systole in the LVOT view (around 110–135°) as the distance from the insertion of the left/non-coronary to the insertion of the right aortic valve cusp. This measurement might be cumbersome in severely calcified valves due to difficulty in identifying the hinge region as well as due to posterior acoustic attenuation.

(3) **Distance from the aortic annulus to the coronary ostia.**
The distance from the aortic annulus to the coronary ostia should be obtained to compare this measurement with the lengths of the aortic valve cusps. These measurements should be acquired in the LVOT view, particularly if the Sapien® valve is used. The length of the aortic valve cusps is usually shorter than the annular-ostial distance. However, these measurements are important since the (calcified) aortic valve cusps are crushed against the aortic wall during the implantation procedure. This might compromise the coronary ostia potentially resulting in life threatening complications.

(4) **Sinus of Valsalva width and height.**
The width and height of the sinus of Valsalva can be measured in the LVOT view. It is assumed that enough space is required to accommodate the native valve cusps to not compromise the coronary ostia. The width of the sinus of Valsalva is measured as the diameter of the aortic root at the midsinusal level. The height of sinus of Valsalva represents the distance between the aortic valve annulus to the level of the sinotubular junction. These measurements are of theoretical concern in particular for the Sapien® valve and should be compared to the dimension of the device intended to implant.

(5) **Diameter of the proximal ascending aorta.**
The diameter of the ascending aorta should be measured at its proximal part about 1 cm distal to the sinotubular junction. This measurement is of importance if the CoreValve®

device is taken into consideration since it contains a broader upper segment that secures the device in the ascending aorta. Thus, in patients with ascending aortic diameters >45 mm, the CoreValve® should not be implanted.

2D transesophageal echocardiography does not accurately depict the actual oval shape of the aortic valve annulus. This is why novel three-dimensional imaging modalities including 3D TEE and MDCT were introduced. Studies comparing 2D TEE to 3D TEE as well as MDCT show significantly larger annular diameters using these novel technologies, suggesting 2D TEE underestimates annular dimensions [1,2].

Aortic annular assessment by 3D transesophageal echocardiography requires the acquisition of a 3D volume. Subsequently, offline analysis with multiplanar reconstruction of this dataset enables the accurate assessment of the shape of the aortic annulus, including its maximum and minimum diameter (Figure 22.3). Husser et al. reported significantly smaller annulus diameters and areas using 3D TEE compared to MDCT. However, 3D TEE sagittal diameters correlated well with MDCT [3].

Although there is no defined gold standard for the acquisition of aortic valve measurements, an increasing number of centers favor performing MDCT scans over echocardiographic measurements. There are a number of advantages using this approach that will be described in the following section.

22.2.1.2 Peri-interventional transesophageal echocardiography

One major advantage of transesophageal echocardiography is its availability during the interventional procedure. In case of doubt, all the abovementioned measurements, including the measurements acquired by 3D TEE, can readily be repeated. Furthermore, several steps of the implantation procedure can be supported by transesophageal echocardiography. First, TEE can assist in balloon and prosthesis sizing and positioning during the implantation procedure. Second, prosthesis function, including residual

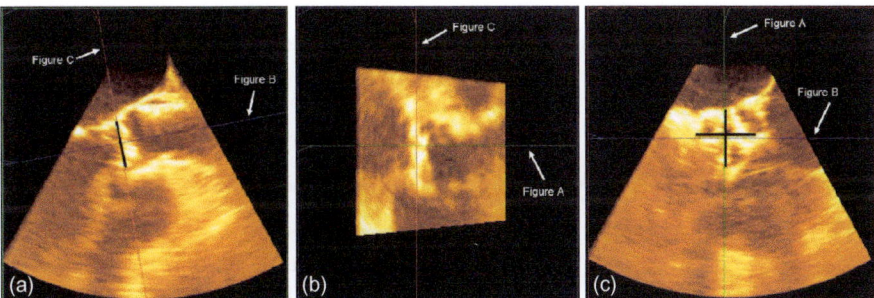

Figure 22.3 Aortic stenosis with 3D aortic annular measurement by means of multiplanar reconstruction. (a) Aortic valve in the sagittal LVOT view where the 3D volume is acquired. Black bar: 2D measurement of aortic annulus. (b) Aortic valve in a transversal view corresponding to the horizontal plane in A. (c) Aortic valve in a coronal view corresponding to the vertical planes in A and B. The vertical plane in A can be moved to the annular level of the aortic valve so that the maximum annular diameter can be measured in the coronal view in addition to the direct measurement in A. Furthermore, the coronal view enables direct planimetry of the aortic annulus area. Black bars: aortic annular measurement.

aortic regurgitation, can be evaluated immediately after implantation. Regarding aortic regurgitation, paravalvular regurgitation can be distinguished from valvular regurgitation, and allows a decision regarding further measures, such as balloon-postdilatation, in particular, in the case of significant paravalvular regurgitation.

However, peri-interventional TEE often necessitates the use of general anesthesia during the implantation procedure. This is why a number of interventionalists prefer performing the TAVI without TEE guidance, irrespective of the valve type intended for use.

22.2.1.3 Follow-up transthoracic echocardiography

Transthoracic echocardiography is used for follow-up evaluation of valve function, including ejection fraction. Usually mean gradients <10 mmHg can be measured in case of proper valve function. Pressure half time is the preferred parameter for the assessment of mostly paravalvular regurgitation. In case of good valve function, yearly follow-up visits should be considered.

22.2.2 Computed tomography

MDCT enables a comprehensive 3D assessment of the aortic valve, aortic root, and the thoracoabdominal aorta as well as its iliofemoral branches for planning purposes prior to TAVI procedures [4]. Therefore, in many centers, MDCT has become a standard modality for this indication. Detailed evaluation of the aortic valve annulus is crucial for accurate sizing of the valve prosthesis. Several studies have demonstrated that the aortic valve annulus is usually oval in shape. The CT examination can be performed in different ways, and there are multiple dimensions that can be measured and reported. So far, there is no single validated CT-methodology for the evaluation of patients referred for TAVI.

22.2.2.1 Image acquisition

A CT examination for TAVI planning needs to cover the aortic root, the entire thoracoabdominal aorta, and the iliac arteries as well as the proximal femoral arteries. If the subclavian arteries are considered for access, then the scan needs to be further extended cranially. Detailed measurements have to be performed, therefore, so the reconstructed slices thickness should be 1.0 mm or less. To allow for a high image quality of the aortic root without major motion artifacts, ECG-synchronized image acquisition is required in this region, either using retrospective ECG gating or prospective ECG triggering. Because a number of studies have shown a larger size of the aortic annulus during systole compared to diastole, systolic image acquisition might be preferable to lower the risk of paravalvular regurgitation. Image data of the remaining parts of the thoracoabdominal aorta and iliofemoral branches do not need to be acquired in an ECG-synchronized fashion, thereby limiting radiation exposure, scan duration, and required amount of contrast agent. The dedicated scan protocol highly depends on the CT system. When using a single-source MDCT system with 64 detectors or fewer, it is reasonable to split the examination into two parts. After an ECG-synchronized scan of the heart and the aortic root, a helical scan of the remaining volume is performed without ECG triggering, which requires a second or long infusion of contrast agent. When using a wide-detector CT system, it might be feasible to image the entire volume with ECG synchronization. Second- and third-generation dual-source CT systems can perform a prospectively ECG-triggered high-pitch spiral scan, which allows a TAVI planning CT examination at a very low radiation and contrast medium exposure. Whereas radiation exposure is not of major concern in TAVI patients, mainly considering their advanced age in general, keeping the amount of contrast agent low is important in patients with severe aortic valve stenosis. First of all, patients with severe aortic valve stenosis have a high risk of cardiac decompensation when subjected to a large amount of injected volume. Second, many patients with severe aortic valve stenosis suffer from renal insufficiency, predisposing them for contrast-induced nephropathy. Typically an amount of 80–120 ml contrast agent is administered for TAVI planning CT. However, it has been shown that the amount of contrast agent might be reduced to 60 ml or even below using dedicated scan protocols [5].

22.2.2.2 Image evaluation

Most importantly, the CT assessment prior to TAVI involves the measurements of the aortic valve annulus for correct prosthesis sizing, its distance to the coronary artery ostia, and evaluation of the thoracoabdominal aorta and its iliofemoral branches.

Exact determination of the aortic valve annulus dimensions is of major importance because the annulus might be too large or too small for available prosthesis sizes. Furthermore, prosthesis undersizing or oversizing might result in complications such as paravalvular regurgitation or rupture of the aortic root. For evaluation of the aortic valve annulus, a double-oblique plane is required that includes all three lowest insertion points of the aortic valve leaflets (Figure 22.4). Using this double-oblique image data, there are three different approaches of deriving the mean diameter of the oval-shaped aortic valve annulus [4] (see Figure 22.4). First, it may be calculated as the average of the long and short diameter. Second, it may be derived from the aortic valve annulus circumference, which is divided by π. Third, it may be calculated from the planimetrically measured annulus area as: $\text{mean diameter} = 2 \times \sqrt{(\text{area} \div \pi)}$. Investigating the reproducibility of aortic annulus assessments, it has been shown that the determination of the area-derived diameter was associated with the best reproducibility, which may indicate that this CT-based method should be preferred over others [6]. Although there is no broad consensus about the ideal timing of CT data acquisition during the heart cycle, and although the quantification of the mean annulus diameter did not differ between diastole and systole, systolic measurements are usually preferred over diastolic measurements [7].

When the transcatheter aortic valve prosthesis is implanted, the native aortic valve leaflets are displaced against the wall of the sinus of Valsalva with the risk of coronary artery occlusion. To minimize the risk of coronary artery occlusion, usually a minimum distance of 11–14 mm between the aortic valve annulus and the coronary artery ostia is generally recommended, depending on prosthesis type and size. Therefore,

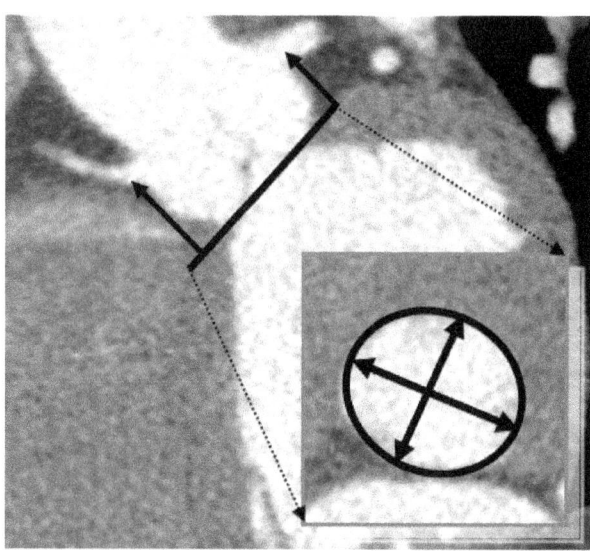

Figure 22.4 Required measurements in the aortic valve annulus plane, which represents a double-oblique plane, including all three lowest insertion points of the aortic valve leaflets. Furthermore, the distances between the aortic annulus plane and the coronary artery ostia are derived.

these distances need to be reported from ECG-synchronized 3D image data of the aortic root (see Figure 22.4). Length or calcification of the aortic valve cusps may also be predictive for coronary artery occlusion.

Commonly, a transfemoral access route is being chosen for the TAVI procedure. Alternatively, a trans-subclavian, transaortic, or transapical (Sapien®) approach may be possible. To determine the optimal access pathway with the lowest risk for vascular complications, a detailed evaluation of the thoracoabdominal aorta and its potential access branches is necessary in every patient. Computed tomography can reliably detect risk factors for vascular complications such as insufficient vessel diameter compared to delivery system, the degree of atherosclerosis, and vessel tortuosity, or kinking. For a transfemoral TAVI approach a minimum vessel diameter between 6 and 8 mm—depending on prosthesis type and size—is required to minimize the risk of vascular complications.

Furthermore, it has been shown that CT image data can be helpful to derive the optimal aortic annulus plane for fluoroscopy. When performing TAVI, a fluoroscopic projection is required in which the valve prosthesis is orthogonal to the native valve plane, preferably with all valve cusps separated. Traditionally, this projection has been derived from repeat aortograms. However, CT offers three-dimensional data of the orientation of the aortic root and therefore is able to predict the optimal fluoroscopic projection for the TAVI procedure. Using CT data has been shown to increase the rate of achieving an optimal fluoroscopic projection angle for implantation [8] and to reduce the number of performed aortic angiograms and amount of contrast agent needed [9].

In addition, CT has been demonstrated to be of prognostic value in TAVI patients. First, the use of CT for aortic annulus sizing was associated with a reduced rate of more than mild paravalvular regurgitation after valve implantation, compared to 2D echocardiography [10]. Second, the extent of aortic valve calcification predicts post-procedural aortic regurgitation, complications during implantation, and 1-year mortality as well as improvement in NYHA-class after TAVI procedure [11].

Today, a variety of dedicated CT software packages are available that facilitate an automated accurate analysis of aortic valve dimensions as well as of vascular tree for preprocedural planning (Figure 22.5). Some software packages also include peri-procedural hybrid CT/fluoroscopic imaging for selection of an optimal fluoroscopic angulation angle and for guiding valve deployment.

22.2.3 Cardiovascular magnetic resonance imaging

Similar to computed tomography, CMR also provides tomographic images of the aortic valve, the aortic valve annulus, and the aortic root, as well as the thoracoabdominal aorta and its iliofemoral branches, but without exposure to ionizing radiation. ECG-gated non-contrast cine CMR sequences allow for a comprehensive assessment of the aortic valve annulus, the aortic root and cardiac function. Furthermore, non-contrast 3D whole-heart MR angiography enable post-acquisition reconstruction of a double-oblique plane of the aortic valve annulus comparable to CT. Gadolinium enhanced MRI angiography of the thoracoabdominal aorta and its iliofemoral branches allow for an accurate evaluation of the vessel lumen, however, with suboptimal assessability of atherosclerotic changes of the vessel wall. However, especially in elderly patients, the long examination time may challenge routine use of CMR in the context of

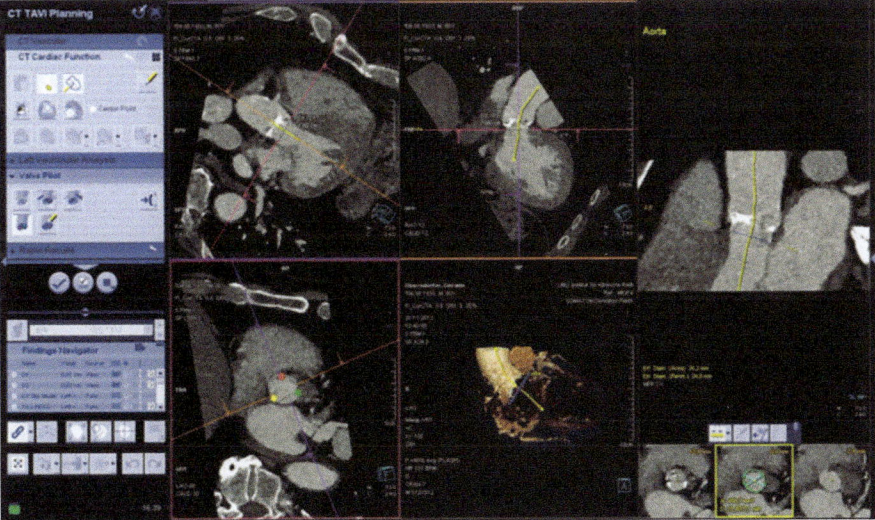

Figure 22.5 Example of a dedicated CT software package for the automated segmentation and analysis of aortic valves.

TAVI planning. Furthermore, the lower spatial resolution of CMR or a reduced image quality in arrhythmic patients can jeopardize the precise evaluation of the aortic annulus and aortic root. Thus at present, MRI is reserved for patients in which adequate preprocedural imaging (including sizing, access pathways) could not be obtained with either CT, echocardiography, or invasive angiography.

MRI is not only applicable pre-interventionally in patients prior to TAVI but also represents a helpful tool in evaluating paravalvular regurgitation in patients post-TAVI. In clinical practice, echocardiography serves as a standard modality for the evaluation of post-TAVI regurgitation. However, recent studies have shown that echocardiography underestimates paravalvular regurgitation in post-TAVI patients when compared to MRI [12]. Therefore, patients after TAVI with suspected paravalvular regurgitation—especially with unclear echocardiographic findings—should be considered to undergo MRI.

22.3 Percutaneous edge-to-edge repair of the mitral valve

Percutaneous edge-to-edge repair of the mitral valve has been shown to be an alternative treatment option in particular for patients who have severe mitral regurgitation (MR) and who are ineligible or at high risk for cardiac surgery (Figure 22.6). Besides the assessment of the grade of MR, a key point for the selection of suitable candidates for mitral valve clipping is a detailed understanding of mitral valve pathology. In this section, we describe standard MR quantification measurements using 2D and 3D transesophageal echocardiography. Furthermore, several steps for the assessment of critical anatomical conditions with focus on 2D as well as 3D TEE are elucidated. Finally the role of transesophageal echocardiography for the guidance of MitraClip® procedures will be illustrated.

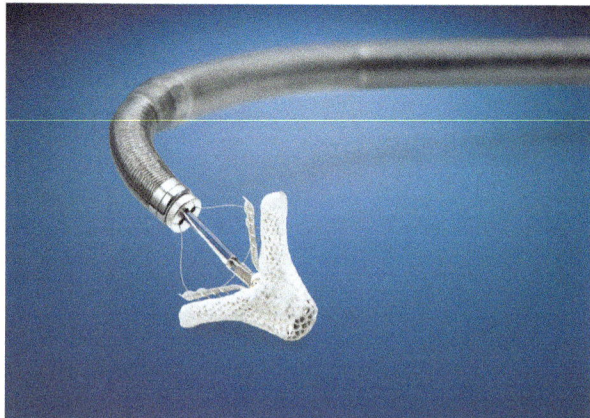

Figure 22.6 The MitraClip® attached to delivery catheter.
Courtesy of Abbott Vascular.

22.3.1 Echocardiography

22.3.1.1 Screening transesophageal echocardiography

First of all, the etiology of MR should be identified. In primary MR (degenerative MR) the mitral valve apparatus per se is diseased. Secondary MR (functional MR) results from left ventricular dilatation and/or restricted leaflet motion.

For both etiologies of MR, the gold standard for the quantification of MR is transesophageal echocardiography. Therefore, MR should be quantified according to current guidelines [13]. The echocardiographic assessment of MR is further detailed in Chapter 16; however, in the context of percutaneous interventions, it is important to re-iterate that the degree of MR depends on volume status, afterload, and heart rhythm and thus can fluctuate over time. The preferred methods of quantification are the determination of vena contracta width in two perpendicular planes as well as measurement of EROA (effective regurgitant orifice area) and regurgitant volume by the PISA (proximal isovelocity surface area) method. In selected cases, direct planimetry of the vena contracta area following multiplane reconstruction of a 3D color volume can be used for MR quantification. However, to date, there are no clear cut-off values for MR quantification. Additional useful criteria are the determination of left atrial regurgitant jet area, the extent of the proximal flow convergence region in the left ventricle, the intensity and shape of the continuous-wave Doppler regurgitant jet signal, and pulmonary vein flow and mitral inflow.

In patients who are ineligible or at high risk for cardiac surgery, the next step is to determine the anatomical prerequisites for a successful clip placement. Optimal conditions were originally defined by the EVEREST studies and developed further based on the developing experience with this novel device [14–17]. Although it is advisable to adhere to the following criteria, experienced centers may take individual decisions for the MitraClip® procedure following a heart team discussion in patients with suboptimal anatomical conditions.

From a procedural perspective, malcoaptation is ideally located in the central mitral valve region (A2/P2) because of the absence of subvalvular chordae tendineae that could complicate the procedure. The location of the malcoaptation should be determined using several imaging modalities. First, the intercommissural two-chamber view visualizing segments P1, A2, and P3 should be applied and 2D as well as live 3D images depicted from the left atrium acquired, as shown in Figure 22.7. This intercommissural view should be used as a reference view and usually enables the localization of the pathological region. Live 3D imaging is considered superior for the detection and localization of flail leaflets, clefts, and perforations. Next, multiplane TEE can be used to gain double cross-sections with imaging planes perpendicular to segment 1, 2, and 3, showing the corresponding three-chamber views. Special attention should be paid on the perpendicular three-chamber view corresponding to the region of malcoaptation. In a second step, the corresponding perpendicular view should be documented directly in a single view to increase the resolution of the images. The four-chamber view is of limited value since it corresponds to an oblique imaging plane reaching from A2/A3 to P1/2. Subsequently, the abovementioned images should be acquired with color Doppler to confirm that the malcoaptation

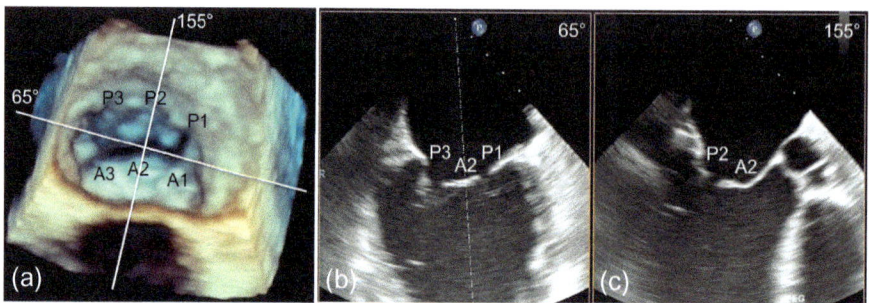

Figure 22.7 (a) Life 3D image of the mitral valve depicted from the left atrium, intersections correspond to the 2D images in (b) and (c). (b) Mitral valve depicted in the intercommissural view. (c) Mitral valve depicted in the three-chamber view. A1/2/3: segment 1, 2, 3 of the anterior mitral valve leaflet. P1/2/3: segment 1, 2, 3 of the posterior mitral valve leaflet.

identified accounts for the resultant regurgitant MR jet. Figure 22.8 depicts images of secondary MR due to flail leaflet of the P3 segment following chordal rupture. The abovementioned images should also be used to assess the structure of the mitral valve leaflets. Ideally, both leaflets should be mobile and thin without calcifications in the grasping region. The mobile length of the smaller posterior mitral leaflet

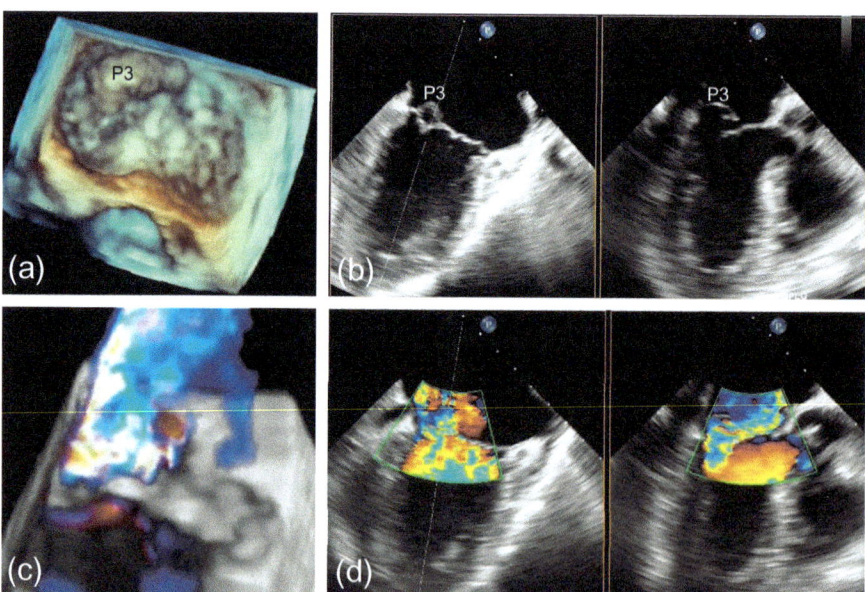

Figure 22.8 (a) Life 3D image of the mitral valve depicted from the left atrium with flail leaflet of the P3 segment due to chordal rupture. (b) Intercommissural view with flail leaflet of segment 3 of the posterior mitral leaflet with corresponding multiplane perpendicular three-chamber view of the pathological region. (c) Color life 3D image of the mitral valve depicted from the left atrium, corresponding to (a). (d) Color intercommissural view with flail leaflet of P3 with corresponding multiplane perpendicular three-chamber view of the pathological region, corresponding to (c).

(PML) should be >10 mm to enable a stable fixation of the leaflet between the clip arm and the corresponding gripper following grasping. Furthermore, in case of flail leaflets, flail height should be <10 mm and flail width <15 mm. Finally, mitral valve orifice area should ideally be >4 cm² to avoid the development of mitral stenosis following clip placement. Mitral valve orifice area should be determined using multiplane reconstruction of a 3D volume acquired in the intercommissural view, as shown in Figure 22.9.

22.3.1.2 Peri-interventional transesophageal echocardiography

Percutaneous edge-to-edge repair of the mitral valve is a primarily TEE guided intervention [18]. In the following section, we describe useful 2D and 3D views that facilitate the successful placement of a MitraClip®. Transseptal puncture plays an important role for the progress and success of the MitraClip® procedure. The puncture site should be located superiorly and posteriorly in the fossa ovalis. Transseptal puncture can be best guided using the bicaval view (100–110°) as well as the corresponding multiplane perpendicular short-axis/four-chamber view (10–20°). The height of the puncture site above the mitral valve annulus should be determined after a tenting can be visualized in the four-chamber view (0°) (Figure 22.10). In degenerative MR due to mitral valve prolapse, the height of the puncture site should be approximately 4–5 cm to allow sufficient maneuverability of the catheter. In functional MR, a height of 3.5–4 cm above the mitral valve annulus is desirable. Following successful transseptal puncture, the introduction of the steerable guide catheter can be best visualized in the short-axis view (40–60°). This view should be maintained for the advancement of the clip delivery system. Perpendicular multiplane imaging with focus on the tip of the closed clip can be useful to guide the steering of the MitraClip® above the mitral valve. As soon as the clip is visible above the mitral valve, the intercommissural view should be used. Following the correct positioning of the clip, the opened clip arms should not be visible in the intercommissural view; however, in the corresponding perpendicular multiplane view, both clip arms should be clearly visible. For the step of clip positioning, live 3D imaging is a useful addition

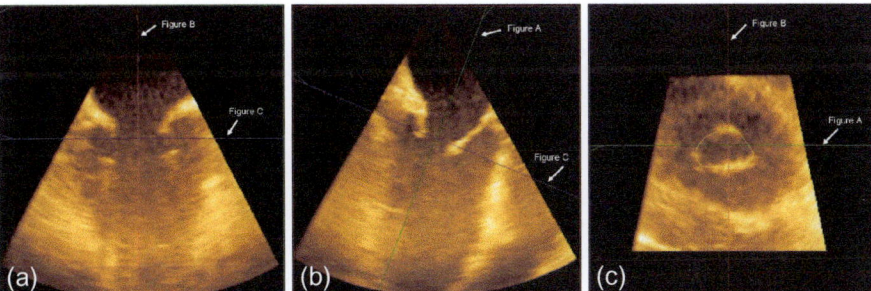

Figure 22.9 Three-dimensional planimetry of mitral valve orifice area. (a) Intercommissural view, vertical plane corresponds to B, horizontal plane corresponds to C. (b) Three-chamber view, vertical plane corresponds to A, horizontal plane corresponds to C. (c) Planimetry of mitral valve orifice area, horizontal plane corresponds to A, vertical plane corresponds to B.

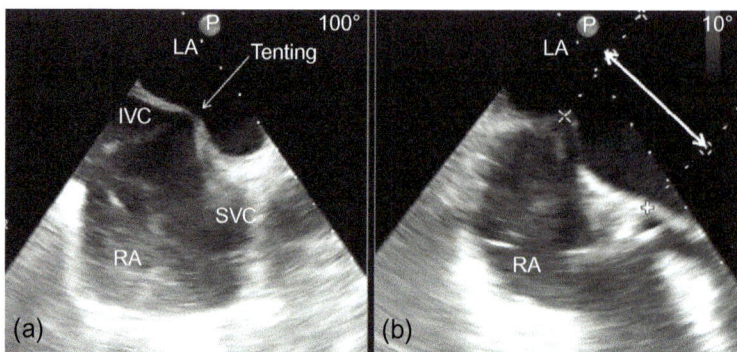

Figure 22.10 Transseptal puncture. (a) Bicaval view. (b) Short-axis/four-chamber view, measurement of the height of the puncture site above the mitral valve annulus. LA, left atrium; RA, right atrium; SVC, superior vena cava; IVC, inferior vena cava.

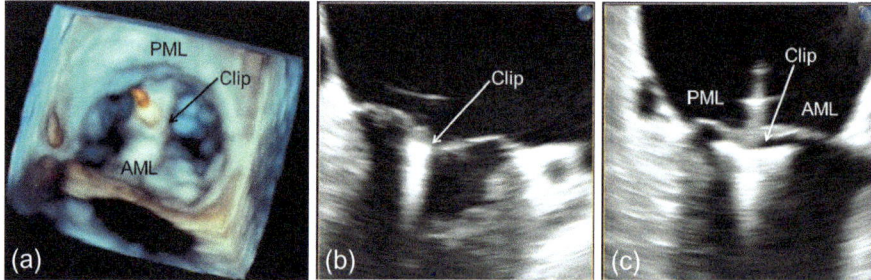

Figure 22.11 (a) Live 3D imaging of clip positioning above the mitral valve. (b) Intercommissural view with desired clip position in the left ventricle. (c) Three-chamber view with desired clip position in the left ventricle. AML, anterior mitral leaflet; PML, posterior mitral leaflet.

that obviates transgastric views (Figure 22.11). The advancement of the MitraClip® into the left ventricle should be done in the intercommissural view with the aid of the corresponding perpendicular multiplane view. After the clip has passed the mitral valve, correct positioning should be controlled in the abovementioned views. For acquisition of meaningful live 3D images, the gain should be down regulated until the clip can be visualized through the mitral leaflets. Grasping is a key step of the procedure, and should be captured in the three-chamber view. For this purpose, the three-chamber view can be captured directly as a single view. An alternative approach is the acquisition of the intercommissural view as well as the three-chamber view as a perpendicular multiplane view (Figure 22.12). The latter approach has the advantage that clip deviations can be rapidly detected in the intercommissural view. It is recommended that during the grasping process, the clip should be closed partially. Full closure of the clip can be done after clip attachment to both leaflets with sufficient leaflet insertion into the clip has been confirmed. Clip attachment to the leaflets can be assessed by traversing the PML in the three-chamber view and the

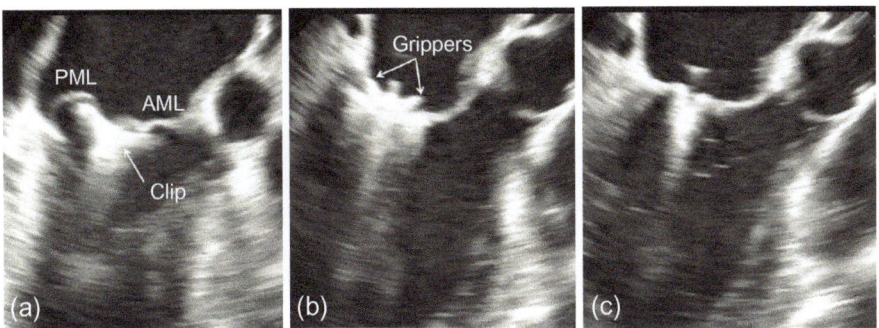

Figure 22.12 Grasping sequence. (a) AML and PML on top of the clip arms. (b) Movement of the grippers toward the clip arms. (c) Closed clip with attached leaflets. AML, anterior mitral leaflet; PML, posterior mitral leaflet.

anterior mitral leaflet in the four-chamber view. However, novel 3D imaging methods for the assessment of clip attachment to the leaflets have been described that might be useful in ambiguous cases [15,16]. In addition to this, the acquisition of a long video loop of the grasping process might be very helpful for the assessment of leaflet insertion. When satisfactory reduction of MR as well as sufficient leaflet insertion has been achieved, the clip can be released. It is noteworthy that after releasing the clip, there might be a slight worsening of MR. Following removal of the clip delivery system, the extent and direction of the residual iatrogenic ASD should be assessed in the bicaval and the short-axis view. Final images should be obtained in the intercommissural and the corresponding perpendicular multiplane view. Furthermore, live 3D imaging should be obtained to compare the final result with the initial MR severity (Figure 22.13) as well as to confirm the establishment of a so-called tissue bridge connecting the anterior and PML. Regular transthoracic echocardiographic follow-up

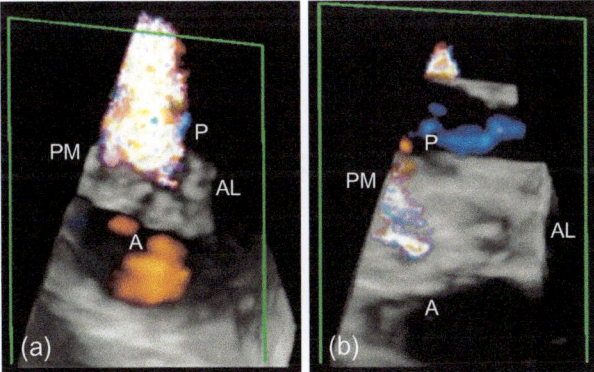

Figure 22.13 (a) Three-dimensional image of severe functional mitral regurgitation depicted from the left atrium before clipping. (b) Three-dimensional image of the same valve after the placement of two MitraClips®. A, anterior; P, posterior; AL, antero-lateral; PM, postero-medial.

examinations are advisable following clipping. In this context, it is important to mention that the placement of MitraClip(s)® usually leads to excentric residual MR jets, making standard MR quantification difficult. Therefore, in uncertain cases, transesophageal echocardiographic follow-up examinations as well as MR quantification using magnetic resonance imaging should be taken into consideration.

Novel, real-time hybrid techniques are available fusing fluoroscopy with real-time transesophageal echocardiography, which allows the interventional cardiologist to work in fluoroscopic projections with simultaneous echo information [19]. This technique may be increasingly used to facilitate complex interventions, such as MitraClip® implantation.

22.3.2 Computed tomography

If ECG-synchronized multi-phase image data are acquired, computed tomography also allows for an evaluation of valvular morphology and function. However, for assessment of the moving cardiac valves, image data from multiple time points of the cardiac cycle are required, which increases radiation exposure.

Other transcatheter mitral valve repair techniques are clinically available or under preclinical investigation [20]. These techniques include direct or indirect anuloplasty devices, implantable neochordae, annular plication, and ventricular remodeling devices. For direct trancatheter anuloplasty (GDS Accucinch, Valtech Cardioband), CT plays an important role in assessing the dimensions and shape of the annulus, identifying the position of the annulus and angulation of the underlying myocardium (to determine the most appropriate angle for anchor insertion), and identifying annular calcifications. Indirect anuloplasty devices (e.g., Carillon, Cardiac Dimensions) exploit the vicinity of the coronary sinus to the mitral annulus by implanting a metallic device in the coronary sinus that exerts tension transmitted to the mitral annulus (Figure 22.14). Unfortunately, in many patients, the coronary sinus is displaced toward the left atrium away and separate from the annulus, which may explain some of the failures observed with these devices. Additionally, in 16–80% of patients, the left circumflex coronary artery courses underneath the coronary sinus and therefore can be dangerously compressed by the contracting device. This can be readily detected by CCTA. With the foreseeable introduction of transcatheter mitral valve prostheses in a few years' time, CT may become more important to size the mitral annulus and provide adequate prosthesis-anulus matching much like it is now in clinical routine with TAVI. Evaluation of heart valves using computed tomography is described in Chapter 16 in more detail.

22.3.3 Cardiovascular magnetic resonance imaging

Imaging of mitral valve pathology is the domain of echocardiography. However, in case of unclear echocardiographic findings, CMR can be useful for assessing mitral valve pathologies. Valve assessment by CMR includes the use of cine imaging for evaluation of cardiac valve anatomy and motion and velocity-encoded imaging for assessment of valvular stenosis and regurgitation. Imaging techniques for evaluation of valvular pathologies are discussed in more detail in Chapter 16.

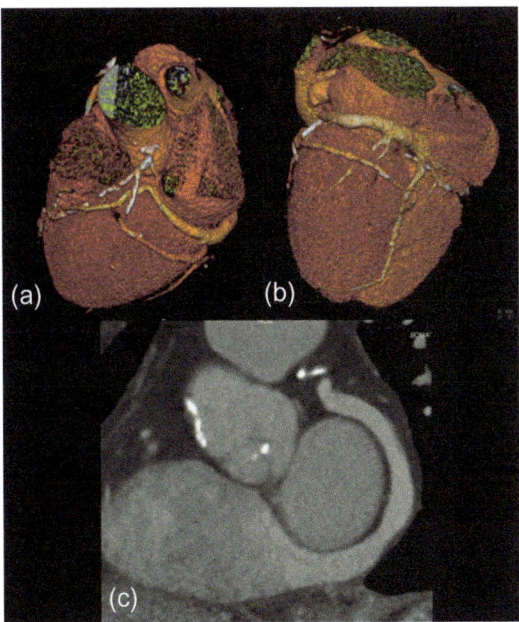

Figure 22.14 CT-based visualization of the anatomic relationship between coronary sinus and coronary arteries using 3-D volume rendering (a and b) and between the coronary sinus and the left atrium using multiplanar reformation (c).

Directly assessing mitral valve regurgitation in CMR can be challenging due to the complex three-dimensional course of movement of the mitral valve; however, with careful planning, in-plane views can usually be obtained. Furthermore, regurgitant mitral volumes can be derived by subtracting the LV stroke volume obtained from a standard cine stack from the aortic forward flow acquired with velocity encoded CMR in the ascending aorta. Prior to mitral valve clipping, CMR, in case of unclear echocardiographic findings, can be useful to determine the exact location and severity of mitral valve regurgitation.

22.4 Occlusion of LAA

Atrial fibrillation (AF) represents the most common supraventricular rhythm disorder (see Chapter 21). Irregular atrial contractions predispose patients to blood stasis favoring atrial thrombus formation. Atrial thrombi are found most frequently in the LAA. Systemic embolization of these thrombi can result in stroke, a life-threating event that occurs in up to 15% of high-risk AF patients per year. Therefore, in clinically asymptomatic patients, the treatment of choice consists of medical rhythm control as well as anticoagulant therapy. The latter has been shown to significantly reduce the risk of stroke. Traditionally, anticoagulation is achieved using vitamin K antagonists, for instance warfarin or acenocoumarol. In recent years, effective novel anticoagulants (i.e., direct thrombin-inhibitor dabigatran, and factor Xa inhibitors rivaroxaban and apixaban) were developed, where frequent laboratory analyses can be omitted. However, all anticoagulants predispose patients to an increased risk of bleeding.

An alternative approach to reduce the risk of stroke is the percutaneous closure of the LAA. For this purpose, the Watchman device (formerly Atritech. Inc., Plymouth, MN, now Boston Scientific) as well as the Amplatzer cardiac plug (formerly AGA Medical, Plymouth, MN, now St. Jude Medical) are currently available (Figure 22.15). It has been shown that percutaneous LAA closure with the Watchman device is non-inferior to warfarin with regard to stroke prevention [21]. This is why these devices might be an alternative for patients with atrial fibrillation and an increased risk of stroke with contraindication to anticoagulant therapy.

A key point for the selection of suitable candidates for LAA occlusion is a detailed understanding of LAA anatomy. In the following sections we describe LAA measurements using 2D and 3D transesophageal echocardiography as well as computed tomography and magnetic resonance imaging. Furthermore, we describe the essential peri-interventional use of transesophageal echocardiography.

22.4.1 Echocardiography

22.4.1.1 Screening transesophageal echocardiography

Transthoracic echocardiography is unsuitable for the assessment of LAA anatomy. Standardized screening transesophageal echocardiography includes measurements of LAA width and depth in four different views: 0°, 45°, 90°, and 135°. There is no clear delineation between left atrium and LAA. This is why a measurement of LAA size depends on the examiner. The required measurements vary for the two available devices. While for the Watchman device, the width of the LAA ostium should be measured, the Amplatzer cardiac plug requires a measurement approximately 5 mm below the ostium where the corpus of this device has to be placed. If the Watchman device is taken into consideration, the measurement of LAA depth should be done perpendicular to the width measurement to account for the relatively inflexible shape of the device. Both LAA width and depth should be correlated with the available Watchman device

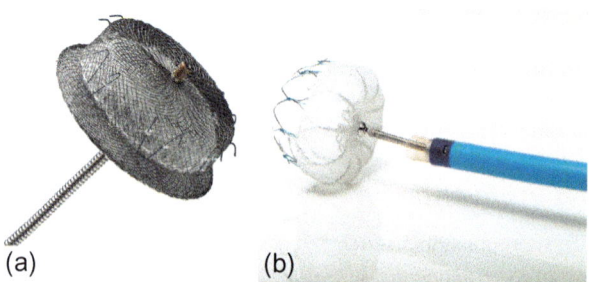

Figure 22.15 (a) Amplatzer Cardiac plug® attached to delivery catheter. Courtesy of St. Jude Medical. (b) Watchman® device attached to delivery catheter.
Courtesy of Boston Scientific.

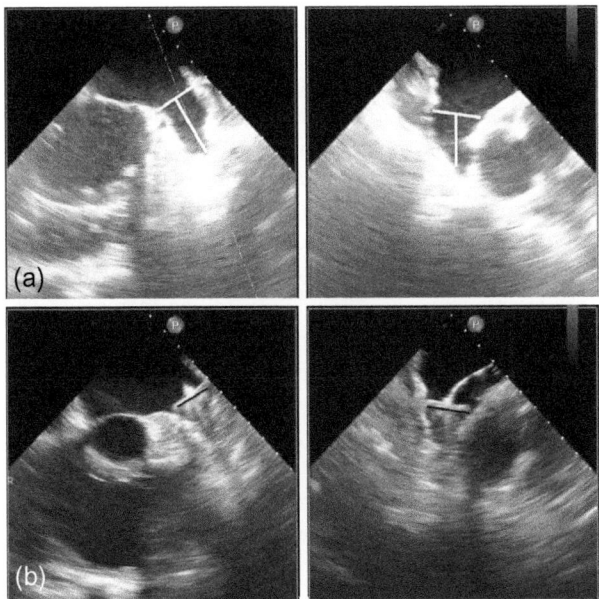

Figure 22.16 (a) LAA measurement of ostium width and LAA depth at 45° and corresponding perpendicular multiplane view (135°). (b) Same patient following implantation of a Watchman device, measurement of device compression at 45° and corresponding perpendicular multiplane view (135°).

sizes (Figure 22.16). First, the Watchman device should be available in a size that allows device compression of approximately 20% (for instance, device size 24 mm for LAA width of 20 mm). Second, the depth of the LAA should be large enough for this device size. If the depth of the LAA is insufficient for the Watchman device, the Amplatzer cardiac plug might be an alternative treatment option, where this criterion is not critical.

The use of 3D TEE is advantageous, since perpendicular multiplane views enables the simultaneous illustration of two views, 0° and 90° as well as 45° and 135°. Thus, it seems easier to get an idea about the three-dimensional LAA structure. Furthermore, unclear structures can often be assigned correctly.

In addition to the abovementioned measurements, extra lobes of substantial size should be described, in particular if they are in close proximity to the LAA ostium. The latter might interfere with a satisfactory LAA closure.

22.4.1.2 Peri-interventional transesophageal echocardiography

In most centers, percutaneous LAA closure is performed under TEE guidance. Alternatively, intracardiac echocardiography has been used. However, due the availability of high-resolution images, including three-dimensional images, TEE should be favored.

One major advantage of TEE for the assessment of LAA size compared to computed tomography is the possibility of reassessing LAA size immediately prior to device implantation, since LAA size can measurably vary depending on the volume status of the patient.

First, analogous to the use of TEE for the MitraClip® procedures, transseptal puncture can be best guided using the bicaval view (100–110°) as well as the corresponding multiplane perpendicular short-axis/four-chamber view (10–20°). The puncture site should be located in the middle or infero-posterior aspect of the fossa ovalis. Following successful transseptal puncture, the introduction of the catheter system can be best viewed in a short-axis view (40–60°). The advancement as well as the positioning of the catheter system in the LAA can usually be guided at 45° along with the perpendicular multiplane view (135°). Following implantation, the key role of echocardiography is to (1) assess the stability of the device position and (2) assess the quality of LAA closure. For both, the device should be visualized again at 0°, 45°, 90°, and 135°. Color Doppler assessment for residual flow should be done at a reduced scale (20 cm/s).

For the Watchman device, the overlap above the ostium as well as gaps close to the device should be minimal. For the assessment of device compression, the device diameter at the level of LAA width should be measured in each view. Device compression should be approximately 20% of the device size. Furthermore, a peri-interventional TEE-guided "tug test" should be performed to assess secure device anchoring. In case of a stable position, no device displacement should be noticed. Previous studies included a 6-week follow-up TEE for the assessment of LAA sealing as well as to exclude thrombotic bearings on the device.

The construction of the Amplatzer cardiac plug containing a flexible sealing disc usually achieves complete occlusion of the LAA, as documented by color Doppler echocardiography. However, device compression cannot be reliably used as a measure of stability since the body of the device is hidden under the disc. Thus stability is assessed by the visual impression of the position of the device.

Following release of the device and removal of the catheter system, the interatrial septum should be assessed in the bicaval as well as the short-axis view.

22.4.2 Computed tomography

22.4.2.1 Image acquisition

Computed tomography offers a 3D dataset for a comprehensive assessment of the left atrium and the LAA. To derive accurate anatomical information about the LAA, image acquisition usually is performed using prospective ECG-triggering or retrospective ECG-gating. Although motion of the left atrium and the LAA can be significantly reduced in patients with atrial fibrillation, image acquisition without ECG-synchronization might result in motion artifacts, however, allowing for a significant reduction of radiation exposure. Prior to implantation of a LAA occlusion device, it is necessary to exclude LAA thrombus. Commonly, this is done using transesophageal echocardiography. However, computed tomography has also been shown to allow for the exclusion of relevant thrombus formation in the LAA. While standard cardiac CT scan protocols show a low specificity (between 44% and 85% [22,23]) for LAA thrombus detection with a high number of false positives due to circulatory stasis in the LAA or artifacts, dedicated scan protocols including delayed imaging (e.g., after 1–2 min) can significantly improve diagnostic accuracy for LAA thrombus evaluation. Furthermore, dual-energy CT may improve discrimination between LAA thrombus and circulatory stasis using iodine mapping.

22.4.2.2 Evaluation of left atrial appendage

An exact three-dimensional model of the LAA anatomy is derived by contrast-enhanced computed tomography. These data are useful for correct sizing of the occlusion device. Analysis of the LAA prior to LAA occlusion includes evaluation of LAA morphology, number of LAA lobes, LAA length, the diameter and shape of the LAA annulus, and its distance to the presumed puncture site and the first LAA bend.

The overall shape of the LAA should be noted. Four different LAA morphologies have been described as shown in Figure 22.17 [24]. When compared to the other morphologies, patients with "chicken wing" morphology have been shown to have a significant lower risk of prior stroke before atrial fibrillation ablation [24].

For optimal positioning of the LAA closure device, it is important to know the presence and exact location of accessory lobes; the distance between the LAA orifice and the first LAA bend should not be too short to allow for a sufficient landing zone. For planning purposes, the distance between the LAA orifice and the assumed location of the transseptal puncture should be reported.

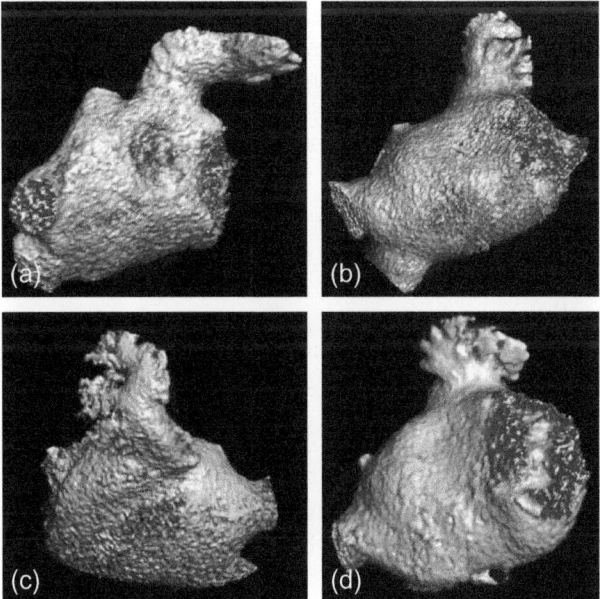

Figure 22.17 Different shapes of the left atrial appendage. (a) Chicken wing; (b) windsock; (c) cactus; (d) cauliflower.

The different occlusion devices are available in different sizes. For an optimal device selection, it is crucial to know the exact diameter and shape of the LAA orifice. In the literature, several different shapes of the LAA orifice have been described including oval, foot-like, triangular, water drop-like, and round. For measuring of the LAA orifice diameter, several methods have been described. Using a basic approach, the diameter is calculated from measurements in axial, sagittal, and coronal image reformations (see Figure 22.18).

Another approach calculates the mean LAA orifice diameter from its long and short axis as derived from a double-oblique plane of the LAA orifice (see Figure 22.19). Alternatively, the mean diameter might be calculated from the LAA perimeter (mean diameter = perimeter $\div \pi$) or area (mean diameter = $2 \times \sqrt{(\text{area} \div \pi)}$). A study by Wang et al. deriving the LAA orifice diameter from its perimeter showed to be the best method for accurate device sizing [25].

Incorrect sizing of the LAA closure device shows a high risk for incomplete occlusion of the LAA. Besides TEE, computed tomography is also able to detect residual blood flow within the LAA, which might prohibit a discontinuation of anticoagulation. Figure 22.20 shows an exemplary cardiac CT examination after LAA occlusion using a watchman device. No residual blood flow was detected in the occluded LAA.

22.4.3 Cardiovascular magnetic resonance imaging

CMR is well suited for imaging of the LAA, as it provides high-resolution three-dimensional tomographic images without ionizing radiation. Pulse sequences used for LAA imaging include cine steady-state free precession and black blood fast spin echo.

With these methods, LAA anatomy can be clearly depicted, and LAA neck diameter, depth, volume, and number of lobes measured. In addition, bright-blood sequences or early and late gadolinium enhancement CMR allow detection of LAA thrombus, although there are only limited data. Some studies showed a very high diagnostic accuracy in evaluating LAA thrombus when compared to TEE [26].

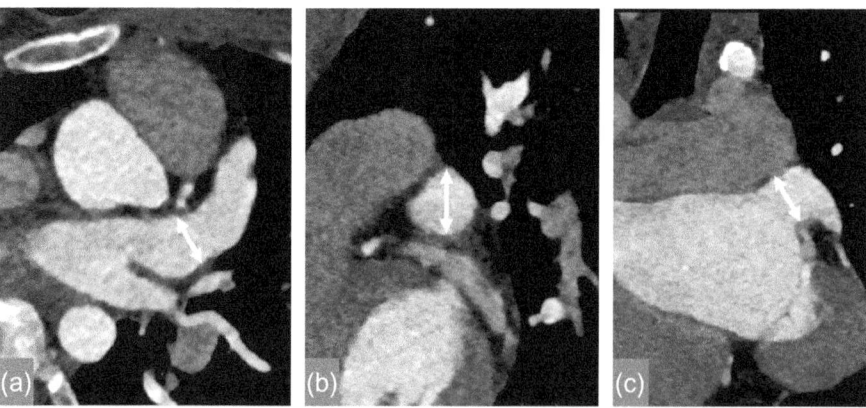

Figure 22.18 Using a basic approach the diameter of the LAA orifice can be derived from axial (a), sagittal (b), and coronal (c) image reconstructions.

Imaging guided interventions 757

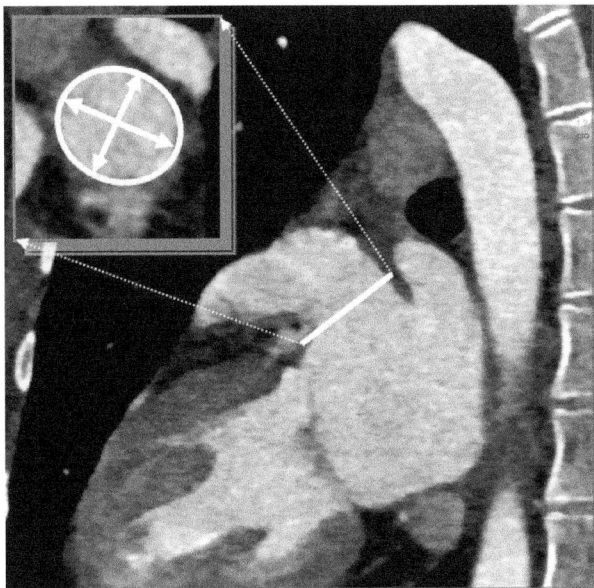

Figure 22.19 The most accurate measurements of the LAA annulus may be derived from a double-oblique plane of its orifice (left upper part of the image).

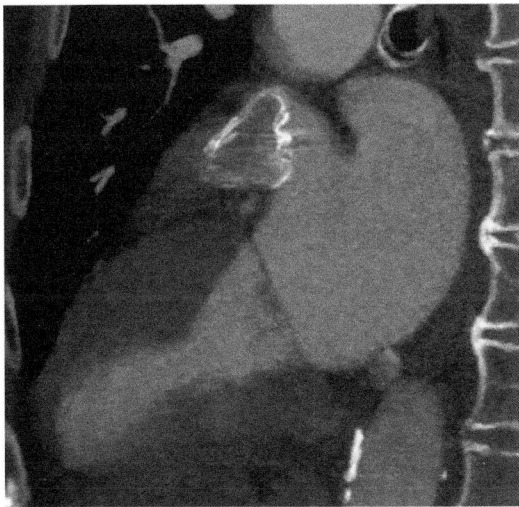

Figure 22.20 An exemplary cardiac CT examination after LAA occlusion using a watchman device. No residual blood flow was detected in the occluded LAA.

22.5 Interventional closure of ASD and PFO

Interventional closure of ASD has the potential to prevent right-sided heart failure due to volume overload. Furthermore, it has been proposed that interventional closure of patent foramen ovale in patients with cryptogenic stroke may prevent recurrent stroke. Randomized trials comparing PFO closure to medical therapy failed to achieve a statistically significant reduction in recurrent stroke. However, in a recent meta-analysis, pooling of the two randomized controlled trials comparing the Amplatzer PFO occluder to medical therapy reported a significant reduction of recurrent stroke in the device group [27]. Therefore, selected patients might benefit from interventional PFO closure.

In the following section, we describe the role of transthoracic and transesophageal echocardiography for screening and implantation of the most commonly used devices, the Amplatzer PFO occluder as well as the Amplatzer septal occluder (Figure 22.21). (The topic is also covered in Chapter 19 of this textbook.)

22.5.1 Echocardiography

22.5.1.1 Screening echocardiography

Transthoracic echocardiography usually cannot directly visualize ASD or PFO. However, the presence of atrial enlargement as well as unexplained right-sided heart failure can be suspicious for ASD.

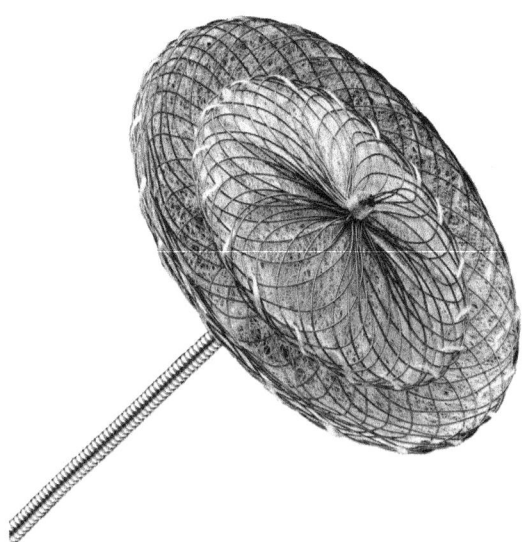

Figure 22.21 Amplatzer PFO occluder attached to delivery catheter. Courtesy of St. Jude Medical.

Transesophageal echocardiography is essential for the detection of ASD or PFO. The key role of this imaging technique is to determine the exact location of the defect. Classification of ASD's into different types according to their location and their underlying embryologic malformation is discussed in detail in Chapter 19. Furthermore, the existence and extent of left-to-right and particularly right-to-left shunt has to be determined. The use of contrast agent, that does not pass the pulmonary vasculature, can be used to detect right-to-left shunt. In case of ASD, the margins of the defect need to be large enough in order to enable an interventional closure of the defect. As a general rule, only ASD type II (ostium secundum defects) are amenable by percutaneous closure, as other types are in too close proximity to vital structures of the heart or have insufficient rim for safe anchoring.

22.5.1.2 Peri-interventional transesophageal echocardiography

In most centers, interventional closure of ASD and PFO is done with the use of TEE guidance. The advancement of the catheter system can be best visualized in a short-axis view (40–60°). Most interventionalists prefer the insertion of a sizing balloon for the assessment of the exact device size. The key role of peri-interventional transesophageal echocardiography is to determine the exact location as well as the size of the defect with and without the sizing balloon. Following the insertion of the double-disc system, both discs have to be closely spaced to the atrial septum. Next, the sealing of the defect needs to be tested with color Doppler using a low velocity scale. In case of unsatisfactory results, the device can be retrieved and placed again. Per instructions for users, Amplatzer ASD occluders should be oversized by 20% of the mean diameter to provide appropriate sealing; however, one may choose to deviate from these recommendations based on individual anatomical characteristics. For PFO, sizing depends on the length of the channel, the presence of a hypermobile atrial septum, and the thickness of the septum secundum. Figure 22.22 depicts an ASD type II with right-to-left shunt before closure using an Amplatzer septal occluder. Figure 22.23 three-dimensionally depicts this ASD type II before and after closure using an Amplatzer septal occluder.

22.6 Interventional closure of paravalvular leaks

Paravalvular leaks (PVL) after surgical valve replacement are cumbersome long-term complications. They can form after incomplete suturing or late dehiscence of prosthetic valves, most commonly in high-pressure (mitral and aortic valves) environments. Infectious endocarditis and paravalvular abscesses may be another source of PVL. PVL may result in variable degrees of paravalvular regurgitation. Additionally, mechanical shear stress from high velocity jets can induce intravascular hemolysis. Percutaneous closure of PVL is feasible using dedicated vascular plugs if the defect is well circumscribed and no active inflammation is present.

TTE and TEE play a crucial role for the detection and quantification of PVL. With mechanical valves, particular attention should be given to the exact site of the PVL jet

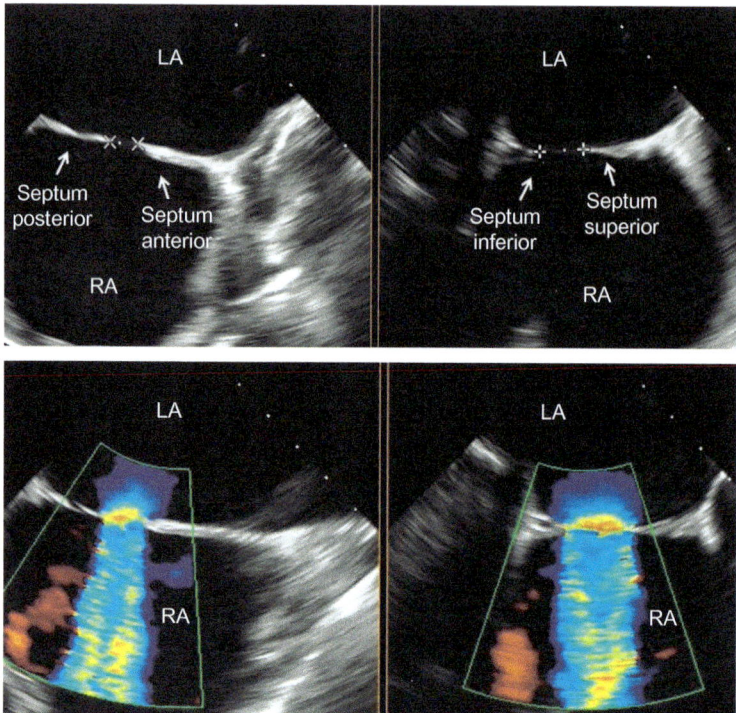

Figure 22.22 (a) TEE image of atrial septal defect type II (left 15°, right corresponding perpendicular 105° view). (b) TEE image of the atrial septal defect type II with right-to-left shunt (left 15°, right corresponding perpendicular 105°). LA, left atrium; RA, right atrium.

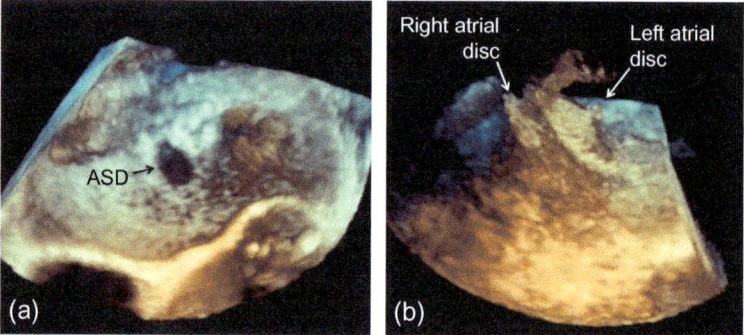

Figure 22.23 (a) Three-dimensional TEE image of atrial septal defect type II depicted from the left atrium (0°). (b) Three-dimensional TEE image of the closed atrial septal defect type II showing left and right atrial disc (65°).

in relation to the prosthesis, as closure devices may otherwise interact with adequate closure or opening of valve leaflets (this is the case in the presence of bi-leaflet or tilting disc prostheses). Thus, in PVL 3D transesophageal echocardiography is advisable to locate the exact position of the PVL within the circumference of the valve and to address

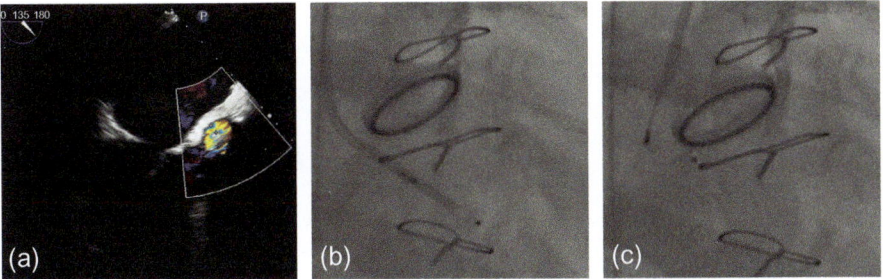

Figure 22.24 (a) Paravalvular leak depicted in the transesophageal LVOT view. (b) Fluoroscopic view after release of the distal part of an Amplatzer vascular plug through the guiding catheter in the left ventricle. (c) Fluoroscopic view after pullback and release of the device into the paravalvular leak.

the proximity to other structures (valve leaflets, neighboring structures, e.g., anterior mitral leaflet for a PVL of the aortic valve). CT may be an alternative to transesophageal echocardiography in patients with poor image quality, and may add information on the orientation of the heart, angulation of valves and other structures, and help to plan the procedure and determine the most appropriate access site (transapical vs. transfemoral vs. transjugular).

During the procedure, TEE guidance (including 3D TEE) is crucial for wiring of the PVL and to assess residual leaks after implantation of vascular plugs (Figure 22.24).

22.7 Pre-interventional imaging in coronary CTO

Coronary chronic total occlusions (CTO) are observed in up to 20% of patients with suspected coronary artery disease. In these patients, successful revascularization of the occluded vessel might result in a reduced cardiac mortality. However, revascularization of CTOs is challenging with success rates ranging between 55% and 80%. Additionally, complication rates are higher than for non-CTO PCI including coronary perforation, pericardial tamponade, stroke, bleeding, and myocardial infarction. Higher contrast agent administration and radiation doses are the source of contrast-induced nephropathy and radiation induced morbidity (radiodermatitis, late stochastic risks).

Consequently, the majority of large volume CTO centers require objective proof of ischemia prior to embarking in potentially difficult CTO procedures. Different imaging techniques for detecting myocardial ischemia are available and extensively discussed in Chapter 9. In patients with minor or no symptoms and low risk ischemic study, the potential benefit of CTO revascularization should be weighed carefully against the risks of the intervention.

Computed tomography provides detailed information about the occluded vessel segment, such as length of occlusion, course of the occluded vessel, side branches, calcifications, or morphology of the vessel stump. Figure 22.25 shows an exemplary

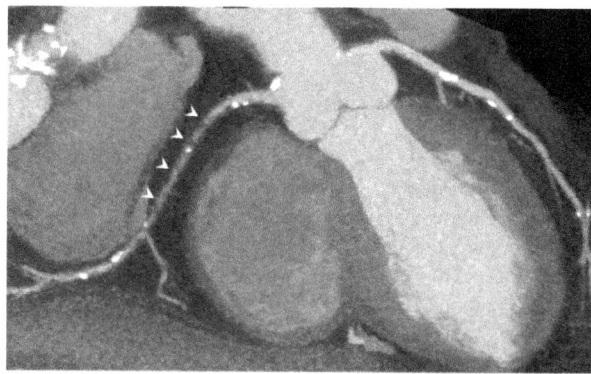

Figure 22.25 Exemplary case of coronary chronic total occlusions of the right coronary artery (white arrowheads).

CCTA of a patient with chronic occlusion of the right coronary artery. Several studies have shown the potential role of CCTA for improving success rates of CTO revascularization. For example, in a recent study in 30 patients and 43 controls [28], the success rate of revascularization was 90% in patients with prior CT angiography and only 63% in patients without.

References

[1] Husser O, Rauch S, Endemann DH, Resch M, Nunez J, Bodi V, et al. Impact of three-dimensional transesophageal echocardiography on prosthesis sizing for transcatheter aortic valve implantation. Catheter Cardiovasc Interv 2013;82(4):E542–51.
[2] Zhang R, Song Y, Zhou Y, Sun L. Comparison of aortic annulus diameter measurement between multi-detector computed tomography and echocardiography: a meta-analysis. PLoS One 2013;8(3), e58729.
[3] Husser O, Holzamer A, Resch M, Endemann DH, Nunez J, Bodi V, et al. Prosthesis sizing for transcatheter aortic valve implantation – comparison of three dimensional transesophageal echocardiography with multislice computed tomography. Int J Cardiol 2013;168(4):3431–8.
[4] Achenbach S, Delgado V, Hausleiter J, Schoenhagen P, Min JK, Leipsic JA. SCCT expert consensus document on computed tomography imaging before transcatheter aortic valve implantation (TAVI)/transcatheter aortic valve replacement (TAVR). J Cardiovasc Comput Tomogr 2013;6(6):366–80.
[5] Bischoff B, Meinel FG, Reiser M, Becker HC. Novel single-source high-pitch protocol for CT angiography of the aorta: comparison to high-pitch dual-source protocol in the context of TAVI planning. Int J Cardiovasc Imaging 2013;29(5):1159–65.
[6] Gurvitch R, Webb JG, Yuan R, Johnson M, Hague C, Willson AB, et al. Aortic annulus diameter determination by multidetector computed tomography. reproducibility, applicability, and implications for transcatheter aortic valve implantation. JACC Cardiovasc Interv 2011;4(11):1235–45.
[7] Bolen MA, Popovic ZB, Dahiya A, Kapadia SR, Tuczu EM, Flamm SD, et al. Prospective ECG-triggered, axial 4-D imaging of the aortic root, valvular, and left ventricular

structures: a lower radiation dose option for preprocedural TAVR imaging. J Cardiovasc Comput Tomogr 2012;6:393–8.
[8] Gurvitch R, Wood DA, Leipsic J, Tay E, Johnson M, Ye J, et al. Multislice computed tomography for prediction of optimal angiographic deployment projections during transcatheter aortic valve implantation. JACC Cardiovasc Interv 2010;3(11):1157–65.
[9] Arnold M, Achenbach S, Pfeiffer I, Ensminger S, Marwan M, Einhaus F, et al. A method to determine suitable fluoroscopic projections for transcatheter aortic valve implantation by computed tomography. J Cardiovasc Comput Tomogr 2012;6(6):422–8.
[10] Binder RK, Webb JG, Willson AB, Urena M, Hansson NC, Norgaard BL, et al. The impact of integration of a multidetector computed tomography annulus area sizing algorithm on outcomes of transcatheter aortic valve replacement: a prospective, multicenter, controlled trial. J Am Coll Cardiol 2013;62(5):431–8.
[11] Leber AW, Kasel M, Ischinger T, Ebersberger UH, Antoni D, Schmidt M, et al. Aortic valve calcium score as a predictor for outcome after TAVI using the CoreValve revalving system. Int J Cardiol 2013;166(3):652–7.
[12] Ribeiro HR, Le Ven F, Larose E, Dahou A, Nombela-Franco L, Urena M, et al. Cardiac magnetic resonance versus transthoracic echocardiography for the assessment and quantification of aortic regurgitation in patients undergoing transcatheter aortic valve implantation. Heart 2014;100(24):1924–32 [Epub ahead of print].
[13] Lancellotti P, Moura L, Pierard LA, Agricola E, Popescu BA, Tribouilloy C, et al. European Association of Echocardiography recommendations for the assessment of valvular regurgitation. Part 2: mitral and tricuspid regurgitation (native valve disease). Eur J Echocardiogr 2010;11(4):307–32.
[14] Boekstegers P, Hausleiter J, Baldus S, von Bardeleben RS, Beucher H, Butter C, et al. Percutaneous interventional mitral regurgitation treatment using the Mitra-Clip system. Clin Res Cardiol 2014;103(2):85–96.
[15] Braun D, Orban M, Michalk F, Barthel P, Hoppe K, Sonne C, et al. Three-dimensional transoesophageal echocardiography for the assessment of clip attachment to the leaflets in percutaneous edge-to-edge repair of the mitral valve. EuroIntervention 2013;8(12):1379–87.
[16] Braun D, Orban M, Tittus J, Nabauer M, Hagl C, Massberg S, et al. [Interventional Mitral valve repair with the MitraClip® procedure. Patient selection criteria]. Herz 2013;38(5):467–73.
[17] Feldman T, Kar S, Rinaldi M, Fail P, Hermiller J, Smalling R, et al. Percutaneous mitral repair with the MitraClip system: safety and midterm durability in the initial EVEREST (Endovascular Valve Edge-to-Edge REpair Study) cohort. J Am Coll Cardiol 2009;54(8):686–94.
[18] Wunderlich NC, Siegel RJ. Peri-interventional echo assessment for the MitraClip procedure. Eur Heart J Cardiovasc Imaging 2013;14(10):935–49.
[19] Corti R, Biaggi P, Gaemperli O, Bühler I, Felix C, Bettex D, et al. Integrated x-ray and echocardiography imaging for structural heart interventions. EuroIntervention 2013;9(7):863–9.
[20] Feldman T, Young A. Percutaneous approaches to valve repair for mitral regurgitation. J Am Coll Cardiol 2014;63(20):2057–68.
[21] Holmes DR, Reddy VY, Turi ZG, Doshi SK, Sievert H, Buchbinder M, et al. Percutaneous closure of the left atrial appendage versus warfarin therapy for prevention of stroke in patients with atrial fibrillation: a randomised non-inferiority trial. Lancet 2009;374(9689):534–42.

[22] Gottlieb I, Pinheiro A, Brinker JA, Corretti MC, Mayer SA, Bluemke DA, et al. Diagnostic accuracy of arterial phase 64-slice multidetector CT angiography for left atrial appendage thrombus in patients undergoing atrial fibrillation ablation. J Cardiovasc Electrophysiol 2008;19(3):247–51.

[23] Kim YY, Klein AL, Halliburton SS, Popovic ZB, Kuzmiak SA, Sola S, et al. Left atrial appendage filling defects identified by multidetector computed tomography in patients undergoing radiofrequency pulmonary vein antral isolation: a comparison with transesophageal echocardiography. Am Heart J 2007;154(6):1199–205.

[24] Di Biase L, Santangeli P, Anselmino M, Mohanty P, Salvetti I, Gili S, et al. Does the left atrial appendage morphology correlate with the risk of stroke in patients with atrial fibrillation? Results from a multicenter study. J Am Coll Cardiol 2012;60(6):531–8.

[25] Wang Y, Di Biase L, Horton RP, Nguyen T, Morhanty P, Natale A. Left atrial appendage studied by computed tomography to help planning for appendage closure device placement. J Cardiovasc Electrophysiol 2010;21(9):973–82.

[26] Rathi VK, Reddy ST, Anreddy S, Belden W, Yamrozik JA, Williams RB, et al. Contrast-enhanced CMR is equally effective as TEE in the evaluation of left atrial appendage thrombus in patients with atrial fibrillation undergoing pulmonary vein isolation procedure. Heart Rhythm 2013;10(7):1021–7.

[27] Capodanno D, Milazzo G, Vitale L, Di Stefano D, Di Salvo M, Grasso C, et al. Updating the evidence on patent foramen ovale closure versus medical therapy in patients with crytogenic stroke: a systematic review and comprehensive meta-analysis of 2303 patients from three randomized trials and 2231 from 11 observational studies. EuroIntervention 2014;9(11):1342–9.

[28] Rolf A, Werner GS, Schuhbäck A, Rixe J, Möllmann H, Nef HM, et al. Preprocedural coronary CT angiography significantly improves success rates of PCI for chronic total occlusion. Int J Cardiovasc Imaging 2013;29(8):1819–27.

Index

Note: Page numbers followed by *f* indicate figures and *t* indicate tables.

A

AA. *See* Aortic root/ascending aorta (AA)
AAS. *See* Acute aortic syndrome (AAS)
Acquired prosthetic valve stenosis
   Doppler-echocardiographic parameters, 544, 546*t*, 547*t*
   endocarditis/chronic process, 544
   quantitative parameters, 545–548, 549*t*, 550*f*, 550*t*
   stress echocardiography, 548
   valve structure and motion, 544, 545*f*, 548*f*
ACS. *See* Acute coronary syndrome (ACS)
Acute aortic syndrome (AAS)
   angiography, 673–674
   aortic dissection, 661–662
   clinical presentation, 662
   CTA, 671, 672*f*
   DeBakey classification, 662
   definition, 661–662
   IMH, 661–662, 663–665, 666*f*, 667*f*
   MRI, 671–673, 673*f*
   PAU, 661–662
   radiography, 665–670
   risk factors, 662–663, 663*t*
   Stanford classification, 662
   Stanford type-A aortic dissection, 663, 665*f*
   Stanford type-B aortic dissection, 663, 664*f*
   structured reporting, 674, 674*t*
   TOE and TTE, 670, 670*f*
Acute coronary syndrome (ACS), 179–180, 274
Acute myocardial infarction (AMI)
   AICD implantation, 279–280
   area at risk (AAR), 277–278, 277*f*
   CMR, 297–303, 299*f*, 302*f*, 303*f*
   DECT, 311–312
   echocardiography, 274, 275*t*, 278, 280–288, 281*f*, 282*f*, 283*f*, 284*f*, 286*f*
   end-systolic volume, 278–279, 279*f*
   LV ejection fraction, 278–280, 279*f*
   microvascular obstruction, 274–277, 277*f*
   multidetector CT, 303–312, 305*f*, 306*f*, 308*t*, 310*f*, 311*f*
   nuclear imaging, 288–297, 290*f*, 292*f*, 294*f*
   pathophysiology of, 271–272, 272*f*, 273*f*, 274*f*, 276*f*
   size quantification, 274
Acute pericarditis, 621–623, 622*f*, 623*f*
Acute pulmonary embolism, 686–687
   clinical presentation, 686–687
   CT, 688–689, 689*f*, 690*f*
   CUS, 688
   echocardiography, 690–691
   MRI, 689
   pulmonary angiography, 690
   radiography, 688
   ventilation-perfusion scintigraphy, 688
Agatston score
   asymptomatic patients, 173–176
   calcific coronary plaque, 173–175
   future adverse outcomes, risk of, 173, 174*f*
   incremental prognostic value, 173–175, 175*f*
   weighting factor, 173–175, 175*t*
AMI. *See* Acute myocardial infarction (AMI)
Amyloidosis, 423–424, 424*f*, 425*f*
Anatomic orifice area (AOA), 503–504, 506*f*
Anderson–Fabry disease, 421, 422–423
Aneurysmatic disease
   bicuspid aortic valve and aneurysmatic dilatation, 697, 698*f*
   clinical presentation, 695, 696*f*
   echocardiography, 699
   fusiform dilatation, 697, 698*f*
   invasive conventional catheter angiography, 702
   MRI, 699–701, 700*f*, 701*f*
   operative repair, 697
   radiography, 699
   structured reporting, 702, 702*t*

Aortic coarctation, 654, 654f
Aortic dissection (AD)
    risk factors, 662–663, 663t
    Stanford type-A aortic dissection, 663, 665f
    Stanford type-B aortic dissection, 663, 664f
Aortic regurgitation (AR)
    aortic valve/root morphology, 503, 504f
    severity of, 503–507, 504f, 505f, 506f, 507f
Aortic root/ascending aorta (AA)
    annular calcification, 491, 491f, 493f
    aortic valve leaflets, 491–493
    sinotubular junction, 493–494
    sizing, 490–491
    SOV, 493–494
    TAVR planning, 489–490, 490f
Aortic stenosis (AS)
    aortic valve/root morphology, 496, 496f, 497f
    severity of, 496–499, 498f, 499f, 500f
    synthesis, 500
Aortic valve leaflets, 491–493
Aortic valve-sparing (AVS), 490–491
Arrhythmia
    CMR, 708t, 720–724, 722f, 723f
    CT, 708t, 717–720, 718f, 719f
    EAM systems, 708t, 724–726, 725f, 726f
    image integration, 727–728, 728f
    intracardiac echocardiography (ICE), 708t, 715f, 717
    radionuclide imaging, 726–727
    routine fluoroscopy, 707, 708t, 710f
    3DRA, 708t, 710
    TOE, 708t, 715–716, 715f
    TTE, 711–714, 712f, 713f
Arrhythmogenic (right) ventricular cardiomyopathy (ARVC), 414–416
Arterial switch surgery, 650–653
Arterial systemic hypertension
    cardiovascular risk factor, 459
    clinical consequences, 459
    CMR, 463
    echocardiographic examination, 459
    E/e' ratio, 460–461
    ESC/ESH guidelines, 460–461, 462t
    GLS, 461–462, 462f
    LV diastolic properties, 459–460
    LV geometry, 459–460

LVM algorithms, 462–463, 463f
LV mass index, 459–460, 460f, 460t
LV systolic function, 459–460
myocardial ischemia, 463–464
PET, 464–465, 464f
symptoms, 459
AS. *See* Aortic stenosis (AS)
ASD. *See* Atrial septal defect (ASD)
Assessment by Coronary Computer Tomography Individuals UndeRgoing InvAsive Coronary AngiographY (ACCURACY), 179
Atherosclerotic plaque
    CCTA, 208–211
    CT, 206–217
    MRI, 212–214
    PET, 214–216
    SPECT, 216–217
    ultrasound, 204–206
Atrial septal defect (ASD)
    Amplatzer PFO occluder, 758, 758f
    CHD, 641–643, 642f, 643f
    TEE, 759, 760f
    TTE, 758
Atrial switch surgery, 650, 651f, 652f
Autoimmune connective tissue disorders, 472–474, 473f
Automated implantable cardioverter defibrillator (AICD), 279–280, 641

B

Balanced steady-state free precession (b-SSFP) sequence, 384
Benign tumours
    fibroelastoma, 586f, 586t, 589t, 601–602, 601f
    fibroma, 586f, 589t, 602–603, 603f
    haemangioma, 586f, 589t, 604, 605f
    lipomas, 586t, 599–601, 600f
    myxomas, 586f, 586t, 597–599, 598f
    rhabdomyoma, 586f, 589t, 603–604
Blood-oxygen-level-dependent (BOLD), 140–141, 140f

C

CABGs. *See* Coronary artery bypass grafts (CABGs)
CAC. *See* Coronary artery calcification (CAC)

Index

CACS. *See* Coronary artery calcium scoring (CACS)
Cadmium-zinc-telluride (CZT) detector
  collimator, 52
  count rate performance, 52
  efficiency, 52–54
  energy discrimination, 52
  function of, 51
  higher resolution of, 52, 54*f*
  miniaturization, 52, 53*f*
  pixels, 51, 51*f*
  shortened acquisition time, 52, 53*f*
  spatial resolution of, 51
Cancer therapeutics-related cardiac dysfunction (CTRCD), 409–411
Cardiac catheterization, CHD, 640, 643
Cardiac computed tomography (CCT)
  CT (*see* Computed tomography (CT))
  sarcoma, 608
Cardiac imaging
  CMR (*see* Cardiovascular magnetic resonance (CMR))
  contrast resolution, 2
  coronary CT angiography (*see* Coronary computed tomography angiography (CCTA))
  CT (*see* Computed tomography (CT))
  echocardiography (*see* Echocardiography)
  evidence-based imaging, 10
  multidisciplinary collaboration, 11
  multimodality imaging, 8–10, 9*f*
  noise level, 2
  nuclear imaging (*see* Nuclear imaging)
  principle purpose of, 1
  temporal and spatial resolution, 2
  trade-offs in, 3*f*
Cardiac implantable electrical devices (CIED), 711–712, 713–714, 716
Cardiac iron overload, 427–428
Cardiac magnetic resonance spectroscopy (CMRS), 227, 244
Cardiac resynchronization therapy (CRT), 351–352, 367–368, 392, 712–713
Cardiac sarcoidosis (CS), 477–478
Cardiac tumours
  cardiac masses (*see* Benign tumours; Malignant primary cardiac tumours; Pseudotumours)
  CCT, 591

  CMR, 588, 589*t*, 590*f*
  echocardiography, 585–587, 587*f*
  nuclear imaging techniques, 591–593, 592*f*
  primary cardiac tumours, 585, 586*f*, 586*t*
  secondary cardiac tumours, 585
Cardio-cerebro-vascular diseases, 469
Cardiomyopathy
  ARVC, 414–416, 415*f*
  cardiac iron overload, 427–428
  classification of, 399
  CMR (*see* Cardiovascular magnetic resonance (CMR))
  CT, 404–405
  definition, 399
  dilated (*see* Dilated cardiomyopathy)
  echocardiography, 401–402
  hypertrophic phenocopies, 421
  infiltrative disease/restrictive (*see* Infiltrative disease/restrictive cardiomyopathy)
  limitations of imaging, 428
  LVNC, 411–413, 412*f*
  non-ischaemic cardiomyopathy, 399
  nuclear imaging, 405–406
  pericardial constriction, 428
  phenotypic description, 399
  stress, 413, 414*f*
  sudden cardiac death, 429
Cardiovascular magnetic resonance (CMR)
  acute and chronic MI, 340–341, 342*f*
  acute pericarditis, 621–623
  advantages, 7, 190–191
  AMI, 297–303, 299*f*, 302*f*, 303*f*
  aortic regurgitation, 505–507
  aortic stenosis, 496, 496*f*, 497*f*
  arrhythmia, 708*t*, 720–724, 722*f*, 723*f*
  arterial systemic hypertension, 463
  ARVC, 414–416
  atrial switch surgery, 650
  blood flow in 3D, 7–8, 7*f*
  cardiac iron overload, 427–428
  cardiac tumours, 588, 589*t*, 590*f*
  clinical applications of, 7
  CoA, 654
  congenital absence, pericardium, 632
  constrictive pericarditis, 626, 627*t*
  contractile function, 367, 383–387
  data collection methods, 135
  DCM, 407–408, 409–411

Cardiovascular magnetic resonance (CMR)
   (Continued)
   delayed enhancement, 341–345, 344*f*
   diagnostic accuracy, 192
   EPI, 137
   gradient stimulation, 136
   hematomas, 630–632
   higher gradient performance, 137
   hyperpolarization, 7–8
   hypertrophic cardiomyopathy, 416–421, 418*f*
   image space *vs.* k-space, 135
   infiltrative disease/restrictive cardiomyopathy, 422–423, 425–427
   ischaemic and non-ischaemic cardiomyopathies, 402
   ischemia assessment, 140–141, 140*f*
   LAA, 756
   "late" phase, 339, 339*f*
   LGE, 428
   LV hypertrophy/wall thickness, causes of, 402–404
   methods, 191–192
   mitral regurgitation, 518–520, 519*f*, 520*f*, 521*f*, 750–751
   multiparametric imaging, 192
   myocardial tissue characterization, 7–8, 8*f*
   myocarditis, 441–442, 447–452
   myocyte death and progressive fibrosis, 339
   navigated methods, 138
   non-compaction cardiomyopathy, 411–412
   parallel imaging techniques, 137–138
   pericardial disease, 428, 629–630
   prognosis, 192
   pulmonary valve disease, 537–539, 538*f*, 539*f*, 539*t*
   real time *vs.* segmentation, 136–137
   resolution and tissue characterisation capability, 340
   safety, 10–11
   SAR, 136
   sarcoidosis, 477–478
   segmental recovery, 340–341, 341*f*
   SNR, 136
   sources, 156–157
   spiral imaging methods, 137
   strengths and weaknesses, 135
   stress cardiomyopathy, 413, 414*f*
   tamponade, 624–626, 625*t*
   TAVI, 743–744
   technical developments, 155–156
   thrombus, 595, 595*t*, 596
   3T imaging, 193
   time acceleration approaches, 138
   TOF, 648
   tricuspid valve, 531–533, 531*f*, 532*f*
   typical image acquisition times, 135
   viability and perfusion chart, 340–341, 343*f*
   viability assessment, 138, 139*f*
Carney complex, 599
Carotid artery ultrasound, 204–206, 205*f*
Carotid intima-media thickness (CIMT)
   cardiovascular risk, 205, 205*f*
   clinical trials, 205, 205*f*
CartoMerge™ system, 727–728, 728*f*
CartoSound® system, 725, 728
CCTA. *See* Coronary computed tomography angiography (CCTA)
CFR. *See* Coronary flow reserve (CFR)
CHD. *See* Congenital heart disease (CHD)
Chest X-ray, CHD, 639
Chronic pericarditis, 623, 624*f*
Chronic total occlusions (CTOs), 761–762, 762*f*
Churg–Strauss syndrome, 477
CIMT. *See* Carotid intima-media thickness (CIMT)
Cine-CMR images, 403
^{11}C-labeled meta-hydroxyephedrine (^{11}C-MHED), 727
CMR imaging. *See* Cardiovascular magnetic resonance (CMR)
Coarctation of the aorta (CoA), 654, 654*f*
Collimators, 48–49, 49*f*
Color-coded tissue Doppler, 382
Color Doppler imaging (CDI), 382
Compression ultrasonography (CUS), 688
Computed tomography (CT)
   acute pericarditis, 621–623, 623*f*
   acute pulmonary embolism, 688–689, 689*f*, 690*f*
   ALARA principle, 106
   aortic regurgitation, 503, 504*f*
   aortic root calcification, 491, 491*f*, 493*f*
   aortic stenosis, 497*f*
   arrhythmia, 717–720, 718*f*, 719*f*
   arterial switch surgery, 653
   ASD and VSD, 645

atherosclerotic plaque, 206–217
attenuation profiles, 99, 99f, 104
CAD, fractional flow reserve, 122–123, 122f
calcium scan, 113, 113f
cardiac tumours, 591
cardiomyopathy, 404–405
CAT scanners, 97
CCTA (see Coronary computed tomography angiography (CCTA))
CoA, 654, 654f
congenital absence, pericardium, 632
constrictive pericarditis, 626, 626f, 627t
contractile function analysis, 114–115
contrast resolution vs. image noise, 107t, 110–111, 111f
coronary arteries, imaging of, 5, 97, 98f
coronary contrast opacification patterns, 120–122
CT number, 104
delayed-enhancement imaging, 115–116, 115f
detector collimation, 99
dual-source CT systems, 100, 106
EBCT technology, 97
ECG-gated spiral mode, 100–102, 100f, 102t
ECG-triggered axial scan mode, 100–101, 100f, 102t, 103
ECG-triggered high-pitch mode, 103
ECG-triggered stationary mode, 103
FBP reconstruction, 104, 105f
Fontan connections, 653
fractional flow reserve, 5–6, 6f
hematoma, 630–632
introduction of, 5
iterative reconstruction, 104–105, 105f
LAA, 754–756, 755f, 756f, 757f
minimally invasive procedures, 5
mitral regurgitation, 750, 751f
multienergy imaging, 106
myocardial perfusion, 5–6, 6f, 106
myocarditis, 452
noncompaction cardiomyopathy, 8–10, 9f
in pediatric patients, 5, 6f
pericardial cysts/diverticula, 629–630
pericardial effusion, 621–623, 622f
prosthetic valves, 558t, 559–560, 559f, 560f, 561f
pulmonary valve disease, 539
qualitative postprocessing tools, 116–117, 116f

radiation and dose reduction, 10–11, 117–119, 118t
rontgen generation, 97–98
safety precautions, 10–11
selective kernels, 105, 105f
SOV, 494
spatial resolution, 5, 107t, 109–110
SPECT, attenuation correction of, 58–59, 59f, 60f
spiral CT, 97
tamponade, 624–626, 625t
TAVI, 735–736, 740–743, 742f, 743f
temporal resolution and heart rhythm, 106–109, 107t, 108f, 109f
Computed tomography coronary angiography (CTCA), 234, 243f, 244–246, 245f
Computerized axial tomography (CAT), 97
Congenital absence, pericardium, 632, 633f
Congenital heart disease (CHD)
  ASD, 641–643, 642f, 643f
  cardiac catheterization, 640
  chest X-ray, 639
  CMR, 637–638, 640–641
  CT, 639, 640–641
  diagnosis and treatment, 635–636
  echocardiography, 636–637
  radionuclide imaging, 639–640
  TGA (see Transposition of the great arteries (TGA))
  TOF, 645–649, 647f, 648f, 649f
  VSD, 643–645, 644f, 645f
Congenitally corrected transposition of the great artery (ccTGA), 653
Constrictive pericarditis
  chronic, 626, 626f, 627t
  effusive, 629, 629f
Contractile function
  CMR, 383–387
  quantitative assessment, 374f, 384–385
  regional, 377f, 386–387
Contrast agents, 23–24, 25t
Contrast echocardiography
  bolus injections, 24
  continuous infusion, 24
  EACVI recommendations, 30–31, 31f
  limitations, 31–32
  LV opacification and endocardial delineation, 27–28, 28f

Contrast echocardiography *(Continued)*
  mechanical index *(see* Mechanical index (MI))
  microbubbles, 24
  molecular imaging, 42–43
  myocardial perfusion, 28–29, 30*f*, 41–42, 42*f*
  safety of, 26
  stress echocardiography, 29–30
  tissue characterization, 28, 29*f*
  ultrasound contrast agents, 23–24, 25*t*
Coronary artery aneurism (CAA), 476
Coronary artery bypass grafts (CABGs)
  anastomotic site, assessment of, 182, 186*f*
  diagnostic accuracy, 182–183
  distal run off, assessment of, 182, 186*f*
  prognosis, 183
Coronary artery calcification (CAC)
  Agatston score *(see* Agatston score)
  atherosclerosis, 173
  coronary artery stenosis, 173, 174*f*
  lumen evaluability, 175–176, 177*f*, 178*f*
  obstructive CAD and MACEs, 173
  zero calcium score, obstructive CAD, 175–176
Coronary artery calcium scoring (CACS)
  cardiovascular risk, 206–207
  clinical trials, 207–208
Coronary artery disease (CAD), 718
  coronary contrast opacification patterns, 120–122
  CTCA, 176
  CT-FFR approach, 122–123, 122*f*
  diabetic patients, 467–468, 469
  high CAC scores, 173
  ICA, 173
  MPI *(see* Myocardial perfusion imaging (MPI))
Coronary artery protective score (CAPS), 183
Coronary computed tomography angiography (CCTA), 2*f*
  after bypass graft surgery, 111, 112*f*
  atherosclerotic plaque, 208–211
  cardiovascular risk, 208–209, 209*f*
  clinical trials, 211
  contrast injection protocol, 111–113
  CTO, 761–762
  ECG-triggered axial scan mode, 111
  emerging tissue and biological characterization techniques, 209–211, 210*f*
  myocardial perfusion, 120, 121*f*
  obstructive CAD, 111
  PET imaging, 71, 87–89, 88*f*, 89*f*
  radiation and dose reduction, 5–6, 119, 119*f*
  RCA and LAD, two-vessel disease of, 5–6, 6*f*
  secondary reconstruction, 113
  and SPECT imaging, 64–67, 66*f*, 67*f*
  TAVI, 750
  thin slices, reconstruction of, 113
Coronary flow reserve (CFR), 30, 64, 234, 235*f*, 236*f*, 466
Coronary magnetic resonance (CMR). *See* Cardiovascular magnetic resonance (CMR)
Coronary vascular resistance
  atheromatosis, 228, 230*f*
  capillary bed, 228, 229*f*
  epicardial branches, 228, 229*f*
  mechanisms of, 228, 229*f*
  microvascular resistance, 228, 231*f*
  microvasculature, 228, 229*f*
  vasorelaxation, 228, 231*f*
Corrected coronary opacification (CCO), 183–184
CT. *See* Computed tomography (CT)
CT coronary angiography (CTCA)
  accuracy, 176–179, 179*t*, 184*f*
  CABG patients *(see* Coronary artery bypass grafts (CABGs))
  clinical use of, 190
  cost/resource utilization, 188
  CT perfusion, 187–188
  emergency department, 189
  fractional flow reserve, 176, 178*f*, 184–187, 187*t*
  iodine contrast medium, 189–190
  obstructive CAD, 176
  PCI patients, 181–182, 185*f*
  plaque characterization, 179–181, 185*f*
  prognostic value of, 181
  TAG and CCO, 183–184
CT dose index (CTDI), 117
CT perfusion (CTP), 187–188
CZT detectors. *See* Cadmium-zinc-telluride (CZT) detector

Index

D

DCM. *See* Dilated cardiomyopathy (DCM)
DeBakey classification, 662
Definity, 24, 25*t*, 26
Degenerative disease, 510
Diabetic cardiomyopathy
  coronary microvascular dysfunction, 466, 467*f*
  diabetes and LV diastolic dysfunction, 465–466
  2 diabetes mellitus (DM2), 465
  diastolic dysfunction, 466–467, 468*f*
  glucose intolerance (GI), 465
  inotropic reserve, diabetic patients, 467–469, 469*f*
Diffusion tensor imaging (DTI), 156, 409–411
Dilated cardiomyopathy (DCM)
  chemotherapy-related cardiomyopathy, 409–411
  CTCA, 409
  diagnosis, 406–408, 407*f*
  prognostic imaging markers, 408–409
Diverticula, 629–630
Dobutamine-stress echocardiography (DSE), 285, 288, 476
Doppler-derived strain rate, 467–468
Doppler-echocardiographic
  acquired prosthetic valve stenosis, 544–548, 545*f*, 546*t*, 547*t*
  prosthetic valve regurgitation, 551, 554*t*, 555*t*
Doppler tissue imaging (DTI), 382
Dose-length product (DLP), 117
Dual-energy CT (DECT), 311–312
Dynamic nuclear polarization (DNP). *See* Hyperpolarization
Dyslipidemia, 470

E

Ebstein anomaly, 531, 531*f*
ECG-gated myocardial perfusion SPECT, 390
Echocardiography
  acquired prosthetic valve stenosis (*see* Acquired prosthetic valve stenosis)
  acute pericarditis, 621–623
  acute pulmonary embolism, 690–691
  AMI, 274, 275*t*, 278, 280–288, 281*f*, 282*f*, 283*f*, 284*f*, 286*f*

aneurysmatic disease, 699
aortic stenosis, 497*f*
arterial switch patient, 650–652
ARVC, 414–416
ASD, 636, 644–645
AV leaflets, 492
benefits, 3
cardiac catheterization, 640
cardiac tumours, 585–587, 587*f*
ccTGA, 653
clinical indices, 43–44
CoA, 654
color Doppler flow imaging, 15
congenital absence, pericardium, 632
constrictive pericarditis, 626, 627*t*
contrast echocardiography (*see* Contrast echocardiography)
cysts and diverticula, 629–630
dilated cardiomyopathy, 406, 408, 409–411
Doppler flow imaging, 15
endocarditis, 574–577, 575*f*, 576*f*, 577*f*
Fontan pathways, 653
fusion imaging, 41
heart failure, 369–374, 371*t*, 374*f*, 377*f*, 378–383, 379*f*, 380*f*, 381*f*
hypertrophic cardiomyopathy, 416–421, 418*f*
ICE, 41
image quality, 39
infiltrative disease/restrictive cardiomyopathy, 422–423, 425
LV opacification, 401
mitral valve movement, assessment of, 3
M-mode recordings, 15
myocarditis, 443–447
non-compaction cardiomyopathy, 411–413
prosthesis-patient mismatch, 543–544
prosthetic valve regurgitation, 550–551, 552*f*, 553*f*, 554*t*, 555*t*
safety, 10–11
SOV, 494
STE strain (*see* Speckle tracking echocardiography (STE))
stress cardiomyopathy, 413
tamponade, 624–626, 625*t*
TDI (*see* Tissue Doppler imaging (TDI))
TGA atrial switch patients, 650
3DE (*see* Three-dimensional (3D) echocardiography)
tissue characterization, 44

Echocardiography *(Continued)*
  TOF, 636–637
  2D imaging, 3, 15
  VSD, 636, 644–645
Echo planar imaging (EPI), 137
Edge-to-edge repair, 571–572, 572*f*
Effective orifice area (EOA), 542
Effective regurgitant orifice area (EROA), 503–504
Effusive constrictive pericarditis, 629, 629*f*
Ehlers–Danlos syndrome, 662–663
Elastography, 44
Electroanatomic mapping (EAM) systems, 724–726, 725*f*, 726*f*, 727, 728*f*
Electron-beam computed tomography (EBCT), 97
Emergency department (ED), 189, 281–284
Endocardial surface area (ESA), 298
Endocarditis
  echocardiography, 574–577, 575*f*, 576*f*, 577*f*
  molecular imaging, 577–579, 578*f*, 579*f*
  MRI, 580
  multislice computed tomography, 579–580, 579*f*
Endomyocardial biopsy (EMB), 441–442
EnSite™ NavX™ system, 724–725, 725*f*
Eosinophilic granulomatosis with polyangiitis (EGPA), 477
Equilibrium contrast cardio-vascular magnetic resonance (EQ-CMR), 143
European Association of Cardiovascular Imaging (EACVI), 27, 30–31, 31*f*
European Society of Cardiology (ESC), 399, 575, 640
Evidence-based imaging, 10
Expectation-maximization (EM), 57–58

F

^{18}F-fluorodexyglucose (^{18}F-FDG), 593
FFR. *See* Fractional flow reserve (FFR)
Fibroelastoma, 586*f*, 586*t*, 589*t*, 601–602, 601*f*
Fibroma, 586*f*, 589*t*, 602–603, 603*f*
Fibroscan system, 44
Filtered back projection (FBP), 56–57, 56*f*, 57*f*, 104, 105*f*
^{18}Fluorine-2-deoxy-D-glucose (FDG), 214–215

Fluoroscopy, 707, 708*t*, 710*f*
Fontan circulation, 653
Fontan procedure, 374–375
Force–frequency relation, 468
Fractional flow reserve (FFR), 5–6, 6*f*, 122–123, 122*f*, 176, 178*f*, 184–187, 187*t*, 230*f*, 234, 236
Framingham Heart Study, 718
Framingham risk score (FRS), 180–181
Frank–Starling law, 376
Frank–Starling mechanism, 376–377
Fulminant myocarditis, 443

G

Gadolinium-based contrast agents, 404
Gated blood pool SPECT, 389–390
Giant cell myocarditis, 443
Global longitudinal strain (GLS), 409–411, 461–462, 462*f*

H

Haemangioma, 586*f*, 589*t*, 604, 605*f*
Half-Fourier acquisition single-shot turbo spin-echo (HASTE), 131, 132*f*
HCM. *See* Hypertrophic cardiomyopathy (HCM)
Heart failure (HF)
  CMR, 367
  coronary artery disease, 367
  CRT, 367–368
  echocardiographic approach, 369–374, 371*t*, 374*f*, 377*f*, 378–383, 379*f*, 380*f*, 381*f*
  ejection fraction, 367
  intra-cardiac defibrillator (ICD), 367
  and ischaemic heart disease (*see* Ischaemic heart disease)
  muscle fibers, 368
  radionuclide techniques (*see* Radionuclide techniques, heart failure)
  RV function, 374–383
  and valvular disease, 352
Heart to mediastinum ratio (HMR), 293
Hematoma, 630–632, 631*f*
Hemorrhage, 621–623
High-field (3T) MR systems, 155–156
Hypereosinophilia, 477
Hyperpolarization

brute force polarization, 151
clinical perspectives, 154–155
hyperpolarized [1-^{13}C]pyruvate, 153, 153f
hyperpolarized [2-^{13}C]pyruvate, 153, 154f
methodology, 152
myocardial infarction and dilated cardiomyopathy, 154, 155f
optical pumping of noble gasses, 151
PHIP, 151
theory, 151–152, 152f
Hyperthyroidism, 475
Hypertrophic cardiomyopathy (HCM), 464–465
diagnosis, 416–421, 418f
echocardiography, 401–402
risk stratification, 421

I

Image acquisition
LAA, 754–755
TAVI, 740–741
Image evaluation
LAA, 755–756, 755f, 756f
TAVI, 741–743, 742f, 743f
^{123}I-meta-iodo-benzylguanidine (^{123}I-mIBG), 55, 293–294, 294f, 708t, 726–727
^{131}I-meta-iodo-benzylguanidine (^{131}I-mIBG), 409, 413
Implantable cardioverter-defibrillator (ICD), 707
Infarct imaging
acute and chronic MI, 340–341, 342f
delayed enhancement CMR, 341–345, 344f
"late" phase, 339, 339f
LGE, 339–340
myocyte death and progressive fibrosis, 339
PET–CT imaging, 338
resolution and tissue characterisation capability, 340
segmental recovery, 340–341, 341f
SPECT MPS, 338
viability and perfusion chart, 340–341, 343f
Infective endocarditis (IE). *See* Endocarditis
Infiltrative disease/restrictive cardiomyopathy
amyloidosis, 423–424, 424f, 425f
sarcoidosis, 425–427, 426f
^{111}In-labeled murine monoclonal antimyosin Fab antibody fragments (R11D10-Fab), 292, 292f, 293
Integrated backscatter signals (IBS), 44
Inter-commissural distance (ICD), 492–493
Intracardial echocardiography (ICE), 41
Intramural hematoma (IMH), 663–665, 666f, 667f
Intravascular ultrasound (IVUS), 179–180, 234
Invasive coronary angiography (ICA), 173
Ischaemic heart disease
cardiac resynchronisation therapy, 351–352
^{18}FDG PET ischaemia/viability assessment, 348t, 349–350
implantable cardiac defibrillator, 351
mortality, 347–349, 348t
STICH study, 348t, 349–350
viability alter medical management, 350–351
Ischemic cascade, 274, 276f, 288, 298
Isovolumic acceleration time (IVA), 382
Iterative reconstruction (IR), 104–105, 105f

K

Kawasaki disease (KD), 475–477

L

Laplace law, 376–377
Late gadolinium enhancement (LGE)-CMR, 138, 139f
Left atrial appendage (LAA), 716, 717, 718–719, 719f, 721
Amplatzer cardiac plug, 752, 752f
atrial thrombi, 751–752
CMR, 756
computed tomography, 754–756, 755f, 756f, 757f
TEE, 752–754, 753f
Watchman device, 752
Left ventricular non-compaction (LVNC), 411–413, 412f
Left ventricular outflow tract (LVOT) obstruction, 417–418
Lipomas, 586t, 599–601, 600f

Look-Locker sequence, 423
Luminity (definity), 24, 25t, 26
Lung perfusion scintigraphy, 640

M

Magnetic resonance imaging (MRI)
  AAS, 671–673, 673f
  acute pulmonary embolism, 689
  aneurysmatic disease, 699–701, 700f, 701f
  atherosclerotic plaque, 212–214
  cardiac strain assessment, 35
  cardiovascular risk, 212–213, 213f
  clinical trials, 213–214
  endocarditis, 580
  KD, 477
  PET imaging, 71, 89, 90, 90f
  prosthetic valves, 562, 563f
Magnetic resonance spectroscopy (MRS)
  diabetes, 150–151
  heart failure, 150
  hyperpolarized ^{13}C MRS, 151
  ischemic heart disease, 150
  limitation, 148
  obesity, 150–151
  7T, 151
  typical ^{31}P spectrum, 148–150, 149f
Major adverse cardiovascular events (MACE), 173, 206–207
Malignant primary cardiac tumours
  cardiac lymphomas, 586f, 589t, 608–609, 609f
  metastatic carcinoid, 589t, 609–610, 611f, 612f
  sarcoma, 589t, 605–608, 606f
Marfan syndrome, 662–663, 695
Maximum intensity projections (MIPs), 116–117
MDCT. See Multidetector computed tomography (MDCT)
Mechanical dispersion, 43–44
Mechanical index (MI)
  EACVI recommendations, 27
  intermittent high MI imaging, 26
  low MI real-time imaging, 27
MediGuide™ system, 725
Metabolic assessment
  BMIPP fatty acid metabolism, 345–347
  ^{18}F FDG imaging, 345
  perfusion and metabolism, 345, 346f
  recovery of segmental contractile function, 328t, 345

Metabolic syndrome, 469–472, 471f
MI. See Myocardial ischemia (MI)
Microvascular obstruction, 274–277, 277f, 284–285, 300
Mitral annular plane systolic excursion (MAPSE), 446–447
Mitral regurgitation (MR), 514t
  aetiology and mechanisms, 510–511, 511f
  CMR, 518–520, 519f, 520f, 521f, 750–751
  computed tomography, 750, 751f
  MitraClip® procedures, 744, 744f
  MSCT, 521–522, 522f
  severity of, 513–516, 515t, 516f, 517f
  TEE, 745–750, 746f, 747f, 748f, 749f
  3DE evaluation, 511–518, 512f, 517f
  2DE evaluation, 511–518, 513f
Mitral stenosis, 19, 20f
Modified Look-Locker Inversion Recovery (MOLLI) method, 141, 420
MPI. See Myocardial perfusion imaging (MPI)
MR angiography (MRA), 156
MRI. See Magnetic resonance imaging (MRI)
MRS. See Magnetic resonance spectroscopy (MRS)
Multi-beat 3D echocardiographic imaging, 17, 18f
Multidetector computed tomography (MDCT)
  AMI, 303–312, 305f, 306f, 308t, 310f, 311f
  cardiomyopathy, 404–405
  prosthetic valves, 558t, 559–560, 559f, 560f, 561f
  pulmonary valve disease, 539
  TAVI, 735–736, 740–743, 742f, 743f
  tricuspid valve, 533
Multiethnic Study of Atherosclerosis (MESA), 206–207
Multigated acquisition (MUGA), 387, 639
Multimodality imaging (MI)
  biphasic response, 333–334, 334f
  dobutamine stress techniques, 335
  functional improvement, 334–335
  infarct (see Infarct imaging)
  LDDSE, 335–336
  metabolic assessment, 328t, 345–347, 346f
  MIBI and tetrofosmin, 336–338, 337f
  morphology, 332–333, 333f
  MPS, 336, 337f
  myocardial responses, 333–334, 335f
Multiplanar reformations (MPR), 116–117

Index 775

Multislice cardiac computed tomography (MSCT)
  endocarditis, 579–580, 579f
  mitral regurgitation, 521–522, 522f
Myocardial AAR, 298–300
Myocardial blood flow (MBF), 331f
Myocardial contrast enhancement (MCE), 284–285, 286–288, 287f
Myocardial deformation imaging (MDI), 280–281
Myocardial fibrosis, 418–419, 418f
Myocardial infarction (MI), 711–712. See also Acute myocardial infarction (AMI)
Myocardial ischemia (MI)
  atheromatosis, 228, 230f
  CAD, 231f, 234
  capillary bed, 228, 229f
  CFR, 234, 235f, 236–238, 236f, 237f
  CTCA, 176–177, 184f
  diagnostic platform, 257f, 259f, 261
  epicardial branches, 228, 229f
  FFR, 230f, 234, 236–238, 237f
  heart team, 238–239
  IHD, 229f, 232, 233f
  ischemic cascade, 232, 233f
  mechanisms of, 228, 229f
  microvascular resistance, 228, 231f
  microvasculature, 228, 229f
  noninvasive imaging modalities (see Noninvasive detection and quantification)
  oxygen demand, 227, 228f
  oxygen supply, 227, 228f
  patient follow-up, 264
  risk stratification and prognosis, 242f, 261–263, 262f, 263t
  vasorelaxation, 228, 231f
  vasospasm, 232
Myocardial Jeopardy Index, 298
Myocardial necrosis, 274, 300
Myocardial Performance Index (MPI/Tei index), 381–382
Myocardial perfusion imaging (MPI)
  AMI, 290f, 291, 295
  cardiac CT exam, 5–6, 6f, 106
  CCTA, 120
  combined SPECT-CT imaging, 4, 5f, 187, 187t
  contrast echocardiography, 28–29, 30f, 41–42, 42f
  dynamic MPI, 120, 121f
  nuclear imaging, 290–291, 290f
  PET imaging, 78–85, 78t, 86–87
  SPECT imaging, 49, 49f
  static perfusion technique, 120
Myocardial perfusion reserve (MPR), 330–331, 331f
Myocardial perfusion scintigraphy (MPS), 336, 337f
Myocardial salvage, 277–278, 277f, 293, 298–301
Myocardial T1-mapping methods
  ECV estimation, 143, 144f
  EQ-CMR, 143
  native T1 mapping, 141–142, 142f
  postcontrast T1 mapping, 143
Myocardial velocity, TDI, 32, 32t
  color Doppler mode, 32–33, 33f
  limitations, 34–35
  pulsed Doppler mode, 33, 34f
Myocardial viability
  assessment, 347–352
  cell death, 329
  clinical setting, 331
  Echo-based techniques, 353
  hibernation, 330–331, 330f, 331f
  hybrid imaging, 353–354, 354f
  ischaemic heart disease and heart failure, 327–329
  MI (see Multimodality imaging (MI))
  speckle tracking, 353
  strengths and weaknesses, 327, 328t
  stunning, 329–330
  viable myocardium, 329
Myocarditis
  aetiology, 439
  clinical presentation, 439
  CMR, 441–442, 447–452
  computed tomography, 452
  coronary angiography, 447
  echocardiography, 443–447
  EMB, 441–442
  follow-up and evolution imaging, 440f, 454
  "natural course" of disease, 439–441
  nuclear imaging, 447
  therapeutic options, 443
Myxoma, 586f, 586t, 597–599, 598f

N

NavX™ fusion system, 727–728
NMR. *See* Nuclear magnetic resonance (NMR)
Noncompaction cardiomyopathy, 8–10, 9*f*
Nongadolinium contrast techniques, 156
Noninvasive coronary angiography
   CMR imaging, 190–193
   coronary artery calcification, 173–176
   CTCA (*see* CT coronary angiography (CTCA))
Noninvasive detection and quantification
   center, 258, 259*f*
   clinical question, 257*f*, 258–259, 259*f*
   CMRS, 242–244
   cost-effectiveness, 260
   CTCA, 243*f*, 244–246, 245*f*
   exercise and pharmacological stressor, 256–258, 256*f*, 257*f*
   hypothetics, 260
   patient, 257*f*, 258–259, 259*f*
   perfusion and function, 243*f*, 246–256, 247*f*, 249*f*, 250*f*, 252*f*, 253*f*, 255*f*
   PET, 244
   PTP, 239–241, 239*f*, 240*f*, 242*f*
   SPECT, 244
   stress ECG, 233*f*, 240*f*, 241, 243*f*
Nuclear imaging
   AMI, 288–297, 290*f*, 292*f*, 294*f*
   cardiac tumours, 591–593, 592*f*
   cardiomyopathy, 405–406
   infarct avid tracers, 291–293, 292*f*
   innervation imaging (^{123}I-mIBG), 293–294, 294*f*
   introduction of, 3
   myocardial perfusion, 4, 5*f*, 290–291, 290*f*
   myocarditis, 447
   prognostic value, AMI, 295–296
   prosthetic valves, 562
   radiation and dose reduction, 10–11
   radiotracer injection and photon emission, 4
   scintigraphy devices, 3–4
   SPECT technique (*see* Single-photon emission computed tomography (SPECT))
Nuclear magnetic resonance (NMR)
   fast-spin-echo/HASTE acquisition, 131, 132*f*
   flow imaging, 133–134
   intrinsic MR contrast, 129–131
   k-space, 128
   MR angiography, 134
   MR contrast agents, 131
   perfusion imaging, 132–133, 134*f*
   spin state, 128
   SSFP cine imaging, 132, 133*f*
   T1 relaxation process, 128, 129*f*
   T2 and T2* relaxation processes, 128, 130*f*
   transverse magnetization, 128
Nuclear medicine, 47

O

Ontario Multicenter CT Angiography Study (OMCAS), 179
Optical coherence tomography (OCT), 234
Optison, 24, 25*t*, 26
Ordered subset expectation maximization (OSEM), 57, 57*f*, 74

P

Paravalvular leaks (PVL), 759–761, 761*f*
Parietal (fibrous) pericardium, 620
Percutaneous coronary intervention (PCI), 181–182, 185*f*
Perfusion gated SPECT, 390–392
Perfusion imaging
   BOLD-CMR, 256
   CT perfusion, 254, 255*f*
   hybrid technique, 254–256
   ischemia assessment, 140–141, 140*f*
   PET perfusion imaging, 248, 249*f*
   SE, 248–251, 250*f*
   sensitivities and specificities, 233*f*, 243*f*, 246–256
   SPECT, 246–248, 247*f*
   stress CMR, 251–254, 252*f*, 253*f*
Pericardial constriction, 428
Pericardial cysts, 596, 597*f*, 629–630, 630*f*
Pericardial diseases
   acute pericarditis, 621–623, 622*f*, 623*f*
   anatomy, 620, 620*f*, 621*f*
   chronic pericarditis, 623, 624*f*
   CMR, 617, 618*t*, 619–620
   congenital absence, 632, 633*f*

Index   777

constrictive pericarditis (*see* Constrictive pericarditis)
  CT, 617, 618*t*, 619
  echocardiography, 617–619, 618*t*, 620
  pericardiocentesis, 624–626
  subacute pericarditis, 623
  tamponade, 624–626, 625*t*
Pericardial effusion (PE), 713–714
Pericardiocentesis, 624–626
Peripheral eosinophilia, 477
Persistent foramen ovale (PFO)
  Amplatzer PFO occluder, 758, 758*f*
  TEE, 759, 760*f*
  TTE, 758
PET. *See* Positron emission tomography (PET)
PFO. *See* Persistent foramen ovale (PFO)
Phase-contrast myocardial velocity imaging, 386, 387
PHT. *See* Pulmonary hypertension (PHT)
15-(*p*-Iodophenyl)-3*R*,*S*-methyl pentadecanoic acid (BMIPP), 244
Polytetrafluoroethylene (PTFE) material, 684, 685*f*
Positron emission tomography (PET), 8–10, 9*f*
  AMI, 296–297
  annihilation photons, 71–74, 73*f*
  arterial systemic hypertension, 464–465, 464*f*
  atherosclerotic plaque, 214–216
  attenuation correction, 75, 76*f*
  biochemical pathways, noninvasive quantification of, 71
  cardiac PET tracers, selection of, 71–74, 72*t*
  cardiomyopathy, 405
  clinical trials, 215–216, 215*f*
  corrections, 75–77, 76*f*
  detector ring, 3–4, 71–74
  ^{18}F-decay, 71–74, 73*f*
  FDG, 214–215
  functions, 71
  hybrid CCTA imaging, 71, 87–89, 88*f*, 89*f*
  inflammation and cardiovascular risk, 214
  line of response (LOR), 71–74
  MPI perfusion tracers, 78–85, 78*t*, 86–87
  MRI imaging, 71, 89, 90, 90*f*
  OSEM reconstructions, 74
  radiotracers, 71, 216–217

  sarcoidosis, 478
  spatial resolution, 77–78, 77*f*
  vs. SPECT, attenuation, 75, 76*f*
  time of flight, 74, 74*f*
  2D/3D acquisition modes, 71–74, 73*f*
Postoperative aorta
  computed tomography, 684–685, 684*f*, 685*f*
  magnetic resonance imaging, 685
  PET-CT, 686
  structured reporting, 686, 686*t*
  surgical interventions and endografts, 681, 682, 683*f*
  TTE and TOE, 684
Pretest probability (PTP)
  clinical PTP, 239–240, 239*f*
  diagnostic test, 239–240, 241
  exercise stress imaging, 241
  high-intermediate PTP, 241
  high/low PTP, 239–240, 240*f*
  intermediate PTP, 239–240, 240*f*
  low-intermediate PTP, 241
  pharmacological stress imaging, 240*f*, 241
  risk determination, 241, 242*f*
Primary cardiac tumours
  benign (*see* Benign tumours)
  malignant (*see* Malignant primary cardiac tumours)
Prosthesis implantation, 568–569
Prosthesis-patient mismatch (PPM), 543–544
Prosthetic heart valves (PHV) implantation, 684
Prosthetic valve regurgitation
  aortic prosthetic valve regurgitation, 551, 554*t*
  mitral, 551, 552*f*, 553*f*, 555*t*
  severity of, 551, 554*t*, 555*t*
  transcatheter aortic valves, 552*f*, 554–557, 554*t*, 556*f*, 557*f*
  TTE and TTE, 551
Prosthetic valves
  cinefluoroscopy, 557–558, 558*t*
  CT, 558*t*, 559–560, 559*f*, 560*f*, 561*f*
  echocardiography, 542–557
  MRI, 562, 563*f*
  nuclear imaging, 562
  quantitative parameters, 545–548
Proximal isovelocity surface area (PISA), 503–505, 513–516

Pseudotumours
  intra-cardiac structures/embryological remnants, 596
  pericardial cysts, 596, 597f
  thrombus, 593–596, 594f
PTP. See Pretest probability (PTP)
Pulmonary artery pressure (PAP), 374–375
Pulmonary embolism (PE), 686–687
Pulmonary hypertension (PHT)
  cardiac MRI, 693
  CT, 691–692, 692f, 693f
  Dana Point classification, 687, 687t
  definition, 687
  echocardiography, 693, 694f
  radiography, 691, 691f
  right-heart catheterization, 693–694
  structured reporting, 694, 695t
Pulmonary valve (PV) disease
  anatomy, 533
  CMR, 537–539, 538f, 539f, 539t
  CT, 539
  pathology, 533
  3DE, 537, 537f, 538f
  2DE, 533–534, 534t
Pulmonary valve replacement, 646

Q

Quantitative mapping techniques
  challenges, 146
  ECV estimation, 143, 144f
  EQ-CMR, 143
  native/precontrast T1 mapping, 141–142, 142f
  postcontrast T1 mapping, 143
  T2 mapping, 142f, 144, 145f
Quantitative perfusion data, 132–133, 134f

R

Radionuclide imaging, 47, 639–640
Radionuclide techniques, heart failure
  gated blood pool SPECT, 389–390
  perfusion gated SPECT, 390–392
  planar equilibrium RNA, 387–389
Radionuclide ventriculography (RNV), 406
Real-time 3D color Doppler echocardiography, 17
Real-time 3D echocardiography (RT3DE), 16, 17, 637

arterial systemic hypertension, 462–463
heart failure, 370, 383
Regional contractile function, 377f, 386–387
Regurgitant fraction (RF), 503–505
Regurgitant volume (RV), 503–505
Restrictive cardiomyopathy, 422–423
Rhabdomyoma, 586f, 589t, 603–604
Rheumatoid arthritis (RA), 472–474, 473f
RV end-diastolic area (RV-EDA), 380
RV end-systolic area (RV-ESA), 380
RV fractional area change (RVFAC), 380
RVOT shortening fraction (RVOT-SF), 379–380

S

Sarcoid/sarcoidosis, 425–427, 426f, 478
Sarcoma, 589t, 605–608, 606f
Saturation-recovery single-shot acquisition (SASHA) sequences, 141
Secondary (functional) mitral regurgitation, 511
Secondary pericardial tumors, 630–632, 632f
Short-tau inversion recovery (STIR) sequences, 403–404
Signal-to-noise ratio (SNR), 136
"Signal void" phenomenon, 531
Single-photon emission computed tomography (SPECT), 216–217
  AMI, 296–297
  atherosclerotic plaque, 216–217
  camera designs, 50–51, 50f
  cardiac tumours, 591–593
  cardiomyopathy, 405
  and CCTA, 64–67, 66f, 67f
  collimators, 48–49, 49f
  CT attenuation correction, 58–59, 59f, 60f
  CZT detectors (see Cadmium-zinc-telluride (CZT) detector)
  dynamic perfusion imaging, 63–64, 65f
  electrocardiogram (ECG)-gated SPECT, 59–62, 61f
  EM/OSEM iterative reconstruction, 57–58
  filtered back projection, 56–57, 56f, 57f
  heart failure, 387
  Kawasaki disease, 476, 478
  list mode acquisition, 62
  low-dose SPECT, 62–63
  myocardial perfusion defects, 49, 49f
  myocarditis, 447

Index

nuclear imaging, 562
 vs. PET, attenuation in, 75, 75*f*
 rotating detector panels, 3–4
 sarcoidosis, 478
 scintigraphy, 47–48
 sodium iodide scintillation detector, 47–48, 48*f*
 tracers, 54–55, 55*t*
 unfiltered back projection, 56–57, 56*f*
Sinotubular junction, 493–494
Sinus of Valsalva (SOV), 493–494
SonoVue, 24, 25*t*
Spatial modulation of magnetization (SPAMM), 387
Specific absorption rate (SAR), 136
Speckle tracking echocardiography (STE), 401–402, 617–619
 arrhythmia, 712–713, 712*f*
 heart failure (HF), 369, 382–383, 383*f*
 limitations, 39
 LV rotation, 32, 32*t*
 vs. TDI strain, 38
 3D STE strain, 39, 40*f*
 2D STE strain, 37, 37*f*, 38*f*, 38*t*
SPECT. *See* Single-photon emission computed tomography (SPECT)
Spin-lattice relaxation time. *See* T1 relaxation time
Spin-spin relaxation time, 129–130
Spin state, 128
Stanford classification, 662
STE. *See* Speckle tracking echocardiography (STE)
Steady-state free-precession (SSFP), 132, 133*f*, 403
 mitral regurgitation, 519–520
 tricuspid valve, 531
ST elevation infarction (STEMI)
 myocarditis, 447
Strain rate (SR), 32, 32*t*
 definition of, 35–36
 limitations, 36
Stress cardiomyopathy, 413
Stress echocardiography
 acquired prosthetic valve stenosis, 548
 contrast, 29–30
 3D echocardiography, 22–23
Subacute pericarditis, 623
Sudden cardiac death (SCD), 711

Surface rendering, 19, 20*f*, 21*f*
Surgical Treatment of IsChaemic Heart failure (STICH) study, 348*t*, 349–350
Systemic diseases
 autoimmune connective tissue disorders, 472–474, 473*f*
 diabetic cardiomyopathy, 465–467, 467*f*, 468*f*, 469*f*
 hypertension (*see* Arterial systemic hypertension)
 metabolic syndrome, 469–472, 471*f*
 systemic vasculitis (*see* Systemic vasculitis)
 thyroid disease, 474–475
Systemic vasculitis
 Churg–Strauss syndrome, 477
 hypereosinophilia, 477
 Kawasaki disease (KD), 475–477
 sarcoidosis, 477–478

T

Takutsubo cardiomyopathy, 301, 303*f*
Tamponade, 624–626, 625*t*
Task Force Criteria for ARVD, 414–416
TAVI. *See* Transcatheter aortic valve implantation (TAVI)
TAVR. *See* Trans-catheter-based AV replacement (TAVR)
^{99m}Tc-glucarate, 292*f*, 293
^{99m}Tc-pyrophosphate, 291, 293
TDI. *See* Tissue Doppler imaging (TDI)
99m-Technetium (^{99m}Tc), 54–55
TEI index, 381–382
Tetralogy of Fallot (TOF), 636–637, 645–649, 647*f*, 648*f*, 649*f*
201-Thallium (^{201}Tl), 54–55, 55*t*
3D color Doppler echocardiography, 22
Three-dimensional (3D) echocardiography, 23
 aortic root calcification, 491, 491*f*, 493*f*
 benefits, 16
 cardiac volumes and mass, assessment of, 16
 cropping, 19
 dropouts, 18
 gating and breath holding, 18
 heart valves, assessment of, 16
 implementation of, 23
 matrix-array transducers, 16
 mitral regurgitation, 511–518, 512*f*, 517*f*

Three-dimensional (3D) echocardiography
    (Continued)
  multi-beat 3D echocardiographic imaging, 17, 18*f*
  myocardial strain imaging, 3, 4*f*
  pulmonary valve disease, 537, 537*f*, 538*f*
  real-time 3D echocardiography, 16, 17
  regurgitant lesions, jets, and shunts, 16
  stress echocardiography, 22–23
  surface rendering, 19, 20*f*, 21*f*
  temporal *vs.* spatial resolution, 17
  3D color Doppler, 22
  3D tomographic slices, 19–22, 21*f*
  tricuspid valve, 530–531, 530*f*
  volume rendering, 19, 20*f*
Three-dimensional rotational angiography (3DRA), 708*t*, 710
Three-dimensional speckle tracking echocardiography (3D STE), 39, 40*f*
Three-dimensional time-resolved (4D) flow
  aorta, 146*f*, 147
  heart, 147–148
  long acquisition time, 148
  software development, 148
Thrombus, 593–596, 594*f*
Thyroid disease, 474–475
Time-activity curves (TAC), 63–64
Time-of-flight positron emission tomography (TF-PET), 74, 74*f*
Tissue Doppler imaging (TDI), 401–402, 637
  clinical use, 37
  displacement, 32, 32*t*, 35
  myocardial velocities (*see* Myocardial velocity, TDI)
  strain and strain rate (SR), 32, 32*t*, 35–36, 36*f*
Transcatheter aortic valve implantation (TAVI)
  CMR, 743–744
  CoreValve® system, 735, 736
  Edwards Sapien® valve, 735, 736, 736*f*
  MDCT, 735–736, 740–743, 742*f*
  TEE, 567–568, 568*f*, 739–740, 739*f*
  TTE, 736–737, 738*f*, 740
  vascular access pathway, 735–736
Trans-catheter-based AV replacement (TAVR), 490*f*
  annular calcification, 491
  annulus (virtual ring) dimensions, 489–490
  aortic stenosis, 496, 497*f*
  computed tomography, 489–490
  para-valvular leak (PVL), 489–490
  SOV, 494
Transesophageal echocardiography (TEE), 3, 16
  aortic stenosis, 496, 496*f*
  ASD, 642, 643*f*, 759, 760*f*
  edge-to-edge repair, 571–572, 572*f*
  endocarditis, 574–577, 575*f*, 576*f*, 577*f*
  LAA, 752–754, 753*f*
  mitral regurgitation, 745–750, 746*f*, 747*f*, 748*f*, 749*f*
  PFO, 759, 760*f*
  prosthetic valves, 542, 542*f*
  prosthetic valve stenosis, 544, 548*f*
  PVR, 569–570, 570*f*
  TAVI, 567–569, 568*f*, 739–740, 739*f*
  TOF, 646, 647*f*
  VSD, 644–645, 645*f*
Transluminal arterial gradient (TAG), 183–184
Transoesophageal echocardiography (TOE)
  AAS, 670, 670*f*
  cardiac tumours, 585–587
  postoperative aorta, 684
Transposition of the great arteries (TGA)
  arterial switch surgery, 650–653
  atrial switch surgery, 650, 651*f*, 652*f*
  ccTGA, 653
  CoA, 654
  Fontan circulation, 653
  univentricular heart, 653
Transthoracic echocardiography (TTE), 16
  AAS, 670, 670*f*
  aortic regurgitation, 496, 503
  aortic stenosis (AS), 496
  arrhythmia, 708*t*, 711–714, 712*f*, 713*f*, 715–716
  ASD/PFO, 758
  cardiac tumours, 585–587, 587*f*
  endocarditis, 574–577, 575*f*, 576*f*, 577*f*
  postoperative aorta, 684
  Prosthetic valve regurgitation, 551, 552*f*
  prosthetic valve stenosis, 544, 545*f*
Transthyretin-related amyloidosis (ATTR), 423, 424, 424*f*
Transverse magnetization, 128
T1 relaxation time, 129
T2 relaxation time, 129–130

Tricuspid annular plane systolic excursion (TAPSE), 380–381, 646
Tricuspid valve (TV)
  anatomy, 526–527, 526f
  CMR, 531–533, 531f, 532f
  CT, 533
  pathology, 527
  3DE, 530–531, 530f
  2DE, 527–530, 527t
Two-dimensional echocardiography (2DE)
  aortic regurgitation, 503
  aortic root calcification, 491, 491f, 493f
  arrhythmia, 711
  mitral regurgitation, 511–518, 513f
  pulmonary valve disease, 533–534, 534t
  tricuspid valve, 527–530, 527t
Two-dimensional speckle tracking echocardiography (2D STE), 37, 37f, 38f, 38t

U

Ultra-high-field (7T) MR systems, 155–156
Ultrashort echo time (UTE) imaging, 156
Univentricular heart, 653

V

Valvular heart disease
  aortic regurgitation, 503–509, 504f, 505f, 506f, 507f, 508t
  aortic root (see Aortic root/ascending aorta (AA))
  aortic stenosis (see Aortic stenosis)
  mitral regurgitation (see Mitral regurgitation)
  prosthetic valves (see Prosthetic valves)
  pulmonary valve (see Pulmonary valve (PV) disease)
  TAVI (see Transcatheter aortic valve implantation (TAVI))
  TV (see Tricuspid valve (TV))
Vascular smooth muscle cells (VSM), 474
Vasculitis
  advantages and disadvantages, 676, 677t
  angiography, 681
  clinical presentation, 675–676, 676t
  computed tomography, 677, 678f
  infectious and non-infectious causes, 675, 675t
  magnetic resonance imaging, 677–681, 679f, 680f
  PET-CT, 681
  radiography, 676
  structured reporting, 681, 682t
  ultrasound, 676
Vena cava stenoses, 650
Ventricular septal defect (VSD), 643–645, 644f
Visceral (serous) pericardium, 620
Volume rendering, 19, 20f

W

Wall motion abnormalities (WMA), 274, 280–282, 297, 298